Oxford Textbook of

Interventional Cardiology

Oxford Textbook of Interventional Cardiology

Edited by

Simon Redwood

Nick Curzen

and

Martyn Thomas

OXFORD
UNIVERSITY PRESS

OXFORD
UNIVERSITY PRESS

Great Clarendon Street, Oxford OX2 6DP

Oxford University Press is a department of the University of Oxford.
It furthers the University's objective of excellence in research, scholarship,
and education by publishing worldwide in

Oxford New York

Auckland Cape Town Dar es Salaam Hong Kong Karachi
Kuala Lumpur Madrid Melbourne Mexico City Nairobi
New Delhi Shanghai Taipei Toronto

With offices in

Argentina Austria Brazil Chile Czech Republic France Greece
Guatemala Hungary Italy Japan Poland Portugal Singapore
South Korea Switzerland Thailand Turkey Ukraine Vietnam

Oxford is a registered trade mark of Oxford University Press
in the UK and in certain other countries

Published in the United States
by Oxford University Press Inc., New York

First edition published 2010

British Library Cataloguing in Publication Data is available

Library of Congress Cataloging in Publication Data is available

Typeset in Minion
by Glyph International, Bangalore, India
Printed in China
on acid-free paper by
C and C Offset Ltd

ISBN 978–0–19–956908–3

10 9 8 7 6 5 4 3 2 1

Oxford University Press makes no representation, express or implied, that the drug dosages in this book are correct. Readers must therefore always check the product information and clinical procedures with the most up-to-date published product information and data sheets provided by the manufacturers and the most recent codes of conduct and safety regulations. The authors and the publishers do not accept responsibility or legal liability for any errors in the text or for the misuse or misapplication of material in this work. Except where otherwise stated, drug dosages and recommendations are for the non-pregnant adult who is not breastfeeding

Preface

The practice of Interventional Cardiology has undergone enormous changes since the first coronary angioplasty performed by Gruentzig in 1977. Angioplasty has evolved from what was a major procedure with unpredictable results and a high likelihood of both acute failure and long-term restenosis, to a routine, often outpatient, procedure with typical success rates in the region of 97% and late recurrence in single figures. With advances in equipment and techniques, there are few lesion and patient subsets not suitable for PCI, such that PCI rates throughout the world continue to rise.

These advances have allowed the development of percutaneous techniques to treat a variety of structural heart defects and this will likely be a major growth area in interventional cardiology over the next few years.

In view of these rapid developments, we carefully selected authors who were not only leaders in their field, but also able to adhere to very strict timelines, resulting in a reference text which is both comprehensive and uniquely up-to-date.

Although this text is primarily aimed at the trainee and practising Interventional Cardiologist, we hope that it will also be of interest to all Cardiologists who have more than a passing interest in interventional procedures. This is particularly true of the expanding structural heart area which inevitably involves close collaboration between several subspecialties, especially imaging.

Being asked to edit this book has been a great privilege, but the successful production of a textbook of this size has required the support and cooperation of numerous individuals. Not only are we grateful to the authors, but also to the staff of Oxford University Press, in particular Helen Liepman and Susan Crowhurst.

Contents

SECTION 3
Percutaneous coronary intervention by clinical syndrome

SECTION 4
Percutaneous coronary intervention by lesion and patient subsets

SECTION 5
Adjunctive therapies in percutaneous coronary intervention

SECTION 6
Complications of percutaneous coronary intervention

List of contributors

Zulfiquar Adam
James Cook University Hospital,
Middlesbrough, UK

David Adlam
Department of Cardiovascular Medicine,
John Radcliffe Hospital,
Oxford, UK

Gurbir Bhatia
Department of Cardiology,
University Hospital of North Staffordshire, UK

Adrian P. Banning
John Radcliffe Hospital,
Oxford, UK

Andreas Baumbach
Bristol Heart Institute,
Bristol, UK

Adam de Belder
Brighton and Sussex University Hospitals, UK

Mark A. de Belder
James Cook University Hospital,
Middlesbrough, UK

Ravinay Bhindi
Department of Cardiovascular Medicine,
University of Oxford,
John Radcliffe Hospital,
Oxford, UK

Eric Brochet
Hôpital Bichat,
Paris, France

Bernard De Bruyne
Cardiovascular Center Aalst,
OLV-Clinic,
Aalst, Belgium

Jonathan Byrne
King's College Hospital,
London, UK

Adriano Caixeta
Center for Interventional Vascular Therapy,
Columbia University Medical Center,
The Cardiovascular Research Foundation,
New York, USA

Patrick A. Calvert
University of Cambridge,
Papworth Hospital NHS Foundation Trust,
Cambridge, UK

Keith M. Channon
Department of Cardiovascular Medicine,
John Radcliffe Hospital,
Oxford, UK

Simon J. Corbett
Wessex Cardiothoracic Unit,
Southampton University Hospitals NHS Trust,
Southampton, UK

Nick Curzen
Wessex Cardiothoracic Unit,
Southampton University Hospitals NHS Trust,
Southampton, UK

George Dangas
Center for Interventional Vascular Therapy,
Columbia University Medical Center,
Cardiovascular Research Foundation,
New York, USA

Carlo Di Mario
Royal Brompton Hospital,
London, UK

Grégory Ducrocq
Hôpital Bichat,
Paris, France

Jean Fajadet
Clinique Pasteur,
Toulouse, France

Bruno Farah
Clinique Pasteur,
Toulouse, France

Pim J. de Feijter
Department of Cardiology and Radiology,
Erasmus MC, Rotterdam, The Netherlands

Peter J. Fitzgerald
Division of Cardiovascular Medicine,
Stanford University Medical Center, USA

Kim F. Fox
Royal Brompton and Harefield NHS Trust, UK

Scot Garg
Department of Interventional Cardiology,
Thoraxcentre, Erasmus Medical Centre,
Rotterdam, The Netherlands

A. H. Gershlick
University Hospitals of Leicester, UK

Philippe Généreux
Center for Interventional Vascular Therapy,
Columbia University Medical Center,
The Cardiovascular Research Foundation,
New York, USA

Youlan L. Gu
Department of Cardiology,
Thorax Center, University Medical
Center Groningen,
University of Groningen,
The Netherlands

Mark Gunning
University Hospital of North Staffordshire,
Stoke-on-Trent, UK

Robert A. Henderson
Consultant Cardiologist, Trent Cardiac Centre,
Nottingham University Hospitals,
Nottingham, UK

David Hildick-Smith
Royal Sussex County Hospital, UK

Dominique Himbert
Hôpital Bichat,
Paris, France

Alex Hobson
Wessex Cardiac Unit,
Southampton University Hospitals NHS Trust,
Southampton, UK

Yasuhiro Honda
Division of Cardiovascular Medicine,
Stanford University Medical Center, USA

Christine Hughes
Clinique Pasteur,
Toulouse, France

Bernard Iung
Hôpital Bichat,
Paris, France

Akhil Kapur
London Chest Hospital, UK

Theodoros D. Karamitsos
Department of Cardiovascular Medicine,
University of Oxford,
John Radcliffe Hospital,
Oxford, UK

Adnan Kastrati
Deutsches Herzzentrum München,
Technische Universität, Munich, Germany

Kenneth Kent
Washington Hospital Center,
Georgetown University School of Medicine,
Washington DC, USA

Charles Knight
London Chest Hospital,
Barts and The London NHS Trust,
London, UK

Neville Kukreja
Royal Brompton Hospital,
London, UK

GertJan Laarman
King's College Hospital,
London, UK

Leong Lee
Trent Cardiac Centre,
Nottingham City Hospital,
Nottingham, UK

Thierry Lefèvre
Institut Cardiovasculaire Paris Sud,
Institut Hospitalier Jacques Cartier,
Massy, France

Tim Lockie
King's College London, St Thomas' Hospital,
London, UK

Yves Louvard
Institut Cardiovasculaire Paris Sud,
Institut Hospitalier Jacques Cartier,
Massy, France

Peter F. Ludman
Queen Elizabeth Hospital,
Birmingham, UK

Philip MacCarthy
King's College Hospital,
London, UK

Michael Mahmoudi
Wessex Cardiothoracic Centre,
Southampton University Hospitals NHS Trust, UK

Iqbal Malik
Imperial College Healthcare NHS Trust, UK

Steffen Massberg
Deutsches Herzzentrum München,
Technische Universität,
Munich, Germany

Peter A. McCullough
Division of Nutrition and Preventive Medicine,
William Beaumont Hospital,
Royal Oak, USA

Julinda Mehilli
Deutsches Herzzentrum München,
Technische Universität,
Munich, Germany

Roxana Mehran
Center for Interventional Vascular Therapy,
Columbia University Medical Center,
Cardiovascular Research Foundation,
New York, USA

Saidi A. Mohiddin
London Chest Hospital,
Barts and The London NHS Trust,
London, UK

Olivier Muller
Cardiovascular Center Aalst,
Onze-Lieve-Vrouw Clinic, Moorselbaan,
Belgium

Aung Myat
University Hospitals of Coventry and
Warwickshire NHS Trust, UK

Stefan Neubaeur
University of Oxford,
Department of Cardiovascular Medicine,
John Radcliffe Hospital,
Oxford, UK

Fabian Nietlispach
St. Paul's Hospital,
University of British Columbia,
Vancouver, BC, Canada

James Nolan
Department of Cardiology,
University Hospital of North Staffordshire, UK

Peter O'Kane
Dorset Heart Centre,
The Royal Bournemouth Hospital,
Bournemouth, Dorset

Hiromasa Otake
Division of Cardiovascular Medicine,
Center for Cardiovascular Technology,
Stanford University Medical Center, USA

Divaka Perera
St. Thomas' Hospital Campus,
Kings College London,
London, UK

Bernard D. Prendergast
Department of Cardio Vascular Medicine,
John Radcliffe Hospital,
Oxford, UK

Katie Qureshi
The London Chest Hospital,
Barts and the London NHS Trust,
London, UK

Bushra S. Rana
Department of Cardiology,
Papworth Hospital NHS Foundation Trust,
Cambridge, UK

Simon Redwood
King's College London,
St. Thomas' Hospital,
London, UK

David H. Roberts
Dept of Cardiovascular Medicine,
Blackpool Victoria Hospital, UK

Helen Routledge
Worcestershire Royal Hospital, UK

Mrinal Saha
Royal Sussex County Hospital, UK

C. Schultz
Department of Cardiology and Radiology,
Erasmus MC, Rotterdam, The Netherlands

Mike Seddon
Wessex Cardiacthoracic Unit,
Southampton University Hospitals NHS Trust,
Southampton, UK

Patrick W. Serruys
Department of Interventional Cardiology,
Thoraxcentre,
Erasmus Medical Centre,
Rotterdam,
The Netherlands

Rod H. Stables
The Liverpool Heart and Chest Hospital,
Liverpool, UK

Julian Strange
Bristol Heart Institute, Bristol, UK

Martyn Thomas
St Thomas' Hospital,
London, UK

Pawel Tyczynski
Royal Brompton Hospital,
London, UK

Alec Vahanian
Hôpital Bichat,
Paris, France

Mariuca Vasa-Nicotera
Glenfield Hospital,
Leicester, UK

William J. van Gaal
The Northern Hospital,
Epping, Victoria,
Australia

John G. Webb
St. Paul's Hospital
University of British Columbia
Vancouver, BC, Canada

Andrew Wiper
Yorkshire Deanery, UK

Joanna J. Wykrzykowska
Department of Interventional Cardiology,
Thoraxcentre,
Erasmus Medical Centre,
Rotterdam,
The Netherlands

Felix Zijlstra
Department of Cardiology
Thorax Center,
University Medical Center Groningen,
University of Groningen,
The Netherlands

SECTION 1

Background and basics

CHAPTER 1

The epidemiology and pathophysiology of coronary artery disease

Robert A. Henderson and Leong Lee

Epidemiology of coronary heart disease

Advances in the prevention and treatment of coronary heart disease (CHD) have led to significant improvements in prognosis and quality of life, but globally CHD remains a leading cause of premature death and disability. In 2001 CHD was responsible for 11.8% of all deaths in low- and middle-income countries and 17.3% in high-income countries, accounting for over 7 million deaths worldwide[1]. By 2020 CHD is projected to be the leading cause of death and disability-adjusted life years[2], reflecting a rapidly increasing prevalence in developing countries and Eastern Europe, and the rising incidence of obesity and diabetes in the Western world.

Mortality

In the United Kingdom around one in five men and one in seven women die from CHD with over 94 000 coronary deaths per annum[3]. CHD is the most frequent cause of premature death (before the age of 75) accounting for almost 31 000 such deaths in 2006, including 19% of premature deaths in men and 10% in women. In the United States in 2005, CHD caused nearly 0.5 million deaths and accounted for one in five of all deaths. Although annual CHD mortality declined by 34.3% from 1995 to 2005 the actual number of deaths fell by only 19.4%[4].

There are regional, social, and ethnic variations in coronary disease-associated mortality, and over the last 25 years death rates from CHD have been consistently higher in Scotland than in other regions in the United Kingdom. The highest coronary deaths rates are reported amongst men of South Asian descent and from 1999 to 2003 mortality rates in men of Bangladeshi origin exceeded rates in the general population by 112%. Death rates from CHD increase during the winter months, and in 2004/2005 winter mortality in England and Wales was 19% higher than at other times of the year[3].

Mortality rates from CHD have been declining in industrialized countries over several decades, but there is currently an epidemic of CHD in Eastern Europe (Fig. 1.1). Over the last decade, coronary mortality in the United Kingdom amongst people aged less than 65 years has fallen by 45%. Nevertheless, reductions in coronary mortality have been slower in the United Kingdom than in most other developed countries, and across Western Europe only Ireland and Finland have higher mortality rates (Fig. 1.2)[3,5].

In recent years the decline in coronary mortality in industrialized countries has been slower in younger than in older age groups. For example, in the United Kingdom from 1997 to 2006 there was a 46% fall in CHD mortality amongst men aged 55–64 years but only a 22% fall among men aged 35–44 years[3]. In the United States the decline in age-adjusted coronary mortality from 1980 to 2002 slowed markedly in adults aged 35–54 years. Moreover, since 1997 the mortality rate among women aged 35–44 years has been increasing by about 1.3% per year[6].

It has been estimated that 58% of the decline in coronary mortality in the United Kingdom between 1981 and 2000 was attributable to reductions in major risk factors, principally smoking, but the remaining 42% was explained by treatment of individuals, including

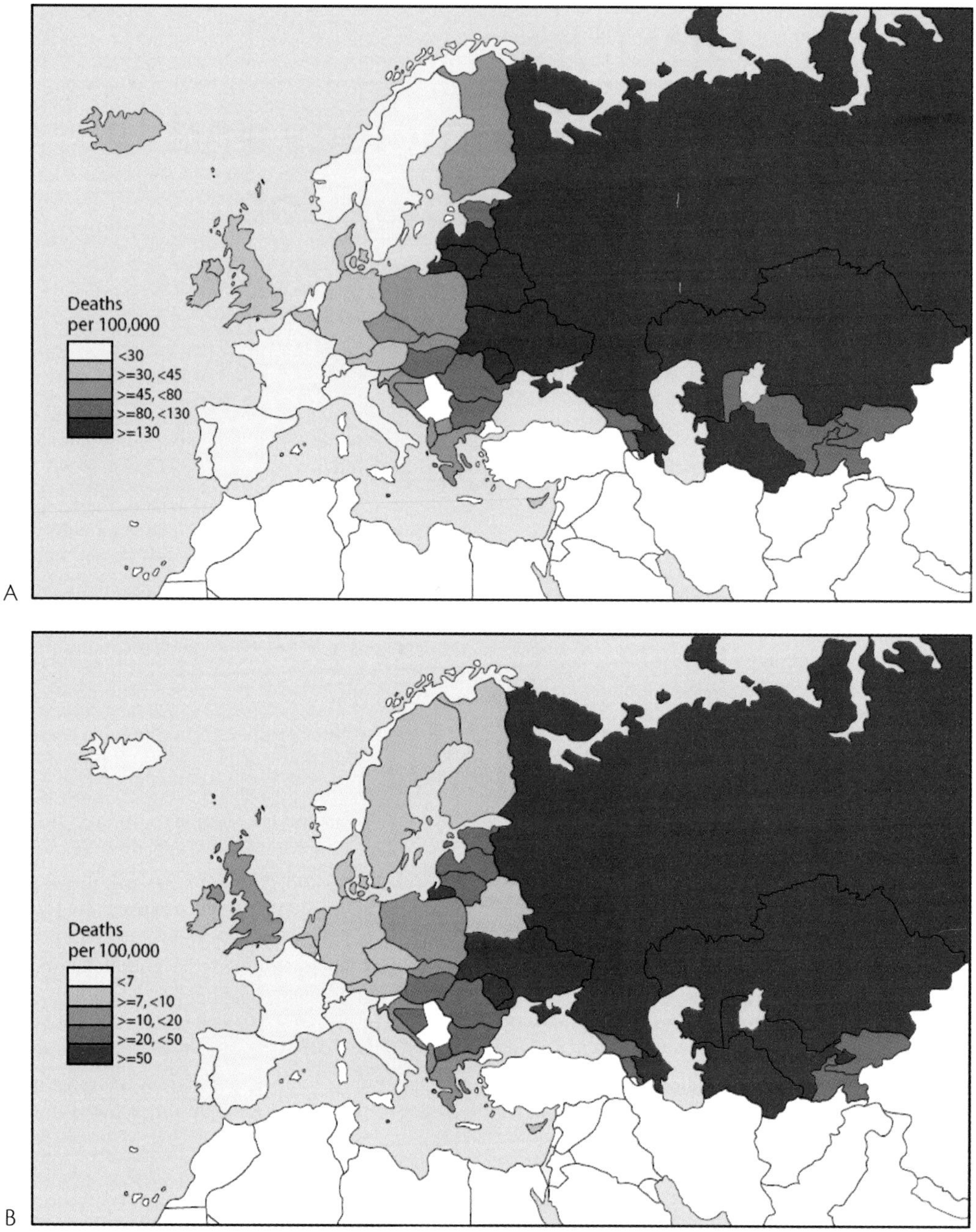

Fig. 1.1 Age-standardized death rates from CHD in Europe: A) men aged 0–64 years; B) women aged 0–64 years. Reproduced with permission from Allender S, Peto V, Rayner M, *et al. European Cardiovascular Disease Statistics 2008*. European Heart Network: Brussels.

secondary prevention[7]. In the United States it has been estimated that 47% of the reduction in CHD mortality from 1980 to 2000 is attributable to treatments and 44% is attributable to modification of risk factors, but this was partially offset by a rise in mortality attributable to increases in body mass index and diabetes prevalence[8]. The WHO-MONICA project examined temporal trends in cardiovascular mortality over the 1980s and 1990s in 21 countries, and demonstrated a strong link between improved care for patients with myocardial

MONICA – monitoring of trends and determinants in CHD.

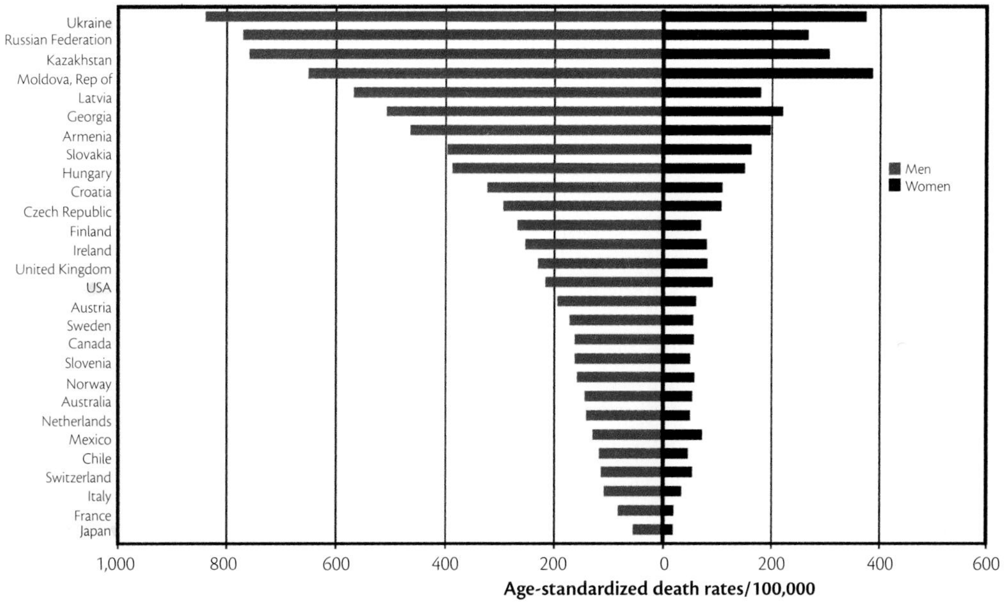

Fig. 1.2 Age-standardized death rates due to coronary heart disease in men and women aged 34–75 years in selected countries (2000). Reproduced with permission from Allender S, Peto V, Scarborough P, Kaur A, Rayner M. *Coronary Heart Disease Statistics*. London: British Heart Foundation, 2008. Also available at www.heartstats.org

infarction and the decline in coronary mortality[9]. An investigation into the potential impact of various preventative and interventional strategies on CHD-related mortality in the United States estimated that delivery of 'perfect care' (through the modification of risk factors and use of all effective therapies) to a hypothetical population (aged 30–84 years) could prevent or postpone around 75% of cardiac deaths[10].

Whilst the rate of CHD-related mortality in developed countries has been steadily declining over recent decades, the global burden of coronary disease has been increasing, particularly in developing countries[11–13]. In Beijing, China, from 1984 to 1999 there was an increase in coronary death rates of approximately 50% in men and 27% in women, primarily attributable to increases in the prevalence of raised total serum cholesterol, smoking, diabetes, and hypertension[11]. Cardiovascular mortality in India is projected to increase rapidly and, if current trends continue, by 2020 India will account for more coronary deaths than either China or the established market economies. As with other emerging economies, urbanization of the Indian population has increased exposure to coronary risk factors, including tobacco use, high blood pressure, elevated blood lipid levels, obesity, diabetes, and sedentary lifestyles[13]. Increasing rates of CHD have also been observed in sub-Saharan Africa and Latin America[14,15].

Morbidity

Coronary artery disease is a chronic degenerative condition, which can present with a wide range of clinical syndromes, including stable angina, acute coronary syndrome, heart failure, arrhythmia, and death. Estimating the incidence and prevalence of coronary disease-related morbidity is therefore challenging and is confounded by changing definitions and diagnostic criteria over time[16,17].

The reported incidence and prevalence of myocardial infarction is higher in men than in women and increases with age. In 2006 the incidence of myocardial infarction in the United Kingdom was estimated to be between 67 000 and 87 000 per year in men of all ages and between 46 000 and 56 000 per year in women of all ages. The Health Survey for England 2006 reported that 4.1% of all men and 1.7% of all women have had a myocardial infarct. In people aged over 35 years, the prevalence of myocardial infarction has been estimated as 970 000 in males and 439 000 in females. As with CHD mortality there are large regional, socioeconomic, and ethnic variations in the incidence and prevalence of myocardial infarction[3]. In the United States in 2006 the prevalence of myocardial infarction in adults aged 20 years or over was estimated at 3.6%, with a prevalence of any coronary disease of 7.6%[4].

Acute coronary syndromes, including unstable angina and myocardial infarction (with and without ST-segment elevation on the electrocardiogram), present a major and growing health burden on industrialized societies. In Scotland in 2000 there were over 9000 admissions to hospital with suspected acute coronary syndrome per million population. These admissions accounted for 19% of all emergency hospitalizations and 12% of medical bed days[18]. The annual incidence of hospitalization with suspected acute coronary syndrome without ST-elevation has been estimated at three per 1000 population[17]. It has been suggested that the ratio of ST-elevation to non-ST-elevation myocardial infarction is decreasing but whether this is due to a real change in disease prevalence, an effect of treatment, or a change in case recognition is unknown[17].

The incidence and prevalence of stable coronary disease is more difficult to estimate. The incidence of angina in the United Kingdom is approximately 96 000 new cases a year, with a higher rate amongst men than women. In 2006 it was estimated that 14% of men and 8% of women aged 65–74 years had experienced angina at some time in their lives[3]. In the United States in 2006 the prevalence of angina in adults aged 20 years or over was estimated at 4.3% in men and 4.5% in women[4]. Paradoxically whilst the rate of mortality from CHD in the developed countries has been declining over the last three decades, rates of CHD-related morbidity appear to be increasing, particularly in the elderly[3].

Risk factors

The INTERHEART study investigated various risk factors for myocardial infarction in 15 152 cases in 52 countries, who were matched to 14 820 controls with no history of heart disease. The mean age of first presentation with myocardial infarction was 8 years younger in men than women and 10 years younger in Africa, the Middle East, and South Asia than the rest of the world. Nine easily measured and potentially modifiable risk factors for myocardial infarction were identified, including smoking, hypertension, diabetes, waist-to-hip ratio, low daily fruit and vegetable consumption, physical inactivity, over-consumption of alcohol, abnormal blood lipid levels, and psychosocial factors. The effect of these risk factors was consistent in both genders and across different ethnic groups and geographic regions. Collectively, the nine risk factors accounted for 90% of the population attributable risk for myocardial infarction in men and 94% in women[19].

Tobacco use, perhaps the most important modifiable risk factor, was associated with a nearly threefold increase in the odds of myocardial infarction (odds ratio (OR) for current smokers 2.95; 95% confidence interval (CI) 2.77–3.14, versus never smokers). This increase in risk of myocardial infarction fell after quitting smoking (OR at 3 years 1.87; CI 1.55–2.24) but remained elevated even after 20 or more years of abstinence (OR 1.22; CI 1.09–1.37). These data suggest that the greatest reduction in global CHD risk could be achieved by preventing smoking and by smoking cessation programmes[20].

A meta-analysis of data from 61 prospective observational studies involving almost 900 000 adults, mostly from Western Europe or North America, confirmed a strong positive relationship between total serum cholesterol and coronary mortality, irrespective of age and the level of blood pressure. Of various simple indices involving measurement of low- (LDL) and high-density lipoprotein (HDL) cholesterol levels, the ratio total/HDL cholesterol was the strongest predictor of coronary mortality[21]. Randomized trials of just a few years of treatment with 3-hydroxy-3-methylglutaryl-coenzyme A reductase inhibitors (statins) have shown that lowering LDL cholesterol by about 1.5mmol/L reduces the incidence of coronary events by about a third[22].

Global reductions in other modifiable risk factors also have the potential to prevent cardiovascular events, but lowering rates of hypertension, obesity, and diabetes will be challenging. Epidemiological evidence suggests that throughout middle and old age usual blood pressure is strongly and directly related to vascular (and total) mortality without any evidence of a threshold down to at least 115/75mmHg[23]. In the United States, however, from 2001 to 2003 state-level age-standardized prevalence of uncontrolled hypertension was estimated to range from 15–21% amongst men and from 21–26% amongst women (Fig. 1.3)[24]. Similarly there is robust evidence that an increase in body mass index of 5kg/m^2 is associated with about a 40% increase in vascular mortality[25], but from 1999 to 2006 the high prevalence of childhood obesity in the United States remained unchanged[26]. Nevertheless, relatively modest downward shifts in the population distribution of modifiable cardiovascular risk factors may have substantial effects on disease prevalence, particularly when compared with prevention strategies directed at high-risk individuals[27].

Pathophysiology

Atherothrombosis

Atherothrombosis, defined as atherosclerosis with superimposed thrombosis, is the principal pathological

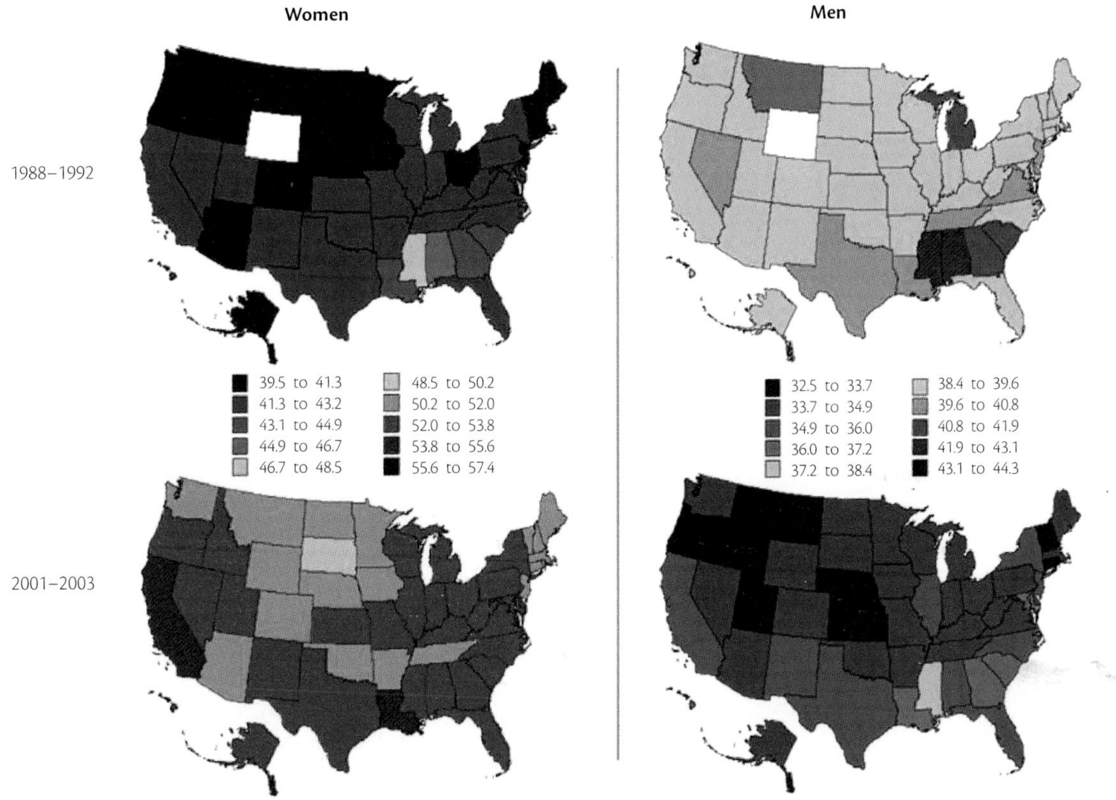

Fig. 1.3 Age-standardized prevalence (in percentage) of uncontrolled hypertension in the United States from 1988 to 1992 and from 2001 to 2003 (men and women ≥60 years of age). Hypertension control decreased in women between the two study periods. Reproduced with permission from Ezzati M, Oza S, Danaei G, Murray CJ. Trends and cardiovascular mortality effects of state-level blood pressure and uncontrolled hypertension in the United States. *Circulation* 2008 Feb 19; **117**(7):905–14.

process underlying the majority of clinical cardiovascular events. Atherosclerosis is a systemic process that involves large and medium-sized elastic and muscular arteries and typically affects the aorta, and coronary, carotid, and peripheral vessels. The epicardial coronary arteries are particularly susceptible, but some arteries including the intra-myocardial arteries are rarely affected.

Atherosclerosis starts in childhood, progresses silently through early adult life, and often manifests in later decades with ischaemia or infarction of the heart, brain, or extremities. The disease is characterized by the development of focal atherosclerotic plaques within the intimal layer of the arterial wall that consist of cells, connective tissue, lipids, and debris. The cellular constituents include endothelial and smooth muscle cells from the vessel wall, and inflammatory and immune cells derived from the circulating blood. As the disease progresses, individual plaque morphology may change abruptly because of plaque rupture and superimposed thrombosis. In addition, secondary changes may develop in the media and adventitia. As a consequence there may be marked heterogeneity in plaque morphology in different vascular territories, even in the same individual. The complex molecular and cellular mechanisms underlying the atherosclerotic disease process are incompletely understood, but it is now recognized that atherosclerosis is an active process involving interplay of cardiovascular risk factors, vascular biology, and chronic inflammation.

Endothelial activation

The vascular endothelium, the innermost cellular layer of blood vessels, has a key role in vascular homeostasis and is critically involved in the development of atherosclerotic disease. In health the endothelium produces a wide range of locally active substances that regulate contractile, secretory, and mitogenic functions of the vessel wall, and influence blood coagulation.

Endothelial physiology

The importance of the endothelium was first demonstrated in studies of vascular tone[28], but it is now recognized that the endothelium releases a range of autocrine and paracrine mediators that control vascular physiology and response to injury. Nitric oxide (NO), the principal endothelium-derived relaxing factor, plays a key role in the maintenance of vascular tone and endothelial reactivity. NO is synthesized from the amino acid L-arginine by the action of endothelial NO synthetase (eNOS). This enzyme requires a critical cofactor, tetrahydrobiopterin, to facilitate endothelial NO production. Following release from endothelial cells NO diffuses into medial smooth muscle cells and activates guanylate cyclase, which results in cyclic guanosine monophosphate (cGMP) mediated vasodilatation. In addition NO maintains the endothelium and medial smooth muscle cells in a non-proliferative state and when released into the blood NO inhibits platelets and leucocytes. An NO-independent pathway also contributes to vasodilator tone but has not yet been fully elucidated[29–31].

The actions of NO are opposed by endothelium-derived vasoconstrictor factors, such as endothelin and vasoactive prostanoids, and by angiotensin-II, which is converted at the endothelial surface from angiotensin-I. These mediators cause vasoconstriction, activate endothelial cells, platelets, and leucocytes, and facilitate thrombosis, directly countering the inhibitory effects of NO[29–31].

Endothelial activation and dysfunction

Exposure to cardiovascular risk factors (including tobacco use, hypertension, hyperlipidaemia, and diabetes) activates mechanisms within endothelial cells that result in expression of chemokines, cytokines, and adhesion molecules programmed to interact with leucocytes and platelets. At a molecular level, risk factor exposure appears to induce a switch from NO-mediated inhibition of endothelial and other cellular processes towards endothelial activation via redox signalling. As part of endothelial activation eNOS, which normally maintains the endothelium in a quiescent state via production of NO, switches to generate reactive oxygen species (ROS). This process is termed eNOS uncoupling and results in superoxide production if there is tetrahydrobiopterin deficiency, and hydrogen peroxide production if levels of L-arginine are inadequate. The resulting oxidative stress within the endothelium leads to increased production of endothelin and other mediators, which promote endothelial activation[30,31]. Recently it has been suggested that the effects of cardiovascular risk factors on endothelial function may be mediated by down-regulation of lysyl oxidase (LOX), a copper-dependent amine oxidase that initiates the covalent cross-linking of collagen and elastin, and plays a crucial role in the maintenance of the tensile and elastic features of connective tissues[32].

Collectively, these processes result in endothelial dysfunction, a systemic disorder affecting all arteries that predisposes to vasoconstriction, increased endothelial cell permeability, expression of adhesion molecules, increased chemokine secretion, leucocyte adherence and migration, vascular smooth muscle cell proliferation, and platelet activation and thrombosis (Fig. 1.4A)[31,33].

Clinical indicators of endothelial activation, such as endothelial vasomotor dysfunction, can predict cardiovascular events in patients with and without overt coronary artery disease[34] but correction of cardiovascular risk factors has been shown to improve endothelial function. For example, treatment of hypercholesterolaemia with statins has been shown to improve or normalize endothelial function in patients with mild coronary artery disease[35]. Angiotensin-converting enzyme inhibitors (ACE-I) also improve endothelial function through a range of mechanisms (antioxidant effects, favourable effect on fibrinolysis, reduction in angiotensin-II, increase in bradykinin), although a direct relationship between these effects and the risk of adverse cardiovascular events has not yet been clearly established[36].

Early stages of atherosclerosis

The mechanisms that underlie the initial stages of atherosclerosis have not been fully elucidated but endothelial activation appears to be integral to the process. Endothelial activation precedes the onset of the disease, facilitates inflammatory processes that lead to atherosclerosis, and promotes mechanisms of disease progression.

Lipid retention and modification

In the earliest stage of atherosclerosis LDL particles probably enter the subendothelial space from the bloodstream. Apolipoprotein in the LDL particles is thought to bind to extracellular proteoglycans (especially biglycan) and other macromolecules, ensuring retention of

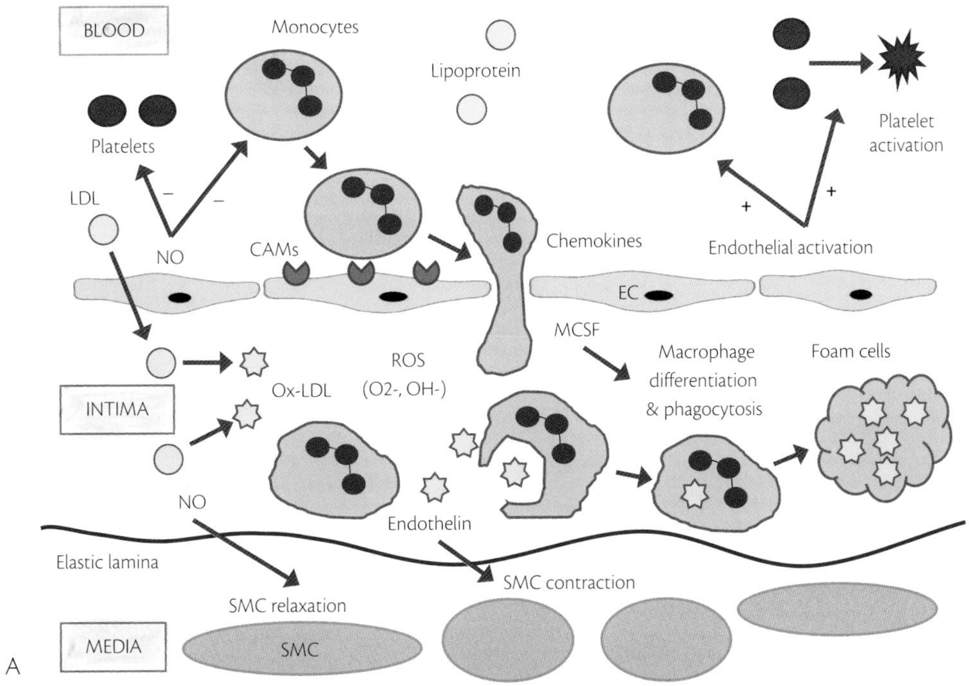

Fig. 1.4A Simplified schematic of atherogenesis. Nitric oxide (NO) secreted by endothelial cells (EC) causes relaxation of smooth muscle cells (SMC) and vasodilatation. NO also inhibits (–) platelets and leucocytes. Low-density lipoprotein (LDL) enters the subendothelial space and is modified, generating oxidized LDL (Ox-LDL). Endothelial activation and dysfunction causes generation of reactive oxygen species (ROS) and endothelin, expression of cell adhesion molecules (CAM) on the endothelial cells, and activation of platelets and monocytes (+). Monocytes adhere to the endothelium and under the influence of chemokines migrate into the subendothelial space. Macrophage colony stimulating factor (MCSF) induces monocyte differentiation into macrophages. Activated macrophages phagocytose lipid and develop into foam cells.

lipid within the extracellular matrix[37,38]. LDL particles may be modified through oxidation and glycation. The precise pathways of this chemical transformation are uncertain but evidence implicates myeloperoxidase, a haem peroxidase enzyme found predominantly in neutrophils, monocytes, and some macrophages. Myeloperoxidase generates numerous reactive oxidants and diffusible radical species that are capable of initiating and promoting peroxidation and other modifications of the lipid[39].

Inflammation

Modified and oxidized LDL contribute to endothelial activation and initiate an inflammatory response in the vessel wall. Activated endothelium expresses several types of cell adhesion molecules (CAMs), which facilitate adhesion of leucocytes rolling along the endoluminal surface of the vessel wall to the endothelium. Chemokines produced in the endothelial cells then stimulate migration of the adherent monocytes and T-cell lymphocytes into the subendothelial space[40–42].

Macrophage colony stimulating factor, a cytokine produced in the activated endothelial cells, stimulates monocytes within the intima to differentiate into macrophages. This transformation is associated with up-regulation of scavenger receptors and Toll-like receptors on the macrophage cell surface that bind modified LDL and oxidized phospholipid. Activation of macrophage Toll-like receptors also induces intracellular signalling and cell activation, with cytoskeletal rearrangements, stimulation of inflammatory cytokine secretion, and production of proteases and cytotoxic oxygen radicals. These processes facilitate endocytosis and destruction of the oxidized LDL particles, but if the lipid cannot be fully metabolized it accumulates as cytosolic droplets and the macrophage transforms into a foam cell[40,43].

Lymphocytes within the intima also produce inflammatory cytokines, chemokines, proteases, and cytotoxic oxygen and nitrogen radical molecules. Cytokines may induce expression of CD40, a transmembrane protein receptor present on inflammatory cells within the plaque. Activation of CD40 by CD40 ligand, derived

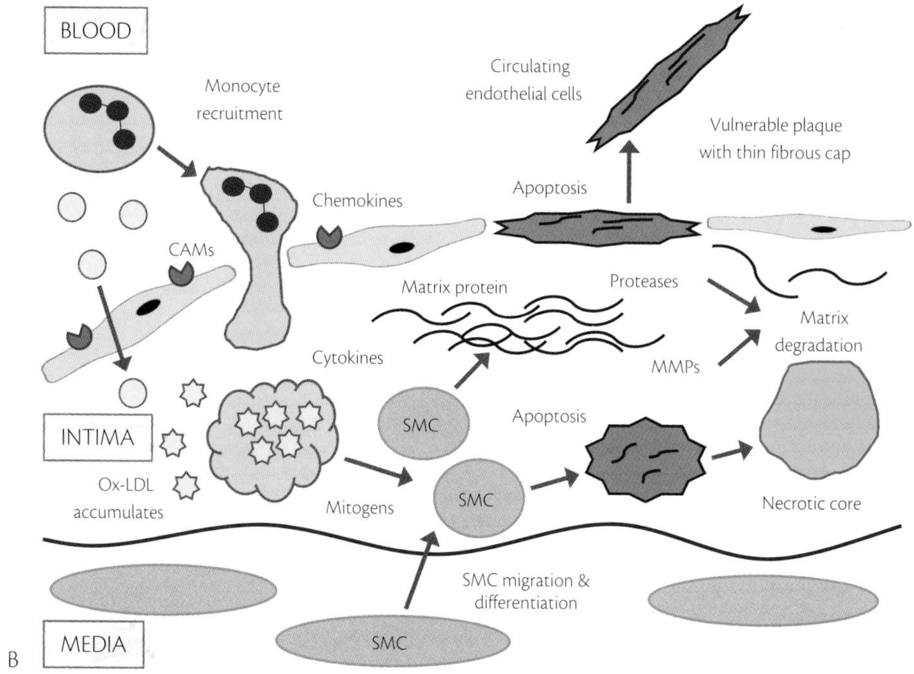

Fig. 1.4B As oxidized lipid accumulates, monocytes are recruited to the developing plaque. Cytokines and mitogens stimulate recruitment and proliferation of smooth muscle cells (SMCs). SMCs produce extracellular matrix, which increases plaque volume. Apoptosis of endothelial cells and impaired endothelial regeneration may lead to plaque erosion. Apoptosis of cells within the plaque leads to the development of a lipid-rich necrotic core. The overlying fibrous cap may be degraded by matrix metalloproteinases (MMPs) and other proteases, increasing the risk of plaque rupture. Other abbreviations as in Fig.1.4A.

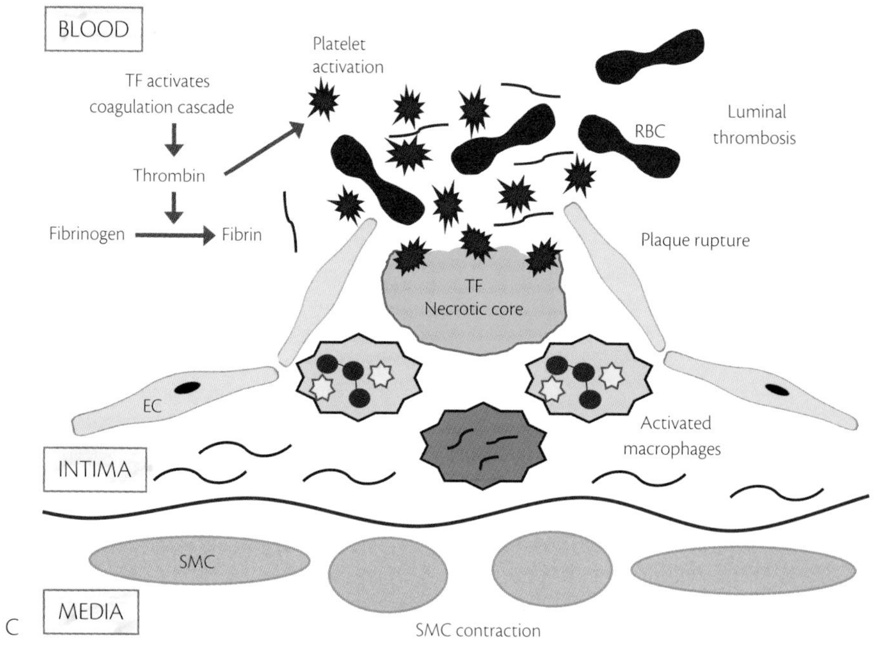

Fig. 1.4C Activated macrophages may cause progressive degradation of the fibrous cap over the lipid core. Plaque rupture exposes the thrombogenic core contents to the circulating blood. Tissue factor (TF) and other thrombogenic factors stimulate the coagulation cascade and cause luminal thrombosis. RBC, red blood cell. Other abbreviations as in Fig.1.4A.

from platelets and other cells, signals upregulation of proinflammatory and atherogenic genes[44]. This process is known to involve the intracellular nuclear factor kappa B transcription pathway, which controls the transcription of genes for many cytokines, chemokines, adhesion molecules, and regulators of apoptosis[45]. These processes augment and perpetuate the inflammatory atherosclerotic process and recruit additional macrophages and medial smooth muscle cells. If the inflammatory response does not remove or neutralize the initiating stimulus it can continue unabated.

The accumulation of lipid-laden monocytes, foam cells and T-cell lymphocytes within the intima leads to the formation of fatty streaks and early atherosclerotic lesions (Fig. 1.5). Fatty streaks are prevalent in young people and are generally considered to be an antecedent of atheroma, but they may also disappear over time[46]. Evidence of early atherosclerosis has been demonstrated in post-mortem studies of young soldiers killed during the Vietnam[47] and Korean[48] wars and in intracoronary ultrasound studies of transplanted hearts retrieved from teenage and young adult donors[49].

Disease progression

Plaque growth

As the atherosclerotic process progresses, the plaque increases in size due to accumulation of inflammatory and smooth muscle cells, production of extracellular matrix, and continuing deposition of lipid in the arterial wall. Vascular smooth muscle cells, stimulated by mitogens and cytokines, differentiate into migratory and secretory cells and migrate into the intima (Fig. 1.4B)[50] Smooth muscle cells produce collagen and other matrix proteins, including gylcosaminoglycans, proteoglycans, elastin, fibronectin, laminin, vitronectin, and thrombospondin[51].

Arterial remodelling

During growth of atherosclerotic plaque the entire vessel can vary in size, a process known as remodelling. Enlargement of the vessel may accommodate the plaque volume without compromising the arterial lumen until the plaque enlarges to over 40% of the vessel area, but thereafter further growth in the plaque causes luminal narrowing[51,52]. Alternatively, the vessel may constrict and further narrow the arterial lumen. The mechanisms

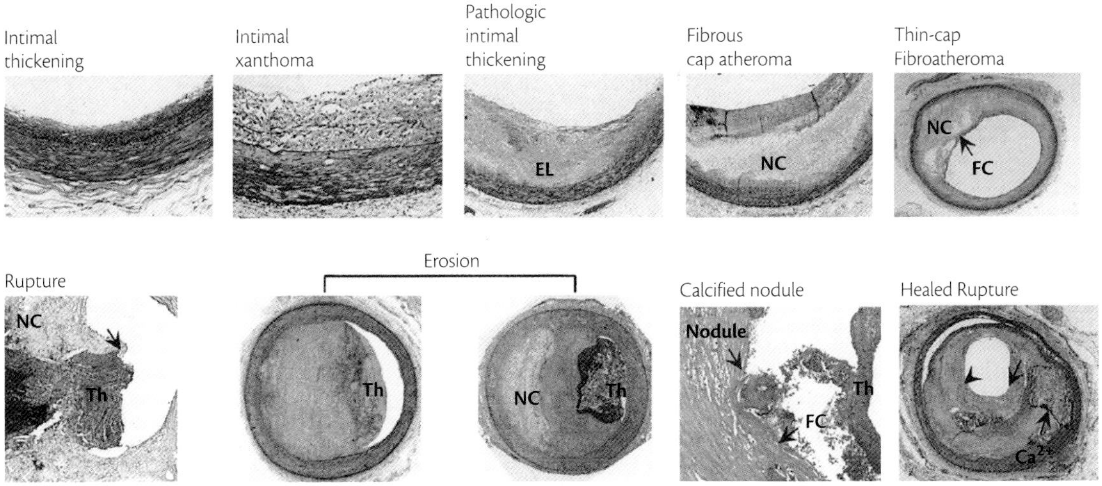

Fig. 1.5 Histopathology of plaque progression. Descriptions begin at top, from left to right. Intimal thickening is normal in all age groups and is characterized by smooth muscle cell accumulation within the intima. Intimal xanthoma corresponds to the fatty streak and denotes the accumulation of macrophages and lymphocytes within the intimal thickening lesion. Pathologic intimal thickening denotes the accumulation of extracellular lipid. Fibrous cap atheroma indicates the presence of a necrotic core under a fibrous cap, which may become thinned (thin-cap atheroma). This lesion may rupture, with exposure of the necrotic core to the lumen. The thrombus of a plaque erosion may overlie pathological intimal thickening (left) or fibrous cap atheroma (right). Calcified nodule is a rare form of coronary thrombus. Acute rupture may progress to healing (healed plaque rupture) without luminal occlusion. EL, extracellular lipid; FC, fibrous cap; NC, necrotic core; Th, thrombus. Reproduced from Frostegard J, Ulfgren AK, Nyberg P, *et al.* Cytokine expression in advanced human atherosclerotic plaques: dominance of pro-inflammatory (Th1) and macrophage-stimulating cytokines. *Atherosclerosis* 1999; **145**(1):33–43 with permission from Elsevier.

regulating remodelling have not been elucidated but may contribute to heterogeneity in the progression and clinical manifestations of arterial disease[53].

Plaque neovascularization

As atheromatous disease advances, new microvessels may develop from the adventitial vasa vasorum, possibly in response to hypoxia and activation of Toll-like receptors within the expanding atherosclerotic plaque. This process appears to be regulated by vascular endothelial growth factor (VEGF) A, which together with angiotensin II can also induce microvascular permeability. These processes may facilitate extravasation of red blood cells and intraplaque haemorrhage. Release of haemoglobin into the extracellular matrix of the plaque exacerbates oxidative stress, amplifying macrophage activation and pro-inflammatory signals, and accelerating the atherosclerotic process[54].

Apoptosis

Apoptosis of the cellular components of the plaque may be mediated by cytokines including interleukin-1, tumour necrosis factor-alpha, and interferon-gamma[55]. Apoptosis has been observed at all stages of atherosclerosis but the consequences for lesion progression may depend on how efficiently the apoptotic cell is cleared by other macrophages. In early lesions phagocytic clearance appears to be efficient, reduces lesion cellularity and atheroma progression. In more advanced lesions phagocytic clearance may be defective, leading to secondary necrosis of the apoptotic cell, further release of inflammatory mediators, and amplification of the inflammatory process. Cumulatively these events may lead to the development of a highly thrombogenic necrotic core within the expanding plaque, which contains cell remnants expressing active tissue factors[56]. As the necrotic lipid-rich core expands, a fibrous cap forms over the luminal surface, creating a barrier between the thrombogenic material within the core and the circulating blood (Fig. 1.4B).

Endothelial cells can also progress to senescence and may detach into the circulation. Whole endothelial cells and microparticles derived from activated or apoptotic endothelial cells can be detected in the circulating blood as markers of endothelial injury and are thought to influence blood thrombogenicity[57]. Restoration of endothelial integrity involves replication of adjacent mature endothelial cells or recruitment of circulating endothelial progenitor cells. Mobilization of endothelial progenitor cells is influenced by NO and may therefore be impaired in individuals with cardiovascular risk factors[31,58]. In animal models restoration of endothelial integrity after balloon injury improves with exercise or statins, which both improve endothelial function[59,60].

Influence of biomechanical forces

Dysfunctional endothelium, fatty streaks, and atheroma all localize preferentially to arterial sites associated with disturbed flow patterns, suggesting an important role for local haemodynamic forces in the development of arterial disease. These sites include branch points on the opposite side of the flow divider, and post-stenotic segments where laminar flow may be disturbed by re-circulation eddies, flow separation, and oscillatory flows. Evidence suggests that exposure of the endothelium to such different biomechanical forces, induces differential expression of specific genes in endothelial cells. Laminar shear stress from the viscous flow of blood against the endothelial cell surface induces eNOS activity, which supports vasoprotective functions in the endothelium. By contrast, reduced or oscillatory shear stress induces endothelial activation, expression of adhesion molecules, and endothelial cell apoptosis[61–65].

Calcification of atheroma

Microscopic areas of calcification may appear within the atherosclerotic plaque, which become denser as the disease advances. The extent of coronary calcification correlates with the severity of luminal narrowing caused by the plaque[66]. The predominant chemical constituent of coronary calcification is identical to hydroxyapatite, the main inorganic constituent of bone[67]. Osteopontin, a gylcosylated protein involved in the formation and calcification of bone is synthesized by macrophages, smooth muscle, and endothelial cells. Endothelial progenitor cells in patients with coronary disease have also been shown to express osteocalcin, an osteoblastic marker[55,68]. The significance of calcification for plaque progression and cardiac events is uncertain, but extensive calcification may impact the outcome of percutaneous coronary intervention. Rarely, eruptive nodular calcification with underlying fibrocalcific plaque is implicated as a cause of coronary thrombosis[69].

Plaque rupture and thrombosis

Most atherosclerotic plaques develop slowly over many years, under the influence of local immune responses and continued exposure to cardiovascular risk factors. Integrity of the fibrous cap overlying the plaque core is maintained by balanced production and degradation of extracellular matrix proteins. If this balance is disturbed, overproduction of matrix may encroach on the arterial lumen, but increased matrix degradation may weaken the plaque cap increasing the risk of plaque rupture.

Matrix metalloproteinases

Matrix protein degradation is mediated by matrix metalloproteinases (MMPs) and other proteases released by inflammatory cells, including macrophages and migrated smooth muscle cells. MMPs are $Zinc^{2+}$-dependent endopeptidases and include collagenases, gelatinases, stromelysins and metalloelastases. MMP activation is controlled at several levels including induction of MMP gene transcription, post-translational activation of MMP proforms, and interaction with specific tissue inhibitors (TIMPs). MMPs may facilitate smooth muscle cell migration through the internal elastic lamina into the intima, are implicated in vascular remodelling, and appear to have a central role in plaque rupture. Expression of MMP activity is influenced by several drugs including the HMG Co-A reductase inhibitors (statins)[51,70,71]. Cysteine proteases, which are induced by certain cytokines and controlled by 'cystatin' inhibitors, also have been implicated in matrix metabolism in atherosclerosis[72].

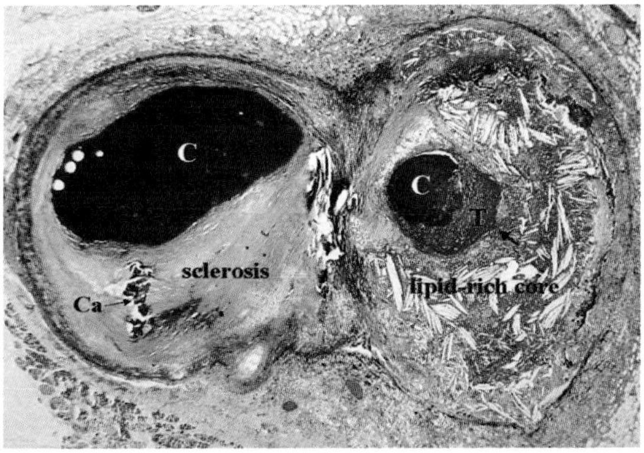

Fig. 1.6 Atherothrombosis: a variable mix of chronic atherosclerosis and acute thrombosis. Cross-sectioned arterial bifurcation illustrating a collagen-rich (blue-stained) plaque in the circumflex branch (left) and a lipid-rich and ruptured plaque (arrow) with a non-occlusive thrombosis superimposed in the obtuse marginal branch (right). C, contrast in the lumen; Ca, calcification; T, thrombosis. Reproduced from Falk E, Prediman S, Fuster V. Coronary plaque disruption. *Circulation* 1995; **92**:657–71.

Plaque rupture

Active degradation and remodelling of the extracellular plaque matrix by macrophages, via release of MMPs and other proteases and by subsequent phagocytosis, inhibits the formation of a stable fibrous cap. Further breakdown of collagen and other proteins within the fibrous cap reduces the structural integrity of the plaque and predisposes to plaque rupture[70,71]. Interaction between CD40 and CD40 ligand may induce MMP production and may play a role in plaque instability[44]. Plaques with a thin fibrous cap, large lipid core, and inflammatory cell infiltrate at the thinnest portion of the cap appear to be particularly vulnerable to rupture (Fig. 1.6)[69]. Inflammatory cells are abundant in the shoulder regions of ruptured plaque and many show signs of activation and inflammatory cytokine production[73,74].

Rupture of a coronary artery plaque causes an acute change in plaque morphology, exposure of tissue factor and other thrombogenic plaque contents to the circulating blood, activation of the coagulation cascade, and coronary thrombosis (Fig. 1.4C). The consequences of plaque rupture are determined by the severity of the plaque injury, local rheology, and the balance between thrombotic and lytic activity at the interface between the plaque and the circulating blood. These factors influence the size and stability of the thrombus, and the severity of the resulting coronary syndrome. Partial or complete thrombotic occlusion of the artery, or thrombus embolism into the distal vessel, may cause myocardial ischaemia and an acute coronary syndrome. More frequently, however, it is thought that plaque disruption occurs silently, and subsequent repair of the vascular injury and fibrotic organization of the thrombus may cause accelerated plaque growth, contributing to progression of the atherothrombotic process[55].

Detailed histopathological examination of coronary arteries in sudden cardiac death victims confirms that rupture of a thin collagenous fibrous cap, with discontinuity of the cap at the site of contact between the thrombus and lipid core, is the cause of coronary thrombosis in the majority of cases. In other cases, however, the coronary thrombosis occurs at the site of a superficial plaque erosion, without involvement of a lipid core. The luminal surface is irregular and devoid of endothelial cells, and the plaque in contact with the thrombus is generally cellular and rich in proteoglycan. Endothelial apoptosis with deficient endothelial repair may be the underlying cause of plaque erosion. Plaque erosion is particularly likely in young women, but with advancing age plaque rupture becomes the dominant cause of coronary thrombosis (Figs. 1.4 and 1.5)[66,69].

Angiographic studies of patients before and after myocardial infarction suggest that the culprit stenosis responsible for the acute coronary syndrome is frequently only of moderate severity[75,76]. Mild or moderate coronary stenoses may be an important cause of acute coronary syndrome because they are much more prevalent than severe stenoses, which are individually at higher risk of causing coronary thrombosis[77].

Systemic markers of inflammation

There is increasing evidence that atherosclerosis is associated with chronic low-grade inflammation in clinically silent plaques throughout the vascular system[40]. Coronary arteriographic studies have demonstrated multiple complex plaques (characterized by thrombus, ulceration, plaque irregularity, and impaired flow) in nearly 40% of patients with recent myocardial infarction, supporting the concept that plaque instability is due to a systemic increase in inflammation[78]. The blood levels of several markers of inflammation including C-reactive protein (CRP), interleukins, soluble CD40 ligand, and tissue factor, are all elevated in patients with acute coronary syndromes, and high levels generally predict worse outcome[79,80]. Elevated levels of CRP, serum amyloid A, interleukin-6, and soluble intercellular adhesion molecule type 1 are also all associated with cardiovascular risk in apparently healthy populations[81]. CRP is an acute phase reactant and is mainly produced in the liver in response to interleukin-6. CRP has therefore been considered an inactive marker of inflammation, but there is increasing evidence that CRP may also play a direct role in atherogenesis[43,79].

Drugs which reduce inflammation may have therapeutic effects in CHD. Aspirin use in otherwise healthy men reduced the risk of first myocardial infarction in those with the highest serum CRP levels[82]. Long-term treatment with pravastatin reduces CRP levels and improves clinical outcome[83,84]. Recently, 17 802 healthy subjects with low LDL-cholesterol levels and elevated high-sensitivity CRP levels were randomized to treatment with rosuvastatin or placebo, but the trial was stopped prematurely because treatment with rosuvastatin reduced serum LDL and CRP levels and the incidence of major cardiovascular events[85].

Summary

CHD remains a leading cause of death and disability across industrialized countries, is prevalent in Eastern Europe, and is a major threat to health in developing countries. Increases in the prevalence of coronary artery disease, both in the developed and developing countries can be largely explained by coronary risk factors, including tobacco use, high blood lipid levels, hypertension, obesity, and diabetes.

Atherothrombosis, the pathological process underlying most cases of CHD, is defined as atherosclerosis with superimposed thrombosis. The molecular and cellular mechanisms of atherothrombosis are incompletely understood, but there is compelling evidence that the disease is due to a chronic inflammatory process in the arterial intima. Exposure to risk factors and deposition of lipoprotein in the intima cause up-regulation of atherogenic and pro-thrombotic processes. Monocytes are recruited into the intima from the circulating blood and a series of inflammatory mechanisms lead to the development of an atherosclerotic plaque. Endothelial apoptosis and inadequate endothelial repair over the plaque may lead to endothelial erosion and arterial thrombosis. Development of a necrotic lipid core within the plaque and degradation of the overlying fibrous cap by proteases, render the plaque vulnerable to disruption. Plaque rupture exposes the core contents to the circulating blood and potent thrombogenic stimuli activate the coagulation cascade, causing arterial thrombosis. In many cases coronary plaque erosion or rupture occur silently, but if the thrombosis impedes coronary blood flow the myocardium may become ischaemic, and the patient may present with an acute coronary syndrome, myocardial infarction, or death. The development of treatment strategies to combat these complex molecular, cellular, and physiological disturbances presents interventional cardiology with the greatest challenge.

References

1. Lopez AD, Mathers CD, Ezzati M, *et al.* Global and regional burden of disease and risk factors, 2001: systematic analysis of population health data. *Lancet* 2006; **367**(9524):1747–57.
2. Murray CJ, Lopez AD. Alternative projections of mortality and disability by cause 1990–2020: Global Burden of Disease Study. *Lancet* 1997; **349**(9064):1498–504.
3. Allender S, Peto V, Scarborough P, *et al. Coronary Heart Disease Statistics*. London: British Heart Foundation, 2008.
4. Lloyd-Jones D, Adams R, Carnethon M, *et al.* Heart Disease and Stroke Statistics – 2009 Update: A Report From the American Heart Association Statistics Committee and Stroke Statistics Subcommittee. *Circulation* 2009; **119**(3):e21–181.
5. Allender S, Scarborough P, Peto V, *et al. European Cardiovascular Disease Statistics 2008*. Brussels: European Heart Network, 2009.
6. Ford ES, Capewell S. Coronary heart disease mortality among young adults in the U.S. From 1980 through 2002: Concealed leveling of mortality rates. *J Am Coll Cardiol* 2007; **50**(22):2128–32.
7. Unal B, Critchley JA, Capewell S. Explaining the decline in coronary heart disease mortality in England and Wales between 1981 and 2000. *Circulation* 2004; **109**(9):1101–7.
8. Ford ES, Ajani UA, Croft JB, *et al.* Explaining the decrease in U.S. deaths from coronary disease, 1980–2000. *N Engl J Med* 2007; **356**(23):2388–98.

9. Tunstall-Pedoe H, Vanuzzo D, Hobbs M, *et al.* Estimation of contribution of changes in coronary care to improving survival, event rates, and coronary heart disease mortality across the WHO MONICA Project populations. *Lancet* 2000; **355**(9205):688–700.
10. Kottke TE, Faith DA, Jordan CO, *et al.* The comparative effectiveness of heart disease prevention and treatment strategies. *Am J Prev Med* 2009; **36**(1):82–8.
11. Critchley J, Liu J, Zhao D, *et al.* Explaining the increase in coronary heart disease mortality in Beijing between 1984 and 1999. *Circulation* 2004; **110**(10):1236–44.
12. Reddy KS, Yusuf S. Emerging epidemic of cardiovascular disease in developing countries. *Circulation* 1998; **97**(6):596–601.
13. Gupta R, Joshi P, Mohan V, *et al.* Epidemiology and causation of coronary heart disease and stroke in India. *Heart* 2008; **94**(1):16–26.
14. Mensah GA. Ischaemic heart disease in Africa. *Heart* 2008; **94**(7):836–43.
15. Lanas F, Avezum A, Bautista LE, *et al.* Risk factors for acute myocardial infarction in Latin America: the INTERHEART Latin American study. *Circulation* 2007; **115**(9):1067–74.
16. Luepker RV, Apple FS, Christenson RH, *et al.* Case Definitions for Acute Coronary Heart Disease in Epidemiology and Clinical Research Studies: A Statement From the AHA Council on Epidemiology and Prevention; AHA Statistics Committee; World Heart Federation Council on Epidemiology and Prevention; the European Society of Cardiology Working Group on Epidemiology and Prevention; Centers for Disease Control and Prevention; and the National Heart, Lung, and Blood Institute. *Circulation* 2003; **108**(20):2543–9.
17. Bassand JP, Hamm CW, Ardissino D, *et al.* Guidelines for the diagnosis and treatment of non-ST-segment elevation acute coronary syndromes: The Task Force for the Diagnosis and Treatment of Non-ST-Segment Elevation Acute Coronary Syndromes of the European Society of Cardiology. *Eur Heart J* 2007; **28**(13):1598–660.
18. MacIntyre K, Murphy NF, Chalmers J, *et al.* Hospital burden of suspected acute coronary syndromes: recent trends. *Heart* 2006; **92**(5):691–2.
19. Yusuf S, Hawken S, Ounpuu S, *et al.* Effect of potentially modifiable risk factors associated with myocardial infarction in 52 countries (the INTERHEART study): case–control study. *Lancet* 2004; **364**(9438): 937–52.
20. Teo KK, Ounpuu S, Hawken S, *et al.* Tobacco use and risk of myocardial infarction in 52 countries in the INTERHEART study: a case–control study. *Lancet* 2006; **368**(9536):647–58.
21. Prospective Studies Collaboration. Blood cholesterol and vascular mortality by age, sex, and blood pressure: a meta-analysis of individual data from 61 prospective studies with 55,000 vascular deaths. [Erratum appears in *Lancet* 2008; **372**(9635):292.] *Lancet* 2007; **370**(9602):1829–39.
22. Baigent C, Keech A, Kearney PM, *et al.* Efficacy and safety of cholesterol-lowering treatment: prospective meta-analysis of data from 90,056 participants in 14 randomised trials of statins. [Erratum appears in *Lancet* 2005; **366**(9494):1358.] *Lancet* 2005; **366**(9493):1267–78.
23. Prospective Studies Collaboration. Age-specific relevance of usual blood pressure to vascular mortality: a meta-analysis of individual data for one million adults in 61 prospective studies. [Erratum appears in *Lancet* 2003; **361**(9362):1060.] *Lancet* 2002; **360**(9349):1903–13.
24. Ezzati M, Oza S, Danaei G, *et al.* Trends and cardiovascular mortality effects of state-level blood pressure and uncontrolled hypertension in the United States. *Circulation* 2008; **117**(7):905–14.
25. Prospective Studies Collaboration. Body-mass index and cause-specific mortality in 900 000 adults: collaborative analyses of 57 prospective studies. *Lancet* 2009; **373**(9669):1083–96.
26. Ogden CL, Carroll MD, Flegal KM. High body mass index for age among US children and adolescents, 2003–2006. *JAMA* 2008; **299**(20):2401–5.
27. Emberson J, Whincup P, Morris R, *et al.* Evaluating the impact of population and high-risk strategies for the primary prevention of cardiovascular disease. *Eur Heart J* 2004; **25**(6):484–91.
28. Furchgott RF, Zawadzki JV, Furchgott RF, *et al.* The obligatory role of endothelial cells in the relaxation of arterial smooth muscle by acetylcholine. *Nature* 1980; **288**(5789):373–6.
29. Verma S, Anderson TJ. Fundamentals of endothelial function for the clinical cardiologist. *Circulation* 2002; **105**(5):546–9.
30. Förstermann U, Münzel T. Endothelial nitric oxide synthase in vascular disease: from marvel to menace. *Circulation* 2006; **113**(13):1708–14.
31. Deanfield JE, Halcox JP, Rabelink TJ. Endothelial function and dysfunction: testing and clinical relevance. *Circulation* 2007; **115**(10):1285–95.
32. Rodriguez C, Martinez-Gonzalez J, Raposo B, *et al.* Regulation of lysyl oxidase in vascular cells: lysyl oxidase as a new player in cardiovascular diseases. *Cardiovasc Res* 2008; **79**(1):7–13.
33. Hink U, Li H, Mollnau H, *et al.* Mechanisms underlying endothelial dysfunction in diabetes mellitus. *Circ Res* 2001; **88**(2):E14–E22.
34. Halcox JP, Schenke WH, Zalos G, *et al.* Prognostic value of coronary vascular endothelial dysfunction. *Circulation* 2002; **106**(6):653–8.
35. Suwaidi JA, Hamasaki S, Higano ST, *et al.* Long-term follow-up of patients with mild coronary artery disease and endothelial dysfunction. *Circulation* 2000; **101**(9):948–54.
36. Anderson TJ, Elstein E, Haber H, *et al.* Comparative study of ACE-inhibition, angiotensin II antagonism, and calcium channel blockade on flow-mediated vasodilation in patients with coronary disease (BANFF study). *J Am Coll Cardiol* 2000; **35**(1):60–6.

37. Khalil MF, Wagner WD, Goldberg IJ. Molecular interactions leading to lipoprotein retention and the initiation of atherosclerosis. *Arterioscler Thromb Vasc Biol* 2004; **24**(12):2211–18.
38. Nakashima Y, Wight TN, Sueishi K. Early atherosclerosis in humans: role of diffuse intimal thickening and extracellular matrix proteoglycans. *Cardiovasc Res* 2008; **79**(1):14–23.
39. Nicholls SJ, Hazen SL. Myeloperoxidase and cardiovascular disease. *Arterioscler Thromb Vasc Biol* 2005; **25**(6):1102–11.
40. Hansson GK. Inflammation, atherosclerosis, and coronary artery disease. *N Engl J Med* 2005; **352**(16):1685–95.
41. Gleissner CA, Leitinger N, Ley K. Effects of native and modified low-density lipoproteins on monocyte recruitment in atherosclerosis. *Hypertension* 2007; **50**(2):276–83.
42. Leitinger N. Oxidized phospholipids as modulators of inflammation in atherosclerosis. *Curr Opin Lipidol* 2003; **14**(5):421–30.
43. Miller YI, Chang MK, Binder CJ, *et al.* Oxidized low density lipoprotein and innate immune receptors. *Curr Opin Lipidol* 2003; **14**(5):437–45.
44. Antoniades C, Bakogiannis C, Tousoulis D, *et al.* The CD40/CD40 ligand system: linking inflammation with atherothrombosis. *J Am Coll Cardiol* 2009; **54**(8): 669–77.
45. de Winther MPJ, Kanters E, Kraal G, *et al.* Nuclear Factor κB signaling in atherogenesis. *Arterioscler Thromb Vasc Biol* 2005; **25**(5):904–14.
46. Stary HC. Evolution and progression of atherosclerotic lesions in coronary arteries of children and young adults. *Arteriosclerosis* 1989; **9**(1 Suppl):I19–I32.
47. McNamara JJ, Molot MA, Stremple JF, *et al.* Coronary artery disease in combat casualties in Vietnam. *JAMA* 1971; **216**(7):1185–7.
48. Virmani R, Robinowitz M, Geer JC, *et al.* Coronary artery atherosclerosis revisited in Korean war combat casualties. *Arch Pathol Lab Med* 1987; **111**(10):972–6.
49. Tuzcu EM, Hobbs RE, Rincon G, *et al.* Occult and frequent transmission of atherosclerotic coronary disease with cardiac transplantation. Insights from intravascular ultrasound. *Circulation* 1995; **91**(6):1706–13.
50. Hedin U, Roy J, Tran PK. Control of smooth muscle cell proliferation in vascular disease. *Curr Opin Lipidol* 2004; **15**(5):559–65.
51. Faxon DP, Fuster V, Libby P, *et al.* Atherosclerotic Vascular Disease Conference: Writing Group III: pathophysiology. *Circulation* 2004; **109**(21):2617–25.
52. Glagov S, Weisenberg E, Zarins CK, *et al.* Compensatory enlargement of human atherosclerotic coronary arteries. *N Engl J Med* 1987; **316**(22):1371–5.
53. Pasterkamp G, de Kleijn DPV, Borst C. Arterial remodeling in atherosclerosis, restenosis and after alteration of blood flow: potential mechanisms and clinical implications. *Cardiovasc Res* 2000; **45**(4):843–52.
54. Moreno PR, Purushothaman KR, Sirol M, *et al.* Neovascularization in human atherosclerosis. *Circulation* 2006; **113**(18):2245–52.
55. Fuster V, Moreno PR, Fayad ZA, *et al.* Atherothrombosis and high-risk plaque: part I: evolving concepts. *J Am Coll Cardiol* 2005; **46**(6):937–54.
56. Tabas I. Consequences and therapeutic implications of macrophage apoptosis in atherosclerosis: the importance of lesion stage and phagocytic efficiency. *Arterioscler Thromb Vasc Biol* 2005; **25**(11):2255–64.
57. Mutin M, Canavy I, Blann A, *et al.* Direct evidence of endothelial injury in acute myocardial infarction and unstable angina by demonstration of circulating endothelial cells. *Blood* 1999; **93**(9):2951–8.
58. Mallat Z, Tedgui A. Current perspective on the role of apoptosis in atherothrombotic disease. *Circ Res* 2001; **88**(10):998–1003.
59. Walter DH, Rittig K, Bahlmann FH, *et al.* Statin therapy accelerates reendothelialization: a novel effect involving mobilization and incorporation of bone marrow-derived endothelial progenitor cells. *Circulation* 2002; **105**(25):3017–24.
60. Laufs U, Werner N, Link A, *et al.* Physical training increases endothelial progenitor cells, inhibits neointima formation, and enhances angiogenesis. *Circulation* 2004; **109**(2):220–6.
61. Chappell DC, Varner SE, Nerem RM, *et al.* Oscillatory shear stress stimulates adhesion molecule expression in cultured human endothelium. *Circ Res* 1998; **82**(5): 532–9.
62. Kinlay S, Libby P, Ganz P. Endothelial function and coronary artery disease. *Curr Opin Lipidol* 2001; **12**(4):383–9.
63. Tricot O, Mallat Z, Heymes C, *et al.* Relation between endothelial cell apoptosis and blood flow direction in human atherosclerotic plaques. *Circulation* 2000; **101**(21):2450–3.
64. Gimbrone MA, Jr, Topper JN, Nagel T, *et al.* Endothelial dysfunction, hemodynamic forces, and atherogenesis. *Ann NY Acad Sci* 2000; **902**:230–40.
65. Dai G, Kaazempur-Mofrad MR, Natarajan S, *et al.* Distinct endothelial phenotypes evoked by arterial waveforms derived from atherosclerosis-susceptible and -resistant regions of human vasculature. *Proc Natl Acad Sci U S A* 2004; **101**(41):14871–6.
66. Burke AP, Virmani R, Galis Z, *et al.* Task force #2 – What is the pathologic basis for new atherosclerosis imaging techniques? *J Am Coll Cardiol* 2003; **41**(11):1874–86.
67. Fitzpatrick LA, Severson A, Edwards WD, *et al.* Diffuse calcification in human coronary arteries. Association of osteopontin with atherosclerosis. *J Clin Invest* 1994; **94**(4):1597–604.
68. Gössl M, Mödder UI, Atkinson EJ, *et al.* Osteocalcin expression by circulating endothelial progenitor cells in patients with coronary atherosclerosis. *J Am Coll Cardiol* 2008; **52**(16):1314–25.

69. Virmani R, Kolodgie FD, Burke AP, *et al.* Lessons from sudden coronary death: a comprehensive morphological classification scheme for atherosclerotic lesions. *Arterioscler Thromb Vasc Biol* 2000; **20**(5):1262–75.
70. Rekhter MD. Collagen synthesis in atherosclerosis: too much and not enough. *Cardiovasc Res* 1999; **41**(2):376–84.
71. Jones CB, Sane DC, Herrington DM. Matrix metalloproteinases: a review of their structure and role in acute coronary syndrome. *Cardiovasc Res* 2003; **59**(4):812–23.
72. Liu J, Sukhova GK, Sun JS, *et al.* Lysosomal cysteine proteases in atherosclerosis. *Arterioscler Thromb Vasc Biol* 2004; **24**(8):1359–66.
73. Kovanen PT, Kaartinen M, Paavonen T, *et al.* Infiltrates of activated mast cells at the site of coronary atheromatous erosion or rupture in myocardial infarction. *Circulation* 1995; **92**(5):1084–8.
74. Frostegard J, Ulfgren AK, Nyberg P, *et al.* Cytokine expression in advanced human atherosclerotic plaques: dominance of pro-inflammatory (Th1) and macrophage-stimulating cytokines. *Atherosclerosis* 1999; **145**(1):33–43.
75. Little WC, Constantinescu M, Applegate RJ, *et al.* Can coronary angiography predict the site of a subsequent myocardial infarction in patients with mild-to-moderate coronary artery disease? *Circulation* 1988; **78**(5):1157–66.
76. Ambrose JA, Tannenbaum MA, Alexopoulos D, *et al.* Angiographic progression of coronary artery disease and the development of myocardial infarction. *J Am Coll Cardiol* 1988; **12**(1):56–62.
77. Falk E, Shah PK, Fuster V. Coronary plaque disruption. *Circulation* 1995; **92**:657–71.
78. Goldstein JA, Demetriou D, Grines CL, *et al.* Multiple complex coronary plaques in patients with acute myocardial infarction. *N Engl J Med* 2000; **343**(13):915–22.
79. Blake GJ, Ridker PM. Inflammatory bio-markers and cardiovascular risk prediction. *J Intern Med* 2002; **252**(4):283–94.
80. Soejima H, Ogawa H, Yasue H, *et al.* Heightened tissue factor associated with tissue factor pathway inhibitor and prognosis in patients with unstable angina. *Circulation* 1999; **99**(22):2908–13.
81. Ridker PM, Hennekens CH, Buring JE, *et al.* C-reactive protein and other markers of inflammation in the prediction of cardiovascular disease in women. *N Engl J Med* 2000; **342**(12):836–43.
82. Ridker PM, Cushman M, Stampfer MJ, *et al.* Inflammation, aspirin, and the risk of cardiovascular disease in apparently healthy men. *N Engl J Med* 1997; **336**(14):973–9.
83. Ridker PM, Rifai N, Pfeffer MA, *et al.* Inflammation, pravastatin, and the risk of coronary events after myocardial infarction in patients with average cholesterol levels. Cholesterol and Recurrent Events (CARE) Investigators. *Circulation* 1998; **98**(9):839–44.
84. Albert CM, Ma J, Rifai N, *et al.* Prospective study of C-reactive protein, homocysteine, and plasma lipid levels as predictors of sudden cardiac death. *Circulation* 2002; **105**(22):2595–9.
85. Ridker PM, Danielson E, Fonseca FA, *et al.* Rosuvastatin to prevent vascular events in men and women with elevated C-reactive protein. *N Engl J Med* 2008; **359**(21):2195–207.

CHAPTER 2

The history of interventional cardiology

Kenneth Kent

The rich history of interventional cardiology is befitting this subspecialty which is now responsible for treating over a million patients each year. These procedures improve quality of lives and reduce mortality. Interventional cardiology recently celebrated its third decade, in September, 2007.

The heart was always regarded as one of the most mysterious organs and was the poorly understood object of earlier anatomists. Galen[1] in the second century, for example, stated that the vessels attached to the heart were all arteries through which blood left the heart and the blood returned from the body by veins which emptied into the liver. However, Vesalius in the 16th century[1] provided the first reasonable presentation of cardiac anatomy. A century passed before William Harvey[2] published his findings on the functional components of the circulatory system with the demonstration of blood flow patterns in the arteries and veins. Subsequent investigations ranged from careful, well planned quantitative approaches with scientific rigor such as Nathan Hales' physiology experiments[3] to chance observations such as Mason Sones, who accidentally performed the first coronary angiogram while imaging the aorta in a patient with tetralogy of Fallot[2]. Hales set out to understand blood flow, pressures, and volumes throughout the circulatory system. One of the most graphic examples is the manometric measurements of the carotid artery pressures in the horse to demonstrate the necessity of pulsatile blood flow in perfusing the brain. Hales' quantitative approach used moulds made from the cardiac chambers which led to calculations of ventricular volumes, stroke volumes, and cardiac outputs.

The most important accidental observation was that made by Mason Sones, a radiologist at the Cleveland Clinic, who was studying a patient with congenital heart disease. While performing an aortogram, the X-ray tube was suspended from the ceiling, the phosphor on which the image appeared was beneath the patient, and the physician was in a 'pit', an opening in the floor beneath the patient. The radiologist, Dr. Sones, was using the fluoroscope to position catheters and obtain X-ray films to record the images. The contrast agent was injected by a power injector at 20mL/s and suddenly the right coronary artery was visualized. It was obvious that the catheter tip had slipped from the aorta into the orifice of the right coronary artery resulting in the power injection of 20mL of contrast. Visualization of the right coronary artery was facilitated by cessation of all cardiac activity. Dr. Sones yelled 'cough' which the patient did and cardiac activity resumed. Years later, Dr. Sones could give no explanation for his reflex to yell 'cough'. From this event, however, it was learned that the coronary arteries could be studied in a beating heart which led to the understanding of obstructive coronary artery disease, risk stratification for patients, and subsequently to a road map for revascularization procedures. One could only imagine how this specialty would have been affected if the asystole induced by the contrast had not been quickly reversed. The shout 'cough' was common in cardiac catheterization laboratories around the world in the 1970–1990s when coronary angiography was performed using ionic contrast agents which frequently led to profound bradycardia and hypotension.

Other wonderful examples of cardiac investigations include Werner Forsmann, a surgical resident in 1929 who demonstrated the feasibility of placing catheters in the heart by passing a urethral catheter through his own brachial vein into his right atrium[2]. To accomplish this feat, he duped a nurse working in the clinic. In order to win her cooperation, he convinced her that he was placing the catheter into her heart. Working behind her, he anaesthetized her antecubital space and then the same to his. He inserted the catheter in his vein and once it was in place, he confessed his trick and the two of them walked down the stairs to the radiology department where a chest X-ray confirmed that the catheter tip was in his heart. This ushered in the subsequent observations of Andre Cournand and Dickinson Richards on cardiac physiology and alterations by diseased states. Forsmann, Richards, and Cournand were awarded the Nobel Prize in 1956.

Rene Favaloro[4] reported the first series of patients with obstructive coronary artery disease in which operative revascularization of the heart was performed using reversed segments of saphenous vein grafts. The saphenous veins have valves which maintain forward flow of blood even in the dependant leg. The conduits were connected to the aorta as the proximal anastomosis and to the coronary artery as the distal anastomosis constructed so that arterial flow kept the valves in the open position. These valves were frequently the site of subsequent obstruction therefore techniques were developed to remove the valves before they were placed as conduits. Prior to Favaloro's reports, there were isolated examples of conduits, saphenous veins, internal mammary arteries, and artificial grafts being used to create aorto-myocardium and subsequently aorto-coronary grafts. Favaloro is credited with perfecting the procedure. Randomized clinical trials (RCTs) were established to test the effectiveness of this procedure. The Coronary Artery Surgery Study (CASS) and a VA Cooperative study of left main disease both demonstrated subgroups of patients in which mortality was reduced in patients after coronary artery bypass grafting (CABG)[5,6]. During the 1970s proliferation of this operation occurred; the operation was done quite well in many centres with documentation of excellent outcomes.

In the 1960s, most of the cardiac catheterization laboratories were focused on haemodynamics and structural heart disease due to congenital and acquired valvular defects. In order to improve the visualization of the coronary arteries for the surgeons, coronary angiography also matured during this time, including improved resolution of radiologic equipment, from 525 to 1050 lines, larger transformers, and subsequently digitization of the images from the phosphor tubes. The major improvement of contrast agents was development of non-ionic and iso-osmolar agents, which contained enough iodine to obtain high contrast angiographic images. There was also improvement in imaging platforms for positioning patients. The initial X-ray examination tables were flat and pillows were used to position patients for angiographic projections. Multidirectional C-arms allowed multiple axial views of the coronary arteries to be obtained. Fortunately, for that which lay ahead, this shift in focus of catheterization laboratories to studying coronary arteries facilitated the anatomical details which would be required for effective operative revascularization and to direct the tiny devices throughout the coronary arteries to perform coronary interventions.

Percutaneous transluminal coronary angioplasty

Much has been written about 'Great Discoveries' and the 'Discoverers'. Andreas Gruentzig (Fig. 2.1) certainly fitted many of the characteristics of a great discoverer. He was charming and charismatic but of strong will and would move forward regardless of the opposition when he felt it was necessary. His conflicts with Hans Peter Krayenbuhl, his Chief of Medicine at University Hospital, Zurich were legendary. He sought collaboration with colleagues who had been working with non-operative techniques, Dotter and Zeitler, he gained the support of Siegenthaler and Senning, Chiefs of Medicine

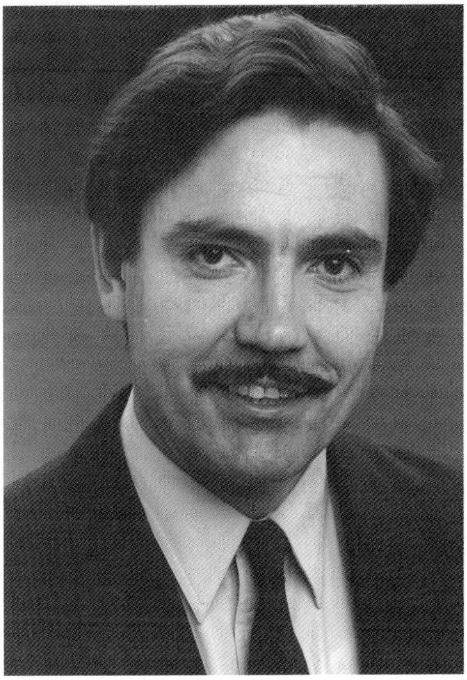

Fig. 2.1 Andreas Roland Gruentzig (1939–1985). Adventurer, creator, inventor, and caring physician, who left many grateful patients and admiring colleagues.

and Surgery, respectively at University Hospital. His intense interest and devotion to this project of non-operative revascularization of the heart coupled with his charm and wit proved successful in overcoming the critics and sceptics.

First, a bit about the man. Andreas Roland Gruentzig was born 25 June 1939 in Dresden, Germany. His father, a high school science teacher, was forced into the meteorology services of the German air-force, and was lost in World War II; his mother escaped to West Germany with Andreas and his brother, Johannes, and subsequently joined her family in Argentina. Because of poor living conditions, they returned to Leipzig, Germany. First Johannes and then Andreas completed medical school in Heidelberg. Following graduation from Medicine, Andreas spent 6 months in London at the School of Hygiene and was intrigued by the statistical approach to medicine and disease patterns. The latter explains his passion for exacting scientific approaches to percutaneous transluminal coronary angioplasty (PTCA) including record keeping, close follow-up of patients, and RCTs. He would certainly be pleased with the maturity of his technique and the thousands of patients who have been subjects in exacting, well controlled RCTs in various aspects of percutaneous coronary intervention. An extensive in-depth discussion of Gruentzig and these early experiences of coronary interventions has been published(7).

Gruentzig landed a training post in Angiology at University Hospital, Zurich. Angiology was the European equivalent of radiology and cardiology, a specialty of studying the vascular structures of the body, coronaries, carotids, aorta, and its major branches and peripheral vessels. He was attracted to Charles Dotter's technique of enlarging peripheral arteries by 'dilating' them with larger and larger catheters. He first introduced the concept of using a tiny balloon to achieve dilatation which had the obvious advantage of working through a small arteriotomy but achieving a larger vessel lumen. With a great deal of trepidation, working under fierce scrutiny by his mostly adversarial chiefs, he performed balloon dilatation of stenoses of the iliac and superficial femoral vessels with reasonable success. However, his passion and dreams were to use this approach to treat coronary arterial obstructions and avoid CABG. The seemingly impossible obstacles placed by Gruentzig's critics were slowly conquered. After this experience with percutaneous transluminal angioplasty in the peripheral arteries and extensive animal experimentation, he was ready to attempt PTCA in a human. The first patient was 38 years old, Dolf Bachmann. He had an isolated left anterior descending artery stenosis, was very symptomatic, and terrified by open heart surgery. The first PTCA was performed in University Hospital on September 16, 1977. Although there are many tales about that first procedure, it was successful. The only glitch was one Andreas hadn't anticipated; Bachmann called the local newspaper the following morning which led to a firestorm of anger by all of Gruentzig's enemies. There were several additional procedures in Zurich but the pessimism and resistance persisted.

Gruentzig travelled to Frankfurt in the next few months and performed PTCA procedures with Martin Kaltenbach at the University Hospital. His experience in Zurich increased. The audiences at the American Heart Association, Miami, November, 1977 heard the first major presentation of his work, four patients treated with PTCA(8). The audience was polarized into those who listened with amazement and praise to those who were sceptical and angry. Those who were impressed by the technique began travelling to Zurich, sometimes bringing patients to Zurich for treatment. He made the bold move of hosting cardiologists from around the world, inviting them to observe this new procedure. He openly reviewed his results, including follow-up angiography which he was routinely obtaining in his patients. These follow-up studies underscored the substantial recurrence rate of about 30% in the first 6 months after the procedures. When the number of visitors became unmanageable, he launched a novel approach; to assemble many physicians in an auditorium and bring them into the catheterization laboratory by closed circuit television. The audience could observe the procedure, talk with Gruentzig, and then have an open discussion with him following the case. This represented a revolutionary idea for launching a new technical procedure, unedited, with complete disclosure of failures and complications. He dwelled on the indications for the procedure underscoring the effectiveness in relieving symptoms but no evidence of improving outcomes. He embraced the National Heart Lung and Blood Institutes PTCA registry(9). He attended the first meeting in 1979 in Bethesda and all subsequent meetings before his death. Since he controlled the distribution of balloon catheters, initially he extracted a promise from the physicians that they would report their experience to the Registry as a condition for sale of the catheter.

Gruentzig's frustration of working in Zurich continued; he found similar hostile environments in other European centres. He then turned his focus to the

United States where he received many offers. His choice was Emory University in Atlanta to which he moved in 1980. His volume of patients increased quickly and he launched the Demonstration Courses at Emory. The initial results of the NHLBI PTCA Registry became available in 1982 which documented safety and initial effectiveness of the procedure, with a mortality of 0.09%, myocardial infarction rate of 5.5%, need for emergency CABG in 6.6%, *but* a first year recurrence rate of almost 30%[10]. Since the physicians performing PTCA were frequently those making the therapeutic decisions for the patients, the enthusiastic acceptance of the procedure was not deterred by these results. Certainly, over one-half of the patients were symptomatically improved at 1 year, without open heart surgery. Furthermore, the recurrent coronary obstructions (restenosis) were usually effectively treated by a second PTCA procedure[11].

During the 1980s the infrastructure for performing PTCA continued to improve. A second balloon dilatation system, developed by John Simpson, brought to market by Advanced Catheter Systems and financed by Ray Williams, gained Food and Drug Administration (FDA) approval in 1981 This was an 'over the wire' system which incorporated a guide wire which could be moved independently from the balloon catheter. Unfortunately, there were no guide wires which were initially developed for this system. The 0.018-inch guide wires developed for paediatric procedures were used and were the first of a long list of 'off label' devices embraced by interventional cardiologists. 1981 also brought approval for reimbursement for PTCA by Health Care Financing Administration (HCFA) in the United States which quickly spread to the other insurance payers. This ushered in an explosion of investments by all of the catheter companies in balloon and guiding catheters, guide wires, dilatation systems, etc. Upgrade of existing imaging systems to achieve better quality, resolution, and most importantly, the ability to store images for 'road mapping'.

Love/hate relationships developed between interventional cardiologists and cardiac surgeons. Since the cardiologists were the primary referral sources of all patients to cardiac surgeons, most cardiac surgeons were supportive. In the early 1980s there was an increase in the need for urgent CABG to about 7%. Most centres performing PTCA developed a system for alerting cardiac surgeons and the operating rooms of patients when difficulties were encountered in the catheterization laboratories. During this time there were major adverse events in patients taken directly from the catheterization laboratory to the operating room including death in about 10% and myocardial infarction in 50% of patients. The improvement in devices was accompanied by improved pharmacology. Although aspirin had been a consistent antiplatelet agent used from the first case of Gruentzig, further interest in platelet inhibition continued. Dextran became a routine agent for platelet inhibition; however that was accompanied by terrible side effects including shock and pulmonary oedema. Dipyridomole (Persantin®), another weak platelet inhibitor showed little promise for important platelet inhibition. The major breakthrough with pharmacologic therapy was introduction of the glycoprotein IIBIIIA inhibitors, the first available being abciximab by Lilly. Clinical trials demonstrated the efficacy of this agent[12] in decreasing adverse cardiac events in the periprocedural interval. Two other IIBIIIA platelet inhibitors, eptifibatide[13] and tirofiban[14], were subsequently introduced. Comparative studies ensued, most of which demonstrated similar improvements of cardiac major adverse cardiac events (MACE) but increased bleeding. However, the one difference was the greater cost of abciximab. During this period of intense competition of these potent platelet inhibitors, the only available anticoagulant was unfractionated heparin, an inexpensive, but far from ideal, anticoagulant which had been in use for decades. Work began with direct thrombin inhibitors primarily because the widespread use of unfractionated heparin had resulted in heparin allergies and heparin-induced thrombocytopenia (HIT). Hirudin and hirulog, both naturally occurring agents were direct thrombin inhibitors. Although these were effective anticoagulants, the production costs were excessive for routine use and after the initial positive clinical studies, these agents sat idle. The Medicines Company discovered a less expensive manufacturing process to produce bivalrudin[15]. This has become a very effective anticoagulant with a better safety profile (decreased bleeding) than unfractionated heparin.

New coronary devices

As these improvements in adjunctive pharmacologic agents were occurring, a great deal of work was underway on new devices to augment or replace balloon dilatation (Fig. 2.2). One of the first new devices was an attempt to harness energy created by the argon laser to create a 'hot tip' system in which the laser energy was focused on a metal catheter tip to create heat[16]. Subsequently an inflated balloon was heated with laser energy to treat the dilated area[16]. Neither of these

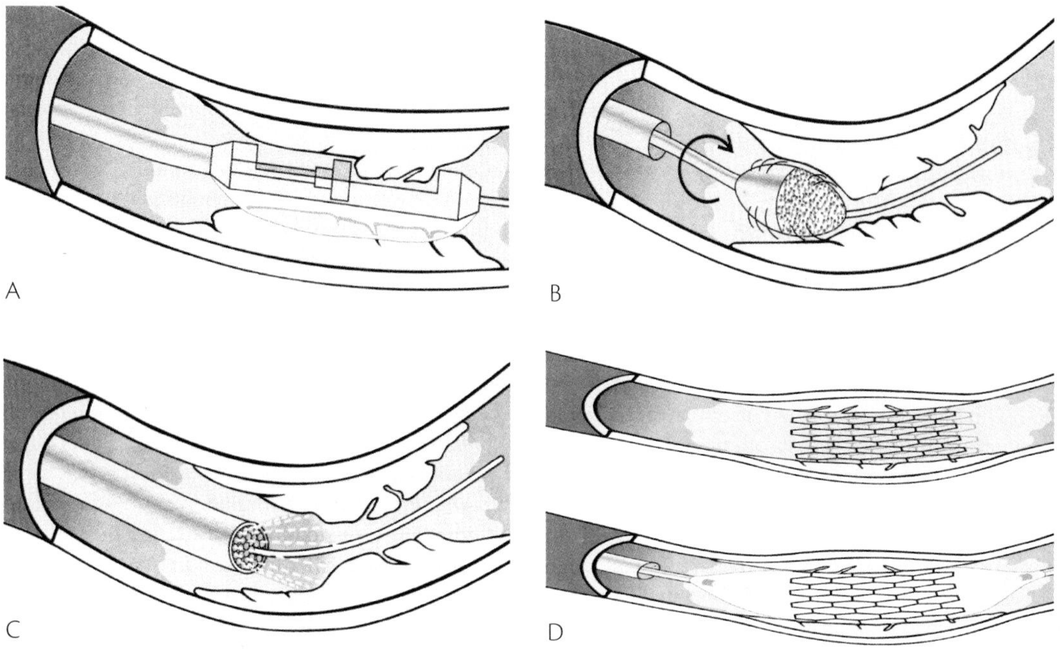

Fig. 2.2 New angioplasty devices. Because of unpredictable initial and disappointing long-term results of balloon angioplasty, new devices were introduced in clinical trials in the 1980s and received FDA approval in the early 1990s. A) Directional coronary atherectomy. B) Rotational atherectomy. C) Excimer laser. D) Stent.

devices were effective but they did demonstrate the deleterious effects of heat in the coronary circulation. Another novel approach was a high speed (150 000–200 000rpm) rotating burr with diamond chips on the leading edge, rotational atherectomy(17). This was effective in removing superficial fibrotic/calcified elements of the coronary plaques. This device, the Rotablator® (Boston Scientific) is still necessary to obtain successful results in plaques with these characteristics. Such plaques occur in 2–5% of patients undergoing PCI. The excimer laser, uses a fibreoptic catheter which directs excimer laser energy through the catheter to a lens at the catheter tip which ablates tissue(18). As opposed to argon energy, this is almost euthermic and led to much less thermal injury. This device has not achieved widespread use in routine coronary interventions, however it is effective in ablating extensive fibrotic plaque, for example, long total occlusions of coronary and peripheral arteries. It has also been found to be an effective thrombolytic device for treating patients with acute myocardial infarction (AMI). Directional atherectomy was also developed by John Simpson(19). This was a microsurgical instrument at the tip of a catheter in which coronary obstructive plaque was forced into a small chamber by dilating a balloon on the opposite side of the catheter. An atherotome was activated which sliced the plaque off the wall of the artery, depositing it in the nose cone at the tip of the catheter. The angiographic results were spectacular since the plaque had been removed instead of disrupted, as occurred with balloons. However, despite the attractive angiographic results, the 6-month recurrence rates were no different than balloon dilatation. The transluminal extraction catheter was another attempt to remove plaque(16). This was a crude system since the entire catheter rotated and the plaque had to be disrupted before it could be extracted. Again, clinical studies demonstrated similar outcomes of this device compared to balloon dilatation.

The coronary intravascular stent was the first device developed during this era which had more predictable and durable results. Although there have been many improvements, the basic concept remains the same. Julio Palmaz had developed these metallic scaffolds to maintain the lumen of diseased peripheral arteries after balloon dilatation. In the mid 1980s, he with Richard Schatz developed an articulated, sheath-covered stent for coronary arteries(20). This Palmaz–Shatz stent™ (Johnson and Johnson) was approved by the FDA for elective stent placement in 1994. Gianturco, a radiologist like Palmaz, worked with Gary Roubin to design a balloon expandable coil stent. The Gianturco–Roubin stent™ (Cook, Inc.) was the first FDA approved stent in 1993 with the indication for threatened or abrupt closure during coronary angioplasty procedures[21]. Of historical interest, the Wiktor stent by Medtronic and the self expanding Wallstent® by Medivent entered small clinical trials but neither emerged as major contenders for this market. Still the only approved stent in the US for elective use was the Palmaz–Schatz stent™. In clinical trials in both the United States and Europe (STRESS and BENESTENT), improved clinical outcomes with reduced restenosis were documented after elective angioplasty[22,23]. The price paid for this benefit, however, was an increase in abrupt closure resulting in AMI due to stent thrombosis. These episodes occurred mostly in the first week after implantation with initial rates of about 5%. As these cases occurred, most interventionalists responded by increasing the intensity of parenteral anticoagulants (heparin), continuing that until warfarin (routinely started after the successful stent placement) would have its effect, usually 3–5 days later. So as the use of anticoagulants increased, the length of hospitalization increased, as did the complications of anticoagulation, groin haematomas, retroperitoneal haematomas, and cerebral vascular accidents. Unfortunately, this vicious cycle continued until more potent antiplatelet agents and improved stent implantation techniques were discovered.

Antonio Columbo[24] was the first to point out that despite the beautiful angiographic appearance of the coronary segments after stent placement, by intravascular ultrasound, the stents were uniformly poorly expanded. The usual maximum inflation pressures at that time were 6–10 atmospheres. The acute and subacute stent thrombosis was substantially reduced when the stents were initially expanded at 14–18 atmospheres during implantation. The evolution of oral antiplatelet agents started with ticlopidine which was effective but had the feared side effect of leucopenia. The study which proved the effectiveness of improved antiplatelet agents was the Stent Anticoagulation Regimen Study (STARS) in which patients after successful stent implantation were randomized to: 1) warfarin/aspirin (the FDA-approved regimen); 2) ticlopidine/aspirin; or 3) aspirin alone[25]. Ticlopidine/aspirin proved to be the best regimen which decreased the bleeding complications of prolonged heparin prior to warfarin's effect and had the lowest stent thrombosis. These alterations in implantation techniques and pharmacology led to substantial improvements in clinical outcomes. Thus, compared to balloon dilatation and the subsequent non-balloon devices, the use of endovascular stents led to predictable results with the ability to correct coronary dissections when they occurred. Most of the unfavourable initial results with stents, prolonged anticoagulation, and stent thrombosis had been solved. The persistent unfavourable long-term outcomes, restenosis requiring repeat procedures, or CABG would be with us for another decade until the dream of a more durable device became reality with the drug eluting stents, released in the United States in 2003.

Percutaneous coronary intervention in acute myocardial infarction

One of the best examples of the impact of interventional cardiology on the improved outcomes in patients with coronary artery disease is the treatment of patients with AMI. One doesn't have to look far back in history to find the rather primitive treatment of this deadly disease. Dwight Eisenhower, following his triumphant return from the Pacific theatre of World War II, was elected President of the United States. In 1955, while playing golf in Colorado, he developed chest pain which he, and his physician, interpreted as gastrointestinal in origin. Enduring this pain for hours, the President's physician gave him morphine and took him to the Fitzsimmons Army Hospital in Denver where the ECG diagnosis of ST-segment elevation myocardial infarction (STEMI) was made. For the next 24h, despite all of the available resources and talented physicians, (including Paul Dudley White), the President of the United States was left with a badly damaged heart. At the time, contemporary care for myocardial infarction was morphine, oxygen, bed rest, and warfarin. Unfortunately, little changed in the care of AMI during the 1960s and early 1970s. Coronary Care Units were established which were very effective in recognizing and treating lethal cardiac arrhythmia. However, the irreversible myocardial damage which inevitably occurs after coronary occlusion continued in these patients. The focus on reperfusion in the setting of AMI was slowed by the confusion of the pathogenesis of AMI. Roberts[26] had examined hundreds of necropsy specimen of patients who died from AMI and had found severe, fixed atherosclerosis with no evidence of 'coronary thrombosis'. Since those observations were made on post-mortem specimens, it is likely that the culprit, intraluminal thrombus, had undergone spontaneous thrombolysis or was lost through the fixation process. As angiographic studies were performed on patients presenting in the first few hours after onset of symptoms, it became obvious that coronary occlusion occurred in most of these patients and the occlusion was due to thrombus. The focus was then directed at opening the obstruction. The initial approach was to use thrombolytic agents; streptokinase was readily available and had been used in peripheral arteries to 'dissolve clots'[27]. The attractiveness of parenteral thrombolytic therapy was that it could be administered in any Emergency Department. The safety and effectiveness of streptokinase and subsequently more thrombin-specific agents were soon proved in RCTs which would soon become the cornerstone of this new subspecialty of 'Interventional Cardiology'. The excitement of administering these agents to individuals writhing in pain, with marked ECG changes, ventricular arrhythmia, and haemodynamic instability with resolution of these signs and symptoms built a global enthusiasm for finally having an effective therapy for this deadly disease.

As exciting as these early results were, intravenous thrombolysis was not perfect. Evidence of reperfusion, resolution of ECG changes, and subsequent improvement of left ventricular function only occurred in about 70% of patients with about 10–15% of these 'successful' patients manifesting early closure of the vessels. Initially these agents were administered intravenously but then, with the emerging experience with coronary angioplasty techniques and catheters, the agents were given selectively into the obstructed artery. Rentrop reported using 'guide wires' to mechanically disrupt the thrombus which could potentially facilitate the action of the lytic agents[28]. Hartzler, an emerging force in the coronary angioplasty field, used balloon dilatation to clear the obstructions[29]. And so, the race was on between medical lytic therapy and direct coronary interventions; the result was that Interventional Cardiologists changed this extraordinarily important problem. The outcomes of these early experiences would usher in a sea change in the treatment of AMI. The TIMI (Thrombolysis in Myocardial Infarction) trials were initially focused on the efficacy of pharmacologic approaches[30].The TAMI (Thrombolysis and Angioplasty in Myocardial Infarction) trials ran in a parallel fashion assessing the efficacy of balloon angioplasty in the treatment of AMI[31]. The 1990s launched the GUSTO (global use of strategies to open occluded coronary arteries) mega-trials enrolling large numbers of patients worldwide[32]. Needless to say, these were very expensive trials but were the foundation of very effective, new approaches to this important worldwide problem (Fig. 2.3). RCTs quickly proved that prompt restoration of coronary flow in an acutely occluded vessel by balloon dilatation was more effective than thrombolytic therapy[33,34] (Fig. 2.4). The effectiveness of balloon angioplasty was enhanced by more potent antiplatelet agents, the IIb/IIIa glycoprotein inhibitors. Platelet aggregation was proved to be important in the reocclusions which occurred after angioplasty with acute coronary syndromes[35]. The obvious limitation of primary angioplasty in AMI was the lack of immediate access to catheterization laboratories and skilled personnel. These logistics led to inevitable delays in re-establishing blood flow.

As evidence mounted on the superiority of angioplasty over thrombolytic therapy, a novel approach to this problem arose. There were large numbers of hospitals in the suburban and rural areas of the United States which had cardiac catheterization laboratories but did not have cardiac surgery services available. Several observations had been established at that time; first, most of the patients presenting with AMI had rather simple coronary anatomy, an occluded or subtotal obstruction of a single coronary artery with or without other coronary lesions. The success rate for opening the occluded vessel was quite high and the complication rates, certainly complications that would require immediate cardiac surgery, were quite low. Thus, the C-PORT (Cardiovascular Patient Outcomes Research Team) trial was launched, which tested the safety and effectiveness of coronary angioplasty in community hospitals without on-site cardiac surgery[36]. Although this was a major departure from usual practice in the United States, it was common in most other countries. This initial clinical trial was successful and this approach has been widely adopted in the United States and elsewhere. Stents were adopted in elective PCI, stents were also demonstrated to improve outcomes in PCI during AMI[37]. Drug eluting stents (DES) have also been studied in this setting. Horizons was a large RCT examining bare metal stents (BMS) versus DES and like all of the comparative trials, DES had less target lesion revascularization (TLR) than BMS[38]. However, it is clear that dual antiplatelet therapy, aspirin and clopidogrel (the latter is currently the most common but will probably be replaced by more effective agents in the future) must be continued for at least a year after implanting the DES. In the setting of AMI, it is frequently difficult to determine whether or not a patient will be able to take the regimen for a year because of compliance, need for surgery, or other bleeding tendencies. Thus, for the small decrease in TLR, the potential complications of interrupting dual antiplatelet therapy must be determined.

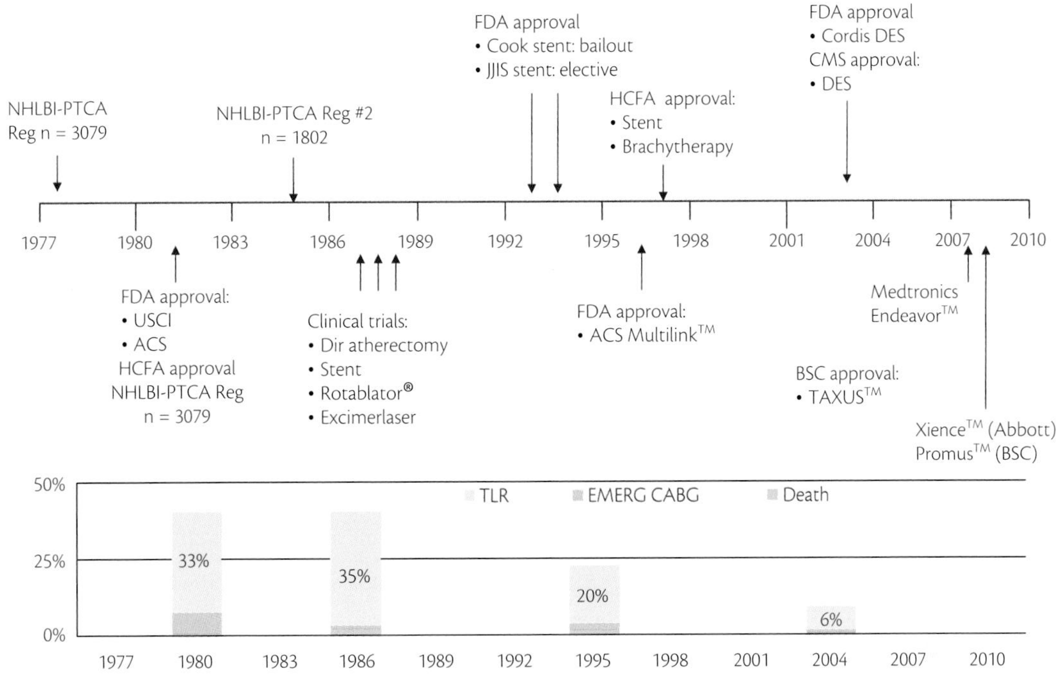

Fig. 2.3 Timeline of events during the first three decades of percutaneous coronary intervention. ACS, Advanced Catheter Systems; BSC, Boston Science Corporation; CMS, Center for Medicare and Medicaid Services; Cook, Cook Inc.; Cordis, Cordis Corporation; DES, drug eluting stents; Dir, directional; FDA, Federal Drug Agency; HCFA, Health Care Financing Administration; JJIS, Johnson and Johnson Interventional Systems; Reg, registry; USCI, United States Catheter Industries.

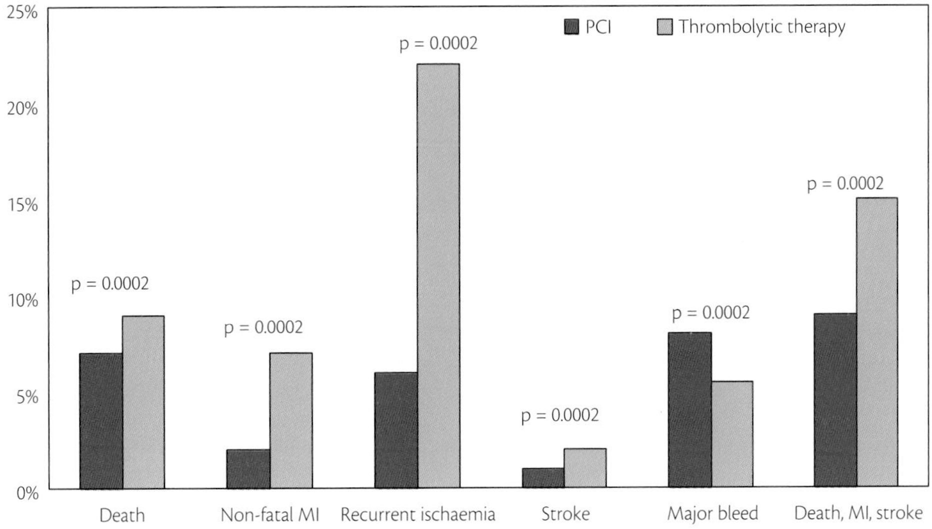

Fig. 2.4 Meta-analysis of clinical trials comparing primary angioplasty versus intravenous thrombolytic therapy in patients with acute ST-segment elevation myocardial infarction.

Continued fine tuning of adjunct pharmacology, newer devices for removing thrombus, and perhaps re-examining distal protection will continue to refine these approaches. There will be exciting new insights from genomics and pharmacogenomics which will improve outcomes. However, this has been an extraordinary success story of medicine. This common disease, AMI, with an in-hospital mortality of 25% has been reduced to a mortality of about 5% over the past three decades. In addition to the reduction of in-hospital mortality, there has been a substantial reduction of hospital stay, readmission for complications, and improved ventricular function at discharge. There is also the probability that the improved left ventricular function at discharge will translate to less congestive heart failure in subsequent years.

References

1. Acierno LJ. *The History of Cardiology*. London: The Parthenon Publishing Group, Inc., 1994.
2. Hurst JW. *The Heart*. New York: McGraw Hill Companies, Inc., 1994.
3. Roth N. Hales' hydraulics: measuring blood pressure, 1706. *Med Instrum* 1981; **15**:1-22.
4. Favaloro RG. Saphenous vein autograft replacement of severe segmental coronary artery occlusion: operative technique. *Ann Thoracic Surg* 1968; **5**:334–39.
5. CASS Principal Investigators and Their Associates. Coronary Artery Surgery Study (CASS): a randomized trial of coronary artery bypass surgery. *Circulation* 1983; **68**:939–50.
6. Peduzzi P, Kamina A, Detre K, *et al.* VA Coronary Artery Bypass Surgery Cooperative Study Group. Twenty-two year follow up of coronary artery bypass surgery for stable angina. *Am J Cardiol* 1998; **81**:1393.
7. Monagan D. *Journey into the Heart*. New York: Gotham Books, Penguin Books (USA), 2007.
8. Gruentzig A, Turina M, Schneider J. Experimental percutaneous dilatation of coronary artery stenosis [abstract]. *Circulation* 1976; **54**:81.
9. Levy RI, Mock MB, Willman VI, *et al.* Percutaneous transluminal coronary angioplasty. *N Engl J Med* 1979; **301**:101–3.
10. Kent KM, Bentivoglio L, Block, LC, *et al.* Percutaneous transluminal coronary angioplasty: Report from the NHLBI Registry. *Am J Cardiol* 1982; **49**:2011–17.
11. Williams DO, Gruentzig AR, Kent KM, *et al.* Efficacy of repeat percutaneous transluminal coronary angioplasty for coronary restenosis. *Am J Cardiol* 1984; **53**:32C–35C.
12. EPIC Investigators. Use of a monoclonal antibody directed against the platelet glycoprotein IIb/IIIa receptor in high risk coronary angioplasty. *N Engl J Med* 1994; **330**:956–61.
13. Tcheng JE, Harrington RA, Kottke-Marchant K, *et al.* Multicenter, randomized, double-blind placebo-controlled trial of the platelet integrin glycoprotein IIb/IIIa blocker integrelin in elective coronary intervention. *Circulation* 1995; **76**:2151–7.
14. The RESTORE Investigators. Effects of platelet glycoprotein IIb/IIIa blockade with tirofiban on adverse cardiac events in patients with unstable angina or acute myocardial infarction undergoing coronary angioplasty. *Circulation* 1997; **96**:1445–53.
15. Lincoff AM. Bittl JA. Harrington RA, *et al.* REPLACE-2 Investigators. Bivalirudin and provisional glycoprotein IIb/IIIa blockade compared with heparin and planned glycoprotein IIb/IIIa blockade during percutaneous coronary intervention: REPLACE-2. *JAMA* 2003; **289**:853–63.
16. Baim DS, Kent KM, King SB, *et al.* Evaluating new devices: Acute (in hospital) results from the New Approaches to Coronary Interventions Registry. *Circulation* 1994; **80**:471–81.
17. Safian RD, Niazi KA, Strzelecki M, *et al.* Detailed angiographic analysis of high-speed mechanical rotational atherectomy in human coronary arteries. *Circulation* 1993; **88**:961–8.
18. Klein LW, Litvack F, Holmes D, *et al.* Six month outcome and determinants of adverse clinical events after successful excimer laser coronary angioplasty. ELCA A.I.S. Multicenter Registry. *J Invasive Cardiol* 1995; **7**:191–9.
19. Hinohara T, Selmon MR, Robertson GC, *et al.* Directional atherectomy. New approaches for treatment of obstructive coronary and peripheral vascular disease. *Circulation* 1990; **81**(3 Suppl):IV79–91.
20. Schatz RA, Palmaz JC, Tio FO, *et al.* Balloon-expandable intracoronary stents in the adult dog. *Circulation* 1987; **76**:450–7.
21. Roubin GS, Cannon AD, Agrawal SK. Intracoronary stenting for acute and threatened closure complicating percutaneous transluminal coronary angioplasty. *Circulation* 1992; **85**:916–27.
22. Fischman DL, Leon MB, Bain DS, *et al.*, for the Stent Restenosis Study investigators. A randomized comparison of coronary-stent placement and balloon angioplasty in the treatment of coronary artery disease. *N Engl J Med* 1994; **331**:496–501.
23. Serruys PW, de Jaegere P, Kiemeneij F, *et al.*, for the Benestent Study Group. A comparison of balloon-expandable-stent implantation with balloon angioplasty in the treatment of coronary artery disease. *N Engl J Med* 1994; **331**:489–95.
24. Colombo A, Hall P, Nakamura S. Intracoronary stenting without anticoagulation accomplished with intravascular ultrasound guidance. *Circulation* 1995; **91**:1676–88.
25. Cutlip DE, Leon MB, Ho KK, *et al.* Acute and nine-month clinical outcomes after "suboptimal" coronary stenting: results from the STent Anti-thrombotic Regimen Study (STARS) registry. *J Am Coll Cardiol* 1999; **34**:698–706.

26. Roberts WC, Buja LM (1972). The frequency and significance of coronary arterial thrombi and other observations in fatal acute myocardial infarction. *Am J Med* 1972; **53**:425–43.
27. Ganz W, Geft I, Shah PK. Intravenous streptokinase in evolving acute myocardial infarction. *Am J Cardiol* 1984; **53**:1209–16.
28. Rentrop P, De Vivie ER, Karsch KR, *et al.* Acute coronary occlusion with impending infarction as an angiographic complication relieved by a guide-wire recanalization. *Clin Cardiol* 1978; **1**:101–6.
29. Hartzler GO, Rutherford BD, McConahay DR. Percutaneous transluminal coronary angioplasty: application for acute myocardial infarction. *Am J Cardiol* 1984; **53**:117C–121C.
30. TIMI Investigators. Early effects of tissue-type plasminogen activator added to conventional therapy on the culprit coronary lesion in patients presenting with ischemic cardiac pain at rest: results of the Thrombolysis in Myocardial Ischemia (TIMI IIIA) trial. *Circulation* 1993; **87**:38–52.
31. Topol EJ, Califf RM, Kereiakes DJ, *et al.* Thrombolysis and Angioplasty in Myocardial Infarction (TAMI) trial. *J Am Coll Cardiol* 1987; **10**:65B–74B.
32. The GUSTO Angiographic Investigators. The effects of tissue plasminogen activator, streptokinase, or both on coronary-artery patency, ventricular function, and survival after acute myocardial infarction. *N Engl J Med* 1993; **329**:1615–22.
33. Williams, DO, Braunwald E, Knatterud G, *et al.* One-year results of the Thrombolysis in Myocardial Infarction Investigation (TIMI) Phase II Trial. *Circulation* 1992; **85**:533–542.
34. Keeley EC, Boura JA, Grimes CL. Primary angioplasty versus intravenous thrombolytic therapy for acute myocardial infarction: a quantitative review of 23 randomised trials. Research Support. *Lancet* 2003; **361**:13–20.
35. EPIC Investigators. Use of a monoclonal antibody directed against the platelet glycoprotein IIg/IIIa receptor in high-risk coronary angioplasty. *N Engl J Med* 1994; **330**:956–61.
36. Aversano T, Aversano LT, Passamani E, *et al.*, for the Atlantic Cardiovascular Patient Outcomes Research Team (C-PORT). Thrombolytic therapy vs primary percutaneous coronary intervention for myocardial infarction in patients presenting to hospitals without on-site cardiac surgery: a randomized controlled trial. *JAMA* 2002; **287**:1943–51.
37. Stone GW, Grines CL, Cox DA, *et al.*, for the Controlled Abciximab and Device Investigation to Lower Late Angioplasty Complications (CADILLAC) Investigators. Comparison of angioplasty with stenting, with or without abciximab, in acute myocardial infarction. *N Engl J Med* 2002; **346**:957–66.
38. Stone GW, Witzenbichler B, Guagliumi G. HORIZONS-AMI Trial Investigators. Bivalirudin during primary PCI in acute myocardial infarction. *N Engl J Med* 2008; **358**:2218–30.

CHAPTER 3

Risk assessment and analysis of outcomes

Peter F. Ludman and Helen Routledge

Introduction

Patient outcomes following percutaneous coronary intervention (PCI) are predominantly determined by two factors: clinical presentation and comorbidities. For example, a patient presenting in cardiogenic shock has a predicted in-hospital mortality in excess of 50%, whereas the corresponding figure for uncomplicated non-ST elevation myocardial infarction (NSTEMI) is less than 1%. A third important factor is the quality of care provided to the patient. Quantification of the relative contribution of these three components to short- and long-term mortality and morbidity is required for several reasons: it informs both the patient and physician in deciding upon the optimal management strategy; it underpins appropriately informed consent; and, by recognizing modifiable elements in the treatment process, it can be used to drive improvements in healthcare delivery.

There has been an increasing interest in monitoring healthcare outcomes, and the publication of these observations. The drivers for this have included the practice of paediatric cardiac surgery in Bristol (United Kingdom) between 1984 to 1995[1], and the string of murders committed by Shipman[2].

Clinical Governance is now embedded in healthcare monitoring. It first appeared prominently in the 'National Health Service (NHS) plan' published in 2000[3] and describes 'a framework through which NHS organizations are accountable for continuously improving the quality of their services and safeguarding high standards of care by creating an environment in which excellence in clinical care will flourish'. Clinical governance is central to the provision of high-quality NHS care, guided by national standards and is supported by professional self-regulation and development. The Commission for Health Improvement was established in 1999 to monitor the quality of services delivered by hospitals.

In addition the Freedom of Information Act allowed previously privileged information to be widely available. In 2005, mortality data for individual surgeons performing coronary artery bypass grafting (CABG) was published despite errors, and an important watershed had been reached. The medical profession began to understand that it was not only essential to disseminate data, but that it must be accurate, and be provided in a way easily understood by the target audience, whether this be patients or providers. In 2008, the NHS Next Stage Review was published[4]. Led by Lord Darzi, this document detailed the vision of quality as the driving force taking the NHS forward. Quality was to be underpinned by audited measurements of clinical performance and patient outcomes. Private and NHS hospital trusts were now mandated to provide this data with the same legal responsibility as their financial accounts.

Alongside legislation has come an explosion of information via the world wide web. Throughout the Darzi review the requirement for data collection and availability was a constant theme. There was a commitment to publish information on quality and performance in order to facilitate patient choice with their healthcare providers, and compel providers to constantly improve their performance through optimal research, management, and regulation.

Professional revalidation is another driving force behind the desire to measure procedural outcomes. Although the General Medical Council (GMC) was set up in 1858, the first link between professional registration and professional competence came with the Merrison report in 1975. Slow to develop, the plans by the GMC to formalize professional revalidation were criticized by Dame Janet Smith in the fifth report of the

Shipman enquiry as 'an expensive rubber-stamping exercise'[2]. The Chief Medical Officer (Sir Liam Donaldson) was assigned the task of 'assuring the safety of patients in situations where a doctor's performance or conduct pose a risk; ensure the operation of an effective system of revalidation [and] modify the role, structure and functions of the GMC'. His report entitled 'Good doctors, safer patients'[5] was endorsed by the 2007 White Paper 'Trust Assurance and Safety – The Regulation of Health Professionals in the 21st Century'. The report contained proposals to strengthen the system, assure and improve the performance of doctors, and to protect the safety of patients. Included were recommendations for a clear and unambiguous set of standards for each area of specialist medical practice. Revalidation would comprise 're-licensing' for all and 're-certification' for professionals wishing to remain on the specialist or General Practice registers. Specialists would have a comprehensive assessment against standards set by their respective society and the Medical Royal Colleges and approved by the GMC. These standards include assessment in three domains: knowledge, skills, and professionalism. The interventional cardiologist would be evaluated on the process, appropriateness, procedure, and outcomes of PCI, with revalidation every 5 years by formal and objective measurement.

In order to calculate expected outcomes, we must first calculate the predicted risk.

Methods of risk assessment

Datasets

Some of the earliest attempts to measure outcome variation were developed for the manufacturing industry[6,7]. The fundamental principles underlying these techniques were to distinguish random variation, or 'common cause variation', from differences caused by extrinsic factors, 'special cause variation'. Translated from healthcare to industry, the aim is to identify outcome variation resulting from healthcare delivery, so that modifiable factors can be targeted to have a favourable impact on patient care. Fixed parameters such as a patient's age or presenting clinical syndrome are important in providing an estimate of overall risk, but cannot be used directly to improve care.

Index cases

The most intuitive method of trying to separate the underlying risk to a patient from the quality of care provided is to restrict analysis to a cohort of patients with very similar clinical features. This homogenous group of patients would be expected to have similar outcomes, allowing straightforward comparisons between different providers. For example, analysis of outcomes only for patients who present with stable angina and have a single lesion in the left anterior descending artery treated by PCI. This use of 'index' cases for comparison has the advantage of simplicity, but the disadvantage that only the treatment of these index case types is assessed. The group assessed must be present in sufficient numbers to allow meaningful comparison, yet it is likely that a more sensitive test of the quality of a healthcare system is in the management of the minority of sicker and more complex patients. It is in the management of such patients that a difference in the quality of care is likely to have the greatest impact on outcome.

Adjustments for case mix

A more encompassing way to assess and compare outcomes involves some form of case-mix adjustment. Models are used from which the expected risk of an adverse outcome can be calculated according to a number of specific features that relate to the patient and their planned treatment. Predicted outcomes can then be compared with observed outcomes, with discrepancies resulting from random fluctuation or differences in the quality of care. Such models have been generated from large datasets containing information on patient characteristics including comorbidities, the procedure itself, and the observed outcomes. Clearly factors not included in the dataset will not be available in the resulting model. If, for example, the dataset fails to include a comorbid condition that influences outcome, this will be missed. Likewise, if the dataset fails to include an important outcome then this outcome cannot be predicted from the model. For example, no current model can predict the influence of platelet reactivity on outcome of PCI, since the most appropriate measure of platelet function is still debated, and no large dataset has included this parameter.

Continuous variables, such as serum creatinine concentration should be used if possible. Dichotomizing at an arbitrary cut off (for example, to greater or less than 200umol/L) reduces the power of the subsequent model. Definitions of all variables in the dataset should be objective, so that the value assigned to the variable is consistent across observers. Unfortunately some of the most important aspects of judgement are impossible to define in an objective manner. The so-called 'end of the bed' test, widely recognized as an extremely important way of judging a patient's risk, is a synthesis of a large number of poorly defined features that have been learned over years of clinical experience. Clinical acumen is hard to replicate with objectively measurable parameters. There is some similarity with the difficulty in generating pattern recognition algorithms for facial recognition or the assessment of abnormal electrocardiographic traces. It is equally difficult to find an objective measure to represent the ease with which a coronary artery will accept a bypass graft, sometimes termed the 'graftability' of a coronary artery. 'Graftability' is not included in EuroSCORE, yet surgeons recognize a patient at higher risk from their angiographic appearances, and also that this increased risk is not captured in the model. For PCI there has been considerable progress made with the development of the 'Syntax score', which does seem to provide some objective assessment of the technical difficulty likely to be encountered in treating a coronary lesion by angioplasty. The term 'three-vessel disease' encompasses a range of coronary anatomy. It describes both the patient with three short discrete lesions in otherwise large smooth arteries, and also the patient with small calibre tortuous and severely calcific diffuse disease including two long chronic total occlusions. Recent studies have also demonstrated the value of the functional assessment of coronary lesions, thus a patient may have three-vessel disease (>50% diameter stenosis in three vessels), but assessment by measurement of fractional flow reserve may demonstrate only one to be obstructive and requiring intervention[8].

As clinicians understand the basis of the variables used for any particular risk model, so there is the possibility both of risk-averse behaviour and of 'gaming the model'. If a patient is recognized as being at higher risk of an adverse outcome than is defined in the known measured parameters (for example, coronary vessels look difficult to graft), there is an anxiety that the actual outcome will be worse than that predicted. The operator will perform less well than the model even if performance is in fact satisfactory.

Subjective features in a model that increase the predicted risk can be over-emphasized, which will tend to make predicted outcomes worse, and observed outcomes relatively better than the model. The accuracy of the data entered in the dataset is critical to the validity and reliability of resulting models. Mortality is the easiest endpoint to measure and validate and as a result is most often included. Many large datasets include in-hospital major adverse cardiovascular and cerebrovascular events (MACCE), and thus several models can estimate risk of this combined outcome.

There have been attempts to determine whether data routinely collected for administrative rather than clinical purposes could be used to generate reliable risk models. Hannan compared the administrative data on the Statewide Planning and Research Cooperative System, with the clinical Cardiac Surgery Reporting System to assess unit-specific mortality following coronary artery bypass surgery in New York State and found the administrative database was considerably inferior, mainly due to three clinical risk factors (ejection fraction, re-operation, and left main stem [LMS] disease)[9]. Ugolini[10] compared administrative datasets with EuroSCORE and found that by adding administrative variables considered a proxy for clinical complexity to the administrative dataset, and linking data across multiple episodes of patient care, they were able to eliminate much of the difference between the clinical and administrative dataset predictions. Certainly there has always been an interest in using routinely collected administrative data to this end, and some have argued that although the data quality in administrative datasets is often very unreliable, once they start to be used in this way, and clinicians engage with the process of data collection and validation, the quality of the data will improve and they may become a valuable way to model outcomes. This may not be particularly relevant in cardiology, where a long tradition of gathering clinical audit data exists, but it may have a role in subspecialties where a focus on data collection has been less prominent.

Statistical methods

Following selection of a dataset, statistical manipulation will generate a model. Bayesian methods have been used, but most models are generated using logistic regression analysis. This technique predicts the binary outcome, such as death or survival, on the basis of variables contained within the dataset. These predictor variables can take any form. They can be continuous, discrete, or dichotomous, and no assumptions are made about their distribution. The variables also need not be independent, though the additional predictive value of a variable already correlated with one in the model will be less.

The dataset is initially analysed using univariate methods to find individual variables that predict outcome. Univariate analysis refers to the simple description of a set of values to assess their central tendency and spread. For example, in a normally distributed group of continuous variables, this might be the mean and standard deviation. Logistic regression is then used to create a model using the identified variables. The goal of logistic regression is to correctly predict the category of outcome for individual cases using the least number of variables. There are a variety of methods used to try to find the minimum number of predictors that give most discriminatory power for a model. Broadly, the variable with the biggest predictive power is added to the model, then multivariate analysis used to find the next most important. An alternative technique involves the creation of a model that includes all the variables, and then variables are sequentially removed to see if their absence reduces the model's discriminatory power.

Once a model has been generated, it is tested to see how well it performs in predicting outcome from a dataset, usually with the Hosmer–Lemeshow technique[11]. The dataset is divided into, say, 10 groups, based on the predicted outcome, ranging from low risk ($p = 0$ to 0.1) to high risk ($p = 0.9$ to 1.0). The predicted outcomes at each risk level are compared with the observed using the chi-squared statistic, and a good model is one that gives an accurate prediction of outcome at each level of risk. A p value of >0.1 usually indicates that the model provides a good fit for the data and that the differences are not statistically significant, but nevertheless does not exclude potentially clinically significant differences between observed and predicted outcomes.

For a model to be clinically useful it should not only work, but also have a high positive and negative predictive accuracy. This is described as its discriminatory power and is usually assessed using receiver operating characteristic (ROC) curves[12,13]. For this analysis a graph of 'sensitivity' on the y axis against '1-specificity' on the x axis is generated for the entire range of cut off values that are used to classify a patient as negative or positive. Let us take the calculation of just one point on an ROC curve to illustrate its construction; consider all the individuals in the dataset with a predicted mortality outcome of 90% or less. We would classify these as 'negative', and those with a predicted risk of more than 90% as positive. The sensitivity and specificity of the model at this cut off is measured and plotted. The process is repeated for all cut off values between 0% and 100% to generate the curve. The area under the curve is called the c statistic and represents the proportion of all possible pairs of patients with different outcomes (e.g. one death and one survivor) for whom the regression model correctly assigns a higher risk to the patient who died. Perfect discrimination gives an area of 1, and no discrimination (no better than the toss of a coin) gives a value of 0.5 (Fig. 3.1). Logistic regression models with a c statistic of about 0.8–0.9 are usually regarded as having high discriminatory ability.

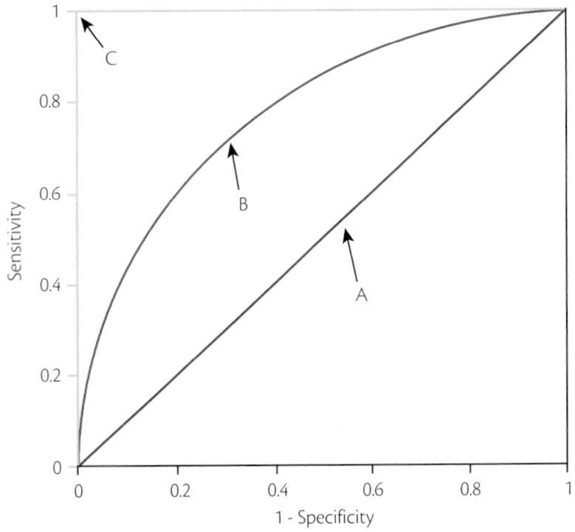

Fig. 3.1 ROC curves. Line A (c statistic = 0.5) shows no discrimination, Line B shows reasonable discrimination (c statistic = 0.8), and as the discriminatory ability of the model improves it moves towards line C, which shows perfect discrimination (c statistic =1).

Important limitations must be recognized with the use of these general statistical methods when they are applied to predict outcome in individual patients. A 'good' model with a c statistic of 0.8 will still miss 20% of patients with an adverse event. Furthermore, even if a model has a perfect fit, the prediction of a 10% mortality in 1000 patients does not highlight the 100 who will die. Box-Jenkins, an industrial statistician, stated that 'all models are wrong, but some are useful'. We do well to bear this in mind.

Models for coronary revascularization

In cardiothoracic surgery, EuroSCORE[14] became the dominant method for calculation of perioperative mortality. Developed from a large clean dataset of a heterogeneous group of patients, the authors created a simple additive score. At a time when computers were far less accessible, it could be readily calculated at the bedside. An alternative based on the Society of Thoracic Surgeons (STS) database in the United States, was unavailable for critical analysis due to intellectual property issues, and so gained less widespread use. The EuroSCORE has been tested in widely differing populations both in Europe[15], Scandavia[16], Japan[17], and in the United States[18], and has consistently worked well despite varying patient demographics and operative techniques. Patients in the United States were older, more often had isolated coronary bypass operations, diabetes (30% versus 17%) and prior cardiac surgery (11% versus 7%)[18], but EuroSCORE still outperformed the STS model. Across Europe EuroSCORE was reliable even though there were particularly large differences in valve surgery (ranging from 18.6% in Finland to 51.5% in Spain)[15].

Though the development of the additive version of EuroSCORE greatly widened its applicability, one of the problems of trying to generate a simple scoring system from the underlying logistic regression equation is that it forces an additive system on one that is essentially multiplicative. In general, as the number of risk factors rises, the logistic score will tend to exceed the additive. This has the effect of making the additive score underestimate risk for high-risk patients, and over-estimating risk for low-risk patients. This effect on the additive EuroSCORE has been well documented[19]. With increasing computing power available at the bedside the full logistic EuroSCORE has been more widely used.

However, the EuroSCORE is now 10 years old and must be updated, as surgeons consistently outperform both the additive and logistic models[20]. Of more concern is that the score is poor at differentiating risk in high risk patients undergoing CABG[21] and aortic valve replacement[22]. Unfortunately it is this minority of high-risk cases that will have the greatest impact on a surgeon's overall measured performance. For developing fields such as transcutaneous aortic valve implantation (TAVI) there are no current models that perform well enough to adequately inform doctors or patients of the relative risks of surgical or the newer alternative. Final models for TAVI should incorporate frailty indices to account for the elderly high risk cohort treated[23].

By comparison, numerous risk assessment systems have been developed for PCI and due to the rapid evolution of PCI technology and adjunctive pharmacological therapy, the more recent models have greater applicability to contemporary PCI (Table 3.1). Kunadian[24] assessed the Mayo Clinical Risk Score[25] and the North West Quality Improvement Programme score[26] in a cohort of over 5000 patients treated between 2002 and 2006 in North West England. Both models had excellent discrimination and calibration, with an area under ROC curve (c index) of ≥0.87 and 0.86 respectively.

Because there is considerable overlap of features that predict risk both from CABG and PCI, EuroSCORE can risk stratify for percutaneous revascularization[27], and PCI risk scores can predict CABG outcome[15,28]. Certain issues, however, are unique to the treatment modality. For PCI the specific characteristics of the lesions treated can weigh heavily in the likely chance of procedural success or adverse outcome. Technological improvements have removed some of the impact of lesion anatomy on early outcomes, but these have been counteracted by the increasing complexity of lesions tackled, which may fair less well in the longer term. Lesion specific issues have been addressed in some models[29,30], but the description of lesion characteristics has been relatively crude.

The Syntax score[31,32] characterizes the coronary vasculature in more detail with respect to number of lesions and their functional impact, location, and complexity. The score is based on modifications and additions to a number of existing systems. The arterial tree is divided into 16 segments, using the classification from the ARTS I and II[33] trials (Fig. 3.2), and the contribution of each segment to total left ventricular blood flow is used as a multiplication factor depending on left or right dominance (Table 3.2).

Only vessels larger than 1.5mm in diameter are included and a lesion is defined as a 50% or more reduction in luminal diameter. The only distinction in lesion severity is between occlusive and non-occlusive stenosis, with a multiplication factor of 2 for non-occlusive lesions and 5 for occlusive lesions reflecting the difficulty of the percutaneous treatment for the latter. All other adverse lesion characteristics have an additive value (Table 3.3).

Tandem lesions are considered a single lesion if they are separated by less than 3 lesion reference diameters.

To classify bifurcation lesions, a synthesis of the Duke[35] and Institut Cardiovasculaire Paris Sud (ICPS)[36] classification systems was employed, and is shown in Fig. 3.3. Thus the Syntax classification has seven types, whereas the previous two systems had six types each. Syntax type G was missing from the Duke system, and type D missing from the ICPS system. In addition, side branch angulation is included in the score on the basis that decreasing angulation (between side branch and distal limb of bifurcation) makes stent coverage of the ostium harder to achieve. Bifurcations are only considered for segment junctions: 5/6/11, 6/7/9, 7/8/10, 11/13/12a, 13/14/14a, and 3/4/16 and 13/14/15 in case of left dominance.

Trifurcations are weighted as in Table 3.3, and only scored for segment junctions 3/4/16/16a, 5/6/11/12, 11/12a/12b/13, 6/7/9/9a, and 7/8/10/10a. Aorto-ostial lesions occur in the LMS (segment 5) and right coronary artery (RCA) (segment 1), unless the left coronary has separate origins, in which case segments 6 and 11 may also score as aorto-ostial. Diffuse disease is a parameter

Table 3.1 Risk assessment systems for PCI

Author	Database/patient source	Date PCIs were performed	Number of patients	Outcome assessed	Outcome time point	Treated with stents (%)	Treated with glycoprotein 2b/3a antagonists (%)	Simplified score system	Comments
Hannan[72]	New York	1991	5827	Death	In-hospital	0%	0%	No	
Hannan[73]	New York	1991–94	62 670	Death	In-hospital	0%	0%	No	Risk model used to assess effect of operator and hospital volume on outcome
Kimmel[74]	SCAI registry	1992–93	10 622	Death/MI/emCABG	In-hospital	0%	0%	Yes	
Ellis[75]	6 hospitals in the United States	1993–94	12 985	Death/MI/CABG	In-hospital			No	
O'Connor[76]	NNE	1994–96	15 331	Death	In-hospital	21.7% (1.8% 1994, 44.95 in 1996)	0.63%	No	
DeBelder[77]	Single centre, London UK	1995–96	1500	Death/MI/emCABG	In-hospital	54%	0.5%	No	Bayesian statistical model
Ellis[29]	Cleveland Clinic	1995–97	6327 (10 907 lesions)	Death/MI/emCABG	In-hospital	40.7%	26.2%	Yes	Focus on angiographic characteristics
Qureshi[78]	William Beaumont Hospital, Michigan	1996–98	9954	Death	In-hospital	Not stated	Not stated	Yes	
Singh[25]	Mayo Clinic	1996–99	5463	Death/MI/emCABG/urCABG/CVA	In-Hospital	82%	41.8%	Yes	Angiographic and clinical features in model
Moscucci[79]	8 Michigan hospitals	1997–99	10 729	Death	In-hospital	70.5%	35%	Yes	
Resnic[80]	Brigham and Women's Hospital, Boston	1997–99	2804	Death/MI/emCABG	In-hospital	77%	42%	Yes	Artificial neural network and logistic modelling
Shaw[46]	ACC-NCDR	1998–2000	50 123	Death	In-hospital	74.7%	55.3%	No	
Grayson[26]	4 hospitals in North West England	2001–03	9914	Death/MI/emCABG/CVA	In-hospital	93%	61.6%	No	
Wu[81]	New York	2002	46 090	Death	In-hospital	Not stated	Not stated	Yes	

(continued)

Table 3.1 (Continued) Risk assessment systems for PCI

Author	Database/patient source	Date PCIs were performed	Number of patients	Outcome assessed	Outcome time point	Treated with stents (%)	Treated with glycoprotein 2b/3a antagonists (%)	Simplified score system	Comments
Valgimigli[32]	Patient from the ARTS II trial[33]	2003	306 (1292 lesions)	Death/MI/CVA/revasc	30/7, and 300/7	99%	33%	No	Angiographic score, multivessel disease
Romagnoli[27]	EuroSCORE applied to PCI procedures	2005–06	1173	Death	In-hospital	Not stated	Not stated	N/A	
Chowdhary[82]	Toronto	2000–08	10 694	Death	In-hospital	94%	79%	Yes	
For STEMI									
De Luca[83]	Zwolle	1994–2001	1791	Death	30-day	49.8%	0%	Yes	Only primary PCI for STEMI. To look at safety of early discharge
Addala[84]	PAMI risk score	Pooled 1990–97	3252	Death	In-hospital, 1 year			Yes	Primary PCI. Pooled data from PAMI-1[85], PAMI-2[86], No-SOS, Stent PAMI[87]

ACC-NCDR, American College of Cardiology–National Cardiovascular Data Registry; CVA, cerebrovascular accident; emCABG; emergency coronary artery bypass grafting; MI: myocardial infarction; NNE, Northern New England Cardiovascular Disease Study Group; PCI, percutaneous coronary intervention; Revasc, coronary revascularization; SCAI, Society for Cardiac Angiography and Interventions; STEMI, ST elevation myocardial infarction; urCABG, urgent coronary artery bypass grafting.

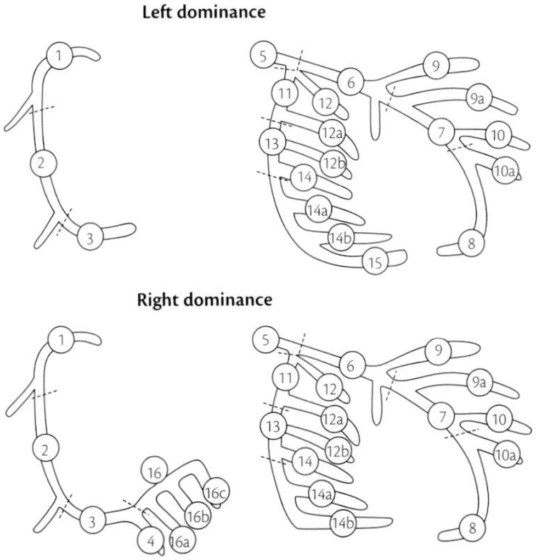

1. RCA proximal: From the ostium to one half the distance to the acute margin of the heart.
2. RCA mid: From the end of first segment to acute margin of heart.
3. RCA distal: From the acute margin of the heart to the orgin of the posterior descending artery.
4. Posterior descending artery: Running in the posterior inverventricular groove.
16. Posterolateral branch from RCA: Posterolateral branch originating from the distal coronary artery distal to the crux.
16a. Posterolateral branch from RCA: First posterolateral branch from segment 16.
16b. Posterolateral brach from RCA: Second posterolateral branch from segment 16.
16c. Posterolateral branch from RCA: Third posterolateral branch from segment 16.
5. Left main: From the ostium of the LCA through bifurcation into left anterior descending and left circumflex branches.
6. LAD proximal: Proximal to and including first major septal branch.
7. LAD mid: LAD immediately distal to origin of first septal branch and extending to the point where LAD froms an angle (RAO view). If this angle is not identifiable this segment ends at one half the distance from the first septal to the apex of the heart.
8. LAD apical: Terminal portion of LAD, beginning at the end of previous segment and extending to or beyond apex.
9. First diagonal: The first diagonal originating from segment 6 or 7.
9a. First diagonal a: Additional first diagonal originating from segment 6 or 7, before segment 8.
10. Second diagonal: Originating from segment 8 or the transition between segment 7 and 8.
10a. Second diagonal a: Additional second diagonal originating from segment 8.
11. Proximal circumflex atery: Main stem of circumflex from its origin of left main and including origin of first obtuse marginal branch.
12. Intermediate/anterolateral artery: Branch from trifurcating left main other than proximal LAD or LCX. It belongs to the circumflex territory.
12a. Obtuse marginal a: First side branch of circumflex running in general to the area of obtuse margin of the heart.
12b. Obtuse marginal b: Second additional branch of circumflex running in the same direction as 12.
13. Distal circumflex artery: The stem of the circumflex distal to the origin of the most distal obtuse marginal branch, and running along the posterior left atrioventricular groove. Caliber may be small or artery absent.
14. Left posterolateral: Running to the posterolateral surface of the left ventricle. May be absent or a division of obtuse marginal branch.
14a. Left posterolateral a: Distal from 14 and running in the same direction.
14b. Left posterolateral b: Distal from 14 and 14 a and running in the same direction.
15. Posterior descending: Most distal part of dominant left circumflex when present. It gives origin to septal branches. When this artery is present, segment 4 is usually absent.

Fig. 3.2 Definition of the segments of the coronary artery tree. Reprinted from Sianos G, Morel M-A, Kappetein AP *et al.* The SYNTAX Score: an angiographic tool grading the complexity of coronary artery disease *EuroIntero*. 2005; **2**: 219–27, with permission from Europa Edition.

introduced to reflect increase difficulty in the creation of a surgical anastomosis, and goes some way to addressing the 'graftability' issue discussed earlier. It is defined as present when at least 75% of the length of the segment distal to the lesion has a vessel diameter of <2mm, irrespective of the presence or absence of disease at that distal segment. These definitions are listed in Table 3.4.

Calculation of the Syntax score is quite demanding, and most easily achieved using a computerized algorithm. The process involves answering a sequence of 12 questions as listed in Table 3.5. The first three questions appear only once (dominance, number of lesions, and number of segments involved per lesion). The maximum number of lesions allowed is 12, but there is no limit on the number of segments that can be involved per lesion. There are then eight questions which are asked for each lesion in turn. The algorithm takes a slightly different course through the questions according to the presence or absence of an occlusion, and whether or not there are side branches of >1.5mm diameter (bifurcations or trifurcations). Finally, the last question is the only one that does not relate to each lesion, since it relates to anatomy beyond the stenosis. It is therefore scored once only for each major arterial territory (LM, LAD, circumflex [Cx], and RCA). The final total Syntax score is the summation of all the scores for each lesion.

Two examples of the calculation of this score are reproduced from Sianos *et al.*[31] in Fig. 3.4.

The hypothesis that higher Syntax scores, indicative of more complex disease, represent a bigger treatment challenge and poorer outcomes has been confirmed in

Table 3.2 Segment weighing factors; based on the 'Leaman' score[34]

Segment No		Right dominance	Left dominance
1	RCA proximal	1	0
2	RCA mid	1	0
3	RCA distal	1	0
4	Posterior descending artery	1	n.a.
16	Posterolateral branch from RCA	0.5	n.a.
16a	Posterolateral branch from RCA	0.5	n.a.
16b	Posterolateral branch from RCA	0.5	n.a.
16c	Posterolateral branch from RCA	0.5	n.a.
5	Left Main	5	6
6	LAD proximal	3.5	3.5
7	LAD mid	2.5	2.5
8	LAD apical	1	1
9	First diagonal	1	1
9a	First diagonal	1	1
10	Second diagonal	0.5	0.5
10a	Second diagonal	0.5	0.5
11	Proximal circumflex artery	1.5	2.5
12	Intermediate/anterolateral artery	1	1
12a	Obtuse marginal	1	1
12b	Obtuse marginal	1	1
13	Distal circumflex artery	0.5	1.5
14	Left posterolateral	0.5	1
14a	Left posterolateral	0.5	1
14b	Left posterolateral	0.5	1
15	Posterior descending	n.a.	1

LAD, left anterior descending artery; RCA, right coronary artery. Reprinted from Sianos G, Morel M-A, Kappetein AP *et al.* The SYNTAX Score: an angiographic tool grading the complexity of coronary artery disease *EuroInterv*. 2005; **2**:219–27, with permission from Europa Edition.

Table 3.3 Segment weighing factors (Syntax scoring system)

Diameter reduction	
Total occlusion	×5
Significant lesion (50–99%)	×2
Total occlusion (T0)	
Age>3 months or unknown	+1
Blunt stump	+1
Bridging	+1
First segment visible beyond T0	+1/per non-visible segment
Side branch (SB) – Yes, SB <1.5mm	+1
– Yes, both SB < & ≥1.5mm	+1
Trifurcations	
1 diseased segment	+3
2 diseased segments	+4
3 diseased segments	+5
4 diseased segments	+6
Bifurcations	
Type A, B, C	+1
Type D, E, F, G	+2
Angulation <70°	+1
Aorto ostial stenosis	+1
Severe tortuosity	+2
Length >20mm	+1
Heavy calcification	+2
Thrombus	+1
'Diffuse disease'/small vessels	+1/per segment number

×: multiplication
+: addition
Reprinted from Sianos G, Morel M-A, Kappetein AP *et al.* The SYNTAX Score: an angiographic tool grading the complexity of coronary artery disease *EuroInterv*. 2005; **2**: 219–27, with permission from Europa Edition.

early studies. Analysis of performance in predicting short- and longer-term risk in patients with multivessel disease is encouraging[32]. Patients with multi-vessel disease treated by PCI in the ARTS II study who were in the highest tertile of syntax score (>26) had a significantly higher event rate than those in the lowest (″18), to 1-year follow up (27.9% versus 8.7%; p = 0.001). This type of score may help predict prognosis and guide decisions regarding CABG or PCI in multi-vessel disease and technically challenging lesion morphologies. The Syntax trial was designed to assess the relative role of PCI and CABG in patients with multi-vessel disease, many including LMS lesions. Initial data analysis to 12-month follow up suggests that individuals with lower Syntax scores may be best treated by PCI, and those with higher scores by CABG[37]. The complexity of lesions treated in this trial was much greater than in ARTS II, with higher tertials of score (lowest ″22, highest >33). In the lowest tertile, the rate of MACCE for CABG versus PCI was 14.7% versus 13.6%, but in the highest tertile the order was reversed, at 10.9% versus 23.4% respectively. As in all previous randomized trials, differences were driven by repeat revascularization procedures rather than mortality, which was equivalent at 1 year. This scoring system will have greatest utility in patients with anatomically complex and multiple lesions.

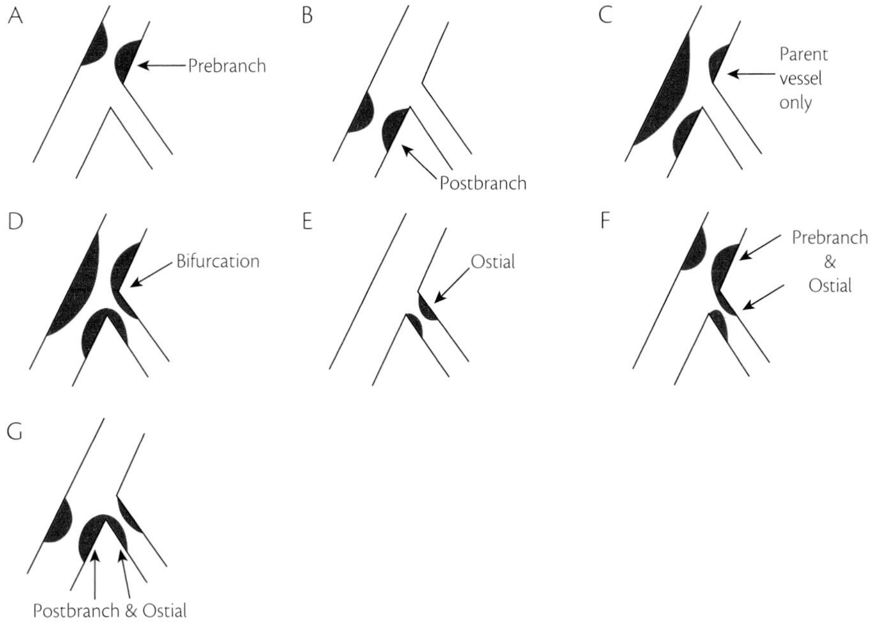

Type A: *Pre-branch stenosis not involving the ostium of the side branch.*
Type B: *Post side branch stenosis of the main vessel not involving the origin of the side branch.*
Type C: *Stenosis encompassing the side branch but not involving its ostium.*
Type D: *Stenosis involving the main vessel and ostium of the side branch.*
Type E: *Stenosis involving only the ostium of the side branch*
Type F: *Stenosis directly involving the main vessel (pre-side branch) and the ostium of the side branch.*
Type G: *Stenosis directly involving the main vessel (post-side branch) and the ostium of the side branch.*

Fig. 3.3 Syntax classification of bifurcation lesions. Reprinted from Sianos G, Morel M-A, Kappetein AP *et al.* The SYNTAX Score: an angiographic tool grading the complexity of coronary artery disease *EuroInterv.* 2005; **2**:219–27, with permission from Europa Edition.

Assessing and displaying outcome data

How data are portrayed visually has important implications to their interpretation.

Periodic assessment

Periodic, also known as cross-sectional or static, assessment compares what would be expected from the model with what was observed at a fixed time period. Results are, by definition, retrospective though there are advantages as there is time for the data to be cleaned and validated. Data may be presented as crude survival or mortality plots, but by using risk models they can also be presented as a comparison between observed and expected numbers of deaths, sometimes expressed as a ratio with a confidence interval to reflect random variation. Examples of this form of analysis and presentation are the New York State's PCI database[38] and New York State's Adult Cardiac Surgery database[39].

The Society for Cardiothoracic surgery in Great Britain and Ireland present their data as a scale, with an arrow pointing to observed mortality, and a green segment of the scale corresponding to the range of expected outcomes for that unit according to the risk-adjusted prediction[40]. Where there is a wish to display comparative rankings of healthcare providers, particularly when a standard against which to judge performance is not available, 'league tables' and 'caterpillar plots' have been used. The implication is that there is a performance difference between alternative providers. But these displays are misleading. Sequential points on the plot visually imply sequential differences between providers where no statistical difference may actually exist (Fig. 3.5). The focus is then on a spurious ranked order of results, with identification of 'best' and 'worst' providers made for an analysis period comprising one snapshot of outcomes. No risk-adjustment system accounts for all aspects of case mix, and calculated ranking systems are simplistic at best and can be counterproductive.

A better way of presenting findings is a statistical process control chart. This assumes that all providers are part of a single system with a similar performance. An example of the use of these charts is in comparing 30-day mortality post myocardial infarction[41].

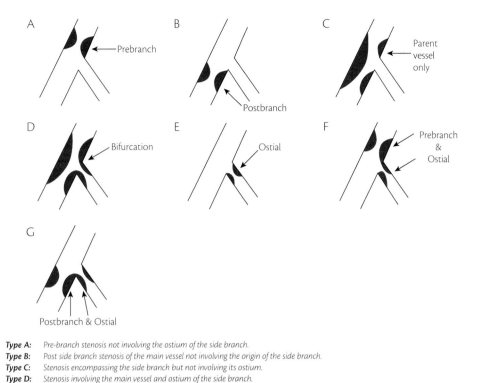

Table 3.4 Definitions used during the calculation of the Syntax score

The SYNTAX score is calculated by a computer programme consisting of sequential and interactive self-guided questions. All the below mentioned definitions are projected in a side window when the signal (i) indicating information, available for each questions, is pointed with the cursor.
Definitions:
Dominance: a) Right dominance: the posterior descending coronary artery is a branch of the right coronary artery (segment 4). b) Left dominance: the posterior descending artery is a branch of the left coronary artery (segment 15). Co-dominance does not exist as an option at the SYNTAX score
Total occlusion: TIMI 0 flow: no perfusion; no antegrade flow beyond the point of occlusion
Bridging collaterals: Small channels running in parallel to the vessel and connecting proximal vessel to distal and being responsible for the ipsilateral collateralization
Trifurcation: A junction of three branches, one main vessel and two side-branches. Trifurcations are only scored for the following segment junctions: 3/4/16/16a, 5/6/11/12, 11/12a/12b/13, 6/7/9/9a and 7/8/10/10a
Bifurcation: A junction of a main vessel and a side branch of at least 1.5mm in diameter. Bifurcations are only scored for the following segment junctions: 5/6/11, 6/7/9, 7/8/10, 11/13/12a, 13/14/14a, 3/4/16 and 13/14/15. Bifurcation lesions may involve one segment (types A, B and E), two segments (types C, F and G) or three segments (type D)
Aorto ostial: A lesion is classified as aorto-ostial when it is located immediately at the origin of the coronary vessels from the aorta (applies only to segments 1 and 5, or to 6 and 11 in case of double ostium of the LCA)
Severe tortuosity: One or more bends of 90° or more, or three or more bends of 45° to 90° proximal of the diseased segment
Length >20mm: Estimation of the length of that portion of the stenosis that has ≥50% reduction in luminal diameter in the projection where the lesion appears to be the longest. (In case of a bifurcation lesion at least one of the branches has a lesion length of >20mm.)
Heavy calcification: Multiple persisting opacifications of the coronary wall visible in more than one projection surrounding the complete lumen of the coronary artery at the site of the lesion
Thrombus: Spheric, ovoid or irregular intraluminal filling defect or lucency surrounded on three sides by contrast medium seen just distal or within the coronary stenosis in multiple projections or a visible embolization of intraluminal material downstream
Diffuse disease/small vessels: More than 75% of the length of the segment has a vessel diameter of 2mm, irrespective of the presence or absence of a lesion

Reprinted from Sianos G, Morel M-A, Kappetein AP *et al*. The SYNTAX Score: an angiographic tool grading the complexity of coronary artery disease *EuroInterv*. 2005; **2**:219–27, with permission from Europa Edition.

Table 3.5 The SYNTAX score algorithm

1. Dominance
2. Number of lesions
3. Segments involved per lesion
Lesion Characteristics
4. Total occlusion
i. Number of segments involved
ii. Age of the total occlusion (>3 months)
iii. Blunt Stump
iv. Bridging collaterals
v. First segment beyond the occlusion visible by antegrade or retrograde filling
vi. Side branch involvement
5. Trifurcation
i. Number of segments diseased
6. Bifurcation
i. Type
ii. Angulation between the distal main vessel and the side branch <70°
7. Aorto-ostial lesion
8. Severe tortuosity
9. Length >20mm
10. Heavy calcification
11. Thrombus
12. Diffuse disease/small vessels
i. Number of segments with diffuse disease/small vessels

Reprinted from Sianos G, Morel M-A, Kappetein AP *et al*. The SYNTAX Score: an angiographic tool grading the complexity of coronary artery disease *EuroInterv*. 2005; **2**: 219–27, with permission from Europa Edition.

The ranking of 37 large acute trusts is demonstrated in Fig. 3.5, with 95% confidence intervals. This use of confidence intervals to differentiate between a significant and insignificant difference will always identify 5% as outliers and for additional reasons has been shown to be rarely appropriate[42]. A control chart constructed from the same information provides a much clearer representation of the data (Fig. 3.6).

There is no inappropriate visual ranking of providers, and the few outliers are easy to identify [19, 32, 35]. Hospital 19 is much more obviously an outlier then can be appreciated from the league table. However, the control limits on this chart do not take account of the fact that confidence intervals surrounding low volume activity will be wider than around high throughput.

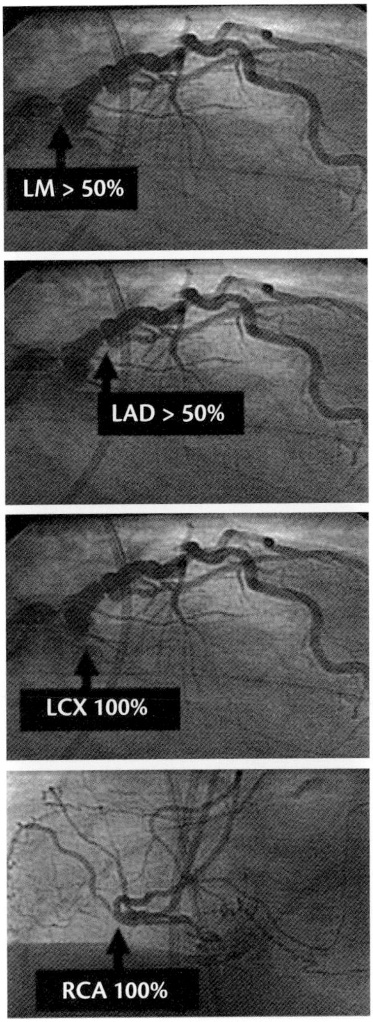

Lesion 1	
Segment 5: 5x2	10
+ Bifurcation Type A	1
+ Heavy calcification	2
Lesion 1 score:	**13**

Lesion 2	
Segment 6: 3,5x2	7
+ Bifurcation Type A	1
+ Angulation <70°	1
+ Heavy calcification	2
Lesion 2 score:	**11**

Lesion 3	
Segment 11: 1,5x5	7,5
Age T.O. is unknown	1
+ Blunt stump	1
+ side branch	1
First segment visualized by contrast: 13	1
+ Heavy calcification	2
+ Length	1
Lesion 3 score: 14,5	

Lesion 4	
Segment 1: 1x5	5
Age T.O. is unknown	1
+ Blunt stump	1
+ side branch	1
first segment visualized by contrast: 4	3
+ Tortuosity	2
+ heavy calcification	2
+ Length	1
core:	**16**

A SYNTAX SCORE 54.5

Fig. 3.4 Two examples demonstrating the calculation of the SYNTAX score. Reproduced with permission from Sianos G, Morel M-A, Kappetein AP, *et al.* The SYNTAX score: an angiographic tool grading the complexity of coronary artery disease. *EuroInterv* 2005; **1**:219–27, with permission from Europa Edition.

This brings us to funnel plots described in some detail by Spiegelhalter[43]. A funnel plot charts the observed rate of an event against the volume of activity. Superimposed are the 95% (approximately two standard deviations) and 99.8% (approximately three standard deviations) prediction limits and the overall mean event rate. The plot is funnel shaped because the random variation in outcomes is higher if fewer procedures are performed. Conversely, in hospitals with high volumes, the confidence intervals are tighter and the degree of certainty about the observed outcomes is greater. These plots are a very useful way to graphically depict large amounts of data, and easily highlight the variations in confidence ranges of the point estimates that exist between different institutions with different levels of activity. The data for in-hospital mortality following CABG in New York State in 1997–1999[44] is displayed in Fig. 3.7. The observed mortality has been divided by expected mortality of each unit to find the standardized mortality rate. This has been multiplied by the overall state wide mortality rate (2.2% in 1997–1999) to obtain a risk-adjusted mortality rate. There is no particularly obvious way to visually analyse these data when presented in this format. Fig. 3.8 is the equivalent funnel plot.

From the latter representation, it is clear that there is a high mortality, low volume hospital, as well as a borderline high volume, low mortality unit. Most units sit well within the funnel, their spurious 'ranking' not

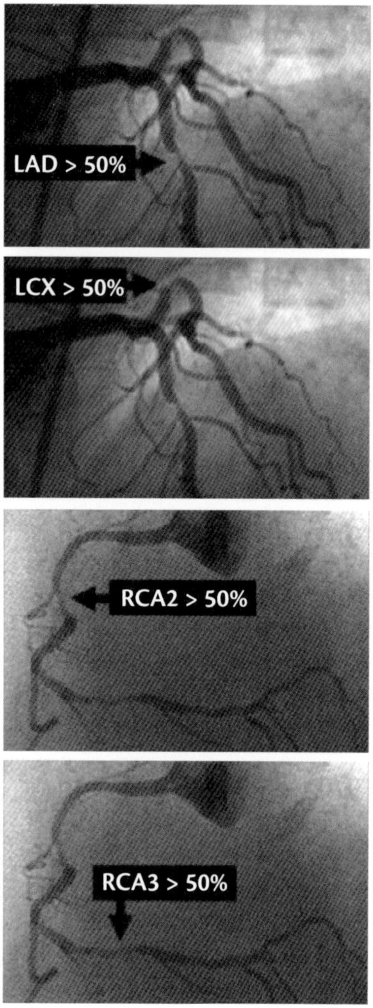

Lesion 1

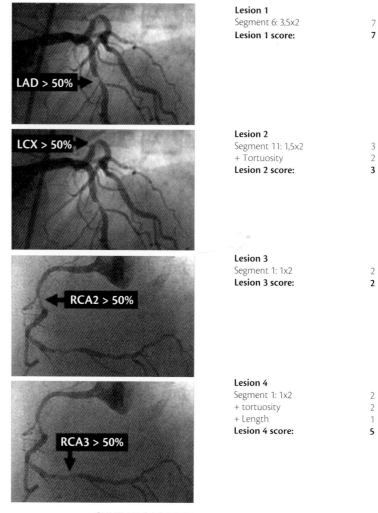

Segment 6: 3,5x2	7
Lesion 1 score:	**7**

Lesion 2

Segment 11: 1,5x2	3
+ Tortuosity	2
Lesion 2 score:	**3**

Lesion 3

Segment 1: 1x2	2
Lesion 3 score:	**2**

Lesion 4

Segment 1: 1x2	2
+ tortuosity	2
+ Length	1
Lesion 4 score:	**5**

SYNTAX SCORE 17

Fig. 3.4 (continued)

being a strong visual signal. The plots also lend themselves to assessment of the relationship between volume and outcome, and there is suggestion of a trend towards lower mortality in higher-volume units. Greater variability in measured outcomes within lower-volume centres is allowed.

Another good example of the comparison of funnels plots to league table analysis was provided in an analysis of the myocardial infarction national audit project (MINAP)[45]. Conventional ranking of performance involved assessing which units attained a predetermined goal (such as door-to-needle times of less than 30min in more than 75% cases), or are within 25% of achieving that goal, or are more than 25% outside this goal. This was compared with a funnel plot analysis which used the mean hospital performance with exact binomial three standard deviation limits, so evaluating hospitals against each other rather than an arbitrary target. Funnel plots could include units with small volumes of activity which had to be excluded from league table analysis. Additionally, league tables overestimated performance at some high-volume hospitals because, while remaining within the set targets, they were underperforming relative to other units. Random variation in performance is greatest when numbers of patients are small, and reduces as these numbers increase. This makes it statistically easier to identify outlier performance in higher-volume hospitals that sit at the right of a

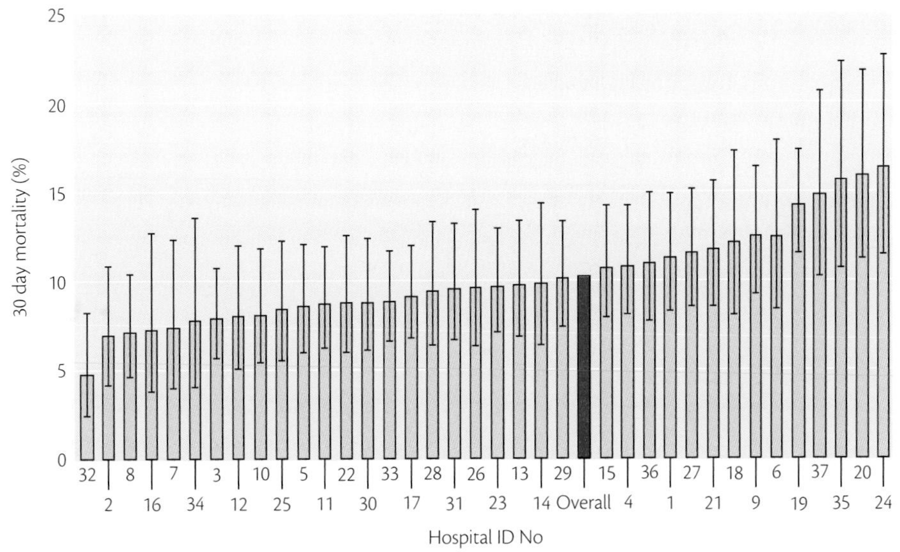

Fig. 3.5 League table for mortality (with 95% confidence interval) in hospital within 30 days of admission for patients admitted with myocardial infarction (patients aged 35–74 years admitted to the very large acute hospitals in England during 1998–1999). Reproduced from Adab P, Rouse AM, Mohammed MA, *et al.* Performance league tables: the NHS deserves better. *BMJ* 2002; **324**(7329):95–8, with permission from BMJ Publishing Group Ltd.

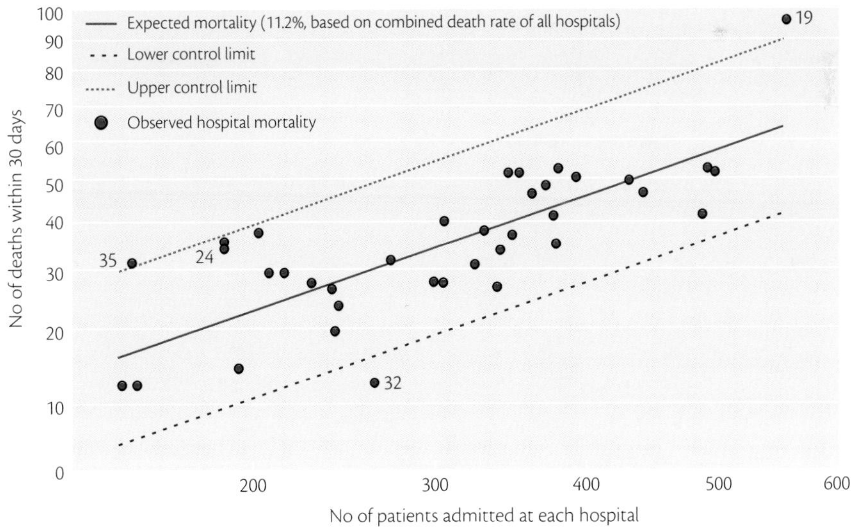

Fig. 3.6 Control chart for number of deaths in hospital within 30 days of admission for patients admitted with myocardial infarction (patients aged 35–74 years admitted to the very large acute hospitals in England during 1998–1999). Reproduced from Adab P, Rouse AM, Mohammed MA, *et al.* Performance league tables: the NHS deserves better. *BMJ* 2002; **324**(7329):95–8, with permission from BMJ Publishing Group Ltd.

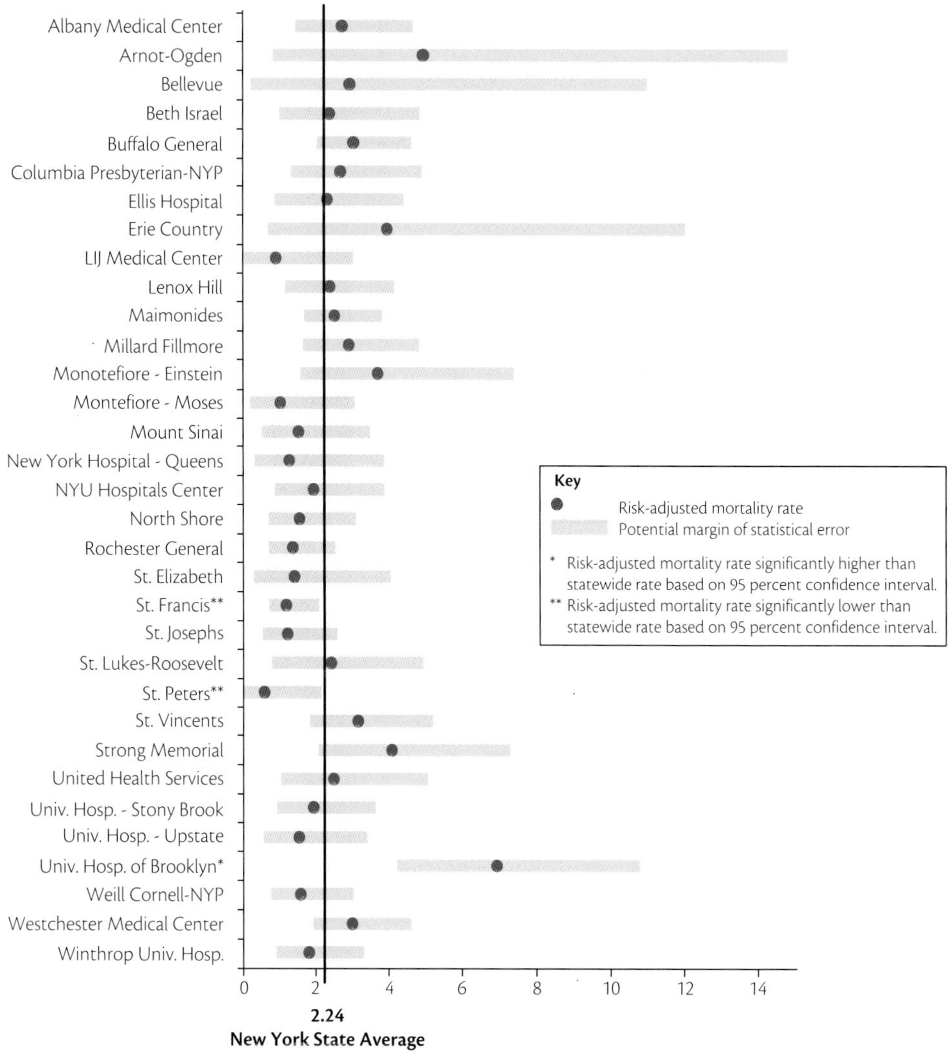

Fig. 3.7 Plot of in hospital mortality following CABG in New York State in 1997–1999.

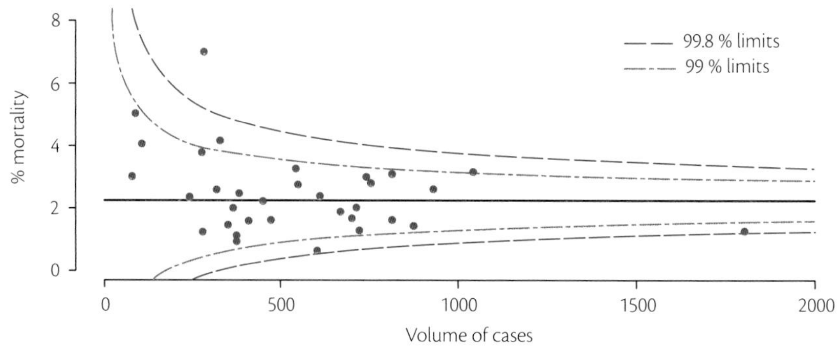

Fig. 3.8 Speigelhalter's funnel plot of in hospital mortality following CABG in New York State in 1997–1999.

funnel plot. In failing to account for the differing variation of measurement with volume, league tables failed to identify some high-volume outliers in the MINAP dataset. Thus the use of league table targets that are independent of case volume can be misleading in the assessment of institutional performance.

Funnel plots do not avoid all the problems of confidence intervals and multiple comparisons. Five per cent of units will fall outside two sigma confidence limits by chance (2.5% appearing to under perform). Wider control limits can be used and different formal statistical tools are needed to address this issue. On repeated plots there will also be regression to the mean, so that an outlier is statistically more likely to move within the funnel on a subsequent assessment.

Sequential assessment

There are several disadvantages with cross-sectional assessments of performance. The findings are always out of date (the New York State PCI data are not available until 3 years after collection) and it is also difficult to detect gradually changing trends. There has been an increasing interest in sequential, or case-by-case monitoring techniques, and a variety of different graphical and statistical process control methodologies have been developed. These methods date back to the 1920s when Shewhart developed graphical displays to try to improve the quality of telephones being manufactured in Bell laboratories[6] and in the case of cumulative sum charts, to clinical chemistry laboratories of the 1950s[46,47].

A key principle behind sequential monitoring charts is intuitive interpretation of the data. However, avoiding misinterpretation requires an understanding of the way they are produced and therefore the assumptions on which they rest. The original Shewhart chart is shown in Fig. 3.9. This shows that if the outcome of interest is 'in control', not deviating from that expected, it marches along the graph in a horizontal line. Random variation will allow this line to deviate up or down, while keeping out of the areas of alarm. Warning limits suggest the system may be out of control, and if the line crosses the upper or lower alarm limit, then there is a high statistical likelihood that the system is out of control and special cause variation has been identified. Almost all the charts described in this section follow the same general principle of a cumulative 'observed–expected' plot with horizontal thresholds.

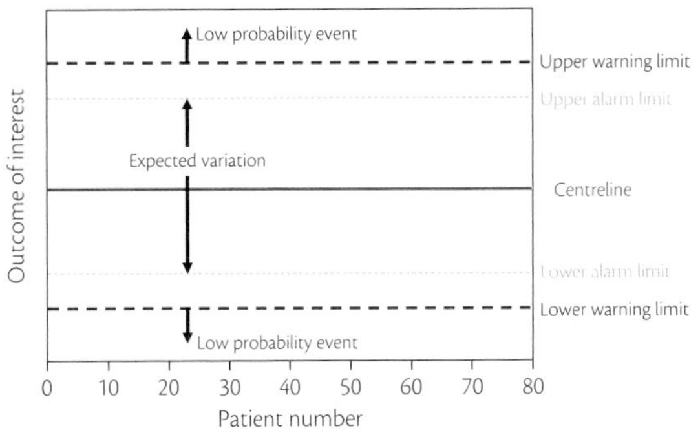

Fig. 3.9 Control chart envisioned by Shewhart.

Cumulative sum (CUSUM)

The Shewhart control charts were designed to monitor batches of results. Cumulative sum charts can be used to assess sequential individual procedures, and were the first group of charting methods widely applied to the assessment of healthcare outcomes. For the following examples let us assume that a procedure is performed, and that the result is either successful or unsuccessful. In its most basic form, the CUSUM chart simply plots success or failure for each successive procedure from zero. Success causes the line to move horizontally, failure causes the line to move up one step (Fig. 3.10).

It is possible to construct boundaries for this chart, based on the expected probability that any procedure will result in success or failure, but this makes the assumption that these probabilities are the same for every procedure. This method was used very effectively in the assessment of neonates undergoing an arterial switch operation[48]. For a more detailed explanation and mathematical derivations see Rogers *et al.*[49].

Risk-adjusted modifications of CUSUM

When attempting to tease out modifiable factors in patient outcome we must account for expected variation based on risk prediction models, and determine whether observed performance is as would be predicted.

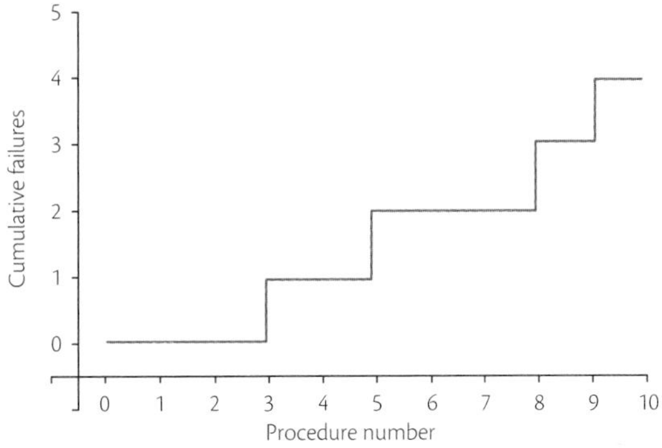

Fig. 3.10 A CUSUM chart showing success following the first two procedures, then failure. Procedure 3 therefore causes line to move up one unit.

To this end, there have been a number of modifications to the fundamental CUSUM chart. One of the earliest described is the variable life-adjusted display (VLAD) chart[50], also called cumulative risk-adjusted mortality (CRAM) [51] and risk-adjusted sequential probability ratio test (SPRT) [52] charts.

The VLAD or CRAM plot is constructed as follows. The graph starts at zero. A successful outcome causes the line to increment, and an unsuccessful outcome causes the line to decrement. The amount the line rises or falls with each case depends on the predicted risk of an adverse outcome before the procedure took place. The calculation is quite simple. If the probability of an adverse outcome (as predicated by the risk model for that particular procedure) is p, then after a case with a successful outcome, then line rises by p. If there was an adverse outcome, then the line falls by 1 − p.

Thus if a high-risk case is carried out without a complication, then a lot of credit is accrued and the line rises more than if a low-risk case is undertaken without complication. Conversely if a low-risk case has an adverse outcome, then the lines falls more than if the adverse outcome occurs in a high-risk case. Overall, after a sequence of cases, if the observed outcomes are similar to the outcomes that would have been predicted by the model, then the line will tend to be horizontal. More failures than predicted by the model will cause the line to fall, and more success will caused it to rise (Fig. 3.11). Interpretation of the display is straightforward but one disadvantage is difficulty in the construction of control limits.

Formal statistical methods for sequential analysis have been developed and are used in risk-adjusted SPRT charts[53–55]. These charts use a running log-likelihood ratio, increased or decreased after each observation by an amount dependant on the observed outcome, and that predicted from the risk model. The risk-adjusted SPRT charts have the advantage providing a formal statistical test of significance, but the chart has a less transparent interpretation. There have been other descriptions of risk adjustment for CUSUM, for example by Steiner *et al.*[56].

Cumulative funnel plots

Recently a method that combines sequential assessment and the advantages of funnel plots has been demonstrated in patients being treated by PCI[57]. Its main advantage over CUSUM styled charts is that while a data on a CUSUM chart combines observed and predicted outcomes, the cumulative funnel plots show observed and expected outcomes as separate lines. This presentation leads to a more intuitive appreciation of the data. The case mix becomes more obvious (evidenced by whether the predicted adverse event rate is high or low), and the way this compares to the observed outcomes is readily apparent. As the number of cases in the sequence rises, the influence of random fluctuation falls and the confidence intervals narrow. To construct these plots the cumulative mean predicted adverse event rate is calculated as each successive case is added to the series, and plotted as a line, with another line drawn from the mean cumulative actual adverse event rate (Fig. 3.12).

For comparison, the same data are plotted in a VLAD plot and cumulative funnel plots in Fig. 3.13.

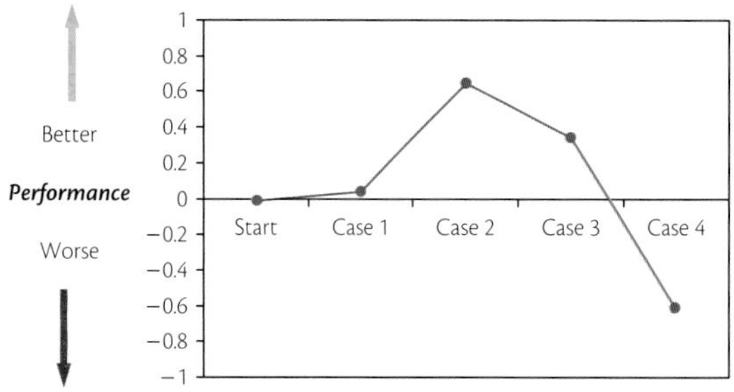

Fig. 3.11 A VLAD plot. Case 1: the risk model predicts the probability of a failed outcome as 5% and the case is successful, the line rises by 0.05. Case 2: the predicted risk of failure is 60% and the procedure was again successful, the line rises more steeply by 0.6. Case 3: predicted risk here was 70% and there was an adverse outcome, the line falls by 0.3 (1 – 0.7). Case 4: predicted risk of 5% was also a failure, the line falls more steeply by 0.95.

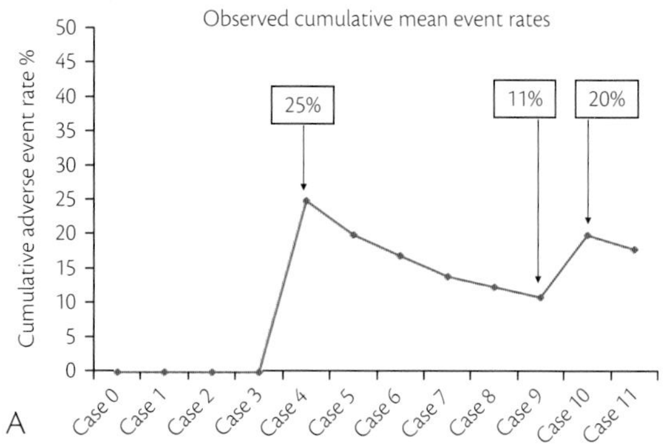

Fig. 3.12A The plot of actual outcomes: the first three procedures occur without an adverse event (running mean event rate = 0%). Case 4 is complicated by an adverse event lifting the running mean from 0 to 25%. The next few cases are uncomplicated so that by Case 9 there has only been 1 adverse event in 9 cases. The running mean has drifted down to 1 in 9, or 11%. Case 10 has a complication, and the running mean rises to 2 in 10, or 20%.

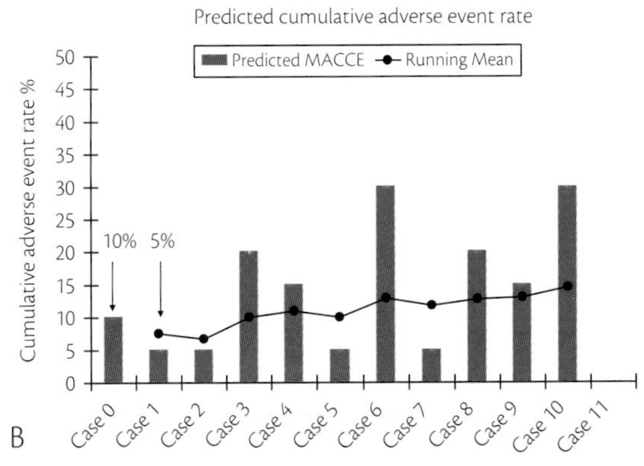

Fig. 3.12B For each case, the adverse event rate predicted from the risk model used is calculated. A running mean is then plotted. If the first 2 cases had a predicted risk of 10% and 5% respectively then the mean predicted risk by case 2 is 7.5% and so on. These 2 running means are then plotted on the same chart. Using an exact binomial method[43], lines are added that delineate the 95% and 99.8% prediction limits. As the number of cases in the sequence rises, so the confidence intervals narrow, giving rise to the characteristic funnel shape of the prediction limit boundaries.

The VLAD plot shows that for the first 60 or more cases, there are no adverse outcomes, and the plot rises as observed outcome exceeds that predicted by the model. Then there is a complication and the plot steps down. The plot then moves up gradually, and then steps up suddenly as a high-risk case is undertaken without a complication. The second downwards step is the result of the second adverse event in this series at procedure 160. As the plot continues, there is an overall downward trend, suggesting that the outcomes are progressively worse than the model would predict.

Compare this with the cumulative plot of the same data. The observed and predicted information is no longer combined into one line, but separated into observed data (coded blue) and predicted (coded red). For the first 60 procedures there are no complications and the mean actual rate (blue line) is 0%. The first adverse event lifts the line to 1.7% (1 case in 60). The mean cumulative observed rates fall again until the second adverse event, so creating the sawtooth pattern. The running mean of the predicted rates (red line)

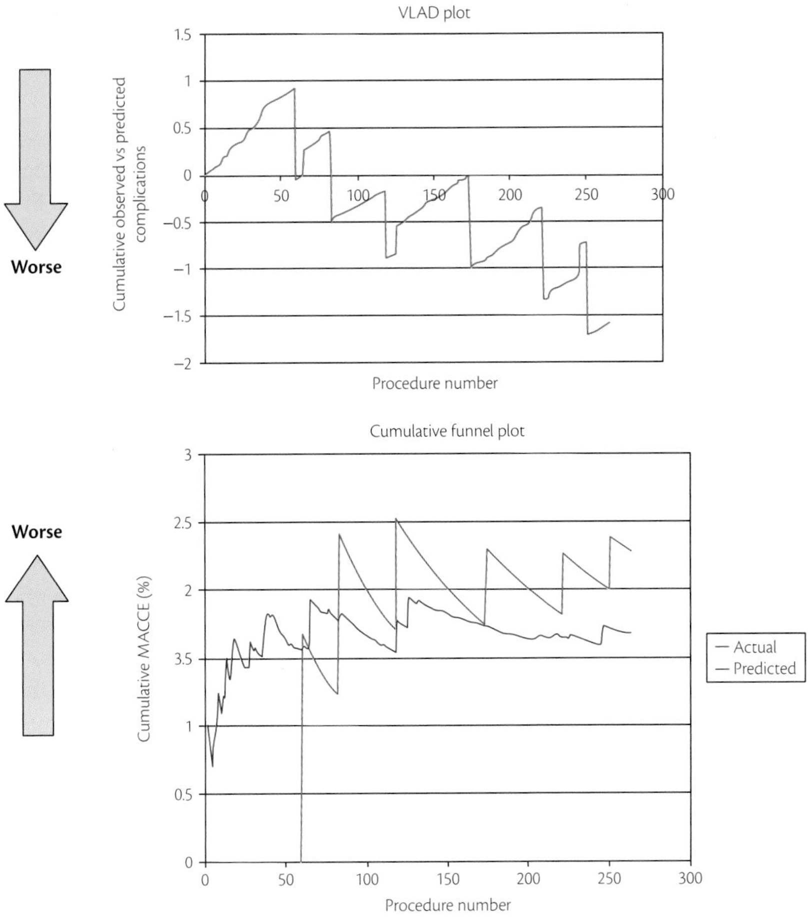

Fig. 3.13 VLAD and cumulative funnel plots of the same data as Fig. 3.12. MACCE, major adverse cardiac and cardiovascular events.

shows again that for the first 60 cases, the observed rate is lower than the predicted. Once the first adverse event has occurred, the mean values are very similar. As the series progresses, and the means are calculated from an ever larger number of procedures, the variations in the lines become less marked (unlike in the corresponding VLAD plot). It can also be appreciated that by the end of this sequence, the outcomes are poorer than the model would have predicted (the observed mean is about 2.4% and the predicted about 1.6%). Unlike the VLAD plot we can see these actual values using the cumulative method. To then gauge whether the observed difference is due to random variation, the confidence intervals are added to create the final part of the funnel (Fig. 3.14). These charts provide a visually intuitive and informative way to evaluate and communicate sequential data, and are being increasingly adopted to aid quality of healthcare delivery.

Statistical process control charts for process

Some aspects of treatment by PCI can be assessed by simply looking at the speed of treatment. For emergency PCI in the treatment of STEMI, delays to provision of PCI must be minimized. Every step in the pathway from a patient's call for help, to the opening of an occluded coronary artery must be as swift as possible. A variety of methods have been used to try to describe these delays, with the intention of minimizing them. A common technique is to describe the percentage of patients treated within a certain target such as

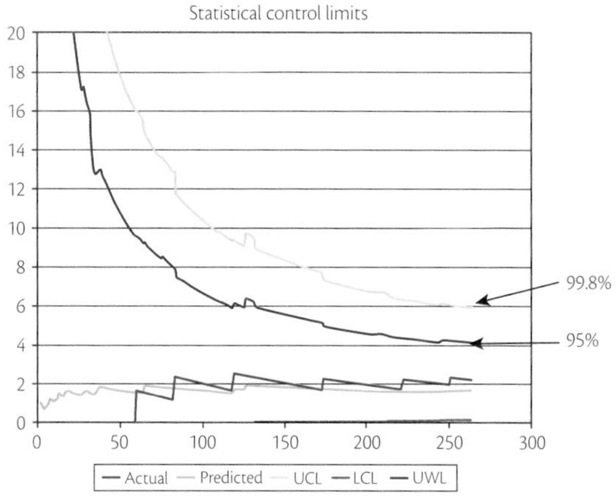

Fig. 3.14 The final cumulative funnel plot. The scale of the axis needs to be modified to accommodate the control limits added (LCL, lower control limit; UWL, upper warning limit) and it is clear that the small differences observed are well within limits or random fluctuation. Evident also in this sequence of 260 patients is that variation in statistically accepted outcome is very large at approximately 0–4%.

door-to-balloon times of less than 90min. Performance can be compared either between different healthcare providers, or within any one provider for different time periods. The resulting statistics are relatively insensitive to the occasional outlier patient, in the same way that a median value is. However, these outliers need to be identified and assessed to find out if there was a preventable problem with the process of care.

Such evaluation is facilitated by data display using statistical process control charts (Fig. 3.15). Successive cases are plotted on the x-axis with the measured time period on the y-axis. Median values for the time points of interest are marked as a horizontal line with confidence intervals added to provide an upper control limit, a statistically defined boundary roughly equivalent to the 99% confidence limit. Individuals with prolonged delays sit well above the control line and so become evident. Overall changes to median times can also be observed.

Unresolved issues regarding statistical process control methods

Memory

CUSUM techniques have no memory loss. A decision needs to be made about when and how to discard past experience, in other words when to reset the chart to zero. If a large amount of 'credit' is built up over a sequence of procedures, then a change to subsequent poorer outcomes will take longer to cross a warning boundary. Yet a shorter series will have wide confidence intervals and little statistical power to detect outliers. There is also the sense that these charts are attempting to provide contemporaneous measurements, and so should reflect current rather than past performance. Rather than taking an arbitrary cut off, an exponential memory loss called 'exponentially weighted moving average' has been proposed[48]. It has also been suggested that SPRT charts are reset whenever an individual crosses the lower boundary line of 'performance as expected', as at that stage monitoring is no longer of interest and it might be appropriate to start a new monitoring period to retain sensitivity to changes in performance line[52]. This approach has been used in the risk-adjusted CUSUM[56]. While similar to the SPRT chart, it is constrained to lie above zero which means that it cannot build up credit, and thus retains sensitivity to under performance. However, the more times the line is restarted, the greater the likelihood of a type 1 statistical error (i.e. rejecting the hypothesis that performance is satisfactory even though it is). Indeed this error becomes a certainty after an infinite number of restarts. Another approach is to try to decide on the 'average run

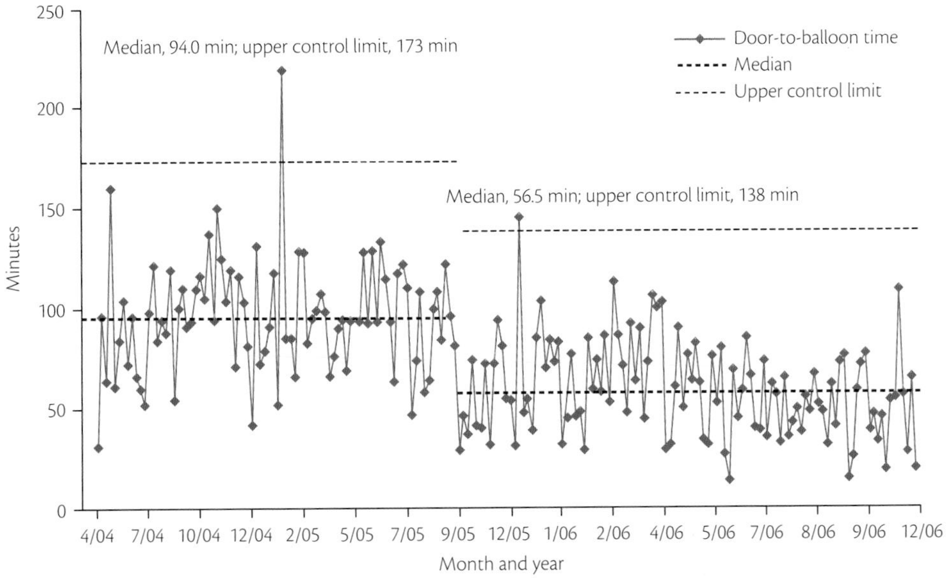

Fig. 3.15 Door-to-balloon times for patients to showing the effect of a procedural change for activation of the cardiac catheterization laboratory[58]. Two intervals are shown, pre- (April 2004 to August 2005) and post- (September 2005 to December 2006) introduction of a single point of contact for activation of the catheterization laboratory. Reproduced from Hall J *et al.* Door-to-Balloon Time in Acute Myocardial Infarction *NEJM* 2009; **356**:1475–79. Copyright © 2009 Massachusetts Medical Society. All rights reserved.

length' for a period of sequential monitoring based on the average number of observations needed before a conclusion can be drawn. The calculations of these run lengths is not straightforward, and will depend on the risk profile being studied. If this changes, then the calculated average run time may no longer be appropriate. Such calculations can be made using the Markov Chain procedure[56,59]. There is no current consensus as to the best way to handle the issue of sequential chart memory.

Multiple comparisons

All these methods are in some senses subject to concerns regarding multiple comparisons. Statistical interpretation depends on how often observations are made but there is debate about the role of multiple comparison corrections in the setting of these process charts.

Conclusions regarding statistical process control plots

These techniques have tremendous value in the assessment and improvement of healthcare delivery. All have their advantages and disadvantages. CUSUM-based methods are very sensitive to subtle shifts away from predicted outcomes but if they prove too sensitive, they will create false alarms and will be discredited. Equipoise must be achieved between systems that are sensitive enough to warn of clinically important changes in outcomes but do not trigger alarms where no clinically important shift exists. Interpretation of these charts must account for their limitations. They should be a guide to monitoring performance which primarily display data, and not used to assess its true statistical significance.

Problems with publication of outcome data

Our ultimate goal in championing these methods is the provision of optimal patient care. We need to measure how well we are treating patients in order to develop strategies to improve this care. Purely clinical components cannot, however, be isolated from political and social factors. The act of reporting data improves a unit's own scrutiny of its performance and increases attention to processes, appropriateness, and quality of care (the Hawthorne effect). Public reporting is intended to nurture a culture of openness and accountability to guarantee quality assurance for patients, commissioners, and regulators. Yet paradoxically there is compelling data that such a mechanism can become deleterious to patient care. Reported advances in outcomes may be due to genuine improvements in patient management, but important factors can suggest apparent improvements where none have taken place. Such illusions occur with alterations in patient selection and manipulation of the risk model. Both have occurred since public reporting and neither is beneficial.

Risk-averse behaviour

The change in patient selection is the most disquieting, as it means that the sickest patients at highest risk of adverse outcomes, but with potentially greatest gains from intervention are turned down for treatment. This is 'risk-averse' behaviour. It is reinforced by difficulties in developing models that adequately account for the severity of illness in extremely sick patients, making them poor at differentiating risk levels within the high-risk cohort. The most studied example of this effect followed the public reporting of outcome for CABG procedures in New York State. Surgeons became reluctant to operate on the sickest patients(60), there was an increase in the number of high-risk patients transferred out of state for their surgery(61), and patients from ethnic minorities were less likely to be offered surgery(62). Across the United Kingdom the public reporting of CABG outcome has also altered patient selection, with surgeons exhibiting risk-averse practice. A recent attempt to measure this objectively failed(63), not least because patients rejected for surgery were not recorded.

Similar behaviour has been observed with PCI. Public reporting seems to be the most compelling explanation for the big differences in case mix and in-hospital mortality between two large quality-controlled regional PCI registries, Michigan (no public reporting) and New York (public reporting)(64). In Massachusetts, public reporting of PCI outcomes was accompanied by a 43% fall in the number of patients being treated with cardiogenic shock (2.28% in 2003, compared to 1.2% in 2005)(65). A retrospective analysis of the SHOCK trial further supports these conclusions. Patients presenting in New York with cardiogenic shock were less likely than those presenting in other regions to be treated by PCI or CABG. After propensity matching the odds ratio for being treated by PCI was 0.51 (95% CI 0.33–0.77, p = 0.002). While there was no significant difference in mortality for patients who did receive revascularization, those untreated had a 1.5-fold higher mortality(66). Resnic describes a useful framework map of relative risks and benefits, and uses this to demonstrate the case selection 'creep' that occurs as high risk patients are left untreated (Figs. 3.16 and 3.17) (67).

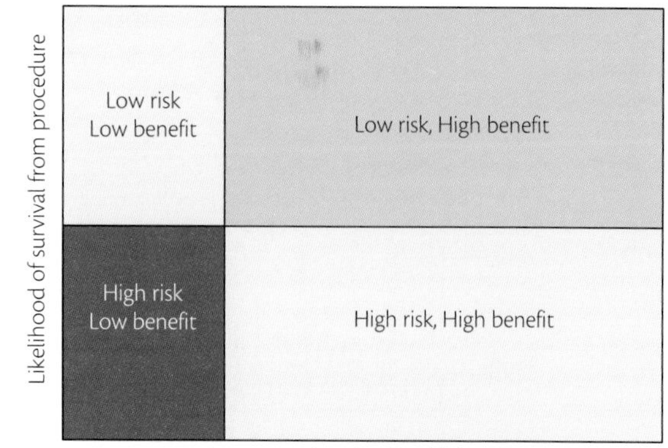

Fig. 3.16 Map of percutaneous coronary intervention risk versus clinical benefit. The vertical axis denotes the risk of the procedure represented as the likelihood of survival to hospital discharge. The horizontal axis denotes the patient benefit represented as the incremental health benefit of having the procedure performed. Reproduced from Resnic FS, Welt FGP. The Public Health Hazards of Risk Avoidance Associated With Public Reporting of Risk-Adjusted Outcomes in Coronary Intervention *JACC* 2009; **53**(10): 825–30 © 2009 American College of Cardiology Foundation. Published by Elsevier Inc

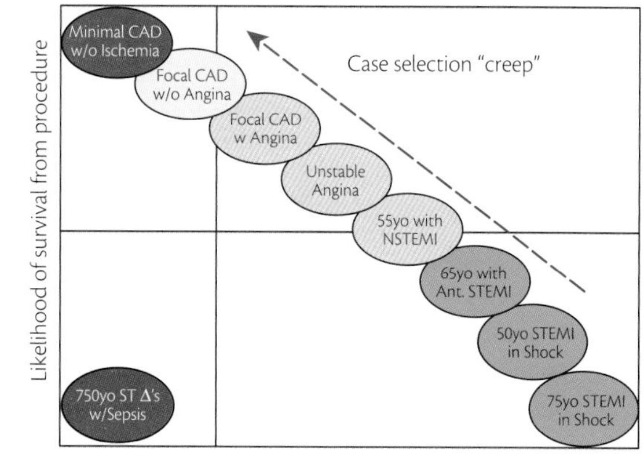

Fig. 3.17 Potential for 'risk avoidance creep'. The map of PCI risk versus clinical benefit (see Fig. 3.16) is shown with illustrative examples. Green ovals indicate scenarios in which clinical benefit is high; grey ovals indicate intermediate risk; and red ovals indicate scenarios in which incremental risk is negligible. The red dashed arrow indicates the 'risk avoidance creep' toward lower-risk cases in the face of public reporting. CAD, coronary artery disease; NSTEMI, non-ST-segment elevation myocardial infarction; STEMI, ST-segment elevation myocardial infarction; yo, years old. Reproduced from Resnic FS, Welt FGP. The Public Health Hazards of Risk Avoidance Associated With Public Reporting of Risk-Adjusted Outcomes in Coronary Intervention *JACC* 2009; **53**(10): 825–30 © 2009 American College of Cardiology Foundation. Published by Elsevier Inc

'Gaming'

There is robust evidence that hospitals have manipulated the predictions of risk models, termed 'gaming'. Following the introduction of the Cardiac Surgery Reporting System in New York, there was a large and sudden increase in the reported prevalence of five key risk factors (renal failure, congestive heart failure, chronic obstructive pulmonary disease [COPD), unstable angina, and low ejection fraction). Thus from 1989 to 1991 reported COPD increased from 6.9% to 17.4%, congestive heart failure from 1.7% to 7.6%, and renal failure from 0.4% to 2.8%. The increase in reported prevalence of 152%, 347%, and 600% could not be explained by a genuine change in patient demographics[(68)].The effect was to artificially elevate predicted risk, making observed outcomes relatively better than predicted, even if there had been no actual change in the quality of the care. Canadian investigators reported that in Ontario, mortality associated with CABG was sharply reduced after providers' results were confidentially disclosed at an institutional level but that public reporting had no added effect on performance[(69)]. Thus performance improvements are accrued though appropriate audit, but there may be little further gain from the extra step of public reporting.

Strategies to mitigate problems with public reporting

Public reporting is here to stay, and so it becomes critical that we do all we can to optimize the benefits, while mitigating the damage it might cause. There are a number of strategies that could be adopted.

All current risk-adjustment models are concentrated on adverse outcomes following intervention, they focus on the 'downside'. A change in design that rewards the treatment of patients who have the most to gain would mitigate against risk-averse behaviour. Such a model would need to compare outcomes between the natural history of the disease process with that achieved if an intervention is performed. A surgical example would be operative correction of critical and otherwise potentially fatal aortic stenosis.

Models are poor at adjusting for outcome in the highest risk patients, so is it possible to improve them, in order to cope with this important group of patients? An analysis of patients treated by PCI in Massachusetts between January 2003 and December 2005 showed that nearly half had at least one severe acute medical condition present before index PCI not accounted for by the risk model. These included advanced malignancy, active infection, acute stroke, and anoxic brain injury[(67)]. Unfortunately an attempt to include these factors in the risk model did not lead to a significant improvement in its performance.

Another strategy, adopted in Massachusetts, is to include the additional composite risk factor 'compassionate-use PCI' in the risk model to accommodate uniquely high-risk patients. A problem with this approach is that it adds a hugely subjective factor to the dataset, which therefore needs to be accompanied by rigorous independent audit.

Adjudicated outcomes are a fourth option, which allow independent assessment of whether or not a death following PCI was considered related to the procedure. 'Unrelated' mortality would then not be counted. This would require the generation of a new risk model, as many high-risk features in current models operate because they predict adverse outcome with PCI as an 'innocent bystander'.

Measures of healthcare performance that are used must be selected with care. A narrow focus risks distorting care in other (unmeasured) areas. Procedures may be completed to minimize acute measured complications but without optimizing long-term consequences. This can be seen in relation to adequate stent deployment, which will have little impact on acute outcomes (to hospital discharge), but may increase the risk of later restenosis.

Peri-procedural MACCE following PCI is very infrequent, and thus a very crude and potentially misleading way to assess the quality of intervention. Later outcomes have been shown to be more determined by disease process than intervention[(70)] and can help to put the relevance of the peri-procedural outcomes into perspective. They also shift the focus onto important issues such as longer-term outcomes and measures of quality of life.

Highlighting appropriateness of care rather than outcomes could reduce patients being turned down for the correct treatment. For example, collecting data on all patients presenting to an institution with STEMI, not just those that receive primary PCI, would allow analysis of patients who should have received angioplasty. Another example is quantification of the proportion of those presenting in cardiogenic shock that are treated by PCI. The development of appropriateness criteria for revascularization by the ACC will facilitate this approach.[71]

Resource allocation towards data collection and validation is mandatory for every strategy.

Conclusions

Selecting patients for procedures is a complex process. As the research base grows, indications for different interventions in a variety of clinical settings are better defined. Interventional techniques evolve and results of earlier trials become redundant. Against this dynamic background, risk assessment must provide patients and physicians with the tools to select optimal management strategies and continually improve delivery of care. Providers will 'game' the model and patients will arrive with risk factors that are not accounted for adequately by any method of risk stratification. Amidst this, mandatory publication of unit- and operator-specific characteristics, intended to cement the goal of optimal patient care, remains omnipresent. Despite its limitations, public reporting will remain and we must navigate a course that never compromises our clinical responsibilities to individual patients.

References

1. BRI Inquiry Panel. *Learning from Bristol: the report of the public inquiry into children's heart surgery at the Bristol Royal Infirmary 1984-1995*. London: The Stationery Office, 2001.
2. Anon. *Fifth report: safeguarding patients, lessons from the past-proposals for the future. Shipman inquiry*. The Shipman Inquiry, 2004.
3. Department of Health. *The NHS Plan*. Crown Copyright, 2000.
4. Department of Health. *NHS Next Stage Review Final Report*. Norwich: The Stationery Office, 2008.
5. Chief Medical Officer. *Good doctors, safer patients. Good doctors, safer patients*. London: Department of Health, 2006.
6. Shewhart WA. *Economic control of quality of manufactured product*. Princeton, NJ: Van Nostrand Reinhold, 1931.
7. Shewhart WA. The application of statistics as an aid in maintaining quality of a manufactured product. *J Am Stat Assoc* 1925; **20**:546–8.
8. Tonino PAL, de Bruyne B, Pijls NHJ, *et al.* Fractional flow reserve versus angiography for guiding percutaneous coronary intervention. *N Engl J Med* 2009; **360**(3):213–24.
9. Hannan EL, Kilburn H, Jr, Lindsey ML, *et al.* Clinical versus administrative data bases for CABG surgery. Does it matter? *Med Care* 1992; **30**(10):892–907.
10. Ugolini C, Nobilio L. Risk adjustment for coronary artery bypass graft surgery: an administrative approach versus EuroSCORE. *Int J Qual Health Care* 2004; **16**(2):157–64.
11. Lemeshow S, Hosmer DW, Jr. A review of goodness of fit statistics for use in the development of logistic regression models. *Am J Epidemiol* 1982; **115**(1):92–106.
12. Hanley JA, Meengs WL. The meaning and use of the area under a receiver operating characteristic (ROC) curve. *Diagn Radiol* 2009; **143**:29–36.
13. Stephan C, Wesseling S, Schink T, *et al.* Comparison of eight computer programs for receiver-operating characteristic analysis. *Clin Chem* 2003; **49**(3):433–9.
14. Nashef SA, Roques F, Michel P, *et al.* European system for cardiac operative risk evaluation (EuroSCORE). *Eur J Cardiothorac Surg* 1999; **16**(1):9–13.
15. Roques F, Nashef SA, Michel P, *et al.* Does EuroSCORE work in individual European countries? *Eur J Cardiothorac Surg* 2000; **18**(1):27–30.
16. Pitkanen O, Niskanen M, Rehnberg S, *et al.* Intra-institutional prediction of outcome after cardiac surgery: comparison between a locally derived model and the EuroSCORE. *Eur J Cardiothorac Surg* 2000; **18**(6): 703–10.
17. Kawachi Y, Nakashima A, Toshima Y, *et al.* Evaluation of the quality of cardiovascular surgery care using risk stratification analysis according to the EuroSCORE additive model. *Circ J* 2002; **66**(2):145–8.
18. Nashef SA, Roques F, Hammill BG, *et al.* Validation of European System for Cardiac Operative Risk Evaluation (EuroSCORE) in North American cardiac surgery. *Eur J Cardiothorac Surg* 2002; **22**(1):101–5.
19. Jin R, Grunkemeier GL, Providence Health System Cardiovascular Study Group. Additive vs. logistic risk models for cardiac surgery mortality. *Eur J Cardiothorac Surg* 2005; **28**(2):240–3.
20. Bhatti F, Grayson AD, Grotte G, *et al.* The logistic EuroSCORE in cardiac surgery: how well does it predict operative risk? *Heart* 2006; **92**(12):1817–20.
21. Bridgewater B, Grayson AD, Jackson M, *et al.* Surgeon specific mortality in adult cardiac surgery: comparison between crude and risk stratified data. *BMJ* 2003; **327**(7405):13–17.
22. Dewey TM, Brown D, Ryan WH, *et al.* Reliability of risk algorithms in predicting early and late operative outcomes in high-risk patients undergoing aortic valve replacement. *J Thorac Cardiovasc Surg* 2008; **135**(1):180–7.
23. Schuurmans H, Steverink N, Lindenberg S, *et al.* Old or frail: what tells us more? *J Gerontol A Biol Sci Med Sci* 2004; **59**(9):M962–M965.
24. Kunadian B, Dunning J, Das R, *et al.* External validation of established risk adjustment models for procedural complications after percutaneous coronary intervention. *Heart* 2008; **94**(8):1012–18.
25. Singh M, Lennon RJ, Holmes DR, Jr, *et al.* Correlates of procedural complications and a simple integer risk score for percutaneous coronary intervention. *J Am Coll Cardiol* 2002; **40**(3):387–93.
26. Grayson AD, Moore RK, Jackson M, *et al.* Multivariate prediction of major adverse cardiac events after 9914 percutaneous coronary interventions in the north west of England. *Heart* 2006; **92**(5):658–63.
27. Romagnoli E, Burzotta F, Trani C, *et al.* EuroSCORE as predictor of in-hospital mortality after percutaneous coronary intervention. *Heart* 2009; **95**(1):43–8.
28. Singh M, Gersh BJ, Li S, *et al.* Mayo Clinic Risk Score for percutaneous coronary intervention predicts in-hospital mortality in patients undergoing coronary artery bypass graft surgery. *Circulation* 2008; **117**(3):356–62.
29. Ellis SG, Guetta V, Miller D, *et al.* Relation between lesion characteristics and risk with percutaneous intervention in the stent and glycoprotein IIb/IIIa era: An analysis of results from 10,907 lesions and proposal for new classification scheme. *Circulation* 1999; **100**(19):1971–6.
30. Krone RJ, Laskey WK, Johnson C, *et al.* A simplified lesion classification for predicting success and complications of coronary angioplasty. Registry Committee of the Society

for Cardiac Angiography and Intervention. *Am J Cardiol* 2000; **85**(10):1179–84.

31. Sianos G, Morel M-A, Kappetein AP, *et al.* The SYNTAX score: an angiographic tool grading the complexity of coronary artery disease. *EuroInterv* 2005; **1**:219–27.
32. Valgimigli M, Serruys PW, Tsuchida K, *et al.* Cyphering the complexity of coronary artery disease using the syntax score to predict clinical outcome in patients with three-vessel lumen obstruction undergoing percutaneous coronary intervention. *Am J Cardiol* 2007; **99**(8):1072–81.
33. Serruys PW, Ong ALT, Morice M-C, *et al.* Arterial Revascularisation Therapies Study Part II – Sirolimus-eluting stents for the treatment of patients with multivessel de novo coronary artery lesions. *EuroInterv* 2005; **1**(2):147–56.
34. Leaman DM, Brower RW, Meester GT, *et al.* Coronary artery atherosclerosis: severity of the disease, severity of angina pectoris and compromised left ventricular function. *Circulation* 1981; **63**(2):285–99.
35. Lansky AJ, Popma JJ. Qualitative and Quantitative Angiography. In Topol EJ (ed) *Textbook of Interventional Cardiology*, pp. 725–47. Philadelphia, PA: W.B. Saunders, 1999.
36. Lefevre T, Louvard Y, Morice MC, *et al.* Stenting of bifurcation lesions: classification, treatments, and results. *Catheter Cardiovasc Interv* 2000; **49**(3):274–83.
37. Serruys PW, Morice MC, Kappetein AP, *et al.* Percutaneous coronary intervention versus coronary-artery bypass grafting for severe coronary artery disease. *N Engl J Med* 2009; **360**(10):961–72.
38. Percutaneous Coronary Interventions (PCI) in New York State 2003–2005. http://www.health.state.ny.us/statistics/diseases/cardiovascular/docs/pci_2003–2005.pdf New York State Department of Health, 2008.
39. Adult Cardiac Surgery in New York State 2003–2005. http://www.health.state.ny.us/diseases/cardiovascular/heart_disease/docs/2003-2005_adult_cardiac_surgery.pdf New York State Department of Health, 2008.
40. Heart Surgery in the United Kingdom: Operations for the year ending March 2007. http://heartsurgery.healthcarecommission.org.uk/Survival.aspx
41. Adab P, Rouse AM, Mohammed MA, *et al.* Performance league tables: the NHS deserves better. *BMJ* 2002; **324**(7329):95–8.
42. Sterne JAC, Smith GD, Cox DR. Sifting the evidence—what's wrong with significance tests? Another comment on the role of statistical methods. *BMJ* 2001; **322**(7280):226–31.
43. Spiegelhalter DJ. Funnel plots for comparing institutional performance. *Stat Med* 2005; **24**(8):1185–202.
44. Adult Cardiac Surgery in New York State 1997–9. http://www.health.state.ny.us/diseases/cardiovascular/heart_disease/ ed. New York State Department of Health, 2002.
45. Gale CP, Roberts AP, Batin PD, *et al.* Funnel plots, performance variation and the Myocardial Infarction National Audit Project 2003–2004. *BMC Cardiovasc Disord* 2006; **6**:34.
46. Shaw RE, Anderson HV, Brindis RG, *et al.* Development of a risk adjustment mortality model using the American College of Cardiology-National Cardiovascular Data Registry (ACC-NCDR) experience: 1998-2000. *J Am Coll Cardiol* 2002; **39**(7):1104–12.
47. Riddick JH, Jr, Giddings NW. Computerized preparation of average CUSUM charts for clinical chemistry. *Clin Biochem* 1971; **4**(3):156–61.
48. de Leval MR, Francois K, Bull C, *et al.* Analysis of a cluster of surgical failures. Application to a series of neonatal arterial switch operations. *J Thorac Cardiovasc Surg* 1994; **107**(3):914–23.
49. Rogers CA, Reeves BC, Caputo M, *et al.* Control chart methods for monitoring cardiac surgical performance and their interpretation. *J Thorac Cardiovasc Surg* 2004; **128**(6):811–19.
50. Lovegrove J, Valencia O, Treasure T, *et al.* Monitoring the results of cardiac surgery by variable life-adjusted display. *Lancet* 1997; **350**(9085):1128–30.
51. Poloniecki J, Valencia O, Littlejohns P. Cumulative risk adjusted mortality chart for detecting changes in death rate: observational study of heart surgery. *BMJ* 1998; **316**(7146):1697–700.
52. Spiegelhalter D, Grigg O, Kinsman R, *et al.* Risk-adjusted sequential probability ratio tests: applications to Bristol, Shipman and adult cardiac surgery. *Int J Qual Health Care* 2003; **15**(1):7–13.
53. Barnard GA. Sequential tests in industrial statistics. *J R Statist Soc* 1946; **8**(suppl):1–26.
54. Wald A. Sequential tests of statistical hypotheses. *Ann Math Statist* 1946; **6**:117–86.
55. Armitage P. Sequential tests in prophylactic and therapeutic trials. *Q J Med* 1954; **23**(91):255–74.
56. Steiner SH, Cook RJ, Farewell VT, *et al.* Monitoring surgical performance using risk-adjusted cumulative sum charts. *Biostatistics* 2000; **1**(4):441–52.
57. Kunadian B, Dunning J, Roberts AP, *et al.* Cumulative funnel plots for the early detection of interoperator variation: retrospective database analysis of observed versus predicted results of percutaneous coronary intervention. *BMJ* 2008; **336**(7650):931–4.
58. Hall J, Roberts T, Belder M. Door-to-balloon time in acute myocardial infarction. *N Engl J Med* 2007; **356**(14):1477–8.
59. Steiner SH, Cook RJ, Farewell VT. Risk-adjusted monitoring of binary surgical outcomes. *Med Decis Making* 2001; **21**(3):163–9.
60. Schneider EC, Epstein AM, Schneider EC, *et al.* Influence of cardiac-surgery performance reports on referral practices and access to care. A survey of cardiovascular specialists.[see comment]. *N Engl J Med* 1996; **335**(4):251–6.
61. Omoigui NA, Miller DP, Brown KJ, *et al.* Outmigration for coronary bypass surgery in an era of public dissemination of clinical outcomes.[see comment]. *Circulation* 1996; **93**(1):27–33.

62. Werner RM, Asch DA, Polsky D, *et al.* Racial profiling: the unintended consequences of coronary artery bypass graft report cards. *Circulation* 2005; **111**(10):1257–63.
63. Bridgewater B, Grayson A, Brooks N, *et al.* Has the publication of cardiac surgery outcome data been associated with changes in practice in Northwest England? An analysis of 25,730 patients undergoing CABG surgery under 30 surgeons over 8 years. *Heart* 2007; **93**(6): 744–8.
64. Moscucci M, Eagle KA, Share D, *et al.* Public reporting and case selection for percutaneous coronary interventions: an analysis from two large multicenter percutaneous coronary intervention databases. *J Am Coll Cardiol* 2005; **45**(11):1759–65.
65. Department of Health Care Policy – Harvard Medical School. Adult percutaneous coronary interventions in the Commonwealth of Massachusetts. http://www.massdac.org/reports/pci.html
66. Apolito RA, Greenberg MA, Menegus MA, *et al.* Impact of the New York State Cardiac Surgery and Percutaneous Coronary Intervention Reporting System on the management of patients with acute myocardial infarction complicated by cardiogenic shock. *Am Heart J* 2008; **155**(2):267–73.
67. Resnic FS, Welt FGP. The public health hazards of risk avoidance associated with public reporting of risk-adjusted outcomes in coronary intervention. *J Am Coll Cardiol* 2009; **53**(10):825–30.
68. Green J, Wintfeld N. Report cards on cardiac surgeons. Assessing New York State's approach. *N Engl J Med* 1995; **332**(18):1229–32.
69. Guru V, Fremes SE, Naylor CD, *et al.* Public versus private institutional performance reporting: what is mandatory for quality improvement? *Am Heart J* 2006; **152**(3):573–8.
70. Singh M, Rihal CS, Roger VL, *et al.* Comorbid conditions and outcomes after percutaneous coronary intervention. *Heart* 2008; **94**(11):1424–8.
71. Patel MR, Dehmer GJ, Hirshfeld JW, *et al.* ACCF/SCAI/STS/AATS/AHA/ASNC 2009 Appropriateness Criteria for Coronary Revascularization: A Report by the American College of Cardiology Foundation Appropriateness Criteria Task Force, Society for Cardiovascular Angiography and Interventions, Society of Thoracic Surgeons, American Association for Thoracic Surgery, American Heart Association, and the American Society of Nuclear Cardiology Endorsed by the American Society of Echocardiography, the Heart Failure Society of America, and the Society of Cardiovascular Computed Tomography. *J Am Coll Cardiol* 2009; **53**(6):530–3.
72. Hannan EL, Arani DT, Johnson LW, *et al.* Percutaneous transluminal coronary angioplasty in New York State. Risk factors and outcomes. *JAMA* 1992; **268**(21):3092–7.
73. Hannan EL, Racz M, Ryan TJ, *et al.* Coronary angioplasty volume-outcome relationships for hospitals and cardiologists. *JAMA* 1997; **277**(11):892–8.
74. Kimmel SE, Berlin JA, Strom BL, *et al.* Development and validation of simplified predictive index for major complications in contemporary percutaneous transluminal coronary angioplasty practice. The Registry Committee of the Society for Cardiac Angiography and Interventions. *J Am Coll Cardiol* 1995; **26**(4):931–8.
75. Ellis SG, Weintraub W, Holmes D, *et al.* Relation of operator volume and experience to procedural outcome of percutaneous coronary revascularization at hospitals with high interventional volumes. *Circulation* 1997; **95**(11):2479–84.
76. O'Connor GT, Malenka DJ, Quinton H, *et al.* Multivariate prediction of in-hospital mortality after percutaneous coronary interventions in 1994-1996. Northern New England Cardiovascular Disease Study Group. *J Am Coll Cardiol* 1999; **34**(3):681–91.
77. de Belder AJ, Jewitt DE, Wainwright RJ, *et al.* Development and validation of a Bayesian index for predicting major adverse cardiac events with percutaneous transluminal coronary angioplasty. *Heart* 2001; **85**(1): 69–72.
78. Qureshi MA, Safian RD, Grines CL, *et al.* Simplified scoring system for predicting mortality after percutaneous coronary intervention. *J Am Coll Cardiol* 2003; **42**(11):1890–5.
79. Moscucci M, Kline-Rogers E, Share D, *et al.* Simple bedside additive tool for prediction of in-hospital mortality after percutaneous coronary interventions. *Circulation* 2001; **104**(3):263–8.
80. Resnic FS, Ohno-Machado L, Selwyn A, *et al.* Simplified risk score models accurately predict the risk of major in-hospital complications following percutaneous coronary intervention. *Am J Cardiol* 2001; **88**(1):5–9.
81. Wu C, Hannan EL, Walford G, *et al.* A risk score to predict in-hospital mortality for percutaneous coronary interventions. *J Am Coll Cardiol* 2006; **47**(3):654–60.
82. Chowdhary S, Ivanov J, Mackie K, *et al.* The Toronto score for in-hospital mortality after percutaneous coronary interventions. *Am Heart J* 2009; **157**(1):156–63.
83. De Luca G, Suryapranata H, van't Hof AW, *et al.* Prognostic assessment of patients with acute myocardial infarction treated with primary angioplasty: implications for early discharge. *Circulation* 2004; **109**(22):2737–43.
84. Addala S, Grines CL, Dixon SR, *et al.* Predicting mortality in patients with ST-elevation myocardial infarction treated with primary percutaneous coronary intervention (PAMI risk score). *Am J Cardiol* 2004; **93**(5):629–32.
85. Grines CL, Browne KF, Marco J, *et al.* A comparison of immediate angioplasty with thrombolytic therapy for acute myocardial infarction. The Primary Angioplasty in Myocardial Infarction Study Group. *N Engl J Med* 1993; **328**(10):673–9.
86. Grines CL, Marsalese DL, Brodie B, *et al.* Safety and cost-effectiveness of early discharge after primary angioplasty in low risk patients with acute myocardial infarction. PAMI-II Investigators. Primary Angioplasty in Myocardial Infarction. *J Am Coll Cardiol* 1998; **31**(5): 967–72.
87. Grines CL, Cox DA, Stone GW, *et al.* Coronary angioplasty with or without stent implantation for acute myocardial infarction. Stent Primary Angioplasty in Myocardial Infarction Study Group. *N Engl J Med* 1999; **341**(26):1949–56.

CHAPTER 4

Vascular access: femoral versus radial

David H. Roberts and Andrew Wiper

Introduction

Gruentzig performed the first intracoronary balloon angioplasty in 1977. In 1993 intracoronary stent deployment became widely accepted. This was in the era before oral dual antiplatelet therapy. The use of intensive antithrombotic therapy at that time led to a dramatic rise in the incidence of femoral arterial access complications. Campeau had already performed the first transradial coronary angiogram in 1989. As the radial artery runs a more superficial course, haemostasis was easier to achieve in a fully anticoagulated patient. Kiemeneij described the first transradial stent deployment in 1995.

In 2007 in the UK, 223 638 diagnostic coronary angiograms and 77 373 percutaneous coronary interventions (PCI) procedures were performed(1). Radial access accounts for less than 10% of procedures performed worldwide and is performed even less frequently in the United States (1%) (Fig. 4.1).

Femoral access

Femoral arterial punctures can be placed into four groups(2) based on their location of vascular entry (Figs. 4.2 and 4.3):

- Group 1: low puncture—at or below the bifurcation of the common femoral artery (CFA) into the superficial femoral artery (SFA) and profunda femoral artery (PFA).
- Group 2: middle puncture—above the femoral bifurcation and below the most inferior border of the inferior epigastric artery (IEA).
- Group 3: high middle puncture—at or above the inferior border of the IEA and below the origin of the IEA.
- Group 4: high puncture—above the origin of the IEA.

The ideal puncture site for the CFA is below the inguinal ligament but above the bifurcation into the PFA and SFA. Using the landmarks of the pubic symphysis and the anterior superior iliac crest, the puncture site is approximately 2cm below the midpoint. A radio-opaque marker such as a pair of scissors or forceps can be used to identify the medial femoral head which is a very reliable marker for the CFA. The inguinal skin lies below the bifurcation in 70% of patients (particularly obese patients) and should not be used as a landmark for common femoral arterial puncture (Fig. 4.4).

Ideally following femoral sheath insertion but prior to PCI, a femoral angiogram should be performed to assess the site of arterial puncture (although this is rarely done). If above the inferior border of the IEA, then there is an increased risk of retroperitoneal haemorrhage following PCI (particularly with the use of glycoprotein IIb/IIIa receptor antagonists) and the procedure should be performed via an alternative access site(2).

Radial access

The radial arterial access site is prepared aseptically in the usual fashion and a 1-m board is placed on the catheter table to support the abducted arm. The wrist is sometimes hyperextended over a roll of gauze. The position of the radial artery at the wrist displays significant inter-individual variability. The best position for arterial puncture is 1cm proximal to the styloid process at the point of maximal pulsation. A common mistake is to attempt to puncture the radial artery in a more distal position over the flexor skin creases. Cannulation at this point is difficult due to a more mobile arterial axis and hinders applying a haemostatic device effectively at the end of the procedure.

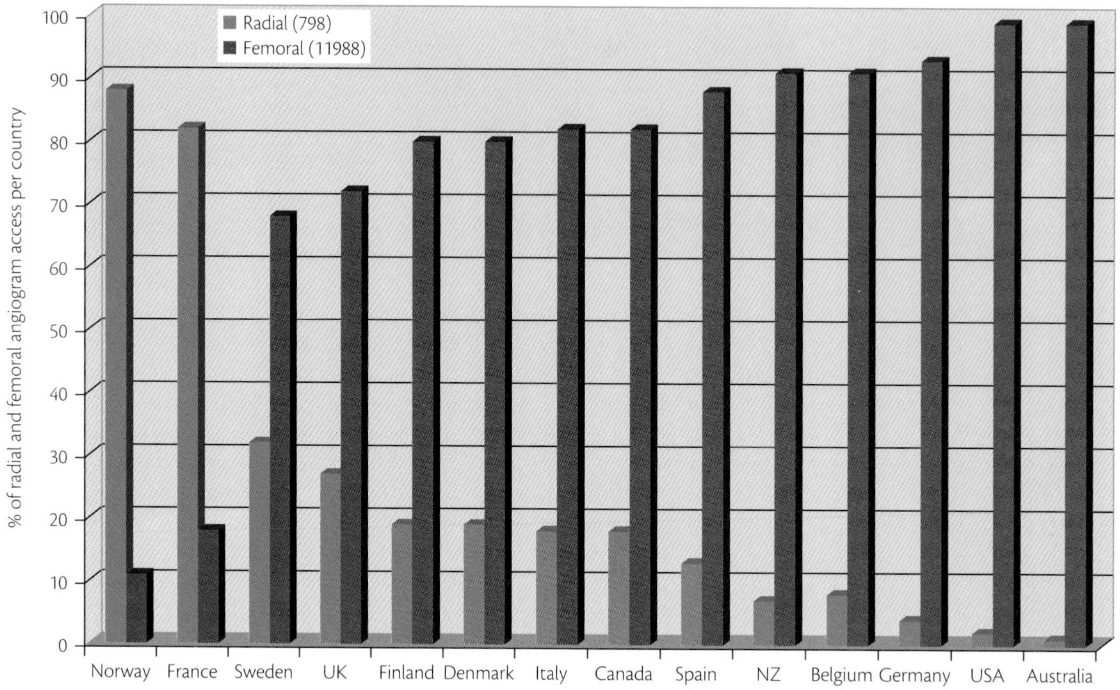

Fig. 4.1 Proportion of femoral and radial coronary angiograms per country (Acuity Access Study, TCT, 2006).

Following intra-arterial sheath placement, a retrograde radial arteriogram may be performed. A mixture of 5mL of contrast diluted with 5mL of blood (to minimize any discomfort with contrast injection) is injected via the radial sheath side port. This aids in identification of any arterial anomalies, thus guiding the operator on potential procedural strategies or indeed ascertaining whether an alternative access site would be more suitable.

Performing radial coronary angiography or PCI is often challenging at first with a steep learning curve[3,4]. When performed by operators experienced in the femoral approach (>200 cases), after approximately 20 radial procedures[4] the procedure duration, fluoroscopy time, and procedural success rate all improve considerably, although 200 procedures are often needed to become completely familiar and competent in the transradial approach.

Left versus right radial arterial access

Catheter advancement via the left radial approach follows a 180–200° curve between the left subclavian artery and the left coronary ostium in contrast to the 90° angle when approaching from the right subclavian artery, when utilizing the right transradial approach. The manipulation of Judkins catheters via the left transradial approach is therefore easier and essentially the same as the transfemoral approach. Saphenous vein graft cannulation is often easier via the left versus right transradial approach. The left internal mammary artery (LIMA) graft is clearly easier to engage via the left transradial approach although the distal tip of most mammary artery catheters is steeply curved and specifically designed radial catheters are available for LIMA cannulation via the left radial approach.

For a left radial approach the operator is on the left side of the patient during the puncture. Following arterial sheath placement, the operator switches to the right side and the arm placed across the patient's body and the procedure thereafter performed in the usual manner.

Limitations and contraindications to femoral access

Peripheral vascular disease

Approximately 10% of patients with cardiovascular disease will have diffuse atherosclerotic disease[5]. In patients with known or presumed peripheral vascular disease (history of intermittent claudication; recent vascular surgical assessment or procedure), the femoral

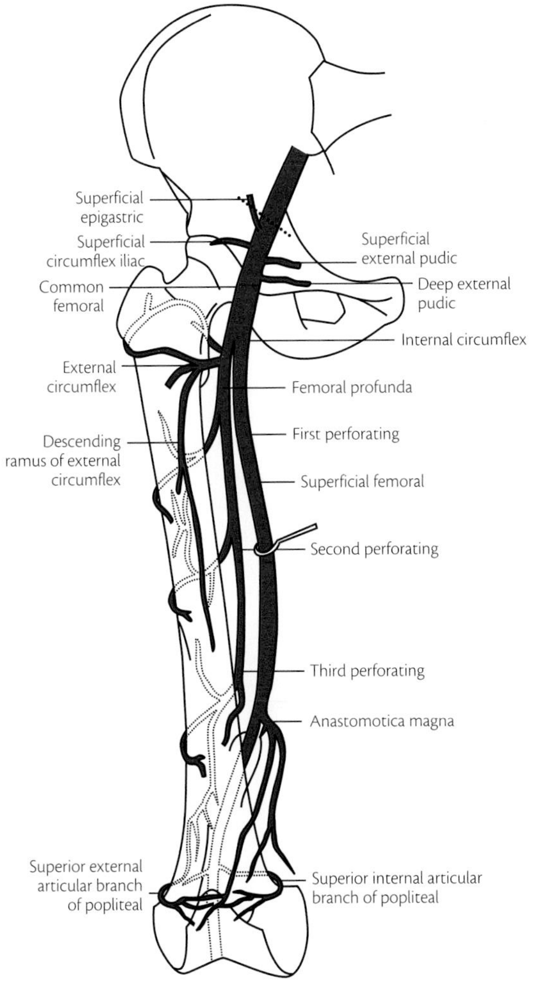

Fig. 4.2 Arterial tree anatomy.

approach has to be used with great caution. Having a very low threshold to use fluoroscopy and hydrophilic coated wires to aid guide wire advancement will reduce the risk of arterial trauma.

Lower limb arterial vascular surgery and abdominal aortic aneurysm (AAA)

In patients who have undergone femoral bypass grafting, the vessel can be punctured below the surgical conduit but there is little data on the safety of this technique for arterial access. This approach should therefore be avoided if at all possible. The femoral approach is also relatively contraindicated in patients with AAA. When traversing the aneurysm, there is a risk of thrombotic disruption or inducing a dissection or even perforation. For these reasons, the femoral approach is best avoided.

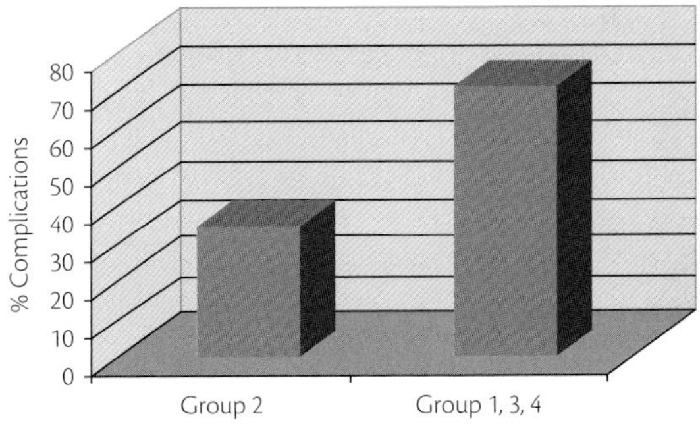

Fig. 4.3 Incidence of complications based on the puncture site location.

Extremes of body mass index

Vascular complications are highest in extremely underweight or morbidly obese patients[(6)]. In very obese patients, there is more difficulty both in obtaining arterial access and in compressing the femoral artery against the femoral head post procedure to obtain haemostasis. The incidence of femoral vascular complications are, however, lowest in the moderately obese patients—the so-called 'obesity paradox'[(6–8)]. One possible explanation is that when an operator is faced with an obese patient, femoral access is obtained more cautiously.

Therapeutic anticoagulation

A standard recommendation for patients anticoagulated with warfarin is to discontinue warfarin for 3–4 days

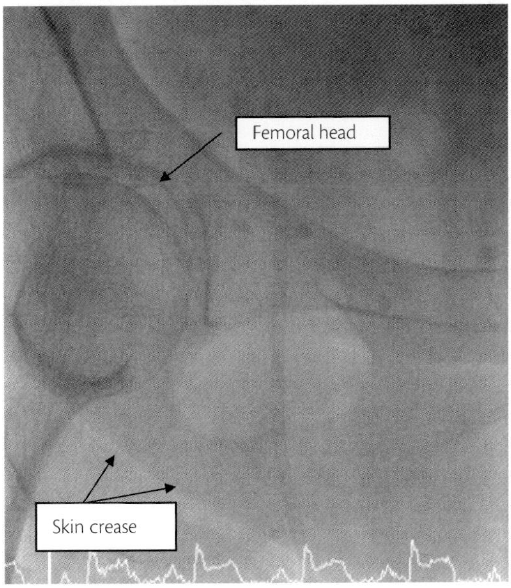

Fig. 4.4 Femoral skin crease and femoral head anatomy in an obese patient.

prior to their elective procedure, aiming for an international normalized ratio (INR) level of <1.8. Despite this approach, vascular complications (especially haematoma formation) are still more likely and the radial approach is much safer to use, including in patients with a therapeutic INR (2–4.5)[9].

Limitations to radial access

Radial diameter

A study examining over 1100 cases of coronary angiography via the radial approach has demonstrated a large variation in the mean radial arterial diameter (RAD)[10]. The mean RAD in men is 2.69mm ± 0.40mm compared to a mean RAD in women of 2.43mm ± 0.38mm ($p < 0.001$). In comparison, the outer diameter of a 5Fr, 6Fr, 7Fr, and 8Fr sheath is approximately 2.28mm, 2.52mm, 2.85mm, and 3.22 respectively[10]. The proportion of mean RAD smaller than 5Fr (2.3mm), 6Fr (2.52mm), and 7Fr (2.85mm), was 17.3%, 43.8%, and 74.4% respectively. The smallest RADs are found in women of small stature (<148cm). This data highlights the value of correct sheath size calculation appropriate to the patient. For example, a 7Fr sheath would be inappropriately large for most patients (74%), with an increased risk of radial spasm, dissection, and occlusion. 7Fr procedures are sometimes needed, however, for certain bifurcation stent procedures (e.g. crush stenting), vein graft PCI using proximal protection (PROXIS) devices, and some operators prefer 7Fr catheters for all bifurcation procedures involving a side branch >2mm diameter for better angiographic visualization during stent deployment. PCI procedures requiring an 8Fr arterial sheath are unusual these days, although intra-aortic balloon pump (IABP) insertion requires 8Fr and femoral access. Sheathless guide catheters are available (e.g. SheathLess Eaucath, Asahi Intecc, Japan) which enable PCI to be performed with a smaller puncture site. For example, a 6.5Fr (2.16mm) sheathless guide catheter possesses approximately the same outer diameter (OD) as a 4Fr (2.00mm) sheath introducer, and a 7.5Fr (2.49mm) as a 5Fr (2.29mm) sheath introducer. A 7.5Fr sheathless guide catheter has a 2.06mm internal diameter and will facilitate a 1.75mm rotablator burr.

Anatomical variations

Radial artery anomalies are seen frequently (13.8%) and are a common cause for procedural failure even in the hands of experienced radial operators[11] (Table 4.1).

Arterial loops (Figs. 4.5 and 4.6) can be a challenging technical issue and are the commonest cause for procedural failure[11], although if the loop is large and the artery of large calibre, the loop can be successfully crossed with a hydrophilic wire and a small calibre catheter (4Fr) used to obtain diagnostic images. Persistent attempts to cross can be very painful for the patient, however, and should prompt swift conversion to an alternative arterial access site.

A particular problem for the right radial operator is the presence of an aberrant right subclavian artery (ARSA) which occurs with a reported incidence of approximately 1.5%. The ARSA arises from the distal and posterior aspect of the horizontal part of the aortic arch at its junction with the descending aorta. The condition is usually asymptomatic and will often cause difficult advancement of the wire or guide catheter into the ascending aorta. The diagnosis can be confirmed by contrast injection. Engagement of the coronary ostia, particularly the left, is often challenging with an ARSA.

Allen's test—is it still relevant?

The hand is supplied by both the radial and ulnar arteries with an anastomosis supplied by both the superficial and deep palmar arch. Thereby if one arterial supply is

Table 4.1 Variations of patients and procedural data in relation to radial artery (RA) anatomy

	Normal anatomy	High bifurcations	RA loops	Tortuous RA	Other anomalies
Patients (n)	1321	108	35	30	39
Women (%)	28	29	49	50	33
Age (years), mean (SD)	63.0 (11.0)	65.5 (10.8)	69.8 (10.4)	72.2 (7.7)	65.1 (11.8)
Procedure duration (min), mean (SD)	41.3 (21.5)	45.2 (23.2)	49.4 (17.1)	41.0 (12.7)	42.1 (19.2)
Fluoroscopy time (min), mean (SD)	9.7 (8.0)	9.3 (6.5)	10.0 (6.6)	10.7 (6.5)	9.6 (7.1)
Failures (%)*	0.9	4.6	37.1	23.3	12.9

*Percentage of failure to radial artery anatomical finding.

Data from Lo TS, Nolan J, Fountzopoulos E, *et al.* Radial artery anomaly and its influence on transradial coronary procedural outcome. *Heart* 2009; **95**: 410–15.

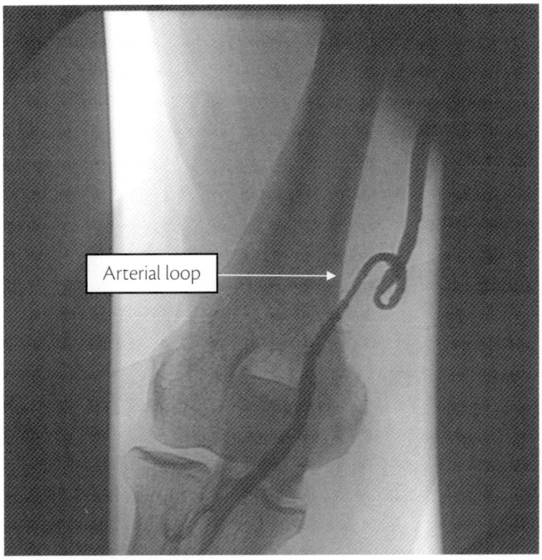

Fig. 4.5 Brachial arterial loop.

severed or reduced, an adequate supply is still maintained by the palmar arches. An inadequate collateral flow has been shown to be present in 8–10% of patients(12).

Edgar Van Nuys Allen (1900–1961) was an American physician with a specialist interest in cardiovascular medicine. His name is lent to the eponymous Allen's test which is used to assess the patency of the palmar arches.

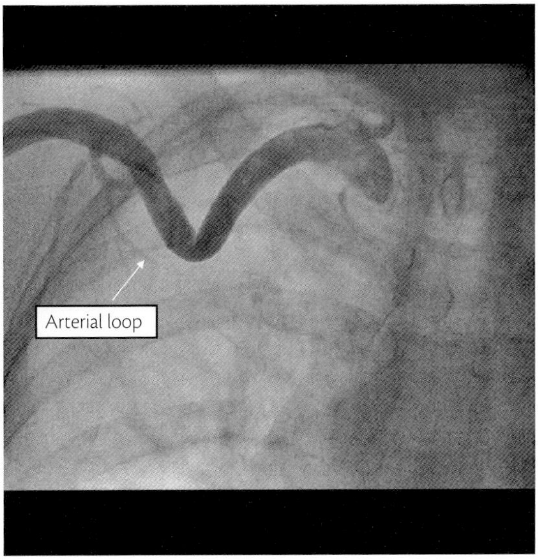

Fig. 4.6 Subclavian arterial loop.

Procedure

1) The hand is elevated and a clenched fist is made for 30s.
2) Digital pressure is placed over both the ulnar and radial arteries so as to occlude distal flow.
3) While still elevated, the hand is opened. It should appear white or blanched (with a typical preservation in colour at the finger nails) (Fig. 4.7a).
4) Pressure over the ulnar artery is then released, and a return to normal colour within the hand should occur within 7–10s—a positive (or non-ischaemic) Allen's test (Fig. 4.7b). A negative (or ischaemic) test implies preservation of pallor for more than 10s (Figs. 4.7c and 4.7d).

It has been shown that in patients with a negative Allen's test, occlusion of the radial artery results in an almost immediate reduction in blood flow to the thumb by 90%, improving to a 75% reduction after 30min of arterial occlusion. Similarly, pulse oximetry gives a strong signal in 0% of patients immediately following radial artery occlusion, rising to 64% at 30min(13).

Additionally, a negative or positive Allen's test does not correlate with distal blood flow as demonstrated by fluorescein dye injections(14) or photoplethysmography(15). *Barbeau's test* is a combination of plethysmography and pulse oximetry used to evaluate the collateral circulation. It has been shown to be more sensitive than Allen's test. In a large cohort, 6.3% of patients were excluded for radial coronary angiography due to an ischaemic Allen's test; however, only 1.5% were excluded when utilizing Barbeau's test(16). The test is simple to perform but as yet is not used routinely in the UK.

The significance of a negative Allen's test is uncertain(17) as there are no documented cases of hand ischaemia and a number of high volume radial operators do not perform this test with no reported adverse clinical events. In patients undergoing a second procedure via the same radial site, a *reverse Allen's test* should be performed, however. In this situation, the operator releases pressure over the radial artery rather than the ulnar. This may detect a proximal radial artery occlusion that may be asymptomatic, thus potentially excluding this access site for a repeat procedure.

Femoral arterial access site complications (Table 4.2)

Retroperitoneal haemorrhage

Retroperitoneal haemorrhage (RPH) is potentially the most serious complication. Several studies have shown

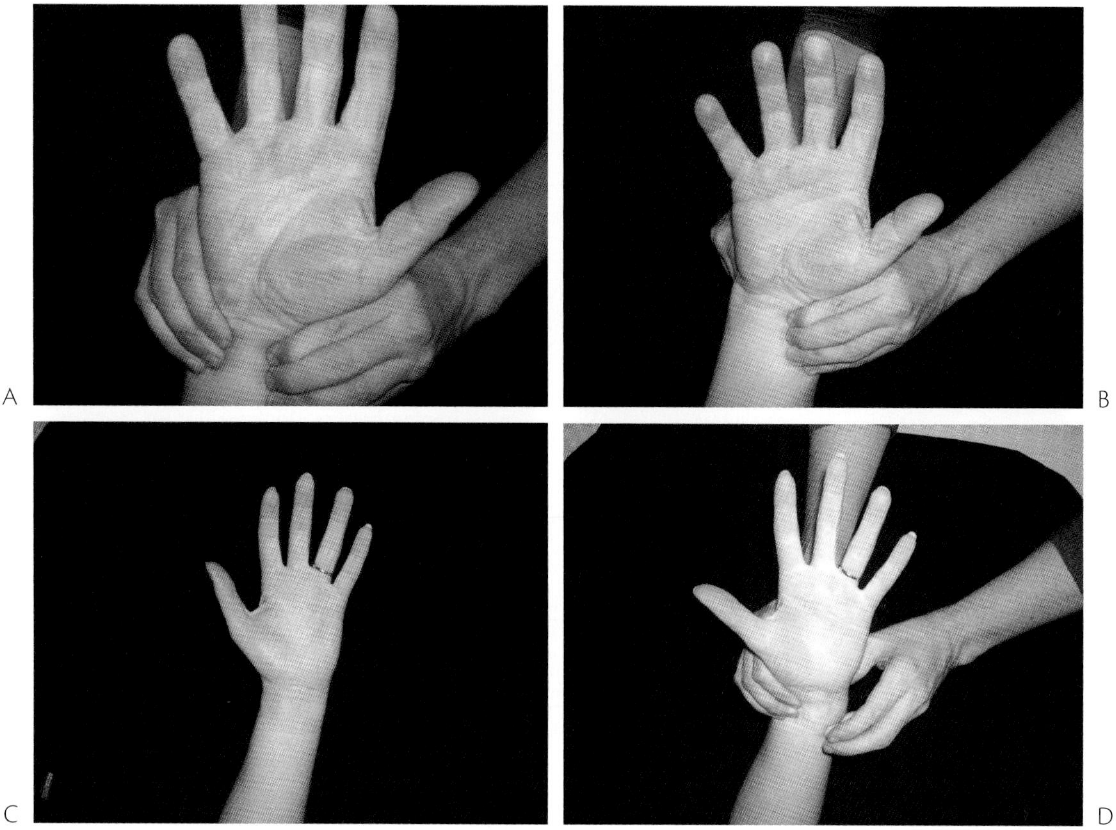

Fig. 4.7 A, B) Non-ischaemic Allen's test. C, D) Ischaemic Allen's test.

Table 4.2 Femoral access vascular complications

	Diagnostic cases (n = 6024)	PCI cases (n = 6913)
	Manual compression (n = 1990)	Manual compression (n = 951)
Groin bleeding	0.3%	1.0%
Haematoma	0.4%	2.5%
Pseudoaneurysm	0.5%	1.0%
Arteriovenous fistula	0%	0.2%
Retroperitoneal haemorrhage	0.1%	0.2%
Limb ischaemia	0.1%	0.1%
Surgical repair	0.3%	0.7%
Any vascular complication	1.1%	4.9%

Other non vascular complications <1%: thickening of perivascular tissues, neuropathy, infection, venous thrombosis, pericatheter thrombus.

Data from Arora N, Matheny ME, Sepke C, *et al.* A propensity analysis of the risk of vascular complications after cardiac catheterization procedures with the use of vascular closure devices. *Am Heart J* 2007; **153**:606–11.

an in-hospital mortality rate of 10%[18]. Arterial puncture above the most inferior border of the inferior epigastric artery has been implicated in all cases of RPH (groups 3 and 4)[2]. Other variables that significantly increase the risk of RPH include the use of GIIb/IIIa receptor antagonists, female gender, peripheral vascular disease, renal impairment, and myocardial infarction, and RPH is inversely related to patient weight[18].

History and clinical examination play a very important role in diagnosis of RPH, although the initial symptoms are often very subtle. In a series of 26 patients[19] who developed an RPH, 46% presented with pain in the groin or hip area with radiation to the lower back and anterior thigh—characteristics of a femoral neuropathy; 42% with abdominal pain; and 23% with back pain. An RPH in close proximity to the iliopsoas muscle will often present with severe muscle spasm resulting in severe pain on any attempt to extend the hip. With an expanding haematoma, femoral nerve compression typically occurs along the iliopsoas gutter with a characteristic pain in the anteromedial thigh. Over 90% of patients with RPH develop hypotension.

Ultrasound may often detect a haematoma but is limited by body habitus, patient discomfort, underlying bowel gas, and operator skill. CT imaging is highly sensitive and readily available and should be requested as an emergency. The definitive treatment of an RPH remains uncertain. All patients should be treated in a high dependency unit or intensive care unit setting with fluid resuscitation, blood products, and normalization of any coagulopathy. Their saturations and urine output should be monitored. If the patient remains haemodynamically stable, conservative therapy will suffice in the majority. The decision of when to intervene with evidence of persistent haemorrhage remains controversial and a vascular surgical consultant should be involved at an early stage. The retroperitoneal haematoma will often have a tamponade effect on the site of persistent haemorrhage. Surgery could potentially reduce the effect of the tamponade with catastrophic consequences. With this in mind, there is a trend towards such techniques as stent-grafts or intra-arterial embolization performed by interventional radiologists to halt the persistent haemorrhage. There is little data available due to the small number performed and this treatment is not universally available. Open surgery should be considered if the patient remains haemodynamically unstable with the above measures being unsuccessful. The transradial approach avoids this potentially catastrophic complication.

Pseudoaneurysm of the femoral artery

Femoral artery pseudoaneurysms (FAPs) are usually seen in arterial punctures that are too low, i.e. at the bifurcation or below (Group 1). The arterial site fails to seal and a haematoma is formed in the surrounding tissues. Marked tenderness, a new bruit, and a pulsatile haematoma are often seen.

Ultrasonography with pulsed and colour Doppler imaging has become the most prevalent investigation for diagnosis (Fig. 4.8).Criteria used to diagnose an FAP include a characteristic 'to and fro' Doppler waveform in the pseudoaneurysm neck, colour flow seen in a lesion separate from the artery, or a tract leading away from the artery consistent with a pseudoaneurysm neck[20].

Several treatment options are available including ultrasound-guided compression, thrombin injection, and surgical repair.

Ultrasound-guided compression

This involves applying manual compression on the pseudoaneurysm neck with the transducer until flow

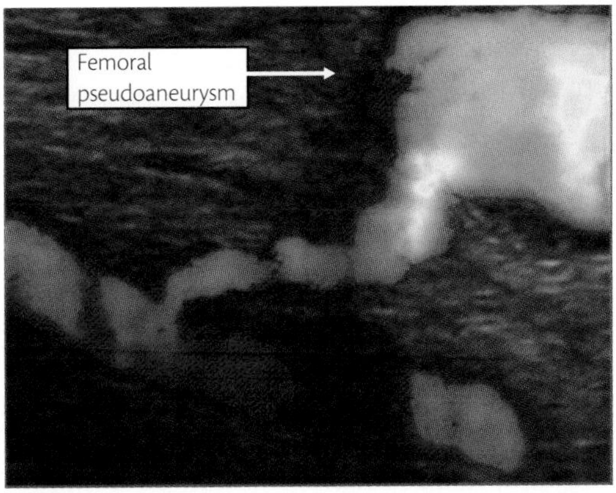

Fig. 4.8 US and colour flow mapping of a femoral pseudoaneurysm.

within the neck is obliterated, and, if possible, the false lumen as well, while still allowing flow down the femoral artery. After approximately 15min both flow and peripheral pulses are reassessed and the procedure repeated a number of times (up to 1h in total length) until successful. It has been shown to be a safe and feasible method with success rates between 74–86%[20,21].The procedure, however, is often very painful, with a reoccurrence rate of approximately 25% and an overall complication rate of 3.6%[20]. These include rupture (1%), FAP enlargement, deep vein thrombosis, and vasovagal syncope.

Thrombin injection

Ultrasound-guided thrombin injection is currently the gold standard treatment. Thrombin converts fibrinogen to fibrin which is then cross-linked by factor XIIIa leading to thrombus formation. The procedure involves injecting thrombin (usually 50–1000IU) under direct ultrasound guidance through the superficial aspect of the pseudoaneurysm until blood flow ceases on colour Doppler ultrasound. The procedure is usually successful on the first attempt, takes seconds to perform, with successful thrombosis formation seen in 86–100% of cases[22–24], with a reoccurrence rate of between 0–9%. Occasionally thrombin may escape into the peripheral circulation with formation of an intra-arterial thrombosis (seen in less than 2% of cases[23]) and is usually managed conservatively. This procedure has several advantages over ultrasound-guided compression—namely a higher success rate, shorter procedural time, and is better tolerated by patients.

Surgery

A profound haemodynamic compromise, femoral neuropathy, or failure of all other measures, are indications for vascular surgery.

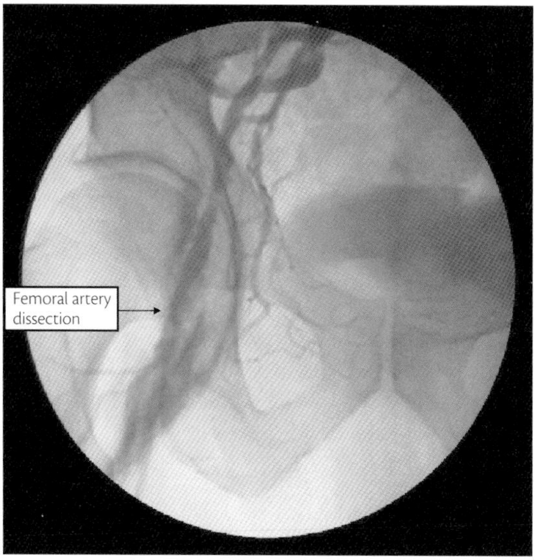

Fig. 4.9 Sheath induced femoral artery dissection.

Femoral artery occlusion/dissection

Femoral artery dissection (Fig. 4.9) is often asymptomatic with a normal ankle–brachial index (ABI). Atherosclerosis, advanced age, and multiple arterial punctures are all risk factors for inducing a dissection. The dissection flap will often seal spontaneously with conservative management. In the event of arterial occlusion, clinical examination will reveal a cold and pulseless limb while the patient will complain of parathesia, pain or decreased movements. Doppler ultrasound and calculating the ABI (<0.5) will confirm the diagnosis. Antegrade femoral angiography via the unaffected contralateral site should be performed with a view to endovascular intervention or surgical repair.

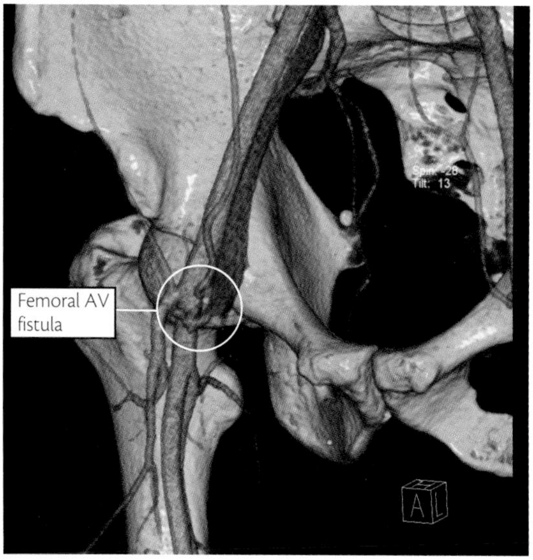

Fig. 4.10 CT imaging of a femoral AV fistula.

Arterio-venous fistula

A new femoral bruit, haematoma, or groin pain the day after coronary angiography or PCI is a typical presentation of an arterio-venous fistula (Fig. 4.10). A small defect will often close spontaneously. Ultrasound-guided compression, endovascular repair (with covered stents and balloon tamponade), and surgical repair are treatment options for larger defects.

Radial arterial access complications

Spasm—including in the brachial and axillary arteries

The reported incidence is approximately 10%. Persistent spasm (Fig. 4.11) may lead to procedural failure due to patient discomfort and an inability to perform catheter manipulation. There are sometimes significant clinical complications with spasm, including risk of vascular sheath or catheter-induced arterial dissection, perforation, and, rarely, avulsion atherectomy.

Prevention, treatment, and management

- If the patient is likely to have a small radial artery (female, <148cm in stature) and/or there is likely to be an equipment/arterial diameter mismatch, then consider performing the procedure through an alternative access site.

Table 4.3 Radial access site complications (in both angiography and PCI)[12,25,33,37]

Radial occlusion	up to 25%
Blood transfusion	<1%
Pseudoaneurysm	<0.2%
AV fistula	<0.2%
Major haematoma	<0.1%
Hand ischaemia	<0.1%
Infection	<0.1%
Neuropathy	<0.1%
Compartment syndrome	<0.01%
Surgery	<0.01%

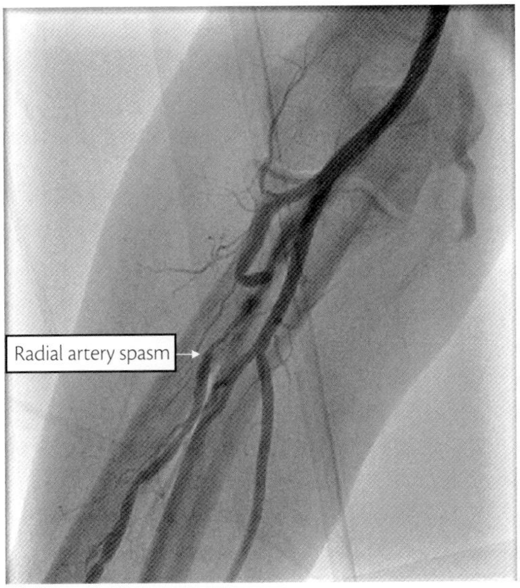

Fig. 4.11 Wire-induced radial artery spasm.

- Explaining the procedure and the anticipated discomfort, along with the use of oral or intravenous anxiolytics (for anxious patients), will minimize the development of spasm.
- A single 'clean' puncture will minimize the risk of spasm formation. If the artery is advertently touched on first attempt, spasm formation may persist for up to 30min, even after withdrawal of all equipment.
- Administration of an intra-arterial 'cocktail'—molsidomine (a nitrate derivative) and verapamil—immediately after sheath insertion is the most commonly used therapy (Fig. 4.12). Some operators omit verapamil if the patient is taking regular oral beta-blockade therapy due to the additional negative inotropic effect, although the synergistic effect is very minimal at most. Studies measuring the maximal pull back force (MPF) as a measure of arterial spasm, and recording patient discomfort on sheath removal, have shown significant benefits for an intra-arterial cocktail when compared to placebo[25]. Other agents such as phentolamine have been suggested but shown no additional benefit. Prophylactic intra-arterial glyceryl trinitrate has also been shown to increase the radial diameter by up to 53%[26].
- Use of a hydrophilic coated sheath has also shown to reduce the incidence of spasm[25].
- A long hydrophilic wire will be able to navigate a tortuous arterial system with easier guide wire exchanges than a short hydrophobic wire. Both these factors will result in a less spasmogenic procedure.
- Very rarely, sheath removal at the end of the procedure may not be possible, despite the use of high-dose intravenous anxiolytics and relaxants. Induction of general anaesthesia (needed very rarely) with profound smooth muscle relaxation will have the required effect.

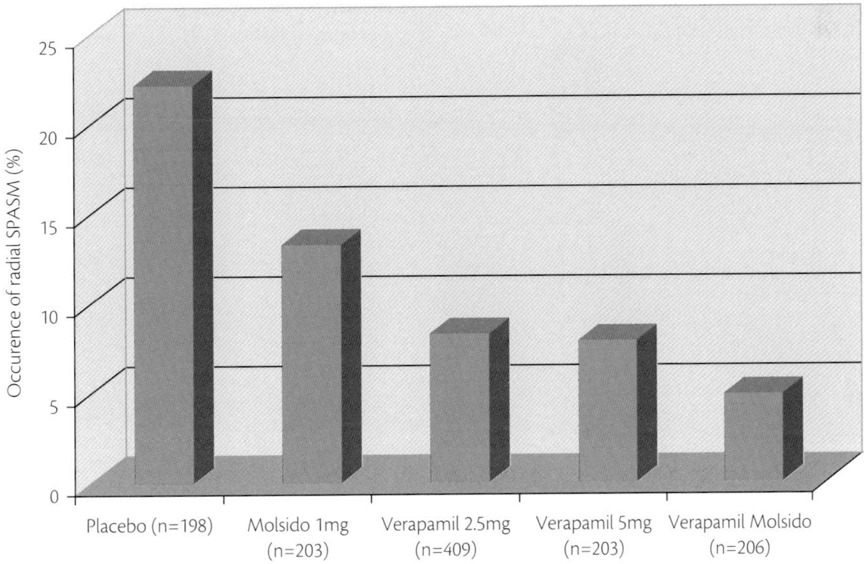

Fig. 4.12 SPASM study (1219 consecutive patients randomized in four groups).

Radial artery dissection and perforation

The incidence of radial artery dissection/perforation following transradial coronary angiography or PCI has been estimated to be around 1%[26]. Arterial tortuosity and looping have been implicated in the aetiology of this rare, but potentially hazardous, complication related to wire and/or sheath trauma. The first symptom of a dissection or perforation is often patient discomfort in the lower forearm. Whenever a patient experiences pain on guide wire or catheter advancement it is wise to stop the procedure temporarily and perform another radial arteriogram via the radial sheath side port. Extravasation of contrast into the area surrounding the artery confirms the diagnosis (Fig. 4.13).

There is no clear consensus on what constitutes optimal management.

An intra-arterial cocktail should be given initially as radial spasm will often coincide. Many operators will abandon the procedure at this point and apply compression while elevating the affected limb. A painful haematoma may subsequently develop; however, any neurovascular deficit (e.g. compartment syndrome) is very rarely seen and surgical management is seldom needed.

However, guide wire manipulation through the dissected radial artery, in to the brachial artery, is sometimes possible. Advancement of a long (20–23cm) sheath over the guide wire, with the tip in the brachial artery, will allow unhindered guide catheter advancement and has been shown to seal the extravasation[27]. One possible theory noted by the authors is that the radial artery may 'shrink' onto the sheath thus sealing the perforation within a matter of minutes.

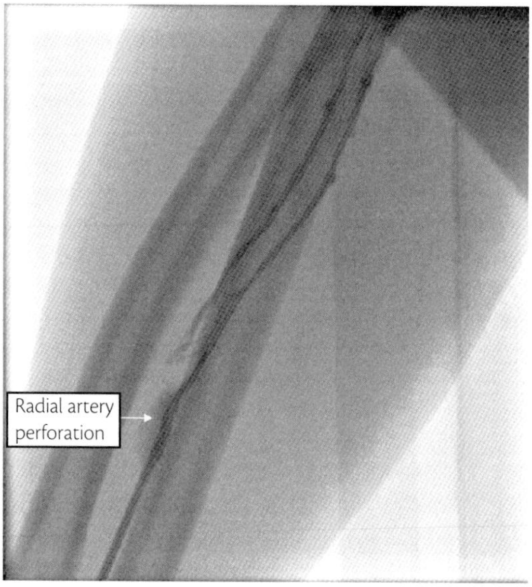

Fig. 4.13 Wire-induced arterial perforation.

Radial artery occlusion

This complication is estimated to occur in up to 25% of cases following radial arterial access although clinical symptoms are seldom seen as a consequence of this[28]. Large sheaths and repeated cannulations are predisposing factors. The use of intra-arterial heparin[29] and hydrophilic-coated sheaths (versus non-hydrophilic) have been shown to reduce the incidence (Fig. 4.14). However it should be noted that the use of hydrophilic-coated sheaths (versus non-hydrophilic) have been associated with a significant excess of patient-reported adverse reactions (14.6% versus 9.6%, p = 0.015)

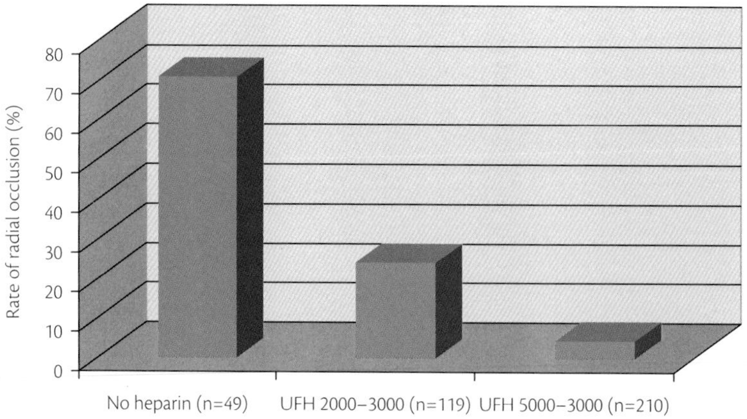

Fig. 4.14 Prevention of radial occlusion anticoagulation. Data from Spaulding C, Lefèvre T, Funck F, *et al.* Left radial approach for coronary radial approach for coronary angiography: results of a prospective study. *Cathet Cardiovasc Diagn* 1996; **39**(4):365–70.

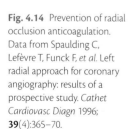

including adverse local reactions, pain, swelling, and non-specific sensory abnormalities[30].

The pathophysiology of arterial occlusion is multifactorial in origin. Following arterial injury, an initiating thrombus formation cascade will lead to chronic occlusion if early arterial recanalization does not occur. Indeed, approximately half of all arterial occlusions will have recanalized at 1 month post procedure[31]. Maintaining radial arterial flow downstream to the site of mechanical pressure following sheath removal has been shown to reduce the incidence of radial arterial occlusion by more than 50%[31].

The radial pulse is frequently present after an occlusion has developed. The artery downstream to the occlusion has been shown to have up to 75% of mean arterial pressure via collaterals from the palmar arch, hence a patent radial pulse does not necessarily mean a patent non-occluded radial artery. Barbeau's test[17] has been shown to be a very reliable and simple technique to detect a radial occlusion, and in these cases, either contralateral radial puncture or a transfemoral approach should be utilized.

Does radial vascular access preclude the use of the radial artery as a conduit for a coronary artery bypass graft?

As most patients are right handed, the left radial artery is more frequently used as a surgical conduit than the right. There is little data to establish whether prior radial access precludes its subsequent use as a surgical conduit. A randomized controlled trial is needed to answer this question.

Arterial site closure

Femoral arterial closure

There are several methods for achieving femoral haemostasis. These include closure devices, assisted manual closure devices (e.g. FemoStop), and manual compression.

Closure devices

Deployment of these devices requires considerable expertise with approximately 20 procedures required before competency is achieved. Device deployment is best taught at the bedside by an experienced operator. Contraindications to Angio-Seal deployment include:

- Arteriotomy site at or below the femoral bifurcation (Fig. 4.15). As this may result in (1) the device anchor catching on the bifurcation and/or (2) collagen deposition into the SFA. Both these events may reduce arterial flow leading to symptoms of distal arterial insufficiency.

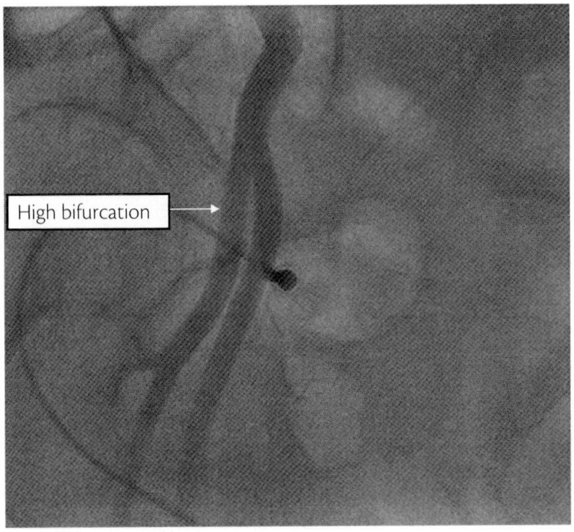

Fig. 4.15 High femoral arterial bifurcation.

- Arteriotomy site proximal to the inguinal ligament (increased risk of retroperitoneal haematoma).
- Greater than 50% stenosis of the common femoral artery due to plaque or calcification.
- A CFA diameter less than 5mm.

Multiple devices are available. The Angio-Seal device has a collagen plug and anchor mechanism which is used to close the arteriotomy site. The collagen will subsequently dissolve over the ensuing months. The Perclose device works by deploying a suture on each side of the arteriotomy site. The suture is non-absorbable. The StarClose Device is an extravascular clip deployed onto the extravascular arterial surface and undergoes primary healing. Other sealing devices include Agiolink EVS, Duett, Elite, Quickseal, Prostar (licensed for 12Fr closure), Vasoseal, and X-site. The sheath size varies from 4–12Fr.

Manual compression and FemoStop

Manual compression is achieved by compressing the femoral artery against the femoral head. Haemostasis, particularly following PCI with anticoagulation and oral antiplatelet therapy, can take up to 20min. Particular attention should be given to the femoral access site following an IABP removal. The device is likely to have been *in situ* for several days, and has a large diameter distal tip. Compression for at least 20min is often needed to secure haemostasis.

The FemoStop device is used to apply a mechanical force to achieve haemostasis. The air cushion is inflated to 30mmHg above the systolic blood pressure and applied continuously for several minutes. The cushion is then gradually deflated and eventually removed. This device is often reported by patients to be uncomfortable and there is a very small incidence of femoral neuropathy or venous thrombosis following prolonged compression. However, it is very useful after complex intervention involving glycoprotein IIb/IIIa receptor antagonists because the device can be left on for several hours at lower pressures in order to minimize haematoma.

Femoral closure devices versus manual compression

An advantage of closure devices is that they have been shown to facilitate earlier patient mobility[32] (2h with closure devices versus 6h with manual compression), reduce hospital stay, reduce staff times with regards to access site compression, and reduce the incidence of occupational health issues (e.g. staff back pain following prolonged manual sheath compression).

Closure device failure has been reported to occur in approximately 5% of cases with complications including incomplete closure with persistent bleeding, thrombus formation, vessel occlusion, embolization of the collagen plug, and late intra-arterial neoplasia proliferation with arterial stenosis.

There is debate concerning whether device closure is superior to manual compression with regards to ensuing vascular complications. A meta-analysis totalling over 35 000 patients, including both diagnostic and interventional procedures with the use of anticoagulation and oral antiplatelet therapy, has shown no superiority to either approach (Fig. 4.16)[33,34].

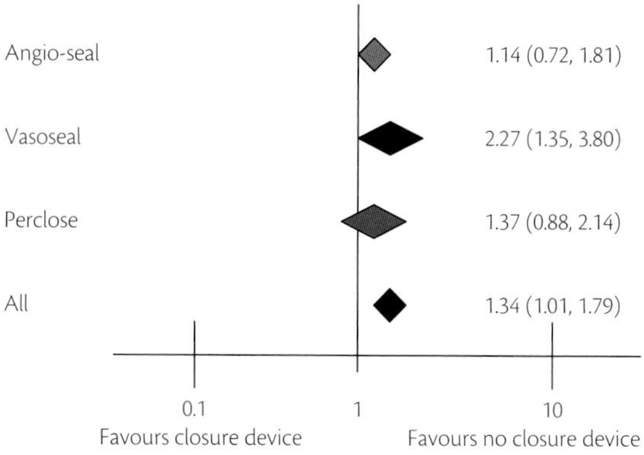

Fig. 4.16 Closure devices versus manual compression. Data from Nikolsky E, Mehran R, Halkin A, *et al.* Vascular complications associated with arteriotomy closure devices in patients undergoing percutaneous coronary procedures: a meta-analysis. *J Am Coll Cardiol* 2004; **44**:1200–9.

Radial arterial closure

The radial sheath is removed at the end of the procedure, typically before the patient leaves the catheterization laboratory. A gentle, constant retractive force is used to remove the sheath while simultaneously applying pressure over the arterial puncture site. Several radial compression systems are available, including the Terumo TR band and the RadiStop devices. These devices have a short learning curve and are very well tolerated.

They are typically left *in situ* for up to 4h, although periods of up to 12h are feasible if high anticoagulation levels or signs of persistent haemorrhage are evident.

The Terumo TR band is very widely used and is available in two band lengths (24cm and 29cm). The arterial sheath is retracted 2–3cm and the green marker on the centre of the compression balloon is placed just proximal to the arteriotomy site. The straps are then secured with the adjustable Velcro fastener. The band must be positioned differently when used on the left or right wrist. The compression balloon is then inflated with the TR band inflator. 15mL of air is injected initially and then the arterial sheath can be removed slowly and with a constant retractive force. Air can then be removed very slowly until a radial arterial flashback is seen and then another 2mL of air inflated to achieve haemostasis while maximizing arterial flow downstream. The device manufacturer recommends that no more than 18mL of air is used to inflate the compression balloon.

Thereafter, 2mL of air is removed with the TR band inflator every 20min until complete haemostasis is achieved.

Radial versus femoral

Procedural time, success rate, and hospital costs—radial versus femoral

A recent large (23 trials) systematic and meta-analysis has shown that radial compared to femoral access was associated with a significantly longer procedural time with a weighted mean difference (WMD) of 3.1min (95% CI 2.4–3.8min; $p < 0.001$). There was a large difference in procedural time in studies performed by low volume radial operators (4.8min; 95% CI 3.7–5.8min) compared to high volume radial operators (1.7min; 95% CI 0.7–2.6min; interaction $p < 0.001$)[35]. The same study also showed that when PCI is performed by experienced radial operators, the success rate of PCI is similar to the femoral approach (OR 1.18; 95% CI 0.77–1.81; p = 0.44), although when performed by non-experienced operators there was a threefold increase in procedure failure rate. These findings are mirrored in multiple studies. In a randomized trial of radial versus femoral diagnostic coronary angiography, hospital stay was significantly shorter (3.6h versus 10.4h; p <0.0001) in the radial group[(36)]. Hospital costs were also lower (£1107 versus £1266; p <0.0001).

Operator radiation exposure—radial versus femoral

A recent large meta-analysis (10 trials) evaluated the fluoroscopy time in both diagnostic and interventional procedures. It was significantly shorter in the transfemoral group (7.8min) when compared to the transradial group (8.9min; WMD 1.05, 95% CI 0.51–1.60; p <0.001)[(37)]. However, measurements of radiation dose, such as fluoroscopy time and dose-area product, have been shown to considerably underestimate the disproportionate rise in radiation exposure. One study (n = 297) measured the operator's radiation exposure via an electronic radiation dosimeter attached to the breast pocket on the outside of the lead apron. For coronary angiography and PCI the measured radiation exposure was up to 100% higher with the transradial approach when compared to the transfemoral[(38)]. Similar, but smaller increases with the transradial approach have been reported in other series. Meticulous use of lead body shielding (including glasses, thyroid collars, and lower limb protection) combined with minimal fluoroscopy screening and maintaining the maximum distance from the radiation source all help to minimize operator exposure. The use of a radiation protection shield is used routinely in some centres. RADPAD (Fig. 4.17) is a sterile, lead free, lightweight, and repositionable radiation protection shield that is placed directly on the patient and can decrease operator exposure to scatter radiation by approximately one-third[(39)]. This very simple device can be used for both femoral and radial procedures.

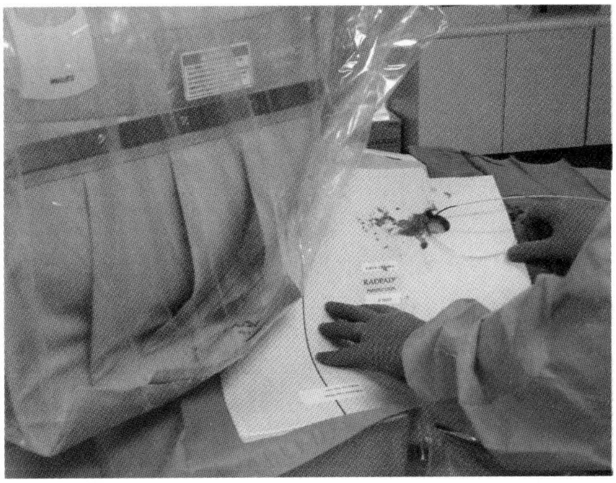

Fig. 4.17 RADPAD scatter radiation protection.

Bleeding and MACE—radial versus femoral

The radial approach virtually eliminates the incidence of haemorrhagic complications when compared to the femoral. It has been hypothesized that there is a correlation between haemorrhage and hard end points such as death, myocardial infarction, and stroke. This correlation between these variables is poorly understood. Several possible mechanisms include (1) interruption of antithrombotic and antiplatelet therapy efficacy; (2) inappropriate activation of the coagulation cascade; and (3) the potential adverse effects of blood product transfusion. Patients who develop an access site haematoma requiring blood product transfusions have an independently increased in-hospital mortality (OR 3.59; 95% CI 1.66–7.77) and 1-year death rate (HR 1.65; 95% CI 1.01–2.70, p = 0.048)[(40)].

A recent large (23 trials) systematic and meta-analysis of randomized trials concluded that radial access reduced the odds of major bleeding by 73% in patients undergoing either diagnostic coronary angiography or PCI when compared to the femoral approach[(35)].The authors noted a trend towards a reduction in the end points of death, myocardial infarction, or stroke (30% decrease), but the study lacked statistical power due to the low incidence of event rates. The MORTAL study[(41)] examined the association between access site (radial or femoral), blood product transfusion, and clinical outcomes in over 32 000 patients undergoing PCI over a period of approximately 6 years. The radial approach was associated with a 50% reduction in blood product transfusion rate (due to the lower incidence of haemorrhagic complications) and a relative reduction in the 30-day and 1-year mortality of 29% and 17% respectively. The OASIS-5 trial (n = 20 078) demonstrated similar results and revealed that following a non-ST segment myocardial infarction, one of every six deaths during the first 30 days occurred in patients who had experienced significant bleeding[(42)].

The PREVAIL study[(43)] examined the peri-procedure outcomes in 1052 patients undergoing either diagnostic coronary angiography or PCI, via the radial (n = 509) or femoral (n = 543) approach, over a 1-month period (Fig. 4.18). In both groups, 40% of patients underwent PCI. The primary outcome was the combined incidence of in-hospital bleeding, stroke, and arterial entry site complications. The secondary outcome was the combined incidence of in-hospital death and myocardial infarction/re-infarction. Multivariate analysis, adjusted for clinical and procedural confounders, demonstrated that the radial approach was significantly and independently associated with a decreased risk of both primary (OR 0.37; 95% CI 0.16–0.84) and secondary endpoints (OR 0.14; 95% CI 0.03–0.62).

Day case PCI and diagnostic angiography—radial versus femoral

Transradial PCI is intuitively attractive as patients are able to mobilize very quickly after their procedure and access complications are very rarely seen. Several retrospective studies have shown a same-day discharge rate of the order of 80–90%[44] with the majority of patients necessitating an overnight stay due to unsuccessful radial access with a switch to the femoral approach.

There is little data concerning femoral day case PCI. The EPOS trial (elective PCI in outpatient study)[45] examined a large cohort of patients for elective femoral PCI. Exclusion criteria included the use of catheters larger than 6Fr, GIIb/IIIa receptor antagonists, and long-term anticoagulation. A decision for same-day discharge was made only after an uncomplicated clinical course of at least 4h. Approximately 80% of patients were deemed suitable for discharge at 4h post procedure with no increased rate of femoral access site complications.

The role of femoral vascular closure devices when compared to manual compression remains uncertain[46,47]; however, the use of such devices has been shown to allow earlier mobilization[35] when compared to manual compression.

Primary PCI—radial or femoral approach

In the setting of ongoing myocardial necrosis, arterial vascular access has to be achieved quickly and safely to facilitate emergency PCI. Most centres in the UK performing primary PCI utilize the femoral approach as opposed to the radial—reasons commonly cited include easier and quicker access, a less tortuous arterial system, and better guide catheter support. Higher dose intravenous heparin and glycoprotein IIb/IIIa receptor antagonists are often used during primary PCI, however. The radial site is far superior in this setting with regards to the incidence of vascular complications (Fig. 4.19). Two large multicentre studies[48,49] demonstrated a non-inferior cannulation and reperfusion time with radial primary PCI when compared to the femoral approach, when performed by experienced radial operators. Conversion to the femoral approach was seldom needed (<2%).

Similarly, rescue PCI is often performed in high-risk, unstable, haemodynamically compromised patients. One small series (n = 105)[50] demonstrated a comparable technical success rate and procedural duration for transradial rescue PCI when compared to a transfemoral approach[51].

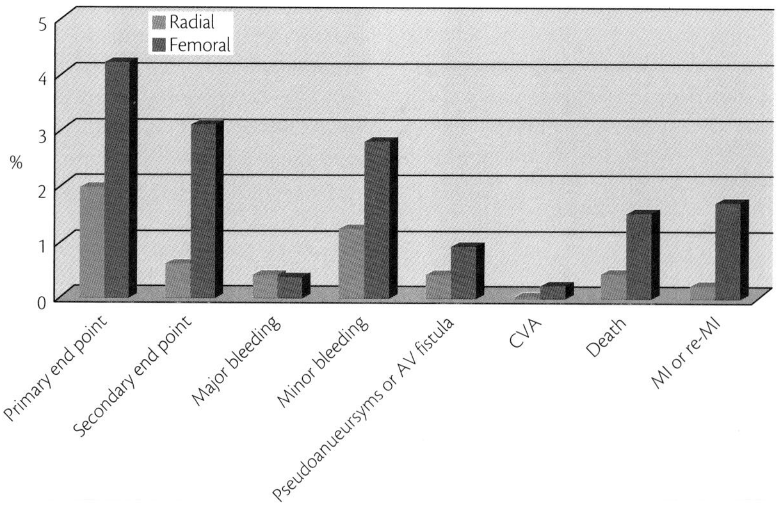

Fig. 4.18 Peri-procedural outcomes in both coronary angiography and PCI—radial versus femoral (PREVAIL study)

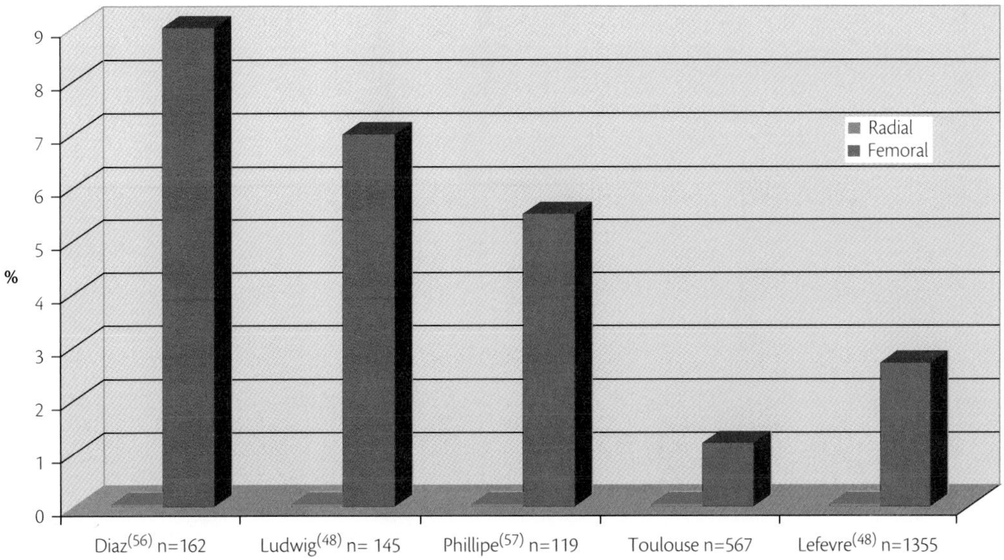

Fig. 4.19 Vascular access complications in primary PCI: radial versus femoral registries.

Radial or femoral approach in the elderly

Advanced age is an independent risk factor for vascular complications, particularly following femoral PCI[52]. In the NHLBI Dynamic Registry over 4500 patients treated with PCI were divided into three age groups and the incidence of femoral vascular access site complications increased with advancing age: 2.6% in patients less than 65 years, 4.8% in patients aged 65–79 years, and 8.8% in patients 80 years or over[53]. The radial approach has been shown to have significantly less vascular complications (1.6% versus 6.5%) without any decrease in the success rate of PCI and only a slight increase in procedure duration[54].

Radial or femoral in the obese

The radial approach has been shown to decrease the rate of vascular complications (0.7% versus 4.0% in patients with femoral access, P = 0.040)[6].

Patient preference—radial versus femoral

In patient surveys the radial approach is typically deemed the preferred site of arterial access in both diagnostic and interventional procedures (Fig. 4.20). The radial puncture site is often claimed to be less painful post procedure[44] with a quicker healing time, and periods of prolonged recumbence are not required.

Alternative arterial access sites

The ulnar artery is used infrequently for vascular access. It is a more mobile artery than the radial. The PCVI-CUBA[55] study, however, has shown that when performed by very experienced operators, the ulnar approach shares similar high success rates and low vascular complications compared to the radial approach. The brachial approach (either by arteriotomy or by direct puncture) is seldom used due to a much higher incidence of neurological and vascular complications (up to 20%). However, in a patient with bilateral absent radial pulses and extensive peripheral vascular disease, this approach may still need to be considered, accepting the increased associated risks.

Future trends

The latest training curricula for the UK and Europe mandate that trainees in interventional cardiology are proficient in both femoral and radial access. Despite a steep learning curve and the perceived technical difficulties, the evidence favouring the transradial approach as the default site for arterial access is overwhelming. The radial approach will likely become the dominant site for coronary intervention. A transfemoral approach should only be considered when the transradial approach

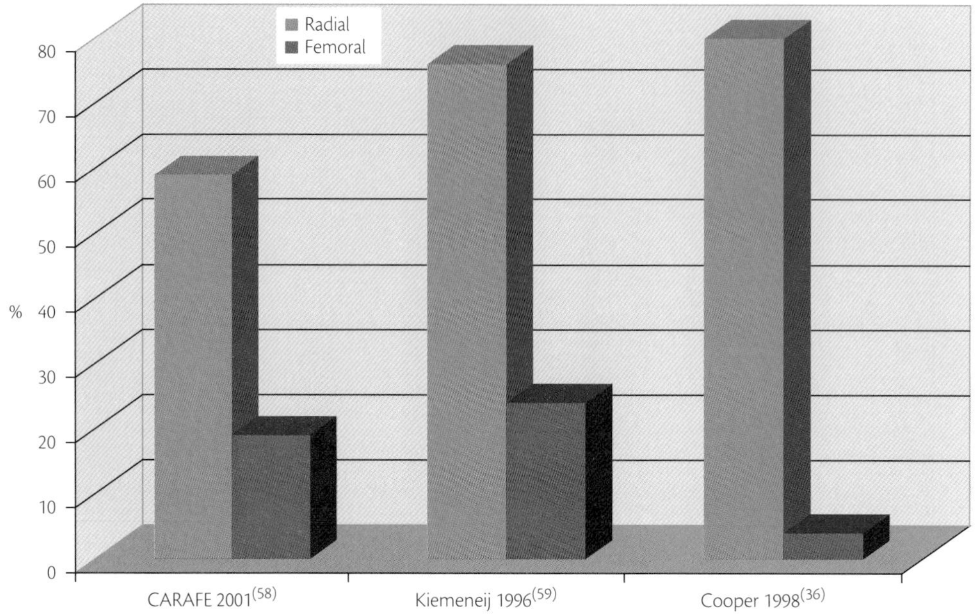

Fig. 4.20 Patient preference: radial versus femoral approach.

has failed or a guide catheter of 7Fr diameter or larger is needed (e.g. IABP), particularly in women of small stature (<148cm) with a small radial arterial diameter.

If transradial catheters larger than 6Fr diameter are needed, ultrasonography should be used to calculate the radial artery diameter. Sheathless radial guide catheters may also be utilized in such cases.

If the femoral approach is utilized, ultrasound-guided femoral puncture (with a 21G 0.81mm micropuncture needle versus 18G 1.27mm conventional needle) and femoral angiography post sheath insertion will ensure 'safe zone' arterial puncture. If an arterial sheath size greater than 8Fr is needed (e.g. for transcutaneous aortic valve implantation or endovascular aortic stenting) and the femoral approach is not deemed suitable, then surgical arteriotomy of the axillary artery is an alternative approach.

Acknowledgements

Dr Roger Bury, Consultant Radiologist; Julie Kelsall and Deborah Forsyth, Senior Radiographers; Lancashire Cardiac Centre, Blackpool, Lancashire, England.

References

1. BCIS data 2007 (http://www.bcis.org:.uk).
2. Sherev DA, Shaw RE, Brent BN. Angiographic predictors of femoral access site complications: Implication for planned percutaneous coronary intervention. *Catheter Cardiovasc Interven* 2005; **65**:196–202.
3. Louvard Y, Krol M, Pezzano M, *et al.* Feasibility of routine transradial coronary angiography: A single operator's experience. *J Invasive Cardiol* 1999; **11**:543–8.
4. Hildick-Smith DJR, Lowe MD, Walsh JT, *et al.* Coronary angiography from the radial artery: Experience, complications and limitations. *Int J Cardiol* 1998; **64**:231–9.
5. Guerrero M, Harjai K, Stone GW, *et al.* Usefulness of the presence of peripheral vascular disease in predicting mortality in acute myocardial infarction patients treated with primary angioplasty (from the Primary Angioplasty in Myocardial Infarction Database). *Am J Cardiol* 2005; **96**(5):649-54.
6. Cox N, Resnic FS, Popma JJ, *et al.* Comparison of the risk of vascular complications associated with femoral and radial access coronary catheterization procedures in obese versus nonobese patients. *Am J Cardiol* 2004; **94**:1174–7.
7. Gurm HS, Whitlow PL, Kip KE, *et al.* The impact of body mass index on short- and long-term outcomes in patients undergoing coronary revascularization. Insights from the Bypass Angioplasty Revascularization Investigation (BARI). *J Am Coll Cardiol* 2002; **39**:834–40.
8. Gurm HS, Brennan DM, Booth J, *et al.* Impact of body mass index on outcome after percutaneous coronary intervention (the obesity paradox). *Am J Cardiol* 2002; **90**:42–5.
9. Hildick-Smith DJ, Walsh JT, Lowe MD, *et al.* Coronary angiography in the fully anticoagulated patient: The transradial route is successful and safe. *Catheter Cardiovasc Interv* 2003; **58**:8–10.

10. Yoo BS, Yoon J, Ko JY, *et al.* Anatomical consideration of the radial artery for transradial coronary procedures: arterial diameter, branching anomaly and vessel tortuosity. *Int J Cardiol* 2005; **101**:421–7.
11. Lo TS, Nolan J, Fountzopoulos E, *et al.* Radial artery anomaly and its influence on transradial coronary procedural outcome. *Heart* 2009; **95**:410–15.
12. Pillow K, Herrick IA. Pulse oximetry compared with Doppler ultrasound for assessment of collateral blood flow to the hand. *Anaesthesia* 1991; **46**:388–90
13. Greenwood MJ, Della-Siega AJ, Fretz EB, *et al.* Vascular communications of the hand in patients being considered for transradial coronary angiography: is the Allen's test accurate? *J Am Coll Cardiol* 2005; **46**:2013–17.
14. McGregor AD. The Allen test – an investigation of its accuracy fluorescein angiography. *J Hand Surg Br* 1987; **12**:82–5.
15. Stead SW, Stirt JA. Assessment of digital blood flow and palmar collateral circulation. *Int J Clin Monit Comput* 1985; **2**:29.
16. Barbeau GR, Arsenault F, Dugas L, *et al.* Evaluation of ulnopalmar arterial arches with pulse oximetry and plethysmography: comparison with the Allen's test in 1010 patients. *Am Heart J* 2004; **147**(3):489–93.
17. Slogoff S, Keats AS, Arlund C. On the safety of radial artery cannulation. *Anesthesiology* 1983; **59**:42–7
18. Ellis SG, Bhatt D, Kapadia S, *et al.* Correlates and outcomes of retroperitoneal hemorrhage complicating percutaneous coronary intervention. *Catheter Cardiovasc Interv* 2006; **67**(4):541–5.
19. Farouque HM, Tremmel JA, Raissi Shabari F, *et al.* Risk factors for the development of retroperitoneal hematoma after percutaneous coronary intervention in the era of glycoprotein IIb/IIIa inhibitors and vascular closure devices. *J Am Coll Cardiol* 2005; **45**:363–8.
20. Eisenberg L, Paulson EK, Kliewer MA, *et al.* Sonographically guided compression repair of pseudoaneurysms: further experience from a single institution. *AJR Am J Roentgenol* 1999; **173**(6):1567–73.
21. Coley BD, Roberts AC, Fellmeth BD, *et al.* Postangiographic femoral artery pseudoaneurysms: further experience with US-guided compression repair. *Radiology* 1995; **194**:307–11.
22. Owen RJ, Haslam PJ, Elliott ST, *et al.* Percutaneous ablation of peripheral pseudoaneurysms using thrombin: a simple and effective solution. *Cardiovasc Intervent Radiol* 2000; **23**:441–6.
23. Paulson EK, Nelson RC, Mayes CE, *et al.* Sonographically guided thrombin injection of iatrogenic femoral pseudoaneurysms: further experience of a single institution. *AJR Am J Roentgenol* 2001; **177**(2):309–16.
24. Olsen DM, Rodriguez JA, Vranic M, *et al.* A prospective study of ultrasound scan-guided thrombin injection of femoral pseudoaneurysm: a trend toward minimal medication. *J Vasc Surg* 2002; **36**:779–82
25. Kiemeneij F, Vajifdar BU, Eccleshall SC, *et al.* Evaluation of a spasmolytic cocktail to prevent radial artery spasm during coronary procedures. *Catheter Cardiovasc Interv* 2003; **58**:281–4.
26. Jeserich M, Just H. Effect of nitrates on arterial blood vessels exemplified by the radial artery. *Z Kardiol* 1998; **87**(2):77–83.
27. Calviño-Santos RA, Vázquez-Rodríguez JM, Salgado-Fernández J, *et al.* Management of iatrogenic radial artery perforation. *Catheter Cardiovasc Interv* 2004; **61**(1):74–8.
28. Nagai S, Abe S, Sato T, *et al.* Ultrasonic assessment of vascular complications in coronary angiography and angioplasty after transradial approach. *Am J Cardiol* 1999; **83**:180–6.
29. Lefevre T, Thebault B, Spaulding C, *et al.* Radial artery patency after percutaneous left radial artery approach for coronary angiography. The role of heparin. *Eur Heart J* 1995; **16**:293.
30. Tharmaratnam D, Webber S, Owens P. Adverse local reactions to the use of hydrophilic sheaths for radial artery cannulation. *Int J Cardiol* 2008; Dec 19 (Epub ahead of print).
31. Pancholy S, Coppola J, Patel T, *et al.* Prevention of radial artery occlusion-patent hemostasis evaluation trial (PROPHET study): a randomized comparison of traditional versus patency documented hemostasis after transradial catheterization. *Catheter Cardiovasc Interv* 2008; **72**(3):335–40.
32. Deuling JH, Vermeulen RP, Anthonio RA, *et al.* Closure of the femoral artery after cardiac catheterization: a comparison of AngioSeal, StarClose, and manual compression. *Catheter Cardiovasc Interv* 2008; **71**(4): 518–23.
33. Dangas G, Mehran R, Kokolis S, *et al.* Vascular complications after percutaneous coronary interventions following percutaneous coronary interventions following haemostasis with manual compression versus arteriotomy closure devices. *J Am Coll Cardiol* 2001; **38**:638–41
34. Nikolsky E, Mehran R, Halkin A, *et al.* Vascular complications associated with arteriotomy closure devices in patients undergoing percutaneous coronary procedures: a meta-analysis. *J Am Coll Cardiol* 2004; **44**:1200–9.
35. Jolly SS, Amlani S, Hamon M, *et al.* Radial versus femoral access for coronary angiography or intervention and the impact on major bleeding and ischemic events: A systematic review and meta-analysis of randomized trials. *Am Heart J* 2009; **157**(1):132–40.
36. Cooper CJ, El-Shiekh RA, Cohen DJ, *et al.* Effect of transradial access on quality of life and cost of cardiac catheterisation: a randomised comparison. *Am Heart J* 1999; **138**:430–6.
37. Agostoni P, Biondi-Zoccai GG, de Benedictis ML, *et al.* Radial versus femoral approach for percutaneous coronary diagnostic and interventional procedures: Systematic overview and meta-analysis of randomized trials. *J Am Coll Cardiol* 2004; **44**(2):349–56.
38. Lange HW, von Boetticher H. Randomised comparison of operator radiation exposure during coronary angiography

and intervention by radial or femoral approach. *Catheter Cardiovasc Interv* 2006; **67**(1):12–16.
39. Germano JJ, Day G, Gregorious D, *et al.* A novel radiation protection drape reduces radiation exposure during fluoroscopy guided electrophysiology procedures. *J Invasive Cardiol* 2005; **17**(9):469–72.
40. Yatskar L, Selzer F, Feit F, *et al.* Access site haematoma requiring blood transfusion predicts mortality in patients undergoing percutaneous coronary intervention: data from the National Heart, Lung, and Blood Institute Dynamic Registry. *Catheter Cardiovasc Interv* 2007; **69**(7):961–6.
41. Chase AJ, Fretz EB, Warburton WP, *et al.* Association of arterial access site at angioplasty with transfusion and mortality. The M.O.R.T.A.L study (Mortality benefit Of Reduced Transfusion after percutaneous coronary intervention via the Arm or Leg). *Heart* 2008; **94**:1019–25.
42. Budaj A, Eikelboom JW, Mehta SR, *et al.* on behalf of Oasis-5 investigators. Improving clinical outcomes by reducing bleeding in patients with non-ST elevation ACS. *Eur Heart J* 2009; **30**(6):655–61.
43. Pristipino C, Trani C, Nazzaro MS, *et al.* Major improvement of percutaneous cardiovascular procedure outcomes with radial artery catheterization: results from the PREVAIL study. *Heart* 2009; **95**:476–82.
44. Wiper A, Kumar S, MacDonald J, *et al.* Day case transradial coronary angioplasty – a four-year single-center experience. *Catheter Cardiovasc Interv* 2006; **68**:549–53.
45. Heyde GS, Koch KT, de Winter RJ, *et al.* Randomized trial comparing same-day discharge with overnight hospital stay after percutaneous coronary intervention. Results of the Elective PCI in Outpatient Study (EPOS). *Circulation* 2007; **115**:2299–306.
46. Koreny M, Riedmuller E, Nikfardjam M, *et al.* Arterial puncture closing devices compared with standard manual compression after cardiac catheterization: systematic review and meta-analysis. *JAMA* 2004; **291**:350–7.
47. Baim DS, Knopf WD, Hinohara T, *et al.* Suture-mediated closure of the femoral access site after cardiac catheterization: results of the Suture to Ambulate and Discharge (STAND I and STAND II) trials. *Am J Cardiol* 2000; **85**(7):864–9.
48. Louvard Y, Ludwig J, Lefèvre T, *et al.* Transradial approach for coronary angioplasty in the setting of acute myocardial infarction: a dual-center registry. *Catheter Cardiovasc Interv* 2002; **55**:206–11.
49. Valsecchi O, Musumeci G, Vassileva A, *et al.* Safety, feasibility and efficacy of transradial primary angioplasty in patients with acute myocardial infarction. *Ital Heart J* 2003; **4**:329–34.
50. Lo TS, Hall IR, Jaumdally R, *et al.* Transradial rescue angioplasty for failed thrombolysis in acute myocardial infarction: reperfusion with reduced vascular risk. *Heart* 2006; **92**:1153–4
51. Sutton AG, Campbell PG, Graham R, *et al.* A randomized trial of rescue angioplasty versus a conservative approach for failed fibrinolysis in ST-segment elevation myocardial infarction: the Middlesbrough early revascularization to limit infarction (MERLIN) trial. *J Am Coll Cardiol* 2004; **44**:287–96
52. Batchelor WB, Anstrom KJ, Muhlbaier LH, *et al.* Contemporary outcome trends in the elderly undergoing percutaneous coronary interventions: results in 7,472 octogenerians. National cardiovascular Network Collaboration. *J Am Coll Cardiol* 2000; **36**:723–30
53. Cohen HA, Williams DO, Holmes DR Jr, *et al.* Impact of age on procedural and 1 year outcome in percutaneous transluminal coronary angioplasty: a report from the NHLBI Dynamic Registry. *Am Heart J* 2003; **146**(3): 513–19.
54. Louvard Y, Benamer H, Garot P, *et al.* Comparison of transradial and transfemoral approaches for coronary angiography and angioplasty in octogenarians (the OCTOPLUS Study). *Am J Cardiol* 2004; **94**:1177–80.
55. Aptecar E, Pernes JM, Chabane-Chaouch M, *et al.* Transulnar versus transradial artery approach for coronary angioplasty: the PCVI-CUBA study. *Catheter Cardiovasc Interv* 2006; **67**(5):711–20.
56. Diaz de la Llera LS, Fournier Andray JA, Gómez Moreno S, et al. Transradial approach for percutaneous coronary stenting in the treatment of acute myocardial infarction. *Rev Esp Cardiol* 2004; **57**(8):732–6.
57. Philippe F, Larrazet F, Meziane T, *et* al. Comparison of transradial vs. transfemoral approach in the treatment of acute myocardial infarction with primary angioplasty and abciximab. *Catheter Cardiovasc Interv* 2004; **61**(1):67–73.
58. Louvard Y, Lefèvre T, Allain A, *et* al. Coronary angiography through the radial or the femoral approach: The CARAFE study. *Catheter Cardiovasc Interv* 2001; **52**(2):181–7.
59. Kiemeneij F. Transradial artery coronary angioplasty and stenting: history and single center experience. *J Invasive Cardiol* 1996; **8**(Suppl D):3D–8D.

CHAPTER 5

Radiation and percutaneous coronary intervention

Gurbir Bhatia and James Nolan

Introduction

Fluoroscopic procedures comprise a major component of the range of diagnostic and therapeutic measures available to the cardiologist. In contemporary practice, coronary angiography and percutaneous coronary intervention (PCI) are performed increasingly frequently. With greater availability of adjunctive techniques, the complexity of PCI procedures has also increased. Against this background, it should be appreciated that the amount of radiation that patients, physicians, and other staff are exposed to will increase accordingly.

Cardiologists should be aware that increasing procedural radiation carries significant risks to both patients and catheter laboratory staff. This is vital in providing informed consent to patients prior to performing PCI procedures. Although there are legal obligations for employers to limit radiation exposure, it may be argued that cardiologists do not receive adequate training in radiation awareness.

This chapter aims to provide an overview of basic radiation physics and biology, and discusses factors influencing procedural radiation doses. Particular attention is given to the potential hazards associated with increasing radiation exposure, and to methods enabling the physician to reduce delivered doses.

X-ray physics

X-rays are a form of ionizing radiation found at the short-wavelength end of the electromagnetic spectrum, in between gamma rays (which have a shorter wavelength) and ultra-violet rays. Typical wavelengths of X-rays are in the range 0.01–10nm, with frequencies between 30×10^{15}–30×10^{18}Hz. In the particle model of electromagnetic radiation, waves are composed of distinct packets (quanta) of energy called photons. When generated, X-rays consist of a spectrum of photon energies, such that the energy range for diagnostic X-rays is typically 5–150keV.

X-ray generation

X-rays are generated in a vacuum tube when electrons are accelerated from a cathode to collide with an anode, in response to a voltage applied across the intervening gap. The anode is typically composed of tungsten, often as an alloy with rhenium. Electrons are emitted from the heated cathode filament. The number of emitted electrons, and consequently the number of X-ray photons produced, is determined by the current at the cathode. The maximal energy of the X-ray photons is a function of the voltage applied across the gap.

As accelerated electrons collide with the anode, energy is liberated, predominantly as heat. A much smaller proportion of energy (around 1%) is released as X-rays, produced by two processes, '*X-ray fluorescence*' and '*Bremsstrahlung*'. When an accelerated electron knocks out an orbiting electron from the inner shell of a metal atom (e.g. in the anode of the X-ray tube), electrons from the higher energy outer shell slot into this gap; X-ray fluorescence refers to the emission of photons when a high-energy electron falls into a vacated, lower energy shell. This process yields a discrete spectrum of X-rays, characterized by the metallic composition of the anode. Bremsstrahlung refers to the process whereby radiation is emitted when an electron is decelerated or scattered by the electrical charge of an atomic nucleus.

X-ray absorption

The penetrative ability of X-rays through a given tissue is determined by their photon energies (determined by the tube voltage), and properties of the tissue, including its atomic make-up, density, and thickness. Important processes that contribute to imaging include *the photoelectric process* and *Compton scattering* (1).

The photoelectric process generally refers to low-energy photons which are completely absorbed by a high atomic number substance (e.g. within bone or X-ray contrast agents), liberating an electron in the process, and ionizing the absorber.

In diagnostic imaging, Compton scattering accounts for most of the interaction between X-rays and tissue. Here, high-energy photons are attenuated by matter to yield a lower energy photon and a recoiling electron. This process provides much of the scattered radiation in a catheter laboratory.

Radiation doses

The radiation dose delivered by a procedure is an important factor in determining its risk of adverse effects. In order to regulate the dose of radiation to patients, the operator, and catheter laboratory staff, it is important to understand the various terms used in its quantification. Definitions of measurements employed are provided in Table 5.1. Regulatory requirements relating to procedural X-ray dose delivery make use of such terms, and will be discussed further in this chapter.

When dealing with emission of X-rays to living tissue, quantification relates better to delivery of *energy* rather than ionizing radiation. Traditional units used for absorbed and effective dose, rad and rem, respectively, have been superseded by the SI units, gray (Gy) and sievert (Sv). The absorbed dose, measured in Gy, refers to the amount of ionizing radiation deposited per unit mass.

Among these parameters, the dose–area–product (DAP) and effective dose (ED) are used commonly. The DAP is a function of entrance dose and field size, and is measured by an ionization chamber integrated within the tube unit. It provides a reasonable estimate of the energy delivered to the patient, and is a useful tool with which operators can monitor their procedural doses. The ED is used to provide an estimate of stochastic (see 'Stochastic effects') risk to the patient or laboratory staff. It is the summation of equivalent doses to organs multiplied by specific tissue-weighting factors, which take into account the inherent sensitivity of tissues. The biological factor to convert absorbed X-ray doses (Gy) to equivalent doses (Sv) is 1.

Whilst it is important for the practitioner to be familiar with these terms, it may be more helpful to consider the radiation doses delivered by various radiological procedures in comparison to other, more basic, procedures. For example, doses of complex procedures can be referred to those typically delivered in obtaining a standard chest X-ray. Alternatively, doses can be referred to the amount of background radiation that subjects are exposed to (e.g. as radon gas or cosmic rays): depending on geographical location, background radiation may impart a dose of 3mSv/year. Table 5.2 allows for a comparison between several radiological procedures with one another, and also estimates the equivalent background dose for each.

Thus, it can be appreciated that a patient undergoing a single-stent PCI will typically receive a DAP of 36Gy.cm^2—equivalent to 450 chest X-rays, or approximately 3.5 years of background radiation exposure!

Adverse effects of radiation

Although X-ray radiation provides undoubted medical benefits, its ionizing capability also creates the potential for harm.

Whilst the number of X-ray-related injuries may be small in the context of the number of procedures

Table 5.1 Quantification of radiation delivery

Measurement	Unit	Definition
Absorbed dose	gray (Gy)	The amount of ionizing radiation deposited per unit mass
Air kerma	gray (Gy)	The dose delivered per unit volume of air
Dose–area–product (DAP)	Gy.cm^2	The air kerma integrated across the X-ray beam from the tube—a surrogate for the entire energy delivered to the patient
Effective dose	sievert (Sv)	The attributable whole-body dose equivalent to the risk of an absorbed dose to particular body part
Entrance skin dose	gray (Gy)	The absorbed dose on the skin at a given location on the patient, including back-scattered radiation
Equivalent dose	sievert (Sv)	The radiation dose applied to a tissue allowing for the effect of that radiation on that tissue
Fluoroscopy time	minutes	The total time fluoroscopy is used during a procedure

Table 5.2 Procedure-related patient doses

Procedure	Effective dose (mSv)	DAP (Gy.cm^2)	Background equivalent
Chest X-ray	0.02	0.08	3 days
Barium meal	2.4	9.6	12 months
IV urogram	2.8	11.3	14 months
Coronary angiogram	5.8	23.5	2.4 years
PCI (single stent)	9.0	36.0	3.7 years
PCI (three stents)	24.6	98 (mean)	10.1 years

Dose–area–product (DAP) data are median doses (except for 3-stent PCI) taken from Hart *et al.* (33)

performed, the absolute number is likely to be underestimated. To some extent, this may simply relate to a lack of awareness of the possibility and nature of radiation-related injuries on the part of both patient and clinician. Other factors may include a latent interval between radiation exposure and recognition of any abnormal symptoms and signs, again for both patient and clinician. Occasionally, a patient may be unaware of any injury, such as a mild skin lesion occurring without discomfort in areas which are difficult to see. Of note, as complex coronary interventional procedures become more frequently performed, and X-ray doses increase, injuries are likely to become more common unless measures ensuring safe practice are implemented.

Adverse effects of radiation can be classified as being *deterministic* or *stochastic*, based upon the presence of a dose threshold underlying the injury.

Deterministic effects

Deterministic adverse effects are *predictable* and *dose-dependent* reactions. They have a critical threshold of radiation exposure, below which injuries do not occur. As doses increase, the injuries will become more severe. Examples of deterministic effects include skin erythema and necrosis, and ocular effects such as cataract formation.

Stochastic effects

Stochastic effects do not have an obvious dose threshold or any relationship between severity and dose. Rather, they are *probabilistic*, with likelihood of stimulation proportional to the dose received. Such effects are brought about by damage to cellular DNA; cancer induction is an example of a stochastic effect.

Skin injuries

Skin injuries are the commonest deterministic adverse effect of fluoroscopic procedures, largely due to the skin receiving the largest dose at the beam entry site. Skin injuries in response to X-ray exposure were first reported in the late 19th century, and have been extensively reported and summarized(2,3) in the modern literature.

Skin injuries are variable, and are determined by the doses received, as well as the innate properties of the tissue. As mentioned earlier, there may be a lag in time before any injuries are apparent; this may be influenced by fractionation of the total dose by performing complex interventions staged over a number of weeks(2). This may allow for tissue repair in between multiple procedures, although injury will occur once the threshold is reached. Threshold skin entrance doses for several skin injuries are shown in Table 5.3(2).

Very early effects include erythema, thought to result from increased capillary permeability in response to histamine-like enzymes. Lesions resemble faint sunburn at the site of beam entry, and the reaction typically peaks at 24h. Depending upon the received dose, injuries may

Table 5.3 Threshold skin entrance doses for various skin injuries

Effect	Dose (Gy)	Typical onset
Early transient erythema	2	Hours
Main erythema	6	~ 10 days
Late erythema	15	~6–10 weeks
Temporary epilation	3	~3 weeks
Permanent epilation	7	~3 weeks
Dry desquamation	14	~4 weeks
Moist desquamation	18	~8 weeks
Secondary ulceration	24	>6 weeks
Ischaemic dermal necrosis	18	>10 weeks
Dermal atrophy (1st phase)	10	>14 weeks
Dermal atrophy (2nd phase)	10	>1 year
Induration	10	
Telangiectasia	10	>1 year
Late dermal necrosis	? >12	>1 year
Skin cancer	Unknown	>5 years

Reproduced from Koenig TR, Wolff D, Mettler FA, *et al.* Skin injuries from fluoroscopically guided procedures: part 1, characteristics of radiation injury. *Am J Roentgenol* 2001; **177**(1):3–11. Reprinted with permission of the American Journal of Roentgenology.

progress to a more marked inflammatory erythema (main erythema) in response to damage to the epidermal basal cell layer. This is often associated with symptoms including discomfort and itch. With large doses, a later, somewhat duskier phase of erythema may be induced.

Hair loss (epilation) can occur within 1 month of exposure in response to depleted germinal layers of hair follicles; such loss may be temporary, but regrowth may be relatively sparse, with discolouration. Melanocytes may be damaged, resulting in areas of hyper- or hypopigmentation, depending on the extent of injury.

More drastic injuries include ischaemic dermal necrosis and frank skin ulceration. The latter may be particularly resistant to healing, and skin grafting following coronary interventions has been reported[(2)].

Interestingly, skin appears to be more radiosensitive in certain areas. The anterior aspect of the neck, the antecubital and popliteal regions, and flexor surfaces of the extremities appeared to be most sensitive. Further, Wagner *et al.* [(4)] noted a possible link between skin reactions following radiotherapy and concurrent connective tissue diseases including scleroderma and systemic lupus erythematosus.

Skin injuries and coronary procedures

There have been several reports of skin injuries after diagnostic and therapeutic coronary procedures. Koenig and colleagues[(2,3)] characterized 73 cases of radiation-induced skin injury from fluoroscopic procedures. The majority of these cases (almost two-thirds) involved coronary procedures, reflecting their frequency in current practice. Chronic ulceration was seen to develop in more than half of these cases, with one-quarter requiring skin grafting. Fluoroscopy times (FT) were only reported for 12 cases of coronary intervention, but the average FT was almost 60min. Causes for such lengthy FT included difficult coronary anatomy, and procedural complications requiring further treatment.

Whilst such injuries are not common, the potential for serious harm is undoubtedly present, and can have severe consequences for all concerned parties. For the patient, the pain and trauma of the skin lesion and its treatment may bring about a loss of confidence in the healthcare service. For the cardiologist and healthcare institution, legal consequences may be damaging[(5)]. In certain instances, e.g. where procedures are likely to be prolonged due to complexity, it could be argued that the possibility of radiation-related injury should be discussed with the patient when obtaining informed consent.

Cataract formation

The lens is relatively sensitive to the effects of ionizing radiation, and cataract formation has been well recognized as a complication of radiation exposure. Such exposure is associated with posterior subcapsular cataracts. However, both the doses necessary to effect cataract formation, and the latent periods between exposure and formation, are uncertain. In a prospective study of a large cohort of radiology technicians in the United States[(6)], the risk of cataract extraction was associated with the total number of X-rays performed on participants. Similarly, cataract extraction was associated with a history of radiotherapy to the head and neck. There was a trend for increased risk of cataract formation among workers in the highest category of occupational dose to the lens of the eye (mean dose, 60.1mGy) compared with counterparts in the lowest category (mean dose, 5.1mGy). The association between occupational dose and cataract risk appeared stronger in subjects diagnosed with cataract aged less than 50 years.

Cancer induction

As discussed earlier, X-rays are capable of ionizing molecules they encounter by effecting displacement of electrons. In biological matter, this can lead to the formation of reactive free radicals, which can initiate damage to cellular DNA. If such damage is not resolved by inherent reparative systems, cancer induction may occur.

Much of what is known about radiation-induced cancer is derived from the longitudinal studies of atom bomb survivors. Survivors exposed to relatively low doses (range 5–150mSv, mean 40mSv) had a significantly increased overall risk of developing cancer[(7–9)]. This is a dose comparable to that of a diagnostic coronary angiogram and subsequent simple PCI.

Information can also be derived from epidemiological data studying cancer risk among radiation workers. For example, in a large cohort of subjects comprising the UK National Registry for Radiation Workers[(10)], the incidences of both leukaemia (excluding chronic lymphocytic leukaemia), and all malignant neoplasms (excluding leukaemia) increased significantly with increasing radiation dose.

Based on a cancer risk of 6% per sievert, and a typical dose of around 10mSv, coronary angiography has a lifetime risk of cancer induction of 0.06%[(11)]; risks for PCI range from 0.1–0.24% based on complexity. Risks are influenced by the patient's age, with younger patients ultimately more sensitive.

Radiation risks to operators and staff

Radiological procedures expose operators and laboratory staff to scattered radiation reflected from the patient and the laboratory walls. Broadly, there appears to be a linear association between fluoroscopic doses delivered to patients and those received by operators of a variety of procedures(12). However, the strength of such correlations is influenced by varying practices in radiation protection (e.g. use of lead shields)(13).

The operator's exposed areas receive about 0.05% of the patient dose, with doses received beneath lead aprons around 10% of exposed areas. Table 5.4a provides estimates of operator doses for 500 diagnostic and interventional procedures.

It is important that operators bear in mind that co-workers are exposed to the radiation scattered in the laboratory. For example, second operators may receive 30% of the operator dose, whereas technicians and radiographers, usually stationed further away from the X-ray tube, may typically receive 1%. Thus, as illustrated in Table 5.4b, over a period of 20 years with a mixed interventional caseload of 500 cases/annum, nurses and radiographers may be exposed to 16 and 0.5 years of background radiation, respectively.

Radiation and cancer risk in medical X-ray workers

In a review of epidemiological studies of radiologists and radiographers undertaken in several countries(14), the most common finding was increased mortality due to leukaemia among those employed before 1950, when radiation exposures were high. While findings on several types of solid cancers were less consistent, several studies provided evidence of a radiation effect for breast cancer and skin cancer. Subsequently, a further study(15) has indicated an increased risk of breast cancer risk in female technicians who experienced long-term, daily low-dose radiation exposures resulting in marked cumulative exposures.

Table 5.4a Operator radiation exposure (500 procedures)

	Exposure (mSv)	Background equivalent (years)
Coronary angiogram	3	1
Simple PCI	6	2
Complex PCI	15	5

Table 5.4b Staff radiation exposure over 20 years*

	Exposure (mSv)	CXR equivalent (n)	Background equivalent (years)
Operator	200	2000	53
Nursing staff	60	600	16
Radiographer	1	20	0.5

*assumes 20 years of mixed interventional experience with 500 cases/annum and 10mSv/annum.

Contemporary interventional cardiology is a relatively young speciality, and there are few data examining the risk of cancer among workers in cardiac catheterization laboratories. Whilst modern equipment and increased radiation awareness may result in lower doses delivered to staff in comparison with those received by earlier workers, the increasing frequency and complexity of procedures may still pose a hazard. Studies among cardiology staff, therefore, are awaited with interest.

Factors affecting radiation exposure to patients and operators

Patient factors

Procedural complexity

As would be expected, more complex interventional procedures are associated with higher radiation doses.

In observational studies, dose parameters have been found to increase incrementally with the number of vessels treated(16) and the number of stents used(16,17). Of course, the number of stents is likely to relate to the number of vessels treated.

Procedural urgency is also an important factor. In one study of over 600 cases (16), emergency PCI in the context of acute myocardial infarction (8% of total cases) was associated with significantly higher dose parameters compared to elective cases. This may have related to a higher number of stents used in acute cases. In current practice, intervention in the emergency situation is more likely to require adjunctive techniques such as thrombus extraction. Employing these techniques is likely to add to procedural dose.

Intervention upon more complex lesions is likely to be more dose-intensive. For example, elective intervention upon chronic total occlusions resulted in higher doses due to more acquisitions as well as longer screening and acquisition times(16). Doses were positively associated with the duration of the occlusion in one study(17). In the same study, intervention upon more tortuous vessels also resulted in higher doses.

Patient size

Body mass index (BMI) is an important predictor of radiation dose in invasive cardiological procedures[18,19]. With increasing patient size, the dose required for satisfactory imaging is increased. The voltage across the cathode–anode gap is increased to provide higher energy photons to compensate for reduced image quality, but this reduces image contrast.

Kuon *et al.* [16] found that among patients undergoing diagnostic and therapeutic coronary procedures, DAP correlated reasonably well with BMI (r = 0.37), and better still with body surface area (r = 0.42). Obesity may be a stronger predictor still in procedures that are likely to be particularly lengthy or complex. For example, among subjects undergoing pulmonary vein isolation, obesity led to exposure to twice the effective dose compared to normal weight subjects[19]. Appreciation of this relationship should be taken into account when assessing suitability for complex coronary intervention, such as chronic total occlusions, and when counselling patients as to procedural risks.

Other factors

Chronic respiratory disorders such as emphysema may influence imaging quality by increasing thoracic cavity dimensions, thereby increasing the distance between the radiation source and image intensifier, and increasing scatter.

The previous radiation exposure of each patient should be considered when listing patients for procedures. Previous exposure may be by way of prior angiography and/or PCI, or may be unrelated, such as that due to radiotherapy for cancer.

Operational factors

Distances

The inverse square law dictates that increasing the distance from an X-ray source by factor x will reduce the radiation dose by factor $1/x^2$. For example, if the distance from the source is doubled, the radiation dose received now will be one quarter of the original dose. This is important when positioning the X-ray tube by altering the table height—placing the tube too near to the patient will ensure that the patient receives a large skin dose. Conversely, it is important to minimize the source to image distance (SID) (or, alternatively, the patient to intensifier distance, PID) by ensuring the image intensifier is as near to the patient as possible. Increasing the SID leads to higher patient doses and greater scattered dose to the attending staff.

The same principle should ensure that the operator (and assistant) is positioned as far from the X-ray tube as is possible. This will significantly reduce the scattered dose received. This can be facilitated by using longer extension tubing (Fig. 5.1) to connect the manifold and the catheter.

Fluoroscopy and acquisition time

Routine coronary interventional practice makes use of two imaging modalities, fluoroscopy and acquisition. Fluoroscopy functions to provide images allowing for appropriate positioning of equipment (e.g. catheters, wires, stents). Subsequently, acquisition produces images providing diagnostic data which can ultimately be archived. Thus, acquisition requires higher quality imaging than simple fluoroscopy, and doses used in acquisition are typically 10–20 times higher than those used during fluoroscopy. Therefore, 60–70% of the DAP during coronary angiography is related to acquisition.

Traditionally, FT has been used as an indication of the radiation dose delivered during coronary procedures. However, it has been shown that halving FT does not confer a similar reduction in procedural DAP[20]. It has been argued[20], therefore, that efforts to reduce radiation doses should concentrate upon reduction in acquisition. Acquisition times can be reduced by limiting the number of cinegraphic runs taken. Also, routine acquisitions should be of short duration; appropriate exceptions to this rule of thumb include the studying of collateralization, graft run-off, or assessment for any contrast entry into the pericardium. Furthermore, choosing less dose-intensive angulations (see later sections) will also reduce overall doses delivered.

Although fluoroscopy has a relatively smaller contribution to overall dose, operators should be aware that

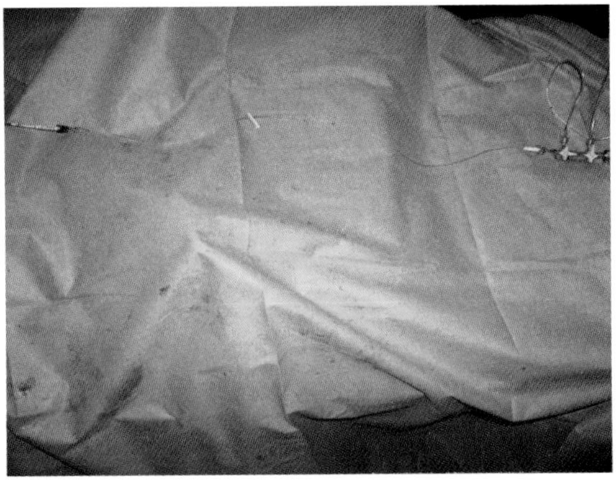

Fig. 5.1 Extension tube. This 90-cm extension tube connects the manifold with the catheter, allowing the operator to stand further away from the X-ray source during contrast injection, thereby reducing radiation exposure.

most modern machines are capable of varying the intensity of dose according to, for example, patient body habitus. For most cases, operators should ensure that the system is set at the lowest dose intensity (Fig. 5.2).

Filtration and collimation

As discussed earlier, X-ray tubes produce photons with varying energies. The lower energy photons are merely absorbed by the patient's skin, and do not contribute to image production, but may ultimately increase the risk of adverse effects. Operators should be aware that modern equipment is capable of filtering out these low-energy rays, by employing aluminium and copper filters. Filtration of the fluoroscopic beam is standard, but additional use of 'wedge' filters may also be possible. The operator should be familiar with the available equipment, and ensure that the wedge filter is used when, for example, the patient's bordering lungs are exposed to the X-ray beam.

Modern equipment allows for collimation, either via multiple blades or an iris diaphragm, which can be partially closed to significantly reduce the image field of view to the region of interest. For example, when positioning angioplasty equipment accurately, 'bringing the cones in' can significantly reduce the size of the irradiated area (Fig. 5.3). This will result in a reduced dose scattered to both the patient and attendant staff; the reduced scatter may even serve to improve image quality.

Some equipment includes computer simulation which allows for *virtual* collimation. This feature enables the physician to bring in the collimator blades without prior application of X-rays to guide position.

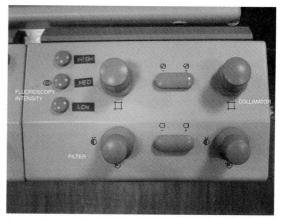

Fig. 5.2 X-ray machine control panel. Operators should be familiar with the X-ray dose-reducing tools available in the lab. Variable fluoroscopic intensity, wedge filters, and collimators are highlighted in this panel.

Shielding

In the contemporary catheter laboratory, lead shielding is employed to reduce radiation exposure to operators and staff. For example, the amount of scattered radiation that is directed toward operators' upper bodies is reduced by lead shields suspended from ceilings. Similarly, the couch may be fitted with a mobile lead drape to absorb radiation that would otherwise reach operators' lower limbs. It has been shown, however, that use of these shields can still allow for 'leaks' in radiation at operators' mid-level. The shielding described

A

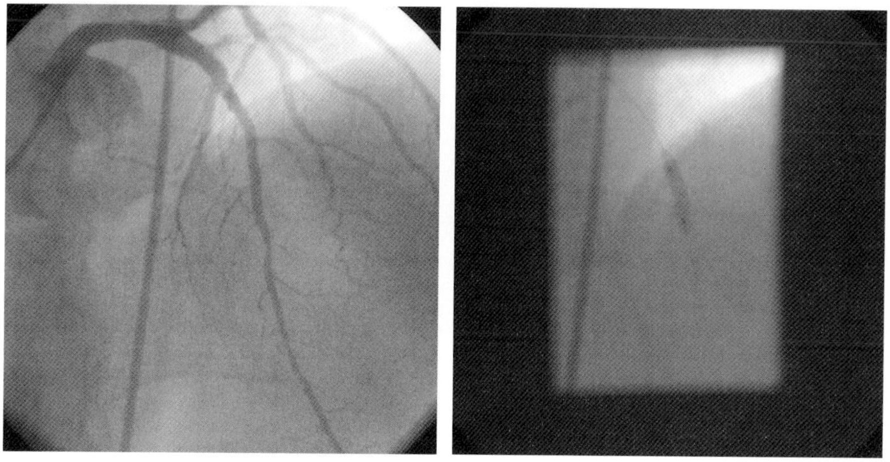

B

Fig. 5.3 Image collimation. A stent is deployed in the mid LAD (A), with subsequent post-dilatation (B). The image was magnified during post-dilatation to aid balloon positioning, with the collimator blades brought in to reduce the size of the irradiated area.

here can be modified by additional lead flaps and this has been shown to augment the reduction in operator exposure[21]. Universal use of such shields can be variable, and may be affected by operator fatigue or emergency peri-procedural complications. However, this can be overcome by well-trained radiographer and nursing colleagues providing 'gentle' reminders.

As well as wearing lead aprons to directly shield the main body, further protection can be obtained by wearing adjunctive garments such as thyroid shields and shin-guards. Doses to the eyes can be further reduced by wearing glasses. Some operators advocate the use of a 0.5-mm lead cap, which further reduces the dose delivered to the head[22].

Angulations

The radiation doses delivered to the patient (and, therefore, those scattered to the operator and staff) are determined by the angulations used during studies. The ideal angulations are those that provide sufficient diagnostic data, but reduce doses to the patient and operator. Left anterior oblique (LAO) angulations, in particular, have been shown to be dose-intensive[23,24].

Kuon *et al.*[24] assessed time-adjusted fluoroscopic doses to a 'phantom' patient and operator according to several angulations, allowing for useful recommendations. The steeper left or right anterior oblique projections (≥60°) were especially dose-intensive, as these views increase the length of the X-ray beam path. For example, when visualizing the distal left main stem (LMS), switching from LAO caudal (60°/20°) to postero-anterior (PA) caudal (0°/30°) angulations led to dose reductions to patient and operator of approximately 60% and 90%, respectively. Similar reductions were possible when switching to a PA cranial (0°/30°) view from LAO caudal to study the LMS ostium, and from the LAO cranial to study LAD /diagonal artery bifurcations.

Clearly, there will be inter-individual variation in determining which angulations provide all of the necessary data, but knowledge of how angulations affect overall doses is invaluable in reducing exposure to patient, operator, and staff.

Access site

Increasingly, more diagnostic and interventional coronary procedures are being performed via the radial route. Advantages for patients include a reduced risk of neurovascular injury and quicker mobilization[25].

However, some, but not all, (mostly observational) data have suggested that the radial route is associated with increased radiation doses to the patient and operator [26–30]. Studies have differed with regards to patient numbers, and have not always controlled for operator experience and use of radiation protection devices; at present, the radial technique should not be denounced on the basis of radiation exposure.

In a pilot study prospectively performed in our centre by two experienced operators[29], standardized angulations were employed, and the operators used the same dose-reduction measures. Radiation exposure during diagnostic angiography for both patient and operator did not differ significantly. Whilst procedural time may have been longer for the radial route, this was offset by a shorter time for patients to mobilize after the procedure. Large-scale randomized studies performed by operators in high-volume centres are required to definitively answer this question.

Fatigue

As more interventional procedures are performed, it is conceivable that operator fatigue may impact upon procedural duration and radiation delivery. In an observational study of a single operator's practice[31], patient radiation exposure from PCI rose significantly in the afternoon after the operator's cumulative workload had exceeded 6 hours. These findings should be confirmed in future studies, with particular attention to the effects of increasing availability of out-of-hours primary PCI.

Technical factors

Numerous advances in angiographic technology and techniques have allowed for reductions in radiation doses.

Pulsed fluoroscopy

With this feature, X-rays are delivered in rapid, successive pulses rather than in a continuous manner. The pulses shorten the time during which X-rays are released, and consequently, the dose can be significantly reduced. Ultimately, the delivered dose is a function of the dose per pulse as well as the pulse frequency.

Last image hold and replay fluoroscopy

This feature of modern machines allows for a reduction in radiation dose. The last image obtained during a fluoroscopy is stored until a new image is produced. As previously discussed, fluoroscopy is less dose-intensive than acquisition. Modern equipment allows for replaying and storage of fluoroscopy runs, limiting the need for acquisition. Where image quality is not vital, fluoroscopy can be stored: for example, balloon inflation or stent deployment can be archived by storing a few frames of a fluoroscopy run.

Frame-grabbing and road-mapping

Frame-grabbing allows the operator to extract and view a specific image from a fluoroscopic series without the necessity of additional radiation. A road-map is created when this image is copied for storage. This allows anatomy to be reviewed without repeat screening or acquisition. This feature may also prevent unnecessary contrast use.

Regulatory bodies and dose reference levels

Regulations governing the medical use of ionizing radiation have been in existence for some time. The background to current guidelines in the UK is well summarized by Wilde *et al.* [32]. The safety of medical staff and the general public who may be exposed to radiation is at the core of the Ionising Radiation Regulations 1999 (IRR99). Similarly, the Ionising Radiation (Medical Exposure) Regulations 2000 (IR(ME)R 2000) relate to the protection of patients undergoing radiological procedures. The latter requires identification of medical staff involved in the patient journey as acting as referrers, practitioners, and operators, justifying the need for the procedure in all cases.

Central to these complementary documents is the principle of keeping delivered doses as low as possible. Moreover, IRR99 stipulates maximum doses for employees and trainees (Table 5.5), which must not be exceeded. Thus, the annual effective occupational effective dose should not exceed 20mSv averaged over a period of 5 years, and no more than 50mSv in any single year.

In a recent survey within the authors' unit, the maximal annual occupational dose was 0.4mSv. By way of comparison, the average annual occupational dose to aircrew in 1991 was 2mSv.

The IR(ME)R 2000 regulations require employers to establish and adhere to dose reference levels (DRLs). It was decided that these could be levels set nationally, or levels adapted according to local audited practice, which should be lower than national limits. The Department of Health DRL Working Party approved DRLs for X-ray procedures based on those recommended by the National Radiological Protection Board (NRPB; this body has now been incorporated into the Radiation Protection Division of the Health Protection Agency). Based upon a review of procedural dose conducted in 2000, the recommended DRLs for coronary angiography included a DAP of 36Gy.cm^2 and FT of 5.6min. A further (larger) review of doses was performed in 2005, and, accordingly, new, lower DRLs have been recently proposed: DAP of 29Gy.cm^2 and FT of 4.5min[33].

For PCI procedures, there appears to be a wide variation in radiation doses, likely related to differing procedural complexity, techniques, and radiation protection awareness. A survey conducted by the European DIMOND (Measures for Optimising Radiological Information and Dose in Digital Imaging and Interventional Radiology) research group, studied dose parameters relating to coronary angiography and PCI across six countries[34]. There was a wide range in DAP for angiography and percutaneous transluminal coronary angioplasty (PTCA): median values ranged from 19.1–39.6 and 27.1–66.9Gy.cm^2, respectively. The group proposed (preliminary) DRLs for each procedure, based on the 75th percentile of all data. Thus, proposed DRLs for PTCA include DAP of 94Gy.cm^2, FT of 16min, and maximal number of frames at 1355. The recently recommended DRLs for (single-stent) PCI based upon the 2005 dose review in the UK were lower: DAP of 50Gy.cm^2, and FT of 13min[33].

Table 5.5 Annual dose limits for employees and members of the public

	Employees	**Trainees**	**Public**
Effective dose (mSv)	20	6	1
Equivalent dose (eye) (mSv)	150	50	15
Equivalent dose (skin) (mSv)	500	150	50
Equivalent dose (hands, forearms, feet, ankles) (mSv)	500	150	50

Reducing radiation exposure

The guiding principle for any radiographic procedure is to use doses as low as reasonably achievable/practicable (ALARA/ALARP). Clearly, this approach will be of benefit to the patient, operator, and attendant staff. Of course, the quality of any study should not be compromised such that imaging data acquired are not of clinical use. However, accepting images that are just of diagnostic quality as opposed to the highest quality images will usually enable a reduction in delivered dose, although this approach may appear to be counter-intuitive.

Practical ways of reducing radiation exposure are shown in Table 5.6.

Employing some of the dose-reducing measures systematically has been shown to cut down patient doses for coronary angiography and both simple and complex

Table 5.6 Ways to reduce radiation exposure

Cut down number and duration of acquisitions
Use low intensity fluoroscopy mode
Collimate to regions of interest
Avoid steep angulations when possible
Use all available lead shielding and wear lead garments
Ensure patient to intensifier distance is minimized
Maximize operator's distance from X-ray source
Try to minimize magnified fluoroscopy and acquisitions
Try to vary angulations during lengthy procedures
Operators to audit their procedural doses against DRLs

PCI procedures[18]. Subsequently, this centre audited their doses in interventional procedures with reference to the DIMOND proposals[16]. Their mean doses for elective PCI procedures were far short of the DIMOND DRLs (e.g. DAP 7.8Gy.cm^2, FT 7.5min, and 146 cinegraphic frames).

It has been shown that providing short tutorials advocating these measures to operators with a wide range of experience led to a reduction in mean doses for angiography[35].

Importantly, it is incumbent upon operators to audit their practice. Modern equipment should facilitate collection of case-related doses, and cardiologists should ensure that their procedural doses fall within their employers' DRLs, and also make every effort to achieve continued improvement.

Within departments, it is vital that equipment is regularly serviced and that quality control checks are frequently undertaken. There is a requirement for trainees to understand the principles underlying good practice (e.g. IR(ME)R 2000 specifications in the United Kingdom). This should be enhanced by 'on the job' training provided by an interactive laboratory staff.

Summary

The increasing frequency and complexity of PCI procedures are associated with an increased risk of radiation-related injury to patients and catheter laboratory staff. It is important that cardiologists are not only aware of these risks, but also strive to improve their day to day practice in reducing radiation exposure. Ultimately, increased radiation awareness will be beneficial to patients, operators, and laboratory staff.

References

1. Hirshfeld JW Jr, Balter S, Brinker JA, *et al.* American College of Cardiology Foundation; American Heart Association/; HRS; SCAI; American College of Physicians Task Force on Clinical Competence and Training. ACCF/AHA/HRS/SCAI clinical competence statement on physician knowledge to optimize patient safety and image quality in fluoroscopically guided invasive cardiovascular procedures: a report of the American College of Cardiology Foundation/American Heart Association/American College of Physicians Task Force on Clinical Competence and Training. *Circulation* 2005; **111**(4):511–32.
2. Koenig TR, Wolff D, Mettler FA, *et al.* Skin injuries from fluoroscopically guided procedures: part 1, characteristics of radiation injury. *Am J Roentgenol* 2001; **177**(1):3–11.
3. Koenig TR, Mettler FA, Wagner LK. Skin injuries from fluoroscopically guided procedures: part 2, review of 73 cases and recommendations for minimizing dose delivered to patient. *Am J Roentgenol* 2001; **177**(1):13–20.
4. Wagner LK, McNeese MD, Marx MV, *et al.* Severe skin reactions from interventional fluoroscopy: case report and review of the literature. *Radiology* 1999; **213**(3):773–6.
5. Berlin L. Radiation-induced skin injuries and fluoroscopy. *Am J Roentgenol* 2001; **177**(1):21–5.
6. Chodick G, Bekiroglu N, Hauptmann M, *et al.* Risk of cataract after exposure to low doses of ionizing radiation: a 20-year prospective cohort study among US radiologic technologists. *Am J Epidemiol* 2008; **168**(6):620–31.
7. Preston DL, Shimizu Y, Pierce DA, *et al.* Studies of mortality of atomic bomb survivors. Report 13: Solid cancer and noncancer disease mortality: 1950–1997. *Radiat Res* 2003; **160**(4):381–407.
8. Pierce DA, Preston DL. Radiation-related cancer risks at low doses among atomic bomb survivors. *Radiat Res* 2000; **154**(2):178–86.
9. Preston DL, Ron E, Tokuoka S, *et al.* Solid cancer incidence in atomic bomb survivors: 1958–1998. *Radiat Res* 2007; **168**(1):1–64.
10. Muirhead CR, O'Hagan JA, Haylock RG, *et al.* Mortality and cancer incidence following occupational radiation exposure: third analysis of the National Registry for Radiation Workers. *Br J Cancer* 2009; **100**(1):206–12.
11. Partridge J. Radiation in the cardiac catheter laboratory. *Heart* 2005; **91**(12):1615–20.
12. Whitby M, Martin CJ. Radiation doses to the legs of radiologists performing interventional procedures: are they a cause for concern? *Br J Radiol* 2003; **76**(905):321–7.
13. Tsapaki V, Kottou S, Vano E, *et al.* Correlation of patient and staff doses in interventional cardiology. *Radiat Prot Dosimetry* 2005; **117**(1–3):26–9.
14. Yoshinaga S, Mabuchi K, Sigurdson AJ, *et al.* Cancer risks among radiologists and radiologic technologists: review of epidemiologic studies. *Radiology* 2004; **233**(2):313–21.
15. Doody MM, Freedman DM, Alexander BH, *et al.* Breast cancer incidence in U.S. radiologic technologists. *Cancer* 2006; **106**(12):2707–15.

16. Kuon E, Empen K, Rohde D, *et al.* Radiation exposure to patients undergoing percutaneous coronary interventions: are current reference values too high? *Herz* 2004; **29**(2):208–17.
17. Tsapaki V, Magginas A, Vano E, *et al.* Factors that influence radiation dose in percutaneous coronary intervention. *J Interv Cardiol* 2006; **19**(3):237–44.
18. Kuon E, Glaser C, Dahm JB. Effective techniques for reduction of radiation dosage to patients undergoing invasive cardiac procedures. *Br J Radiol* 2003; **76**(906):406–13
19. Ector J, Dragusin O, Adriaenssens B, *et al.* Obesity Is a Major Determinant of Radiation Dose in Patients Undergoing Pulmonary Vein Isolation for Atrial Fibrillation. *J Am Coll Cardiol* 2007; **50**:234–42.
20. Kuon E. Radiation exposure in invasive cardiology. *Heart* 2008; **94**(5):667–74.
21. Kuon E, Schmitt M, Dahm JB. Significant reduction of radiation exposure to operator and staff during cardiac interventions by analysis of radiation leakage and improved lead shielding. *Am J Cardiol* 2002; **89**(1):44–9.
22. Kuon E, Birkel J, Schmitt M, *et al.* Radiation exposure benefit of a lead cap in invasive cardiology. *Heart* 2003; **89**(10):1205–10.
23. Pitney MR, Allan RM, Giles RW, *et al.* Modifying fluoroscopic views reduces operator radiation exposure during coronary angioplasty. *J Am Coll Cardiol* 1994; **24**(7):1660–3.
24. Kuon E, Dahm JB, Empen K, *et al.* Identification of less-irradiating tube angulations in invasive cardiology. *J Am Coll Cardiol* 2004; **44**(7):1420–8.
25. Jolly SS, Amlani S, Hamon M, *et al.* Radial versus femoral access for coronary angiography or intervention and the impact on major bleeding and ischemic events: a systematic review and meta-analysis of randomized trials. *Am Heart J* 2009; **157**(1):132–40.
26. Sandborg M, Fransson SG, Pettersson H. Evaluation of patient-absorbed doses during coronary angiography and intervention by femoral and radial artery access. *Eur Radiol* 2004; **14**(4):653–8.
27. Geijer H, Persliden J. Radiation exposure and patient experience during percutaneous coronary intervention using radial and femoral artery access. *Eur Radiol* 2004; **14**(9):1674–80.
28. Lange HW, von Boetticher H. Randomized comparison of operator radiation exposure during coronary angiography and intervention by radial or femoral approach. *Catheter Cardiovasc Interv* 2006; **67**(1):12–6.
29. Lo TS, Fountzopoulos E, Freestone B, *et al.* Radiation exposure and procedural duration: implications for transradial and transfemoral coronary angiography. *Heart* 2007; **93**(Suppl 1):A5–A105.
30. Brasselet C, Blanpain T, Tassan-Mangina S, *et al.* Comparison of operator radiation exposure with optimized radiation protection devices during coronary angiograms and ad hoc percutaneous coronary interventions by radial and femoral routes. *Eur Heart J* 2008; **29**(1):63–70.
31. Kuon E, Dahm JB, Schmitt M, *et al.* Short communication: time of day influences patient radiation exposure from percutaneous cardiac interventions. *Br J Radiol* 2003; **76**(903):189–191
32. Wilde P, Pitcher EM, Slack K. Radiation hazards for the patient in cardiological procedures. *Heart* 2001; **85**(2):127–30.
33. Hart D, Hillier MC, Wall BF. National reference doses for common radiographic, fluoroscopic and dental X-ray examinations in the UK. *Br J Radiol* 2009; **82**(973):1–12.
34. Neofotistou V, Vano E, Padovani R, *et al.* Preliminary reference levels in interventional cardiology. *Eur Radiol* 2003; **13**(10):2259–63.
35. Kuon E, Empen K, Robinson DM, *et al.* Efficiency of a minicourse in radiation reducing techniques: a pilot initiative to encourage less irradiating cardiological interventional techniques (ELICIT). *Heart* 2005; **91**(9):1221–2.

CHAPTER 6

The 'golden rules' of percutaneous coronary intervention

Rod H. Stables

Introduction

In the practice of percutaneous coronary intervention (PCI), the usual aim is to deliver maximum clinical gain—at the lowest possible risk—achievable in that specific clinical setting. Most interventionists will accept that PCI has established limitations. The enthusiasm to recommend and perform this form of therapy should be tempered in the light of this reality.

- Clinical gain can be real but is often modest.
- Performance can be associated with morbidity and mortality.
- Alternative therapeutic options exist and are effective.

Other chapters in this textbook will seek to guide on case selection, to refine technique, and to provide an appreciation of available technologies and pharmacotherapy. I believe, however, that substantial improvements in both elements of the 'risk:benefit' ratio can be achieved with a re-examination and more universal application of some core, fundamental principles underpinning optimal PCI practice. A talk describing my 'golden rules of PCI' has been well-received, by trainees and experienced operators alike, at educational meetings over the last decade and most recipients come to accept my assertion that almost all procedure-related adverse events or suboptimal outcomes can be traced back to a breach of these core concepts.

All who seek to assume a lead operator role need to accept that, to all intents and purposes, everything that happens in PCI is as a direct result of the actions of the leader and the clinical team. Very little is beyond the control of the operator and, short of catastrophic failure of the power supply or imaging equipment, everything that goes wrong will be related to an action, omission, or decision on their part. I have grown tired of case review sessions when operators recount events in detached and passive terms. A few examples with my proposed alternative (in brackets) are as follows:

- 'The wire position was lost . . .' (Through sloppy handling and poor attention to detail I managed to pull the guide wire back proximal to the lesion.)
- 'The stent fell off the balloon . . .' (As I tried to withdraw the undeployed stent back into the guide catheter, my failure to ensure coaxial alignment resulted in my stripping the stent off its delivery balloon.)
- 'The guide catheter pinged and I had to reposition the catheter and wire . . .' (Because I was not paying attention to the guide catheter as I tried to force the balloon through the occlusion segment, I caused the catheter to prolapse into the left ventricle, taking the guide wire into the same unfortunate position. I was very lucky and was able to re-establish catheter and wire position without adverse incident.)

This type of realistic, reflective practice is an important element of self-development as an operator. We are fortunate that major adverse events are very infrequent in routine PCI practice but should continue to strive towards their elimination. I am sure we could profit by paying more attention to 'near miss' events (like the loss of wire position) that are so often the prelude to subsequent mishap. The promotion and sharing of best practice has been a key feature of the PCI community and here is my 'back to basics' contribution.

Preparation of the case

Know the patient and the details of the case

The self-evident truth that an optimum PCI procedure can only be planned and performed with a complete appreciation of all relevant facts is, sadly, perhaps the most neglected golden rule in modern practice. I am sure most operators will recognize uncomfortable events of this nature:

- Completing a long, complex but successful PCI to then realise (900mL of contrast later) that the patient is diabetic with established and significant renal dysfunction.
- When the patient remarks that he is not surprised that you did not gain access from the right leg as two other cardiologists had also failed over recent years—ever since he had that failed peripheral angioplasty for common femoral occlusion.
- Mid way through a PCI on a patient with previous coronary grafting asking 'How many grafts did you have?' whilst dispatching a junior doctor to find copies of the original surgical record.
- In an acute case when angiography reveals a number of potential target lesions asking, 'Where were those ECG changes again?'
- Implanting multiple drug-eluting stent devices into a patient who then thanks you on the subsequent ward round as they will now be able to have their proposed surgical resection of a newly-diagnosed carcinoma.

One key element of preparation is to achieve a complete appreciation of the coronary anatomy. Even in the most acute cases it is wise to evaluate all elements of the vascular supply before moving with a guide catheter to the suspected culprit vessel. In primary PCI for acute myocardial infarction, chronic occlusion with retrograde filling or incorrect dominance assumptions can result in operators tacking the wrong lesion or failing to appreciate the true scale, scope, and risk of a procedure.

In elective settings, if initial diagnostic studies are inadequate then deficiencies should be highlighted and resolved before committing to a PCI procedure. Additional angiographic or intravascular ultrasound images and tests of functional significance can often be performed with an option to proceed to PCI at the same sitting. In other cases, however, additional information on viability, graft persistence, or aberrant anatomy may require distinct imaging procedures. Current experience in the management of chronic occlusions suggests that we will see an expanding role for multimodality imaging in the planning of coronary intervention.

Planning the strategic approach—establish the desired aim or end-point

Observation of case review sessions over many years has led me to believe that a number of PCI procedures are undertaken without any initial, established concept of the desired final result. To quote the teachings of the British Army in its consideration of the principles of war, 'selection and maintenance of the aim' should be the core strategic approach. Decide what is best and then do it. If it happens to go well, be grateful and do not be tempted into a procedural extension to more lesions of more marginal potential value or higher risk.

When the desired end result has been established it is then possible to plan the broad strategic approach to the case. This phase may, for example, include (but is by no means limited to) a consideration of:

- Lesion sequencing: it usually makes sense to tackle occlusions first and to, when possible, tackle lesions from distal to proximal. Exceptions to these rules do exist but they are, in reality, very rare.
- Options for stopping or staging: it is wise to set pre-specified options or limits. In a patient with impaired renal function the contrast dose used should be considered between individual target lesions to allow sensible staging for renal protection. In another case, failure to re-open an important but occluded vessel may serve as the trigger to discontinue the procedure and recommend surgery, rather than performing incomplete revascularization with a 'consolation angioplasty' at a lesion in another territory.
- Special equipment requirements: is there the correct stock, in the correct sizes, and the required skill mix in the allocated team? Some examples might include:
    - Heavy calcification suggesting rotational atherectomy.
    - Over-the-wire or long shaft balloons for specialist occlusion work.
    - Large-calibre guide catheters for specialist equipment or multiple simultaneous stent deployment
- Side branch preservation plans: there is often value in deciding an approach to side branches (taking their origin within the segments to be treated) prior to starting the procedure. The recognition that a tributary has a significant myocardial distribution and should be preserved will drive a very different approach than that used for small branches considered to be of no outcome significance.

The skilled and effective operator will need to retain some flexibility in response. To continue the military theme, Von Moltke the Elder (who was chief of staff of the Prussian armies for 30 years) declared that 'No battle plan survives contact with the enemy'. Nevertheless, deviations from the proposed strategy should be reserved for substantial and unforeseen events rather than a failure to appreciate, define, or deliver a logical and well-chosen endpoint.

Meet the patient (and sometimes the family)

'I had never seen Dr X until (s)he appeared half way through my angioplasty procedure . . .' This never sounds good when subsequently related and is the basis of much patient disquiet, often fuelling dissatisfaction with other aspects of a procedure or its outcome. There is no substitute for a meaningful interaction with the patient prior to a procedure. This interaction should be a dialogue and include a consideration of the patient's wishes and expectations. Operators should be involved in the formal consent process, especially if the case has unusual features or exceptional risk. In cases with these latter characteristics, there is merit in including other family members in the discussion of risk and benefit to guide their perception in the advent of a tragedy.

Ensure optimum scheduling

It is unwise to introduce external distractions or limitations into a list that has not been adjusted for their accommodation. Interventional cardiologists often delude themselves that they thrive in a multitasking environment, and to their credit, many do increase apparent productivity with this approach. If I, however, were a patient on the table, I would like to think that my angioplasty had the undivided attention of my cardiologist rather than hear him or her conducting an unrelated meeting during its performance with one eye on the clock because of the need to catch a flight to a different continent at 1800 hours.

Operators must assume responsibility for key elements of the case scheduling process. The provision of adequate time for pre- and postprocedural care is but one element of this task. Certain procedures may need extra time or demand access to specialized equipment, supporting staff with particular skills, or a high dependency nursing environment for the recovery phase. Adequate planning and good communication will allow all elements for procedural success to be brought together in the right place and at the right time.

Poor planning creates unnecessary pressures and drives poor decision-making. In an over-populated list, many important lesions will be judged as 'probably not significant' and the failure rate for occluded vessels will be more substantial than usual. An abundance of time may prompt the performance of procedures, or the extension of procedures, with questionable value. Availability should not drive 'spur of the moment' decisions.

Performance of the procedure

Never compromise on the guide catheter stability and guide wire position

In my experience there are few complications of angioplasty that cannot be effectively corrected if the operator has the security of a sound guide catheter and a guide wire in the true lumen, towards the distal end of the main target vessel. Procedural failure, abrupt vessel closure, resulting myocardial infarction, and death are usually the result of the loss of control of one or both of these key elements of PCI equipment. Manipulation and movement of stents and balloons along coronary vessels is subject to the laws of physics. The fact that static friction is greater than dynamic friction will be familiar to any operator trying to advance a stalled balloon through tortuous and tight anatomy. More important, however, is Newton's third law of motion stating that 'action and reaction are equal and opposite'. Movements of the guide catheter, wire, and balloon catheter (or other device) are inter-related. Continued introduction of the shaft of a balloon, when the leading tip is impacted and static in a lesion will result in changes in the line and curvature of the guide catheter (as it seeks to accommodate the additional length of the angioplasty device). Sudden and sometimes catastrophic disengagement of the guide catheter can result.

I ask my trainees to imagine sitting on a classic office chair, their feet supported on a bar, above the wheeled base. They are asked to open a door by pushing on the door surface with an outstretched hand. At this point either the door opens or they, and their chair, move backwards. It all depends on the balance of forces. The stability of the guide catheter is the key to the ability to project force and advance angioplasty equipment. It is possible to make most catheter shapes engage most coronary ostia to some degree but the temptation to think, 'This will do' or 'I can make it fit' should be avoided. Never compromise on the guide catheter and be prepared to modify an initial choice *before* initial treatment of a lesion.

The guide wire should be manipulated with care and precision. Any substantial buckling of the tip segment or backing out of the guide catheter is a clue to injudicious handling. Wire-induced trauma can result in dissection and abrupt closure, which may involve vessels or segments not targeted for intervention, and can be difficult to correct if it proves impossible to ever gain the true distal lumen. As a general rule, start with the softest and least traumatic wire available before escalating to more aggressive designs. Try to keep the wire in the desired target vessel with minimal excursion into other branches. Such deviations should be promptly recognized and corrected. Bi-plane imaging or regular camera rotation can be very valuable in this respect. It is important *in every case* to check the final wire position in two planes of X-ray projection. A single image may be very persuasive that the wire is in the correct place but only because of vessel overlap. This important rule is often ignored. It is indeed rare that an operator is fooled into an incorrect stent deployment or balloon inflation. Nevertheless, I maintain a library of images recording the inevitable reality that, with enough activity, disregard of this rule will result in adverse outcomes.

Select a final wire position in a distal portion of the largest and most important branch of the target vessel. Invest time and effort to secure the optimal position. You can only protect the vessel that contains the wire. If you allow the wire to be in a second diagonal during a proximal left angioplasty, then a spiral dissection could close the main vessel beyond repair. In a dominant right, the choice of vessel for wiring beyond the principal bifurcation should be the subject of intelligent thought and not random chance.

The wire should be as distal as possible without risking trauma to vessels that are very small in calibre, tortuous, or subject to substantial motion with cardiac systole. The presence of the wire may induce substantial change in the angiographic appearance of the target vessel and one's perception of the lesion location and morphology. Be prepared to reacquire reference or road-map images to better reflect current reality.

Define the target lesion segment with multiple observations

The target lesion segment must be identified and characterized. If you cannot see it, you cannot treat it. Sometimes a PCI may not be advisable, simply because it proves impossible to define the true nature of the target in any angiographic image. In all cases, a number of different projections (sometimes combined with adjunctive imaging modalities) should be examined. Bifurcations and ostial lesions demand specific care to avoid foreshortening and identify the true carina of vessel separation. Avoid the temptation to work in the plane that provides the most favourable angiographic image; an alternative view may be less pleasing but provide greater insight about the true problem.

Think about vessel calibre and the potential for underestimation because of spasm or, more commonly, reduced flow mediated dilation in arteries that have been occluded or under filled for some time. Vessels that run for a long distance on the epicardial surface, and bear branches are rarely small. Predilatation, vasodilators, and time can create an encouraging response before the selection of a final treatment device.

Once the treatment segment is characterized consider the specific imaging requirements for the distal and proximal portions as these may be different. An angiographic projection that best resolves the origin of a diagonal branch of the left anterior descending artery will not be ideal for a proximal stent landing zone close to the left main bifurcation. In the absence of bi-plane imaging, camera movement will be required during placement.

Work with precision

Maintain a clean and orderly working area

Keep your hands and the exposed length of wires free of contrast and other debris that might prevent easy manoeuvre of equipment. Remove unnecessary items and packaging from the trolley and table and place them in a bin. Employ a standard system and ensure that important items (like the torque device) are kept in a specific and secure location. If the wire is displaced and needs urgent repositioning will the key tools immediately be to hand?

Find, and use in a consistent manner, strategies to avoid confusion in more complex cases—for example, multiple wires. There are many approaches to these types of problem and personal preference is important here. I like to have the distal end of the wires marked (for example, with a small bend in the wire serving the more minor vessel) and clear separation of wires at the haemostatic valve (by having the non-active wire running under a wet swab). I try to avoid fixed clipping of the wires, as any movement of patient or drapes will then result in wire displacement.

Use 'natural downtime' to perform these housekeeping tasks; this generates valuable product from what otherwise may have seemed like a frustrating wait for the arrival of a specific size of device.

Commit to quality at every stage of every procedure—rehearse excellence

Most operators will have experienced the disappointment of finding the guide wire proximal to the target lesion after a balloon exchange. In the vast majority of cases, after a tut and a sigh, the wire is rapidly repositioned and the case continues. Guide catheter displacements are often accepted in the same dismissive manner. In so doing, a valuable learning opportunity is lost as a 'near miss event' passes without appropriate acknowledgement consideration and corrective intervention. Instead, think why this handling error has occurred:

- Poor attention to detail and sloppy movements?
- Incoordination between operator and assistant?
- Sticky fingers pulling the wire at the wrong time?
- Wire falling off the edge of the table?

Measure what can be measured

Woodworkers are trained on the maxim 'Measure twice, cut once.' PCI operators should follow this lead. One key element of science is the desire to measure and characterize. If the guide catheter enters the left ventricle, do not pull it out in disgust without first having noted at least the end-diastolic pressure as a measure of immediate cardiac performance. Do not 'trust' anticoagulant drugs if their anticoagulant effect can be measured and recorded, guiding your response at key stages of the procedure.

One cannot estimate the diameter of the target vessel if the guide catheter is not in the picture. It is very common to see an operator remove from a lesion, a balloon of known and precise dimensions and then spend time pondering the desired stent length. One image with the 'ruler' in place would allow improved precision. Accuracy is of course improved if the initial balloon selection is made so that the chosen length will be close to (but, of course, less than) that thought best for the final stent device. Stent length choices can be critical if the treated segment is to avoid branches at its start and/or end. When placing overlapping stents, the initial devices must be selected with care to avoid leaving double mesh overlap zones at obvious side branches, and to avoid excessive vessel tortuosity that might make the passage of the nose of the new stent into the tail of the previous stent more difficult.

For key decisions or actions you may choose to modify the setup of the working angiographic image. Magnification and field size reduction (by coning) will improve image quality. Doubling the frame rate will improve resolution and can be very useful for detecting the location of deployed stent devices (during post-dilatation, for example) or visualizing minor dissections.

Predict key stages or threats and plan to ensure success

Some individual stages of each procedure will have special significance or risk. You must know the moments of real threat and mobilize all your assets to achieve success. Examples would be the sequential inflation of stent delivery systems in a crush stent procedure or the retrieval of an undeployed stent back into the guide catheter. It is important to allow additional preparation of oneself and the team prior to these 'crux' events. Be sure that all know their role. Key equipment should be marked and identified, the guide catheter and wire in sound positions, and the image line-up, contrast reservoir, and patient status should be optimum. I have a particular failing in that I find it hard to remember to remove a buddy wire before deployment of a stent. The relief that the chosen device has, at last and often after a struggle, made it to the desired position generates an overwhelming desire to grab the inflation device and get the stent implanted. Knowledge of this unfortunate tendency allows me to seek the aid of my team who will intervene to remind me of the correct sequence of actions.

To improve overall procedure speed, think first about the elimination of downtime. Try to be doing something productive all the time. Cleaning and tidying have been mentioned earlier but angiographic review, case discussion, or balloon preparation are other examples of tasks that can be performed while 'waiting' for some other process or piece of equipment. More time can be saved by employing a more logical sequence for routine activities. If you are planning to give nitrates after a balloon predilatation (for more accurate stent sizing) then administer the drug before the removal of the balloon. This allows time for the vasodilator to work while you perform the monorail exchange. If the balloon is removed first then few operators can demonstrate sufficient patience and the key images for sizing may be acquired too early.

Avoid lesion obsession—keep an eye on the big picture

I have already stressed the need to maintain awareness and control of the guide catheter and distal wire position. If the current angiographic images do not allow continuous review then the operator will need to make frequent and specific checks on their status. The heart rate and phasic blood pressure profile are critical in understanding the impact of the intervention on immediate haemodynamics. The operator should review these parameters on a regular basis and encourage colleagues to feel free to report even minor changes in the recordings, as they occur. Damping or ventricularization of the pressure waveform is always important and demands explanation and often some intervention. Finally be prepared to consider possible changes or problems in non-target coronary vessels. Although rare such events do occur and tend to be recognized too late to effect an ideal correction.

Never give up an asset until a better one is secured

In searching to improve the status of their equipment, some operators end up moving in a retrograde direction. A classic example would be the desire to replace a guide wire with a more supportive, stiffer model. If the current wire is removed, the ability to protect and treat the target vessel is interrupted and the patient enters a period of unnecessary additional risk. Passage of the new wire could cause occlusive dissection and abrupt vessel closure that cannot then be fixed.

Another, lesser example is the immediate removal of a balloon directly after its use. The next angiographic acquisition may show abrupt closure, vessel perforation, or merely doubt about the lesion length for stent selection. In all of these cases the ability to advance the balloon sitting in the guide catheter will be a distinct advantage. If all is well the balloon can be removed in the natural downtime as the chosen stent is fetched.

Always study your last pictures the most

At the end of a long and complex procedure it is tempting to rip off the gloves and be grateful that a successful conclusion has been reached. This must be avoided. The final images represent the status in which the patient must fare over the coming hours, days, and months. Failure to recognize a stent-edge dissection or trauma to the left main stem induced by the guide catheter is inexcusable. The final views should be obtained in at least two planes and with the guide wire removed. Guide wires can splint small dissections and render them undetectable. Wire stiffness can mask unnatural vessel flexion at the end of a rigid stented segment.

A systematic review can be helpful:

- Overall status of vessel and quality of flow?
- Stent inflow?
- Stent outflow?
- Stented segment and minimal luminal diameter review?
- Side branches?
- Distal wire trauma or perforation?
- Guide catheter injury?

In a crisis there is always time to think

Very few events require immediate response. Do not make thing worse by guessing:

- Stop.
- Gather information.
- Establish problem.
- Seek opinions.
- Consider options.
- Take action.

Conclusions

Intelligence is the ability to profit from experience. Teaching and learning affords us the ability to profit from the experience of others. We have the potential to predict and plan to avoid bad experiences. Despite this, it would appear that the human brain has an imperfect memory for pain as PCI operators will make the same mistakes over and over again for want of a more fastidious application of the basic principles underpinning optimum practice. Treat every procedure as if the patient were your nearest and dearest and as if the fate of the operator would follow the patient. The golden rules of PCI will not let you down.

CHAPTER 7

Routine management after percutaneous coronary intervention

Jonathan Byrne, GertJan Laarman, and Philip MacCarthy

Introduction

Following a technically successful procedure, it is the post-procedural care of the patient that will often dictate both short- and long-term outcomes. Post-procedural care involves close monitoring of the patient for early complications, which may be secondary to the procedure itself or the presenting complaint. Immediate complications following percutaneous coronary intervention (PCI) may occur due to bleeding, most commonly at the access site, or due to early cardiac complications, often related to technical issues during the procedure (see Section 6). Non-cardiac complications, such as the development of contrast nephropathy, will become apparent in the hours or days following the initial procedure. Prompt and accurate identification of post-procedural complications is essential if they are to be managed effectively, and identification of the 'at risk' patient may also facilitate early identification of problems when they do occur. Complication rates are higher in patients with acute coronary syndromes, often exacerbated by aggressive antithrombotic regimens, and also in older patients with comorbid conditions. The type of care and length of stay will also vary according to the clinical context and needs to be carefully considered once the PCI has been performed. Following discharge, the longer-term management of residual coronary disease and recurrent ischaemia along with appropriate secondary prevention may all affect longer-term outcome. This chapter will examine the issues surrounding the immediate and longer-term care of the patient following PCI.

Immediate post-procedural care

Access site management

The main aim of access site management following PCI is to achieve adequate haemostasis and avoid major bleeding complications and vascular injury. Vascular access can be achieved via transfemoral, transradial, or transbrachial routes, although the transbrachial route is rarely used in contemporary practice, and has a high complication rate in inexperienced hands[1]. The transfemoral route remains the routine approach in most centres, although the transradial approach offers the distinct advantage of lower vascular access site complications, albeit at a slightly increased risk of technical failure[2].

Transfemoral haemostasis

Haemostasis can be achieved following angiography/PCI by manual compression or using a number of vascular closure devices (VCDs). Manual haemostasis remains the gold standard for achieving haemostasis; however, the need for early mobilization and patient preference has led to a dramatic increase in the numbers of devices facilitating haemostasis. Despite their popularity and ease of use, they are not associated with a reduction in femoral access site complications. Indeed, they may even increase access site complication rates[3]. Infections, femoral artery stenosis/compromise, arterial laceration, uncontrolled bleeding, pseudoaneurysm, arteriovenous fistula, as well as device embolism and critical limb ischaemia have all been reported after their use. Furthermore, their use is limited by the presence of significant atherosclerosis and vessel calcification.

A large number of different devices have been developed using a variety of mechanisms including collagen plugs, clips, or suture closure at the arteriotomy site. All achieve haemostasis, with varying degrees of efficacy.

Collagen-based closure devices

On exposure to blood, bovine collagen plugs cause platelet adherence and aggregation, thereby achieving haemostasis. An extraluminal collagen plug has the distinct advantage that haemostasis is rapidly achieved, but the collagen plug itself will remain in the vessel wall and biodegrade over a period of time. Repuncture above or below the initial site can be safely performed before the collagen plug has dissolved if re-access is required[4]. These devices should not be used in patients who are due to undergo surgical cut-down procedures on the vessel, in view of the risk of disruption and embolization of the collagen plug. Commercially available devices include Angio-Seal® (St Jude Medical, Minnesota), VasoSeal® (Datascope, New Jersey), and Duett Pro® (Vascular Solutions, Minnesota).

Suture-based closure devices

These devices immediately close the artery by passage of a suture through the arterial wall and have the advantage that no intravascular device is deployed and the suture remains in the wall of the vessel. Furthermore, the devices also allow closure of larger holes, particularly relevant when carrying out procedures which require large-bore devices such as transcatheter aortic valves and percutaneous left ventricular assist devices. Perclose® (Abbott Vascular, California), X Site®, (Datascope, New Jersey), and SuperStich® (Sutura, California) are commercially available.

Staples/clips

These devices remain *in situ* following deployment. They are deployed extraluminally; commercially available devices include StarClose® (Abbott Vascular) and Angiolink EVS (Medtronik, Minneapolis).

Transradial haemostasis

After removal of the sheath the radial artery access site should be compressed to achieve haemostasis. Whichever method is used it is important only to apply enough pressure to stop bleeding which should be gradually released; haemostasis is usually achieved within 2–3h, including after PCI using adjunctive antiplatelet pharmacotherapy. This improves radial patency rates and reduces very rare complications such as chronic regional pain syndromes (which seem to be related to prolonged compression causing neural oedema and ischaemia[5]). Flow-limiting compression has recently been found to be a strong predictor of radial artery occlusion, reinforcing the benefit of avoiding excessive compression[6].

Vascular access site complications

Access site bleeding

Access site haematoma following transfemoral procedures is the most common periprocedural complication occurring in 0.5–12% of cases[7,8]. The precise incidence varies largely due to the non-uniform definitions of bleeding and access site haemorrhage used across many randomized trials, and the incidence is higher in most retrospective series. Small bruises are common and do not require specific management other than observation. Larger haematomas are more problematic and often lead to delayed mobilization and a more prolonged hospital stay. More significant access site haematomas may require transfusion, and although less common (<2%) are associated with adverse clinical outcomes and lower procedural success rates[9].

Bleeding may be insidious and missed, particularly in those with an elevated body mass. The presence of blood in the femoral compartment may lead to compression of adjacent structures. If puncture of the posterior wall occurs above the inguinal ligament, bleeding may extend into the retroperitoneum. Rarely, laceration of the inferior epigastric artery anterior to the femoral artery can also lead to retroperitoneal blood accumulation[10]. Retroperitoneal blood loss is an important, but relatively infrequent, complication of transfemoral PCI. The clinical presentation is often delayed until a large volume of blood is lost into the retroperitoneal cavity with features of hypovolaemia and haemodynamic compromise. Associated flank pain is often, but not invariably, seen. Other clinical features that may be observed include suprainguinal tenderness and, rarely, femoral neuropathy. The incidence of retroperitoneal haemorrhage following PCI is small (0.5–1%) but potentially serious with a 4% mortality and a 12–16% requirement for urgent surgical repair[11,12]. Hypovolaemia may also cause a reduction in cardiac output leading to myocardial ischaemia and the potential for stent thrombosis, all of which serve to increase patient risk. Furthermore, temporary discontinuation of antiplatelet therapy may also be necessary following an acute bleed and this will substantially increase the risk of early stent thrombosis. Peri-procedural bleeding is a powerful independent predictor of in-hospital, 30-day and 1-year mortality after PCI[13]. What remains unclear is whether the adverse outcome associated with bleeding is due to PCI-related complications, or relates to an effect of transfusion itself. Important pathophysiological effects of transfusion may explain this[14,15], and recent data have shown that red cells stored for prolonged periods have a direct effect on both short- and long-term outcome. Where possible, transfusion of blood products following PCI should be avoided.

The risk of major access site bleeding after PCI is dependent upon a number of procedural and demographic features listed in Table 7.1. Adjunctive pharmacology also plays an important role with a higher prevalence seen over the past decade with the use of more aggressive adjunctive antiplatelet agents[16]. Recent data have suggested that the use of bivalarudin, a hirudin analogue, results in significantly lower access site bleeds at the expense of a slight increase in ischaemic complications[17].

Management of major access site bleeding is usually conservative with a small proportion requiring vascular surgical exploration and repair.

Pseudoanuerysm and atrioventricular fistulae

A pseudoaneurysm comprises blood flow from the arterial lumen into an encapsulated haematoma and may develop after any form of arterial access. Suboptimal haemostasis may predispose to formation but the clinical sequelae will depend on the size and extent of any vascular or neurological compromise. Small pseudoaneurysms (<3cm) are rarely of clinical significance and can often be conservatively managed. When treatment is required, a variety of techniques can be attempted. Ultrasound-guided compression is simple and is usually attempted first. Local thrombin injection, coils, and covered stents have all been used with some success although for persistent, large pseudoaneurysms surgical repair may be necessary.

Post-procedural cardiac biomarkers: when should they be measured and how should they be managed?

Small post-procedural elevations of CK-MB are relatively common following non-emergent PCI, occurring in 5–30% of patients[18]. Troponin elevation is even more common given the sensitivity of this marker for detecting myocardial damage. Considerable debate has focused on the importance of post-procedural enzyme rises. Concerns were initially raised following the EPIC (Evaluation of 7E3 for the Prevention of Ischemic Complications) trial where increased late mortality was observed with an increase in CK-MB levels threefold above baseline[19]. A large number of early studies, including extensive retrospective analyses, have shown an association between cardiac enzyme release (whether CK-MB or troponin) and long-term outcomes, particularly when levels are much increased compared to baseline[20]. This had led many to advocate close observation and delayed discharge when CK or troponin levels are elevated following PCI. However, the clinical relevance of small troponin or CK-MB leaks remains unclear; elevated levels appear to impact on long-term rather than short-term prognosis, supporting the hypothesis that these elevations are reflective of the individual burden of atherosclerotic disease rather than microembolization at the time of the initial interventional procedure. It is also important to distinguish between unforeseen enzyme leaks, and those which occur following a procedural complication; a study of 5850 patients suggested that the increase in 1-year mortality risk of peri-procedural CK-MB elevation was restricted to the 2% of patients with unsuccessful stent procedures[21]. It is likely that this disease burden drives future cardiac events[22]. In a large cohort of 5487 patients who underwent non-emergent PCI, pre-procedural troponin elevation identified a group with adverse clinical characteristics and who had greater atherosclerotic burden, and it also appeared that troponin rise was a marker of lesion complexity[23]. In this study procedural success was lower with a higher incidence of angiographic complications and an adverse long-term prognosis.

The data on post-procedural biomarker elevation remains conflicting, and it is not routine practice to check levels in all patients after PCI. Indeed, the 2005 ACC/AHA/SCAI guidelines recommended checking levels only in patients suspected of having a procedural myocardial infarction, with a weaker emphasis on routine CK or troponin analysis[24].

It is certainly reasonable at present to selectively measure biomarkers in higher risk clinical situations, including no-reflow, side-branch occlusion, and prolonged peri-procedural haemodynamic instability, all conditions which preclude early or same-day discharge. PCI for acute infarction should be considered separately,

Table 7.1 Risk factors for access site bleeding

Patient related	Procedure related
Body mass; morbidly obese/underweight	High femoral arterial puncture
Female gender	Glycoprotein IIb/IIIa inhibitor use
Age >70 years	Multiple/difficult puncture
Marked hypertension	Prolonged procedure time
	Intra-aortic balloon pump use

where routine post-procedural biomarker measurement gives important clinical information regarding the timing of the acute event along with infarct size, and has prognostic importance.

The practicalities of routine biomarker measurement following PCI have become more difficult because an increasing proportion of PCI is performed for the treatment of patients with acute coronary syndromes, who will already have raised biomarkers pre-PCI. Interpreting post-PCI levels in this setting becomes very difficult and such investigations will not usually change management. Elective PCI is increasingly performed as a day-case procedure, adding to the practical difficulty of routine biomarker measurement.

Renal injury following PCI (see Chapter 27)

Contrast-induced nephropathy is most widely defined as a 25% increase in serum creatinine following PCI. The reported incidence of contrast-induced nephropathy (CIN) varies among studies, due to differences in definition and background risk of the study populations; in those at very high risk the incidence can be as high as 50%. It is of critical importance to identify those patients at higher risk of CIN since its development has important prognostic implications[(25)]. Patients at risk include those with pre-existing renal impairment, diabetics, and those receiving high volumes of peri-procedural contrast (>3mL/kg)[(26)]. In these higher-risk groups, prevention, in the form of adequate peri-procedural hydration, discontinuation of nephrotoxic drugs, and close attention to contrast loads during the intervention, are likely to be the most effective means of avoidance. Use of additional agents, such as N-acetylcysteine and sodium bicarbonate, have led to heterogeneous results in numerous studies but certainly appear to do little harm and are commonly used in addition to peri-procedural hydration in at-risk populations[(27–29)]. The type of contrast agent is also important. Ionic contrast agents have been replaced by low or iso-osmolar non-ionic solutions which are associated with less nephrotoxicity[(30)]. Whether iso-osmolar solutions have a further advantage over hypo-osmolar contrast agents in preventing contrast nephropathy remains less certain, although a recent meta-analysis of 16 randomized studies comparing these agents did show lower rates of CIN among high-risk populations and suggest that this more expensive agent should be targeted at higher-risk groups[(31)]. A reduction in the volume of contrast used can also be achieved by careful planning, and staging of multivessel intervention.

Currently biomarkers other than creatinine are being studied as alternatives to detecting CIN. The concentration of cystatin C (protein derived from nucleated cells) and neutrophil gelatinase-associated lipocalin (NGAL), have promise as measures of glomerular filtration rate (GFR) and may allow earlier identification of CIN following PCI[(32)].

Clinical features and treatment of CIN

CIN usually occurs within the first 12–24h following contrast exposure, and in the majority of cases will recover within 3–5 days. Additional insults during the PCI procedure, such as prolonged hypotension or pre-procedural nephrotoxic drugs, can complicate the picture with the development of acute tubular necrosis and oliguric renal failure. Most therapy is supportive with a small proportion requiring permanent renal replacement (<1% in an unselected population but clearly much increased in the high-risk groups); this is most likely to occur in those with a baseline creatinine of more than 350mmol/L. The development of late or prolonged renal impairment may suggest renal atheroembolic disease, and may be associated with other evidence of embolic complications. Although rare (<2% of biopsy specimens) it often follows a prolonged course with limited recovery of renal function[(33)].

Management of high-risk patients following PCI

As the nature of interventional cardiology changes and the average age of patients investigated/treated invasively increases, PCI has become increasingly complex. Technological advances have facilitated the treatment of more difficult lesions and decreased the risk of these procedures. PCI can be 'high risk' because of: 1) *patient factors* (e.g. advanced age, morbid obesity, comorbidity); 2) *anatomical/coronary factors* (e.g. left main stem, bifurcation, calcified disease); and 3) *clinical factors* (e.g. ST-elevation myocardial infarction [STEMI], cardiogenic shock), or a combination of two or more of these factors. Patients who have undergone high-risk PCI with any of these features need close attention in the period following revascularization because early identification and prompt management of complications have a significant impact on survival. The increasing use of primary PCI in the setting of STEMI has led to a change in coronary care, with patients bypassing smaller district hospitals as they are rapidly transferred to larger 'Heart Attack Centres'. These larger centres should have more sophisticated catheter laboratories and high-dependency areas, capable of multiorgan support with easy access to ventilation, haemofiltration, left ventricular support, and cardiac surgery.

Intra-aortic balloon pump (see Chapter 17)

Intra-aortic counter-pulsation decreases LV afterload and increases coronary flow, thus conferring stabilizing haemodynamic benefits on the 'high risk' PCI patient. Intra-aortic balloon pumps (IABPs) can be placed prior to high-risk PCI to provide haemodynamic support during the procedure and in this case, the contralateral femoral artery is used (or the right femoral artery in radial cases). However, the IABP is also often used as a supportive measure when haemodynamic instability occurs during PCI. In this situation, the patient can be left with the IABP in the femoral access site of the PCI. Clearly, puncturing both femoral arteries increases the chance of a vascular complication. Most operators advocate 'sheathless' introduction to minimize the size of the femoral arteriotomy.

Post PCI, such patients should be cared for by nurses experienced with this form of haemodynamic support. In some centres, perfusionists still advise about the optimal settings on the IABP console. Close observation of the femoral artery site will identify any bleeding, which often occurs around the IABP and can be managed with pressure dressings and occasional judicious use of light compression with devices such as the FemoStop®. Caution should be taken with this approach, however, as trauma/thrombosis of the femoral artery is possible.

Adjunctive pharmacology is often challenging in this setting. Patients with IABPs *in situ* should be anticoagulated and intravenous unfractionated heparin is the most common agent used. Robust antiplatelet regimens (e.g. glycoprotein IIb/IIIa inhibitors) are often used in high-risk PCI which increase bleeding risk and when this is the case, commencement of heparin can be delayed by 12–24h. With contemporary IABP devices the risk of thrombosis is low and bleeding is more of a threat. As a general principle, and in order to minimize risks of vascular compromise and sepsis, the length of time that the IABP is in place should be kept to a minimum.

Left ventricular assist devices

Left ventricular assist devices (LVADs) are becoming increasingly sophisticated and can be used when IABP support is not sufficient in high-risk PCI. The principal problem with these devices has been the size and the consequent risk of vascular complications. The Impella Recover® is showing promise as an adjunct to high-risk PCI with encouraging early studies and a suggestion that haemodynamic support may be superior to IABP[34]. Several trials are currently recruiting to address this question in more detail.

The key to successful management of patients with these devices is meticulous attention to the arterial access site and competence/experience in the use of the console. Such devices should only be used in units experienced in this form of haemodynamic support with adequately trained perfusion staff to maintain optimal console settings.

Care of the ventilated patient after PCI

The number of ventilated patients undergoing PCI is increasing with more widespread use of primary PCI as the preferred mode of revascularization in STEMI. In this clinical setting, cardiac arrest due to ventricular arrhythmia may lead to intubation/ventilation before arrival at the catheter laboratory or during primary PCI. The priority remains adequate and timely coronary reperfusion but neurological recovery can be difficult to predict. Successful management in this scenario depends on seamless communication between intensivists and cardiologists to jointly discuss difficult management issues which can include:

- Removal of arterial sheaths/IABPs/temporary pacing wires.
- The weaning of circulatory support.
- Adjunctive pharmacology (including the importance of continuous dual antiplatelet therapy).
- Frequent echocardiographic assessment in the haemodynamically unstable patient.
- Assessment of neurological status and end-of-life decisions.

Such patients benefit from a multidisciplinary approach and cannot be successfully or effectively managed without this.

Same-day discharge after PCI

Rationale of same-day discharge after PCI

Patients should not be kept in hospital longer than needed in terms of safety, psychosocial reasons, adequate mobilization, and patient comfort. In many tertiary centres with a busy PCI programme, insufficient bed capacity is an ongoing concern. Moreover, it seems obvious that shorter hospital stay will lead to significant cost reduction.

Early events after PCI

In order to determine whether same-day discharge after PCI is feasible and safe one should identify the events that might threaten the patient as well as the timing of occurrence of such events.

The possible events occurring early after PCI are: cardiac complications (unstable angina pectoris, myocardial infarction, pump failure, supra-ventricular and ventricular arrhythmias); non-cardiac complications, such as renal failure in certain high-risk patients, and bleeding complications (access-site related bleedings, and other sources of bleeding [e.g. gastrointestinal], and cerebral bleeding, including stroke).

Life-threatening arrhythmias, such as ventricular tachycardia or fibrillation, predominantly occur in the first minutes to hours after the onset of ischaemia and seldom occur later in the absence of failed PCI or pump failure.

Very little is known about the exact timing of events in the very early phase after initially successful PCI, as the literature mainly describes predictors of 30-day mortality. A practical score for risk stratification, that incorporates these predictors, could distinguish low-risk from high-risk patient groups, but is less helpful in the decision-making regarding when exactly the patient can be discharged.

Defining an acceptable incremental risk of same-day discharge is difficult; to minimize this, careful consideration is crucial and, if there is any doubt, the patient should not be discharged the same day.

In the early 1990s it was demonstrated that same-day discharge after balloon angioplasty using 6Fr catheters via the brachial approach was safe and feasible[35]. Patients were selected with a limited risk of events (stable angina pectoris, suitable, non-complex lesion morphology, a limited region at risk, and normal renal function). There was a post-PCI triage after 2h of observation close to the catheterization laboratory. Patients with a successful PCI, in the absence of dissection or acute occlusion, repeat PCI, or clinical signs of myocardial infarction, were triaged to outpatient treatment. During follow-up in the first 24h the clinical course in all patients was uneventful. These early observations are partly obsolete as major changes have been made in PCI with respect to devices and adjunctive medication. Stent implantation is associated with an improvement in both early and late outcomes, as compared with balloon angioplasty alone, predominantly as a result of a reduction in early vessel closure and late target-vessel revascularization. Kiemeneij and colleagues demonstrated that using careful selection criteria, outpatient transradial stent implantation was entirely safe[36].

In larger series from the same institution it could be confirmed that uneventful same-day discharge could be achieved in over 60% of all patients undergoing PCI[37,38].

Regarding drug treatment, the combination of aspirin, a thienopyridine (clopidogrel or prasugrel), a glycoprotein IIb/IIIa inhibitor (abciximab), or a direct thrombin inhibitor (bivaluridin) have improved early and late clinical outcomes after PCI, at the cost of an increased bleeding tendency[39,40]. A preferential use of the transradial approach using small-bore guiding catheters has been proposed to further decrease the incidence of access-site related bleeding[41,42]. Protocols with longer infusion of certain antithrombotic drugs after PCI will preclude same-day discharge.

It can be concluded that in patients with an optimal result after transradial PCI with stent-implantation, an uneventful 3–4-h observation period, and suitable social circumstances, same-day discharge is not only feasible and safe, but should be the preferred treatment in modern interventional cardiology.

Post-discharge care

Role of stress testing following PCI

There has been considerable debate regarding the utility of stress testing following PCI. If effective, post-procedural testing will identify the presence of clinically important restenosis and/or confirm the functional significance of residual disease following the index procedure. However, in low-risk subgroups, and particularly those with single vessel coronary artery disease (CAD), routine stress testing has little clinical use. Nevertheless, restenosis does remain a significant problem in specific subgroups and this underlies the current stance of the ACC, which does not recommend functional testing routinely, but suggests that this is reserved for 'high-risk' cohorts; diabetics, and those with multivessel or left main stem disease or impaired left ventricular function[43]. Exercise testing, myocardial perfusion imaging, stress echocardiography, and magnetic resonance imaging (MRI) stress perfusion imaging are all utilized with highly variable test performance among heterogeneous study populations.

Exercise testing following PCI

Exercise testing is routinely used but has low sensitivity and specificity, particularly in the presence of one-vessel disease, and this limits its clinical utility. The use of exercise testing is widespread[44], but it must be remembered that, despite the obvious limitations, this investigation provides important information regarding symptoms, exercise capacity, and cardiorespiratory fitness that remain very relevant to long-term prognosis. With the limitations of exercise, more sensitive forms of functional imaging offer distinct technical advantages but at higher cost which must be balanced with their undoubted clinical utility.

Myocardial perfusion imaging and stress echocardiography following PCI

The clinical utility of myocardial perfusion imaging (MPI) and stress echocardiography (both exercise and dobutamine) to identify restenosis has been shown to have a much higher sensitivity and specificity than exercise testing. In a meta-analysis of studies examining the three techniques from the era of balloon angioplasty, the sensitivity of exercise testing was 53% compared to 82% and 83% for stress echocardiography and MPI respectively[(42)]. Specificity was similar between all three modalities (approximately 80%). More limited data are available from the stent era, but those studies which have been performed suggest similar efficacy of both techniques. Stress MRI, using adenosine or dobutamine, is a potentially superior modality due to improved image quality, but both availability of the technique along with the study time (often over 1h) limit widespread use[(45)]. Choice of each particular imaging modality will depend largely on local expertise. Accuracy will also depend on the study population and patient characteristics.

Timing of non-invasive testing

Both the timing and application of non-invasive testing following PCI remains a hotly debated issue. Symptoms occurring in the first few days or weeks following PCI may be suggestive of subacute stent thrombosis and usually warrant early repeat angiography. Timing of functional testing largely depends upon the clinical indication, whether to assess the functional significance of residual disease or recurrent symptoms.

Early testing (within a few weeks)

Although clinically important restenosis is highly unlikely at such an early stage following intervention, functional testing may be of value in determining the significance of residual coronary disease and incomplete revascularization. This has particular relevance following primary PCI for STEMI but data are currently lacking. Very early stress testing in the days and weeks following intervention has previously been shown to give misleading results. Studies from the pre-stent era demonstrated sequential changes in perfusion studies and exercise tests, with early evidence of reversible ischaemia in the territory of the treated vessel that normalized over subsequent months[(46,47)]. It has been postulated that these early abnormalities are related to vessel trauma or coronary vasospasm early post procedure that improve with time, but it is also possible that the performance of balloon angioplasty itself may have contributed to these findings, with higher rates of untreated vessel dissection and vessel recoil. In general, the occurrence of significant or unstable symptoms early after PCI is suggestive of subacute thrombosis and warrants early angiography and re-intervention. This risk of thrombosis depends largely on the patient population and procedural complexity. In general, incidence varies according to the population, ranging from <1.5–3%[(48–50)]. Rates are higher following acute myocardial infarction, after treatment of bifurcation lesions or those with long segments of stent deployed. Incidence is also related to age and reduced left ventricular function[(49,50)].

Functional testing in the first few months

Recurrent symptoms suggestive of restenosis will usually occur within the first 6 months, although there is an incident rate between 6–12 months which should not be ignored[(51)]. Functional testing is useful for those patients with recurrent or atypical symptoms several months following PCI and it may also be useful following the coincidental finding of asymptomatic in-stent restenosis at the time of repeat angiography (e.g. during research). The more widespread use of functional testing following PCI is more controversial, and current guidelines do not support the use of routine stress testing for all following PCI, but favour a more selective approach. The ACC recommend routine stress testing post PCI in 'high-risk' subgroups including diabetics (due to the high incidence of silent ischaemia), those with decreased left ventricular function, multivessel CAD, and suboptimal PCI results[(43)]. The rationale for these recommendations stems from the bare metal stent era, where a positive functional test identified asymptomatic patients with an adverse long-term prognosis[(52)]; however the evidence base for this rests upon relatively small prospective studies and requires further evaluation in larger randomized studies. An algorithm for stress testing following PCI is shown in Fig. 7.1.

Surveillance coronary angiography

The use of routine surveillance angiography has primarily been advocated following left main stem PCI. Early studies noted an ominous proportion of patients who died unexpectedly in the first few months following the procedure, possibly due to aggressive, early in-stent restenosis and angiography has been recommended early

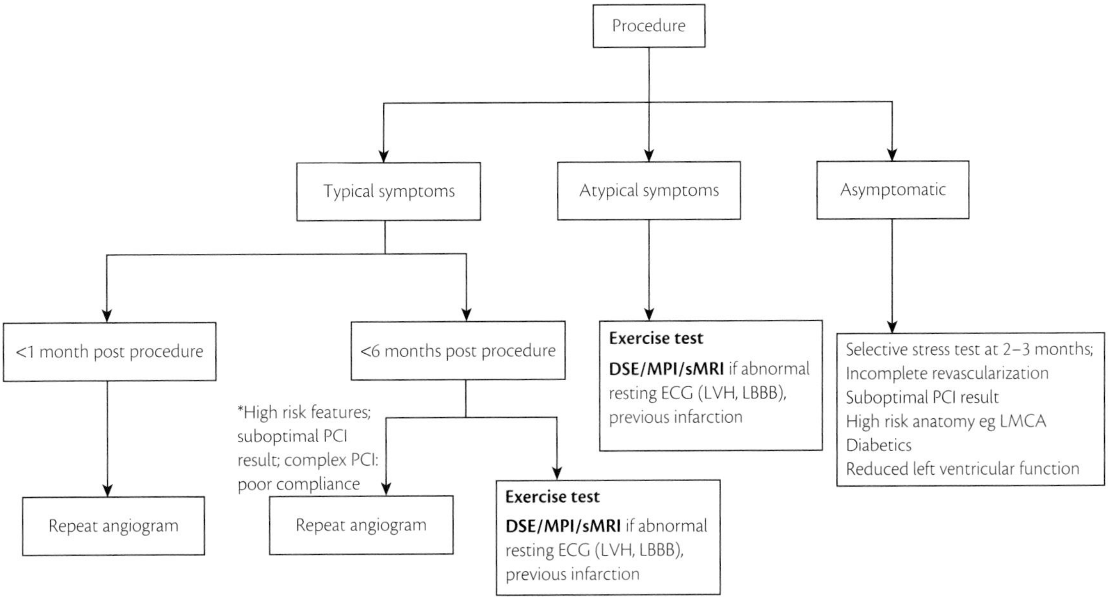

Fig. 7.1 Suggested algorithm for stress testing following PCI. LBBB, left bundle branch block; LMCA, left main coronary artery; LVH, left ventricular hypertrophy; MPI, myocardial perfusion imaging; sMRI, structural magnetic resonance imaging.

(at 3–6 months) to identify those at potential risk(53). However, surveillance angiography may expose an asymptomatic patient to the potential risk of an unnecessary invasive procedure. There are relatively little data in the literature to guide the interventional cardiologist but repeat surveillance angiography in this clinical setting remains a Class IIa recommendation in the ACC/AHA guidelines(24). Nevertheless, in the absence of symptoms it is entirely reasonable to obtain an appropriate functional test before proceeding to repeat invasive angiography. If anatomical information is required at serial follow-up, multislice cardiac computed tomography may be useful to exclude the development of in-stent restenosis in this, and other high risk patient subgroups(54).

Subsequent intervention: management of residual coronary disease

The management of residual coronary disease following the initial PCI procedure remains an important and unresolved dilemma for the interventional cardiologist. Multivessel disease is common in the population undergoing PCI, particularly in those who present with acute myocardial infarction, ranging from 40–71% in contemporary studies(55,56). The benefits of complete revascularization have been suggested by largely historical reports in the surgical literature, with most studies showing improved long-term outcome when compared to an incomplete procedure(57–59). Interpretation of the data is somewhat complicated; incomplete surgical revascularization may be due to the presence of extensive atherosclerotic disease with poor surgical targets, or ungrafted vessels may supply infarcted territories. These characteristics are associated with an adverse clinical outcome and may lead to considerable bias in these retrospective data. Furthermore, complete revascularization, even with a coronary artery bypass graft (CABG), can be difficult to achieve; in the recent SYNTAX (SYNergy between percutaneous coronary intervention with TAXus and cardiac surgery) study comparing three-vessel disease treated with either surgery or PCI, the rates of complete revascularization in either arm was surprisingly low: 63.2% in the surgical cohort compared to 56.7% in the PCI group(60). It is likely that this figure reflects the anatomic complexity of the patient population involved; in the older ARTS (Arterial Revascularization Therapies Study) trial 84.1% compared to 70.5% of patients treated with CABG and PCI respectively, received complete revascularization(61). There are few data regarding the benefits of complete revascularization in patients treated percutaneously, and most of the studies are observational in design, and the majority were performed in the pre-stent era (62–64). In general terms, these studies have failed to show a clear advantage of complete revascularization, although most were performed in the era of balloon angioplasty and are less likely to be relevant to current clinical practice. In the ARTS study, those patients who achieved complete revascularization had a lower 1-year event rate, an observation which was attributable to increased CABG in those who underwent incomplete revascularization[61]. In a large retrospective study of the New York registry, Hannan and colleagues demonstrated an adverse 1-year survival in those who had incomplete procedures, even after adjustment for baseline patient risk[64].In the single, small, randomized trial to date, no clinical benefit of complete revascularization was demonstrated, with similar event rates seen in both groups at 1 year[65]. Complete functional, rather than anatomical, revascularization is an attractive concept, and recent data from the FAME (Fractional Flow Reserve versus Angiography for Multivessel Evaluation) study has shown a clear clinical benefit for fractional flow reserve-guided revascularization in patients with multi-vessel disease[66].

The decision to undertake further PCI in order to achieve complete revascularization will continue to be made on an individual patient basis and will often depend on the clinical context. Following primary PCI for STEMI it is reasonable to treat significant residual coronary disease in order to achieve full revascularization, although the timing of this remains debatable. Ideally this should be done with evidence of ischaemia (via invasive or non-invasive means) and/or symptoms. It is likely that further data to guide us will emerge in the near future. Whether revascularization should be performed by surgical or percutaneous means will usually be determined by the extent and anatomical nature of the residual disease.

Conclusion

Careful management of the patient following PCI is essential to ensure immediate and long-term success. Early recognition of acute complications, particularly in high-risk subgroups, is essential if they are to be managed effectively. As well as immediate supportive care, it is also essential to ensure that the patient is treated in a holistic fashion, with close attention paid to risk factor management, secondary prevention, and appropriate management of residual coronary disease in order to maintain an optimal long-term outcome.

References

1. Hildick-Smith DJ, Khan ZI, Shapiro LM, *et al.* Occasional operator percutaneous brachial coronary angiography: first, do no harm. *Catheter Cardiovasc Interv* 2002; **57**:161–5.
2. Agostoni P, Biodi-Zoccai GG, de Benedictus ML, *et al.* Radial versus femoral approach for percutaneous diagnostic and interventional procedures; systematic overview and meta-analysis of randomised trials. *J Am Coll Cardiol* 2004; **44**:349–56.
3. Exaire JE, Tcheng JE, Dean J. *et al.* Closure devices and vascular complications among percutaneous coronary intervention patients receiving enoxaparin, glycoprotein IIb/IIIa inhibitors, and clopidogrel. *Catheter Cardiovasc Interv* 2005; **64**:369–72.
4. Applegate RJ, Rankin KM, Little WC, *et al.* Restick following initial AngioSeal® use. *Catheter Cardiovasc Interv* 2003; **58**:181–4.
5. Sanmartin M, Gomez M, Rumoroso JR, *et al.* Interruption of blood flow during compression and radial artery occlusion after transradial catheterization. *Catheter Cardiovasc Interv* 2007; **70**:185–9.
6. Hall IR, Lo TS, Nolan J. Deep vein thrombosis in the arm following transradial cardiac catheterization: an unusual complication related to hemostatic technique. *Catheter Cardiovasc Interv* 2004; **62**:346–8.
7. Dangas G, Mehran R, Kokolis S, *et al.* Vascular complications after percutaneous coronary interventions following hemostasis with manual compression versus arteriotomy closure devices. *J Am Coll Cardiol* 2001; **38**:638–641.
8. Berry C, Kelly J, Cobbe SM, *et al.* Comparison of femoral bleeding complications after coronary angiography versus percutaneous coronary intervention. *Am J Cardiol* 2004; **94**:361–3.
9. Yatskar L, Selzer F, Feit F, *et al.* Access site hematoma requiring blood transfusion predicts mortality in patients undergoing percutaneous coronary intervention: data from the National Heart, Lung, and Blood Institute dynamic registry. *Catheter Cardiovasc Interv* 2007; **69**: 961–6.
10. Kawamura A, Piemonte TC, Nesto RW, *et al.* Retroperitoneal haemorrhage from inferior epigastric artery: Value of femoral angiography for detection and Management. *Catheter Cardiovasc Interv* 2006; **68**:267–70.
11. Farouque HMO, Tremmel JA, Shabari FR, *et al.* Risk factors for the development of retroperitoneal hematoma after percutaneous coronary intervention in the era of glycoprotein IIb/IIIa inhibitors and vascular closure devices. *J Am Coll Cardiol* 2005; **45**:363–8
12. Kent KC, Moscucci M, Mansour KA, *et al.* Retroperitoneal hematoma after cardiac catheterization: prevalence, risk factors, and optimal management A prospective evaluation of surgically treated groin complications following percutaneous cardiac procedures. *J Vasc Surg* 1994; **20**:905–10.
13. Kinnaird TD, Stabile E, Mintz GS, *et al.* Incidence, predictors, and prognostic implications of bleeding and blood transfusion following percutaneous coronary interventions. *Am J Cardiol* 2003; **92**:930–5.

14. Rao SV, Eikelboom JA, Granger CB, *et al.* Bleeding and blood transfusion issues in patients with non-ST-segment elevation acute coronary syndromes. *Eur Heart J* 2007; **28**:1193–204.
15. Rao SV, Jollis JG, Harrington RA, *et al.* Relationship of blood transfusion and clinical outcomes in patients with acute coronary syndromes. *JAMA* 2004; **292**:1555 –62
16. Blankenship JC, Hellkamp AS, Aguirre FV, *et al.* Vascular access site complications after percutaneous coronary intervention with abciximab in the Evaluation of c7E3 for the Prevention of Ischemic Complications (EPIC) trial. *Am J Cardiol* 1998; **81**:36–40.
17. Manoukian SV, Feit F, Mehran R, *et al.* Impact of major bleeding on 30-Day mortality and clinical outcomes in patients with acute coronary syndromes: an analysis from the ACUITY trial. *J Am Coll Cardiol* 2007; **49**:1362 –8.
18. Nallamothu BK, Bates ER. Periprocedural myocardial infarction and mortality: causality versus association. *J Am Coll Cardiol* 2003; **42**:1412 –14.
19. EPIC Investigators. Use of a monoclonal antibody directed against the platelet glycoprotein IIb/IIIa receptor in high-risk coronary angioplasty. *N Engl J Med* 1994; **330**:956 –61.
20. Stone GW, Mehran R, Dangas G, *et al.* Differential impact on survival of electrocardiographic Q-wave versus enzymatic myocardial infarction after percutaneous intervention. *Circulation* 2001; **104**:642 –7
21. Jeremias A, Baim DS, Ho KK, *et al.* Differential mortality risk of postprocedural creatine kinase-MB elevation following successful versus unsuccessful stent procedures. *J Am Coll Cardiol* 2004; **44**(6):1210–14.
22. Califf RM, Abdelmeguid AE, Kuntz RE, *et al.* Myonecrosis after revascularization procedures. *J Am Coll Cardiol* 1998; **31**(2):241–51.
23. Prasad A, Rihal CS, Lennon RJ, *et al.* Significance of periprocedural myonecrosis on outcomes after percutaneous coronary intervention. An analysis of preintervention and postintervention troponin T levels in 5487 patients. *Circ Cardiovasc Intervent* 2008; **1**:10–19.
24. Smith SC Jr, Feldman TE, Hirshfeld JW Jr, *et al.* ACC/AHA/SCAI 2005 Guideline Update for Percutaneous Coronary Intervention—summary article: a report of the American College of Cardiology/American Heart Association Task Force on Practice Guidelines (ACC/AHA/SCAI Writing Committee to Update the 2001 Guidelines for Percutaneous Coronary Intervention). *Circulation* 2006; **113**:156–75.
25. Gruberg, L, Mintz, G, Mehran, R, *et al.* The prognostic implications of further renal function deterioration within 48h of interventional coronary procedures in patients with pre-existent chronic renal insufficiency. *J Am Coll* Cardiol 2000; **36**(5):1542–8.
26. McCullough PA, Adam A, Becker CR, *et al.* Risk prediction of contrast-induced nephropathy. *Am J Cardiol* 2006; **98**(Suppl):27K–36K.
27. Tepel M, Van der Giet M, Schwarzfeld C, *et al.* Prevention of radiographic-contrast-agent-induced reductions in renal function by acetylcysteine. *N Engl J Med* 2000; **343**:180–4.
28. Brar SS, Shen A Y-J, Jorgensen MB, *et al.* Sodium bicarbonate vs sodium chloride for the prevention of contrast medium-induced nephropathy in patients undergoing coronary angiography: a randomized trial. *JAMA* 2008; **300**(9):1038–46.
29. Briguori C, Airoldi F, D'Andrea D, *et al.* Renal insufficiency following contrast media administration trial (REMEDIAL): a randomized comparison of 3 preventive strategies. *Circulation* 2007; **115**:1211–17.
30. Lautin EM, Freeman NJ, Schoenfeld AH, *et al.* Radiocontrast-associated renal dysfunction: a comparison of lower-osmolality and conventional high-osmolality contrast media. *Am J Roentgenol* 1991; **157**(1):59–65.
31. McCullough PA, Bertrand ME, Brinker JA, *et al.* A meta-analysis of the renal safety of isosmolar iodixanol compared with low-osmolar contrast media. *J Am Coll Cardiol* 2006; **48**(4):692–9.
32. Bachorzewska-Gajewska H, Malyszko J, Sitniewska E, *et al.* Could neutrophil gelatinase-associated lipocalin and cystatin C predict the development of contrast-induced nephropathy after percutaneous coronary interventions in patients with stable angina and normal serum creatinine values? *Kidney Blood Press Res* 2007; **30**: 408–15.
33. Rudnick MR, Berns JS, Cohen RM, *et al.* Nephrotoxic risks of renal angiography: contrast-media associated nephrotoxicity and atheroembolism — A critical review. *Am J Kidney Dis* 1994; **24**(4):713–27.
34. Seyfarth M, Sibbing D, Bauer I, *et al.* A randomized clinical trial to evaluate the safety and efficacy of a percutaneous left ventricular assist device versus intra-aortic balloon pumping for treatment of cardiogenic shock caused by myocardial infarction. *J Am Coll Cardiol* 2008; **52**(19):1584–8.
35. Laarman GJ, Kiemeneij F, van der Wieken LR, *et al.* A pilot study of coronary angioplasty in outpatients. *Br Heart J* 1994; **72**:12–15.
36. Kiemeneij F, Laarman GJ, Slagboom T, *et al.* Outpatient coronary stent implantation. *J Am Coll Cardiol* 1997; **29**:323–7.
37. Slagboom T, Kiemeneij F, Laarman GJ, *et al.* Actual outpatient PTCA: results of the OUTCLAS pilot study. *Catheter Cardiovasc Interv* 2001; **53**:204–8.
38. Slagboom T, Kiemeneij F, Laarman GJ, *et al.* Outpatient coronary angioplasty: feasible and safe. *Catheter Cardiovasc Interv* 2005; **64**:421–7.
39. Stone GW, Brent T, McLaurin, *et al.* Bivalirudin for patients with acute coronary syndromes. *N Engl J Med* 2006; **355**:2203–16.
40. Wiviott SD, Braunwald E, McCabe CH, *et al.* Prasugrel versus clopidogrel in patients with acute coronary syndromes. *N Engl J Med* 2007; **357**:2001–15.
41. Agostoni P, Biondi-Zoccai GG, de Benedictis ML. Radial versus femoral approach for percutaneous coronary diagnostic and interventional procedures; systematic

overview and meta-analysis of randomized trials. *Am J Cardiol* 2004; **44**:349–56.

42. Jolly S, Amlani S, Hamon M. Radial versus femoral access for coronary angiography or intervention and the impact on major bleeding and ischemic events: a systematic review and meta-analysis of randomized trials. *Am Heart J* 2009; **157**:132–40.
43. ACC/AHA 2002 Guideline Update for Exercise Testing: Summary Article: A Report of the American College of Cardiology/American Heart Association Task Force on Practice Guidelines (Committee to Update the 1997 Exercise Testing Guidelines). *Circulation* 2002; **106**: 1883–92.
44. Eisenberg MJ, Schechter D, Lefkovits J, *et al.* Use of routine functional testing after percutaneous transluminal coronary angioplasty: results from the ROSETTA Registry. *Am Heart J* 2001; **141**(5):837–41.
45. Nagel, E, Lehmkuhl, HB, Bocksch, W, *et al.* Noninvasive diagnosis of ischemia-induced wall motion abnormalities with the use of high-dose dobutamine stress MRI: Comparison with dobutamine stress echocardiography. *Circulation* 1999; **99**:763–70.
46. Scholl JM, Chaitman BR, David PR, *et al.* Exercise electrocardiography and myocardial scintigraphy in the serial evaluation of the results of percutaneous transluminal coronary angioplasty. *Circulation* 1982; **66**:380–90.
47. Manyari DE, Knudtson M, Kloiber R, *et al.* Sequential thallium-201 myocardial perfusion studies after successful percutaneous transluminal coronary artery angioplasty: delayed resolution of exercise-induced scintigraphic abnormalities. *Circulation* 1988; **77**:86–95.
48. Schuhlen H, Kastrati A, Pache J, *et al.* Incidence of thrombotic occlusion and major adverse cardiac events between two and four weeks after coronary stent placement: analysis of 5,678 patients with a four-week ticlopidine regimen. *J Am Coll Cardiol* 2001; **37**(8): 2066–73.
49. Stone GW, Witzenbichler B, Guagliumi G, *et al.* Bivalirudin during primary PCI in acute myocardial infarction. *N Engl J Med* 2008; **358**:2218–30.
50. Mak KH, Belli G, Ellis SG, *et al.* Subacute stent thrombosis: evolving issues and current concepts. *J Am Coll Cardiol* 1996; **27**(2):494–503.
51. Cutlip DE, Chauhan MS, Baim DS, *et al.* Clinical restenosis after coronary stenting: perspectives from multicenter clinical trials. *J Am Coll Cardiol* 2002; **40**(12):2082–9.
52. Giedd KN, Bergmann SR. Myocardial perfusion imaging following percutaneous coronary intervention: the importance of restenosis, disease progression, and directed reintervention. *J Am Coll Cardiol* 2004; **43**(3):328–36.
53. Tan WA, Tamai H, Park SJ, *et al.*; ULTIMA Investigators. Long-term clinical outcomes after unprotected left main trunk percutaneous revascularization in 279 patients. *Circulation* 2001; **104**(14):1609–14.
54. Van Mieghem CA, Cademartiri F, Mollet NR, *et al.* Multislice spiral computed tomography for the evaluation of stent patency after left main coronary artery stenting: a comparison with conventional coronary angiography and intravascular ultrasound. *Circulation* 2006; **114**(7):645–53.
55. Andersen HR, Nielsen TT, Rasmussen K, *et al.* A comparison of coronary angioplasty with fibrinolytic therapy in acute myocardial infarction. *N Engl J Med* 2003; **349**:733–42.
56. Zijlstra F, Beukema WP, van't Hof AW, *et al.* Randomized comparison of primary coronary angioplasty with thrombolytic therapy in low risk patients with acute myocardial infarction. *J Am Coll Cardiol* 1997; **29**(5): 908–12.
57. Jones EL, Craver JM, Guyton RA, *et al.* Importance of complete revascularization in performance of the coronary bypass operation. *Am J Cardiol* 1993; **51**:7–12.
58. Bell MR, Gersh BJ, Schaff HV, *et al.* Effect of completeness of revascularization on long-term outcome of patients with drug-eluting stent in multivessel disease. A report from the coronary artery surgery study (CASS) registry. *Circulation* 1992; **86**:446–57.
59. Kleisli T, Cheng W, Jacobs MJ, *et al.* In the current era, complete revascularization improves survival after coronary artery bypass surgery. *J Thorac Cardiovasc Surg* 2005; **129**:1283–91.
60. Serruys PW, Morice MC, Kappetein AP, *et al.*; SYNTAX Investigators. Percutaneous coronary intervention versus coronary-artery bypass grafting for severe coronary artery disease. *N Engl J Med* 2009; **360**(10):961–72.
61. Van den Brand MJ, Rensing BJ, *et al.* The effect of completeness of revascularization on event-free survival at one year in the ARTS trial. *J Am Coll Cardiol* 2002; **19**:559–64.
62. Bourassa MG, Yeh W, Holubkov R, *et al.*; for the Investigators of the NHLBI PTCA Registry. Long-term outcome of patients with incomplete vs. complete revascularization after multivessel PTCA: A report from the NHLBI Registry. *Eur Heart J* 1998; **19**:103–11.
63. McLellan CS, Ghali WA, Labinaz M, *et al.* Association between completeness of percutaneous coronary revascularization and postprocedure outcomes. *Am Heart J* 2005; **150**:800–6.
64. Hannan EL, Racz M, Holmes DR, *et al.* Impact of completeness of percutaneous coronary intervention revascularization on long-term outcomes in the stent era. *Circulation* 2006; **113**:2406–12.
65. Ijsselmuiden AJ, Ezechiels J, Westendorp IC, *et al.* Complete versus culprit vessel percutaneous coronary intervention in multivessel disease: A randomized comparison. *Am Heart J* 2004; **148**:467–74.
66. Tonino PA, De Bruyne B, Pijls NH, *et al.*; FAME Study Investigators. Fractional flow reserve versus angiography for guiding percutaneous coronary intervention. *N Engl J Med* 2009; **360**(3):213–24.

SECTION 2

Percutaneous coronary intervention-related imaging

CHAPTER 8

Angiography: indications and limitations

David Adlam and Bernard D. Prendergast

Angiography

The technique of coronary angiography provides and records an instantaneous real-time fluoroscopic assessment of coronary luminal anatomy. It is used both as a diagnostic tool for the assessment of coronary disease and to provide the images which guide percutaneous coronary intervention (PCI). The procedure involves the injection of a bolus of radio-opaque contrast agent through a catheter placed in the coronary ostium, thereby delineating the luminal structure of the epicardial coronary arteries when viewed using simultaneous fluoroscopy. Angiography allows the identification of areas of intimal atheroma which impinge on the vessel lumen with potential to impair blood flow. In conjunction with clinical assessment and non-invasive investigation, the number, extent, location, and distribution of these coronary stenoses are pivotal in determining the optimal revascularization strategy, whether by surgical or percutaneous techniques.

Indications for coronary angiography

Coronary angiography is currently a prerequisite for coronary revascularization and is also useful for clarification in cases where diagnostic uncertainty exists but revascularization is not planned and in the assessment of other forms of cardiac disease (e.g. valve disease or cardiomyopathy). However, given the small but demonstrable risks of diagnostic angiography (see later sections) and radiation exposure (see Chapter 5), careful selection of patients is essential.

Stable chest pain syndromes

Formal clinical assessment is the first and most important aspect of assessing patients with possible ischaemic heart disease and provides a powerful predictor of future coronary events[1]. The sensitivity and specificity of all subsequent investigations depends on the pretest probability of coronary disease established during this process. Careful assessment of the clinical history (including evaluation of coronary risk factors), a thorough physical examination and baseline investigation, including blood tests (full blood count, renal profile, clotting if relevant, fasting glucose and cholesterol, and haemoglobin A1c), and an electrocardiogram (ECG), should be undertaken. These assessments may suggest an alternative aetiology for the patient's symptoms which may be either cardiac (e.g. valvular heart disease) or non-cardiac (e.g. chest or gastrointestinal disease). This assessment is also an opportunity to obtain crucial baseline data on relevant comorbidities prior to subsequent coronary angiography. A clinical finding of peripheral vascular disease, for example, may be relevant to the future route of arterial access. Baseline haemoglobin (see Chapter 3) and renal function (see Chapter 27) both impact on subsequent procedural risk.

Rapid access chest pain clinics

Referral of stable patients for coronary angiography may be initiated in a conventional out-patient setting. However, a model of early assessment (within 2 weeks) by either a doctor or specialist nurse and physiologist in a 'rapid access chest pain clinic' has been validated as an improved screening tool for new patients referred from primary care with possible angina. In a study of 6496 patients referred to such a clinic, those given a diagnosis of angina had a 16.5% (14.9–18.3%) rate of cardiac events over 3 years follow-up, compared with a rate of 2.7% (2.3–3.3%) in those with a diagnosis of non-cardiac chest pain. This difference would be magnified if those with a diagnosis of angina were left untreated. However, despite their effectiveness, this study also illustrates that these clinics remain an imperfect screening tool with a significant number of events occurring in those patients not attributed a diagnosis of cardiac disease[2,3].

Further investigations prior to coronary angiography

In patients with stable symptoms, decision-making on whom may benefit from diagnostic angiography may be enhanced using one or more of a number of non-invasive tests. These enhance the pretest probability of significant stenotic coronary disease prior to angiography and, more importantly, identify patients with a low probability of significant coronary disease and good prognosis who are probably best managed medically without recourse to angiography. The investigations also provide important functional information on the extent and anatomical location of myocardial ischaemia which may guide future revascularization strategies.

Exercise electrocardiography

Physical exercise increases myocardial oxygen demand and may provoke myocardial ischaemia. A supervised period of incremental exercise either on a bicycle or treadmill is safe (risk of death or myocardial infarction [MI] 1:2500 tests[4]). Continuous monitoring of patient symptoms, blood pressure, heart rate, and ECG changes is required during exercise and the recovery period. A normal exercise ECG confers a low risk of death during prolonged follow-up, whilst a positive test (Fig. 8.1)

A

B

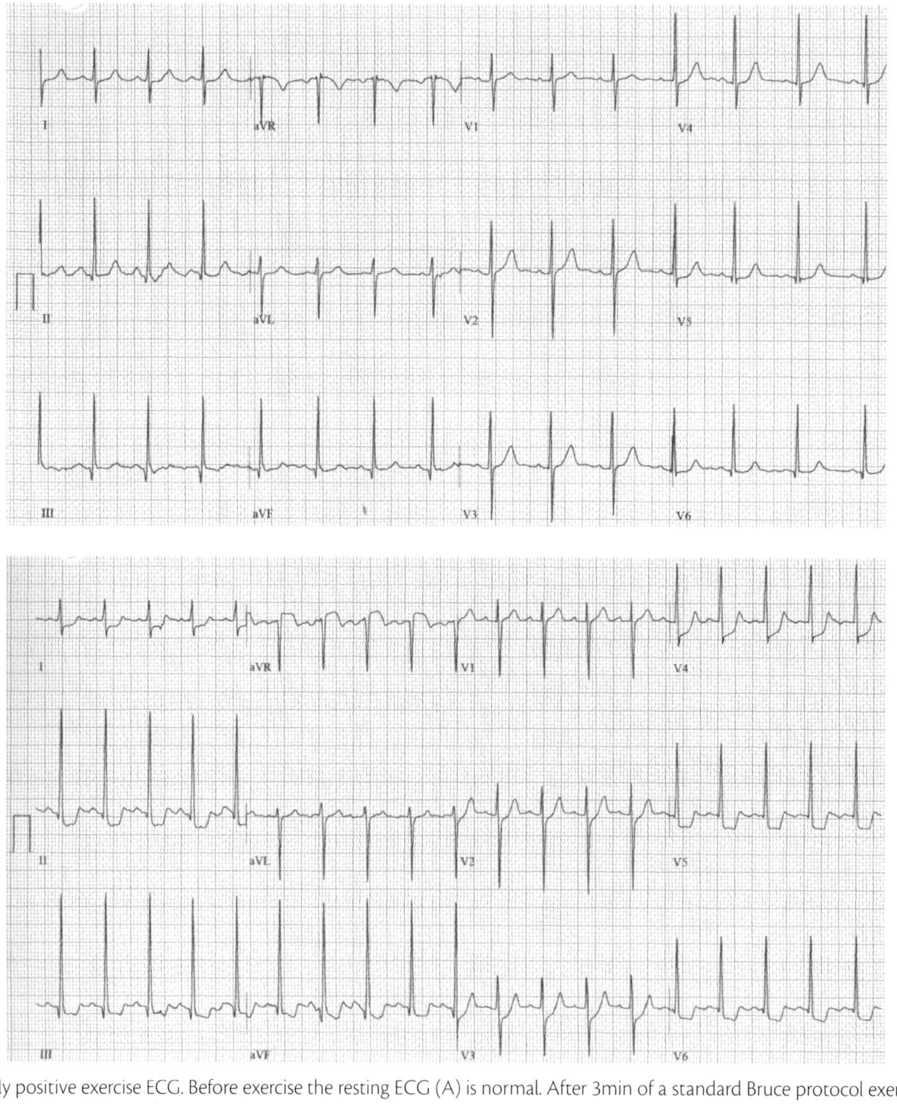

Fig. 8.1 Strongly positive exercise ECG. Before exercise the resting ECG (A) is normal. After 3min of a standard Bruce protocol exercise test there is marked inferolateral down-sloping ST depression (B).

is an independent predictor of adverse outcome[5,6]. The sensitivity and specificity of exercise testing depends on the pretest probability of coronary disease. Tables 8.1a and 8.1b illustrate how exercise testing alters the probability of significant coronary disease in symptomatic patients[7]. Although of inferior sensitivity and specificity to functional stress imaging, the exercise ECG is of low cost and relatively simple to perform and interpret. It therefore remains the most popular screening test for stable coronary disease and is

Table 8.1a Exercise testing and the pre-test probability of underlying coronary artery disease[7]

Age (years)	Typical angina		Atypical angina		Non-anginal chest pain	
	Male	Female	Male	Female	Male	Female
30–39	69.7 ± 3.2	25.8 ± 6.6	21.8 ± 2.4	4.2 ± 1.3	5.2 ± 0.8	0.8 ± 0.3
40–49	87.3 ± 1.0	55.2 ± 6.5	46.1 ± 1.8	13.3 ± 2.9	14.1 ± 1.3	2.8 ± 0.7
50–59	92.0 ± 0.6	79.4 ± 2.4	58.9 ± 1.5	32.4 ± 3.0	21.5 ± 1.7	8.4 ± 1.2
60–69	94.3 ± 0.4	90.1 ± 1.0	67.1 ± 1.3	54.4 ± 2.4	28.1 ± 1.9	18.6 ± 1.9

Table 8.1b Exercise testing and the post-test probability of underlying coronary artery disease [7]

Age (years)	ST depression (mV)	Typical angina		Atypical angina		Non-anginal chest pain		Asymptomatic	
		Male	Female	Male	Female	Male	Female	Male	Female
30–39	0.00–0.04	25	7	6	1	1	<1	<1	<1
	0.05–0.09	68	24	21	3	5	1	2	4
	0.10–0.14	83	42	38	9	10	2	4	<1
	0.15–0.19	91	59	55	15	19	3	7	1
	0.20–0.24	96	79	76	33	39	8	18	3
	>0.25	99	93	92	63	68	24	43	11
40–49	0.00–0.04	61	22	16	3	4	1	1	<1
	0.05–0.09	86	53	44	12	13	3	5	1
	0.10–0.14	94	72	64	25	26	6	11	2
	0.15–0.19	97	84	78	39	41	11	20	4
	0.20–0.24	99	93	91	63	65	24	39	10
	>0.25	>99	98	97	86	87	53	69	28
50–59	0.00–0.04	73	47	25	10	6	2	2	1
	0.05–0.09	91	78	57	31	20	8	9	3
	0.10–0.14	96	89	75	50	37	16	19	7
	0.15–0.19	98	94	86	67	53	28	31	12
	0.20–0.24	99	98	94	84	75	50	54	27
	>0.25	>99	99	98	95	91	78	81	56
60–69	0.00–0.04	79	69	32	21	8	5	3	2
	0.05–0.09	94	90	65	52	26	17	11	7
	0.10–0.14	97	95	81	72	45	33	23	15
	0.15–0.19	99	98	89	83	62	49	37	25
	0.20–0.24	99	99	96	93	81	72	61	47
	>0.25	>99	99	99	98	94	90	85	76

routinely used as part of the assessment protocol in rapid access chest pain clinics.

Functional stress imaging

Imaging during either physical or pharmacological stress can further enhance the positive and negative predictive value of assessment prior to coronary angiography. Physical stress can be induced using treadmill or bicycle exercise. Pharmacological stress can be used in patients who are physically unable to exercise to the required level. The latter approach involves incremental dose infusions of agents which increase myocardial blood flow and/or oxygen demand. Dobutamine (a positive inotropic and chronotropic agent) may be used alone or in combination with atropine[(8)] and dipyridamole or adenosine (vasodilator agents) are frequent alternatives—all have a good safety record with low complication rates[(9–11)]. These investigations have improved sensitivity and specificity for the detection of coronary disease[(12)] and can be particularly useful in patients with baseline ECG changes (e.g. left bundle branch block) which challenge interpretation during exercise[(13,14)]. Functional imaging may also be used to identify areas of hibernating myocardium in patients with ischaemic cardiomyopathy where revascularization holds the potential to improve contractile function[(15)]. The major disadvantage is the relative time, expertise, and expense required to perform these investigations and interpret their results.

Stress echocardiography

Echocardiography allows the assessment of myocardial thickening during left ventricular systole—endocardial definition may be further enhanced by use of echocontrast agents[(16–18)]. Myocardial infarction leads to permanent regional wall motion abnormalities whereas myocardial ischaemia may lead to reversible impairment of regional wall contraction. The location of these changes in myocardial thickening will depend on the coronary territory affected. For example, ischaemia or infarction in the left anterior descending (LAD) coronary artery may lead to abnormalities in the anteroseptal myocardium whereas the inferior wall will be affected if the right coronary artery (RCA) is involved. Stress echocardiography involves the assessment of regional wall motion during a period of physical or pharmacological stress. Comparison is made between baseline regional contraction and that during moderate and peak stress with differences indicating coronary ischaemia (Fig. 8.2). Stress echocardiography is both sensitive and specific for the detection of coronary disease[(12,19,20)] and has long-term prognostic value[(20–23)]. However, the technique is inherently limited by the quality of the available sonographic windows and some patients with inadequate image quality will be unsuitable for this investigation. Even in optimal circumstances, the rapid acquisition of good quality images following a period of peak exercise requires considerable experience and expertise.

Nuclear imaging

The uptake of blood-soluble radioisotopes by the myocardium is perfusion dependent; infarcted myocardium will not take up radiotracer whilst ischaemic myocardium may take up tracer at rest but not during physical or pharmacological stress. Thallium 201 or technetium 99m radiotracers are imaged using ECG-gated single photon emission computed tomography (SPECT) before and after exercise or pharmacological stress (Fig. 8.3). Comparison of the images demonstrates

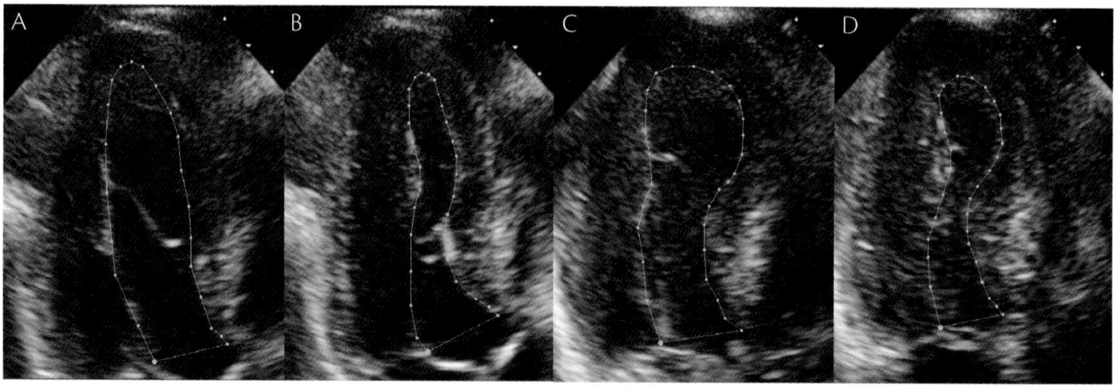

Fig. 8.2 Positive stress echocardiogram. Apical three-chamber view at rest in systole (A) and diastole (B) showing normal contraction and at peak stress in systole (C) and diastole (D) showing impaired anteroapical function consistent with a left anterior descending coronary lesion. Images courtesy of Dr Jim Newton.

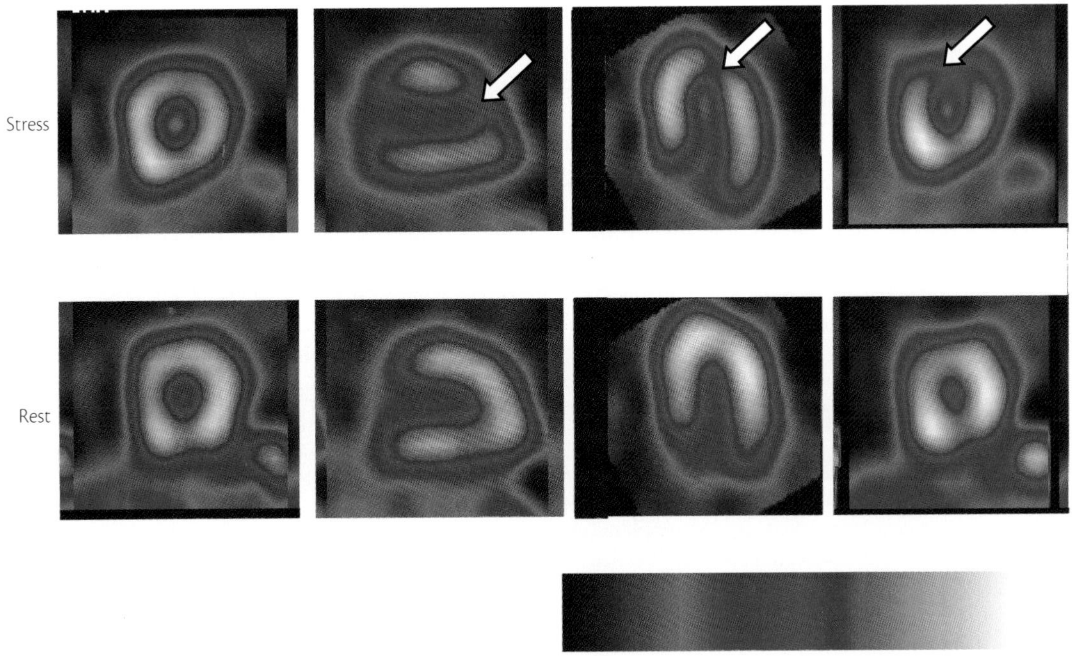

Fig. 8.3 Positive nuclear perfusion study demonstrating distal anterior and apical reversible ischaemia (arrowed) consistent with a severe stenosis of the mid-distal left anterior descending coronary artery. Images courtesy of Dr Nik Sabharwal.

areas of infarction or ischaemia and provides an assessment of overall myocardial function. Nuclear perfusion imaging has a high sensitivity and specificity for the detection of significant coronary artery disease(24) and is a reliable predictor of prognosis(25,26). It may be used as a primary diagnostic tool in patients who are unable to perform an exercise ECG and for those in whom baseline ECG abnormalities render interpretation difficult. It is also useful in patients whose exercise ECG is non-diagnostic, those with intermediate outcome, and when the result does not match the pretest probability(27). Futhermore, this technique can be used in patients with established coronary disease to establish the functional and prognostic importance of coronary lesions prior to revascularization(27). The main specific limitation is the expertise required for image interpretation and handling of radioisotopes.

Cross sectional imaging

Magnetic resonance imaging (MRI). Cardiac magnetic resonance pharmacological stress imaging can provide an assessment of changes in both regional contractile motion and myocardial perfusion(28,29). It also has a greater consistency of image quality in comparison with stress echocardiography(30). Although not yet widely used for the de novo assessment of chest pain syndromes, cardiac MRI is increasingly used in patients with complex coronary artery disease when questions of potential regional myocardial viability determine revascularization strategy. Cardiac MRI is discussed in more detail in Chapter 13.

Cardiac computed tomography (CT). There have been recent rapid technological advances in the use of CT to assess coronary artery disease. The upgrade from 16- to 64-slice scanning has enabled greater spatial resolution allowing more detailed assessment of coronary structure and disease. This has enabled the use of CT to assess unusual coronary anatomy(31) and increasingly to investigate the presence or absence of atheromatous coronary disease. CT has reasonable positive predictive value for the assessment of stenoses in proximal and larger calibre coronary vessels, such as vein grafts. It also has high negative predictive value (>96%) and its greatest current use is the non-invasive exclusion of significant coronary disease(32). This approach has been validated in patients with a low probability of coronary artery disease prior to valve surgery. Limitations in the universal use of cardiac CT as the primary diagnostic tool for coronary disease include difficulties in the assessment of smaller calibre vessels, the challenges of artefact from coronary calcification, and the assessment of in-stent disease. However, with continued development CT may ultimately supersede angiography as the primary diagnostic tool. Cardiac CT is discussed in more detail in Chapter 12.

Acute coronary syndromes

The selection of patients with an acute coronary syndrome for angiography and possible revascularization requires an assessment of the balance of risks—those of an adverse outcome if the patient is managed medically compared with the risks and outcome of coronary angiography and subsequent revascularization. Detailed consideration is beyond the scope of this chapter and this topic is discussed in detail in Chapters 15 and 16.

Risks of coronary angiography

Coronary angiography is a low-risk procedure. However, as with any invasive technique it is associated with occasional serious adverse events. A clear explanation of these risks prior to the procedure is a vital aspect of informed patient consent[33].

In a multicentre study of 211 645 diagnostic angiograms in the 1990s, the complication rate was 0.74%, with a mortality of 0.07%[34]. Specific complications and their incidence are listed in Table 8.2. Temporal trends during the decade of this study demonstrated progressive reduction in rates of complication and mortality, suggesting that improvements in angiographic techniques have a positive impact on outcome. Since publication of this dataset there have been further refinements, including the greater use of smaller calibre catheters and increased use of the radial approach. These developments may further reduce the rate of complications during and following coronary angiography[35].

When considering procedural risk it is important to appreciate the interaction of factors specific to an individual patient. For example, the risk of coronary angiography in an octogenarian arteriopath with known cerebrovascular and peripheral vascular disease may greatly exceed those presented in Table 8.2. Predictors of major complications during diagnostic cardiac catheterization identified in a multivariate analysis of 58 332 procedures are shown in Tables 8.3a and 8.3b[36].

Complications related to arterial access, contrast nephropathy, and PCI are addressed elsewhere (Chapters, 4, 27 and Section 3) and the important issue of radiation protection is discussed in Chapter 5.

Table 8.2 The incidence of complications associated with diagnostic coronary angiography

All adult diagnostic angiography N = 211 645	Complication (%) 1560 (0.74%)	Death (%) 155 (0.073%)
Allergy	53 (0.025%)	0
Arrhythmia	533 (0.25%)	18 (0.0085%)
Cerebrovascular accident	137 (0.065%)	8 (0.0038%)
Coronary dissection	71 (0.034%)	6 (0.0028%)
Haemodynamic collapse	94 (0.044%)	29 (0.014%)
Intramyocardial injection of contrast	16 (0.0075%)	0
Ischaemia	178 (0.084%)	74 (0.035%)
Myocardial infarction	12 (0.0057%)	5 (0.0024%)
Vascular	335 (0.16%)	7 (0.0033%)
Miscellaneous	25 (0.012%)	5 (0.0024%)
Unknown	86 (0.041%)	3 (0.0014%)

Management of patients prior to coronary angiography

Patients in whom the pretest probability of coronary disease is high should be initiated on appropriate medical therapy (aspirin, lipid-lowering agents, and anti-anginal therapy—usually including a beta-blocker) prior to coronary angiography. If PCI is planned as a possible follow-on procedure in conjunction with diagnostic angiography, a loading dose of clopidogrel should be followed by daily maintenance doses in the run-up to the procedure. Non-pharmacological interventions such as smoking cessation and lifestyle modification advice are also appropriate. The routine management of patients before and after PCI is discussed in Chapter 7.

Practical aspects of coronary angiography

The catheter laboratory team

Successful coronary angiography (and indeed all coronary procedures) requires a dedicated and highly specialist team. At minimum, this team consists of: an operator, who performs the procedure; a catheter lab nurse; responsible for administration of drugs to the patient and (usually) as a scrubbed assistant to the operator; a radiographer, responsible for the fluoroscopy equipment; and a physiologist, responsible for monitoring the ECG and cardiac pressures during the procedure. A schematic representation of the layout of a typical catheter laboratory and position of the team members is shown in Fig. 8.4.

Table 8.3a Univariate predictors of major complications of diagnostic angiography

Variable	OR (95% CI)	Variable	OR (95% CI)
Age (>60 years)	1.33 (1.12–1.89)	S/P thrombolysis	1.02 (0.57–1.81)
Gender (M/F)	0.97 (0.82–1.16)	S/P PTCA	0.65 (0.46–1.04)
NYHA Class I	1.0	S/P CABG	0.16 (0.90–1.50)
Class II	1.05 (0.86–1.29)	Diabetes	1.45 (1.17–1.80)
Class III	1.02 (0.85–1.23)	Hypertension	1.57 (1.33–1.85)
Class IV	1.58 (1.32–1.89)	Renal insufficiency	1.93 (1.30–2.85)
Previous catheter	0.94 (0.78–1.12)	Dialysis	2.15 (0.95–4.88)
Out-/in-patient	0.81 (0.67–0.98)	Shock	3.52 (2.04–6.07)
Coronary artery disease	1.25 (0.99–1.57)	Acute MI (<24h)	0.52 (0.19–1.39)
Valcular heart disease	1.19 (0.83–1.71)	Moribund	12.9 (4.95–33.8)
Cardiomyopathy	0.45 (0.20–1.01)	Unstable angina	1.43 (1.19–1.71)
Acute MI (<14 days)	1.28 (0.95–1.71)	Congestive heart failure	1.67 (1.26–2.20)
Mitral valve disease	1.59 (1.18–2.15)	Aortic valve disease	1.67 (1.20–2.32)

CABG, coronary artery bypass graft; CI, confidence interval; F, female; M, male; MI, myocardial infarction; NYHA, New York Heart Association; OR, odds ratio; PTCA, percutaneous transluminal coronary angioplasty; S/P, status post.

Table 8.3b Multivariate predictors of major complications of diagnostic angiography

Variable	Coefficient	OR (95% CI)
Moribund	−1.902	10.22 (3.77–27.76)
NYHA Class:	−0.151	
Class I		1.00
Class II		1.15 (0.94–1.4)
Class III		1.32 (0.92–1.51)
Class IV		1.52 (1.16–1.74)
Hypertension	−0.375	1.45 (1.22–1.73)
Shock	−1.086	6.52 (4.18 – 10.18)
Aortic valve disease	−0.356	2.72 (2.02 – 3.66)
Out-/in-patient	0.336	0.63 (0.52–0.76)
Renal insufficiency	−0.431	3.30 (2.39–4.55)
Unstable angina	−0.244	1.42 (1.16–1.74)
Mitral valve disease	−0.301	2.33 (1.76–3.08)
Acute MI (<24h)	0.975	4.03 (2.61–6.21)
Congestive heart failure	−0.319	2.22 (1.71–2.90)
Cardiomyopathy	0.787	3.29 (3.23–4.86)

CI, confidence interval; MI, myocardial infarction; NYHA, New York Heart Association; OR, odds ratio.

Monitoring during coronary angiography

Throughout the procedure, the patient is monitored continuously for changes in ECG and oxygen saturations. Blood pressure is transduced from the inserted sheath or catheters. Local rather than general anaesthesia is usually used and intravenous sedation may be administered. This allows continuous assessment of patient symptoms during the procedure. Full resuscitation facilities are always available in any catheter laboratory and access to an intra-aortic balloon pump is desirable should haemodynamic complications arise.

Vascular access

There are three established routes of vascular access for coronary angiography: femoral, radial, and brachial. A detailed discussion of their relative merits is presented in Chapter 4.

Seldinger technique

Many aspects of both coronary angiography and subsequent coronary intervention make use of the fundamentals of the Seldinger technique. This involves the passage of an appropriately thin-calibre guide wire into and along a vessel. By over-riding this guide wire, larger-calibre catheters (or other equipment) can be safely guided along the wire into the desired position (see Fig. 8.5).

During a coronary angiogram, the first Seldinger process is the insertion of a sheath into the selected

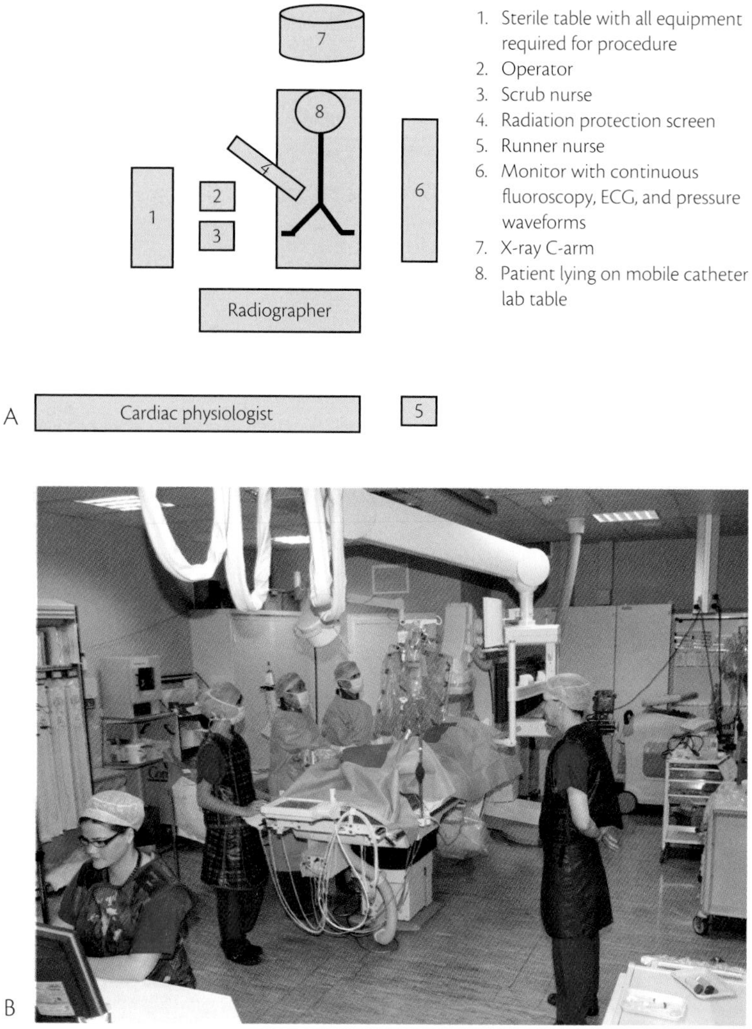

Fig. 8.4 A) Schematic representation of the catheter laboratory layout. B) The catheter lab team

access artery. Following puncture with a cannula, a guide wire is passed into the artery and advanced smoothly, with or without fluoroscopic guidance. The needle is then removed and an arterial sheath of appropriate calibre is passed over the guide wire into the arterial lumen. Finally, the guide wire is withdrawn and the sheath left in position.

For diagnostic angiography, 4, 5, or 6 French diameter catheters are commonly used (1 French = 1/3mm). More complex intervention procedures may require larger diameter catheters and hence larger calibre sheaths. Specialist sheaths are available for radial access and longer sheaths may be useful in the presence of iliofemoral tortuosity.

Catheter passage into the aortic root

Once the sheath is *in situ*, a guide wire is passed into the descending aorta. The angiography catheter is then passed onto the guide wire and both catheter and wire are advanced under fluoroscopic screening until the guide-wire tip is positioned in the ascending aorta. The wire position is then fixed to prevent further movement, the catheter advanced over its tip, and the guide wire withdrawn.

Passage of the guide wire within the aorta may be difficult. From the femoral route, iliofemoral atheroma or tortuosity may hinder advancement and this may be detected by resistance to free guide-wire manipulation.

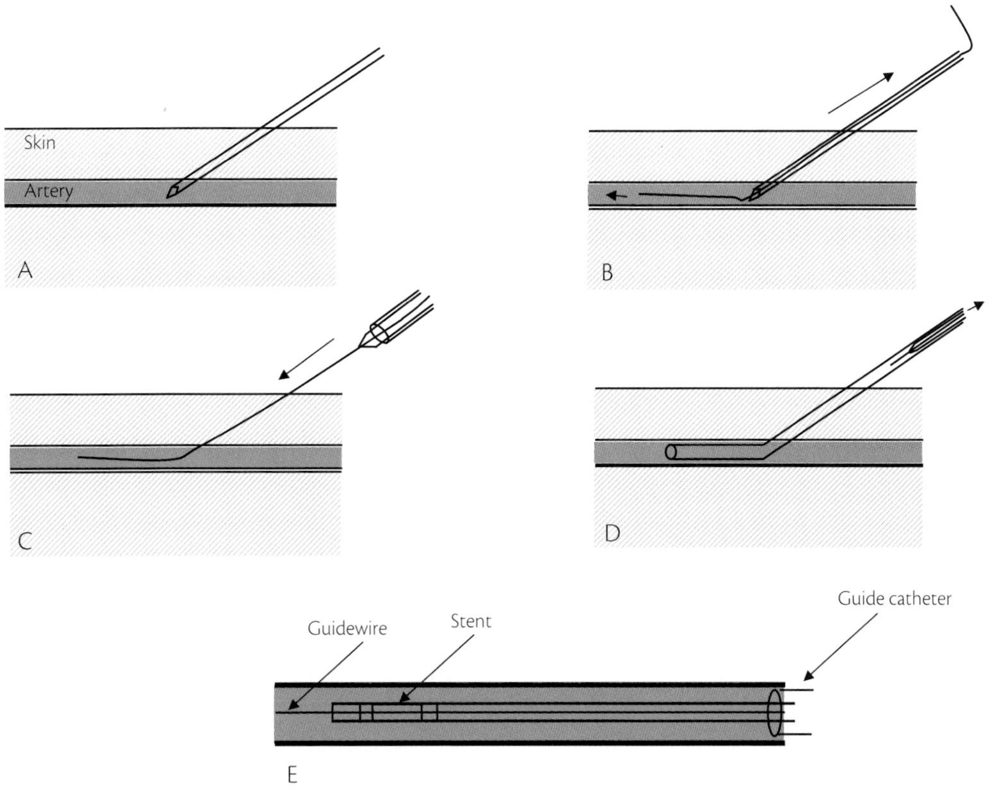

Fig. 8.5 The Seldinger technique. A) A cannula is introduced into the arterial lumen. B) A guide wire is then passed through the needle into the vessel lumen and the needle is removed (C). D) A sheath mounted on a dilator is railroaded over the guide wire and passed into the vessel lumen. E) The dilator and guide wire are then removed. A guide wire passed from a guide catheter into a coronary artery can be used in a similar way to railroad a stent mounted on a deployment balloon into the correct position for deployment.

In these circumstances, direct fluoroscopy may be used to identify the position of the wire tip. Careful passage of a catheter to the point of resistance with subsequent contrast injection may allow visualization of the arterial lumen and identification of the cause of obstruction (Fig. 8.6). If passage with a standard 0.038-inch 150cm J wire is not possible, a hydrophilic wire (e.g. Turumo®) may be useful in finding the luminal route. For atheroma or tortuosity confined to the iliac system, a long sheath may be used to protect and straighten this area and improve catheter torque. Following such challenging guide-wire passage into the aortic root, a longer (260cm) 'exchange' wire may be used during subsequent catheter exchanges. The extra length allows the tip of the wire to be fixed by the operator in the aortic root during catheter exchanges and prevents repeated guide-wire passage (with potential injury) through difficult or potentially diseased areas of the peripheral arterial system.

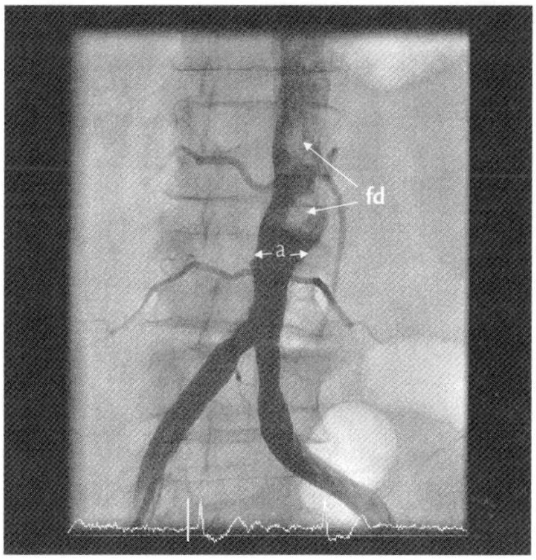

Fig. 8.6 Aortofemoral angiogram taken using a long sheath positioned in the right femoral artery. A standard guide wire would not easily pass through the distal descending aorta. Both a small aneurysmal area (a) and filling defect (fd) are seen indicating severe atherosclerotic disease. A Turumo® wire was passed through the diseased area and the case completed using a long exchange wire.

The radial approach offers similar and additional challenges. The incidence of arterial spasm may be reduced by using a single arterial puncture and reducing catheter manipulation to a minimum. Spasm may be treated with intra-arterial vasodilators (often administered prophylactically), adequate analgesia, and sedation. Vascular tortuosity may be overcome using a hydrophilic guide wire and subsequent exchange wire. If the guide wire preferentially enters the descending aorta from the brachiocephalic trunk, a carefully timed inspiration is often effective in redirecting the advancing guide wire into the aortic root. Patients undergoing radial angiography are routinely heparinized to maintain radial artery patency. Radial angiography and PCI are discussed in detail in Chapter 4.

Coronary anatomy: normal variants

Usual coronary anatomy consists of two coronary ostia, one in the left coronary sinus and the other in the right coronary sinus. The left main stem (LMS) arises from the left coronary ostium and bifurcates into the left anterior descending (LAD) and circumflex (Cx) coronary arteries. The right coronary artery (RCA) arises from the right coronary ostium.

Dominance

The posterior descending coronary artery (PDA) arises from the Cx in 10% of subjects (left dominant) and from the RCA in 70% (right dominant). The remaining 20% of subjects are said to have codominant supply to this territory from both the Cx and RCA.

Variations in coronary ostia

The most common variation is the separate origin of LAD and Cx vessels. In these patients there is no LMS but instead the LAD and Cx arise from separate ostia. Selective intubation of each origin is required during angiography (Fig. 8.7).

Other variations include ectopic origins of the coronary arteries and common ostia. These are rare but can pose challenges during angiography with particular reference to catheter selection. Rarely, aberrant coronary anatomy may be associated with an increased risk of sudden death or symptomatic ischaemia as a result of external arterial compression by the great vessels.

Catheter selection

The catheters used in coronary angiography are preshaped to fit the aortic root and coronary ostia (Fig. 8.8). Different sizes and shapes may be selected depending on the anatomy of the aortic root and location of the coronary ostia.

Catheter engagement

The coronary ostia are engaged by careful advancement and torque of the appropriate catheter and this is a critical moment during any coronary procedure. Several potential serious complications may occur at this time:

Coronary dissection

Intubation of the coronary ostium can rarely disrupt the vessel wall with resultant dissection (Fig. 8.9). This disastrous complication is most likely to occur in the presence of pre-existing ostial disease and may result from poorly controlled ostial intubation, especially with a catheter which is malaligned or undersized. Subsequent high-pressure contrast injection into a catheter whose tip is angulated into the ostial vessel wall is potentially catastrophic as an extending dissection flap can obstruct

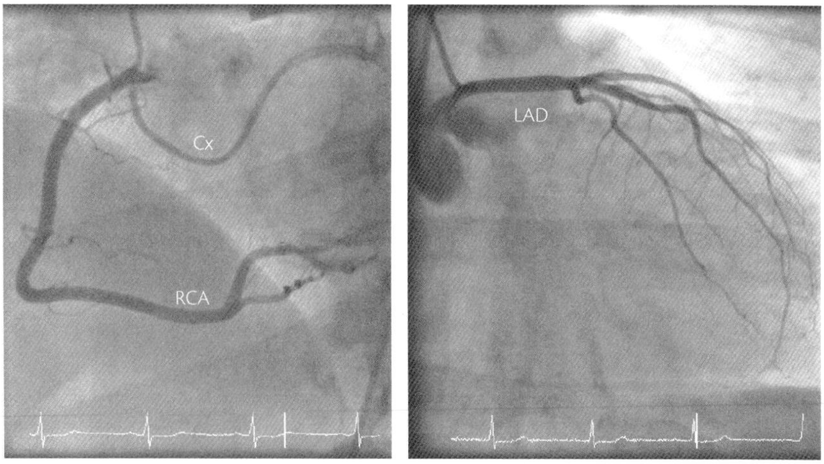

Fig. 8.7 An aberrant circumflex coronary artery. In this case, the circumflex (Cx) arises from the right coronary sinus close to the right coronary artery (RCA). The left coronary injection shows only the left anterior descending system (LAD) giving the typical appearance of an abnormally long left main stem.

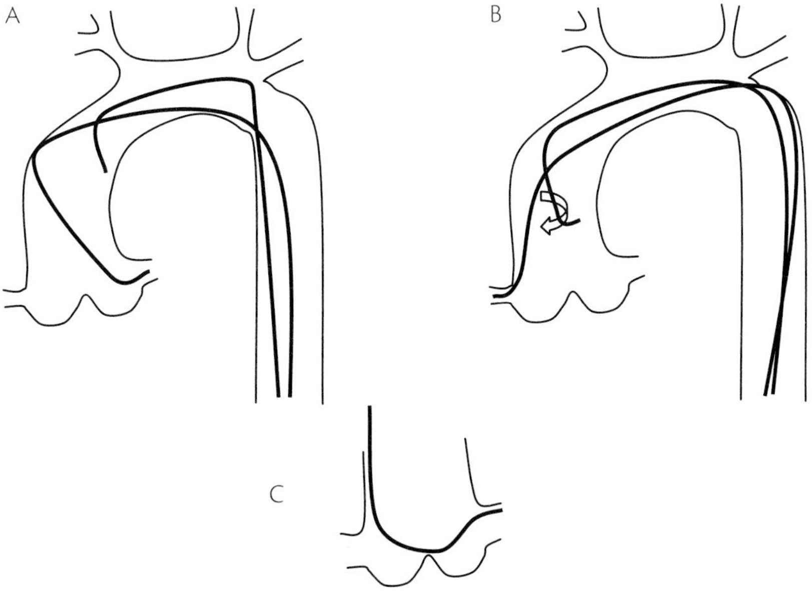

Fig. 8.8 Positioning and shape of catheters within the aortic root. A) The Judkins left 4 catheter is shaped to enter the left coronary ostium. B) The Judkins right coronary catheter requires careful clockwise rotation prior to engagement of the right coronary ostium. C). The Amplatz catheter is shaped differently and sits across the aortic root.

luminal flow and may progress to aortic root dissection or perforation.

Pressure damping

If there is significant ostial coronary disease (Fig. 8.10) (or simply a small-calibre artery), coronary intubation may effectively abolish blood flow in that vessel. This is usually immediately apparent by loss of arterial pressure upon engagement. Subsequent contrast injection will reveal the extent of ostial disease usually with little back flow of contrast into the aortic root. Even a short period of catheter-mediated obstruction of coronary flow may lead to significant ischaemia with risk of arrhythmia. In this context, the catheter must be left

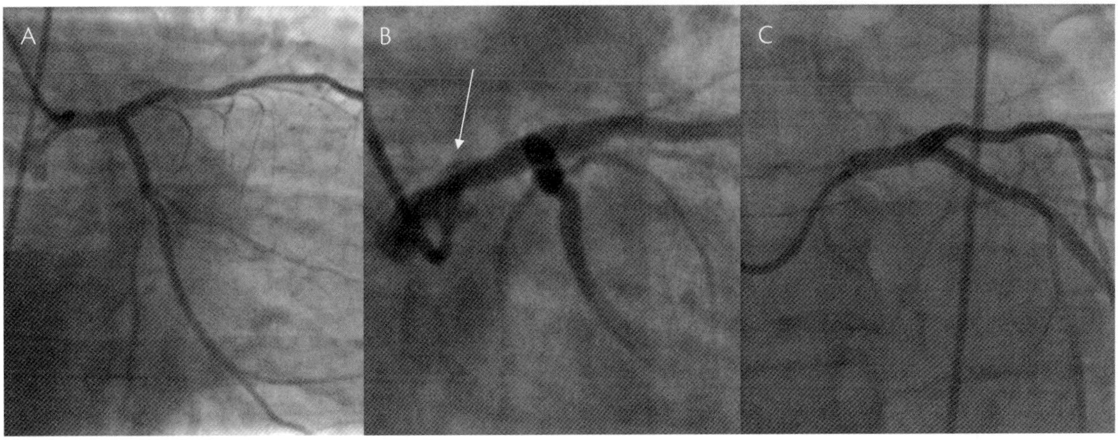

Fig. 8.9 Catheter-induced left main stem dissection (arrow). A) Initial left coronary angiogram obtained using a Judkins shaped catheter. The catheter tip is not coaxial but directed upwards into the wall of the left main stem. B) Injection of contrast during angiography leads to extravasation of contrast into an intimal dissection (arrow). C) This case was managed conservatively. Subsequent angiography (this time with an Amplatzer shaped catheter) confirmed complete healing of the dissection flap.

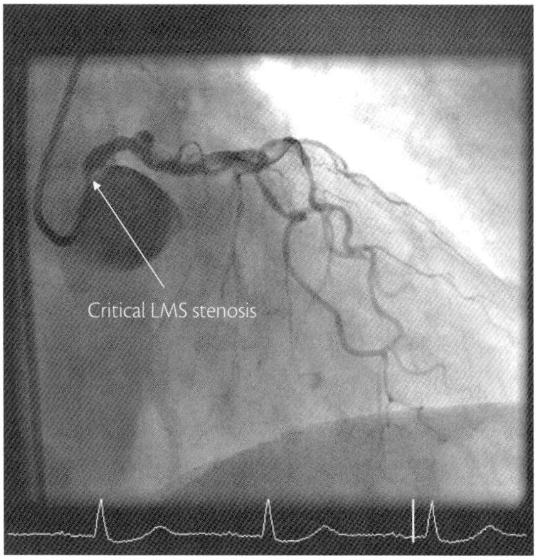

Fig. 8.10 Critical ostial left main stem disease. Upon engagement of the Judkins left 4 diagnostic catheter there was severe pressure damping.

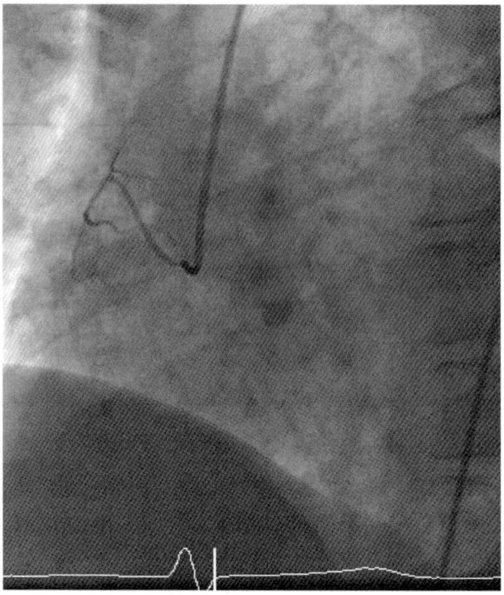

Fig. 8.11 Conus injection during right coronary intubation.

engaged for a minimal period to ensure rapid restoration of coronary perfusion.

Conal injection and ventricular arrhythmia

Special additional care must be taken following intubation of the right coronary ostium. Depending on the relative angles of the catheter tip and proximal vessel, it is possible for the catheter tip to selectively enter the conus branch (Fig. 8.11). This is often, but not always, heralded by pressure damping and subsequent injection of contrast can induce ventricular arrhythmia. Similar problems may arise following injection of an excessive volume of contrast into a small RCA. For this reason, injection of a small test shot of contrast is recommended following intubation and exclusion of pressure damping to ensure correct positioning.

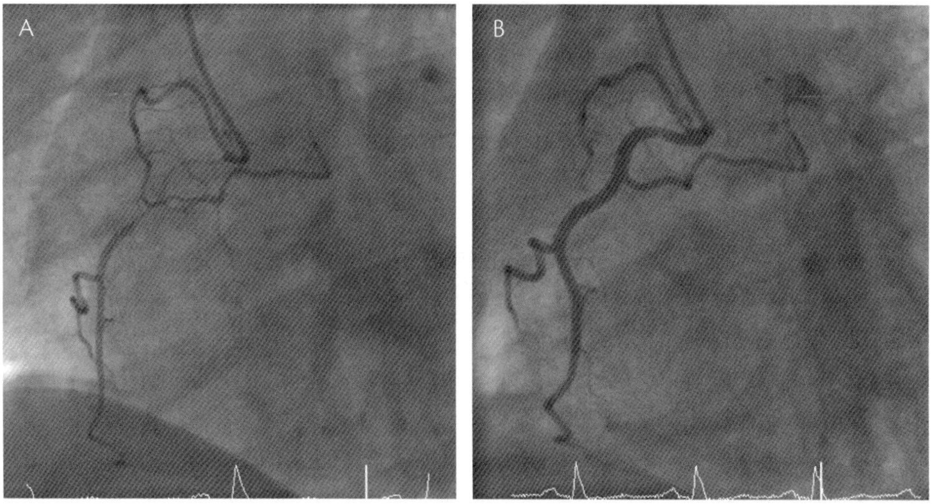

Fig. 8.12 Severe spasm in the proximal right coronary artery. Right coronary angiogram before (A) and after (B) injection of intracoronary nitrate.

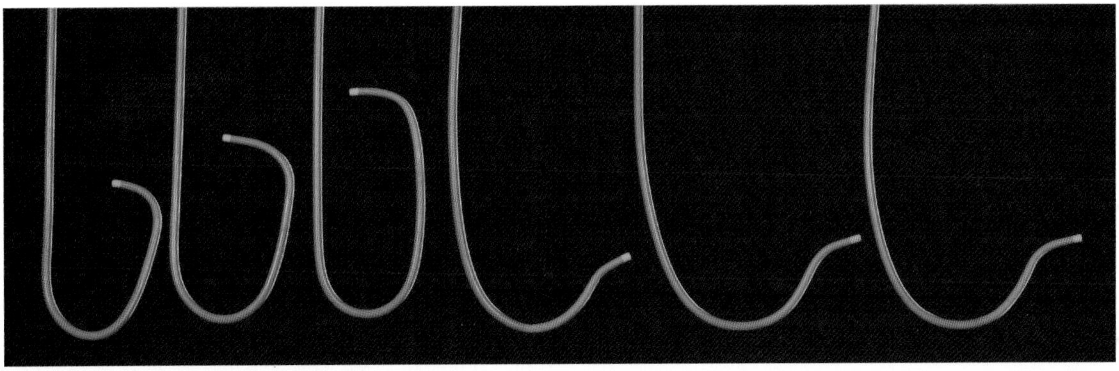

Fig. 8.13 Catheters for intubation of the left coronary artery. From left to right; Judkins left 3.5, 4, 5, Amplatz left 1, 1.5, 2.

Coronary spasm

Coronary arteries are not simply a passive conduit for blood but have a reactive smooth muscle media which can alter vessel calibre. Focal areas of coronary muscle 'spasm' can be provoked by catheter or guidewire contact and may also occur spontaneously with resultant angina and even MI. However, provocation testing at angiography with ergonovine or acetylcholine is now rarely performed. Areas of coronary spasm can appear angiographically similar to stenotic atheromatous lesions but will usually resolve with an intracoronary bolus of nitrate vasodilator (Fig. 8.12). It is important to distinguish spasm from disease as there is little evidence that percutaneous intervention to areas of spasm is a useful therapeutic strategy[37].

Catheters for the left coronary ostium

Engagement of the left coronary ostium is usually performed in the postero-anterior (PA) or left anterior oblique projection (LAO, see below). The diagnostic catheters most commonly used are the Judkins left catheters (Fig. 8.13). Larger aortic roots generally require a broader hooked section at the catheter tip and alternatives include the Amplatz catheters (Fig. 8.13).

Catheters for the right coronary ostium

Engagement of the right coronary ostium is usually performed in the LAO projection. Following location of the catheter in the aortic root, gentle clockwise rotation is used to engage the ostium. Judkins right catheters are commonly used with the 3DRC (Williams) catheter a popular alternative. A number of other shapes are available for difficult ostial locations (Fig. 8.14).

Catheters for saphenous vein grafts

The location of vein graft ostia is highly variable according to surgical technique and aortic root anatomy. In general, right coronary vein grafts can be accessed with a Judkins right 4, right coronary vein graft, multipurpose or Sones catheters (Fig. 8.15A). Left coronary vein grafts can be intubated using a Judkins right 4, left coronary vein graft or Amplatz catheter (Fig. 8.15B). Location of vein graft ostia may be facilitated by aortography (see below), although undue dependence on this approach should be avoided since patent grafts are not always identified.

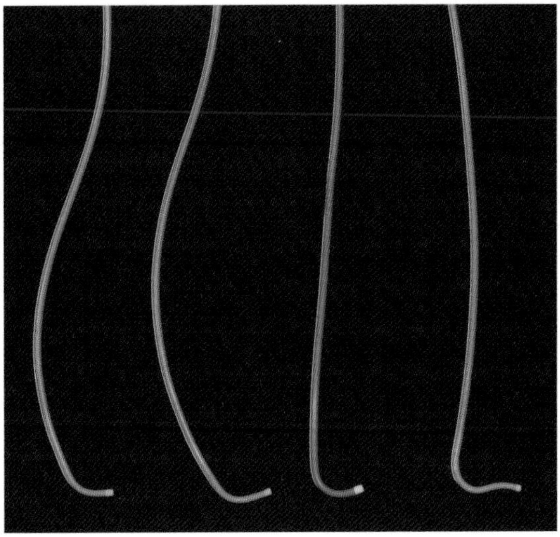

Fig. 8.14 Catheters for right coronary intubation. From left to right; Judkins right 3.5 and 4, 3DRC (Williams), Amplatz right modified.

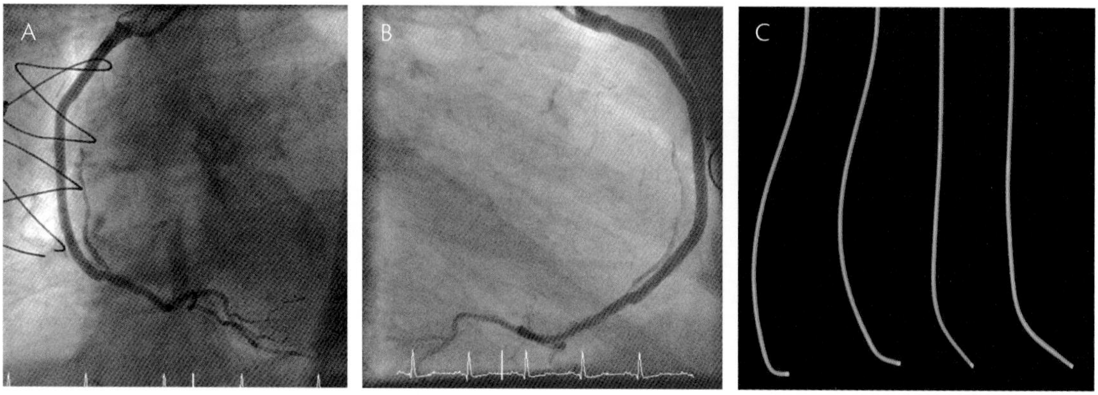

Fig. 8.15A A) and B) Right coronary vein graft angiography using two orthogonal views. C) Catheters for intubation of the right coronary vein graft. From left to right; Judkins right 4, right coronary bypass catheter, Multipurpose 1 catheter, Sones 1 catheter.

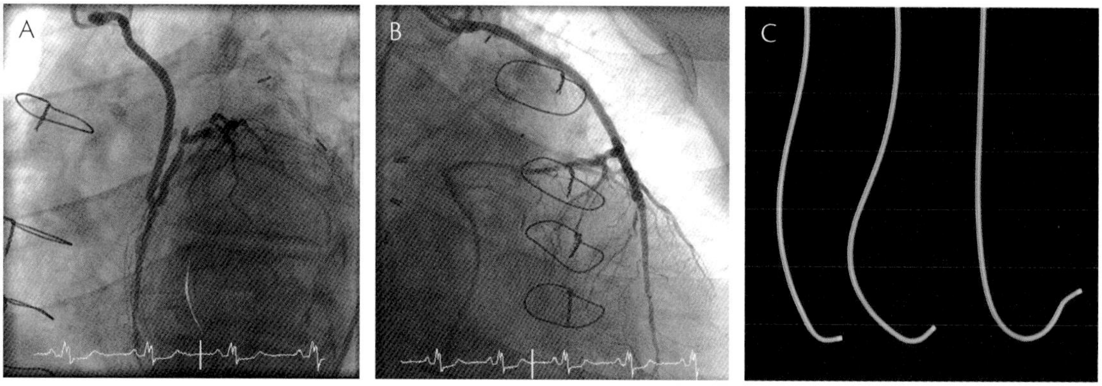

Fig. 8.15B A) and B) Saphenous vein graft to the left anterior descending coronary artery in two orthogonal views. C) Catheters for intubation of left coronary vein grafts. From left to right; Judkins right 4, left coronary bypass catheter, Amplatz left 1 catheter.

Catheters for the left internal mammary artery

The left internal mammary artery (LIMA) is the most common arterial conduit used for surgical revascularization—the right internal mammary artery (RIMA) is more rarely used. The LIMA is accessed by passage of a Judkins right 4 or dedicated LIMA catheter from the aortic arch into the left subclavian artery (Fig. 8.16). A non-selective injection is often adequate to visualize the LIMA and the territory it supplies and selective engagement carries a small risk of ostial dissection. Simultaneous inflation of a left arm blood pressure cuff to suprasystolic pressure may improve LIMA visualization during non-selective angiography. LIMA grafts which are difficult to access are more easily approached from the left radial route.

Radial catheters

The standard catheters used in femoral angiography may also be used when the radial route is employed. There are also an increasing number of specific catheters designed for the radial approach (Fig. 8.17) which allow sequential intubation of both left and right coronary ostia without the need for catheter exchange.

Fundamentals of fluoroscopy: limitations of angiography

It is important to appreciate that the image produced during coronary angiography is a two-dimensional representation of a three-dimensional structure. i.e. the coronary arteries are in reality running a complex course around the epicardial surface of the heart rather than lying in a single imaging plane perpendicular to the angle of projection (as appears on the viewing screen). This understanding is fundamental to the production of an adequate series of coronary angiographic images and critical to the use of fluoroscopy to guide PCI procedures. A series of images must be obtained in

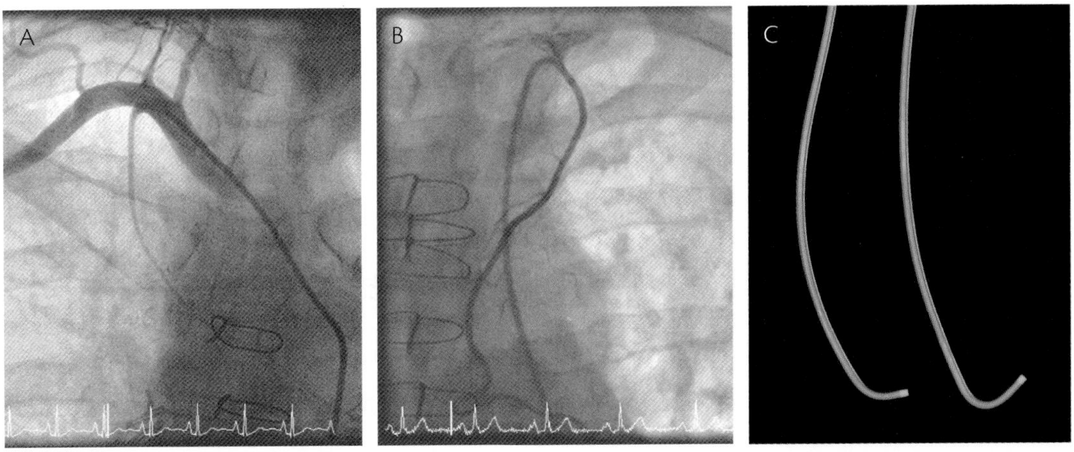

Fig. 8.16 Right internal mammary (RIMA) (A) and left internal mammary (LIMA) (B) angiography. C) Catheters used to intubate mammary arteries. From left to right; Judkins right 4 catheter, LIMA catheter.

which all segments of the coronary arteries are adequately visualized in at least two orthogonal projections. Common pitfalls are as follows:

Overlapping coronary arteries

Coronary arteries which lie at different depths in the imaging plane will appear as overlapping vessels. Overlapping segments have the potential to conceal potentially important areas of disease and may confuse the operator as to the relationship between branch vessels and the major epicardial coronary arteries (Fig. 8.18). During the acquisition of an angiographic series, great care must be taken to ensure that all overlapping segments have been adequately demonstrated. As well as overlapping vessels, the contrast-filled catheter will also overlap the coronary arteries in some projections and care should be taken to ensure this does not conceal an area of important disease (Fig. 8.19).

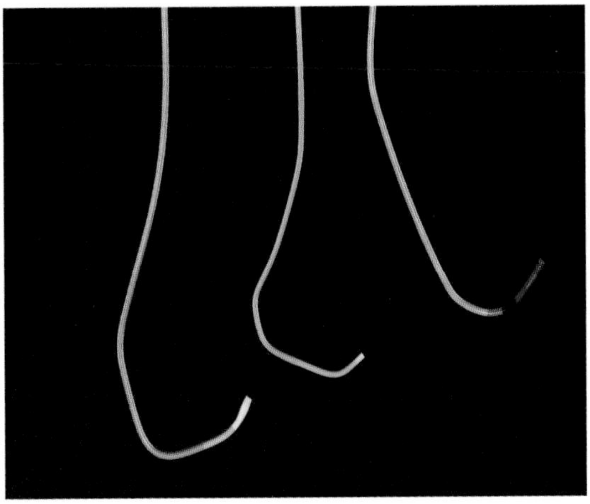

Fig. 8.17 Typical catheter shapes for left and right coronary intubation using the transradial approach: From left to right; Kimny, Tiger, IKARI.

Foreshortening

Coronary arterial segments which are progressing towards or away from the plane of imaging (rather than perpendicular to it) will appear foreshortened. This has the potential to obscure significant areas of disease and may also lead to an underestimation of lesion length and misrepresentation of the precise relationship between segments of disease and important branch vessels (Fig. 8.20). This information is essential for planning PCI strategy and, in particular, the determination of stent length.

Bifurcation points

Issues of vessel overlap and foreshortening are particularly relevant at bifurcation points where disease is common and easily missed. Every effort should be made to generate angiographic images which maximally diverge the vessels at major bifurcation points to ensure these sites are adequately assessed (Fig. 8.21).

Eccentric plaque

The coronary lumen is also represented in only two dimensions and this is not a concern if plaque burden is uniformly and concentrically distributed. However, eccentric plaque may only be seen in profile from

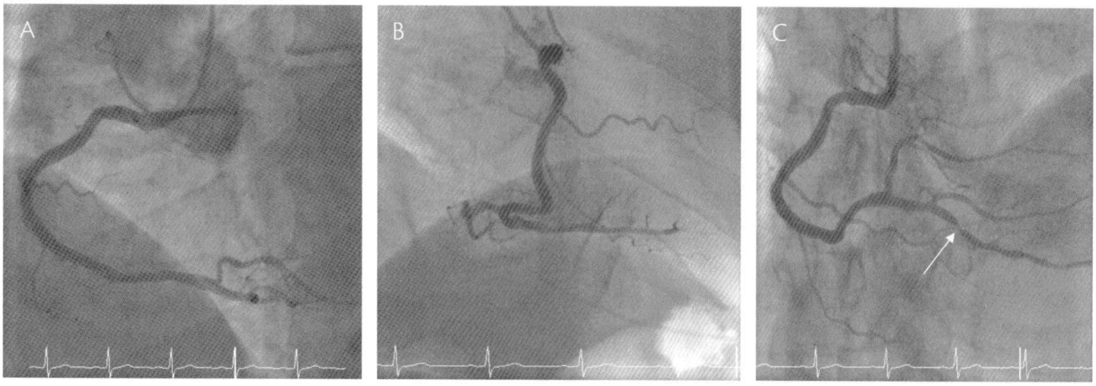

Fig. 8.18 Overlapping vessels. In these views of the right coronary artery, the discrete stenosis in the posterior descending branch (arrowed) is only clearly demonstrated in the PA cranial view (C) but is obscured by overlapping vessels in both the LAO (A) and RAO (B) projections.

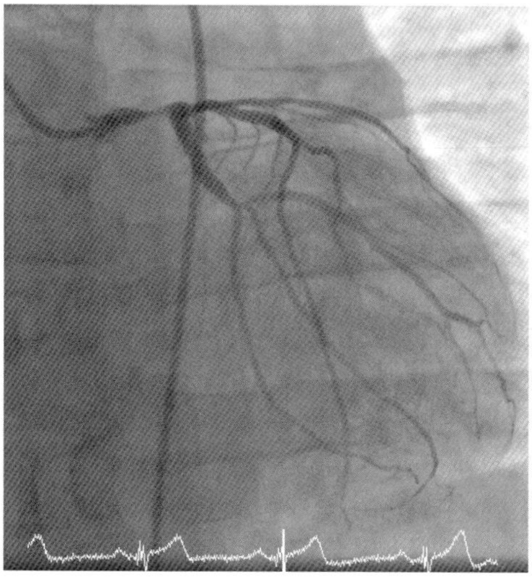

Fig. 8.19 Modified projection from PA to shallow RAO caudal ensures the catheter in the descending aorta does not overlie the severe LMS stenosis. Further projections will be required to allow complete assessment of the proximal LAD territory.

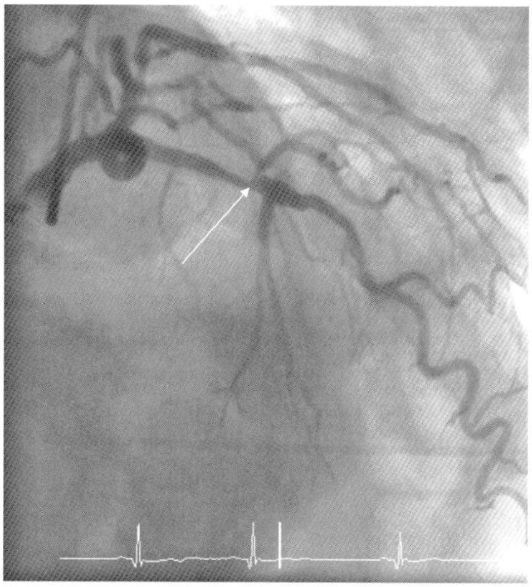

Fig. 8.21 Bifurcation disease. In this PA cranial projection the relationship between the proximal LAD disease and a severe stenosis at the origin of the first diagonal branch (arrowed) is clearly delineated. Careful modification of standard projections is often required to adequately demonstrate bifurcation disease.

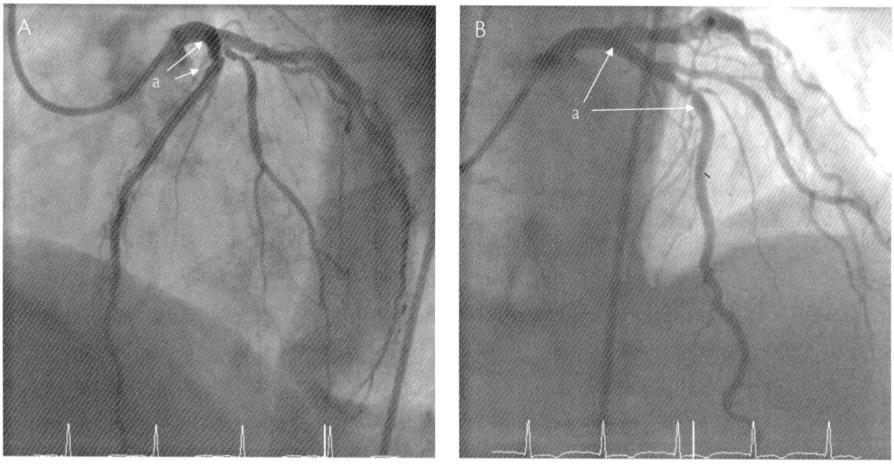

Fig. 8.20 Foreshortening. In the LAO projection (A) the proximal segment of the left anterior descending coronary artery (a) is significantly foreshortened as demonstrated in the PA cranial projection (B). In this example, the severity and length of the LAD stenosis and its relationship to the diagonal branches can only be appreciated in the non-foreshortened projection.

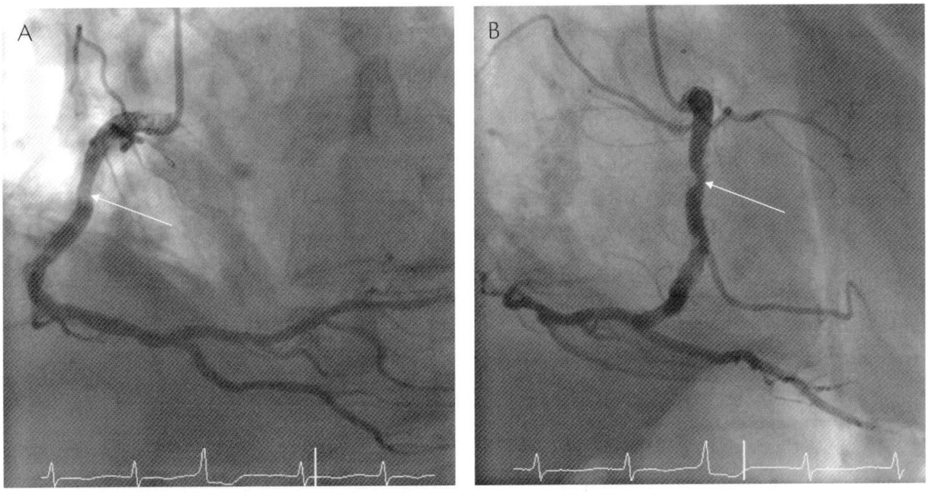

Fig. 8.22 Eccentric plaque (arrowed) in the proximal right coronary artery. In the LAO view (A) contrast opacification is reduced although there is minimal apparent stenosis. However, in the RAO view (B) a discrete eccentric plaque is evident.

particular fluoroscopic projections where the encroachment of plaque into the vessel lumen can be fully appreciated. In those projections where plaque impingement of the vessel lumen is superficial or deep to the plane of imaging, the outline of the vessel may appear unaltered (although there may be some variation in the relative opacification of the lumen at this site) (Fig. 8.22). Intravascular ultrasound (IVUS) and optical coherence tomography (OCT) are useful techniques for complete demonstration of cross-sectional luminal anatomy in cases where the severity of stenosis is uncertain (Fig. 8.23) (see Chapter 11). An alternative strategy, which assesses the functional effect of an equivocal stenosis, is provided by measurement of intracoronary pressure or flow. This is discussed in Chapter 9.

Negative remodelling

Coronary angiography delineates coronary luminal anatomy and is therefore an excellent tool for the identification of stenotic or occlusive coronary disease. However, it is now recognized that coronary stenosis is only the luminal manifestation of a more extensive

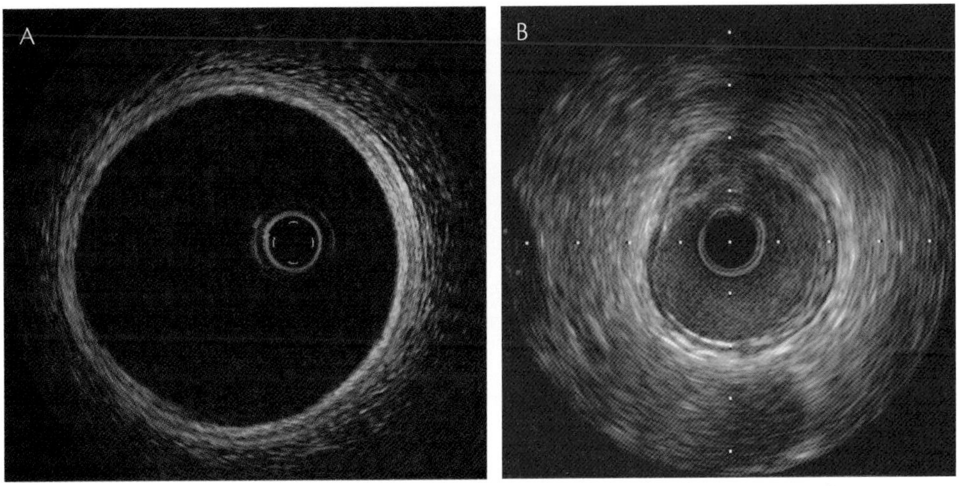

Fig. 8.23 OCT (A) and IVUS (B) intracoronary images.

disease of the coronary intima. Thus, atheromatous plaque may also project towards the outer surface of the coronary artery (so called negative remodelling) and this will not be readily evident from the luminal angiogram. This issue of non-stenotic coronary disease is of particular relevance in acute coronary syndromes where plaque rupture events may occur in apparently undiseased vessels. Furthermore, an acute coronary syndrome in the context of multivessel disease may present difficulties in accurately identifying the culprit lesion, particularly if the ECG does not localize the plaque rupture event. A number of techniques, including IVUS and OCT (Fig. 8.23), have been developed to allow visualization and assessment of non-luminal coronary disease and these are discussed in detail in Chapter 11.

Flow

Angiographic flow is graded according to the TIMI (Trombolysis in Myocardial Infarction trial) scale (Table 8.4) and is a useful marker of distal perfusion. The course of chronically occluded coronary arteries can be revealed via antegrade or retrograde collaterals demonstrated during left or right coronary injections (Fig. 8.24). However, one of the principal challenges during PCI of chronic total occlusions is that the location and course of the occluded vessel(s) may not be demonstrable by coronary angiography (see Chapter 20).

Table 8.4 The TIMI classification of intracoronary flow

TIMI score	Definition
TIMI 0	No antegrade flow
TIMI 1	Contrast penetration of an obstruction but failure to opacify the distal coronary bed
TIMI 2	Contrast penetration of an obstruction with delayed passage and/or clearance from the distal vessel
TIMI 3	Normal flow throughout with no difference in contrast penetration and clearance when compared to an uninvolved coronary bed

Optimal imaging

Adequate imaging of all segments of the epicardial coronary tree is the central tenant of good coronary angiography. This requires imaging during contrast injection into the left and right coronary ostia in a number of projections. Commonly used projections and their relative merits are illustrated in Fig. 8.25 and discussed below. Of fundamental importance is the understanding that the range of views used and fluoroscopic angles utilized should be adjusted for each patient in order to obtain optimal images and minimize exposure to contrast (see Chapter 27) and radiation (see Chapter 5).

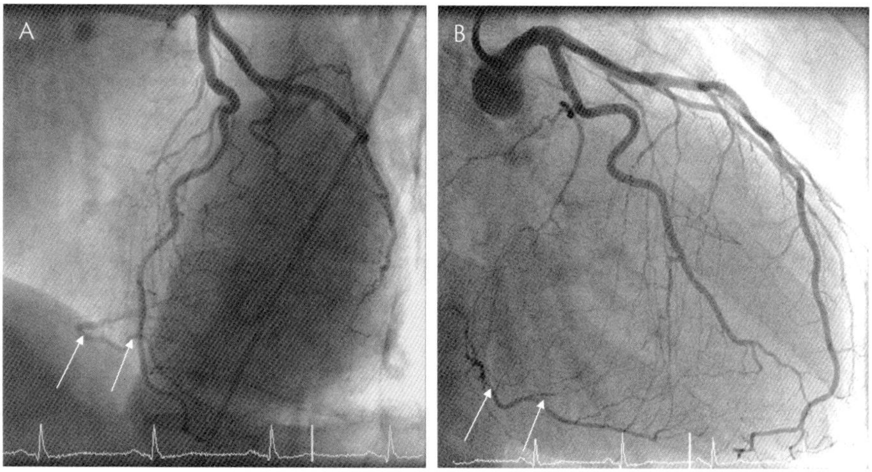

Fig. 8.24 Collateral filling of occluded coronary arteries. A) Left coronary injection in the LAO cranial projection. The right coronary artery fills retrogradely via collaterals (arrowed). B) The RAO caudal projection demonstrates right coronary collateralization from the circumflex (arrowed).

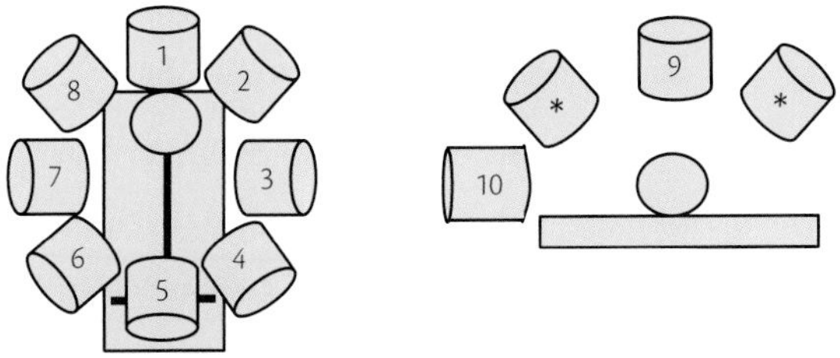

Fig. 8.25 X-ray cone standard positions. (1) PA cranial, (2) LAO cranial, (3) LAO, (4) LAO caudal (spider), (5) PA caudal, (6) RAO caudal, (7) RAO, (8) RAO cranial. These views are taken at an angle to the horizontal (*) with the exception of PA (9) which is taken vertically, and lateral (10) which is taken from the patient's side.

Positioning of the angiographic image, magnification, filters, and coning

Following engagement of the coronary ostium and prior to acquisition of the angiogram, the radiographer, guided by the operator, will magnify the image. The position of the patient relative to the camera is then optimized so that minimal subsequent camera movement is required (Fig. 8.26). X-ray filters are used to cover areas of lung which would otherwise appear unduly bright (Fig. 8.27) and the boundaries of the image may be cropped ('coning') to minimize the area of exposure to regions of interest.

Biplane imaging

Use of two imaging cones during each contrast injection allows the simultaneous acquisition of two projections, thereby reducing the volume of contrast used to obtain an adequate angiographic series[38] (Fig. 8.28).

Left coronary projections

PA (Fig. 8.29)

Most operators take their first projection in the straight PA projection. This provides an image of the LMS, proximal LAD, and Cx coronary arteries. The mid LAD and the diagonal (D) branches, as well as the obtuse marginal (OM) branches of the Cx, may be variably concealed by overlapping vessels. Subtle movement to a shallow right anterior oblique (RAO) or shallow RAO caudal position avoids projection of the catheter in the descending aorta over the LMS.

The following sequence (or local variation thereof) is then followed:

RAO caudal (Fig. 8.30)

The LMS, proximal LAD, and Cx are often well delineated. The greater separation of the LAD and Cx in this projection allows better visualization of the OM branches of the Cx. The LAD and its diagonal branches may be variably concealed by overlapping but some segments will be clearly delineated.

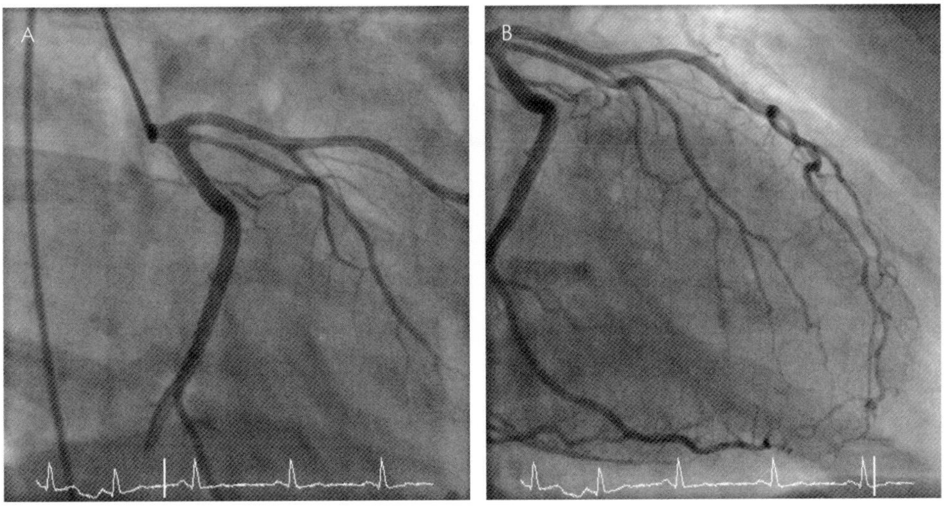

Fig. 8.26 Poor positioning during diagnostic angiography. A) The catheter tip is placed too centrally in this RAO caudal shot. As a result, the distal LAD and Cx territories are not demonstrated without camera movement. The catheter tip should be placed closer to the top left hand corner in this view. B) The catheter tip is absent during image acquisitionas a result, the left main stem is not demonstrated and part of the distal Cx is not shown.

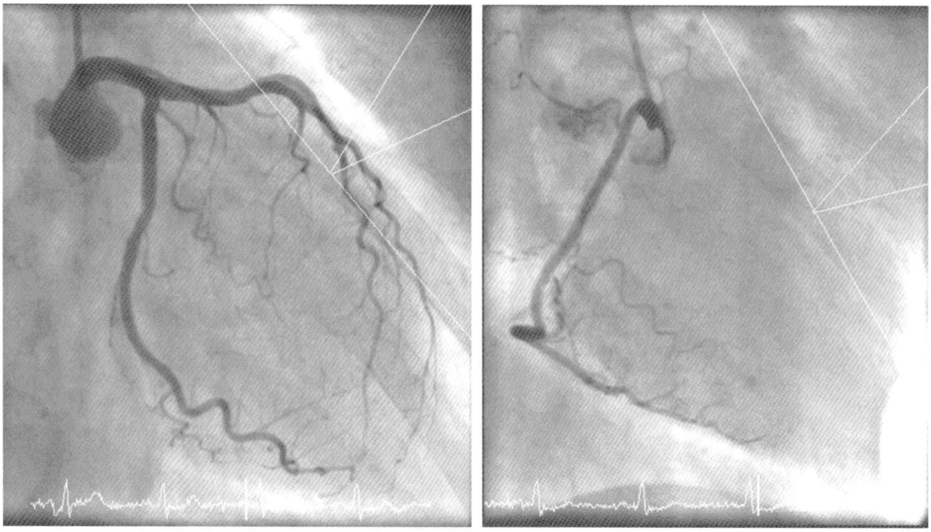

Fig. 8.27 The use of filters during diagnostic coronary angiography. Filters are wedge shaped and positioned to prevent image degradation in areas of higher X-ray penetration (e.g. lung tissue).

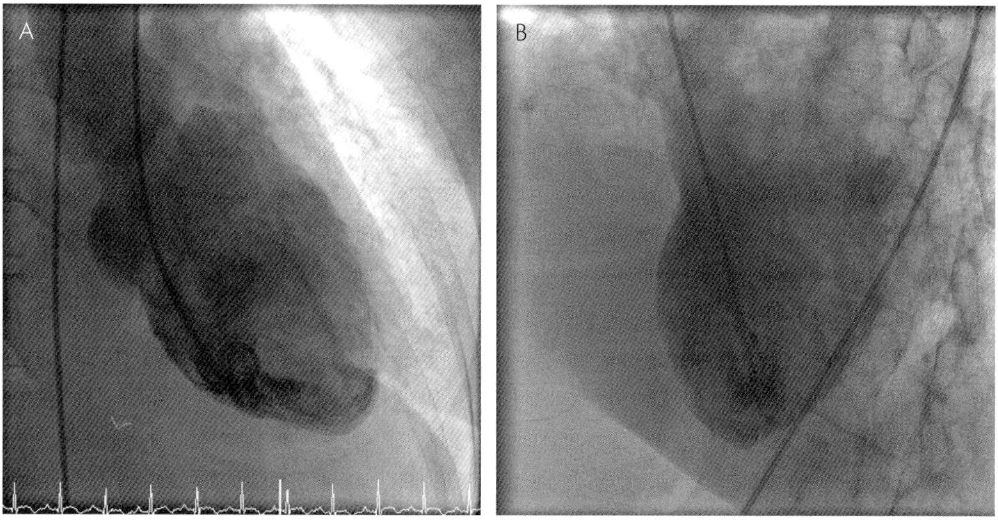

Fig. 8.28 Biplane imaging limits contrast and X-ray exposure during a single acquisition. In this example, left ventriculography in (A) RAO and (B) LAO allows more detailed assessment of regional wall motion than single plane imaging.

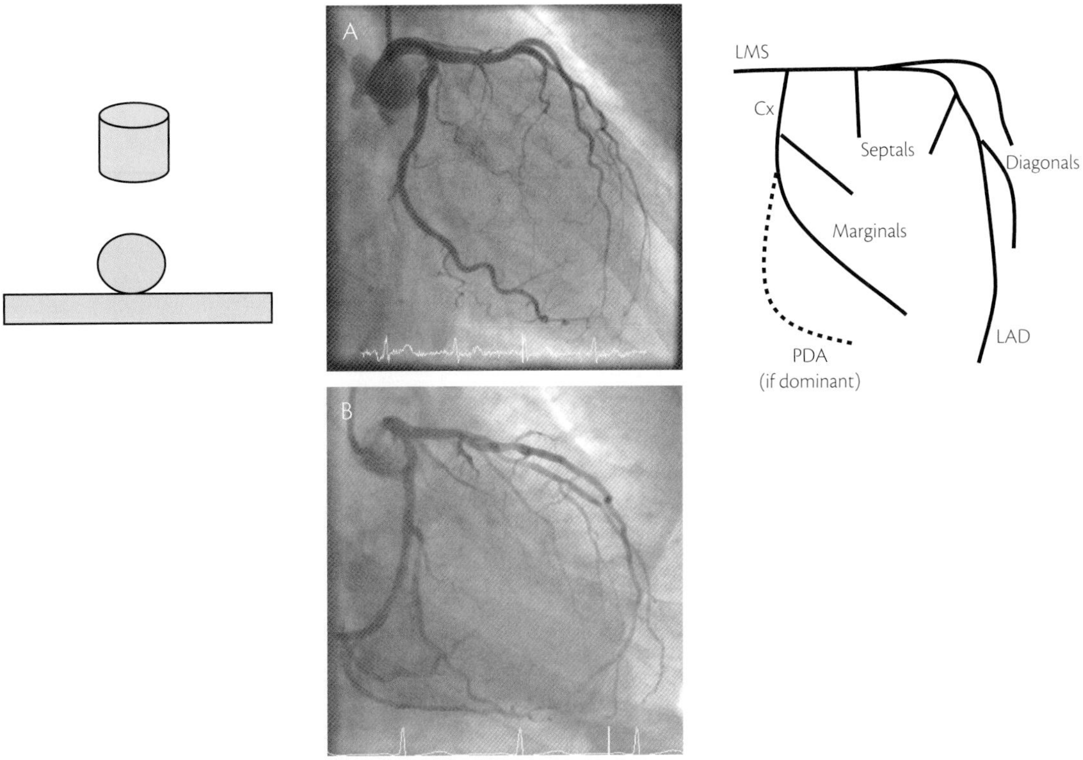

Fig. 8.29 PA or shallow RAO caudal projection. A) Non-dominant circumflex; B) dominant circumflex system. Cx, circumflex; LAD, left anterior descending; LMS, left main stem; PDA, posterior descending artery.

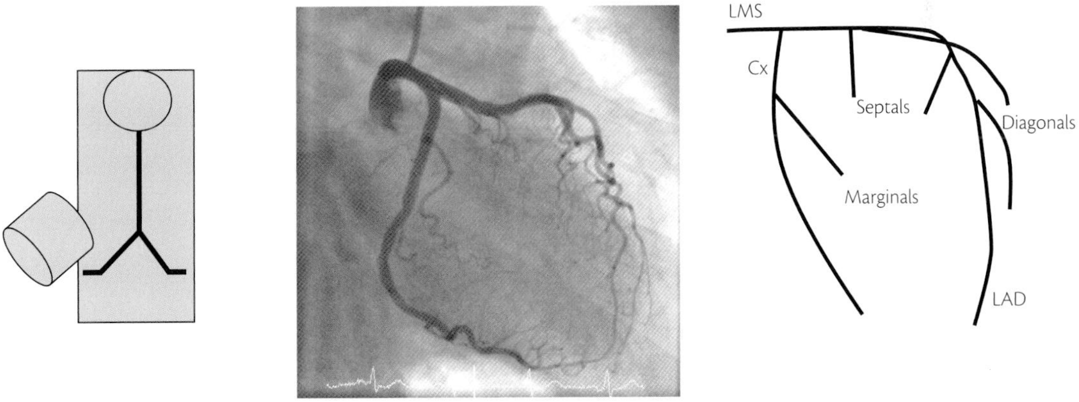

Fig. 8.30 Left coronary artery RAO caudal projection. Cx, circumflex; LAD, left anterior descending; LMS, left main stem.

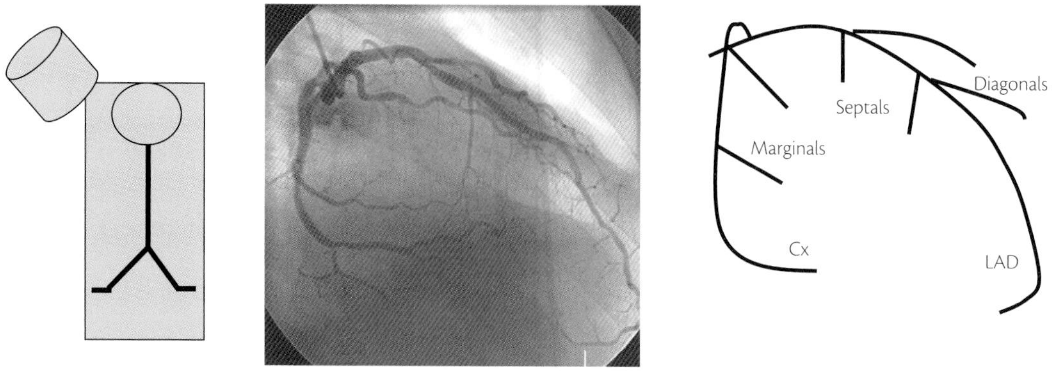

Fig. 8.31 Left coronary artery RAO cranial projection. Cx, circumflex; LAD, left anterior descending.

***RAO cranial* (*Fig. 8.31*)**

This view is generally chosen for imaging the proximal and mid LAD and its diagonal branches. The ostial and very proximal LAD segments are often overlapped by the Cx but LAD/D segments distal to this are usually well demonstrated. The Cx is poorly demonstrated in this projection.

***LAO cranial* (*Fig. 8.32*)**

The mid and distal LAD and the bifurcating diagonal and septal branches are well demonstrated in this view. The proximal LAD may be foreshortened and overlapped by the Cx. This view is also occasionally useful for assessment of the distal Cx territory, particularly the distal PDA when it is the anatomically dominant vessel.

***LAO caudal—'Spider'* (*Fig. 8.33*)**

Commonly referred to as the 'spider' view, the LAO caudal provides an image of the LMS bifurcation into the proximal LAD and Cx (or trifurcation when there is a large intermediate vessel). Adjustment of the relative degree of angulation is often required to obtain an optimal image of this important anatomical location. This view is also useful for assessing the proximal and mid Cx. The LAD is generally foreshortened after the bifurcation from the LMS but this view can sometimes be useful in demonstrating the LAD/D1 bifurcation.

***PA cranial* (*Fig. 8.34*)**

This is an alternative to the RAO cranial for viewing the LAD and its branches. It may be useful if important segments of the LAD are affected by foreshortening or overlap in other cranial projections.

***PA cadual* (*Fig. 8.35*)**

This is an alternative view which is useful for the LAD/Cx bifurcation and the proximal Cx if other caudal views are affected by foreshortening or overlap.

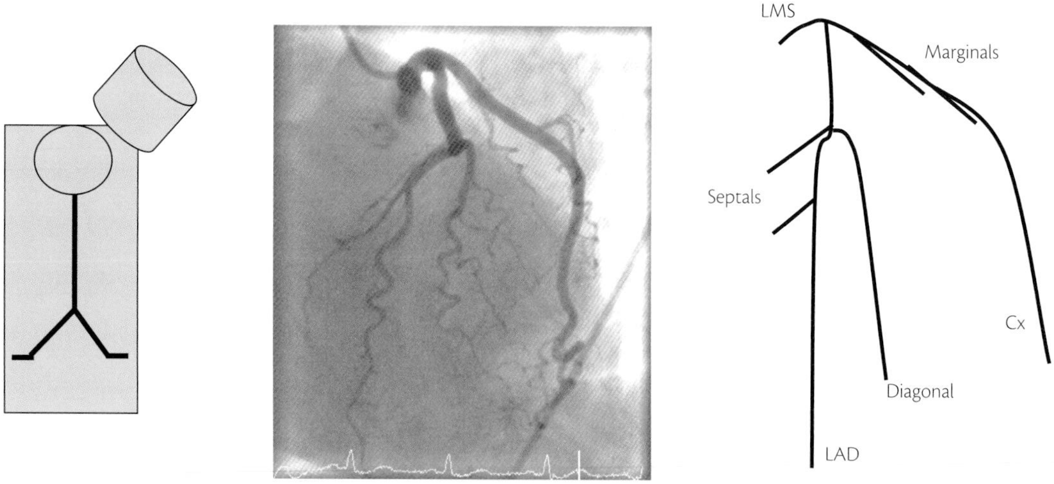

Fig. 8.32 Left coronary artery LAO cranial projection. Cx, circumflex; LAD, left anterior descending; LMS, left main stem.

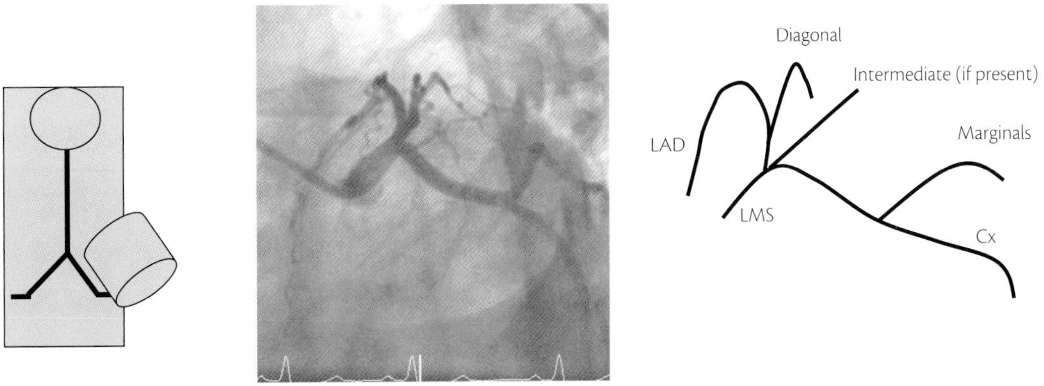

Fig. 8.33 Left coronary artery LAO caudal (spider) projection. Cx, circumflex; LAD, left anterior descending; LMS, left main stem.

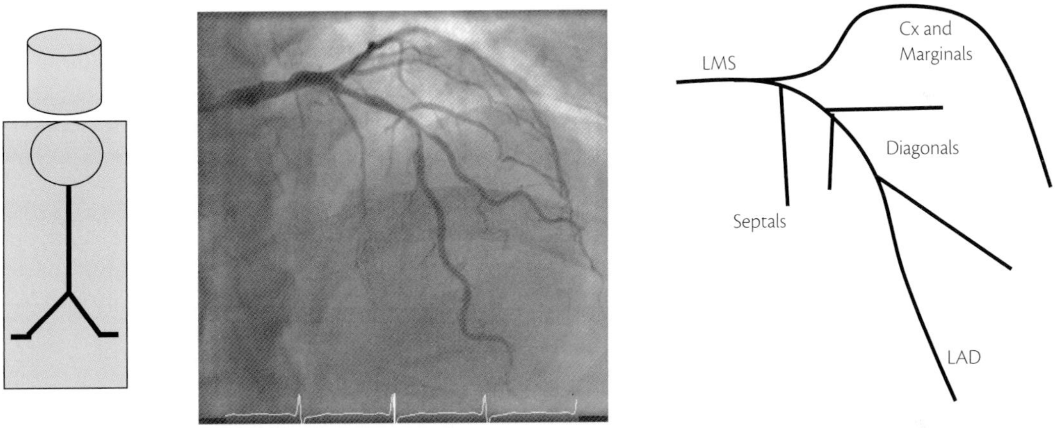

Fig. 8.34 Left coronary artery PA cranial projection. Cx, circumflex; LAD, left anterior descending; LMS, left main stem.

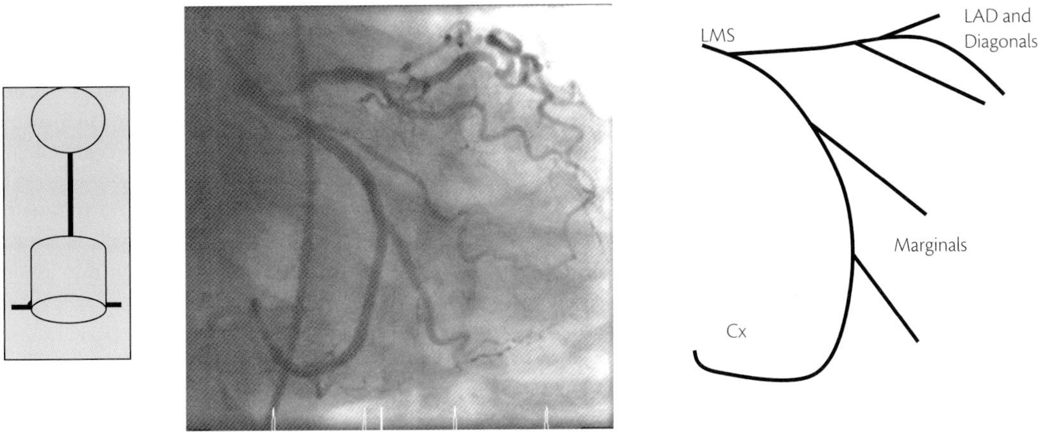

Fig. 8.35 Left coronary artery PA caudal projection. Cx, circumflex; LAD, left anterior descending; LMS, left main stem.

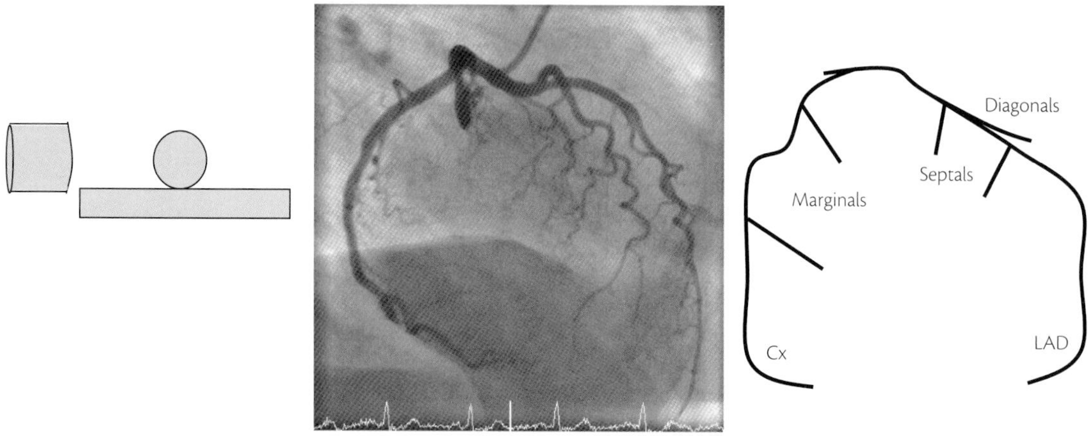

Fig. 8.36 Left coronary artery right lateral projection. Cx, circumflex; LAD, left anterior descending.

***Lateral** (Fig. 8.36)*

The lateral projection widely separates the LAD and Cx territories and is minimally affected by foreshortening (with the exception of the very proximal segments) although either vessel may be affected by overlapping branches. This view is particularly useful for assessing the relative position of the LAD, especially if it is occluded, as the vessel runs a consistent course along the sky-line of the cardiac shadow in this projection.

Right coronary projections

***LAO** (Fig. 8.37)*

Acquisition in this position will show the RCA throughout its course with a variable amount of overlap of the distal branches.

***RAO** (Fig. 8.38)*

The ostium and proximal vessel are foreshortened in this projection but the mid vessel is shown well and the full length of the distal PDA is demonstrated.

***PA cranial** (Fig. 8.39)*

If the LAO projection fails to adequately demonstrate the bifurcation of the PDA and posterior left ventricular branches this view will often separate these and show the relationship of disease to the bifurcation. An LAO cranial may also provide the same information.

***Lateral** (Fig. 8.40)*

This is a good alternative view which may be used if the more usual projections are inadequate.

Imaging coronary bypass grafts

Saphenous vein grafts are generally intubated in the LAO projection although the lateral and RAO projections are also helpful. The precise projections used for image acquisition will vary depending on the course of the graft, the native coronary anatomy beyond its insertion and the location of any disease. At least two orthogonal views should be obtained (see Fig. 8.15).

The left internal mammary pedicle is accessed via the left subclavian artery in the PA projection. Two orthogonal views might include the RAO caudal and LAO cranial projections but chosen angles will vary as described earlier (see Fig. 8.16).

Non-coronary assessment during coronary angiography

In addition to delineation of the coronary anatomy, further information may be obtained during a coronary angiogram according to the clinical context.

Left ventricular angiogram

Injection of a 30–40-mL bolus of contrast via a mechanical pump and pigtail catheter within the left ventricular cavity can be used to assess left ventricular function and detect regional wall-motion abnormalities. Left ventricular angiography is usually performed in the RAO projection which also allows assessment of the degree of mitral regurgitation and demonstration of the aortic root (Fig. 8.41). Crossing the aortic valve with a catheter is also an opportunity to directly measure pressure within the left ventricle. Subsequent careful withdrawal allows assessment of the peak-to-peak transaortic valve gradient. Paradoxically, this is not usually performed in patients with known severe aortic stenosis when echocardiographic data are available because of the risk of embolic stroke associated with trauma to a

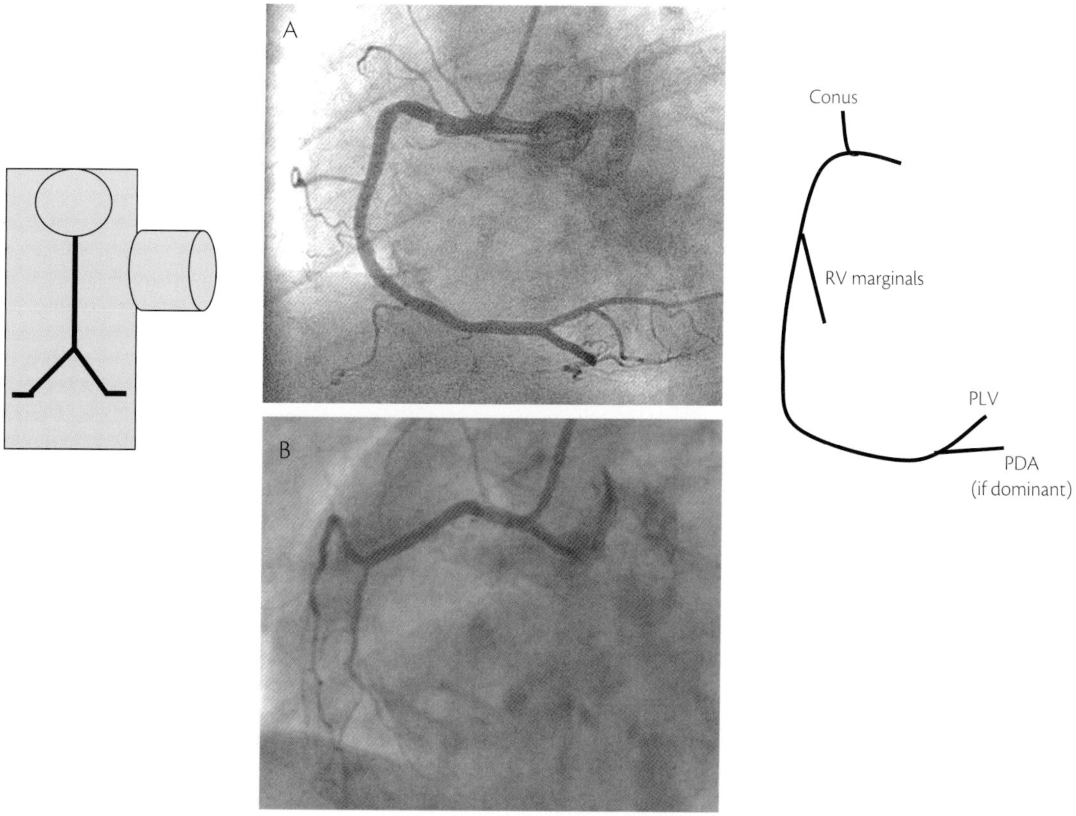

Fig. 8.37 Right coronary artery in LAO projection (A) dominant (B) non-dominant anatomy. PDA, posterior descending artery; PLV, posterior left ventricular branch; RV, right ventricular branch.

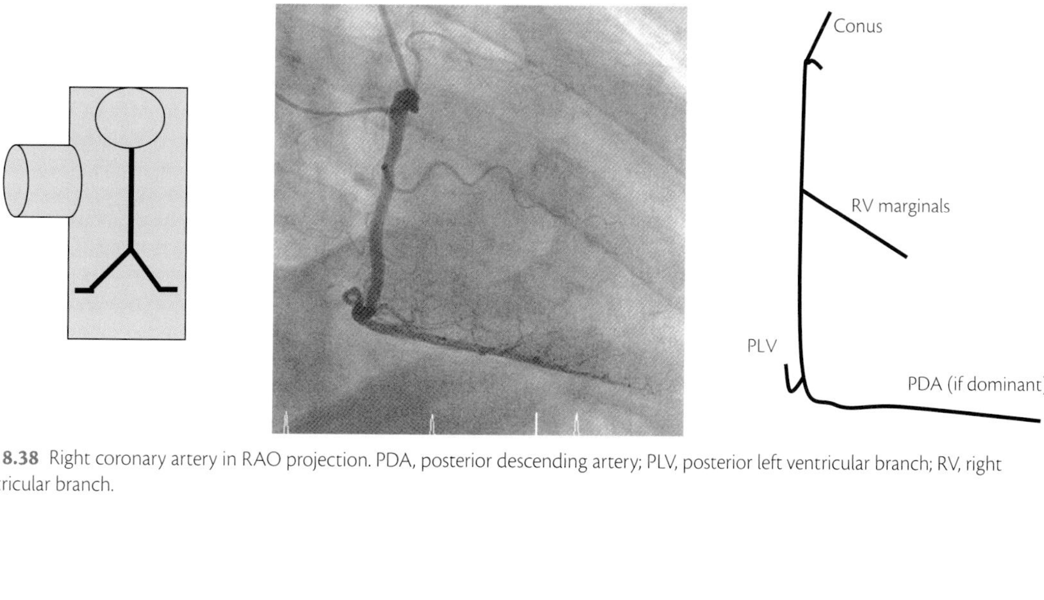

Fig. 8.38 Right coronary artery in RAO projection. PDA, posterior descending artery; PLV, posterior left ventricular branch; RV, right ventricular branch.

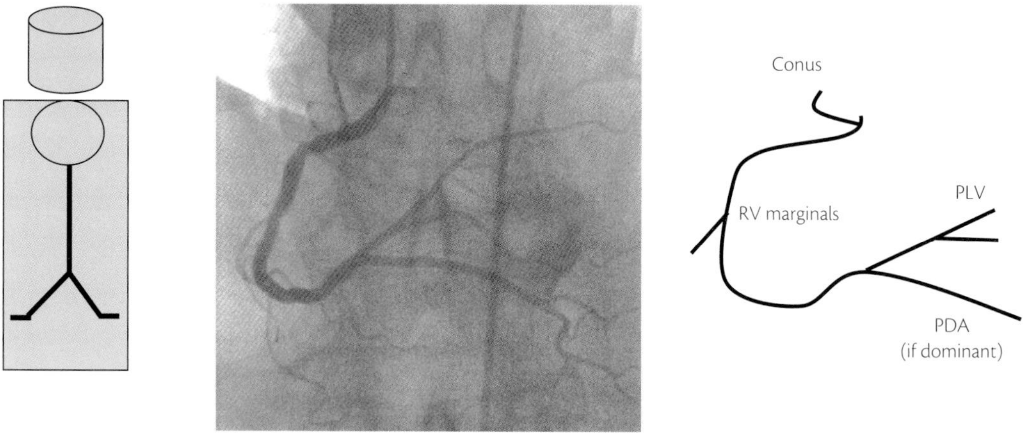

Fig. 8.39 Right coronary artery in RAO cranial projection. PDA, posterior descending artery; PLV, posterior left ventricular branch; RV, right ventricular branch.

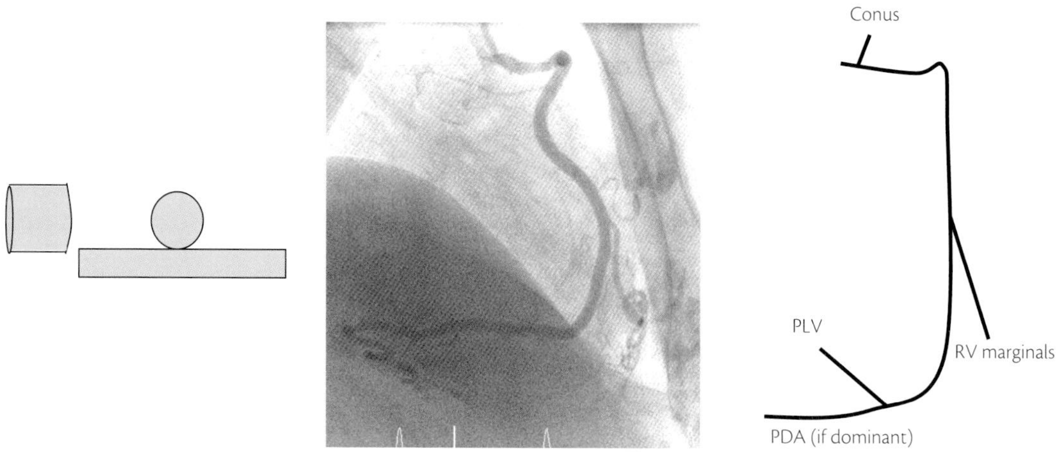

Fig. 8.40 Right coronary artery in lateral projection. PDA, posterior descending artery; PLV, posterior left ventricular branch; RV, right ventricular branch.

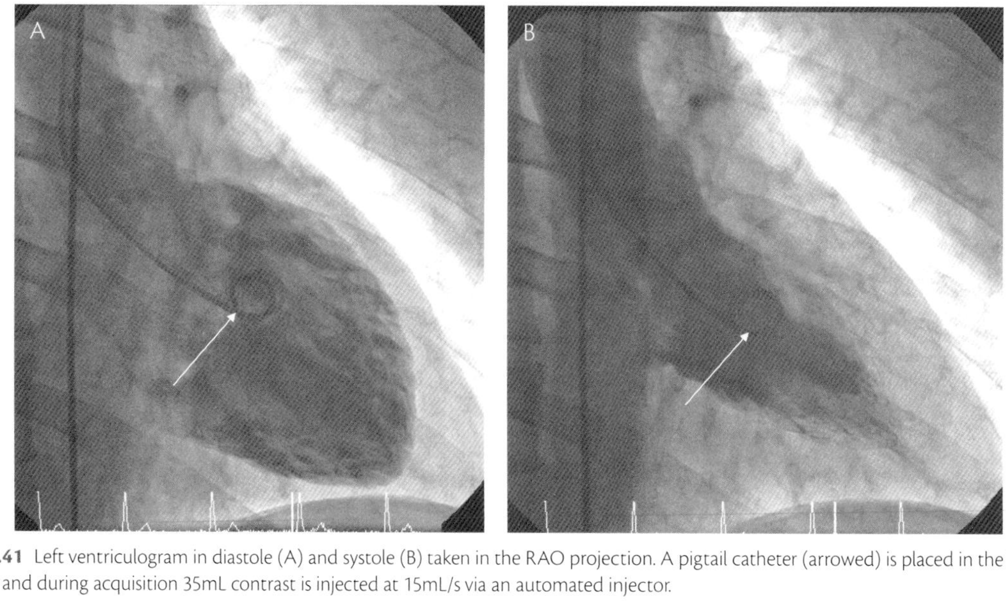

Fig. 8.41 Left ventriculogram in diastole (A) and systole (B) taken in the RAO projection. A pigtail catheter (arrowed) is placed in the LV cavity and during acquisition 35mL contrast is injected at 15mL/s via an automated injector.

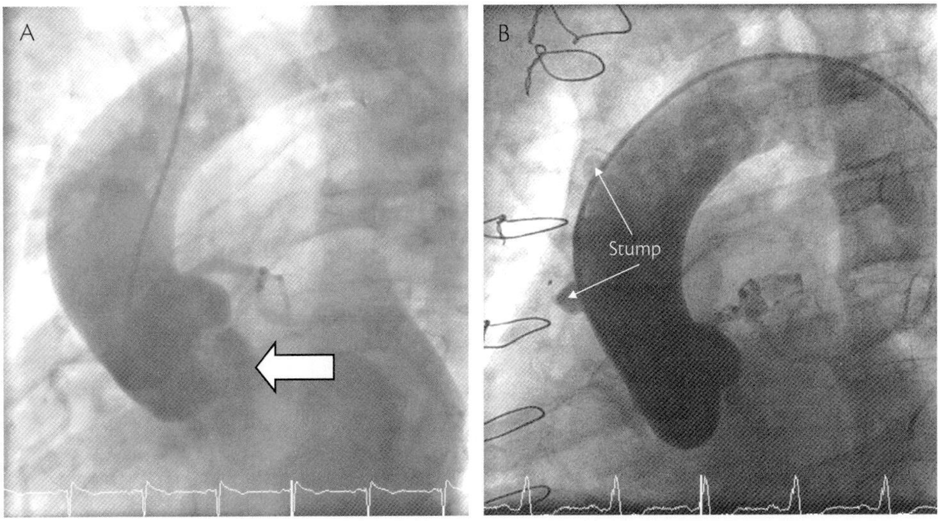

Fig. 8.42 Aortography. A pigtail catheter is positioned in the aortic root: (A) radial approach (B) femoral approach. During acquisition in the LAO projection 40mL of contrast is injected at 20mL/s using an automated injector. (A) Significant aortic regurgitation (arrowed) into the left ventricular cavity. (B) Sternal wires following previous coronary bypass grafting and the stumps of two occluded saphenous vein grafts (arrowed) are demonstrated.

heavily diseased valve. Nevertheless, the technique remains useful in cases of diagnostic uncertainty and is a prerequisite during the interventional procedure of trans-catheter aortic valve implantation (TAVI; see Chapter 39).

Aortogram

Injection of a 30–40-mL bolus of contrast (usually in the LAO projection) via a mechanical pump and pigtail catheter positioned in the aortic root can be used to demonstrate the anatomy of the root, ascending aorta, and aortic arch (Fig. 8.42). Aortography is particularly important in the assessment of patients with aortic valve disease being considered for surgery, in patients with aortic stenosis prior to TAVI, and in locating the origins of bypass grafts (see earlier sections).

Right heart catheterization

Passage of a multipurpose catheter via a venous sheath into the right heart allows the measurement of pulmonary capillary wedge pressure (an indirect measure of left atrial pressure), and pressure within the pulmonary artery, right ventricle, and right atrium. Oxygen saturations can also be measured at different sites to determine cardiac output and investigate the possibility of intracardiac shunting. The technique and interpretation of right heart catheterization findings are beyond the scope of this chapter. Aspects related to non-coronary percutaneous interventions are discussed in Section 8.

Angiography during PCI

Coronary angiography is, of course, more than a diagnostic tool alone—the fundamental principles are also essential for PCI. Indeed, many angiographic procedures in the modern era are performed as an immediate preamble to PCI if the clinical findings support that revascularization strategy. The basic tenants of coronary angiography and PCI are therefore the same. Selection of the optimal catheter shape for stable and coaxial tip position is of equal importance for good, safe angiography and for guide catheter selection during PCI. Identification of optimal orthogonal views of the target stenosis which are free of the effects of vessel overlap and foreshortening are critical elements of diagnostic angiography precisely because these are the images which the interventional operator will use to approach the lesion targeted for PCI. Even when it is performed as a separate diagnostic procedure, coronary angiography should therefore be regarded as a continuum with PCI ensuring that the quality of the images is adequate for full decision-making on all aspects of optimal revascularization.

References

1. Sekhri N, Feder GS, Junghans C, *et al.* Incremental prognostic value of the exercise electrocardiogram in the initial assessment of patients with suspected angina: cohort study. *BMJ* 2008; **337**:a2240.
2. Sekhri N, Feder GS, Junghans C, *et al.* How effective are rapid access chest pain clinics? Prognosis of incident angina and non-cardiac chest pain in 8762 consecutive patients. *Heart* 2007; **93**(4):458–63.
3. Boyle RM. Value of rapid-access chest pain clinics. *Heart* 2007; **93**(4):415–16.
4. Stuart RJ Jr, Ellestad MH. National survey of exercise stress testing facilities. *Chest* 1980; **77**(1):94–7.
5. Marwick TH, Case C, Vasey C, *et al.* Prediction of mortality by exercise echocardiography: a strategy for combination with the duke treadmill score. *Circulation* 2001; **103**(21):2566–71.
6. Mark DB, Shaw L, Harrell FE Jr, *et al.* Prognostic value of a treadmill exercise score in outpatients with suspected coronary artery disease. *N Engl J Med* 1991; **325**(12): 849–53.
7. Fox K, Angeles A, Garcia A, *et al.* Guidelines on the management of stable angina pectoris: executive summary: The Task Force on the Management of Stable Angina Pectoris of the European Society of Cardiology. *Eur Heart J* 2006; **27**(11):1341–81.
8. Tsutsui JM, Dourado PM, Falcão SN, *et al.* Prognostic value of dobutamine stress echocardiography with early injection of atropine with versus without chronic beta-blocker therapy in patients with known or suspected coronary heart disease. *Am J Cardiol* 2008; **102**(10): 1291–5.
9. Lette J, Tatum JL, Fraser S, *et al.* Safety of dipyridamole testing in 73,806 patients: the Multicenter Dipyridamole Safety Study. *J Nucl Cardiol* 1995; **2**(1):3–17.
10. Cortigiani L, Picano E, Coletta C, *et al.* Safety, feasibility, and prognostic implications of pharmacologic stress echocardiography in 1482 patients evaluated in an ambulatory setting. *Am Heart J* 2001; **141**(4):621–9.
11. Secknus MA, Marwick TH. Evolution of dobutamine echocardiography protocols and indications: safety and side effects in 3,011 studies over 5 years. *J Am Coll Cardiol* 1997; **29**(6):1234–40.
12. Schinkel AF, Bax JJ, Geleijnse ML, *et al.* Noninvasive evaluation of ischaemic heart disease: myocardial perfusion imaging or stress echocardiography? *Eur Heart J* 2003; **24**(9):789–800.
13. Higgins JP, Williams G, Nagel JS, *et al.* Left bundle-branch block artifact on single photon emission computed tomography with technetium Tc 99m (Tc-99m) agents: mechanisms and a method to decrease false-positive interpretations. *Am Heart J* 2006; **152**(4):619–26.
14. Yetkin E, Turhan H, Tandogan I. Left bundle branch block: a diagnostic challenge in cardiology. *Am J Cardiol* 2007; **99**(8):1179–80.
15. Schinkel AF, Bax JJ, Poldermans D, *et al.* Hibernating myocardium: diagnosis and patient outcomes. *Curr Probl Cardiol* 2007; **32**(7):375–410.
16. Shaikh K, Chang SM, Peterson L, *et al.* Safety of contrast administration for endocardial enhancement during stress echocardiography compared with noncontrast stress. *Am J Cardiol* 2008; **102**(11):1444–50.
17. Aggeli C, Giannopoulos G, Roussakis G, *et al.* Safety of myocardial flash-contrast echocardiography in combination with dobutamine stress testing for the detection of ischaemia in 5250 studies. *Heart* 2008; **94**(12):1571–7.
18. Timperley J, Mitchell AR, Thibault H, *et al.* Safety of contrast dobutamine stress echocardiography: a single center experience. *J Am Soc Echocardiogr* 2005; **18**(2): 163–7.
19. Picano E, Molinaro S, Pasanisi E. The diagnostic accuracy of pharmacological stress echocardiography for the assessment of coronary artery disease: a meta-analysis. *Cardiovasc Ultrasound* 2008; **6**:30.
20. Sicari R, Nihoyannopoulos P, Evangelista A *et al.* Stress echocardiography expert consensus statement: European Association of Echocardiography (EAE) (a registered branch of the ESC). *Eur J Echocardiogr* 2008; **9**(4):415–37.
21. Poldermans D, Fioretti PM, Boersma E, *et al.* Long-term prognostic value of dobutamine-atropine stress echocardiography in 1737 patients with known or suspected coronary artery disease: A single-center experience. *Circulation* 1999; **99**(6):757–62.
22. Steinberg EH, Madmon L, Patel CP, *et al.* Long-term prognostic significance of dobutamine echocardiography in patients with suspected coronary artery disease: results of a 5-year follow-up study. *J Am Coll Cardiol* 1997; **29**(5):969–73.
23. Kamaran M, Teague SM, Finkelhor RS, *et al.* Prognostic value of dobutamine stress echocardiography in patients referred because of suspected coronary artery disease. *Am J Cardiol* 1995; **76**(12):887–91.
24. Underwood SR, Anagnostopoulos C, Cerqueira M, *et al.* Myocardial perfusion scintigraphy: the evidence. *Eur J Nucl Med Mol Imaging* 2004; **31**(2):261–91.
25. Iskandrian AS, Chae SC, Heo J, *et al.* Independent and incremental prognostic value of exercise single-photon emission computed tomographic (SPECT) thallium imaging in coronary artery disease. *J Am Coll Cardiol* 1993; **22**(3):665–70.
26. Hachamovitch R, Berman DS, Shaw LJ, *et al.* Incremental prognostic value of myocardial perfusion single photon emission computed tomography for the prediction of cardiac death: differential stratification for risk of cardiac death and myocardial infarction. *Circulation* 1998; **97**(6):535–43.
27. Marcassa C, Bax JJ, Bengel F, *et al.* Clinical value, cost-effectiveness, and safety of myocardial perfusion scintigraphy: a position statement. *Eur Heart J* 2008; **29**(4):557–63.

28. Jerosch-Herold M, Kwong RY. Optimal imaging strategies to assess coronary blood flow and risk for patients with coronary artery disease. *Curr Opin Cardiol* 2008; **23**(6):599–606.
29. Jahnke C, Nagel E, Gebker R, *et al.* Prognostic value of cardiac magnetic resonance stress tests: adenosine stress perfusion and dobutamine stress wall motion imaging. *Circulation* 2007; **115**(13):1769–76.
30. Nagel E, Lehmkuhl HB, Bocksch W, *et al.* Noninvasive diagnosis of ischemia-induced wall motion abnormalities with the use of high-dose dobutamine stress MRI: comparison with dobutamine stress echocardiography. *Circulation* 1999; **99**(6):763–70.
31. Zeina AR, Blinder J, Sharif D, *et al.* Congenital coronary artery anomalies in adults: non-invasive assessment with multidetector CT. *Br J Radiol* 2009; 82(975):254–61.
32. Stein PD, Yaekoub AY, Matta F, *et al.* 64-slice CT for diagnosis of coronary artery disease: a systematic review. *Am J Med* 2008; **121**(8):715–25.
33. Docherty A, Oldroyd KG. Percutaneous coronary intervention: obtaining consent and preparing patients for follow-on procedures. *Heart* 2001; **86**(6):597–8.
34. West R, Ellis G, Brooks N. Complications of diagnostic cardiac catheterisation: results from a confidential inquiry into cardiac catheter complications. *Heart* 2006; **92**(6):810–14.
35. Ammann P, Brunner-La Rocca HP, *et al.* Procedural complications following diagnostic coronary angiography are related to the operator's experience and the catheter size. *Catheter Cardiovasc Interv* 2003; **59**(1):13–18.
36. Laskey W, Boyle J, Johnson LW. Multivariable model for prediction of risk of significant complication during diagnostic cardiac catheterization. The Registry Committee of the Society for Cardiac Angiography & Interventions. *Cathet Cardiovasc Diagn* 1993; **30**(3): 185–90.
37. Adlam D, Azeem T, Ali T, *et al.* Is there a role for provocation testing to diagnose coronary artery spasm? *Int J Cardiol* 2005; **102**(1):1–7.
38. Kane GC, Doyle BJ, Lerman A, *et al.* Ultra-low contrast volumes reduce rates of contrast-induced nephropathy in patients with chronic kidney disease undergoing coronary angiography. *J Am Coll Cardiol* 2008; **51**(1):89–90.

CHAPTER 9

Coronary physiology in clinical practice

Olivier Muller and Bernard De Bruyne

Introduction

The goal of any treatment is to improve patients' prognosis and/or symptoms. Accordingly, the goal of any diagnostic tool is to guide decision-making to apply optimal treatment in individual patients. Any diagnostic tool not fulfilling these requirements should not be used in patients. Keeping this in mind, this chapter will briefly review what is often referred to as 'invasive coronary physiology'.

As opposed to anatomical (also referred to as 'morphologic') approaches, physiological ('functional') measurements assess the function of the coronary circulation. The function of the coronary arterial circulation is to provide nutrients to the myofibrils. Accessorily, the coronary arteries play a role in diastolic function (turgor effect). No other organ is so dependent on the function of the organ it perfuses.

The combination of an accurate anatomic assessment and precise functional information is indispensable to tailor the treatment of patients with suspected or known coronary artery disease.

Anatomical considerations

Three-layer histology of the coronary arteries

Normal arteries have a well-developed trilaminar structure, the intima, media, and the adventitia. The endothelial cells of the tunica intima constitute the barrier with blood and play an important role in the regulation of haemostasis and vascular tone. The strategic location of the endothelium allows it to sense changes in haemodynamic forces and blood-borne signals and to respond by releasing vasoactive substances. A balance between endothelium-derived relaxing (i.e. nitric oxide) and contracting factors (i.e. endothelin) maintains vascular homeostasis. When this balance is disrupted (i.e. atherosclerosis), it predisposes the vasculature to vasoconstriction and, thus, to disturbance in coronary blood flow[1].

The size of the arteries is proportional to myocardial mass

In normal individuals, there is a close correlation between the lumen cross-sectional area of a coronary artery at each point along its length and the corresponding regional myocardial mass. In contrast, in patients with coronary atherosclerosis, measured coronary artery lumen area is diffusely 30–50% too small for distal myocardial bed size compared with normal subjects[2]. Fig. 9.1 shows the relation between the size of a given artery and the mass of myocardium perfused by this artery. In patients with coronary artery disease, the dimension of a given artery is too small for the mass of myocardium. This relation will be important when considering a stenosis in a large artery (i.e. left anterior descending) compared to a smaller one.

Physiological considerations

A detailed review of myocardial flow regulation is beyond the scope of this chapter. Yet, a reminder of a number of aspects is useful to understand the basics of the physiological assessment of the coronary circulation.

A few basic concepts

Flow, pressure, and resistance

The main parameters of the circulatory function are flow, pressure, and resistance:

$$Q = \Delta P/R$$

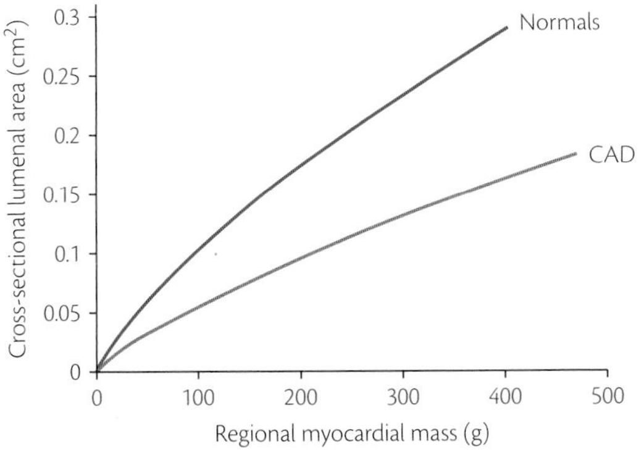

Fig. 9.1 Relation between the size of epicardial coronary artery and myocardial mass in normal an in patients with coronary artery disease. Modified from Seiler C, Kirkeeide RL, Gould KL. Basic structure-function relations of the epicardial coronary vascular tree. Basis of quantitative coronary arteriography for diffuse coronary artery disease. *Circulation* 1992; **85**(6):1987–2003. Copyright © 2003 American Heart Association. All rights reserved.

Measuring absolute coronary blood flow (in mL/min) and absolute resistance (in mmHg/mL/s) sounds like the 'alpha and the omega' of vascular physiology. However, even if absolute flow and resistance were to be measured easily and reliably in patients, it is most likely that their impact on clinical decision-making would be rather modest. Flow—and therefore resistance—both depend on the myocardial mass to be perfused. Therefore, there is no unequivocal normal value for coronary flow and resistance. In contrast, under normal conditions, coronary pressure equals central aortic pressure over the entire length of the epicardial arteries, even during hyperaemia. This unique characteristic of coronary pressure gives the interventionalist an unequivocal reference value: whatever the myocardial mass, the size of the artery, the systemic haemodynamics, the age of the patient, the status of the microvasculature, etc., the pressure in the distal part of an epicardial artery should be identical to central aortic pressure. If this is not the case, i.e. in case of a pressure gradient, it necessarily implies that the resistance of the epicardial artery is abnormal.

Coronary flow and myocardial contractions

Due to the squeezing effect of the contracting ventricles, coronary blood flow occurs mainly during diastole. This diastolic pre-eminence of coronary blood flow is most pronounced at rest (as compared to hyperaemia) and in the left coronary artery. In case of epicardial stenosis, the pressure gradient will therefore be mainly diastolic ('no flow, no gradient').

Flow–function relationship

Myocardial blood flow represents approximately 5% of cardiac output. Due to its constant work, resting myocardial oxygen demand is high and the extraction of oxygen by the myocardium is close to its maximum, much higher than in other organs. Oxygen saturation of the coronary sinus venous blood is close to 20% (as a comparison, the oxygen saturation in the renal vein is 85%). Hence, since extraction cannot increase much further, the coronary circulation can only meet oxygen demand by fine tuning myocardial blood flow. In addition, as soon as myocardial flow decreases below 90% of its normal resting levels, myocardial function starts to decrease (Fig. 9.2). It is obvious that the control of myocardial blood flow must be remarkably tight to avoid wall-motion abnormalities. Conversely, this also implies that when myocardial wall motion is normal, its resting perfusion must be normal.

The control of myocardial flow

The regulation of myocardial blood flow is multifactorial. These neurohumoral, endothelial, endo- and

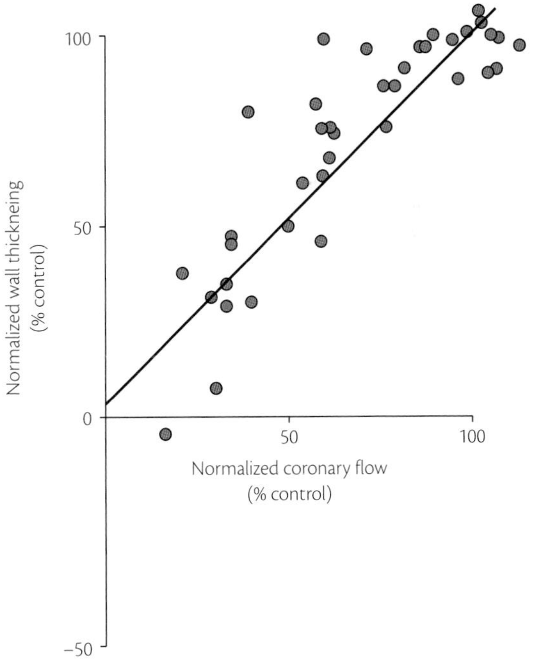

Fig. 9.2 Plots of the relation between reductions in endocardial flow and both wall thickening reductions. Modified from Canty JM, Jr. Coronary pressure-function and steady-state pressure-flow relations during autoregulation in the unanesthetized dog. *Circ Res* 1988; **63**(4):821–36. Copyright © 1988 American Heart Association. All rights reserved.

paracrine, metabolic, and physical factors are largely non-linear, cumulative, and interacting. It is therefore very difficult to study these factors individually.

To simplify, the coronary circulation can be considered a two-compartment model. The first compartment consists of epicardial vessels, which are also referred to as 'conductance vessels' because they do not oppose any resistance to blood flow. The second compartment consists of arteries smaller than 400 microns, or 'resistive vessels' (Fig. 9.3); when no stenosis is present, myocardial flow is primarily controlled by resistive vessels[3], as they are able to vasodilate under physiological and pharmacological stress. At coronary angiography they are not clearly delineated but appear as a myocardial blush of contrast medium. During exercise or any other form of increased oxygen demand, the resistance of the microvasculature decreases allowing for an increased blood flow. Similarly, when a stenosis is present in the epicardial artery, this increased epicardial resistance is compensated by an equivalent decrease in microvascular resistance. This results in a maintained total resistance to blood flow and a preserved resting flow, with residual—albeit reduced—coronary flow reserve. When the epicardial stenosis progresses further, its relative contribution to total resistance increases. At the extreme, when the stenosis becomes 'critical', the compensation capacity of the microvascular circulation is exhausted. Any additional increase in epicardial resistance will result in an increase in total resistance and in a decrease in myocardial flow.

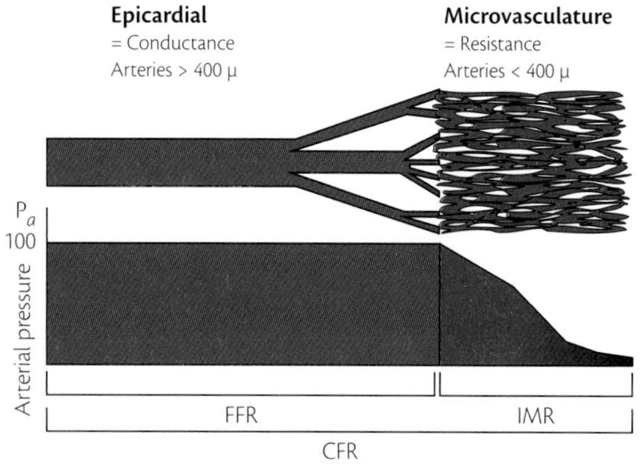

Fig. 9.3 Since the epicardial vessels contribute only a minimal fraction of the total vascular resistance there is no significant pressure drop along the conductance vessels. In contrast passage through the resistive vessels produces a large drop in pressure.

Physiological indices of the coronary circulation

Since the seminal work of K.L. Gould[4], several indices of coronary physiology have been proposed to guide clinical decision-making. Fractional flow reserve (FFR) is the best validated index. Therefore, we will briefly describe the other indices before focusing on FFR.

Coronary flow reserve

Coronary flow reserve (CFR) is defined as the ratio of hyperaemic blood flow (Q_{max}) to resting myocardial blood flow (Q_{rest}).

$$CFR = Q_{max}/Q_{rest}$$

Its normal value is between 4–6, which means that microvascular resistance can decrease by a factor 4–6. Since absolute myocardial flow is not easy to determine, surrogates of flow are commonly used: flow velocities assessed by the Doppler wire (FloWire®, Volcano Inc, Rancho Cordova, California, USA) or mean transit time (T_{mn}) assessed by the PressureWire® (RadiMedical Systems Inc, Uppsala, Sweden). Regardless of technical/practical aspects, the concept of CFR has several limitations: (1) resting flow which appears, at the denominator, is very variable; (2) hyperaemic flow is directly dependant on systemic blood pressure; (3) the hyperaemic and resting measurements are not performed simultaneously but successively; and (4) CFR is not specific for the epicardial stenosis. Stated another way, when CFR is too low, it is impossible to tell whether this abnormal value is related to a stenosis in the epicardial artery, to microvascular disease, or to a combination of both. For these reasons, CFR is of limited value for clinical decision-making[5].

The index of microvascular resistance

The resistance of a vascular system is given by the ratio of the pressure gradient to the flow across that particular system. Accordingly, the resistance (R) of the coronary microvascular compartment is the ratio of

$$R = (P_d - P_v)/Q$$

where P_d is distal coronary arterial pressure and P_v coronary venous pressure, or right atrial pressure. In the coronary circulation P_v is often almost negligible. Fearon and colleagues introduced the concept of index of microvascular resistance (IMR) considering that the mean transit time during maximal hyperaemia is inversely proportional to hyperaemic flow.

Therefore, during maximal hyperaemia

$$IMR = P_d/1/T_{mn} = P_{d.}\ T_{mn}$$

where P_d *is the distal coronary pressure and* T_{mn} *is the mean transit time.* IMR is specific for the microcirculation and is simple to obtain as P_d and T_{mn} can be obtained simultaneously with the PressureWire®. It has been well validated in animals[6] and was recently used in the setting of acute coronary syndromes to predict clinical outcomes[7] and assess the effect of treatment[8].

Hyperaemic stenosis resistance

The resistance an epicardial stenosis can be given by the ratio of the pressure gradient and the flow across that particular stenosis. Accordingly, Meuwissen and colleagues introduced the concept of hyperaemic stenosis resistance (HSR) which can be calculated as the ratio of trans-stenotic gradient ($P_a - P_d$) to average peak flow velocity (Vel) during maximal hyperaemia:

$$HSR = (P_a - P_d)/Vel$$

This measurement requires both a flow and a pressure sensor (ComboWire®, Volcano Inc, Rancho Cordova, California, USA) and is specific for the epicardial stenosis[9,10]

Fractional flow reserve

Definition

FFR is the ratio of maximal myocardial blood flow depending on a stenotic artery to maximal myocardial blood flow if that same artery were to be normal. In other words, it is a fraction of the maximal normal flow assuming that these measurements are obtained when the microvasculature resistance is minimal and constant (maximal hyperaemia)[11,12].

FFR represents the extent to which maximal myocardial blood flow is limited by the presence of an epicardial stenosis. If FFR is 0.60, it means that maximal myocardial blood flow reaches only 60% of its normal value. Conversely, FFR provides the interventionalist with the exact extent to which optimal stenting of the epicardial stenosis will increase maximal myocardial blood flow. An FFR of 0.60 implies that stenting the focal stenosis responsible for this abnormal FFR should bring FFR to 1.0, which represents an increase in maximal myocardial blood flow of 67%.

Calculation

FFR is a ratio of two flows. It has been shown, however, that this ratio of two flows can be derived from two pressures (distal coronary pressure and aortic pressure), provided they are both measured during maximal hyperaemia. The theoretical explanation of this relationship between hyperaemic flows and hyperaemic pressures is displayed in Fig. 9.4.

Equipment

Catheters

The use of diagnostic catheters is technically feasible[13]. Yet, due to higher levels of friction hampering wire manipulation, the smaller internal calibre prejudicing pressure measurements, and the inability to perform

1. Fractional flow reserve is the ratio of hyperaemic myocardial flow in the stenotic territory (Q_S^{max}) to normal hyperaemic myocardial flow (Q_N^{max})

$$FFR = \frac{Q_S^{max}}{Q_N^{max}} \quad \text{(Empiric definition)}$$

2. Since the flow (Q) is the ratio of the pressure (P) difference across the coronary system divided by its resistance (R), Q can be substituted as following:

$$FFR = \frac{(P_d - P_v)/R_S^{max}}{(P_a - P_v)/R_N^{max}}$$

3. Since the measurements are obtained under maximal hyperaemia, resistances are minimal and therefore equal, and thus they cancel out;

$$FFR = \frac{(P_d - P_v)}{(P_a - P_v)}$$

4. In addition P_v is negligible as compared to P_a or P_d, therefore,

$$FFR = \frac{P_d}{P_a} \quad \text{(Practical measurement)}$$

A

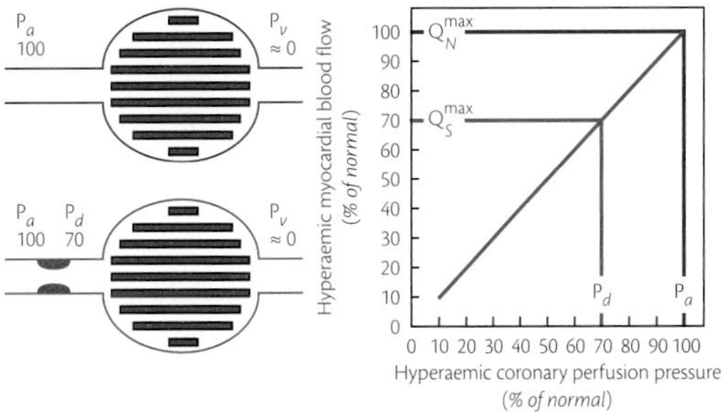

B

Fig. 9.4 A) Simplified theoretical explanation illustrating how a ratio of two flows can be derived from a ratio of two pressures provided these pressures are recorded during maximal hyperaemia. B) Concept of fractional flow reserve (FFR) measurements. When no epicardial stenosis is present (blue lines) the driving pressure Pa determines a normal (100%) maximal myocardial blood flow. In case of stenosis responsible for a hyperaemic pressure gradient of 30mmHg (red lines), the driving pressure will no longer be 100mmHg but 70mmHg (P_d). Since during maximal hyperaemia the relationship between driving pressure and myocardial blood flow is linear, myocardial blood flow will only reach 70% of its normal value. This numerical example shows how a ratio of two pressures (P_d/P_a) corresponds to a ratio of two flows (Q_S^{max} / Q_N^{max}). It also illustrates how important it is to induce maximal hyperaemia.

ad hoc percutaneous coronary intervention (PCI) using diagnostic catheters, the use of guiding catheters is highly recommended.

Wires

Measuring intracoronary pressure requires the use of a specific solid state sensor mounted on a floppy-tipped guide wire. In mainstream practice two such systems are available at his time, namely the PressureWire® and the Volcano WaveWire® (Volcano Inc, Rancho Cordova, California, USA). The sensor is located 3cm from the tip, at the junction between the radiopaque and the radiolucent portions. The last generations of these 0.014-inch wires have similar handling characteristics to most standard angioplasty guide wires.

Hyperaemia

To measure FFR, it is absolutely essential to achieve maximal vasodilatation of the two vascular compartments of the coronary circulation, namely the conductance arteries (epicardial) and the resistance arteries (microvasculature). The pharmacological agents most often used to induce hyperaemia are listed in Table 9.1[14–16].

The epicardial arteries: a bolus of 200mg isosorbide dinitrate (or any other form of intracoronary nitrates) allows the abolition of any form of epicardial vasoconstriction. It is good clinical practice to give intracoronary nitrates when performing coronary angiograms, especially when a wire is manipulated in the coronary tree. In addition, it is important to realize that all the data on FFR and its relation with non-invasive stress modalities or with clinical outcome have been obtained after intracoronary administration of nitrates.

Microvascular circulation: inducing maximal hyperaemia to obtain physiological information about a stenosis might be compared to placing the stenosis in a wind tunnel. From a theoretical point of view, the concept of FFR is based on achieving minimal microvascular resistance (Fig. 9.4). Therefore, expressions like 'baseline FFR' or 'FFR at rest' are physiological nonsense. This also extends to all other circulations. Even when the resting pressure gradient is large we recommend the induction of hyperaemia because it allows us to evaluate the residual resistance reserve.

An example of a typical coronary pressure tracing during the administration of intravenous adenosine is shown in Fig. 9.5.

Anticoagulation

As soon as a device is advanced into the coronary tree, the use of the same anticoagulation regimens as employed during a PCI procedure are recommended: heparin adjusted to weight, validated by a monitored activated coagulation time (ACT) of at least 250s. Patients are supposedly under aspirin.

Unique characteristics of FFR

FFR has a number of unique characteristics that make this index particularly suitable for functional assessment of coronary stenoses and clinical decision-making in the catheterization laboratory.

FFR has a 'universal' normal value of 1

An unequivocally normal value is easy to refer to but is rare in clinical medicine. Since in a normal epicardial artery there is virtually no decline in pressure, not even during maximal hyperaemia, it is obvious that P_d/P_a will equal or be very close to unity. FFR was obtained in 37 arteries in 10 individuals without atherosclerosis (group I) and in 106 non-stenotic arteries in 62 patients with arteriographic stenoses in another coronary artery (group II). In group I, the FFR was near unity (0.97 ± 0.02; range, 0.92–1), indicating no resistance to flow in truly normal coronary arteries, but it was significantly

Table 9.1 Importance of epicardial and microvascular vasodilatation when measuring fractional flow reserve

	Plateau(s)	Half-life (min)	Dose
Epicardial vasodilation: Isosorbide dinitrate			At least 200mg IC bolus, at least 30s before the first measurements
Microvascular vasodilation:			
Adenosine IC	5–10	0.5–1	50mg IC bolus
Adenosine IV	60–120	1–2	140mg/kg/min*
Papaverine IC	30–60	2	8mg in the RCA, 12mg in the LCA
Nitroprusside IC	20	1	0.6mg/kg in bolus

LCA, left coronary artery; RCA, right coronary artery.
*preferably through a central venous (e.g. femoral) line

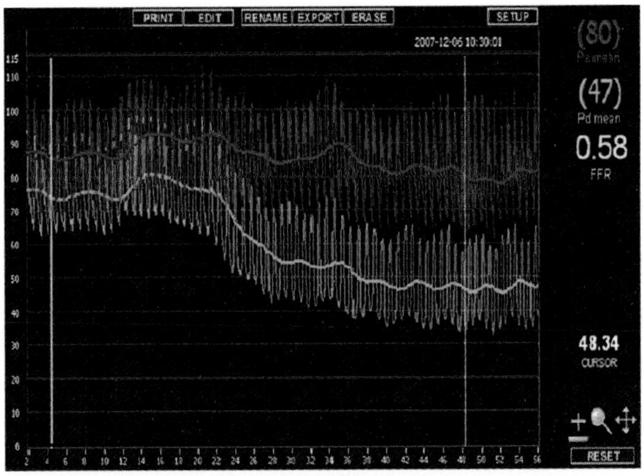

Fig. 9.5 Typical example of simultaneous aortic pressure (P_a) and distal coronary pressure (P_d) recordings at rest and during maximal steady state hyperaemia as induced by an intravenous infusion of adenosine. Soon after starting the infusion, the decrease in distal pressure is preceded by a transient increase in aortic pressure.

lower (0.89 ± 0.08; range, 0.69–1) in group II, indicating a higher resistance to flow[3].

Thus, it is important to realize that in normal-looking coronary arteries in patients with proven atherosclerosis elsewhere, the epicardial coronary arteries may contribute to total resistance to coronary blood flow even though there is no discrete stenosis visible on the angiogram. In approximately 50% of these arteries, FFR is lower than the lowest value found in strictly normal individuals. In approximately 10% of atherosclerotic arteries, FFR will be lower than the ischaemic threshold. Practically speaking, this finding implies that myocardial ischaemia might be present in atherosclerotic patients in the absence of discrete stenoses[3,17].

FFR has a well defined cut-off value

Cut-off or threshold values are values that distinguish normal from abnormal levels for a given measurement. To enable adequate clinical decision-making in individual patients, it is paramount that any level of uncertainty is reduced to a minimum. Cut-off value for FFR has been evaluated in several studies and compared to several decision-making modalities; among them, radionuclide perfusion was the most used[5]. Stenoses with FFR measurement of <0.75 are almost invariably able to induce myocardial ischaemia (cut-off with a specificity of 100%, a sensitivity of 88%, a positive predictive value of 100%, and an overall accuracy of 93%). Stenoses with an FFR >0.80 are almost never associated with exercise induced ischaemia (Table 9.2). This means that the 'grey zone' for FFR (between 0.75–0.80) spans over 6–7% of the entire range of FFR values.

FFR is not influenced by systemic haemodynamics

In the catheterization laboratory systemic pressure, heart rate and left ventricular contractility are prone to change. In contrast to many other indices measured in the catheterization laboratory, changes in systemic haemodynamics do not influence the value of FFR in a given coronary stenosis[18]. This is due not only to the fact that aortic and distal coronary pressures are measured simultaneously, but also to the extraordinary capability of the microvasculature to repeatedly vasodilate to exactly the same extent. In addition, FFR measurements are extremely reproducible and FFR has been shown to be independent of gender and risk factors such as hypertension and diabetes[19]. These characteristics contribute to the accuracy of the method and to the trust in its value for decision-making.

FFR takes into account the contribution of collaterals

Whether myocardial flow is provided antegradely by the epicardial artery, or retrogradely through collaterals, does not really matter for the myocardium. Distal coronary pressure during maximal hyperaemia reflects

Table 9.2 Cut-off values for fractional flow reserve

Authors (reference)	Patients	No.	Test	Threshold
De Bruyne *et al.*[54]	1-VD	60	Bicycle ECG	0.72*
Pijls et al.[17]	1-VD pre + post PCI	60	Bicycle ECG	0.74*
Pijls *et al.*[20]	1-VD, intermediate stenosis	45	Bicycle ECG, thallium + dobutamine echo	0.75*
Bartunek *et al.*[55]	1-VD	75	Dobutamine echo	0.78*
Chamuleau *et al.*[56]	MVD	127	MIBI-SPECT	0.74**
Abe *et al.*[57]	1-VD	46	Thallium	0.75*
De Bruyne *et al.*[37]	Post-MI	57	MIBI-SPECT	0.75–0.80*

MI, myocardial infarction; MVD, multivessel disease; PCI, percutaneous coronary intervention; VD, vessel disease. *100% specificity; **optimal cut-off value.

both antegrade and retrograde flow according to their respective contribution. This holds for the stenoses supplied by collaterals but also for stenosed arteries providing collaterals to another more critically diseased vessel (Fig. 9.6).

FFR specifically relates the severity of the stenosis to the mass of tissue to be perfused

The larger the myocardial mass subtended by a vessel, the larger the hyperaemic flow, and in turn, the larger the gradient and the lower the FFR. This explains why a stenosis with a minimal cross-sectional area of $4mm^2$ has totally different haemodynamic significance in the proximal left anterior descending artery (LAD) versus the second marginal branch. It also explains FFR measurements of collaterals, where the mass supplied by an artery can change after revascularization of the retrograde supplied vessel.

FFR has unequalled spatial resolution

The exact position of the sensor in the coronary tree can be monitored under fluoroscopy, and documented angiographically. Pulling back the sensor under maximal hyperaemia (usually adenosine IV) gives the operator an instantaneous assessment of the abnormal resistance of the arterial segment located between the guide catheter and the sensor. While other functional tests reach a 'per patient' accuracy (exercise ECG) or, at best, a 'per vessel' accuracy (myocardial perfusion imaging), FFR reaches a 'per segment' accuracy with a spatial resolution of a few millimetres.

Clinical applications

FFR in angiographically dubious stenoses

The main general indication for FFR is the precise assessment of the functional consequences of a given

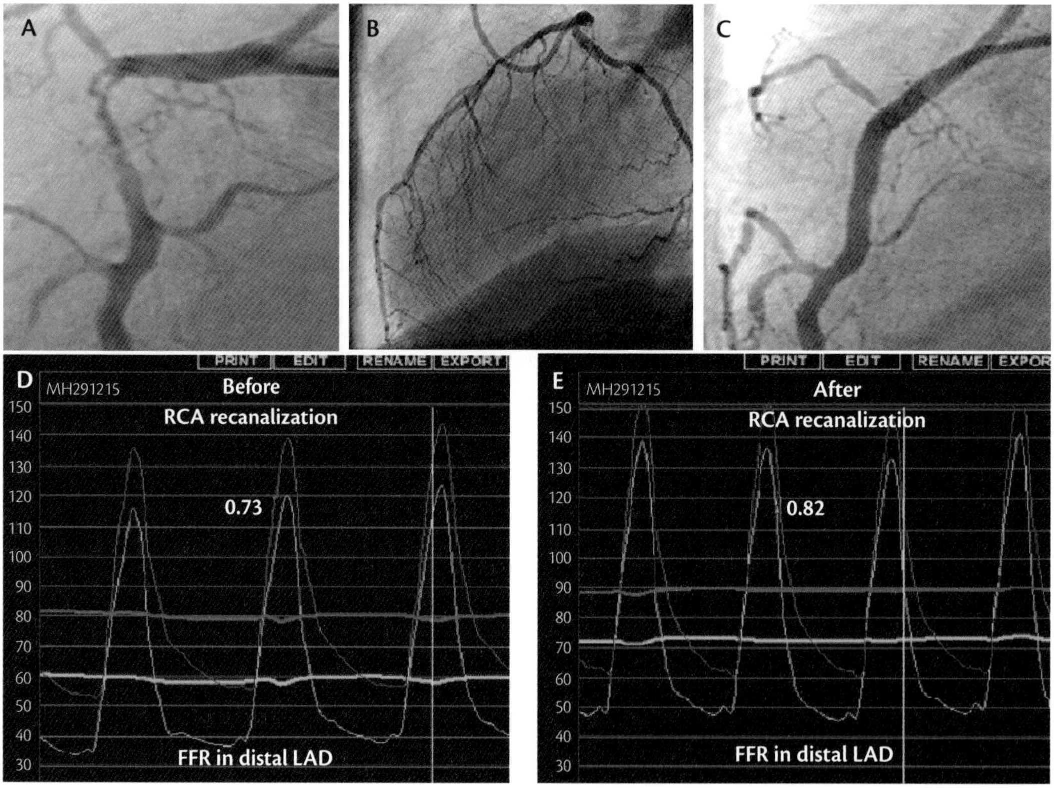

Fig. 9.6 Example of the influence of collaterals on fractional flow reserve (FFR) measurements in a 76-year-old man with a critical stenosis in the proximal right coronary artery (RCA) (A) and collaterals supplied by the left coronary artery (B). The FFR in the distal left anterior descending artery (LAD) was measured first before recanalization of the RCA (A and D) and after recanalization of the RCA (C and E). When antegrade flow was restored in the RCA, the LAD had no longer to supply blood to the territory of the RCA. Therefore, hyperaemic flow in the LAD was lower than before and the FFR increased from 0.76 to 0.82. This example also illustrates the relationship between FFR and the myocardial mass supplied by the artery: the larger the myocardial mass, the greater the hyperaemic flow, and the lower the FFR for a given stenosis.

coronary stenosis with unclear haemodynamic significance[20]. Cardiologists describe angiographic coronary narrowings with uncertain functional consequences as mild-to-moderate stenoses, dubious lesions, intermediate stenoses, non-flow limiting, etc. Angiographic assessment of such stenoses produce insufficient information to determine whether a stenosis is haemodynamically significant or not. Moreover, angiographic assessment is often the only decision-making modality to perform an angioplasty. Even if a clinical cardiologist is offered many options and techniques for non-invasive functional evaluation, it has been reported that up to 71% of PCIs are being performed in the absence of any sort of functional evaluation[21]. This scenario, often referred to as the *oculostenotic reflex*, is even more worrisome now that safety concerns associated with late stent thrombosis have been identified[22].

Direct translesional pressure measurements correlate well with non-invasive assessment of coronary artery disease. In a study of 45 patients with angiographically dubious stenoses it was shown that FFR has a much larger accuracy in distinguishing haemodynamically significant stenoses than exercise ECG, myocardial perfusion scintigraphy, and stress echocardiography taken separately[20]. Furthermore, the results of these non-invasive tests are often contradictory, which renders appropriate clinical decision-making difficult (Fig. 9.7). In addition, the clinical outcome of patients in whom PCI has been deferred, because the FFR indicated no haemodynamically significant stenosis, is very favourable. In this population the risk of death or myocardial infarction is approximately 1% per year, and this risk is not decreased by PCI[23]. These results strongly support the use of FFR measurements as a guide for decision-making about the need for revascularization in 'intermediate' lesions. Fig. 9.8 illustrates how two angiographically similar stenoses may have a completely different haemodynamic severity. One of them should be revascularized, the other not. Based solely on the angiogram, the decision should be identical in both cases, which would lead to an inappropriate interventional decision in one of these patients.

FFR in left main stem disease

The presence of a significant stenosis in the left main stem is of critical prognostic importance[24]. Conversely, revascularization of a non-significant stenosis in the left main may lead to atresia of the conduits, even when internal mammary arteries are used[25]. Furthermore, the left main is among the most difficult segments to assess by angiography[26]. Non-invasive testing is often non-contributive in patients with a left main stenosis. Perfusion defects are often seen in only one vascular territory, especially when the right coronary artery is significantly diseased[27]. In addition, tracer uptake may be reduced in all vascular territories ('balanced ischaemia') giving rise to false negative studies[28]. Several studies have shown that FFR could be used safely in left main stenosis and that the decision not to operate on left main stenosis with an FFR >0.75 is safe[29–31]. In addition, angiographic assessments of left main lesions with an FFR <0.75 were no different from those with an FFR >0.75, further reinforcing the importance of physiological parameters in case of doubt. Therefore, patients with an intermediate left main stenosis deserve physiologic assessment before blindly taking a decision about

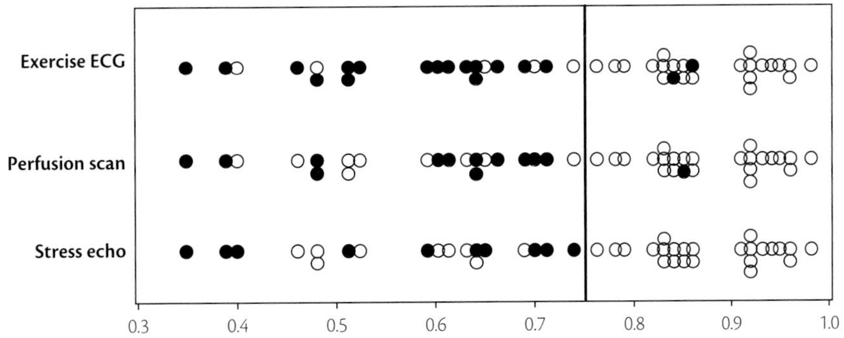

Fig. 9.7 Plots of the fractional flow reserve (FFR) in 45 patients with an angiographically intermediate stenosis according to the results of non-invasive testing. The hollow circles represent negative tests. The black dots represent positive tests. Tests were considered positive only if they were positive before revascularization and reversed to negative after revascularization. Among the 21 patients with an FFR <0.75, only four showed concordant results of non-invasive tests. Reproduced with permission from Pijls NH, De Bruyne B, Peels K, et al. Measurement of fractional flow reserve to assess the functional severity of coronary-artery stenoses. *N Engl J Med* 1996; **334**(26):1703–8. Copyright © 1996 Massachusetts Medical Society. All rights reserved.

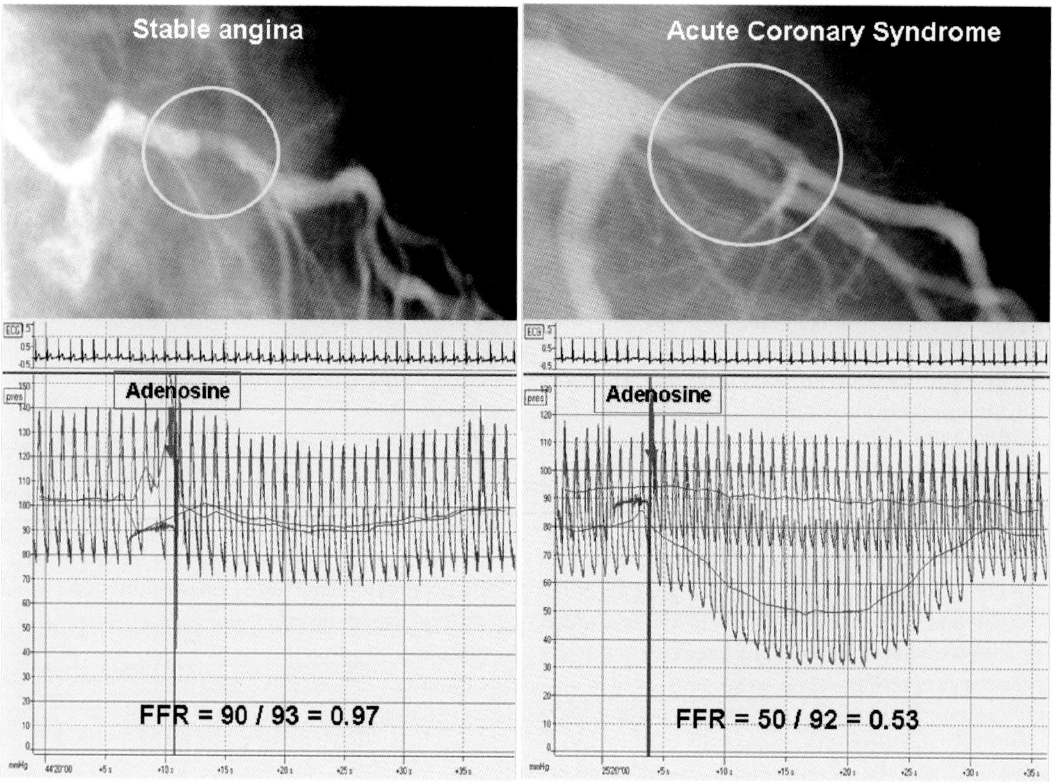

Fig. 9.8 Example of two patients presenting with different clinical syndromes, and in whom an angiographically similar stenosis is found in the proximal left anterior descending coronary artery. In the left example the lesion has no haemodynamic significance and does not need any form of mechanical revascularization. In the right example the stenosis is haemodynamically very significant and deserves an intervention.

the need for revascularization. Two examples shown in Fig. 9.9 illustrate how FFR measurements in the left main may drastically influence the type of treatment in these patients. Left main disease is rarely isolated. When tight stenoses are present in the LAD or in the left circumflex artery (LCx) the presence of these lesions will tend to increase the FFR measured across the left main. The influence of an LAD/LCx lesion on the FFR value of the left main will depend on the severity of this distal stenosis but, even more, on the vascular territory supplied by this distal stenosis. For example, if the distal stenosis is in the proximal LAD, its presence will notably impact the stenosis in the left main. If the distal stenosis is located in a small second marginal branch, its influence on the left main stenosis will be minimal (Fig. 9.10).

FFR in multivessel disease

Patients with 'multivessel disease' actually represent a very heterogeneous population. Their anatomical features (number of lesions, their location, and their respective degree of complexity) may vary tremendously and have major implications for the revascularization strategy. Moreover, there is often a large discrepancy between the anatomic description and the actual severity of each stenosis. For example, a patient may have 'three-vessel disease' based on the angiogram, but actually have only two haemodynamically significant stenoses; vice versa, a patient can be considered as having one-vessel disease of the right coronary artery (RCA) but actually have a haemodynamically significant stenosis of the left main. Fig. 9.11 shows a typical example of a patient in whom the RCA and the LCx are critically narrowed and in whom the mid-LAD shows a mild stenosis. Myocardial perfusion imaging showed a reversible perfusion defect in the inferolateral segments and a normal flow distribution in the segments supplied by the LAD. In contrast, FFR shows that all three vessels are significantly narrowed but to a different extent. This has a major implication as far as revascularization is concerned. Preliminary FFR-guided revascularization strategies in patients with

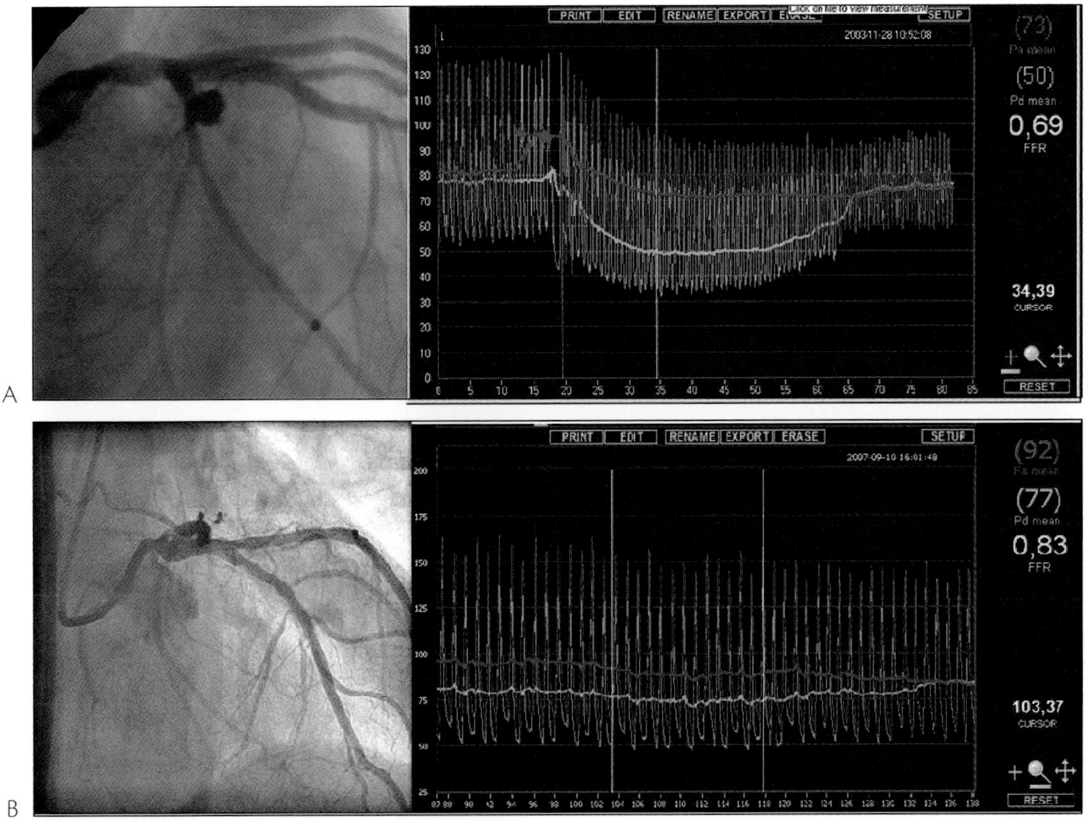

Fig. 9.9 Example of two patients in whom fractional flow reserve (FFR) measurements in an 'intermediate' ostial left main stenosis changed the therapeutic strategy. The first (A) represents a 67-year-old man with massive mitral regurgitation who was scheduled for minimally invasive (port access) mitral valvuloplasty. The coronary angiogram showed an 'intermediate' ostial left main stenosis. The FFR of the left main stenosis was 0.69. Accordingly, this patient underwent conventional coronary artery bypass grafting and mitral valvuloplasty via a median sternotomy. The second (B) represents an 89-year-old man with critical aortic stenosis, referred for aortic valve replacement and bypass surgery because of the presence of an ostial left main stenosis. FFR of the left main stem was 0.83. Accordingly, only a percutaneous aortic valve implantation was performed and the left main stenosis was left alone.

multivessel disease were very encouraging[32–34]. Tailoring the revascularization according to the functional significance of the stenoses rather than on their mere angiographic appearance may decrease costs and avoid the need for surgical revascularization. A recent randomized multicenter study (FAME [Fractional Flow Reserve versus Angiography for Multivessel Evaluation] study) in 1000 patients showed that routine measurement of FFR during PCI with drug-eluting stents in patients with multivessel disease, when compared to current angiography guided strategy reduces the rate of the composite endpoint of death, myocardial infarction, re-PCI, and coronary artery bypass grafting at 1 year by approximately 30% and reduces mortality and myocardial infarction at 1 year by approximately 35 %. Moreover, the FFR-guided strategy reduces the number of stents used, decreases the amount of contrast agent used, does not prolong the procedure, and is cost-saving[35,36].

FFR after myocardial infarction

After a myocardial infarction, previously viable tissue is partially replaced by scar tissue. Therefore, the total mass of functional myocardium supplied by a given stenosis in an infarct-related artery will tend to decrease[37]. By definition, hyperaemic flow and thus hyperaemic gradient will both decrease as well. Assuming that the morphology of the stenosis remains identical, FFR must therefore increase. This does not mean that FFR underestimates lesion severity after myocardial infarction. It simply illustrates the relationship that exists between

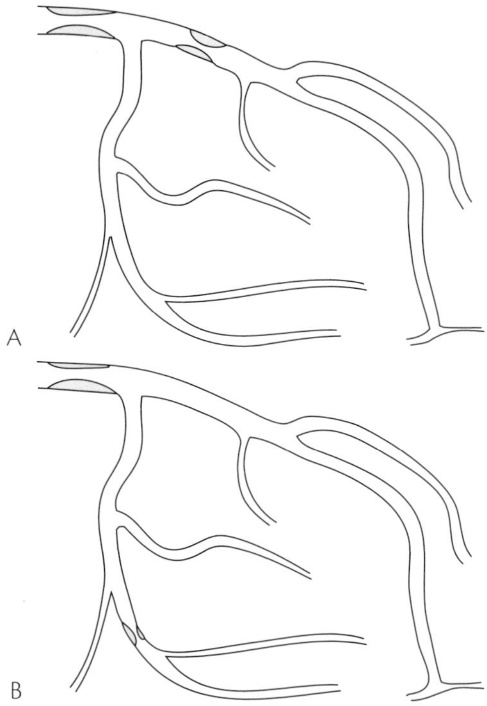

Fig. 9.10 DraSchematic wing of a left main coronary stenosis associated with a proximal left anterior descending stenosis (A) or with a stenosis in the distal circumflex coronary artery (B). The influence of a second stenosis distal on the fractional flow reserve value of the left main will depend on the severity of this distal stenosis and on the vascular territory supplied by this distal stenosis

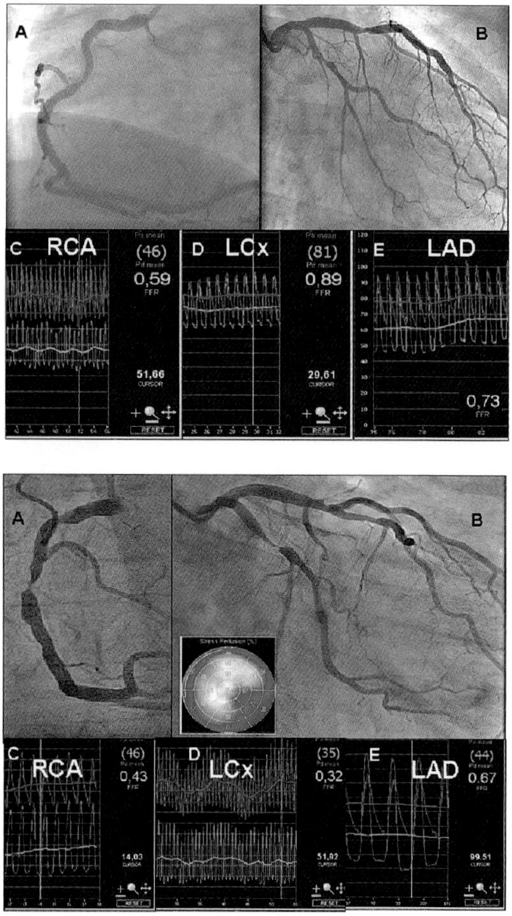

Fig. 9.11 Example of two patients with multivessel disease. Upper panel: a 46-year-old man with stable angina and angiographic three-vessel disease, but functional two-vessel disease (LAD, RCA). Lower panel: a 69-year-old man with severe angina. Myocardial perfusion imaging (MPI) showed a reversible defect in the inferolateral segments. From the angiogram it is obvious that the RCA and the LCx are significantly narrowed (no pressure measurements are needed). However, the mid-LAD stenosis, considered 'non-significant' on the angiogram, appears to be haemodynamically significant. This LAD stenosis was undetected by MPI because the uptake of tracer is notably worse in the LCx territory than in the LAD territory. LAD, left anterior descending artery; LcX, left circumflex artery; RCA, right coronary artery.

flow, pressure gradient, and myocardial mass, and, conversely, illustrates that the mere morphology of a stenotic segment does not necessarily reflect its functional importance. This principle is illustrated in Fig. 9.12. Recent data confirm that the hyperaemic myocardial resistance in viable myocardium within the infarcted area remains normal[38]. This further supports the application of the established FFR cut-off value in the setting of partially infarcted territories. Earlier data had suggested that microvascular function was abnormal in regions remote from a recent myocardial infarction[39,40]. However, more recent work taking into account distal coronary pressure indicates that hyperaemic resistance is normal in these remote segments[41]. These data support the use of FFR to evaluate stenoses remote from a recent myocardial infarction.

FFR in diffuse disease

Histopathology studies and, more recently, intravascular ultrasound have shown that atherosclerosis is diffuse in nature and that a discrete stenosis in an otherwise normal artery is actually rare. The concept of a focal lesion is a mainly angiographic description but does not reflect pathology. Until recently it was believed that when no focal narrowing of greater than 50% was seen at the angiogram no abnormal resistance was present in the epicardial artery. It was therefore assumed that distal pressure was normal and thus that 'diffuse mild disease without focal stenosis' could not cause myocardial

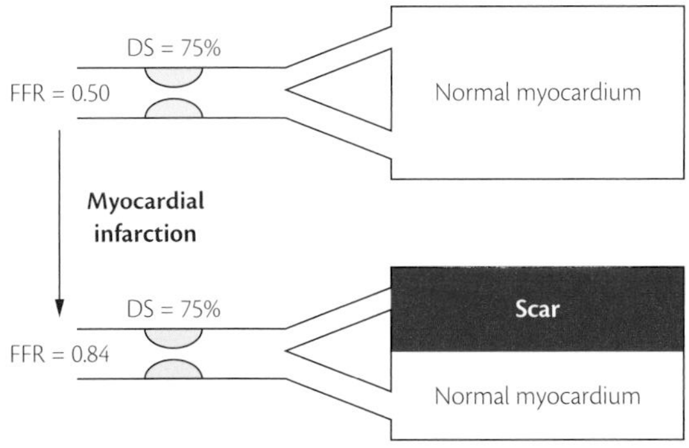

Fig. 9.12 Schematic representation of the relationship between fractional flow reserve (FFR) and myocardial mass before and after myocardial infarction. See text for details. DS, diameter stenosis.

ischaemia. This paradigm has recently been shifted: the presence of diffuse disease is often associated with a progressive decrease in coronary pressure[3] and flow[42], and this cannot be predicted from the angiogram. In contrast, this decline in pressure correlates with the total atherosclerotic burden[43]. In approximately 10% of patients this abnormal epicardial resistance may be responsible for reversible myocardial ischaemia. In these patients chest pain is often considered non-coronary because no single focal stenosis is found, and the myocardial perfusion imaging is wrongly considered false positive ('false false positive')[44]. Such diffuse disease and its haemodynamic impact should always be kept in mind when performing functional measurements. In a large multicentre registry of 750 patients, FFR was obtained after technically successful stenting. A post-PCI FFR value <0.9 was still present in almost one-third of patients and was associated with a poor clinical outcome[45]. The only way to demonstrate the haemodynamic impact of diffuse disease is to perform a careful pullback manoeuvre of the pressure sensor under steady-state maximal hyperaemia (Fig. 9.13).

FFR in sequential stenoses

When several stenoses are present in the same artery, the concept and the clinical value of FFR is still valid to assess the effect of all stenoses together. Yet, it is important to realize that when several discrete stenoses are

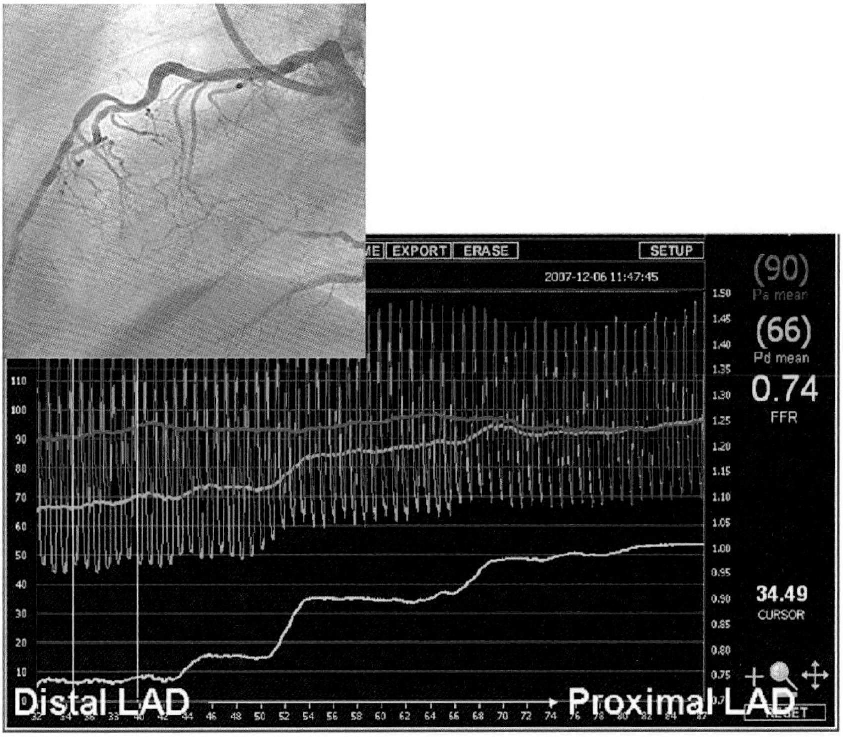

Fig. 9.13 A 73-year old man with angina related to a tight stenosis in the proximal right coronary artery (RCA). The distal P_d/P_a ratio in the left anterior descending artery (LAD) is 0.74. The pressure pullback tracing under steady state maximal hyperaemia shows that the distal pressure increases progressively in three or four 'steps'. This indicates that the abnormal fractional flow reserve (FFR) value is due to diffuse disease, rather than to one focal stenosis (red arrow) that was the intended target of percutaneous coronary intervention.

present in the same coronary artery, each of them will influence hyperaemic flow and therefore the pressure gradient across the other one. The influence of the distal lesion on the proximal is more important than the reverse. The FFR can theoretically be calculated for each stenosis individually[46,47]. However, this is neither practical nor easy to perform and therefore of little use in the catheterization laboratory. Practically, as for diffuse disease, a pullback manoeuvre under maximal hyperaemia is the only way to appreciate the exact location and physiological significance of sequential stenoses.

FFR in bifurcation lesions

Overlapping of vessel segments as well as radiographic artefacts render bifurcation stenoses particularly difficult to evaluate at angiography, while PCI of bifurcations is often more challenging than for regular stenoses. The principle of FFR-guided PCI applies in bifurcation lesions even though clinical outcome data are currently limited. Two recent studies by Koo and colleagues[48,49] used FFR in the setting of bifurcation stenting. The results of these studies can be summarized as follows: (1) after stenting the ostium of the side branch looks often 'pinched'. Yet such stenoses are grossly overestimated by angiography—none of these ostial lesions where the diameter stenosis was estimated as, 75% were found to have an FFR below 0.75. (2) When kissing balloon dilation was performed only in ostial stenoses with an FFR <0.75, the FFR at 6 months was >0.75 in 95% of all cases.

FFR and coronary artery bypass graft lesions

Assessment of stenosis severity in coronary artery bypass grafts by FFR is technically very easy. In addition, all theoretical assumptions underlying the concept of FFR hold in cases of bypasses. There is no reason to believe that another threshold value should be found even though this has not being formally investigated in large series[50]. Stated another way, FFR is able to define

Table 9.3 Tips and tricks in FFR measurements

Handling the coronary pressure wire	Be careful with the sensor that is located at the junction between the radiopaque and radiolucent part of the wire
Introducer needles	Use thin needles (should be tested before, do not use if significant backflow). Valve of the Y-connector should be tightly closed
Equalization	The aortic pressure transducer should be positioned at a height 5cm below the patient's sternum, which is estimated to be the location of the aortic root. After calibration of aortic pressure and microchip of the PressureWire®, the PressureWire® is advance into the proximal part of the target artery, located at the tip of the guiding in order to equalize electronically both pressure
Drift	After a long procedure, differences may sometimes occur between aortic and coronary pressures. Morphology of the distal pressure can make the difference between true pressure gradient (ventricularized) and drift (exactly the same morphology). Drift in right coronary artery is more difficult to recognize. One should suspect drift if aortic notch is maintained in a presence of a large gradient
Whipping	When the guide wire sensor hits the coronary wall, an increase in the pressure signal can be seen. Pull back (or advance) the wire a few mm
Accordion effect	This artefact is due to folds of the vessel wall when tortuous coronary segment is stretched by the guide wire, inducing a false pressure gradient. When the wire is pulled back the folds immediately disappear
Guiding catheter in the ostium	The presence of a guiding catheter in the coronary ostium may induce a pressure drop (especially during hyperaemia) which can be recognized by ventricularization of the guiding pressure signal. Pull the guiding catheter back a few mm into the aorta
Catheter with sides holes	The guiding pressure will result in a pressure 'somewhere in between' coronary and aortic pressure (side holes and end-hole). Intracoronary administration of drugs is unreliable. One should avoid using a side-holes catheter for FFR measurements
Disconnection and reconnection of the wire	On the proximal end of PressureWire®, three flat electrodes can be seen. This part (approximately 2.5cm) of the wire should ideally be kept dry and free of blood and contrast medium. In practice, this is often impossible as balloons, stents, and other catheters have to be advanced over the wire. It is therefore advisable, when the pressure wire has been disconnected, to wipe the electrodes with wet gauze and to dry them with dry gauze afterwards

whether or not a stenosis in a bypass graft is capable of inducing ischaemia. In contrast, there are no clinical outcome data obtained in patients in whom decisions regarding revascularization have been based on FFR. It seems common sense to admit that in patients with an FFR <0.75, the revascularization of this lesion might be beneficial for the patient. However, deferring the revascularization procedure because on the basis of an FFR value >0.75 is not proven. Therefore, FFR should be used with caution in bypass graft.

One important study by Botman *et al.* has investigated the relationship between stenosis severity in native arteries and graft patency after 6 months. The authors showed that the rate of occlusion was approximately three times higher when the bypass was placed on a native artery with a haemodynamically non-significant stenosis(51). These results corroborate the data reported by Berger *et al.* who showed that internal mammary arteries placed on mildly diseased native arteries showed a very high attrition rate(25).

Tips and tricks

Since this book is intended to be as practical as possible, a list of tips and tricks is given in Table 9.3.

Conclusion: towards a new diagnostic algorithm for patients with known or suspected coronary artery disease

Pressure-derived FFR is a theoretically robust and practically simple means of assessing the functional consequences of epicardial coronary atherosclerosis. With minimal experience the technique of FFR measurements is simple, swift, and safe. Only a pressure wire and a bolus of hyperaemia-inducing medication are required. Its invasive nature is counterbalanced by its unequalled spatial resolution, offering functional information down to the 'per centimetre' level, while non-invasive tests operate, at best, at the 'per vascular territory' level. Clinical outcome data of patients in whom the revascularization strategy has been based on FFR measurements are very encouraging. Accordingly, FFR can be considered as the interventional cardiologist's 'pocket myocardial perfusion imaging' modality. This is true with some important qualifications: (1) FFR is more accurate in intermediate lesions; (2) FFR has a better spatial resolution; (3) combined with the index of myocardial resistance (IMR), FFR is able to distinguish epicardial and myocardial resistance(6); and (4) it is available in the catheterization laboratory, as FFR is performed in conjunction with coronary angiography. Therefore, it is the only true 'all-in-one' approach for patients with suspected or known coronary artery disease as it combines unequalled physiological information, the best possible anatomical information, and the possibility of immediate revascularization if needed.

We therefore believe that the diagnostic work-up of patients with known or suspected coronary artery disease might be drastically shortened (Fig. 9.14). The conventional teaching(52) is that patients with suspected coronary stenosis should first undergo non-invasive functional testing, the so-called 'gate-keepers' of the catheterization laboratory. Patients are referred for diagnostic coronary angiography if (and only if) these

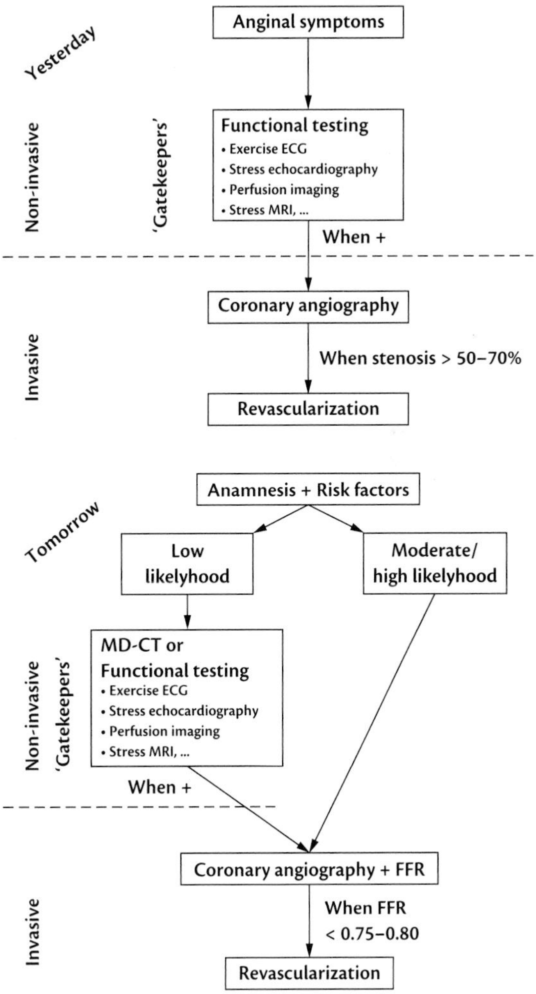

Fig. 9.14 Two plots to show how fractional flow reserve (FFR) might change the current appraisal of coronary artery disease.

tests indicate reversible myocardial ischaemia. At angiography, a 50–70% stenosis is often considered a justification for revascularization. We have seen, however, how often the results of non-invasive functional tests performed sequentially are inaccurate and/or contradictory. In addition, the angiographic degree of stenosis is a battered gold standard, leading to a large number of inappropriate decisions regarding revascularization[22]. Finally, non-invasive testing is actually performed in only a minority of patients undergoing angioplasty[21].

In contrast to this conventional approach, we propose to put more emphasis on a careful interrogation of the patients including a precise analysis of his/her risk factors. If, on this basis, an experienced cardiologist comes to the conclusion 'this person might well have significant coronary artery stenoses' we believe it is more efficacious to send the patient directly to the catheterization laboratory *if and only if*, in the catheterization laboratory, FFR measurements can be obtained *and* the revascularization strategy is guided by the integration of clinical, anatomic (angiographic), and functional (FFR) information.

References

1. Verma S, Anderson TJ. Fundamentals of endothelial function for the clinical cardiologist. *Circulation* 2002; **105**(5):546–9.
2. Seiler C, Kirkeeide RL, Gould KL. Basic structure-function relations of the epicardial coronary vascular tree. Basis of quantitative coronary arteriography for diffuse coronary artery disease. *Circulation* 1992; **85**(6): 1987–2003.
3. De Bruyne B, Hersbach F, Pijls NH, *et al.* Abnormal epicardial coronary resistance in patients with diffuse atherosclerosis but "normal" coronary angiography. *Circulation* 2001; **104**(20):2401–6.
4. Gould KL, Lipscomb K, Hamilton GW. Physiologic basis for assessing critical coronary stenosis. Instantaneous flow response and regional distribution during coronary hyperemia as measures of coronary flow reserve. *Am J Cardiol* 1974; **33**(1):87–94.
5. Kern MJ, Lerman A, Bech JW, *et al.* Physiological assessment of coronary artery disease in the cardiac catheterization laboratory: a scientific statement from the American Heart Association Committee on Diagnostic and Interventional Cardiac Catheterization, Council on Clinical Cardiology. *Circulation* 2006; **114**(12):1321–41.
6. Fearon WF, Balsam LB, Farouque HM, *et al.* Novel index for invasively assessing the coronary microcirculation. *Circulation* 2003; **107**(25):3129–32.
7. Fearon WF, Shah M, Ng M, *et al.* Predictive value of the index of microcirculatory resistance in patients with ST-segment elevation myocardial infarction. *J Am Coll Cardiol* 2008; **51**(5):560–5.
8. Sezer M, Oflaz H, Goren T, *et al.* Intracoronary streptokinase after primary percutaneous coronary intervention. *N Engl J Med* 2007; **356**(18):1823–34.
9. Siebes M, Verhoeff BJ, Meuwissen M, *et al.* Single-wire pressure and flow velocity measurement to quantify coronary stenosis hemodynamics and effects of percutaneous interventions. *Circulation* 2004; **109**(6): 756–62.
10. Meuwissen M, Siebes M, Chamuleau SA, *et al.* Hyperemic stenosis resistance index for evaluation of functional coronary lesion severity. *Circulation* 2002; **106**(4):441–6.
11. Pijls NH, van Son JA, Kirkeeide RL, *et al.* Experimental basis of determining maximum coronary, myocardial, and collateral blood flow by pressure measurements for assessing functional stenosis severity before and after percutaneous transluminal coronary angioplasty. *Circulation* 1993; **87**(4):1354–67.
12. De Bruyne B, Baudhuin T, Melin JA, *et al.* Coronary flow reserve calculated from pressure measurements in humans. Validation with positron emission tomography. *Circulation* 1994; **89**(3):1013–22.
13. Legalery P, Seronde MF, Meneveau N, *et al.* Measuring pressure-derived fractional flow reserve through four French diagnostic catheters. *Am J Cardiol* 2003; **91**(9):1075–8.
14. De Bruyne B, Pijls NH, Barbato E, *et al.* Intracoronary and intravenous adenosine 5'-triphosphate, adenosine, papaverine, and contrast medium to assess fractional flow reserve in humans. *Circulation* 2003; **107**(14):1877–83.
15. McGeoch RJ, Oldroyd KG. Pharmacological options for inducing maximal hyperaemia during studies of coronary physiology. *Catheter Cardiovasc Interv* 2008; **71**(2): 198–204.
16. Parham WA, Bouhasin A, Ciaramita JP, *et al.* Coronary hyperemic dose responses of intracoronary sodium nitroprusside. *Circulation* 2004; **109**(10):1236–43.
17. Pijls NH, Van Gelder B, Van der Voort P, *et al.* Fractional flow reserve. A useful index to evaluate the influence of an epicardial coronary stenosis on myocardial blood flow. *Circulation* 1995; **92**(11):3183–93.
18. de Bruyne B, Bartunek J, Sys SU, *et al.* Simultaneous coronary pressure and flow velocity measurements in humans. Feasibility, reproducibility, and hemodynamic dependence of coronary flow velocity reserve, hyperemic flow versus pressure slope index, and fractional flow reserve. *Circulation* 1996; **94**(8):1842–9.
19. Murtagh B, Higano S, Lennon R, *et al.* Role of incremental doses of intracoronary adenosine for fractional flow reserve assessment. *Am Heart J* 2003; **146**(1):99–105.
20. Pijls NH, De Bruyne B, Peels K, *et al.* Measurement of fractional flow reserve to assess the functional severity of coronary-artery stenoses. *N Engl J Med* 1996; **334**(26):1703–8.
21. Topol EJ, Ellis SG, Cosgrove DM, *et al.* Analysis of coronary angioplasty practice in the United States with an insurance-claims data base. *Circulation* 1993; **87**(5): 1489–97.

22. Wijns W, De Bruyne B, Vanhoenacker PK. What does the clinical cardiologist need from noninvasive cardiac imaging: is it time to adjust practices to meet evolving demands? *J Nucl Cardiol* 2007; **14**(3):366–70.
23. Pijls NH, van Schaardenburgh P, Manoharan G, *et al.* Percutaneous coronary intervention of functionally nonsignificant stenosis: 5-year follow-up of the DEFER Study. *J Am Coll Cardiol* 2007; **49**(21):2105–11.
24. Chaitman BR, Fisher LD, Bourassa MG, *et al.* Effect of coronary bypass surgery on survival patterns in subsets of patients with left main coronary artery disease. Report of the Collaborative Study in Coronary Artery Surgery (CASS). *Am J Cardiol* 1981; **48**(4):765–77.
25. Berger A, MacCarthy PA, Siebert U, *et al.* Long-term patency of internal mammary artery bypass grafts: relationship with preoperative severity of the native coronary artery stenosis. *Circulation* 2004; **110** (11 Suppl 1):II36–40.
26. Lindstaedt M, Spiecker M, Perings C, *et al.* How good are experienced interventional cardiologists at predicting the functional significance of intermediate or equivocal left main coronary artery stenoses? *Int J Cardiol* 2007; **120**(2):254–61.
27. Lima RS, Watson DD, Goode AR, *et al.* Incremental value of combined perfusion and function over perfusion alone by gated SPECT myocardial perfusion imaging for detection of severe three-vessel coronary artery disease. *J Am Coll Cardiol* 2003; **42**(1):64–70.
28. Ragosta M, Bishop AH, Lipson LC, *et al.* Comparison between angiography and fractional flow reserve versus single-photon emission computed tomographic myocardial perfusion imaging for determining lesion significance in patients with multivessel coronary disease. *Am J Cardiol* 2007; **99**(7):896–902.
29. Bech GJ, Droste H, Pijls NH, *et al.* Value of fractional flow reserve in making decisions about bypass surgery for equivocal left main coronary artery disease. *Heart* 2001; **86**(5):547–52.
30. Jasti V, Ivan E, Yalamanchili V, *et al.* Correlations between fractional flow reserve and intravascular ultrasound in patients with an ambiguous left main coronary artery stenosis. *Circulation* 2004; **110**(18):2831–6.
31. Leesar MA, Mintz GS. Hemodynamic and intravascular ultrasound assessment of an ambiguous left main coronary artery stenosis. *Catheter Cardiovasc Interv* 2007; **70**(5):721–30.
32. Botman KJ, Pijls NH, Bech JW, *et al.* Percutaneous coronary intervention or bypass surgery in multivessel disease? A tailored approach based on coronary pressure measurement. *Catheter Cardiovasc Interv* 2004; **63**(2): 184–91.
33. Berger A, Botman KJ, MacCarthy PA, *et al.* Long-term clinical outcome after fractional flow reserve-guided percutaneous coronary intervention in patients with multivessel disease. *J Am Coll Cardiol* 2005; **46**(3):438–42.
34. Wongpraparut N, Yalamanchili V, Pasnoori V, *et al.* Thirty-month outcome after fractional flow reserve-guided versus conventional multivessel percutaneous coronary intervention. *Am J Cardiol* 2005; **96**(7): 877–84.
35. Fearon WF, Tonino PA, De Bruyne B, *et al.* Rationale and design of the Fractional Flow Reserve versus Angiography for Multivessel Evaluation (FAME) study. *Am Heart J* 2007; **154**(4):632–6.
36. Tonino PA, De Bruyne B, Pijls NH, *et al.* Fractional flow reserve versus angiography for guiding percutaneous coronary intervention. *N Engl J Med* 2009; **360**(3):213–24.
37. De Bruyne B, Pijls NH, Bartunek J, *et al.* Fractional flow reserve in patients with prior myocardial infarction. *Circulation* 2001; **104**(2):157–62.
38. Marques KM, Knaapen P, Boellaard R, *et al.* Microvascular function in viable myocardium after chronic infarction does not influence fractional flow reserve measurements. *J Nucl Med* 2007; **48**(12):1987–92.
39. Uren NG, Crake T, Lefroy DC, *et al.* Reduced coronary vasodilator function in infarcted and normal myocardium after myocardial infarction. *N Engl J Med* 1994; **331**(4):222–7.
40. Claeys MJ, Vrints CJ, Bosmans J, *et al.* Coronary flow reserve during coronary angioplasty in patients with a recent myocardial infarction: relation to stenosis and myocardial viability. *J Am Coll Cardiol* 1996; **28**(7): 1712–9.
41. Marques KM, Knaapen P, Boellaard R, *et al.* Hyperaemic microvascular resistance is not increased in viable myocardium after chronic myocardial infarction. *Eur Heart J* 2007; **28**(19):2320–5.
42. Gould KL, Nakagawa Y, Nakagawa K, *et al.* Frequency and clinical implications of fluid dynamically significant diffuse coronary artery disease manifest as graded, longitudinal, base-to-apex myocardial perfusion abnormalities by noninvasive positron emission tomography. *Circulation* 2000; **101**(16):1931–9.
43. Fearon WF, Nakamura M, Lee DP, *et al.* Simultaneous assessment of fractional and coronary flow reserves in cardiac transplant recipients: Physiologic Investigation for Transplant Arteriopathy (PITA Study). *Circulation* 2003; **108**(13):1605–10.
44. Aarnoudse WH, Botman KJ, Pijls NH. False-negative myocardial scintigraphy in balanced three-vessel disease, revealed by coronary pressure measurement. *Int J Cardiovasc Intervent* 2003; **5**(2):67–71.
45. Pijls NH, Klauss V, Siebert U, *et al.* Coronary pressure measurement after stenting predicts adverse events at follow-up: a multicenter registry. *Circulation* 2002; **105**(25):2950–4.
46. De Bruyne B, Pijls NH, Heyndrickx GR, *et al.* Pressure-derived fractional flow reserve to assess serial epicardial stenoses: theoretical basis and animal validation. *Circulation* 2000; **101**(15):1840–7.
47. Pijls NH, De Bruyne B, Bech GJ, *et al.* Coronary pressure measurement to assess the hemodynamic significance of serial stenoses within one coronary artery: validation in humans. *Circulation* 2000; **102**(19):2371–7.

48. Koo BK, Kang HJ, Youn TJ, *et al.* Physiologic assessment of jailed side branch lesions using fractional flow reserve. *J Am Coll Cardiol* 2005; **46**(4):633–7.
49. Koo BK, Park KW, Kang HJ, *et al.* Physiological evaluation of the provisional side-branch intervention strategy for bifurcation lesions using fractional flow reserve. *Eur Heart J* 2008; **29**(6):726–32.
50. Aqel R, Zoghbi GJ, Hage F, *et al.* Hemodynamic evaluation of coronary artery bypass graft lesions using fractional flow reserve. *Catheter Cardiovasc Interv* 2008; **72**(4):479–85.
51. Botman CJ, Schonberger J, Koolen S, *et al.* Does stenosis severity of native vessels influence bypass graft patency? A prospective fractional flow reserve-guided study. *Ann Thorac Surg* 2007; **83**(6):2093–7.
52. Bugiardini R, Bairey Merz CN. Angina with "normal" coronary arteries: a changing philosophy. *JAMA* 2005; **293**(4):477–84.
53. Canty JM, Jr. Coronary pressure-function and steady-state pressure-flow relations during autoregulation in the unanesthetized dog. *Circ Res* 1988; **63**(4):821–36.
54. De Bruyne B, Bartunek J, Sys SU, *et al.* Relation between myocardial fractional flow reserve calculated from coronary pressure measurements and exercise-induced myocardial ischemia. *Circulation* 1995; **92**(1):39–46.
55. Bartunek J, Marwick TH, Rodrigues AC, *et al.* Dobutamine-induced wall motion abnormalities: correlations with myocardial fractional flow reserve and quantitative coronary angiography. *J Am Coll Cardiol* 1996; **27**(6):1429–36.
56. Chamuleau SA, Meuwissen M, van Eck-Smit BL, *et al.* Fractional flow reserve, absolute and relative coronary blood flow velocity reserve in relation to the results of technetium-99m sestamibi single-photon emission computed tomography in patients with two-vessel coronary artery disease. *J Am Coll Cardiol* 2001; **37**(5):1316–22.
57. Abe M, Tomiyama H, Yoshida H, *et al.* Diastolic fractional flow reserve to assess the functional severity of moderate coronary artery stenoses: comparison with fractional flow reserve and coronary flow velocity reserve. *Circulation* 2000; **102**(19):2365–70.

CHAPTER 10

The role of intravascular ultrasound in percutaneous coronary intervention

Hiromasa Otake, Yasuhiro Honda, and Peter J. Fitzgerald

Contrast angiography has been used in routine clinical practice to evaluate coronary and peripheral artery disease. However, angiography provides only indirect information about the vessel wall structure, possibly misguiding operators in catheter-based interventions. In contrast, intravascular ultrasound (IVUS) has been the first widely-applied clinical imaging technology to directly visualize atherosclerosis and other pathologic conditions within the vessel wall. Its ability to image the entire arterial cross-section in real time offers better understanding of the process of atherosclerosis, as well as improvement of the precision of interventional procedures. This chapter reviews current clinical evidence established by IVUS technology, with an overview of basic image interpretation and IVUS-based assessment of coronary lesions.

Principles and procedures

IVUS imaging systems use reflected sound waves to visualize the vessel wall in a two-dimensional, tomographic format, analogous to a histologic cross-section. Compared to non-invasive echocardiography, significantly higher frequencies of the miniaturized IVUS transducers achieve higher radial resolutions (150 microns for the coronary catheters) at the expense of limited beam penetration (4–8mm from the catheter tip). Current IVUS catheters used in the coronary arteries have centre frequencies ranging from 20–45MHz, providing theoretical lower limits of resolution (calculated as half the wavelength) of 31 microns and 19 microns respectively. In practice, the radial resolution is at least two to five times poorer, as determined by factors such as the length of the emitted pulse and the position of the imaged structures relative to the transducer.

Imaging systems

There are two basic catheter designs—solid-state or mechanical—both generating a 360-degree, cross-sectional image plane perpendicular to the catheter tip. In the solid-state approach, the individual elements of a circumferential array of transducer elements are mounted near the tip of the catheter and activated with different time delays, to create an ultrasound beam that sweeps the circumference of the vessel (Fig. 10.1A). Complex miniaturized integrated circuits in the catheter tip control the timing and integration of the transducer activation, and route the resulting echo information to a computer where cross-sectional images are reconstructed and displayed in real time. In the mechanical approach, a single transducer element is rotated inside the tip of a catheter via a flexible torque cable spun by an external motor drive unit attached to the proximal end of the catheter (Fig. 10.1B). Images from each angular position of the transducer are collected by a computerized image array processor, which synthesizes a cross-sectional ultrasound image of the vessel.

One advantage of the solid-state systems is the absence of any moving parts within the catheter, precluding non-uniform rotational distortion (NURD) occasionally observed with the mechanical transducers. This artefact is represented as a wedge-shaped, smeared

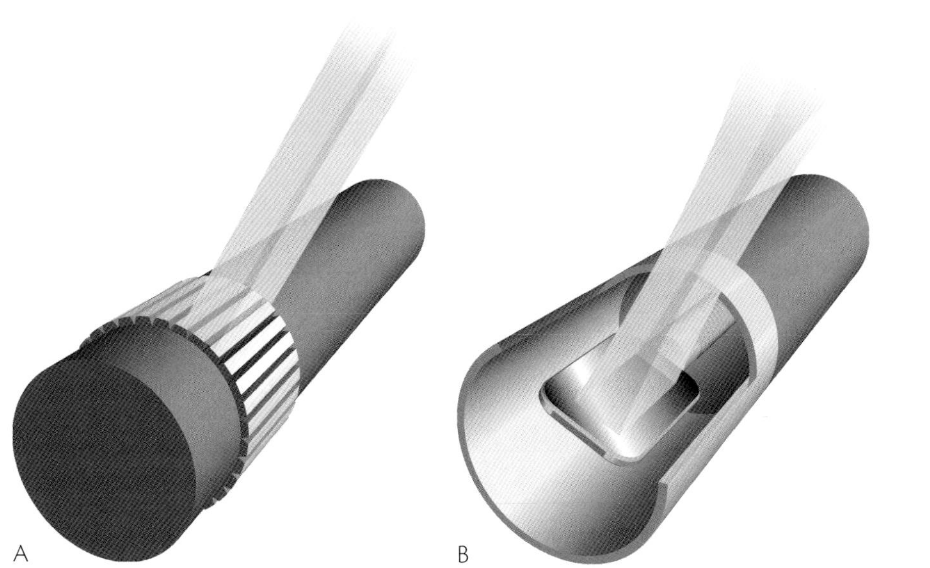

Fig. 10.1 Diagrams of the two basic imaging catheter designs, solid state (A) and mechanical (B).

image to appear in one or more segments of the image (Fig. 10.2D), and can occur when the mechanical catheter is placed in tortuous anatomy or with overtightening of a haemostatic valve. On the other hand, the mechanical transducers have traditionally offered advantages in image quality compared to the solid-state systems. Also, the mechanical catheters with a stationary outer sheath are easy to use with a motorized pullback device, allowing the transducer to be moved through a segment of interest in a precise and controlled manner. With both systems, still frames and video images can be digitally archived on local storage memory or a remote server using DICOM Standard 3.0.

Imaging procedures

Prior to IVUS imaging, intravenous heparin (5000–10 000 units) or equivalent anticoagulation should be administered, as well as intracoronary nitroglycerin (100–300mcg) to reduce the potential risk of spasm. The image integrity should be checked before inserting the catheter. Mechanical catheters require flushing with saline to remove the residual microbubbles from inside the catheter. Insufficient flushing can result in poor image quality once the catheter is inserted (Fig. 10.2A). The solid-state catheter requires an extra step to mask 'ring-down' artefact prior to being inserted into the coronary artery. This masking process is accomplished by pressing a button on the system, while the catheter tip is disengaged from the ostium and the tip of the imaging catheter positioned in the aorta.

Using standard interventional techniques with a 0.014-inch angioplasty guide wire, the imaging element is advanced distal to the area of interest. When NURD is observed (mechanical IVUS), the operator should attempt to straighten the catheter and motor drive assembly, lessen guiding catheter tension, or loosen the haemostatic valve of the Y-adapter. The length of the target vessel is then scanned by retracting the transducer manually or mechanically within a stationary outer sheath (mechanical IVUS), or by moving the catheter itself (solid-state IVUS). Image acquisition is recommended to include at least 10mm of distal vessel, lesion site, and the entire proximal vessel, back to the aorta. Automated motorized pullback at a constant speed (0.5–1mm/s) is strongly recommended, since it enables precise longitudinal distance measurements or registration of a given cross-section for repeat studies. This also allows longitudinal image display or three-dimensional reconstruction of a vessel segment[1,2]. Use of negative contrast may be considered when abnormal lesion morphologies, such as tears, thrombus, and incomplete stent apposition are suspected.

Safety

As with other interventional procedures, the possibility of spasm, dissection, and thrombosis exists when IVUS

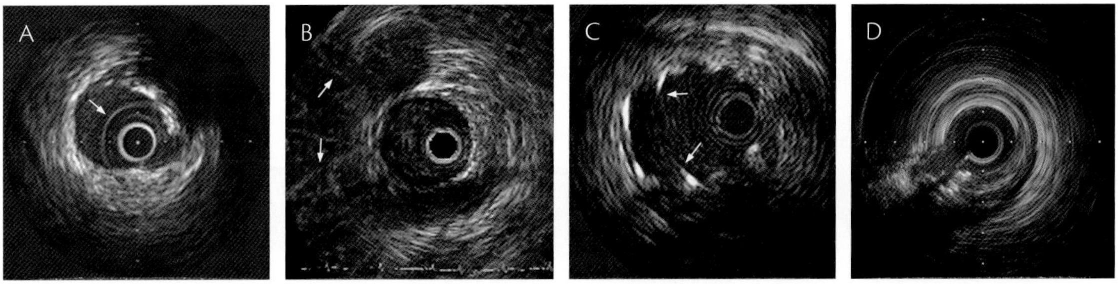

Fig. 10.2 Common image artefacts. A) A 'halo' or a series of bright rings immediately around the mechanical intravascular ultrasound (IVUS) catheter is generally caused by air bubbles that need to be flushed out. B) Radiofrequency noise appears as alternating radial spokes or random white dots in the far-field. The interference is usually caused by other electrical equipment in the catheterization laboratory. C) 'White cap' artefacts due to side-lobe echoes originate from a strong reflecting surface, such as metal stent struts and calcification. The smearing of the strut image can lead to the mistaken impression that the struts are protruding into the lumen, potentially interfering with area measurements and the assessment of apposition, dissection, etc. D) Non-uniform rotational distortion (NURD) results in a wedge-shaped, smeared appearance in one or more segments of the image.

catheters are used. A retrospective study of 2207 patients identified spasm in 2.9% of patients and other complications including dissection, thrombosis, and abrupt closure with 'certain relation' to IVUS in 0.4%[3]. This study was performed with first-generation catheters in the early 1990s, and it is likely that the incidence of complications is substantially lower with the current generation catheters.

Basics of image interpretation

Three-layered appearance of arterial wall

In muscular arteries such as the coronary tree, the media may stand out as a thin dark band, since it contains much less echo-reflective material (collagen and elastin) than the neighbouring intima and adventitia, providing a characteristic three-layered (bright–dark–bright) appearance on IVUS images (Fig. 10.3)[4,5]. However, the stronger echo-reflectivity of the intimal layer often causes a spillover effect, known as 'blooming', resulting in a slight overestimation of the intimal thickness with a corresponding underestimation of the medial thickness. Also, this three-layered appearance may be undetectable in truly normal coronary arteries of which the intimal thickness is below the effective resolution of IVUS[6]. In atherosclerotic disease where the media has been destroyed, the media may not appear as a distinct layer around the full circumference of the vessel[7–9]. In the proximal vessel segments and at branch points, the media contains relatively high amounts of collagen and elastin, frequently causing it to blend with the surrounding layers[10]. Even in these cases, however, the boundary between the outer media and adventitia (the outer perimeter of plaque-plus-media zone) is accurately identifiable due to a step-up in echo reflectivity at this boundary without blooming. For these reasons, the plaque-plus-media area is adopted as a surrogate measure for plaque area alone. The adventitia and peri-adventitial tissues are similar enough in echo reflectivity that a clear outer adventitial border cannot be defined.

Quantitative measurements

Unlike angiography, IVUS has an intrinsic distance calibration, provided as a grid on the image or as tag information of DICOM files. Electronic caliper (diameter) and tracing (area) measurements can be performed at the tightest cross-section, as well as at reference segments located proximal and distal to the lesion[11]. In general, the reference segment is selected as the most normal-looking (largest lumen with smallest plaque burden) cross-section within 10mm from the lesion with no intervening major side branches. Quantitative IVUS assessment should not be attempted in the presence of significant NURD.

Vessel and lumen diameter measurements are important in everyday clinical practice where accurate sizing of devices is needed. The maximum and minimum diameters (the major and minor axes of an elliptical cross-section) are the most widely used. The ratio of maximum to minimum diameter defines a measure of symmetry. Area measurements are performed with computer planimetry; lumen area is determined by tracing the leading edge of the blood/intima border, while vessel (or external elastic membrane, EEM) area is defined as the area enclosed by the outermost interface

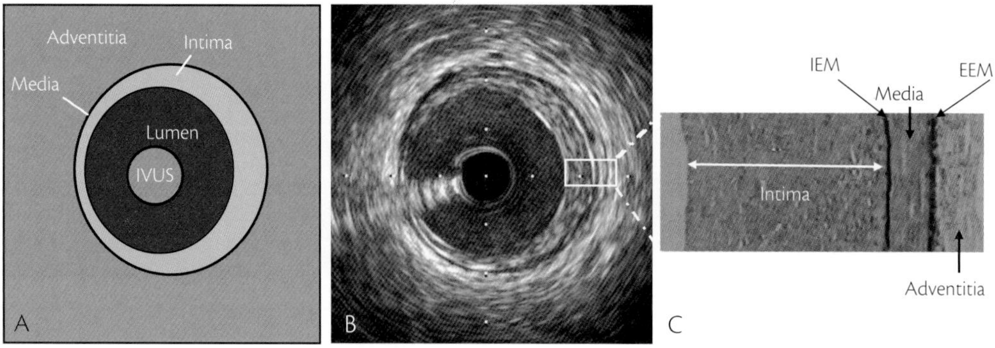

Fig. 10.3 A schematic diagram (A) and intravascular ultrasound (IVUS) image (B) with the corresponding histologic section (C), demonstrating the classic three-layered appearance of intima (plaque), media, and adventitia. In many cases, the media can be difficult to resolve clearly in some portion of the image, but in this particular image, it stands out in all sectors. Note the speckled appearance of the blood within the lumen, particularly near the luminal border. EEM, external elastic membrane; IEM, internal elastic membrane.

between media and adventitia. Plaque area (or plaque-plus-media area) is calculated as the difference between vessel and lumen areas; the ratio of plaque to vessel area is termed either the percent plaque area, plaque burden, or percent cross-sectional narrowing. With the use of motorized pullback, area measurements can be added to calculate volumes using Simpson's rule.

Qualitative assessment

Calcification is recognized as an intensely bright interface that overlies an acoustic shadow extending radially outward[7,12–14]. Shadowing precludes determination of the thickness of a calcific deposit as well as visualization of vessel structures behind the calcium. It is often accompanied by 'reverberation' (multiple ghost images of the leading calcium interface spaced at regular intervals radially). Densely fibrous plaque is also echogenic and can cause signal attenuation or partial acoustic shadowing. The extent of shadowing depends on the thickness and density of the fibrotic component as well as the transducer power. Fatty plaque has less echoreflectivity than fibrous plaque, and the brightness of the adventitia can be used as a gauge to discriminate predominantly fatty from fibrous plaque. In some cases, IVUS can identify the presence of a lipid pool from the appearance of a dark region within the plaque[7,15]. However, the sensitivity and specificity of IVUS for the detection of lipid accumulations are both relatively low[15]. False channels within the plaque can give a similar appearance and, occasionally, shadowing from an adjacent calcified or fibrous region can mimic the appearance of a lipid pool[16]. Newly developed imaging modalities, such as spectroscopy [17], optical coherence tomography (OCT)[18], and intravascular magnetic resonance imaging (MRI)[19], promise to offer more accurate identification of lipid pool within plaques.

One of the major limitations of IVUS in tissue identification is the difficulty in discriminating thrombus from soft plaque[20]. In some cases, several IVUS findings can be clues to the presence of thrombus. Fresh thrombus can exhibit a scintillating tissue appearance that is fairly characteristic. Thrombus is much more likely than soft plaque to have the appearance of clefts or microchannels. In favourable cases, a thrombus has an undulating motion during the pulse cycle that is not seen with plaque.

Image orientation

One important aspect of image interpretation is determining the position of the imaging plane within the artery. The IVUS beam penetrates beyond the artery, providing images of perivascular structures, such as the cardiac veins, the myocardium, and the pericardium[21]. These structures have a characteristic appearance when viewed from different positions within the arterial tree, so they provide useful landmarks regarding the position of the imaging plane (Fig. 10.4). The branching patterns of the arteries are also distinctive and help identify the position of the transducer. In the left anterior descending (LAD) system, for example, the septal perforators generally branch at a wider angle than the diagonals, so that on the IVUS scan, the septals appear to bud away from the LAD much more abruptly than the diagonals. The combination of perivascular landmarks and branching patterns allows the experienced operator to identify the vessel and segment from the IVUS image

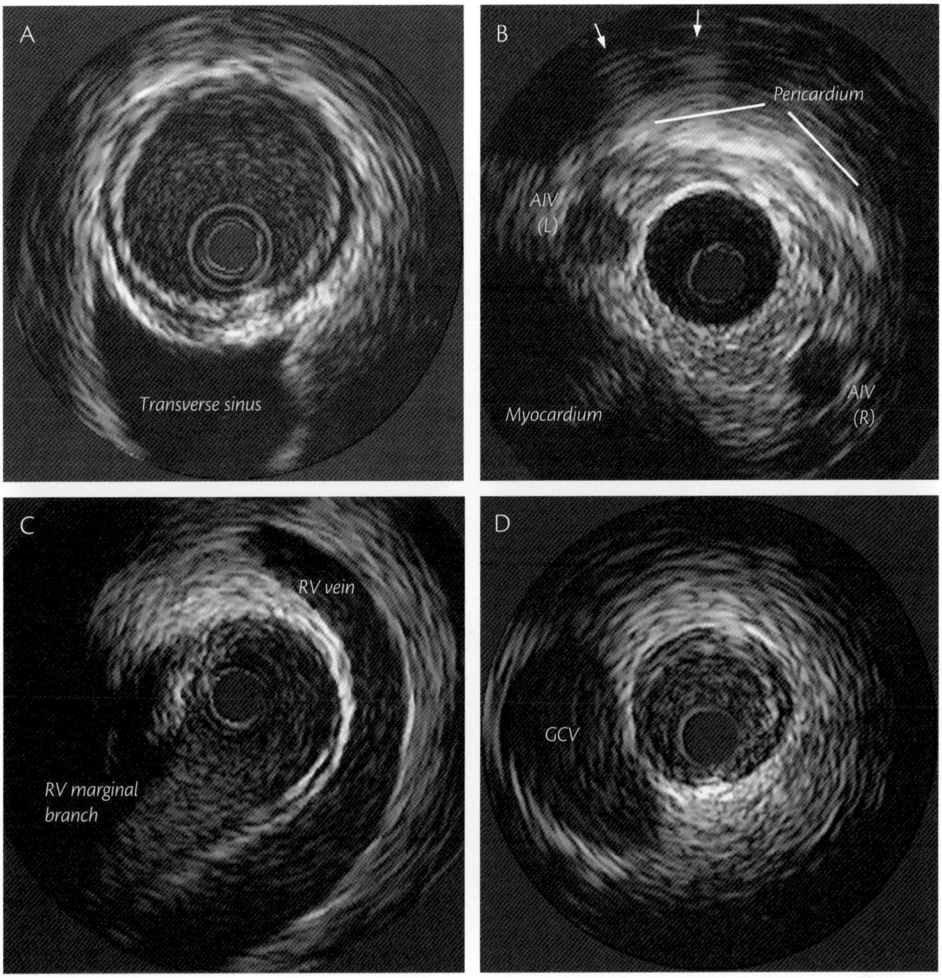

Fig. 10.4 Representative ultrasound image of perivascular landmarks. A) In the proximal portion of the left main coronary artery, a clear echo-free space filled with pericardial fluid, called the transverse sinus, is found adjacent to the artery, immediately outside of the left lateral aspect of the aortic root. B) In this distal cross-section from the LAD, the right and left branches of the anterior interventricular vein (AIV) are seen to straddle the coronary artery. The pericardium appears as a typical bright stripe with rays emitting from it (arrows). C) At the level of the mid right coronary artery, the veins arc over the artery, typically at a position just adjacent to the right ventricular (RV) marginal branches. D) The great cardiac vein (GCV), running superiorly to the left circumflex coronary artery (LCx), appears as a large low-echoic structure with fine blood speckle. The recurrent atrial branches emerge from the LCx in an orientation directed toward the GCV, while the obtuse marginal branches emerge opposite the GCV and course inferiorly to cover the lateral myocardial wall.

alone. It is also important to understand that with current systems, the rotational orientation of an IVUS image as presented on the screen is arbitrary and can vary between imaging runs. Here again, the branching pattern and perivascular landmarks, once understood, can provide a reference to the actual orientation of the image in space.

Common interventional applications

Pre-interventional imaging

Pre-interventional IVUS has been used to assess the severity and morphology of coronary artery stenosis, especially when angiography is equivocal or difficult to interpret (Fig. 10.5; Table 10.1). For intermediate

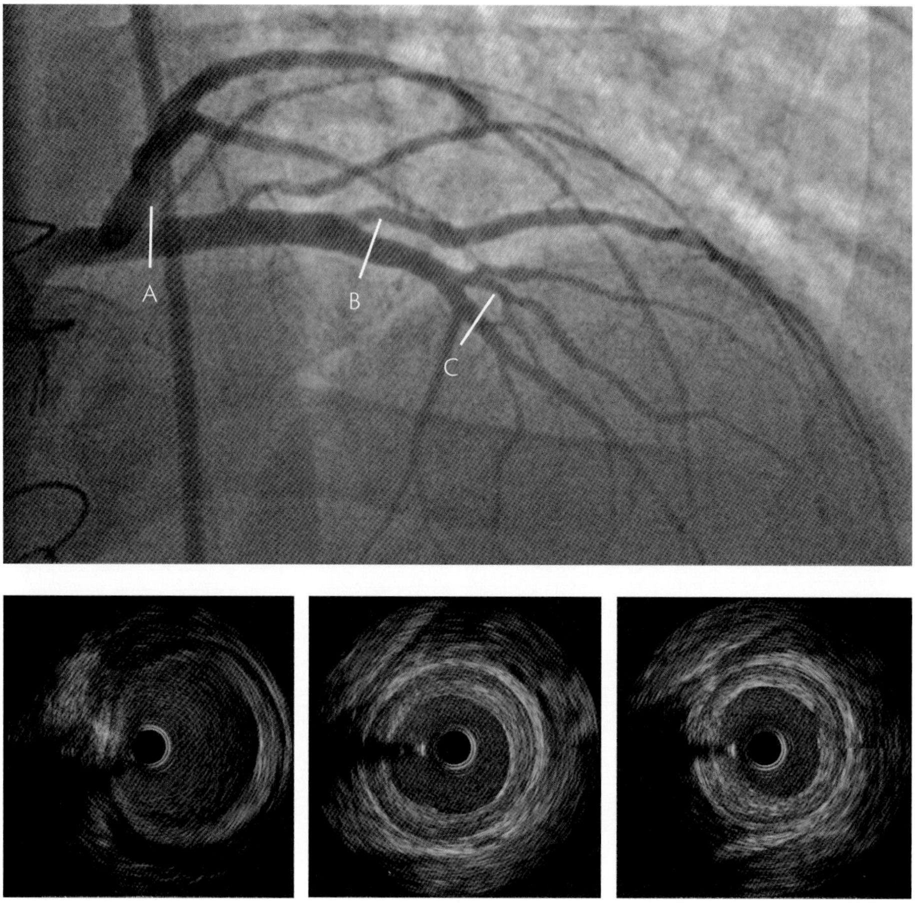

Fig. 10.5 Angiographic and intravascular ultrasound (IVUS) images from a transplant patient. The IVUS image from the proximal left anterior descending coronary artery (A) shows minimal plaque accumulation, while the angiogram showed almost normal-appearing. The IVUS images from cross-section (B) and (C) on the angiogram show greater amount of concentric plaque that also is not detectable on the angiogram.

lesions, careful IVUS measurement is made of the minimum lumen area (MLA) compared to the reference lumen areas. Using physiological assessments such as fractional flow reserve, coronary flow reserve, and stress scintigraphy, the ischaemic MLA threshold has been reported as 3–4mm^2 for major epicardial coronaries[(22–25)] and as 5.5–6mm^2 for the left main coronary artery[(26)].

Left main disease

In the assessment of left main coronary disease, angulations, calcification, or spasm in this location can lead to poor catheter engagement and confounded angiographic interpretation. Several investigators showed that high percentages of patients with angiographically normal left main coronary artery had disease by IVUS[(27–30)]. Conversely, a recent IVUS study demonstrated that only less than half of angiographically ambiguous left main stenosis had a significant stenosis[(31)]. This was especially true for ostial left main coronary disease where only 36.4% of the lesions had a significant stenosis and 40.5% had plaque burden <50% by IVUS. IVUS can also differentiate between true ostial and 'pseudo-ostial' lesions. Thus, patients with left main coronary disease deserve IVUS or physiologic assessment before blindly deciding treatment strategy, since the result of detailed evaluation can dramatically alter therapeutic strategies.

Bifurcation lesions

Plaque is commonly encountered at the outside edge (hips) and inseam of coronary bifurcations due to uneven flow patterns and differential shear conditions.

Table 10.1 Practical IVUS check points for stent implantation in the catheterization laboratory

Purpose	Location	Check point	Parameter	Details
Before stenting				
To assess lesion severity	Target lesion	Lumen size	MLA	Minimum lumen CSA
		Amount of disease	%P+M CSA	P+M CSA/EEM CSA
To assess lesion morphology	Target lesion	Eccentricity	Plaque Eccentricity Index	(Max – Min) P+M CSA/Max P+M CSA
	Target lesion and reference site	Remodelling	Remodelling Index	Lesion EEM CSA/Reference EEM CSA, Positive >1.0–1.05; Negative <0.95–1.0
	Target lesion	Plaque composition		Soft, fibrous, calcific, mixed, thrombus
		Calcification		Size (the arcs) Location (superficial, deep, mixed)
		Plaque distribution		Diffuse, focal
		Relation to the branch		Plaque encroachment of side branch orifice
For device sizing	Target lesion	Lumen and vessel size	Lumen and EEM CSA	
		Lesion length		
	Reference site	Amount of disease	%P+M CSA	P+M CSA/EEM CSA
		Lumen and vessel size	Lumen and EEM CSA	
For safe device delivery	Proximal vessel	Occult stenosis	MLA	Minimum lumen CSA
		Calcification		Size (the arcs) Location (superficial, deep, mixed)
During and after stenting				
To assess stent expansion	Stented site	Stent expansion	Stent Expansion Index % Stent expansion	Min stent CSA/ Predefined reference area
		ISA		Size and location (body and/or edge)
		Stent eccentricity	Stent Eccentricity Index	(Max-Min) stent diameter/Max stent diameter, or Min stent diameter/Max stent diameter
To assess complications	Stented site	Prolapse		Longitudinal length and Extent of luminal encroachment
		Relation to the branch		Presence of jailed side branch
	Stented and reference sites	Haematoma		Location (intra- or extra-vascular), longitudinal length, and extent of luminal encroachment
	Reference site	Edge dissection		Size and severity (intimal or medial)
Follow-up				
To assess the restenosis	Stented site	In-stent restenosis	In-lesion MLA	In-lesion minimum lumen CSA
		Original stent under-expansion	MSA	Min stent CSA
		Neointimal proliferation	Max % cross sectional narrowing	Max (neointimal CSA/stent CSA)
		Longitudinal distribution of neointima		
	Reference site	Edge restenosis	In-segment MLA	In-segment minimum Lumen CSA

(Continued)

Table 10.1 (Continued) Practical IVUS check points for stent implantation in the catheterization laboratory

Purpose	Location	Check point	Parameter	Details
To assess abnormal morphology	Stented site	ISA		Persistent, resolved, or late acquired
		Non-uniform stent strut distribution		
		Stent strut discontinuity (fracture)		
	Reference site	Edge dissection (haematoma)		Healed or unhealed

CSA, cross-sectional area; EEM, external elastic membrane; MLA, minimum lumen area; MSA, minimum stent area; P+M; plaque + media.

The extent of side-branch involvement can be difficult to assess by angiography alone, and the decision to pursue catheter-based treatment or surgical revascularization is often dependent on unambiguous demonstration of these complex lesions. The combination of plaque and carina shift following balloon dilatation or stenting may produce severe narrowing or occlusion of a side branch, particularly in the presence of a pre-existing ostial narrowing. Such anatomical situations are responsible for a majority of creatine kinase elevations following stent implantation[(32)]. Accurate measurements of side-branch EEM, lumen, and plaque dimensions require direct imaging of the branch. Nevertheless, plaque deposition in the ostial lesion of a side branch can often be appreciated by looking across from the parent artery into the ostium of the branch.

Plaque type and distribution

Pre-interventional IVUS is also useful in determining appropriate catheter-based intervention strategy by providing detailed information about the circumferential and longitudinal extent of plaque, as well as the character of the tissue involved. When observed by IVUS, angiographically hazy lesions represents a spectrum of morphologies, including calcium, dissection, thrombus, and excessive plaque burden with extreme remodelling. Especially, the presence, location, and extent of calcium can significantly affect the results of balloon angioplasty, atherectomy, and stent deployment. Precise measurements of lesion length and vessel size can guide the optimal sizing of devices to be employed. Accurate assessment of plaque eccentricity, which cannot be achieved by angiography[(33,34)], may also have important clinical implications, particularly when considering atherectomy, intracoronary brachytherapy, or other new catheter-based biologic treatment techniques targeting the plaque or adventitia of coronary arteries.

The assessment of remodelling is clinically important, not only for optimal therapeutic device sizing, but for risk stratification regarding plaque rupture or procedural and long-term outcomes of intervention. The term 'arterial remodelling' refers to a change in vessel size during the development of atherosclerosis. This phenomenon was first described in human coronary specimens by the pathologist Glagov, who reported a positive correlation between vessel size and atheroma area (positive or compensatory remodelling). Subsequent IVUS studies have demonstrated that this remodelling response is in fact bidirectional, with some segments showing negative remodelling, or constriction, in the area of lumen stenosis (Fig. 10.6). Although remodelling was originally conceptualized as a vessel change over time, measurements of reference sites are often used as a surrogate for vessel size before it became diseased. A remodelling index (the ratio of vessel area at the lesion site versus the reference site) as a continuous variable may also be used, in combination with the categorical classifications (positive remodelling = remodelling index >1.0 or 1.05; negative remodelling = remodelling index <1.0 or 0.95). The culprit lesions responsible for unstable angina or acute coronary syndromes usually represent extensive positive remodelling[(35–40)]. Several studies have also shown that pre-interventional positive remodelling predicts no-reflow phenomena, target lesion revascularization, and in-hospital complications following coronary interventions[(41–48)]. Although its predictive value in the context of stenting has not been established with certainty[(44,45,49–52)], cumulative evidence have suggested that positively remodelled lesions are more biologically active than intermediate or negatively remodelled lesions.

Post-interventional imaging

IVUS can frequently clarify angiographically hazy lesions that impact on the therapeutic strategy. In fact, haziness seen at a stent border after the deployment often prompts the operator to additional dilation or

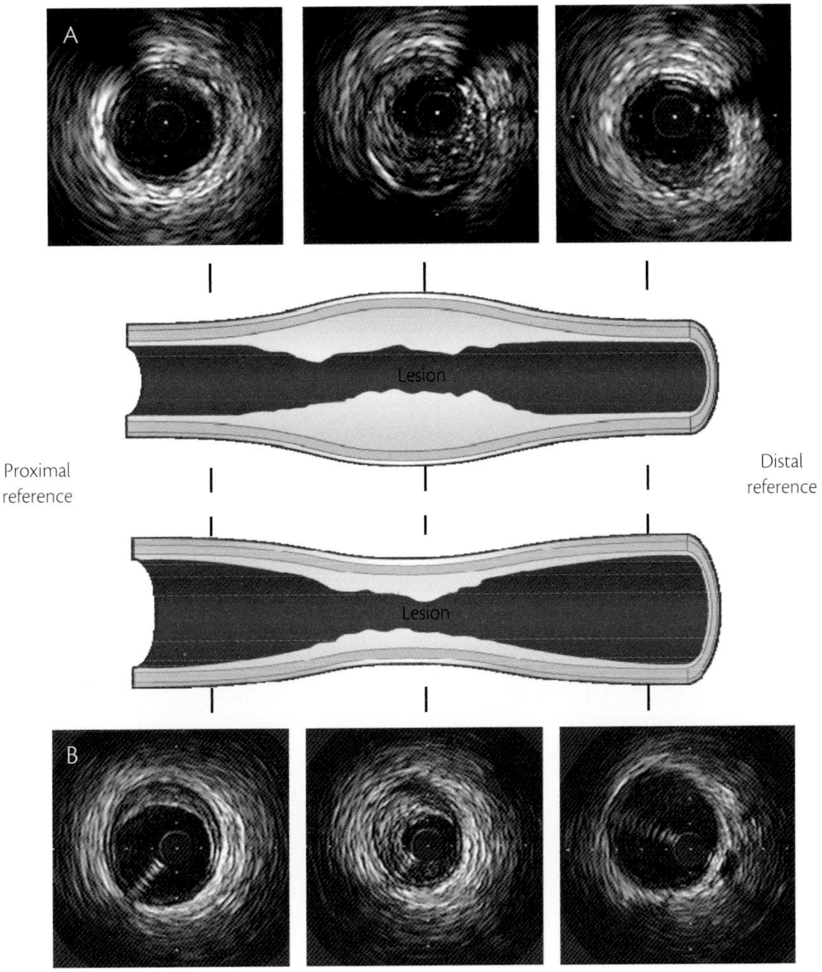

Fig. 10.6 Intravascular ultrasound (IVUS) images with schematic diagram showing remodelling. A) Glagov remodelling, in which there is localized expansion of the vessel in the area of plaque accumulation. B) Negative remodelling or shrinkage, in which the lesion has a smaller media-to-media diameter than the adjacent, less diseased sites.

stent placement, driven by the concern for angiographically occult dissection or unrecognized reference plaque. Angiographic hazy lesions can represent a spectrum of during- and post-intervention anatomic morphologies, including calcium, dissection, thrombus, haematoma, and excessive plaque burden with extreme remodelling at reference segment[53,54]. The incidence of persistent haziness is 15% of patients after high-pressure coronary stent deployment[55] and its aetiology can be quickly and precisely defined by IVUS.

IVUS has a higher sensitivity than contrast angiography for detecting both spontaneous and post-intervention tears or dissection in the vessel wall, and can also demonstrate the precise location(s) and severity of dissection flaps[56]. In addition to overall size and length of the dissection, the location of the dissection can be important for risk of extension. Dissections on the free wall side may have a higher likelihood of propagating antegrade or retrograde through to the vessel wall when located on the free wall (same side as pericardium) versus the mural wall where the surrounding muscle constrains further propagation. Other criteria of vulnerable dissection are large, moving flaps and extensive medial tears occupying greater than 50% of the vessel circumference (onion skin-like appearance). Identification of these patients at high risk of abrupt closure, who require prophylactic treatment such as (additional) stent implantation, is often possible and augments the angiographic findings.

Specific interventional applications

Non-stent angioplasty

Mechanism of action

IVUS studies have shown that acute lumen gain achieved by conventional balloon angioplasty consists of two

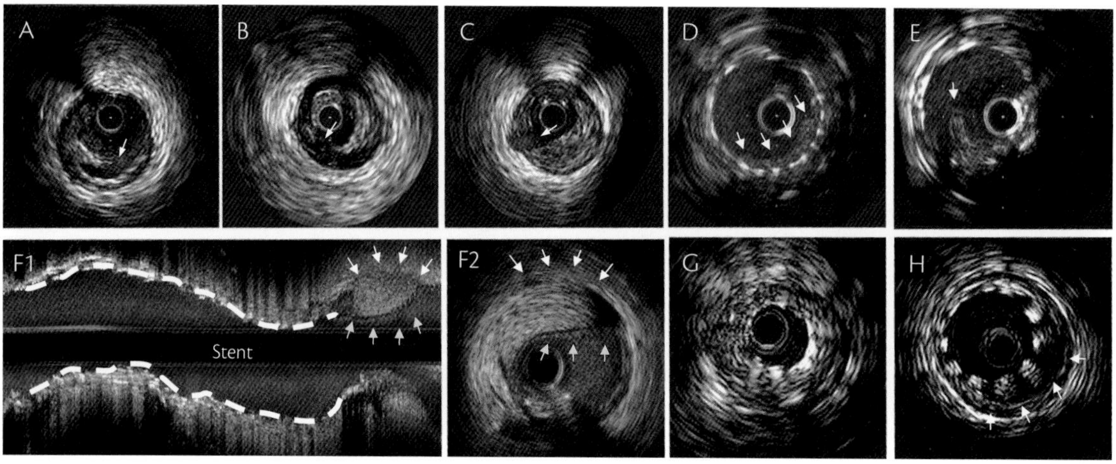

Fig. 10.7 Problems seen immediately after percutaneous coronary intervention detectable by intravascular ultrasound (IVUS). A) A superficial (intimal) dissection starting at 6 o'clock and extending clockwise. The dissection flap does not extend far into the lumen. B) A deeper (medial) dissection with a flap extending into the lumen may compromise flow or precede abrupt closure. Injection of contrast in this setting can demonstrate free fluid flow behind the flap to better define the extent of tear. C) Eccentric plaque with a deep (adventitial) dissection at 8 o'clock that penetrates the external elastic lamina and extends into the adventitia. D) and E) Two examples of IVUS images showing plaque protrusion after stenting (white arrows). F) A Longitudinal (F1) and cross-sectional IVUS image (F2) of intramural haematoma. Intramural haematoma appears as an accumulation of blood within the medial space starting from the distal edge of the stent, displacing the internal elastic membrane inward (yellow arrows) and external elastic membrane outward (white arrows). G) An example of incomplete stent expansion relative to the ends of the stent and the reference segments. H) incomplete apposition, where there is a gap between a portion of the stent and the vessel wall (white arrows).

major components, namely, plaque redistribution and additional vessel stretching with dissection(57–59). IVUS imaging of balloon angioplasty sites demonstrate plaque disruption or dissection more often than angiography (40–70% versus 20–45% of cases by angio)(34,59–63). Dissections are often observed at the junction of calcified and non-calcified plaque (where shear forces from dilation are high)(64–66) or at the junction between eccentric plaque and normal vessel wall (as the elastic, non-diseased wall separates away from the more rigid plaque) (Fig. 10.7A–C).

In directional coronary atherectomy (DCA), IVUS studies demonstrated that plaque removal accounts for up to 60–70% of lumen gain, with the remainder due to mechanical expansion by the device and balloon dilatation(67,68). As in the case of balloon angioplasty, the presence and location of calcium within the lesion has a significant impact on the performance of the DCA device. On the other hand, rotational atherectomy is highly effective in treating superficial calcification. IVUS studies have shown that in hard plaque, the neolumen created by the device is round and regular, with essentially the same diameter as the definitive burr(69–71). Conversely, in soft plaque, the post-procedure lumen is typically less round and may be significantly smaller than the burr used, perhaps due to some combination of less effective debulking and spasm.

Serial IVUS studies demonstrated that the majority of late lumen loss following non-stent angioplasty was due to negative arterial remodelling (a decrease in vessel cross-sectional area), with only about a quarter of the late loss due to tissue proliferation(72–74).

IVUS-guided procedures

A direct approach to balloon sizing, based on IVUS images, was pursued in the Clinical Outcomes with Ultrasound Trial (CLOUT), where IVUS-guided balloon sizing was performed with the average of the reference lumen and media-to-media diameters for cases without extensive calcification(75). This strategy led to an average 0.5-mm 'oversizing' of the balloon compared to the standard angiographic guidance, resulting in a low post-procedure residual stenosis without increased complication rates, and a late adverse event (death, myocardial infarction, or target lesion revascularization) rate of 22% at 1 year(76). More recently, this IVUS-guided aggressive PTCA strategy was expanded and confirmed by two single-centre studies of provisional stenting that demonstrated equivalent long-term outcomes to elective stenting(77,78).

A practical issue in applying IVUS to DCA is how to orient the atherectomy catheter toward the maximal accumulation of plaque(79). In practice, the location of branches on the ultrasound scan is the most useful cue for orienting the device. A branch near the plaque is identified on the ultrasound image, and the rotational orientation of the deepest portion of the plaques is gauged, relative to the branch. Once the atherectomy device is inserted, the housing is rotated the corresponding degrees clockwise or counterclockwise from the branch. Serial IVUS examination with repeated orientation is required for aggressive debulking.

Device-specific IVUS insights

In addition to the final lumen dimensions, residual plaque burden has been demonstrated as a powerful IVUS predictor of long-term outcomes following balloon angioplasty and atherectomy. A single-centre study of 360 non-stented native coronary lesions showed that the percentage plaque area (plaque area divided by vessel area, %) as assessed by IVUS was a more powerful and consistent predictor of binary restenosis, follow-up diameter stenosis, and late lumen loss than clinical or angiographic risk factors(80). Phase II of the GUIDE trial confirmed these findings by the analysis of 524 follow-up studies obtained from 22 institutions in the United States and Europe(81).

A series of DCA trials with IVUS investigation also provided a composite picture of the impact of residual plaque burden on the long-term outcomes. In the Optimal Atherectomy Restenosis (OARS) trial, residual plaque burden was thus 57% with a restenosis rate of 29%(68), while an average post-procedure plaque burden of 46% in the Adjunctive Balloon Angioplasty following Coronary Atherectomy Study (ABACAS) trial resulted in a 6-month angiographic restenosis of 21%(82). These findings were confirmed in the contemporary series of the Stent versus Directional Coronary Atherectomy Randomized Trial (START)(83). When considered together, a technique that could effectively remove relatively large amounts of plaque (with a residual of 50% or less) appear to have restenosis rates that are competitive with stenting.

In the era of drug-eluting stents (DES), however, the role of atherectomy appears to be changing from aggressive plaque reduction to plaque modification in order to achieve optimal stent results and/or to avoid unfavourable events during the procedure. A recent IVUS registry suggested that DCA before DES implantation with non-aggressive strategy (average residual plaque burden 56%) can possibly provide a better long-term outcome in patients with bifurcation lesions by avoiding complex stenting(84). Another study retrospectively examined the outcomes of patients who underwent sirolimus-eluting stent implantation for the treatment of heavily calcified coronary lesions with versus without rotational atherectomy(85). Despite the more complex lesion characteristics at pre-intervention, the lesions requiring rotational atherectomy to facilitate stent delivery and expansion achieved equivalent outcomes to those that could be stented without the need for plaque modification with rotational atherectomy.

Intracoronary radiation

Mechanism of action

Intracoronary radiation therapy (ICRT), the first biological treatment targeting excessive proliferative response of vascular smooth muscle cells to mechanical intervention, underwent extensive clinical testing with IVUS characterization. Regardless of radiation sources or delivery platforms, most IVUS studies of ICRT in PTCA, stenting, and treatment of in-stent restenosis have shown significant in-lesion or in-stent efficacy(86–95). Serial IVUS investigations have confirmed that these beneficial effects are primarily derived from decreased neointimal hyperplasia. An accelerated positive remodelling has also been reported at the irradiated segment(86,96).

IVUS-guided procedures

IVUS has revealed that a combination of increased neointimal hyperplasia and either negative remodelling or absence of compensatory remodelling, accounts for the unfavourable edge effect of ICRT(97–99). Since, in catheter-based ICRT (not radioactive stents), most edge effects are related to inadequate coverage of injured edge segments (geographic miss)(100), IVUS guidance greatly enhances the safety and efficacy of this highly geographically specific technique. Several investigator groups also developed detailed dosimetric analysis algorithms, based on dose–volume histograms derived from three-dimensional IVUS(101–107), for optimal dose prescription.

Device-specific IVUS insights

Unusual IVUS observations following ICRT include unhealed dissections, late-acquired incomplete stent apposition, and echolucent neointimal tissue (so-called 'black hole'). Delayed healing is commonly seen after ICRT (up to 50% of dissections), while dissections seen after non-radiation intervention normally heal within 6 months(108–110). Late-acquired incomplete stent apposition after ICRT is primarily a result of excessive positive remodelling of the underlying vessel wall combined with significant neointimal inhibition(111,112). The acoustic or 'black hole' consists of echolucent neointimal tissue and has been seen in all types of ICRT(113). Post-ICRT specimens retrieved with DCA show large myxoid areas, with interspersed smooth muscle cells, scattered in a proteoglycan-containing extracellular matrix—findings which are compatible with a weak backscattering of echoes and a dark appearance on IVUS. These IVUS findings post ICRT are unique but their exact clinical implications remain unknown.

Bare-metal stents

Mechanism of action

Stents essentially scaffold the diseased vessel wall against the force of vessel recoil. According to the previous IVUS studies, axial extrusion of non-calcified plaque into the adjacent reference zone may also contribute to lumen gain following stent implantation(114–117). Although a similar phenomenon was demonstrated in balloon angioplasty(118), the extrusion effect in stenting may be more prominent, commensurate with the increased ability of the stent to enlarge and hold open the treated segment. This phenomenon may partly account for the angiographic step-up/step-down appearance seen after stenting, as well as some of the side branch encroachment after stent deployment.

At follow-up, the primary mechanism of stent restenosis is exaggerated neointimal hyperplasia, while chronic stent recoil and strut fracture can also be observed infrequently. IVUS can provide not only a total amount of neointimal hyperplasia but also the information on longitudinal distribution of neointimal hyperplasia.

IVUS-guided procedures

IVUS has identified several stent deployment issues, including incomplete expansion and incomplete apposition (see Fig. 10.7G, H). Incomplete expansion occurs when a portion of the stent is inadequately expanded compared to the distal and proximal reference dimensions, as may occur where dense fibrocalcific plaque is present. Incomplete apposition occurs when part of the stent structure is not fully in contact with the vessel wall, possibly increasing local flow disturbances and the potential risk for subacute thrombosis in certain clinical settings. An early clinical study demonstrated an unexpectedly high percentage of these IVUS-detected stent deployment issues even after angiographically successful results. These observations led to the concept of the current high-pressure stent deployment technique with IVUS guidance(119,120).

In 10–15% of stent cases, IVUS may show tears at the edge of the stent (Fig. 10.11)(121-123). These tears have been attributed to result from both the shear forces created at the junction between the metal edge of the stent and the adjacent, more compliant tissue, and to the effect of balloon expansion beyond the edge of the stent (the 'dog-bone' phenomenon). Minor non-flow-limiting edge dissections do not appear to impact on late angiographic in-stent restenosis. In fact, 75% heal when imaged at follow-up—a frequency similar to balloon angioplasty(124). However, significant residual dissections can lead to an increased risk of early major adverse cardiac events(125,126). The practical strategy is to make a determination from the IVUS image whether the tear appears to be flow-limiting (i.e. whether there is an extensive tissue arm projecting into the lumen). If this is the case, an additional stent is placed to cover this region.

Over the past decade, a number of studies have shown that IVUS-guided stent placement improves the clinical outcome of bare-metal stents(127–135). In the Multicenter Ultrasound guided Stent Implantation in Coronaries (MUSIC) trial, IVUS guided stenting required: (1) complete apposition over the entire stent length; (2) in-stent minimum stent area (MSA) greater than or equal to 90% of the average of the reference areas or 100% of the smallest reference area; and (3) symmetric stent expansion with minimum/maximum lumen diameter greater than or equal to 0.7(136). Subacute thrombosis of less than 2% was felt to represent a reduction over non-guided deployment, although with current antiplatelet regimens, similar results can usually be achieved by high pressure post dilation without IVUS confirmation. Nevertheless, a number of studies have suggested a link between suboptimal stent implantation and stent thrombosis, including the Predictors and Outcomes of Stent Thrombosis (POST) registry that demonstrated that 90% of thrombosis patients had suboptimal IVUS results—incomplete apposition (47%), incomplete expansion (52%), and evidence of thrombus (24%)—even though only 25% of patients had abnormalities on angiography(137). These observations were replicated in a more recent study by Cheneau and colleagues, suggesting that mechanical factors continue to contribute to stent thrombosis, even in this modern stent era, with optimized antiplatelet regimens(138). Although the use of IVUS in all patients for the sole purpose of reducing thrombosis is clearly not warranted from a cost standpoint, IVUS imaging should be considered in patients at particularly high risk for thrombosis (e.g. slow flow) or in whom the consequences of thrombosis would be severe (e.g. left main coronary artery or equivalent).

MSA, as measured by IVUS, is one of the strongest predictors for both angiographic and clinical restenosis following bare-metal stenting(139–143). Kasaoka and colleagues indicated that the predicted risk of restenosis

Table 10.2 IVUS versus angiographic guidance of bare-metal stent implantation

	Population	Study design	IVUS criteria for optimal expansion	Criteria fulfilled	Endpoints	Results
Albiero *et al.*[129] (N = 312)	De novo Native	Multicentre Registry	Complete apposition, No ref disease MSA ≥60% of average ref VA (early phase) or MSA ≥ distal ref LA (late phase)	NA	6-month angio	IVUS better (early phase)
Blasini, *et al.*[128] (N = 212)	De novo and restenotic Native and SVG	Single centre Registry	Complete apposition, No residual dissection, MSA >8mm^2 and/or 90% of average ref LA	50%	6-month angio	IVUS better
Choi, *et al.*[130] (N = 278)	De novo Native	Single centre Registry	Complete apposition, No residual dissection, MSA ≥80% of distal ref LA	NA	Acute closure 6-month MACE	IVUS better
Gaster, *et al.*[233] (N = 108)	De novo and restenotic Native	Single centre Randomized	MUSIC criteria	64%	6-month angio, CFR, FFR, TVR 2.5-year MACE	IVUS better
AVID[127] (N = 759)	De novo Native and SVG	Multicentre Randomized	MUSIC criteria	NA	12-month TLR	IVUS better (subset analysis)
CRUISE[131] (N = 499)	De novo and restenotic Native	Multicentre Non-randomized	Discretion of individual institutional practice	–	9-month TVR	IVUS better
OPTICUS[234] (N = 550)	De novo and restenotic Native	Multicentre Randomized	MUSIC criteria	56%	6-month angio 12-month MACE	No difference
PRESTO[145] (N = 9070)	De novo and restenotic Native	Multicentre Non-randomized	Discretion of individual institutional practice	–	9-month MACE	No difference
RESIST[133,235] (N = 155)	De novo Native	Multicentre Randomized	MSA >80% of average ref LA	80%	6-month angio 18-month MACE	IVUS better (non-significant reduction)
SIPS[132] (N = 269)	De novo and restenotic Native	Single centre Randomized	MLA >65% of average ref LA	69%	6-month angio 2-year TLR	IVUS better (2-year TLR)
TULIP[135] (N = 144)	Long lesions >20mm	Single centre Randomized	Complete apposition, MLD ≥80% of average ref diameter MSA ≥ distal ref LA	89%	6-month angio 12-month MACE	IVUS better

CFR, coronary flow reserve; FRR, fractional flow reserve; LA, lumen area; MACE, major adverse cardiac events; MLD, minimum lumen diameter; MSA, minimum stent area; TLR, target-lesion revascularization; TVR, target-vessel revascularization.

decreases 19% for every 1-mm^2 increase in MSA, and suggested that stents with MSA >9mm^2 have a greatly reduced risk of restenosis[142]. In the Can Routine Ultrasound Improve Stent Expansion (CRUISE) trial, IVUS guidance by operator preferences increased MSA from 6.25 to 7.14mm^2, leading to a 44% relative reduction in target vessel revascularization at 9 months, compared with angiographic guidance alone[131]. In the Angiography vs. IVUS-Directed stent placement (AVID) trial, IVUS-guided stent implantation resulted in larger acute dimensions than angiography alone (7.54 versus 6.94mm^2) without an increase in complications, and lower 12-month TLR rates for vessels with angiographic reference diameter <3.25mm, severe stenosis at pre-intervention (>70% angiographic diameter stenosis), and vein grafts[127]. However, controversial results were also reported in some IVUS-guided stent trials[144,145], presumably due to differing procedural endpoints for IVUS-guided stenting, as well as various adjunctive treatment strategies that were utilized in these trials in response to suboptimal results (Table 10.2). Overall, a meta-analysis of nine clinical studies (2972 patients) demonstrated that IVUS-guided stenting significantly lowers 6-month angiographic restenosis (odds ratio, 0.75; 95% CI, 0.60–0.94; P = 0.01) and target vessel revascularizations (odds ratio, 0.62; 95% CI, 0.49-0.78; P = 0.00003) with a neutral effect on death and non-fatal MI, compared to an angiographic optimization[146].

Device-specific IVUS insights

In-stent restenosis is primarily due to intimal proliferation rather than chronic stent recoil[73,147]. Growth of neointima is generally greatest in the areas with the largest plaque burden[45,148,149], and the intimal growth process seems to be more aggressive in patients with diabetes or hyperinsulinaemia[150,151]. In the treatment of in-stent restenosis, IVUS can be helpful to differentiate pure intimal ingrowth from poor stent expansion. A serial IVUS analysis immediately before and after balloon angioplasty for in-stent restenosis have demonstrated that, in 1090 consecutive in-stent restenosis lesions, 38% of lesions had a MSA <6.0mm^2[152]. Stent under-expansion can result in clinically significant lumen compromise even with minimal neointimal hyperplasia. For this type of in-stent restenosis, mechanical optimization will be appropriate in most cases.

IVUS can also track the response to treatment, with evidence that angioplasty of in-stent restenosis is followed by early lumen loss due to decompression[153] and/or reintrusion[154] of tissue immediately after intervention. This phenomenon was more prominent in longer lesions and those with greater in-stent tissue burden, which may partially help explain the worse long-term outcomes in diffuse in-stent restenosis as compared with focal in-stent restenosis. Several investigators have subsequently reported a considerable reduction in angiographic and/or clinical recurrence of in-stent restenosis in patients with diffuse in-stent restenosis treated with ablative therapies (DCA, rotational atherectomy, or laser angioplasty) compared with PTCA alone[155–161].

Drug-eluting stents

Mechanism of action

In antiproliferative DES technology, IVUS studies have demonstrated a striking reduction of in-stent neointimal hyperplasia, while mechanical performances of these new stents are similar to those of conventional bare-metal stents[162–166]. Additionally, both statistical and geographic distributions of neointimal hyperplasia can be significantly different between the biologic (DES) and mechanical (bare-metal) stents. In general, neointimal volume (as a percentage of stent volume) within bare-metal stents follows a near-Gaussian or normal frequency distribution, with a mean value of 30–35%. The standard deviation of this statistical distribution represents biologic variability in vascular response to acute and chronic vessel injury by interventions. In contrast, biologic modifications by DES often result in a non-Gaussian frequency distribution, with variable degrees of the tail ends. Since restenosis corresponds to the right tail end of the distribution curve, a discrepancy between mean neointimal volume versus binary or clinical restenosis can be observed in DES trials (Fig. 10.8)[162,167,168]. Similarly, bare-metal stents show a wide individual variation in geographic distribution of neointima along the stented segment[169], while some types of DES demonstrate predilection of in-stent neointimal hyperplasia for specific locations (e.g. proximal stent edge)[170].

Among the several conventional risk factors, diabetes mellitus remains an important determinant for unfavourable clinical outcome after DES implantation[171]. The smaller vessel size, longer lesion length, accelerated form of atherosclerosis, and exaggerated neointimal proliferation after stenting presents in diabetics may be important contributors to increased restenosis after stent implantation[150]. Although there are some observational registry data, reporting no significant difference in MACE between the first-generation DES

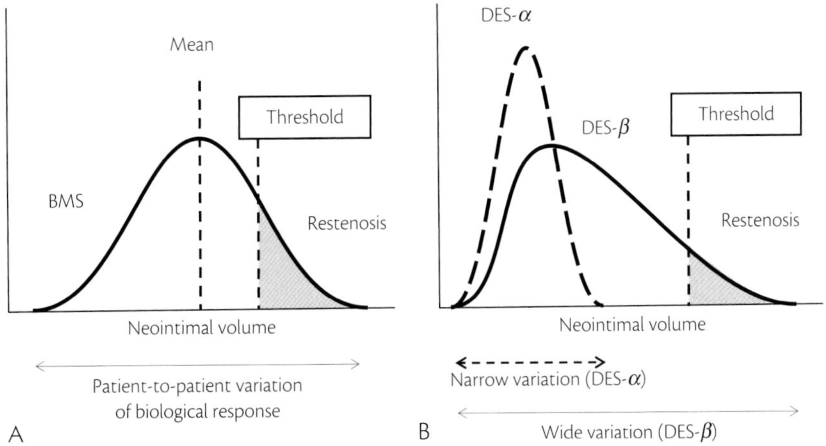

Fig. 10.8 Frequency distributions of neointimal hyperplasia following stent implantation. A) Neointimal volume within bare-metal stents (BMS) follows a near-Gaussian or normal frequency distribution, where the width of the distribution curve indicates individual variation in biological response. The right tail end of the curve above a threshold of tolerable neointima (grey area) represents patients with restenosis. Achieving a larger acute lumen gain increases the tolerable amount of neointima (i.e. shifts the threshold toward the right), leading to a reduced restenosis rate. B) Drug-eluting stents (DES) can cause a markedly skewed or deformed frequency distribution due to the biological effects of pharmacologic agents. A larger acute lumen gain would continue to help reduce the restenosis rate, if the DES shows a wide variation with a relatively long right tail end (DES-ß), regardless of the mean value.

(paclitaxel versus sirolimus)[172–175], angiographic randomized trials have consistently shown significantly less late lumen loss and MACE rate with sirolimus-eluting stents in the treatment of diabetics[176–178]. A recent 130-diabetic patient randomized multicentre IVUS study has supported these findings by showing that sirolimus-eluting stents inhibited neointimal hyperplasia more effectively with more focal pattern of neointimal distribution than paclitaxel-eluting stents[179].

IVUS-guided procedures

Although MSA is one of the strongest predictors for restenosis following stenting, its diagnostic accuracy is often blunted due to a wide variety of neointimal proliferation seen among patients treated with bare-metal stents. In DES, however, the drugs dramatically reduce the variability of the biologic response (neointimal proliferation), and therefore, the prognostic value of the MSA is magnified as a powerful predictor for in-stent restenosis[180–184]. For instance, in an IVUS study of de novo coronary lesions, sirolimus-eluting stents showed a stronger correlation between baseline MSA and 8-month MLA, compared to control bare-metal stents[182].

Currently, most interventional cardiologists rely on a compliance chart provided by stent manufactures for the selection of stent size and inflation pressure. With this method, however, a recent IVUS study has shown that the first-generation DES (sirolimus and paclitaxel) achieved only 75% of predicted minimum stent diameter and 66% of predicted MSA *in vivo*[166]. In addition to the adjunctive use of high-pressure, non-compliant balloon post dilatation[185], the utility of IVUS to assure adequate stent expansion cannot be overemphasized in daily practice, particularly when there are clinical risk factors for DES failure (e.g. diabetes, renal failure).

In this context, plaque composition assessment by pre-interventional IVUS can also provide useful information to assure the adequate DES deployment. In particular, identification of calcified plaque is important, since the presence, degree, and location of calcium within the target vessel can substantially affect the delivery and subsequent deployment of coronary stents[186,187]. One important advantage of on-line IVUS guidance is the ability to get precise information on calcium deposit within a plaque, such as the extent and distance from the lumen. For example, lesions with extensive superficial calcium may require rotational atherectomy prior to stenting[186,188]. Conversely, even for the lesion with significant calcification on fluoroscopy, IVUS may find to be distributed in a deep portion of the vessel wall or to have a lower degree of calcification (calcium arc <180°). In these cases, stand-alone stenting is generally adequate to achieve a lumen expansion large enough for DES.

The discovery of 'edge effects' associated with ICRT raised the concern of lumen narrowing in adjacent reference segments as a potential limitation of DES. To date, however, clinical experience with DES has shown no accelerated edge restenosis overall, when compared to conventional bare-metal stents. Serial IVUS analyses from multiple clinical trials suggest that the favourable edge effect of DES is primarily due to the lack of vessel shrinkage, despite similar amounts of plaque proliferation compared to bare-metal stents(165,189–191). On the other hand, some early DES trials demonstrated relatively high incidence of restenosis at the proximal edge segment compared to the distal edge, which led to an important clue for optimal deployment of DES. In an IVUS substudy of the Sirolimus-Eluting Stent in De Novo Coronary Lesions (SIRIUS) trial, lesions with peri-stent edge stenosis (>50% diameter stenosis) at 8-months had greater reference plaque burden (61% versus 49%, p = 0.03) (Fig. 10.9A) and a higher overexpansion index (maximum stent area/reference MLA: 1.8 versus, 1.5, P = 0.03) at baseline, compared to those without edge stenosis(192). More recently, the Stent

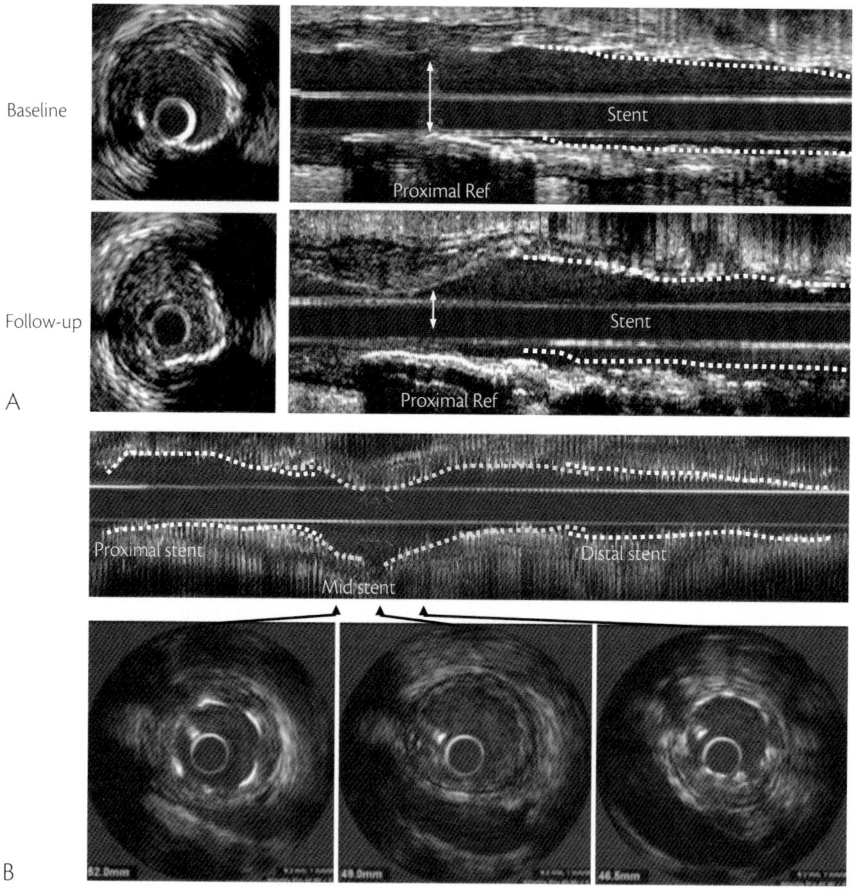

Fig. 10.9 Problems seen at follow-up intravascular ultrasound (IVUS) study. A) Proximal disease development seen 8 months following drug-eluting stent implantation. In this example, the new stenosis at the proximal peri-stent margin is primarily due to plaque proliferation, despite minimal neointimal hyperplasia observed inside the stent. Baseline IVUS reveals a significant residual plaque at the corresponding uncovered segment. B) Stent strut discontinuity (fracture) observed 8 months after deployment of three overlapping drug-eluting stents. On the cross-sectional IVUS image (lower, middle), an abnormal paucity of stent struts, not seen at implantation, is detected at a portion of the mid stent. The longitudinal IVUS image (upper) shows an acute-angled bend at the corresponding segment. In this particular case, however, the strut discontinuity is not associated with increased intimal hyperplasia, at least as of this time point.

Deployment Techniques on Clinical Outcomes of Patients Treated with the Cypher® Stent (STLLR) trial also demonstrated that geographic miss (defined as the length of injured or stenotic segment not fully covered by DES) had a significant negative impact on both clinical efficacy (target vessel and lesion revascularization) and safety (myocardial infarction) at 1 year following sirolimus-eluting stent implantation(193). Therefore, complete coverage of reference disease with less aggressive stent dilatation is currently recommended. On the other hand, although angiographic studies with mid-term clinical follow-up suggest that long drug-eluting stenting with multiple overlapping strategy is clinically feasible(194–197), longer stent length is independently associated with DES thrombosis and restenosis(181). Furthermore, significant under-expansion and incomplete strut apposition may also result in unfavourable outcomes. On-line IVUS guidance can facilitate both the determination of appropriate stent size and length as well as optimal procedural endpoint, achieving the goal of covering significant pathology with reasonable stent expansion, while anchoring the stent ends in relatively plaque-free vessel segments.

To date, there is only one large study that assessed the impact of IVUS guidance during DES implantation on clinical outcomes. In this single-centre study of 884 cases treated with IVUS-guided DES implantation versus matched control population with angiographic guidance alone, a higher rate of definite stent thrombosis was seen in the angio-guided group at both 30 days (0.5 versus 1.4%; p = 0.046) and 12 months (0.7 versus 2.0%; p = 0.014). Although there were no major differences in late stent thrombosis and MACE (14.5 versus 16.2%; p = 0.33) at 12 months, a trend was observed in favour of IVUS guidance in target lesion revascularization (5.1 versus 7.2%; p = 0.07)(198).

Device-specific IVUS insights

Because of the low incidence of DES failure, clarification of the exact mechanisms responsible for DES failure still awaits the cumulative analysis of large clinical studies. Nevertheless, previous studies consistently implied that procedure-related factors appear to remain important contributors to the development of both restenosis and thrombosis. Particularly, the most consistent risk factor is stent underexpansion, the incidence of which has been reported as 60–80% of DES failures(184,199,200). In a study of 670 native coronary lesions treated with sirolimus-eluting stents, the only independent predictors of angiographic restenosis were post-procedural final MSA <5.5mm^2 and IVUS-measured stent length >40mm (odds ratio, 0.586 and 1.029, respectively)(181). Recurrent restenosis following DES implantation for bare-metal stent restenosis was also investigated using IVUS. In a series of 48 in-stent restenosis lesions treated with sirolimus-eluting stents, 82% of recurrent lesions had a MSA <5.0mm^2 versus 26% of non-recurrent lesions (P = 0.003)(200). In addition, a gap between sirolimus-eluting stents was identified in 27% of recurrent lesions versus 5% of non-recurrent lesions. These observations emphasize the importance of procedural optimization at the DES implantation for both de novo and in-stent restenosis lesions.

Although published data on DES thrombosis are further limited, two small single-centre IVUS studies have reported stent underexpansion and significant residual reference disease as risk factors of acute, subacute, or late DES thrombosis(201). For very late DES thrombosis (>12 months), another investigator group also suggested smaller stent expansion and incomplete stent apposition as possible risk factors(202).

Serial IVUS studies have added the concept of classification of incomplete stent apposition according to the time course (Fig. 10.10). The incidence of post-procedural incomplete stent apposition with DES has been reported comparable to that with BMS (7.0–16.2%)(203,204), whereas the frequency of late-acquired incomplete stent apposition with DES has been reported to be relatively higher than that of bare-metal stents (bare-metal stents 5.4% versus drug-eluting stents 8.7–12.1%)(203,205,206). This phenomena has been reported in both experimental

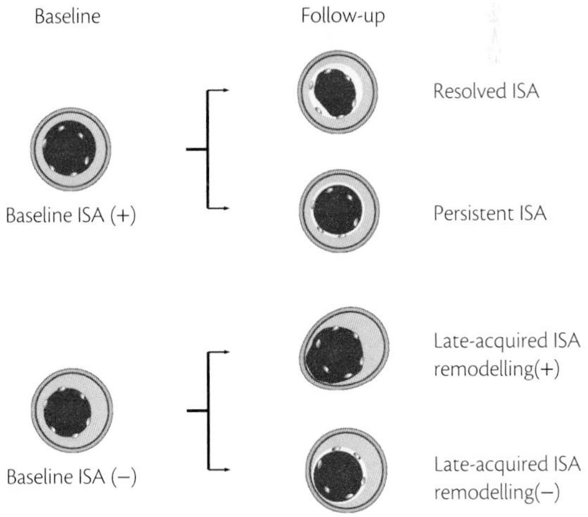

Fig. 10.10 Classification of incomplete stent apposition (ISA). Baseline ISA can either be resolved (resolved ISA) or remains (persistent ISA) at follow-up. Late-acquired ISA without vessel expansion is typically seen in thrombus-containing lesions, while late-acquired ISA with focal, positive vessel remodelling is more characteristic to brachytherapy and drug-eluting stents.

(paclitaxel)[207] and clinical studies (sirolimus and paclitaxel)[163,165,203,204] (Fig. 10.10), and detailed IVUS analysis indicated the predominant mechanism is regional, positive vessel remodelling, as previously reported after brachytherapy[163,203,208]. In addition, there is a strong suggestion that incompletely apposed struts are seen primarily in eccentric plaques, and that the gaps develop mainly on the disease-free side of the vessel wall. The combination of mechanical vessel injury during stent implantation and biological vessel injury with pharmacologic agents or polymer[209,210] in the setting of little underlying plaque may predispose the vessel wall to chronic, pathological dilatation. Given the low incidence of late stent thrombosis, however, enough statistical power to detect a direct link of this finding with long-term clinical events requires considerably larger patient sample sizes. To circumvent this problem, a meta-analysis of multiple clinical trials was recently conducted, demonstrating a significantly higher risk of late or very-late stent thrombosis in patients with late stent apposition, compared with those without this IVUS finding (OR, 6.51; 95% CI 1.34–34.91). The potential impact of this morphologic abnormality on long-term clinical outcomes needs to be carefully assessed over an extended period of time.

Other IVUS-detected conditions that may be of importance in DES include non-uniform stent strut distribution (Fig. 10.9B), branch jailing, and strut fractures following implantation[180,211–213]. Theoretically, all abnormalities can reduce the local drug dose delivered to the arterial wall, as well as mechanical scaffolding of the affected lesion segment. A recent IVUS study of 24 sirolimus-eluting stent restenoses identified the number of visualized struts (normalized for the number of stent cells) and maximum interstrut angle as the independent multivariate IVUS predictors of both neointimal hyperplasia and MLA[180]. In contrast, the exact incidence and clinical implications of strut fractures remain to be investigated[214,215]. Finally, the clinical implications of jailing major side branches with DES may differ from those of conventional bare-metal stenting due to delayed stent strut endothelialization. Several clinical trials confirmed bifurcation stenting as a multivariate predictor of stent thrombosis in sirolimus- and paclitaxel-eluting stent implantation[216–218].

Early results of second-generation drug-eluting stents

Currently there are two types of the second generation DES approved by the United States Food and Drug Administration (FDA): zotarolimus-eluting stents with phosphoryl-choline (PC) coating technology and everolimus-eluting stents.

The zotarolimus-eluting stents demonstrated significantly improved effectiveness and equivalent safety compared with bare-metal stents in ENDEAVOR II[168]. A detailed IVUS analysis of this trial revealed that, as observed in the first-generation DES, zotarolimus-eluting stents had a strong positive correlation between follow-up MLA and post-procedure MSA ($r = 0.73$; $p < 0.0001$), with post-procedure MSA $<6.0mm^2$ associated with a steep decrease in follow-up stent patency[219]. Overall, however, subsequent IVUS studies showed slightly less effectiveness in inhibiting neointimal hyperplasia than sirolimus-eluting stents (percent neointimal volume: zotarolimus-eluting stents 16.1% versus sirolimus-eluting stents 2.7% in ENDEAVOR III)[219]. On the other hand, uniform neointimal coverage and extremely low incidence of late acquired incomplete stent apposition (0% in ENDEAVOR II and 0.5% in ENDEAVOR III) appear to represent unique safety profile of this DES. A rapid and uniform vascular healing with less inflammation has also been confirmed in a preclinical rabbit model comparing zotarolimus-eluting stents with sirolimus- and paclitaxel-eluting stents[220].

At present, relatively limited data are available on the IVUS findings of everolimus-eluting stents. In a recent 1002-patient multi-centre randomized trial (SPIRIT III), everolimus-eluting stents has shown a significant reduction in angiographic in-segment late loss at 8 months and a fewer major adverse cardiac events during 1-year follow-up as compared with paclitaxel-eluting stents[221]. These findings have been confirmed by an IVUS substudy, demonstrating greater reduction of neointimal hyperplasia by everolimus-eluting stents as compared with paclitaxel-eluting stents without any adverse vessel response detected by IVUS (percent neointimal volume: 7.0% versus 11.1%, $p = 0.004$)[222]. Additional real-world investigations are warranted to further characterize the property of this DES.

Future directions

Recently, IVUS has begun to be installed directly into the cine angiogram system (Boston Scientific Corp, Natick, MA; Volcano Corp, Rancho Cordova, CA), enabling operators quickly and easily to incorporate IVUS interrogations into their procedures. With this pre-installed IVUS system, IVUS is always on and ready, and there is no need to transport a console from lab to lab. Additionally, the system's tableside controller gives physicians control of the device within the sterile field, so that operators can easily investigate the exact location of lesion of interest during the procedure.

Another intriguing area of current IVUS development is the attempt to identify tissue components using computer-assisted analysis of raw radiofrequency signals in the reflected ultrasound beam. This is primarily based on the fact that there is greater information contained in the backscattered ultrasound signal than is revealed by the conventional amplitude-based image presentation alone. To date, a variety of signal parameters and mathematical modelling have been proposed and shown to enhance the tissue discrimination (see Fig. 10.11)[223]. One investigator group demonstrated that integrated backscatter values, calculated as the average power of the backscattered ultrasound signal from a sample tissue volume, were significantly different among tissue types (calcification, fibrous tissue, mixed lesion, lipid core or intimal hyperplasia, and thrombus) (Fig. 10.11A)[224]. Other investigators, including the authors' group, utilize unique ultrasound wave properties from different tissue types (e.g. signal attenuation slopes, statistical frequency distribution,

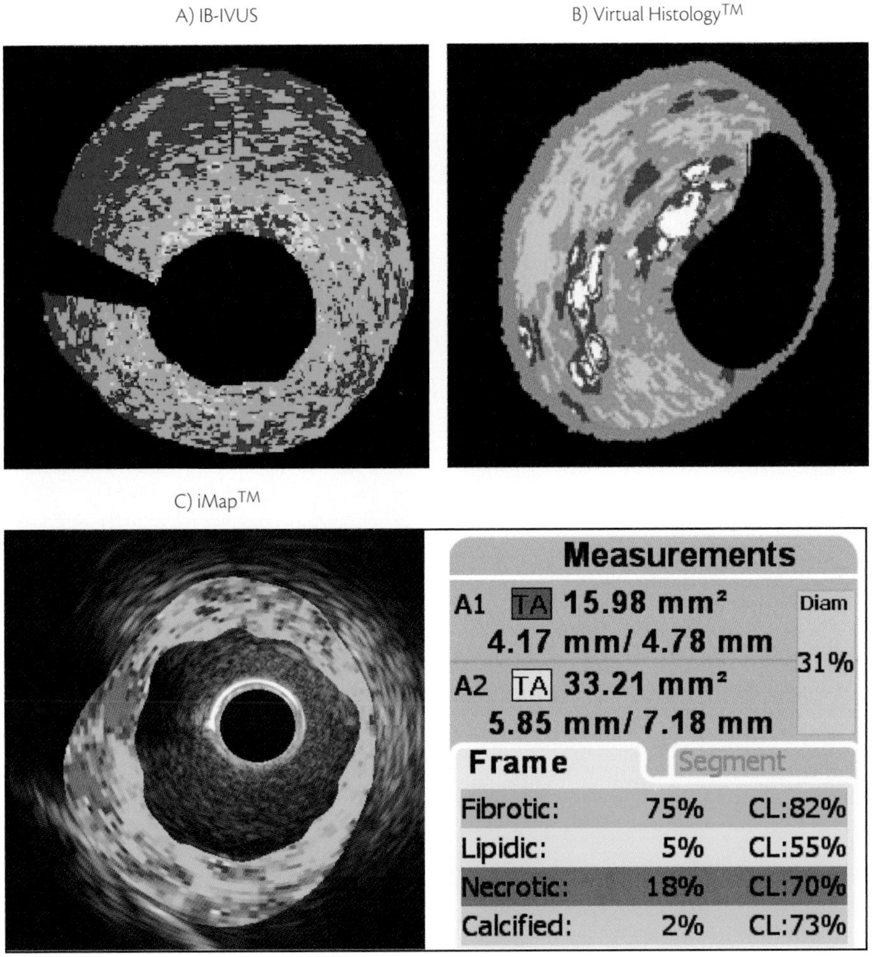

Fig. 10.11 Examples of plaque characterization by radiofrequency IVUS analysis. A) A colour-mapped presentation of integrated backscatter values (IB-IVUS. YD Co., Ltd.). Blue, lipid pool; green, fibrous; yellow, dense fibrous; red, calcification. (Courtesy of Yoshihiro Morino, MD.) B) Virtual Histology™ (Volcano Therapeutics, Inc.). Plaque components are determined using spectral radiofrequency signal analyses with a classification algorithm. Dark green, fibrous; light green, fibrofatty; white, calcium; red, necrotic core. C) iMap™ (Boston Scientific, Corp.) employs the concept of spectral similarity. It characterizes tissue type by comparing the spectrum originating from backscatter from a specified area on the vessel to entries in a library of spectra corresponding to known tissue types. In addition to delivering a colorized tissue map superimposed on the gray-scale image (left), this method provides a confidence level (CL) assessment of each plaque component (right).

and angle-dependent echo-intensity variation)[225–229]. Wavelet analysis, a mathematical model for assessing local wave patterns within a complex signal, has also been proposed, demonstrating accurate *in vitro* and *in vivo* discrimination of lipid-rich from fibrous plaques[230].

To date, one system (Virtual Histology™, Volcano Therapeutics, Inc., Rancho Cordova, CA) has been commercialized in the United States, utilizing spectral radiofrequency analyses with a classification algorithm developed from *ex vivo* coronary data sets[231]. The pattern recognition algorithm generates colour-mapped images of the vessel wall, with a distinct colour for each of the fibrous, necrotic, calcific and fibrofatty categories (Fig. 10.11B). An initial clinical study has shown a significant correlation of IVUS-determined plaque compositions with corresponding histopathology of the coronary specimens obtained by directional atherectomy[232]. Current technical limitations include limited spatial resolution (100–250µm), no classifications for thrombus, blood, or intimal hyperplasia, and potential errors due to poor ultrasound penetration through extensive calcification. Several multicentre studies have been initiated worldwide, and its roles in the detection of rupture-prone plaques and/or the guidance of interventions await the accumulation of clinical evidence.

References

1. Fuessl RT, Mintz GS, Pichard AD, *et al.* In vivo validation of intravascular ultrasound length measurements using a motorized transducer pullback system. *Am J Cardiol* 1996; **77**:1115–18.
2. Nissen SE, Yock P. Intravascular ultrasound: novel pathophysiological insights and current clinical applications. *Circulation* 2001; **103**:604–16.
3. Hausmann D, Erbel R, Alibelli CM, *et al.* The safety of intracoronary ultrasound. A multicenter survey of 2207 examinations. *Circulation* 1995; **91**:623–30.
4. Tobis JM, Mallery J, Mahon D, *et al.* Intravascular ultrasound imaging of human coronary arteries in vivo. Analysis of tissue characterizations with comparison to in vitro histological specimens. *Circulation* 1991; **83**: 913–26.
5. Siegel RJ, Chae JS, Maurer G, *et al.* Histopathologic correlation of the three-layered intravascular ultrasound appearance of normal adult human muscular arteries. *Am Heart J* 1993; **126**:872–8.
6. Fitzgerald PJ, St Goar FG, Connolly AJ, *et al.* Intravascular ultrasound imaging of coronary arteries. Is three layers the norm? *Circulation* 1992; **86**:154–8.
7. Gussenhoven EJ, Essed CE, Lancee CT, *et al.* Arterial wall characteristics determined by intravascular ultrasound imaging: an in vitro study. *J Am Coll Cardiol* 1989; **14**:947–52.
8. Gussenhoven EJ, Frietman PA, The SH, *et al.* Assessment of medial thinning in atherosclerosis by intravascular ultrasound. *Am J Cardiol* 1991; **68**:1625–32.
9. Isner JM, Donaldson RF, Fortin AH, *et al.* Attenuation of the media of coronary arteries in advanced atherosclerosis. *Am J Cardiol* 1986; **58**:937–9.
10. Maheswaran B, Leung CY, Gutfinger DE, *et al.* Intravascular ultrasound appearance of normal and mildly diseased coronary arteries: correlation with histologic specimens. *Am Heart J* 1995; **130**:976–86.
11. Mintz GS, Nissen SE, Anderson WD, *et al.* American College of Cardiology Clinical Expert Consensus Document on Standards for Acquisition, Measurement and Reporting of Intravascular Ultrasound Studies (IVUS). A report of the American College of Cardiology Task Force on Clinical Expert Consensus Documents. *J Am Coll Cardiol* 2001; **37**:1478–92.
12. Mintz GS, Popma JJ, Pichard AD, *et al.* Patterns of calcification in coronary artery disease. A statistical analysis of intravascular ultrasound and coronary angiography in 1155 lesions. *Circulation* 1995; **91**: 1959–65.
13. Mintz GS, Douek P, Pichard AD, *et al.* Target lesion calcification in coronary artery disease: an intravascular ultrasound study. *J Am Coll Cardiol* 1992; **20**:1149–55.
14. Tuzcu EM, Berkalp B, De Franco A, *et al.* The dilemma of diagnosing coronary calcification: angiography versus intravascular ultrasound. *J Am Coll Cardiol* 1996; **27**: 832–8.
15. Potkin BN, Bartorelli AL, Gessert JM, *et al.* Coronary artery imaging with intravascular high-frequency ultrasound. *Circulation* 1990; **81**:1575–85.
16. Yock PG, Fitzgerald PJ, Linker DT, *et al.* Intravascular ultrasound guidance for catheter-based coronary interventions. *J Am Coll Cardiol* 1991; **17**:39B–45B.
17. Caplan JD, Waxman S, Nesto RW, *et al.* Near-infrared spectroscopy for the detection of vulnerable coronary artery plaques. *J Am Coll Cardiol* 2006; **47**:C92–6.
18. Yabushita H, Bouma BE, Houser SL, *et al.* Characterization of human atherosclerosis by optical coherence tomography. *Circulation* 2002; **106**:1640–5.
19. Correia LC, Atalar E, Kelemen MD, *et al.* Intravascular magnetic resonance imaging of aortic atherosclerotic plaque composition. *Arterioscler Thromb Vasc Biol* 1997; **17**:3626–32.
20. Pandian NG, Kreis A, Brockway B. Detection of intraarterial thrombus by intravascular high frequency two-dimensional ultrasound imaging in vitro and in vivo studies. *Am J Cardiol* 1990; **65**:1280–3.
21. Fitzgerald PJ, Yock C, Yock PG. Orientation of intracoronary ultrasonography: looking beyond the artery. *J Am Soc Echocardiogr* 1998; **11**:13–19.
22. Abizaid A, Mintz GS, Pichard AD, *et al.* Clinical, intravascular ultrasound, and quantitative angiographic determinants of the coronary flow reserve before and after percutaneous transluminal coronary angioplasty. *Am J Cardiol* 1998; **82**:423–8.

23. Takagi A, Tsurumi Y, Ishii Y, *et al.* Clinical potential of intravascular ultrasound for physiological assessment of coronary stenosis: relationship between quantitative ultrasound tomography and pressure-derived fractional flow reserve. *Circulation* 1999; **100**:250–5.
24. Briguori C, Anzuini A, Airoldi F, *et al.* Intravascular ultrasound criteria for the assessment of the functional significance of intermediate coronary artery stenoses and comparison with fractional flow reserve. *Am J Cardiol* 2001; **87**:136–41.
25. Nishioka T, Amanullah AM, Luo H, *et al.* Clinical validation of intravascular ultrasound imaging for assessment of coronary stenosis severity: comparison with stress myocardial perfusion imaging. *J Am Coll Cardiol* 1999; **33**:1870–8.
26. Jasti V, Ivan E, Yalamanchili V, *et al.* Correlations between fractional flow reserve and intravascular ultrasound in patients with an ambiguous left main coronary artery stenosis. *Circulation* 2004; **110**:2831–6.
27. Hermiller JB, Buller CE, Tenaglia AN, *et al.* Unrecognized left main coronary artery disease in patients undergoing interventional procedures. *Am J Cardiol* 1993; **71**:173–6.
28. Yamagishi M, Hongo Y, Goto Y, *et al.* Intravascular ultrasound evidence of angiographically undetected left main coronary artery disease and associated trauma during interventional procedures. *Heart Vessels* 1996; **11**:262–8.
29. Gerber TC, Erbel R, Gorge G, *et al.* Extent of atherosclerosis and remodeling of the left main coronary artery determined by intravascular ultrasound. *Am J Cardiol* 1994; **73**:666–71.
30. Davies SW, Winterton SJ, Rothman MT. Intravascular ultrasound to assess left main stem coronary artery lesion. *Br Heart J* 1992; **68**:524–6.
31. Sano K, Mintz GS, Carlier SG, *et al.* Assessing intermediate left main coronary lesions using intravascular ultrasound. *Am Heart J* 2007; **154**:983–8.
32. Di Mario C, DeGregorio J, Kobayashi Y, *et al.* Atherectomy for ostial LAD stenosis: 'a cut above'. *Cathet Cardiovasc Diagn* 1998; **43**:101–4.
33. Mintz GS, Popma JJ, Pichard AD, *et al.* Limitations of angiography in the assessment of plaque distribution in coronary artery disease: a systematic study of target lesion eccentricity in 1446 lesions. *Circulation* 1996; **93**:924–31.
34. Fitzgerald PJ, Yock PG. Mechanisms and outcomes of angioplasty and atherectomy assessed by intravascular ultrasound imaging. *J Clin Ultrasound* 1993; **21**:579–88.
35. Schoenhagen P, Ziada KM, Kapadia SR, *et al.* Extent and direction of arterial remodeling in stable versus unstable coronary syndromes: an intravascular ultrasound study. *Circulation* 2000; **101**:598–603.
36. Smits PC, Pasterkamp G, Quarles van Ufford MA, *et al.* Coronary artery disease: arterial remodelling and clinical presentation. *Heart* 1999; **82**:461–4.
37. Kaji S, Akasaka T, Hozumi T, *et al.* Compensatory enlargement of the coronary artery in acute myocardial infarction. *Am J Cardiol* 2000; **85**:1139–41, A9.
38. Jeremias A, Spies C, Herity NA, *et al.* Coronary artery compliance and adaptive vessel remodelling in patients with stable and unstable coronary artery disease. *Heart* 2000; **84**:314–9.
39. Gyongyosi M, Yang P, Hassan A, *et al.* Arterial remodelling of native human coronary arteries in patients with unstable angina pectoris: a prospective intravascular ultrasound study. *Heart* 1999; **82**:68–74.
40. Nakamura M, Nishikawa H, Mukai S, *et al.* Impact of coronary artery remodeling on clinical presentation of coronary artery disease: an intravascular ultrasound study. *J Am Coll Cardiol* 2001; **37**:63–9.
41. Dangas G, Mintz GS, Mehran R, *et al.* Preintervention arterial remodeling as an independent predictor of target-lesion revascularization after nonstent coronary intervention: an analysis of 777 lesions with intravascular ultrasound imaging. *Circulation* 1999; **99**:3149–54.
42. Okura H, Hayase M, Shimodozono S, *et al.* Impact of pre-interventional arterial remodeling on subsequent vessel behavior after balloon angioplasty: a serial intravascular ultrasound study. *J Am Coll Cardiol* 2001; **38**:2001–5.
43. Okura H, Morino Y, Oshima A, *et al.* Preintervention arterial remodeling affects clinical outcome following stenting: an intravascular ultrasound study. *J Am Coll Cardiol* 2001; **37**:1031–5.
44. Endo A, Hirayama H, Yoshida O, *et al.* Arterial remodeling influences the development of intimal hyperplasia after stent implantation. *J Am Coll Cardiol* 2001; **37**:70–5.
45. Shiran A, Weissman NJ, Leiboff B, *et al.* Effect of preintervention plaque burden on subsequent intimal hyperplasia in stented coronary artery lesions. *Am J Cardiol* 2000; **86**:1318–21.
46. Tanaka A, Kawarabayashi T, Nishibori Y, *et al.* No-reflow phenomenon and lesion morphology in patients with acute myocardial infarction. *Circulation* 2002; **105**: 2148–52.
47. Kotani J, Mintz GS, Castagna MT, *et al.* Usefulness of preprocedural coronary lesion morphology as assessed by intravascular ultrasound in predicting Thrombolysis In Myocardial Infarction frame count after percutaneous coronary intervention in patients with Q-wave acute myocardial infarction. *Am J Cardiol* 2003; **91**:870–2.
48. Wexberg P, Gyongyosi M, Sperker W, *et al.* Pre-existing arterial remodeling is associated with in-hospital and late adverse cardiac events after coronary interventions in patients with stable angina pectoris. *J Am Coll Cardiol* 2000; **36**:1860–9.
49. Hoffmann R, Mintz GS, Kent KM, *et al.* Serial intravascular ultrasound predictors of restenosis at the margins of Palmaz-Schatz stents. *Am J Cardiol* 1997; **79**:951–3.
50. Dangas G, Mintz GS, Mehran R, *et al.* Stent implantation neutralizes the impact of preintervention arterial remodeling on subsequent target lesion revascularization. *Am J Cardiol* 2000; **86**:452–5.

51. Hong MK, Park SW, Lee CW, *et al.* Preintervention arterial remodeling as a predictor of intimal hyperplasia after intracoronary stenting: a serial intravascular ultrasound study. *Clin Cardiol* 2002; **25**:11–15.
52. Mintz GS, Kimura T, Nobuyoshi M, *et al.* Relation between preintervention remodeling and late arterial responses to coronary angioplasty or atherectomy. *Am J Cardiol* 2001; **87**:392–6.
53. White CJ, Ramee SR, Collins TJ, *et al.* Ambiguous coronary angiography: clinical utility of intravascular ultrasound. *Cathet Cardiovasc Diagn* 1992; **26**:200–3.
54. Lee DY, Eigler N, Luo H, *et al.* Effect of intracoronary ultrasound imaging on clinical decision making. *Am Heart J* 1995; **129**:1084–93.
55. Ziada KM, Tuzcu EM, De Franco AC, *et al.* Intravascular ultrasound assessment of the prevalence and causes of angiographic 'haziness' following high-pressure coronary stenting. *Am J Cardiol* 1997; **80**:116–21.
56. Kearney P, Erbel R, Ge J, *et al.* Assessment of spontaneous coronary artery dissection by intravascular ultrasound in a patient with unstable angina. *Cathet Cardiovasc Diagn* 1994; **32**:58–61.
57. Potkin BN, Keren G, Mintz GS, *et al.* Arterial responses to balloon coronary angioplasty: an intravascular ultrasound study. *J Am Coll Cardiol* 1992; **20**:942–51.
58. Tenaglia AN, Buller CE, Kisslo KB, *et al.* Mechanisms of balloon angioplasty and directional coronary atherectomy as assessed by intracoronary ultrasound. *J Am Coll Cardiol* 1992; **20**:685–91.
59. Braden GA, Herrington DM, Downes TR, *et al.* Qualitative and quantitative contrasts in the mechanisms of lumen enlargement by coronary balloon angioplasty and directional coronary atherectomy. *J Am Coll Cardiol* 1994; **23**:40–8.
60. Tobis JM, Mallery JA, Gessert J, *et al.* Intravascular ultrasound cross-sectional arterial imaging before and after balloon angioplasty in vitro. *Circulation* 1989; **80**:873–82.
61. Baptista J, Umans VA, Di Mario C, *et al.* Mechanisms of luminal enlargement and quantification of vessel wall trauma following balloon coronary angioplasty and directional atherectomy. *Eur Heart J* 1995; **16**:1603–12.
62. Baptista J, Di Mario C, Ozaki Y, *et al.* Impact of plaque morphology and composition on the mechanisms of lumen enlargement using intracoronary ultrasound and quantitative angiography after balloon angioplasty. *Am J Cardiol* 1996; **77**:115–21.
63. Honye J, Mahon DJ, Jain A, *et al.* Morphological effects of coronary balloon angioplasty in vivo assessed by intravascular ultrasound imaging. *Circulation* 1992; **85**:1012–25.
64. Fitzgerald PJ, Ports TA, Yock PG. Contribution of localized calcium deposits to dissection after angioplasty. An observational study using intravascular ultrasound. *Circulation* 1992; **86**:64–70.
65. Lee RT, Richardson SG, Loree HM, *et al.* Prediction of mechanical properties of human atherosclerotic tissue by high-frequency intravascular ultrasound imaging. An in vitro study. *Arterioscler Thromb* 1992; **12**:1–5.
66. Richardson PD, Davies MJ, Born GV. Influence of plaque configuration and stress distribution on fissuring of coronary atherosclerotic plaques. *Lancet* 1989; **2**:941–4.
67. Nakamura S, Mahon DJ, Leung CY, *et al.* Intracoronary ultrasound imaging before and after directional coronary atherectomy: in vitro and clinical observations. *Am Heart J* 1995; **129**:841–51.
68. Simonton CA, Leon MB, Baim DS, *et al.* 'Optimal' directional coronary atherectomy: final results of the Optimal Atherectomy Restenosis Study (OARS). *Circulation* 1998; **97**:332–9.
69. Dussaillant GR, Mintz GS, Pichard AD, *et al.* Effect of rotational atherectomy in noncalcified atherosclerotic plaque: a volumetric intravascular ultrasound study. *J Am Coll Cardiol* 1996; **28**:856–60.
70. Kovach JA, Mintz GS, Pichard AD, *et al.* Sequential intravascular ultrasound characterization of the mechanisms of rotational atherectomy and adjunct balloon angioplasty. *J Am Coll Cardiol* 1993; **22**:1024–32.
71. Mintz GS, Potkin BN, Keren G, *et al.* Intravascular ultrasound evaluation of the effect of rotational atherectomy in obstructive atherosclerotic coronary artery disease. *Circulation* 1992; **86**:1383–93.
72. Kimura T, Kaburagi S, Tamura T, *et al.* Remodeling of human coronary arteries undergoing coronary angioplasty or atherectomy. *Circulation* 1997; **96**:475–83.
73. Mintz GS, Popma JJ, Hong MK, *et al.* Intravascular ultrasound to discern device-specific effects and mechanisms of restenosis. *Am J Cardiol* 1996; **78**:18–22.
74. Mintz GS, Popma JJ, Pichard AD, *et al.* Arterial remodeling after coronary angioplasty: a serial intravascular ultrasound study. *Circulation* 1996; **94**: 35–43.
75. Stone GW, Hodgson JM, St Goar FG, *et al.* Improved procedural results of coronary angioplasty with intravascular ultrasound-guided balloon sizing. The CLOUT pilot trial. *Circulation* 1997; **95**:2044–52.
76. Stone GW, Frey A, Linnemeier T, *et al.* 2.5 year follow-up of the CLOUT study. Long-term implications for an aggressive IVUS guided balloon angioplasty strategy. *J Am Coll Cardiol* 1999; **33**:81A.
77. Schroeder S, Baumbach A, Haase KK, *et al.* Reduction of restenosis by vessel size adapted percutaneous transluminal coronary angioplasty using intravascular ultrasound. *Am J Cardiol* 1999; **83**:875–9.
78. Abizaid A, Pichard AD, Mintz GS, *et al.* Acute and long-term results of an intravascular ultrasound-guided percutaneous transluminal coronary angioplasty/ provisional stent implantation strategy. *Am J Cardiol* 1999; **84**:1298–303.
79. Kimura BJ, Fitzgerald PJ, Sudhir K, *et al.* Guidance of directed coronary atherectomy by intracoronary ultrasound imaging. *Am Heart J* 1992; **124**:1365–9.
80. Mintz GS, Popma JJ, Pichard AD, *et al.* Intravascular ultrasound predictors of restenosis after percutaneous

transcatheter coronary revascularization. *J Am Coll Cardiol* 1996; **27**:1678–87.

81. The GUIDE trial investigators. IVUS-determined predictors of restenosis in PTCA and DCA: final report from the GUIDE trial, phase II (abstract). *J Am Coll Cardiol* 1996; **27**:156A.
82. Suzuki T, Hosokawa H, Katoh O, *et al.* Effects of adjunctive balloon angioplasty after intravascular ultrasound-guided optimal directional coronary atherectomy: the result of Adjunctive Balloon Angioplasty After Coronary Atherectomy Study (ABACAS). *J Am Coll Cardiol* 1999; **34**:1028–35.
83. Tsuchikane E, Sumitsuji S, Awata N, *et al.* Final results of the STent versus directional coronary Atherectomy Randomized Trial (START). *J Am Coll Cardiol* 1999; **34**:1050–7.
84. Tsuchikane E, Aizawa T, Tamai H, *et al.* Pre-drug-eluting stent debulking of bifurcated coronary lesions. *J Am Coll Cardiol* 2007; **50**:1941–5.
85. Clavijo LC, Steinberg DH, Torguson R, *et al.* Sirolimus-eluting stents and calcified coronary lesions: clinical outcomes of patients treated with and without rotational atherectomy. *Catheter Cardiovasc Interv* 2006; **68**:873–8.
86. Kay IP, Sabate M, Costa MA, *et al.* Positive geometric vascular remodeling is seen after catheter-based radiation followed by conventional stent implantation but not after radioactive stent implantation. *Circulation* 2000; **102**:1434–9.
87. Albiero R, Adamian M, Kobayashi N, *et al.* Short- and intermediate-term results of (32)P radioactive beta-emitting stent implantation in patients with coronary artery disease: The Milan Dose-Response Study. *Circulation* 2000; **101**:18–26.
88. Bhargava B, Mintz GS, Mehran R, *et al.* Serial volumetric intravascular ultrasound analysis of the efficacy of beta irradiation in preventing recurrent in-stent restenosis. *Am J Cardiol* 2000; 85:**651**:3, A10.
89. Mintz GS, Weissman NJ, Teirstein PS, *et al.* Effect of intracoronary gamma-radiation therapy on in-stent restenosis: An intravascular ultrasound analysis from the gamma-1 study. *Circulation* 2000; **102**:2915–18.
90. Raizner AE, Oesterle SN, Waksman R, *et al.* Inhibition of restenosis with beta-emitting radiotherapy: Report of the Proliferation Reduction with Vascular Energy Trial (PREVENT). *Circulation* 2000; **102**:951–8.
91. Sabate M, Marijnissen JP, Carlier SG, *et al.* Residual plaque burden, delivered dose, and tissue composition predict 6-month outcome after balloon angioplasty and beta-radiation therapy. *Circulation* 2000; **101**:2472–7.
92. Popma JJ, Suntharalingam M, Lansky AJ, *et al.* Randomized trial of 90Sr/90Y beta-radiation versus placebo control for treatment of in-stent restenosis. *Circulation* 2002; **106**:1090–6.
93. Silber S, Popma JJ, Suntharalingam M, *et al.* Two-year clinical follow-up of 90Sr/90 Y beta-radiation versus placebo control for the treatment of in-stent restenosis. *Am Heart J* 2005; **149**:689–94.
94. Teirstein PS, Massullo V, Jani S, *et al.* Catheter-based radiotherapy to inhibit restenosis after coronary stenting. *N Engl J Med* 1997; **336**:1697–703.
95. Waksman R, White RL, Chan RC, *et al.* Intracoronary gamma-radiation therapy after angioplasty inhibits recurrence in patients with in-stent restenosis. *Circulation* 2000; **101**:2165–71.
96. Sabate M, Serruys PW, van der Giessen WJ, *et al.* Geometric vascular remodeling after balloon angioplasty and beta- radiation therapy: A three-dimensional intravascular ultrasound study. *Circulation* 1999; **100**:1182–8.
97. Albiero R, Nishida T, Adamian M, *et al.* Edge restenosis after implantation of high activity (32)P radioactive beta-emitting stents. *Circulation* 2000; **101**:2454–7.
98. Ahmed JM, Mintz GS, Waksman R, *et al.* Serial intravascular ultrasound analysis of edge recurrence after intracoronary gamma radiation treatment of native artery in-stent restenosis lesions. *Am J Cardiol* 2001; **87**:1145–9.
99. Okura H, Lee DP, Handen CE, *et al.* Contribution of vessel remodeling to 'edge effect' following intracoronary beta-radiation therapy: a serial volumetric intravascular ultrasound study (abstract). *Circulation* 1999; **100**:I–511.
100. Sabate M, Costa MA, Kozuma K, *et al.* Geographic miss: A cause of treatment failure in radio-oncology applied to intracoronary radiation therapy. *Circulation* 2000; **101**:2467–71.
101. Kirisits C, Wexberg P, Gottsauner-Wolf M, *et al.* Dose-volume histograms based on serial intravascular ultrasound: a calculation model for radioactive stents. *Radiother Oncol* 2001; **59**:329–37.
102. Carlier SG, Marijnissen JP, Coen VL, *et al.* Guidance of intracoronary radiation therapy based on dose-volume histograms derived from quantitative intravascular ultrasound. *IEEE Trans Med Imaging* 1998; **17**:772–8.
103. Kozuma K, Costa MA, Sabate M, *et al.* Relationship between tensile stress and plaque growth after balloon angioplasty treated with and without intracoronary beta-brachytherapy. *Eur Heart J* 2000; **21**:2063–70.
104. Crocker I, Fox T, Carlier SG. IVUS based dosimetry and treatment planning. *J Invasive Cardiol* 2000; **12**:643–8.
105. Morino Y, Kaneda H, Fox T, *et al.* Delivered dose and vascular response after beta-radiation for in-stent restenosis: retrospective dosimetry and volumetric intravascular ultrasound analysis. *Circulation* 2002; **106**:2334–9.
106. Kaneda H, Honda Y, Morino Y, *et al.* Safety of beta radiation exposure to the non-target segment: an intravascular ultrasound dosimetric analysis. *J Invasive Cardiol* 2006; **18**:309–12.
107. Maehara A, Patel NS, Harrison LB, *et al.* Dose heterogeneity may not affect the neointimal proliferation after gamma radiation for in-stent restenosis: a volumetric intravascular ultrasound dosimetric study. *J Am Coll Cardiol* 2002; **39**:1937–42.
108. Alfonso F, Hernandez R, Goicolea J, *et al.* Coronary stenting for acute coronary dissection after coronary

angioplasty: implications of residual dissection. *J Am Coll Cardiol* 1994; **24**:989–95.

109. Di Mario C, Gorge G, Peters R, *et al.* Clinical application and image interpretation in intracoronary ultrasound. Study Group on Intracoronary Imaging of the Working Group of Coronary Circulation and of the Subgroup on Intravascular Ultrasound of the Working Group of Echocardiography of the European Society of Cardiology. *Eur Heart J* 1998; **19**:207–29.
110. Meerkin D, Tardif JC, Bertrand OF, *et al.* The effects of intracoronary brachytherapy on the natural history of postangioplasty dissections. *J Am Coll Cardiol* 2000; **36**:59–64.
111. Kozuma K, Costa MA, Sabate M, *et al.* Late stent malapposition occurring after intracoronary beta-irradiation detected by intravascular ultrasound. *J Invasive Cardiol* 1999; **11**:651–5.
112. Okura H, Lee DP, Lo S, *et al.* Late incomplete apposition with excessive remodeling of the stented coronary artery following intravascular brachytherapy. *Am J Cardiol* 2003; **92**:587–90.
113. Kay IP, Ligthart JM, Virmani R, *et al.* The black hole: a new IVUS observation after intracoronary radiation (abstr). *Circulation* 2000; **102**:II–568.
114. Honda Y, Yock CA, Hermiller JB, *et al.* Longitudinal redistribution of plaque is an important mechanism for lumen expansion in stenting (abstract). *J Am Coll Cardiol* 1997; **29**:281A.
115. Ahmed JM, Mintz GS, Weissman NJ, *et al.* Mechanism of lumen enlargement during intracoronary stent implantation: An intravascular ultrasound study. *Circulation* 2000; **102**:7–10.
116. Maehara A, Takagi A, Okura H, *et al.* Longitudinal plaque redistribution during stent expansion. *Am J Cardiol* 2000; **86**:1069–72.
117. von Birgelen C, Mintz GS, Eggebrecht H, *et al.* Preintervention arterial remodeling affects vessel stretch and plaque extrusion during coronary stent deployment as demonstrated by three-dimensional intravascular ultrasound. *Am J Cardiol* 2003; **92**:130–5.
118. Mintz GS, Pichard AD, Kent KM, *et al.* Axial plaque redistribution as a mechanism of percutaneous transluminal coronary angioplasty. *Am J Cardiol* 1996; **77**:427–30.
119. Nakamura S, Colombo A, Gaglione A, *et al.* Intracoronary ultrasound observations during stent implantation. *Circulation* 1994; **89**:2026–34.
120. Colombo A, Hall P, Nakamura S, *et al.* Intracoronary stenting without anticoagulation accomplished with intravascular ultrasound guidance. *Circulation* 1995; **91**:1676–88.
121. Schwarzacher SP, Metz JA, Yock PG, *et al.* Vessel tearing at the edge of intracoronary stents detected with intravascular ultrasound imaging. *Cath Cardiovasc Diagn* 1997; **40**:152–5.
122. Metz JA, Mooney MR, Walter PD, *et al.* Significance of edge tears in coronary stenting: Initial observations from the STRUT registry (abstract). *Circulation* 1995; **92**:I–546.
123. Goldberg SL, Colombo A, Nakamura S, *et al.* Benefit of intracoronary ultrasound in the deployment of Palmaz-Schatz stents. *J Am Coll Cardiol* 1994; **24**: 996–1003.
124. Sheris SJ, Canos MR, Weissman NJ. Natural history of intravascular ultrasound-detected edge dissections from coronary stent deployment. *Am Heart J* 2000; **139**:59–63.
125. Nishida T, Colombo A, Briguori C, *et al.* Outcome of nonobstructive residual dissections detected by intravascular ultrasound following percutaneous coronary intervention. *Am J Cardiol* 2002; **89**:1257–62.
126. Hong MK, Park SW, Lee NH, *et al.* Long-term outcomes of minor dissection at the edge of stents detected with intravascular ultrasound. *Am J Cardiol* 2000; **86**: 791–5, A9.
127. Russo R, Silva P, Teirstein P, *et al.* A randomized controlled trial of angiography versus intravascular ultrasound-directed bare-metal coronary stent placement (The AVID Trial). *Circulation Cardiovasc Interv* 2009; **113**:123.
128. Blasini R, Neumann FJ, Schmitt C, *et al.* Restenosis rate after intravascular ultrasound-guided coronary stent implantation. *Cathet Cardiovasc Diagn* 1998; **44**:380–6.
129. Albiero R, Rau T, Schluter M, *et al.* Comparison of immediate and intermediate-term results of intravascular ultrasound versus angiography-guided Palmaz-Schatz stent implantation in matched lesions. *Circulation* 1997; **96**:2997–3005.
130. Choi JW, Goodreau LM, Davidson CJ. Resource utilization and clinical outcomes of coronary stenting: a comparison of intravascular ultrasound and angiographical guided stent implantation. *Am Heart J* 2001; **142**:112–8.
131. Fitzgerald PJ, Oshima A, Hayase M, *et al.* Final results of the Can Routine Ultrasound Influence Stent Expansion (CRUISE) study. *Circulation* 2000; **102**:523–30.
132. Frey AW, Hodgson JM, Muller C, *et al.* Ultrasound-guided strategy for provisional stenting with focal balloon combination catheter: results from the randomized Strategy for Intracoronary Ultrasound-guided PTCA and Stenting (SIPS) trial. *Circulation* 2000; **102**:2497–502.
133. Schiele F, Meneveau N, Seronde MF, *et al.* Medical costs of intravascular ultrasound optimization of stent deployment. Results of the multicenter randomized 'REStenosis after Intravascular ultrasound STenting' (RESIST) study. *Int J Cardiovasc Intervent* 2000; **3**:207–13.
134. Schiele F, Meneveau N, Gilard M, *et al.* Intravascular ultrasound-guided balloon angioplasty compared with stent: immediate and 6-month results of the multicenter, randomized Balloon Equivalent to Stent Study (BEST). *Circulation* 2003; **107**:545–51.
135. Oemrawsingh PV, Mintz GS, Schalij MJ, *et al.* Intravascular ultrasound guidance improves angiographic and clinical outcome of stent implantation for long coronary artery stenoses: final results of a randomized comparison with angiographic guidance (TULIP Study). *Circulation* 2003; **107**:62–7.

136. de Jaegere P, Mudra H, Figulla H, *et al.* Intravascular ultrasound-guided optimized stent deployment. Immediate and 6 months clinical and angiographic results from the Multicenter Ultrasound Stenting in Coronaries Study (MUSIC Study). *Eur Heart J* 1998; **19**:1214–23.
137. Uren NG, Schwaxzacher SP, Metz JA, *et al.* Predictors and outcomes on stent thrombosis: an intravascular ultrasound registry. *Eur Heart J* 2002; **23**:124–32.
138. Cheneau E, Leborgne L, Mintz GS, *et al.* Predictors of subacute stent thrombosis: results of a systematic intravascular ultrasound study. *Circulation* 2003; **108**:43–7.
139. Hoffmann R, Mintz GS, Mehran R, *et al.* Intravascular ultrasound predictors of angiographic restenosis in lesions treated with Palmaz-Schatz stents. *J Am Coll Cardiol* 1998; **31**:43–9.
140. Ziada KM, Tuzcu EM, De Franco AC, *et al.* Absolute, not relative, post-stent lumen area is a better predictor of clinical outcome (abstract). *Circulation* 1996; **94**:I–453.
141. Moussa I, Moses J, Di Mario C, *et al.* Does the specific intravascular ultrasound criterion used to optimize stent expansion have an impact on the probability of stent restenosis? *Am J Cardiol* 1999; **83**:1012–17.
142. Kasaoka S, Tobis JM, Akiyama T, *et al.* Angiographic and intravascular ultrasound predictors of in-stent restenosis. *J Am Coll Cardiol* 1998; **32**:1630–5.
143. Morino Y, Honda Y, Okura H, *et al.* An optimal diagnostic threshold for minimal stent area to predict target lesion revascularization following stent implantation in native coronary lesions. *Am J Cardiol* 2001; **88**:301–3.
144. Mudra H, di Mario C, de Jaegere P, *et al.* Randomized comparison of coronary stent implantation under ultrasound or angiographic guidance to reduce stent restenosis (OPTICUS Study). *Circulation* 2001; **104**: 1343–9.
145. Orford JL, Denktas AE, Williams BA, *et al.* Routine intravascular ultrasound scanning guidance of coronary stenting is not associated with improved clinical outcomes. *Am Heart J* 2004; **148**:501–6.
146. Casella G, Klauss V, Ottani F, *et al.* Impact of intravascular ultrasound-guided stenting on long-term clinical outcome: a meta-analysis of available studies comparing intravascular ultrasound-guided and angiographically guided stenting. *Catheter Cardiovasc Interv* 2003; **59**:314–21.
147. Hoffmann R, Mintz GS, Dussaillant GR, *et al.* Patterns and mechanisms of in-stent restenosis. A serial intravascular ultrasound study. *Circulation* 1996; **94**: 1247–54.
148. Prati F, Di Mario C, Moussa I, *et al.* In-stent neointimal proliferation correlates with the amount of residual plaque burden outside the stent: an intravascular ultrasound study. *Circulation* 1999; **99**:1011–4.
149. Hibi K, Suzuki T, Honda Y, *et al.* Quantitative and spatial relation of baseline atherosclerotic plaque burden and subsequent in-stent neointimal proliferation as determined by intravascular ultrasound. *Am J Cardiol* 2002; **90**:1164–7.
150. Kornowski R, Mintz GS, Kent KM, *et al.* Increased restenosis in diabetes mellitus after coronary interventions is due to exaggerated intimal hyperplasia. A serial intravascular ultrasound study. *Circulation* 1997; **95**:1366–9.
151. Takagi T, Yoshida K, Akasaka T, *et al.* Hyperinsulinemia during oral glucose tolerance test is associated with increased neointimal tissue proliferation after coronary stent implantation in nondiabetic patients: a serial intravascular ultrasound study. *J Am Coll Cardiol* 2000; **36**:731–8.
152. Castagna MT, Mintz GS, Leiboff BO, *et al.* The contribution of 'mechanical' problems to in-stent restenosis: An intravascular ultrasonographic analysis of 1090 consecutive in-stent restenosis lesions. *Am Heart J* 2001; **142**:970–4.
153. Albertal M, Abizaid A, Munoz JS, *et al.* A novel mechanism explaining early lumen loss following balloon angioplasty for the treatment of in-stent restenosis. *Am J Cardiol* 2005; **95**:751–4.
154. Shiran A, Mintz GS, Waksman R, *et al.* Early lumen loss after treatment of in-stent restenosis: an intravascular ultrasound study. *Circulation* 1998; **98**:200–3.
155. Dauerman HL, Baim DS, Cutlip DE, *et al.* Mechanical debulking versus balloon angioplasty for the treatment of diffuse in-stent restenosis. *Am J Cardiol* 1998; **82**:277–84.
156. Mehran R, Mintz GS, Satler LF, *et al.* Treatment of in-stent restenosis with excimer laser coronary angioplasty: mechanisms and results compared with PTCA alone. *Circulation* 1997; **96**:2183–9.
157. Mahdi NA, Pathan AZ, Harrell L, et al. Directional coronary atherectomy for the treatment of Palmaz-Schatz in-stent restenosis. *Am J Cardiol* 1998; **82**:1345–51.
158. Lee SG, Lee CW, Cheong SS, *et al.* Immediate and long-term outcomes of rotational atherectomy versus balloon angioplasty alone for treatment of diffuse in-stent restenosis. *Am J Cardiol* 1998; **82**:140–3.
159. Sharma SK, Kini A, Mehran R, *et al.* Randomized trial of Rotational Atherectomy Versus Balloon Angioplasty for Diffuse In-stent Restenosis (ROSTER). *Am Heart J* 2004; **147**:16–22.
160. Radke PW, Klues HG, Haager PK, *et al.* Mechanisms of acute lumen gain and recurrent restenosis after rotational atherectomy of diffuse in-stent restenosis: a quantitative angiographic and intravascular ultrasound study. *J Am Coll Cardiol* 1999; **34**:33–9.
161. Dahm JB, Kuon E. High-energy eccentric excimer laser angioplasty for debulking diffuse in-stent restenosis leads to better acute- and 6-month follow-up results. *J Invasive Cardiol* 2000; **12**:335–42.
162. Moses JW, Leon MB, Popma JJ, *et al.* Sirolimus-eluting stents versus standard stents in patients with stenosis in a native coronary artery. *N Engl J Med* 2003; **349**:1315–23.
163. Serruys PW, Degertekin M, Tanabe K, *et al.* Intravascular ultrasound findings in the multicenter, randomized,

double-blind RAVEL (RAndomized study with the sirolimus-eluting VElocity balloon-expandable stent in the treatment of patients with de novo native coronary artery Lesions) trial. *Circulation* 2002; **106**: 798–803.

164. Tanabe K, Serruys PW, Degertekin M, *et al.* Chronic arterial responses to polymer-controlled paclitaxel-eluting stents: comparison with bare metal stents by serial intravascular ultrasound analyses: data from the randomized TAXUS-II trial. *Circulation* 2004; **109**: 196–200.
165. Weissman NJ, Koglin J, Cox DA, *et al.* Polymer-based paclitaxel-eluting stents reduce in-stent neointimal tissue proliferation: a serial volumetric intravascular ultrasound analysis from the TAXUS-IV trial. *J Am Coll Cardiol* 2005; **45**:1201–5.
166. de Ribamar Costa J, Jr, Mintz GS, Carlier SG, *et al.* Intravascular ultrasound assessment of drug-eluting stent expansion. *Am Heart J* 2007; **153**:297–303.
167. Stone GW, Ellis SG, Cox DA, *et al.* A polymer-based, paclitaxel-eluting stent in patients with coronary artery disease. *N Engl J Med* 2004; **350**:221–31.
168. Fajadet J, Wijns W, Laarman GJ, *et al.* Randomized, double-blind, multicenter study of the Endeavor zotarolimus-eluting phosphorylcholine-encapsulated stent for treatment of native coronary artery lesions: clinical and angiographic results of the ENDEAVOR II trial. *Circulation* 2006; **114**:798–806.
169. Weissman NJ, Wilensky RL, Tanguay JF, *et al.* Extent and distribution of in-stent intimal hyperplasia and edge effect in a non-radiation stent population. *Am J Cardiol* 2001; **88**:248–52.
170. Hirohata A, Morino Y, Ako J, *et al.* Comparison of the Efficacy of Direct Coronary Stenting With Sirolimus-Eluting Stents Versus Stenting With Predilation by Intravascular Ultrasound Imaging (from the DIRECT Trial). *Am J Cardiol* 2006; **98**:1464–7.
171. Abizaid A, Kornowski R, Mintz GS, *et al.* The influence of diabetes mellitus on acute and late clinical outcomes following coronary stent implantation. *J Am Coll Cardiol* 1998; **32**:584–9.
172. Stankovic G, Cosgrave J, Chieffo A, *et al.* Impact of sirolimus-eluting and Paclitaxel-eluting stents on outcome in patients with diabetes mellitus and stenting in more than one coronary artery. *Am J Cardiol* 2006; **98**:362–6.
173. Buch AN, Javaid A, Steinberg DH, *et al.* Outcomes after sirolimus- and paclitaxel-eluting stent implantation in patients with insulin-treated diabetes mellitus. *Am J Cardiol* 2008; **101**:1253–8.
174. Daemen J, Garcia-Garcia HM, Kukreja N, *et al.* The long-term value of sirolimus- and paclitaxel-eluting stents over bare metal stents in patients with diabetes mellitus. *Eur Heart J* 2007; **28**:26–32.
175. Billinger M, Beutler J, Taghetchian KR, *et al.* Two-year clinical outcome after implantation of sirolimus-eluting and paclitaxel-eluting stents in diabetic patients. *Eur Heart J* 2008; **29**:718–25.
176. Dibra A, Kastrati A, Mehilli J, *et al.* Paclitaxel-eluting or sirolimus-eluting stents to prevent restenosis in diabetic patients. *N Engl J Med* 2005; **353**:663–70.
177. Lee SW, Park SW, Kim YH, *et al.* Drug-eluting stenting followed by cilostazol treatment reduces late restenosis in patients with diabetes mellitus the DECLARE-DIABETES Trial (A Randomized Comparison of Triple Antiplatelet Therapy with Dual Antiplatelet Therapy After Drug-Eluting Stent Implantation in Diabetic Patients). *J Am Coll Cardiol* 2008; **51**:1181–7.
178. Tomai F, Reimers B, De Luca L, *et al.* Head-to-head comparison of sirolimus- and paclitaxel-eluting stent in the same diabetic patient with multiple coronary artery lesions: a prospective, randomized, multicenter study. *Diabetes Care* 2008; **31**:15–19.
179. Jensen LO, Maeng M, Thayssen P, *et al.* Neointimal hyperplasia after sirolimus-eluting and paclitaxel-eluting stent implantation in diabetic patients: the Randomized Diabetes and Drug-Eluting Stent (DiabeDES) Intravascular Ultrasound Trial. *Eur Heart J* 2008; **29**: 2733–41.
180. Takebayashi H, Mintz GS, Carlier SG, *et al.* Nonuniform strut distribution correlates with more neointimal hyperplasia after sirolimus-eluting stent implantation. *Circulation* 2004; **110**:3430–4.
181. Hong MK, Mintz GS, Lee CW, *et al.* Intravascular ultrasound predictors of angiographic restenosis after sirolimus-eluting stent implantation. *Eur Heart J* 2006; **27**:1305–10.
182. Sonoda S, Morino Y, Ako J, *et al.* Impact of final stent dimensions on long-term results following sirolimus-eluting stent implantation: serial intravascular ultrasound analysis from the sirius trial. *J Am Coll Cardiol* 2004; **43**:1959–63.
183. Cheneau E, Pichard AD, Satler LF, *et al.* Intravascular ultrasound stent area of sirolimus-eluting stents and its impact on late outcome. *Am J Cardiol* 2005; **95**: 1240–2.
184. Kim SW, Mintz GS, Escolar E, *et al.* An intravascular ultrasound analysis of the mechanisms of restenosis comparing drug-eluting stents with brachytherapy. *Am J Cardiol* 2006; **97**:1292–8.
185. Brodie BR. Adjunctive balloon postdilatation after stent deployment: is it still necessary with drug-eluting stents? *J Interv Cardiol* 2006; **19**:43–50.
186. Hoffmann R, Mintz GS, Popma JJ, *et al.* Treatment of calcified coronary lesions with Palmaz-Schatz stents. An intravascular ultrasound study. *Eur Heart J* 1998; **19**: 1224–31.
187. Hodgson JM. Oh no, even stenting is affected by calcium! *Cathet Cardiovasc Diagn* 1996; **38**:236–7.
188. Henneke KH, Regar E, Konig A, *et al.* Impact of target lesion calcification on coronary stent expansion after rotational atherectomy. *Am Heart J* 1999; **137**:93–9.
189. Kataoka T, Grube E, Honda Y, *et al.* Three-dimensional IVUS assessment of edge effects following drug-eluting stent implantation. *J Am Coll Cardiol* 2002; **39**:70A.

190. Hong MK, Mintz GS, Lee CW, *et al.* Paclitaxel coating reduces in-stent intimal hyperplasia in human coronary arteries: a serial volumetric intravascular ultrasound analysis from the ASian Paclitaxel-Eluting Stent Clinical Trial (ASPECT). *Circulation* 2003; **107**:517–20.
191. Serruys PW, Degertekin M, Tanabe K, *et al.* Vascular responses at proximal and distal edges of paclitaxel-eluting stents: serial intravascular ultrasound analysis from the TAXUS II trial. *Circulation* 2004; **109**:627–33.
192. Sakurai R, Ako J, Morino Y, *et al.* Predictors of edge stenosis following sirolimus-eluting stent deployment (a quantitative intravascular ultrasound analysis from the SIRIUS trial). *Am J Cardiol* 2005; **96**:1251–3.
193. Costa MA. *Impact of stent deployment techniques on long-term clinical outcomes of patients treated with sirolimus-eluting stents: results of the multicenter prospective S.T.L.L.R. trial.* Transcatheter Cardiovascular Therapeutics, Washington DC, 2006.
194. Tsagalou E, Chieffo A, Iakovou I, *et al.* Multiple overlapping drug-eluting stents to treat diffuse disease of the left anterior descending coronary artery. *J Am Coll Cardiol* 2005; **45**:1570–3.
195. Degertekin M, Arampatzis CA, Lemos PA, *et al.* Very long sirolimus-eluting stent implantation for de novo coronary lesions. *Am J Cardiol* 2004; **93**:826–9.
196. Aoki J, Ong AT, Rodriguez Granillo GA, *et al.* 'Full metal jacket' (stented length > or =64 mm) using drug-eluting stents for de novo coronary artery lesions. *Am Heart J* 2005; **150**:994–9.
197. Lee CW, Park KH, Kim YH, *et al.* Clinical and angiographic outcomes after placement of multiple overlapping drug-eluting stents in diffuse coronary lesions. *Am J Cardiol* 2006; **98**:918–22.
198. Roy P, Steinberg DH, Sushinsky SJ, *et al.* The potential clinical utility of intravascular ultrasound guidance in patients undergoing percutaneous coronary intervention with drug-eluting stents. *Eur Heart J* 2008; **29**:1851–7.
199. Takebayashi H, Kobayashi Y, Mintz GS, *et al.* Intravascular ultrasound assessment of lesions with target vessel failure after sirolimus-eluting stent implantation. *Am J Cardiol* 2005; **95**:498–502.
200. Fujii K, Mintz GS, Kobayashi Y, *et al.* Contribution of stent underexpansion to recurrence after sirolimus-eluting stent implantation for in-stent restenosis. *Circulation* 2004; **109**:1085–8.
201. Fujii K, Carlier SG, Mintz GS, *et al.* Stent underexpansion and residual reference segment stenosis are related to stent thrombosis after sirolimus-eluting stent implantation: an intravascular ultrasound study. *J Am Coll Cardiol* 2005; **45**:995–8.
202. Cook S, Wenaweser P, Togni M, *et al.* Intravascular ultrasound in very late DES-stent thrombosis. *J Am Coll Cardiol* 2006; **47**:9B.
203. Ako J, Morino Y, Honda Y, *et al.* Late incomplete stent apposition after sirolimus-eluting stent implantation: a serial intravascular ultrasound analysis. *J Am Coll Cardiol* 2005; **46**:1002–5.
204. Tanabe K, Serruys PW, Degertekin M, *et al.* Incomplete stent apposition after implantation of paclitaxel-eluting stents or bare metal stents: insights from the randomized TAXUS II trial. *Circulation* 2005; **111**:900–5.
205. Hong MK, Mintz GS, Lee CW, *et al.* Incidence, mechanism, predictors, and long-term prognosis of late stent malapposition after bare-metal stent implantation. *Circulation* 2004; **109**:881–6.
206. Hong MK, Mintz GS, Lee CW, *et al.* Late stent malapposition after drug-eluting stent implantation: an intravascular ultrasound analysis with long-term follow-up. *Circulation* 2006; **113**:414–19.
207. Drachman DE, Edelman ER, Seifert P, *et al.* Neointimal thickening after stent delivery of paclitaxel: change in composition and arrest of growth over six months. *J Am Coll Cardiol* 2000; **36**:2325–32.
208. Siqueira DA, Abizaid AA, Costa Jde R, *et al.* Late incomplete apposition after drug-eluting stent implantation: incidence and potential for adverse clinical outcomes. *Eur Heart J* 2007; **28**:1304–9.
209. John MC, Wessely R, Kastrati A, *et al.* Differential healing responses in polymer- and nonpolymer-based sirolimus-eluting stents. *JACC Cardiovasc Interv* 2008; **1**:535–44.
210. Nakazawa G, Ladich E, Finn AV, *et al.* Pathophysiology of vascular healing and stent mediated arterial injury. *EuroIntervention* 2008; **4**(Suppl C):C7–10.
211. Sano K, Mintz GS, Carlier SG, *et al.* Volumetric intravascular ultrasound assessment of neointimal hyperplasia and nonuniform stent strut distribution in sirolimus-eluting stent restenosis. *Am J Cardiol* 2006; **98**:1559–62.
212. Lemos PA, Saia F, Ligthart JM, *et al.* Coronary restenosis after sirolimus-eluting stent implantation: morphological description and mechanistic analysis from a consecutive series of cases. *Circulation* 2003; **108**:257–60.
213. Halkin A, Carlier S, Leon MB. Late incomplete lesion coverage following Cypher stent deployment for diffuse right coronary artery stenosis. *Heart* 2004; **90**:e45.
214. Aoki J, Nakazawa G, Tanabe K, *et al.* Incidence and clinical impact of coronary stent fracture after sirolimus-eluting stent implantation. *Catheter Cardiovasc Interv* 2007; **69**(3):380–6.
215. Lee MS, Jurewitz D, Aragon J, *et al.* Stent fracture associated with drug-eluting stents: Clinical characteristics and implications. *Catheter Cardiovasc Interv* 2007; 69: 387–94.
216. Kuchulakanti PK, Chu WW, Torguson R, *et al.* Correlates and long-term outcomes of angiographically proven stent thrombosis with sirolimus- and paclitaxel-eluting stents. *Circulation* 2006; **113**:1108–13.
217. Iakovou I, Schmidt T, Bonizzoni E, *et al.* Incidence, predictors, and outcome of thrombosis after successful implantation of drug-eluting stents. *JAMA* 2005; **293**:2126–30.
218. Ong AT, Hoye A, Aoki J, *et al.* Thirty-day incidence and six-month clinical outcome of thrombotic stent

occlusion after bare-metal, sirolimus, or paclitaxel stent implantation. *J Am Coll Cardiol* 2005; **45**:947–53.

219. Sakurai R, Bonneau HN, Honda Y, Fitzgerald PJ. Intravascular ultrasound findings in ENDEAVOR II and ENDEAVOR III. *Am J Cardiol* 2007; **100**:71M–76M.
220. Nakazawa G, Finn AV, John MC, *et al.* The significance of preclinical evaluation of sirolimus-, paclitaxel-, and zotarolimus-eluting stents. *Am J Cardiol* 2007; **100**: 36M–44M.
221. Stone GW, Midei M, Newman W, *et al.* Comparison of an everolimus-eluting stent and a paclitaxel-eluting stent in patients with coronary artery disease: a randomized trial. *JAMA* 2008; **299**:1903–13.
222. Yamasaki M, Tsujino I, Sakurai R, *et al.* Comparison of everolimus-eluting stents with paclitaxel-eluting stents in de novo native coronary artery lesions: Intravascular ultrasound results from the SPIRIT III trial. *Circulation* 2007; **116**:615.
223. Kawasaki M, Takatsu H, Noda T, *et al.* Noninvasive quantitative tissue characterization and two-dimensional color-coded map of human atherosclerotic lesions using ultrasound integrated backscatter: comparison between histology and integrated backscatter images. *J Am Coll Cardiol* 2001; **38**:486–92.
224. Kawasaki M, Sano K, Okubo M, *et al.* Volumetric quantitative analysis of tissue characteristics of coronary plaques after statin therapy using three-dimensional integrated backscatter intravascular ultrasound. *J Am Coll Cardiol* 2005; **45**:1946–53.
225. Wilson LS, Neale ML, Talhami HE, *et al.* Preliminary results from attenuation-slope mapping of plaque using intravascular ultrasound. *Ultrasound Med Biol* 1994; **20**:529–42.
226. Spencer T, Ramo MP, Salter DM, *et al.* Characterisation of atherosclerotic plaque by spectral analysis of intravascular ultrasound: an in vitro methodology. *Ultrasound Med Biol* 1997; **23**:191–203.
227. Komiyama N, Berry GJ, Kolz ML, *et al.* Tissue characterization of atherosclerotic plaques by intravascular ultrasound radiofrequency signal analysis: An in vitro study of human coronary arteries. *Am Heart J* 2000; **140**:565–74.
228. Hiro T, Fujii T, Yasumoto K, *et al.* Detection of fibrous cap in atherosclerotic plaque by intravascular ultrasound by use of color mapping of angle-dependent echo-intensity variation. *Circulation* 2001; **103**:1206–11.
229. Nair A, Kuban BD, Obuchowski N, *et al.* Assessing spectral algorithms to predict atherosclerotic plaque composition with normalized and raw intravascular ultrasound data. *Ultrasound Med Biol* 2001; **27**:1319–31.
230. Murashige A, Hiro T, Fujii T, *et al.* Detection of lipid-laden atherosclerotic plaque by wavelet analysis of radiofrequency intravascular ultrasound signals: in vitro validation and preliminary in vivo application. *J Am Coll Cardiol* 2005; **45**:1954–60.
231. Nair A, Kuban BD, Tuzcu EM, *et al.* Coronary plaque classification with intravascular ultrasound radiofrequency data analysis. *Circulation* 2002; **106**: 2200–6.
232. Nasu K, Tsuchikane E, Katoh O, *et al.* Accuracy of in vivo coronary plaque morphology assessment: a validation study of in vivo virtual histology compared with in vitro histopathology. *J Am Coll Cardiol* 2006; **47**:2405–12.
233. Gaster AL, Slothuus Skjoldborg U, Larsen J, *et al.* Continued improvement of clinical outcome and cost effectiveness following intravascular ultrasound guided PCI: insights from a prospective, randomised study. *Heart* 2003; **89**:1043–9.
234. Mudra H, Macaya C, Zahn R, *et al.* Interim analysis of the 'OPTimization with ICUS to reduce stent restenosis' (OPTICUS) trial (abstr). *Circulation* 1998; **98**:I–363.
235. Schiele F, Meneveau N, Vuillemenot A, *et al.* Impact of intravascular ultrasound guidance in stent deployment on 6-month restenosis rate: a multicenter, randomized study comparing two strategies–with and without intravascular ultrasound guidance. RESIST Study Group. REStenosis after Ivus guided STenting. *J Am Coll Cardiol* 1998; **32**:320–8.

CHAPTER 11

Virtual histology intravascular ultrasound and optical coherence tomography in percutaneous coronary intervention

Ravinay Bhindi and Keith M. Channon

Background

The inadequacies of angiography to identify and characterize coronary atherosclerosis were not fully appreciated until pathologic studies revealed that coronary atherosclerosis in patients with fatal myocardial infarction was typically diffuse and in many cases was accompanied by positive remodelling, without luminal stenosis. Pathologic studies also identified the critical pathophysiological role of plaque rupture in coronary thrombosis, and the appreciation that plaque biology and composition, rather than luminal stenosis alone, were more critical determinants of plaque behaviour. Clinical and experimental studies have shown that the vulnerable plaque, prone to rupture, is characterized by a large lipid core rich in inflammatory cells, a thin fibrous cap, and by positive remodelling.

The development of novel intracoronary imaging techniques has enabled a greater appreciation of plaque composition in the pathogenesis of coronary artery disease in living patients. In particular, advances in intravascular ultrasound (IVUS) to provide 'virtual histology' of coronary plaque components, and optical coherence tomography (OCT) to define plaque composition in exquisite detail have provided new insights into the relationships between coronary plaque, the risk of clinical events, and the response of the vessel wall to percutaneous intervention.

Virtual histology intravascular ultrasound

Greyscale IVUS has been widely adopted as a clinical modality to evaluate coronary atheroma. However, greyscale IVUS has limited ability to discriminate between tissues within the plaque, particularly in the assessment of low echogenic regions, in relation to plaque components that are critical determinants of plaque biology, such as the lipid core. Virtual histology IVUS (VH-IVUS) is an approach which combines conventional IVUS imaging with a mathematical autoregressive spectral analysis of back-reflected radiofrequency ultrasound signals, that provides a more accurate characterization of coronary plaque composition(1). The VH software processes IVUS pull-back information in real time and generates a colour-coded topogram which can be adjusted to overlay the greyscale pullback image, thus providing a 'virtual histology' sectional image of the vessel wall.

Validation of VH-IVUS for analysis of plaque composition

Correlation of VH-IVUS images with *ex vivo* histopathological specimens of atheroma reveals a 80–92% accuracy in identification of plaque components(1). Based on *ex vivo* validation, VH-IVUS identifies four types of tissue within atheroma: fibrous tissue (encoded dark green); necrotic core (encoded red); fibrofatty (encoded light green); and dense calcium (encoded white). VH-IVUS plaque characterization of coronary atheroma has also been correlated with histological analysis of coronary atherectomy specimens, with predictive accuracies of 87.1% for fibrous tissue, 87.1% for fibrofatty tissue, 88.3% for necrotic core, and 96.5% for dense calcium regions[2].

Clinical applications of VH-IVUS for plaque characterization

Several clinical studies have demonstrated the feasibility and utility of VH-IVUS in both characterizing atheromatous plaques and predicting outcomes following coronary intervention. The VH-IVUS hallmark of a vulnerable plaque is defined by the thin-capped fibrous atheroma (TCFA), a combination of necrotic core of more than 10% without overlying fibrous tissue (i.e. contiguous with the lumen) and a percentage atheroma volume of greater than 40% in at least three consecutive frames. TFCA could be detected in non-culprit coronary vessels in patients with acute coronary syndrome (ACS), and occurred more commonly in patients with ACS compared with stable angina, with the majority occurring within 20mm of the ostium of the vessel[3]. Another VH-IVUS study of culprit coronary lesions found, however, that patients with an ACS had plaques with a smaller necrotic core size and more fibrous tissue compared with stable angina patients[4], contradicting commonly held perceptions about plaque vulnerability.

Three-vessel VH-IVUS in patients with ACS has demonstrated a higher frequency of culprit and non-culprit TCFA compared with stable angina[5] Lipid core size detected within atheroma of vessels has been shown to be inversely proportional to the distance from the ostium of the vessel by VH-IVUS[6]. As there is proximal spatial preponderance of angiographic occlusion following STEMI[7], this finding supports the notion that the lipid core size is an important factor in plaque instability.

A multicentre VH-IVUS registry found that a necrotic core/dense calcium ratio of greater than 3 was associated with risk factors for sudden cardiac death including smoking and a total cholesterol/high-density lipoprotein ratio greater than 5 and may therefore be associated with an adverse prognosis[8]. Similar findings were also reported in a separate study with relative necrotic core size and necrotic core/dense calcium ratio correlating with high-risk ACS presentations[9].

VH-IVUS has also been used to evaluate the relationship between plaque composition and coronary arterial remodelling, although there are conflicting reports in this area. Fujii and colleagues[10] found a linear correlation between fibrofatty plaque area and positive remodelling. In contrast, Rodriguez-Granillo and colleagues found a direct correlation between lipid core size and positive remodelling whilst fibrous content was associated with negative remodelling. The study also found that positively remodelled vessels had a higher frequency of plaques with VH-IVUS features of plaque instability compared to negatively remodelled plaques[11]. By using VH-IVUS to assess plaque composition at the narrowest luminal point of the atheroma, Surmely and colleagues[12] found that lesions with positive remodelling had significantly lower necrotic core percent area compared with intermediate or negatively remodelled lesions.

VH-IVUS may also help to establish possible relationships between plaque composition and the occurrence of no-reflow following percutaneous ccoronary intervention (PCI). In the setting of STEMI, Kawaguchi and colleagues found that a necrotic core volume of greater than 33.4mm^3 (sensitivity of 81.7% and specificity of 63.6%) was the only IVUS parameter to correlate with the likelihood of distal embolization resulting in no-reflow following PCI[13]. In contrast, Bae *et al.* [14] found that no-reflow was associated with a large fibrofatty volume, more positive vessel remodelling, larger plaque area, larger fibrous area and fibrofatty area. In a separate study by Hong and colleagues[15], necrotic core volume and presence of TCFA were found to be independent predictors of no-reflow following stent deployment in patients with ACS, including ST elevation myocardial infarction (STEMI). In stable patients, necrotic core size was also an independent predictor of high-risk microvascular embolization following stent implantation[16].

Predicitive value of VH-IVUS for clinical events and response to therapy

Systematic plaque characterization using VH-IVUS, in combination with other plaque imaging modalities, has been undertaken to determine whether the plaque characteristics identified by VH-IVUS, in particular TFCAs, are predictors of future coronary events. The PROSPECT (Providing Regional Observations to Study Predictors of Events in the Coronary Tree) study undertook systematic VH-IVUS images of all three proximal coronary arteries in patients presenting with ACS, treated with PCI. In the 166 ± 70mm of coronary artery imaged by VH-IVUS in 616 patients, 266 TFCAs were identified, ranging between 0 and 5 TFCAs per patient; almost 30% of patients had 1 or more TFCAs. The clinical follow-up of these patients is currently in progress.

VH-IVUS has also been used to evaluate the potential change in coronary plaque composition in response to novel treatments that could reduce plaque instability. The IBIS-2 study tested the effects of the Lp-PLA2 inhibitor, darapladib, in a randomized, placebo-controlled trial in 330 patients who underwent index PCI following presentation with ACS.

A substudy of the IBIS trial in 239 patients prospectively assessed plaque composition using VH-IVUS at baseline and at repeat angiography after 12 months[17]. In placebo-treated patients on standard medical therapy, VH-IVUS revealed a small but significant increase in plaque necrotic core volume, and a reciprocal decrease in fibrotic tissue, despite no overall change in plaque size. In contrast, there was no increase in necrotic core in patients treated with darapladib. Despite the change in necrotic core volume associated with PLA2 inhibition, other plasma biomarkers such as CRP, IL-6, and MMP9 did not differ between treatment group, suggesting that quantification of necrotic core by VH-IVUS is a sensitive and specific marker of response to plaque stabilization treatments.

Limitations of VH-IVUS

Current iterations of VH-IVUS are subject to technical and practical limitations. IVUS technology only allows imaging to 100–200μm resolution, which is insufficient to directly image the fibrous cap of TCFAs, which are less than 65 microns thick. Definition of TFCA using VH-IVUS relies instead on apparent confluence between lumen and necrotic core, without evaluation of fibrous cap rupture or erosion. Image distortion arising from calcium shadowing makes accurate plaque composition analysis difficult in the obscured plane. Automatic edge detection software which generates VH-IVUS analysis is not entirely reliable and problems such as discrimination between stent struts and calcified plaque require time-consuming manual correction. Accurate characterization of low echogenic signals, e.g. thrombus compared with soft atheroma, remains an area of potential improvement despite current radiofrequency spectral analysis algorithms.

These factors combined with the inherent variability in morphology of vulnerable plaques and the dynamic nature of the plaque rupture and healing as well as methodological differences between operators may account for the variability and conflicting data reported in *in vivo* studies.

Optical coherence tomography

Background

Coronary artery OCT is a high-resolution imaging modality, often described as the optical analogue of IVUS. It generates real-time images of biological tissue by transmitting infrared light to the target and indirectly analysing back-reflected light intensity and delay, using low-coherence inferometry to determine relative distance.

In vivo human application of OCT imaging was first reported in the early 1990s[18,19] where investigators reported the accuracy and feasibility of imaging the anterior chamber of the eye and retina.

The potential use of OCT for imaging the vascular wall to characterize plaque atheroma was first assessed *ex vivo* using post-mortem specimens. Technical modifications to the system used in the ophthalmological application needed to be made to overcome the relative differences between transparent ocular tissue and non-transparent vascular tissue. OCT imaging relies on the optical reflectance of tissues, however whilst vascular material absorbs visible light it reflects infrared light making this spectrum of light a viable option for imaging. The depth of imaging is then limited by light scattering which can be increased by lengthening the wavelength of imaging infrared light. Brezinski and colleagues incorporated these principles in their imaging catheter and were able to image both aortic and coronary atheromatous plaques with good spatial resolution in human autopsy specimens[20,21]. *Ex vivo* studies also confirmed the ability of OCT to accurately measure fibrous cap thickness of lipid-rich plaques[22] and quantify fibrous cap macrophage density[23]. Further *in vitro* imaging of post-mortem aortic samples using OCT demonstrated superior contrast and resolution compared with IVUS in detecting vascular microstructures[24].

A catheter was subsequently developed to facilitate high speed *in vivo* imaging of non-transparent tissues and the feasibility of this system was demonstrated by Tearney and colleagues in respiratory and gastrointestinal tract applications in the rabbit[25]. A key issue impacting on ready application of OCT in *in vivo* intravascular imaging is the presence of moving blood which casts shadows and interferes with image quality. Fujimoto and colleagues overcame this by displacing blood with saline injections and were able to successfully image the rabbit aorta *in vivo*[26].

Validation of OCT to characterize plaque characteristics

A number of subsequent *ex vivo* human studies validated OCT's capacity to identify atheromatous plaque composition. OCT criteria for three types of plaque were proposed and validated using histology with high sensitivity and specificity: 1) fibrous-signal rich; 2) fibrocalcific-signal poor with sharp upper and lower borders; and 3) lipid rich–signal poor with diffuse borders and signal-rich upper border(27). OCT has also been shown to be superior in comparison to IVUS in detecting and characterizing such plaques(28,29).

A balloon occlusion system using a compliant balloon was developed to transiently obstruct coronary flow, followed by an injection of saline through the balloon catheter to facilitate visualization of the vessel wall was first successfully applied *in vivo* to image the rabbit aorta by Fujimoto *et al.*(26) Prati and colleagues have subsequently demonstrated the safety and feasibility of a non-occlusive approach to OCT imaging by flushing the vessel lumen with a viscous iso-osmolar contrast solution(30).

The first systematic study reporting the use of OCT in human coronary arteries was undertaken by Jang and colleagues(31) who demonstrated the feasibility and safety of using such a system. In the study, patients with acute myocardial infarction (AMI) or ACS had a higher incidence of TCFA (defined as cap thickness of less than 65μm with lipid in two or more quadrants) compared with stable angina pectoris, although despite a trend toward a difference in lipid pool size, this did not achieve statistical significance(31).

With its ability to provide high-resolution imaging up to 20μm, OCT is presently the only imaging modality able to detect thin fibrous caps(22) (less than 65μm) which have been shown in autopsy studies to be a marker of plaque vulnerability(32). Jang's group(33) subsequently assessed macrophage density within coronary atheroma using OCT and found a correlation between systemic white cell count and local coronary fibrous cap macrophage density. Furthermore, plaques classified as TCFA had a higher macrophage density compared with non-TCFA plaques, consistent with histopathological studies.

OCT has been used to assess angioscopically-detected yellow plaques which are considered vulnerable. Takano *et al.* found that yellow plaques frequently contained lipid material covered by thin fibrous caps and that plaques which were more intensely yellow had thinner fibrous caps(34). In comparison to an earlier *ex vivo* study(35) which found OCT could detect intracoronary thrombus and distinguish red and white clot, this study found that OCT could misclassify red coronary thrombus as lipid plaques. Kubo and colleagues(36) compared OCT, IVUS, and coronary angiosopy in assessing culprit lesion morphology in patients with AMI and found OCT superior to the other modalities in detecting plaque rupture, fibrous cap erosion, and TCFA.

Consistent with *ex vivo* studies which have demonstrated that positive coronary lesion remodelling is associated with histopathologic markers of plaque vulnerability, *in vivo* OCT imaging has also found that positively-remodelled plaques are more likely contain a lipid-rich core, thin fibrous cap, and a higher fibrous-cap macrophage density compared with absent or negatively remodelled plaques(37). Serial OCT imaging has also shown that statin therapy in patients presenting with AMI and hyperlipidaemia, significantly increases fibrous-cap thickness, supporting the notion that statins stabilize coronary atheroma(38).

Combining OCT and VH-IVUS may improve the ability to detect and characterize TCFA. Using previously validated histopathological criteria for TCFA for each modality, one study found that that neither OCT nor VH-IVUS was adequate alone in detecting TCFA and the authors proposed that a system which allowed concurrent IVUS and OCT imaging may be more precise(39). Using OCT to evaluate culprit atheroma following AMI, Tanaka and colleagues found that in patients in whom physical exertion had been a precipitant of the infarct, the fibrous cap was thicker and the plaque rupture site was more likely to be at the shoulder region, compared with patients where physical exertion was not an identifiable precipitant, suggesting that OCT can provide insights in to the mechanisms of plaque rupture in acute MI(40).

OCT to evaluate stent coverage and restenosis

In the setting of PCI, OCT is highly sensitive in evaluating stent expansion, identifying individual stent struts and strut apposition or malapposition, side-branch origins, prolapsed plaque material or thrombi, and small dissections (Fig. 11.1). Bouma *et al.* compared OCT with IVUS to assess coronary arteries following stent implantation and found that OCT was more sensitive in identifying tissue prolapsed between struts, stent apposition, and vessel dissection(41). Using a rabbit model of carotid stenting, Prati *et al.* used histopathological correlation to confirm that OCT could both identify and quantify stent strut coverage by tissue, at only 11 days after stent implantation(42). In follow-up studies, particularly in relation to the potential concerns

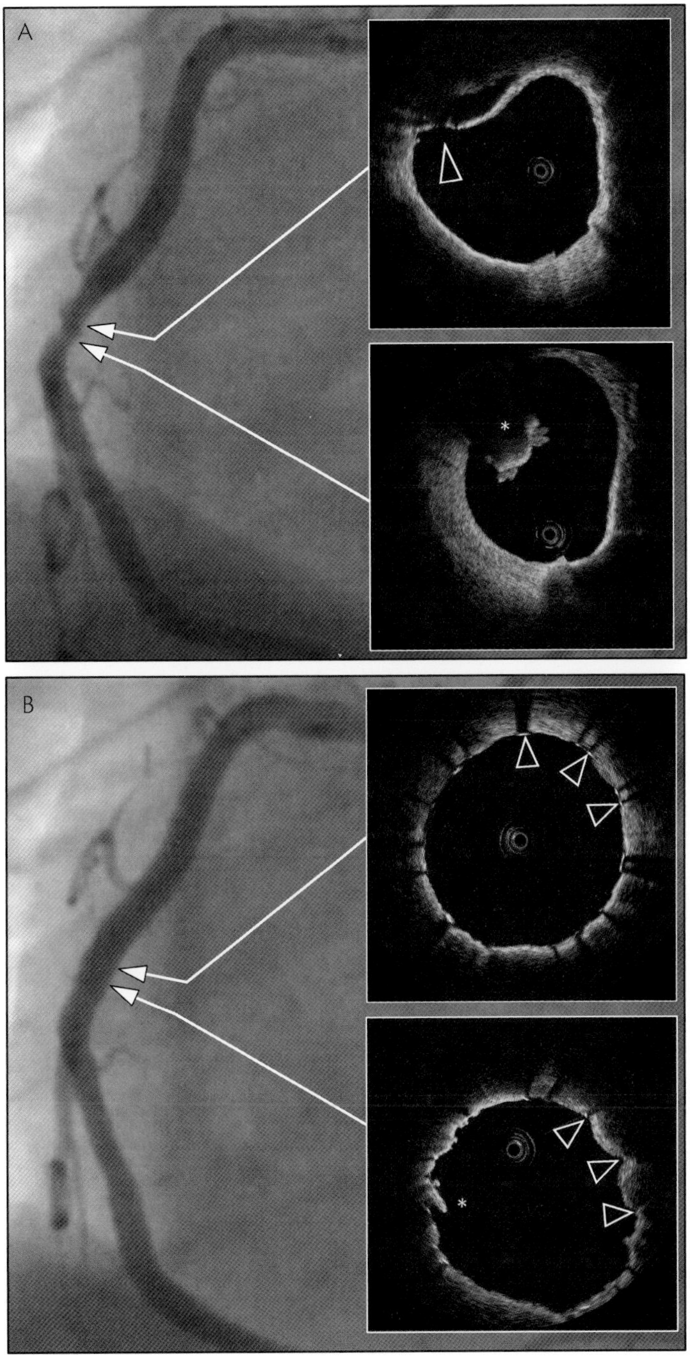

Fig. 11.1 OCT imaging of acute plaque rupture. A) The angiographic image shows a hazy lesion in the mid right coronary artery (white arrows) in a 56-year-old male who had presented with an acute inferior myocardial infarction. Angiography did not suggest significant stenosis or flow limitation. However, OCT imaging using the flush technique revealed a proximal plaque rupture (upper panel, white arrowhead) and an adherent luminal thrombus immediately downstream (lower panel, asterisk). B) The lesion was treated by administration of abciximab and by direct stenting, with a good angiographic result. OCT confirmed good stent expansion and strut apposition (upper panel, arrowheads), although within the segment corresponding to the plaque rupture (lower panel), there was moderate prolapse of plaque material between the stent struts (arrowheads) and a disrupted fragment within the vessel lumen (asterisk).

over impaired re-endothelialization with drug-eluting stents, OCT has been used to assess both stent restenosis and as well as healing. Several OCT studies have shown a higher incidence of incomplete stent coverage and strut malapposition following implantation of sirolimus-eluting stents compared with bare-metal stents[43–45]. These features appear to be more frequent in patients with unstable coronary lesions than stable disease[46]. OCT has also been used in conjunction with angiography, IVUS, and multislice CT to characterize the vascular responses following implantation of bioabsorbable everolimus-eluting coronary stent system[47], revealing early strut malapposition but subsequent resorption of the stent material, with favourable vessel remodelling by 2 years.

An OCT sub-study of the HORIZONS-AMI study found low rates of stent malapposition and uncovered struts 13 months after the implantation of paclitaxel-eluting stents for AMI[48]. The OCTAMI and OCTAXUS studies (NCT00704561 and NCT00704145, respectively) are currently underway, assessing completeness of strut coverage and vessel wall response after STEMI following implantation of zotarolimus- and paclitaxel-eluting stents, respectively[49,50]. The Optical Coherence Tomography for Drug Eluting Stent Safety (ODESSA) study (NCT00693030) will evaluate the long-term outcome of overlapped drug-eluting stents in long lesions.

Thus, OCT has proven to be the imaging modality of choice in the evaluation of short- and long-term results of stenting, including the detailed evaluation of strut coverage and stent apposition following use of drug-eluting stents.

Limitations of OCT

Use of current OCT systems is hampered by technical and practical limitations. The OCT imaging 'wire' is a delicate fibreoptic that is fragile and, compared with coronary guide wires, difficult to steer in tortuous or branching coronary arteries. The use of a separate procedure wire with over-the-wire balloon exchange of the OCT wire is cumbersome and time consuming, compared with the monorail IVUS catheter. A major limitation of OCT is the need to clear the lumen of blood to allow imaging of the vessel wall. The balloon occlusion method of imaging is time consuming and not suited for very proximal lesions, although this problem can be overcome by using the non-occlusive flush technique. However, the acquisition rate of current systems is slow (0.5–3.0mm/s), so multiple sequential pullbacks with large-volume flushes to clear the lumen may be required.

Furthermore, OCT has a limited depth of penetration, limiting visualization of plaques and the vessel wall to small–medium vessels, but cannot adequately acquire images of the whole vessel when the luminal diameter is greater than 3.5mm. This presents a problem following stent implantation and for imaging of large vessels including vein grafts.

Future developments

The next generation of OCT systems are currently being developed to overcome some of the problems with the first generation of machines. A major advance is the utilization of Fourier or frequency-domain analysis, instead of conventional time-domain analysis. This approach uses a wavelength-swept laser source instead of broadband light that results in better sensitivity, improved signal-to-noise ratio, and much faster image acquisition compared with conventional OCT systems[51]. The rapid pullback, using a monorail-type imaging catheter analogous to IVUS, will allow long acquisitions during a short flush of saline or contrast to transiently clear the arterial lumen, obviating the need for large-volume flushes or balloon occlusion to enable long pullbacks. Other applications being developed with OCT include: polarization-sensitive OCT to image collagen fibre and smooth muscle content of atheromatous plaques; OCT elastography to measure plaque strength;

Table 11.1 Comparison of VH-IVUS and OCT imaging for plaque characterization and PCI

	VH-IVUS	OCT
Technical features:		
Catheter type	Monorail	Single wire/ Monorail
Pullback speed	0.5mm/s	0.5–3mm/s
Resolution	100–200 microns	25 microns
Imaging depth	4–8mm	3–4mm
Imaging medium	Blood	Saline/contrast
Flushing required	No	Yes
Plaque imaging:		
Fibrous cap	+/–	++
Lipid core	++	+
Plaque rupture	+	++
Thrombus	+/–	++
Systematic algorithm	+++	–
Quantification	++	+/–
Stent and PCI imaging:		
Plaque characteristics, length	++	++
Lumen diameter	++	++
Stent expansion	++	+++
Strut apposition	+/–	+++
Small dissections	+/–	++
Strut coverage	+	++
Neointima	+	+++
Thrombus	+/–	++

Doppler OCT to evaluate plaque microvascular flow; and molecular imaging[52].

Conclusions

OCT and VH-IVUS are evolving as useful tools in the characterization of coronary atheroma and the identification of plaque vulnerability. Clinically they are having an increasing role in identification and characterization of culprit lesions, assessing lesion response to PCI, predicting downstream myocardial injury, and in the evaluation of immediate and long-term PCI results. OCT and VH-IVUS have contrasting strengths and weaknesses that makes their respective roles complementary rather than competitive (Table 11.1). Continued technical advances and an expanding scientific research basis will together ensure that VH-IVUS and OCT imaging play central roles in PCI clinical practice and research.

References

1. Nair A, Kuban BD, Tuzcu EM, *et al.* Coronary plaque classification with intravascular ultrasound radiofrequency data analysis. *Circulation* 2002; **106**:2200–6.
2. Nasu K, Tsuchikane E, Katoh O, *et al.* Accuracy of in vivo coronary plaque morphology assessment: a validation study of in vivo virtual histology compared with in vitro histopathology. *J Am Coll Cardiol* 2006; **47**:2405–12.
3. Rodriguez-Granillo GA, Garcia-Garcia HM, Mc Fadden EP, *et al.* In vivo intravascular ultrasound-derived thin-cap fibroatheroma detection using ultrasound radiofrequency data analysis. *J Am Coll Cardiol* 2005; **46**:2038–42.
4. Surmely JF, Nasu K, Fujita H, *et al.* Coronary plaque composition of culprit/target lesions according to the clinical presentation: a virtual histology intravascular ultrasound analysis. *Eur Heart J* 2006; **27**:2939–44.
5. Hong MK, Mintz GS, Lee CW, *et al.* A three-vessel virtual histology intravascular ultrasound analysis of frequency and distribution of thin-cap fibroatheromas in patients with acute coronary syndrome or stable angina pectoris. *Am J Cardiol* 2008; **101**:568–72.
6. Valgimigli M, Rodriguez-Granillo GA, Garcia-Garcia HM, *et al.* Distance from the ostium as an independent determinant of coronary plaque composition in vivo: an intravascular ultrasound study based radiofrequency data analysis in humans. *Eur Heart J* 2006; **27**:655–63.
7. Wang JC, Normand SL, Mauri L, *et al.* Coronary artery spatial distribution of acute myocardial infarction occlusions. *Circulation* 2004; **110**:278–84.
8. Missel E, Mintz GS, Carlier SG, *et al.* In vivo virtual histology intravascular ultrasound correlates of risk factors for sudden coronary death in men: results from the prospective, multi-centre virtual histology intravascular ultrasound registry. *Eur Heart J* **29**:2141–7.
9. Missel E, Mintz GS, Carlier SG, *et al.* Necrotic core and its ratio to dense calcium are predictors of high-risk non-ST-elevation acute coronary syndrome. *Am J Cardiol* 2008; **101**:573–8.
10. Fujii K, Carlier SG, Mintz GS, *et al.* Association of plaque characterization by intravascular ultrasound virtual histology and arterial remodelling. *Am J Cardiol* 2005; **96**:1476–83.
11. Rodriguez-Granillo GA, Serruys PW, Garcia-Garcia HM, *et al.* Coronary artery remodelling is related to plaque composition. *Heart* 2006; **92**:388–91.
12. Surmely JF, Nasu K, Fujita H, *et al.* Association of coronary plaque composition and arterial remodelling: a virtual histology analysis by intravascular ultrasound. *Heart* 2007; **93**:928–32.
13. Kawaguchi R, Oshima S, Jingu M, *et al.* Usefulness of virtual histology intravascular ultrasound to predict distal embolization for ST-segment elevation myocardial infarction. *J Am Coll* Cardiol 2007; **50**:1641–6.
14. Bae JH, Kwon TG, Hyun DW, *et al.* Predictors of slow flow during primary percutaneous coronary intervention: an intravascular ultrasound-virtual histology study. *Heart* 2008; **94**:1559–64.
15. Hong YJ, Jeong MH, Choi YH, *et al.* Impact of plaque components on no-reflow phenomenon after stent deployment in patients with acute coronary syndrome: a virtual histology-intravascular ultrasound analysis. *Eur Heart J* 2009; Feb 19. [Epub ahead of print]
16. Kawamoto T, Okura H, Koyama Y, *et al.* The relationship between coronary plaque characteristics and small embolic particles during coronary stent implantation. *J Am Coll Cardiol* 2007; **50**:1635–40.
17. Rodriguez-Granillo GA, Serruys PW, McFadden E, *et al.* First-in-man prospective evaluation of temporal changes in coronary plaque composition by in vivo intravascular ultrasound radiofrequency data analysis: an Integrated Biomarker and Imaging Study (IBIS) substudy. *Eurointervention* 2005; **1**:282–8
18. Izatt JA, Hee MR, Swanson EA, *et al.* Micrometer-scale resolution imaging of the anterior eye in vivo with optical coherence tomography. *Arch Ophthalmol* 1994; **112**:1584–9.
19. Hee MR, Izatt JA, Swanson EA, *et al.* Optical coherence tomography of the human retina. *Arch Ophthalmol* 1995; **113**:325–32.
20. Brezinski ME, Tearney GJ, Bouma BE, *et al.* Optical coherence tomography for optical biopsy. Properties and demonstration of vascular pathology. *Circulation* 1996; **93**:1206–13.
21. Brezinski ME, Tearney GJ, Bouma BE, *et al.* Imaging of coronary artery microstructure (in vitro) with optical coherence tomography. *Am J Cardiol* 1996; **77**:92–3.
22. Kume T, Akasaka T, Kawamoto T, *et al.* Measurement of the thickness of the fibrous cap by optical coherence tomography. *Am Heart J* 2006; **152**:755 e1–4.
23. Tearney GJ, Yabushita H, Houser SL, *et al.* Quantification of macrophage content in atherosclerotic plaques by optical coherence tomography. *Circulation* 2003; **107**:113–19.
24. Brezinski ME, Tearney GJ, Weissman NJ, *et al.* Assessing atherosclerotic plaque morphology: comparison of optical

coherence tomography and high frequency intravascular ultrasound. *Heart* 1997; **77**:397–403.

25. Tearney GJ, Brezinski ME, Bouma BE, *et al.* In vivo endoscopic optical biopsy with optical coherence tomography. *Science* 1997; **276**:2037–9.
26. Fujimoto JG, Boppart SA, Tearney GJ, *et al.* High resolution in vivo intra-arterial imaging with optical coherence tomography. *Heart* 1999; **82**:128–33.
27. Yabushita H, Bouma BE, Houser SL, *et al.* Characterization of human atherosclerosis by optical coherence tomography. *Circulation* 2002; **106**:1640–5.
28. Rieber J, Meissner O, Babaryka G, *et al.* Diagnostic accuracy of optical coherence tomography and intravascular ultrasound for the detection and characterization of atherosclerotic plaque composition in ex-vivo coronary specimens: a comparison with histology. *Coron Artery Dis* 2006; **17**:425–30.
29. Kume T, Akasaka T, Kawamoto T, *et al.* Assessment of coronary arterial plaque by optical coherence tomography. *Am J Cardiol* 2006; **97**:1172–5.
30. Prati F, Cera M, Ramazzotti V, *et al.* From bench to bedside: a novel technique of acquiring OCT images. *Circ J* 2008; **72**:839–43.
31. Jang IK, Tearney GJ, MacNeill B, *et al.* In vivo characterization of coronary atherosclerotic plaque by use of optical coherence tomography. *Circulation* 2005; **111**:1551–5.
32. Burke AP, Farb A, Malcom GT, *et al.* Coronary risk factors and plaque morphology in men with coronary disease who died suddenly. *N Engl J Med* 1997; **336**:1276–82.
33. Raffel OC, Tearney GJ, Gauthier DD, *et al.* Relationship between a systemic inflammatory marker, plaque inflammation, and plaque characteristics determined by intravascular optical coherence tomography. *Arterioscler Thromb Vasc Biol* 2007; **27**:1820–7.
34. Takano M, Jang IK, Inami S, *et al.* In vivo comparison of optical coherence tomography and angioscopy for the evaluation of coronary plaque characteristics. *Am J Cardiol* 2008; **101**:471–6.
35. Kume T, Akasaka T, Kawamoto T, *et al.* Assessment of coronary arterial thrombus by optical coherence tomography. *Am J Cardiol* 2006; **97**:1713–17.
36. Kubo T, Imanishi T, Takarada S, *et al.* Assessment of culprit lesion morphology in acute myocardial infarction: ability of optical coherence tomography compared with intravascular ultrasound and coronary angioscopy. *J Am Coll Cardiol* 2007; **50**:933–9.
37. Raffel OC, Merchant FM, Tearney GJ, *et al.* In vivo association between positive coronary artery remodelling and coronary plaque characteristics assessed by intravascular optical coherence tomography. *Eur Heart J* 2008; **29**:1721–8.
38. Takarada S, Imanishi T, Kubo T, *et al.* Effect of statin therapy on coronary fibrous-cap thickness in patients with acute coronary syndrome: assessment by optical coherence tomography study. *Atherosclerosis* 2009; **202**:491–7.
39. Sawada T, Shite J, Garcia-Garcia HM, *et al.* Feasibility of combined use of intravascular ultrasound radiofrequency data analysis and optical coherence tomography for detecting thin-cap fibroatheroma. *Eur Heart J* 2008; **29**:1136–46.
40. Tanaka A, Imanishi T, Kitabata H, *et al.* Morphology of exertion-triggered plaque rupture in patients with acute coronary syndrome: an optical coherence tomography study. *Circulation* 2008; **118**:2368–73.
41. Bouma BE, Tearney GJ, Yabushita H, *et al.* Evaluation of intracoronary stenting by intravascular optical coherence tomography. *Heart* 2003; **89**:317–20.
42. Prati F, Zimarino M, Stabile E, *et al.* Does optical coherence tomography identify arterial healing after stenting? An in vivo comparison with histology, in a rabbit carotid model. *Heart* 2008; **94**:217–21.
43. Matsumoto D, Shite J, Shinke T, *et al.* Neointimal coverage of sirolimus-eluting stents at 6-month follow-up: evaluated by optical coherence tomography. *Eur Heart J* 2007; **28**:961–7.
44. Xie Y, Takano M, Murakami D, *et al.* Comparison of neointimal coverage by optical coherence tomography of a sirolimus-eluting stent versus a bare-metal stent three months after implantation. *Am J Cardiol* 2008; **102**:27–31.
45. Chen BX, Ma FY, Luo W, *et al.* Neointimal coverage of bare-metal and sirolimus-eluting stents evaluated with optical coherence tomography. *Heart* 2008; **94**:566–70.
46. Tanaka A, Imanishi T, Kitabata H, *et al.* Morphology of exertion-triggered plaque rupture in patients with acute coronary syndrome: an optical coherence tomography study. *Circulation* 2008; **118**:2368–73.
47. Serruys PW, Ormiston JA, Onuma Y, *et al.* A bioabsorbable everolimus-eluting coronary stent system (ABSORB): 2-year outcomes and results from multiple imaging methods. *Lancet* 2009; **373**:897–910.
48. Guagliumi G, Costa M, Musumeci G, *et al.* Long-Term Strut Coverage of Paclitaxel Eluting Stents Compared with Bare-Metal Stents Implanted During Primary PCI in Acute Myocardial Infarction: A Prospective, Randomized, Controlled Study Performed with Optical Coherence Tomography. HORIZONS-OCT. In American Heart Association's Scientific Sessions. New Orleans, 2008.
49. Guagliumi G. Early Coverage and Vessel Wall Response of the Zotarolimus Drug-Eluting Stent Implanted in AMI Assessed by Optical Coherence Tomography (OCTAMI). In ClinicalTrialsgov, 2008. http://clinicaltrials.gov/ct2/show/NCT00704561
50. Guagliumi G. Optical Coherence Tomography Following Paclitaxel Eluting Stent Implantation in Multivessel Coronary Artery Disease (OCTAXUS). In: *ClinicalTrialsgov*, 2008. http://clinicaltrials.gov/ct2/show/study/NCT00704145
51. Yun SH, Tearney GJ, Vakoc BJ, *et al.* Comprehensive volumetric optical microscopy in vivo. *Nature Med* 2006; **12**:1429–33.
52. Raffel OC, Akasaka T, Jang IK. Cardiac optical coherence tomography. *Heart* 2008; **94**:1200–10.

CHAPTER 12

Coronary computed tomography for the interventionalist

P.J. de Feijter and C. Schultz

Introduction

In recent years coronary computed tomography (CT) has developed as a spectacular non-invasive technique to visualize the coronary arteries and its manifestations of coronary atherosclerosis[1–5]. The coronary CT scanner has rapidly evolved from the initial 4-and 16-slice CT scanners, to the now considered state-of-the-art 64-slice CT scanners, while 256- and 320-slice CT-prototype scanners have now been introduced for clinical evaluation. It is expected that the CT technique will further evolve and eventually will become of sufficient diagnostic quality that it may replace invasive coronary angiography (CA) to reliably assess both non-obstructive and obstructive coronary lesions.

CT CA scanning protocols

There are two protocols to scan the beating heart[6–8]. First, the electrocardiogram (ECG)-triggered prospective sequential mode protocol (step-and-shoot mode) whereby scanning is triggered by the ECG (timing based on lengths of previous heart cycles) during a pre-selected phase (usually the end-diastolic, relatively motion-free phase) of the cardiac cycle, while the patient (table) does not move. After image acquisition the table is moved (along the z-axis) to the next position for the next scan and the procedure is repeated until the whole heart is scanned (Fig. 12.1). This mode is associated with considerably less radiation exposure but a disadvantage is that the acquisition window is fixed, and in case of motion, artefacts cannot be corrected by selection of other cardiac phases with less motion blurring.

Second, the ECG-gated retrospective spiral mode (helical scanning) whereby the patient table moves continuously through the gantry with continuous data acquisition (Fig. 12.1). Retrospectively (after scanning) images can be reconstructed from ECG-gated data from different cardiac phases allowing the flexibility to select a cardiac phase with no or minimal motion artefacts. An advantage of this mode is the robustness in case of heart rate variability during scanning or other causes of motion artefacts but the disadvantage is the rather high associated radiation exposure.

Coronary CT angiography: temporal and spatial resolution

The coronary arteries exhibit rapid motion and to ‘freeze’ the coronary arteries a very rapid acquisition time is required. The motion velocity of the left anterior descending artery (LAD) is 22.4 ± 4.0mm/s, of the left circumflex artery (LCx) 48.4 ± 15mm/s, and of the right coronary artery (RCA) 69.5 ± 22.5mm/s[9,10]. Ideally the temporal resolution of CT CA should be less than 50ms to capture motion-free coronary images. The temporal resolution of CT scanners used for CT CA is equal to half the rotation speed of the X-ray tube (gantry) and ranges from 83–165ms, and therefore may still cause image blurring (cardiac motion artefacts), in particular during higher heart rates (greater than 65–70bpm). To decrease the chance of image blurring the heart rate is lowered (to less than 60bpm) to increase the relatively motion-free diastolic phase of the heart cycle, during which period the data acquired are used

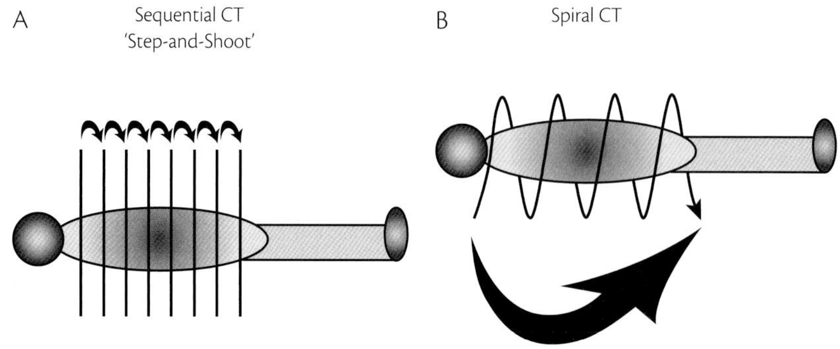

Fig. 12.1 A) ECG-triggered prospective sequential mode. B) ECG-gated retrospective spiral mode.

for reconstruction of the coronary images. Prescan high heart rates (greater than 65bpm) should be reduced by beta-receptor blocking agents prior to scanning to (ideally) less than 60bpm. The relatively small coronary arteries and acquired coronary atherosclerotic changes require detailed assessment with high spatial resolution. The spatial resolution in the z-axis of the heart (longitudinal axis) is determined by the slice thickness and current CT scanners in a phantom setting have a spatial resolution of 0.4 × 0.4 × 0.4mm (x,y,z-axis) but in clinical practice this is estimated to be 0.6–0.7mm.

CT CA contrast agent

To increase the contrast difference between the coronaries and surrounding structures administration of an iodine contrast medium is required. Current 64-slice CT CA protocols recommend using a bolus injection of 80–100mL contrast medium at an injection rate of 4–6mL/s. Only patients with normal renal function are selected for CT CA.

CT CA radiation exposure

Using prototype 64-slice CT CA was associated with an effective dose ranging from 13–15mSv for men and 18–21mSv for women, which is considerably higher than the effective dose of 3–6mSv during invasive CA. Radiation exposure reduction techniques such as ECG-controlled tube current modulation (decrease of nominal tube current to 20% outside data-reconstruction window in diastole) have significantly reduced the effective dose to 10–14mSv[(11)] and a prospective ECG-triggered CT data acquisition technique (step-and-shoot protocol) has dramatically reduced the effective dose to less than 3.0m Sv[(12)] but its use requires a very stable heart rate during scanning.

CT CA to detect or rule out coronary artery disease

Sixty-four slice CT CA is now considered the state-of-the art CT technology. Three recent meta-analyses, including 19–28 studies, concerning 875–2045 patients, with stable angina and prevalence of significant coronary artery disease (CAD) of approximately 60%, who were referred for invasive CA, demonstrated that 64-slice CT CA had a high negative predictive value as well in patient-based analysis or segment-based analysis and hence was reliable in ruling out the presence of CAD (Fig. 12.2; Table 12.1)[(13–15)]. Similar results were achieved in patients with acute coronary syndromes (Fig. 12.3; Table 12.2)[(16)]. The diagnostic performance of the fastest CT-scanner, the dual-source 64-slice CT scanner, was also excellent, and this accuracy was achieved without the use of beta-blockade to reduce to the heart rate (Tables 12.3 and 12.4)[(17–24)]. The diagnostic accuracy of a positive CT scan is not sufficiently high and is associated with a rather high number of false positive outcomes and therefore multislice CT (MSCT) can not replace invasive CA. A significant problem remains coronary calcification which, if extensive, does not allow the scoring of coronary segments underlying these calcifications or often may lead to overestimation of the severity of a coronary stenosis. Another problem is the often occurring mismatch between the severity of a coronary stenosis as seen on CT (i.e. diameter stenosis greater than 50%) and the presence of ischaemia as can be observed by non-invasive perfusion imaging, or invasive fractional flow reserve measurements which is particularly problematic with intermediate lesions[(25,26)]. This mismatch is due mainly to the limited spatial resolution of current CT technology, but in addition other factors such as presence of

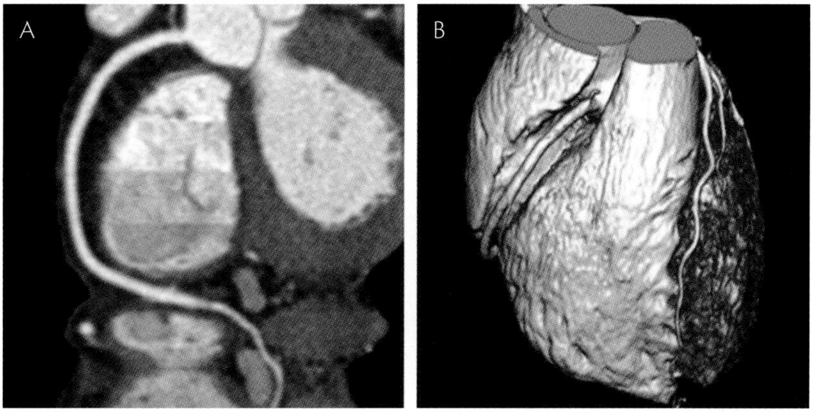

Fig. 12.2 Normal right coronary artery (RCA). A) Multiplanar reconstruction RCA. B) Volume-rendered RCA and left anterior descendens coronary artery.

Table 12.1 Meta-analysis of diagnostic accuracy of 64-slice CT CA in patients with stable angina

Analysis	Studies	N of patients	N of segments	Non-evaluable patients/segment %	Prevalence CAD %	Sensitivity %	Specificity %	PPV %	NPV %
Patient analysis									
Abdulla[13]	19	875	–	1.2	57.5	97.5	91	93.5	96.5
Mowatt[14]	28	1268	–	2.0	58	99	89	93	100
Stein[15]	23	2045	–	–	61	98	88	93	96
Segment analysis									
Abdulla[13]	19	1251	17695	4.0	19	86	96	83	96.5
Mowatt[14]	28	1268	14199	8.0	–	90	97	76	99
Stein[15]	23	2045	32046	–	–	90	96	73	99

CAD, coronary artery disease; CI, confidence interval; NPV, negative predictive value; PPV; positive predictive value.

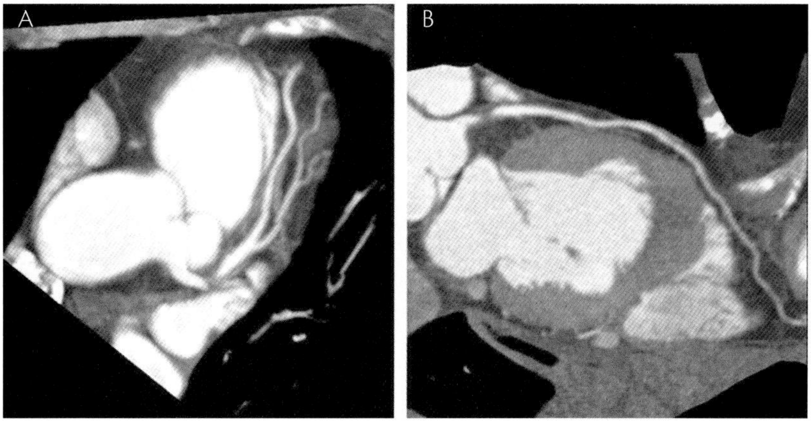

Fig. 12.3 Severe lesion in proximal left anterior descendens coronary artery of a patient with an acute coronary syndrome visible in two different multiplanar reconstructions.

Table 12.2 Meta-analysis of diagnostic accuracy of 16-, 64-slice CT-coronary angiography in patients with ACS (excluded ST-segment elevation MI)

Sensitivity	Specificity	LR	LR
%	%	+	–
95	90	8.6	0.12

Table 12.3 Diagnostic performance of 64-slice dual-source CT CA—per patient analysis

Author	N of patients	Prevalence CAD %	Non-evaluable patients %	Sensitivity %	Specificity %	PPV %	NPV %
Scheffel[17]	30	50	0	93	100	100	94
Weustink[18]	100	77	0	99	87	96	95
Leber[19]	90	30	2	95	90	74	99
Heuschmid[20]	51	75	0	97	73	90	92
Ropers[21]	100	41	3	98	84	80	98
Brodoefel[22]	100	73	0	100	82	94	100
Johnson[23]	35	48	0	100	89	89	100
Achenbach[24]	100	47	3	98	90	87	98

NPV, negative predictive value; PPV; positive predictive value.

Table 12.4 Diagnostic performance of 64-slice dual-source CT CA—per segment analysis

Author	N segments	Non-evaluable segments %	Sensitivity %	Specificity %	PPV%	NPV %
Scheffel[17]	420	1.4	97	98	86	99.4
Weustink[18]	1489	0	95	95	75	99
Leber[19]	1216	1.3	90	98	81	89
Heuschmid[20]	663	4.7	96	87	61	99
Ropers[21]	1343	4.0	90	98	79	99
Brodoefel[22]	1229	1.6	91	92	76	98
Johnson[23]	481	2.0	88	98	78	99
Achenbach[24]	1337	3.5	93	99	84	99

NPV, negative predictive value; PPV, positive predictive value.

collateral circulation, serial stenoses, or diffuse coronary artery disease play a role. In general, patients with atrial fibrillation should not be referred for CT CA because of the high chance of the generation of unsharp coronary images, although in some cases the CT scan produces assessable coronary images[27].

CT for coronary artery bypass graft assessment

The detection of a total occlusion of an arterial or venous bypass graft is very reliable with an almost 100% success rate. The detection of more than 50% stenosis

Table 12.5 Diagnostic accuracy of 64-slice CT angiography for bypass-graft disease—per segment analysis

Author	Number of patients	Graft type		Excluded segments %	Stenosis or occlusion (>50%)			
		Arterial (N)	Venous (N)		Sensitivity %	Specificity %	PPV %	NPV %
Pache[28]	31	23	73	6	98	89	90	98
Ropers[29]	50	37	101	0	100	94	92	100
Malagutti[30]	52	45	64	0	100	98	98	100
Meyer[31]	138	147	259	2	97	97	93	99
Onuma[32]	54	72	74	6	100	98	94	100

NPV, negative predictive value; PPV, positive predictive value.

(including also a total occlusion) is more difficult but the diagnostic accuracy is still high (Table 12.5)[28–32]. However, the evaluation of a symptomatic post-bypass graft surgery patient is more difficult and should include assessment of the native non-grafted coronary segment and the grafted distal run-off coronary segments. These segments are often small, diffusely diseased, and severely calcified, all of which contribute to misdiagnosis of disease. Also the blooming effects of surgical clips hamper correct diagnosis of underlying disease.

CT CA for in-stent restenosis

The metal struts of the stent cause a significant blooming artefact, which often prevents accurate visualization of the lumen within the stent (Fig. 12.4) The diagnostic accuracy of 64-slice CT CA is reasonably good for the evaluation of larger stents, more than 3.0mm in diameter, but often fails in smaller stent sizes (Table 12.6)[33–40]. Currently, use of CT scanning post-stent implantation cannot be recommended.

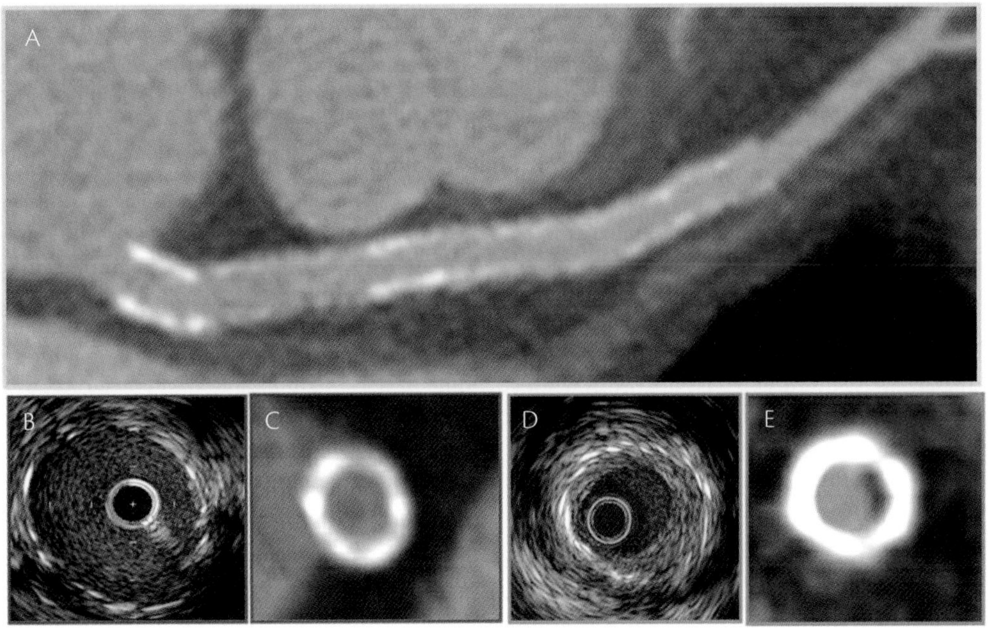

Fig. 12.4 MSCT – Stents A) Overlapping stents in left main and proximal and mid left anterior descendens coronary artery without in-stent restenosis. B) and C) Ultrasound of stent with corresponding MSCT stent (note blooming). D) and E) Ultrasound in-stent-restenosis with corresponding CT: note strong blooming effect with dark non contrast enhanced rim (in-stent restenosis)

Table 12.6 Diagnostic performance of 64-multislice CT for in-stent restenosis

Author	Number of Patients	Stents (N)	Not assessable	Sensitivity %	Specificity %	PPV %	NPV %
Van Mieghem[33]	70	162	0	100	91		
Oncel[34]	30	39	0	89	95	94	90
Rixe[35]	64	102	42	86	98	86	98
Ehara[36]	81	163	12	91	93	77	98
Cademartiri[37]	182	192	7	95	93	63	99
Carbone[38]	41	88	28	79	84		
Pugliese[39]*	100	247	5	94	92	77	98
Rist[40]	25	46	2	75	92	67	94

*dual source CT-CA.
NPV, negative predictive value; PPV, positive predictive value.

CT CA for stenosis detection: recommendations

CT CA is attractive as it suggests that it provides similar information as invasive CA, while this information is retrieved in a patient-friendly non-invasive manner. Yet, there is still a rather great gap between the spatial and temporal resolution of CT CA and invasive CA in favour of the latter and therefore CT CA cannot replace invasive CA. The clinical use of CT CA focuses on its ability to rule out the presence of significant coronary artery stenoses. According to a report of the Writing Group of the Working Group Nuclear Cardiology and Cardiac CT of the European Society of Cardiology and European Council of Nuclear Cardiology, CT CA may be recommended for:

- Patients at intermediate risk of CAD in whom the clinical presentation—stable or acute chest pain—requires evaluation of possible underlying CAD.
- CT CA is not recommended for in-stent restenosis evaluation except in large-sized stents (greater than 3mm in diameter).
- CT CA may be useful in selected patients in whom only bypass graft evaluation is required, but should not be recommended in the evaluation of post-bypass patients.

The role of multislice CT in cardiac intervention

Aberrant or difficult anatomy

MSCT is the method of choice for determining an aberrant coronary anatomy (Fig. 12.5). This also applies when vessels have been unsuccessfully or inadequately intubated during CA as can occasionally be the case with vein grafts or native vessels where the aorta is excessively tortuous or the aortic root severely dilated and rotated[41]. MSCT may facilitate the shape selection of the guide catheter and provide optimal C-arm angulation for coronary intubation in cases where the take-off of the vessel is unusual.

Ostial lesions

The percutaneous treatment of ostial lesions has a lower success rate and a higher restenosis rate when compared to non-ostial lesions[42–46]. Geographic miss may be one of the factors contributing to higher restenosis rates both for aorto-ostial and branch ostial lesions[4–6]. The selection of an optimal angiographic view that separates branches and displays the ostium without foreshortening or overlap is fundamental to optimal stent or balloon positioning. Alternatively the stent may over protrude into the aorta which may increase the difficulty and risks of future re-intubation or the coronary artery[47,48]. Multiple contrast injections may be required, particularly when the heart has an unusual orientation in the chest or vessels are highly tortuous and with multiple branches, to obtain an angiographic projection that meets these criteria. In contrast the optimal C-arm angulation for viewing a specific coronary segment may be selected before the start of a procedure by evaluating an MSCT-derived, three-dimensional (3D) virtual coronary tree (Fig. 12.6). Some MSCT analysis software facilitate the process by quantifying the degree of foreshortening at a region of interest in any particular view and may even suggest more suitable views (Fig. 12.7)[49].

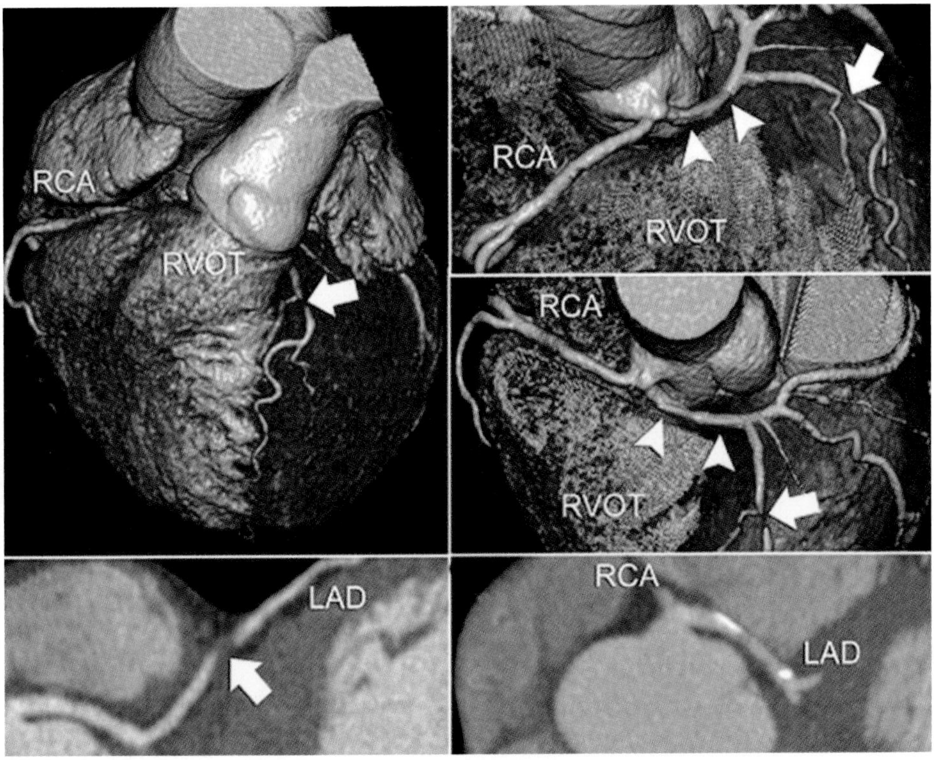

Fig. 12.5 Aberrant course of left coronary artery which originated from the right coronary cusp and runs between the aorta and right ventricular outflow track (RVOT) (arrowheads). Note also severe stenosis in LAD (arrow). LAD, left anterior descending coronary artery; RCA, right coronary artery.

Bifurcations

The treatment of bifurcations shares the complexities of ostial lesions discussed in the preceding section, including lower treatment success and higher restenosis rates than for non-bifurcation lesions[50,51]. Visualizing all three arms of the bifurcation without overlap or foreshortening is important and may be guided by pre-procedural MSCT[49]. The bifurcation angle between the main branch and side branch may be an independent predictor of outcome in bifurcation stenting. A high bifurcation angle (>50°) may be associated with an adverse outcome with certain two-stent techniques (Culotte and Crush)[52,53]. Knowledge of the bifurcation angle before the procedure could inform decisions on optimal treatment strategy. Measuring a 3D bifurcation angle on a two-dimensional (2D) modality such as cine-angiography is frequently inaccurate with low reproducibility, whereas MSCT is a 3D-imaging modality that may accurately and reproducibly measure bifurcation angles[54]. MSCT also provides additional information on the distribution of calcification and plaque in bifurcations[55].

Chronic total occlusions

MSCT may also provide additional information for the treatment of chronic total occlusions (CTO) that may be useful to the interventionalist (Fig. 12.8). Despite recent advances in guide-wire technology and the development of new treatment strategies, such as the retrograde approach, the percutaneous treatment of CTO remains technically challenging, time consuming, associated with high radiation exposure to both patient and operator, and the use of high volumes of iodated contrast medium[56–58]. Despite these costs the procedural success rates remain disappointingly low, around 70% in the majority of centres, and stand in stark contrast to that of percutaneous coronary intervention (PCI) of other lesions where it approaches 99%[59–61].

The difficulties in treating CTOs follow largely from failing to visualize the occluded segment by CA and also

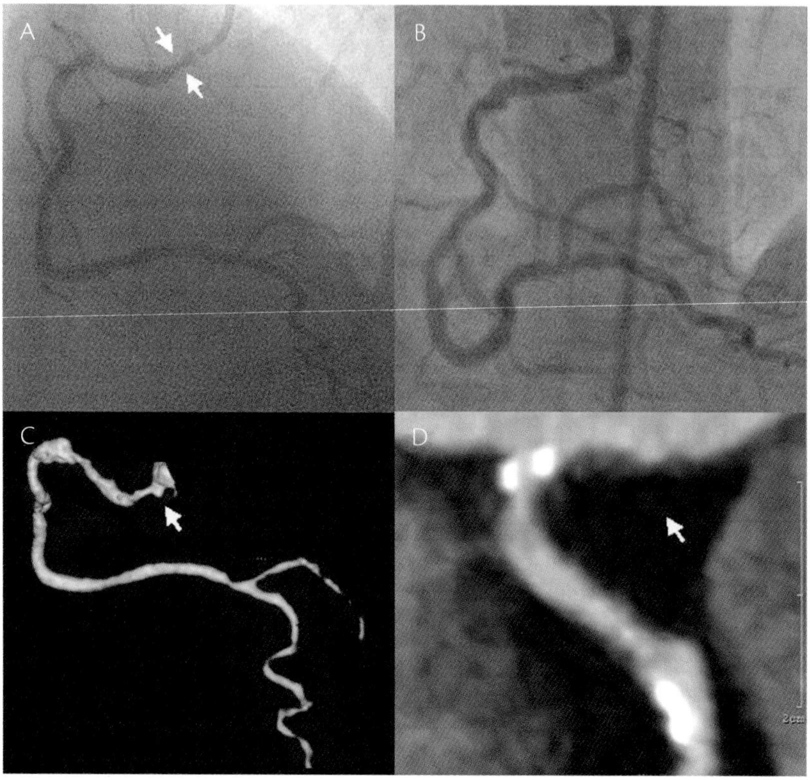

Fig. 12.6 During coronary angiography ostial lesions may be missed by being ascribed to catheter-induced spasm or due to a position of catheter tip beyond the lesion (A). Both of these pitfalls may avoided with MSCT (C and D). Cine-angiography after stent placement is shown (B).

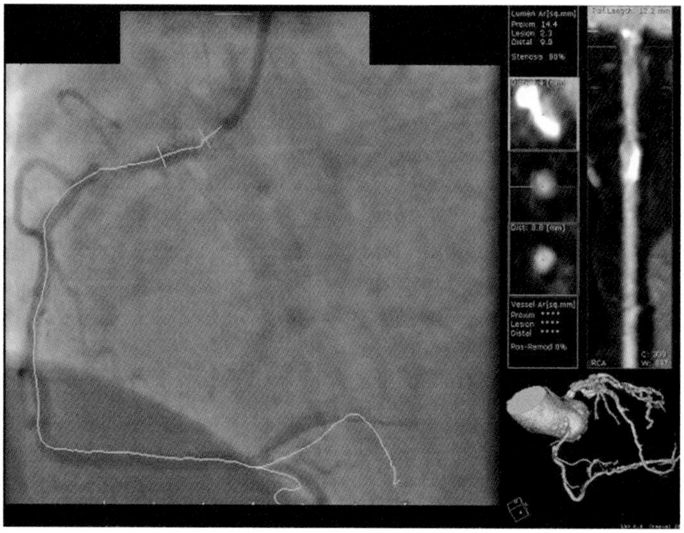

Fig. 12.7 Increasingly sophisticated software is available to integrate MSCT in the interventional catheter laboratory. Current versions (Shina systems) allow coregistration of an MSCT coronary artery (right upper and lower panels) with a still frame from cine-angiography. The 3D view on MSCT (right lower panel) is then orientated to reflect the C-arm position. By moving a slider (red, green, and yellow lines) along the image (main panel) plaque and quantitative MSCT angiography information are provided at any region of interest. The least foreshortened angiographic view for the region of interest is automatically suggested in the 3D view. This may be especially helpful for tortuous anatomy, bifurcations, or ostial lesions as in the example shown.

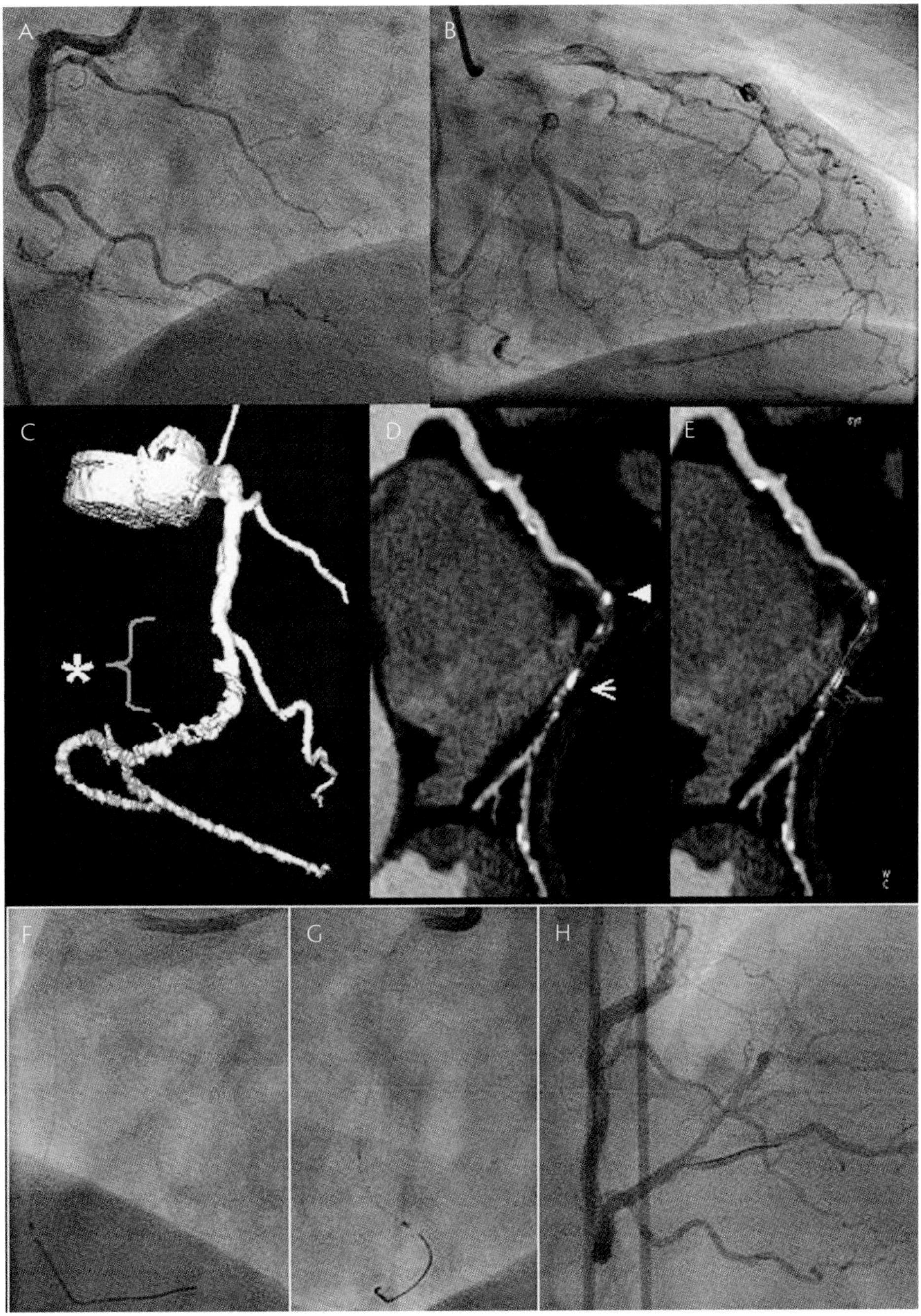

Fig. 12.8 Cine-angiogram of a potentially challenging chronic occlusion of the right coronary artery filled retrogradely via left epicardial collaterals (A and B). Additional data seen only on MSCT included a chicane within the occluded segment (star, panel C), a calcified proximal (closed arrow) and distal (open arrow) cap (D), and the true 3D occlusion length (E). The guide wire is shown negotiating the chicane in biplane (F and G) with the final result (H).

from obstruction of passage of the guide wire through the occluded segment by tough fibrocalcific tissue. Tortuosity and angulation within the occluded segment that cannot be anticipated from CA may contribute to wire exit and procedural failure.

MSCT is able to non-invasively image the occluded segment as well as the distal vessel and can provide information about the lesion length, distribution of calcium, 3D-vessel trajectory, and more (Fig. 12.8). These data may help the interventionalist to anticipate difficulties before embarking on a recanalization procedure and to devise successful treatment strategies. Registries of patients where MSCT was available to interventionalists before PCI of CTOs have reported that the more powerful predictor of procedural failure is heavy calcification in the occluded segment[62,63]. In one of these series the procedural success was higher when pre-informed by MSCT imaging of the occluded segment when compared to other CTOs treated contemporarily[63]. However, other registries did not see any difference in procedural success in patients who received an MSCT pre-procedure when compared to historical controls[64,65].

Beyond the strong predictive value of heavy calcification in the occluded segment (defined as occupying more than 50% of the lumen) on procedural success it is not possible to draw conclusions about the potential benefits of informing CTO treatment with pre-procedural MSCT because the studies were non-randomized and retrospective. A further limitation is that the MSCT data were available only for pre-procedural planning and not as a roadmap and guide in the catheter lab to fill in the missing segment.

MSCT as guidance of intervention

The 3D coronary roadmap provided by MSCT may also serve as a static roadmap for intra-procedural guidance of PCI, which can be either passive using the Shina systems (Fig. 12.7) or active using the magnetic navigation system (MNS) (Fig. 12.9).

The MNS is an innovative system that combines the ability for omni-directional steering of the tip of a magnetically enabled guide wire *in vivo* with the ability to integrate 3D roadmaps of the coronary tree, including those derived from MSCT, onto the live fluoroscopy

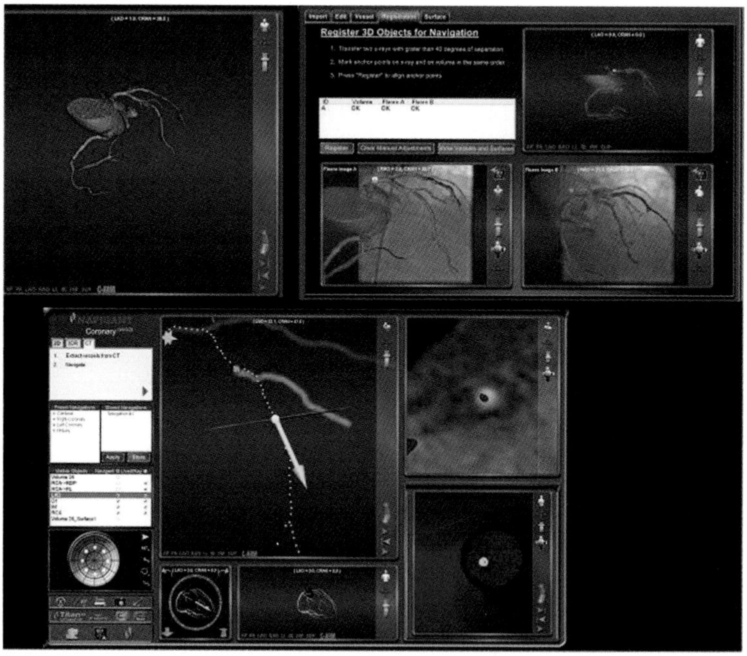

Fig. 12.9 Integration of MSCT datasets into the Navigant 3.0 magnetic navigation software allows extraction of 3D vessel centrelines (top left panel). The MSCT dataset is then coregistered on two perpendicular angiographic images to match the orientation of the patient's anatomy (top right panel). 3D vectors (arrow) for guidance of a magnetically enabled guide wire are then provided at any point along the vessel (lower panel) and can be combined with axial MSCT images, which provide information on the vessel lumen and plaque composition (lower panel). The vectors and centreline can be overlaid on the live fluoroscopy screen orientated to the C-arm to provide further guidance.

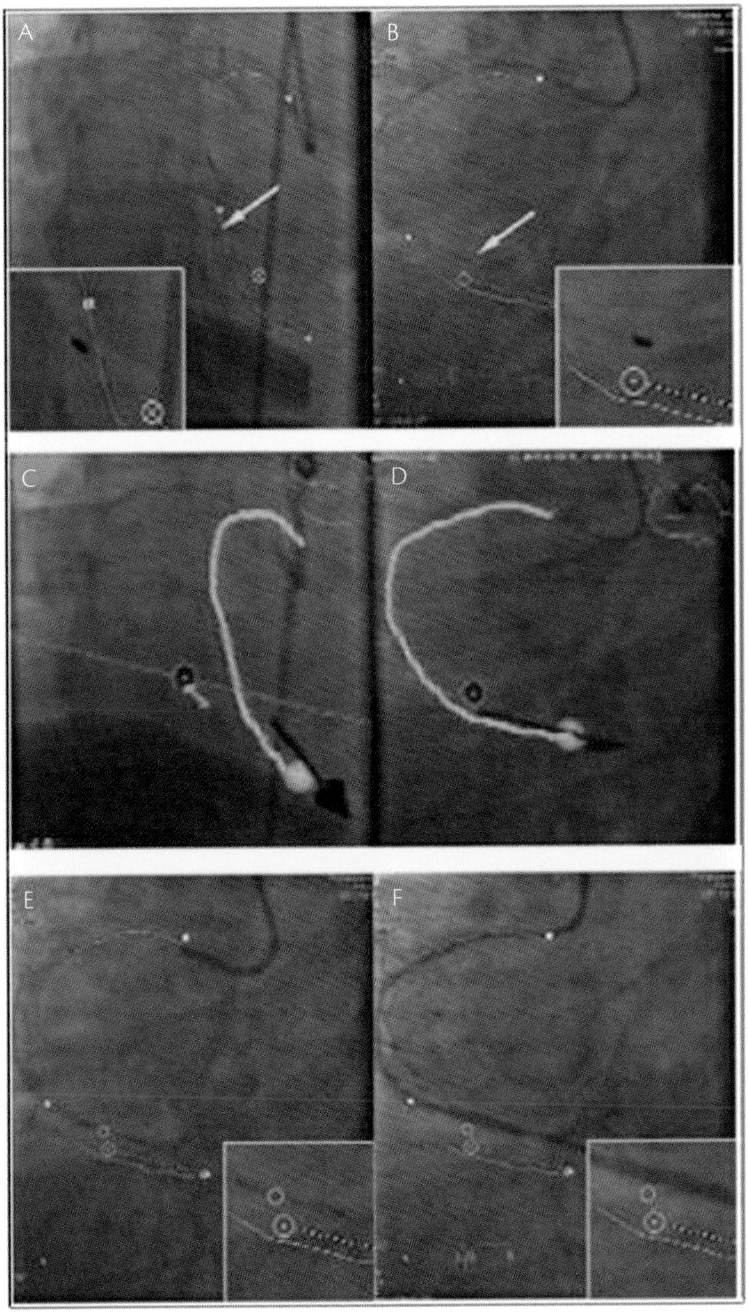

Fig. 12.10 Integration of MSCT data into the Navigant, Stereotaxis system allows positioning of a magnetically-enabled guidewire without the use of iodated contrast. IVUS was used to decide on stent size and position without requiring contrast. By positioning the radiographic marker on the tip IVUS catheter in the middle of the lesion the optimal stent position was marked on two orthogonal fluoroscopic views (A and B), thereby coregistering a new reference point (green circle, panels C and D) in the 3D dataset. The stent was positioned according to the reference point overlayed on live fluoroscopy without the use of contrast (E). A minimal amount of contrast was used in this proof of concept study to verify correct position before stent deployment (F). Reproduced from Ramcharitar S, Pugliese F, Schultz C, *et al.* Integration of multislice computer tomography with magnetic navigation facilitates percutaneous coronary interventions without contrast agents–A proof of concept paper. *J Am Coll Cardiol* 2010; **53**:742–6, with permission of Elsevier.

screen in order to provide real-time guidance during PCI (Fig. 12.9)[66–68]. The system makes use of a powerful (0.09 Tesla) directional magnetic field generated by two movable magnets positioned on either side of the patient. Manipulation of the magnetic field vector by precise control of the position of these magnets allows steering of a magnetically-enabled guide wire in three dimensions. The vectors used for steering the tip can be generated manually or either from 3D quantitative CA based on angiographic views 40° apart or from MSCT-acquired 3D coronary anatomy. During PCI the centreline of the target vessel is displayed on the live fluoroscopy screen in the same orientation as the C-arm. A small target circle (TC) indicates the position along the vessel centreline where the vector is being calculated and an additional arrow indicates the direction of the vector. Additionally, an axial multiplanar reformatted (MPR) image from MSCT shows calcification and plaque distribution with similarities to IVUS although at a lower resolution (500 × 500μm for modern MSCT scanners) at the point of the active vector (Fig. 12.9)

The MNS takes slightly more time than conventional PCI for guide wire crossing of simple lesions with only a minimal saving in contrast use, but may have application for the treatment of complex lesions such as those with excessive tortuosity or angulation or when recrossing during bifurcation stenting is required, especially when conventional PCI has failed[68,69]. Conceptually the MNS is also attractive for the treatment of CTO because the centreline roadmap and axial visualization of the occluded segment has obvious advantages that should facilitate success. A study that treated 43 patients with CTO with MNS reported a procedural success rate of 56%. In failed cases, conventional PCI succeeded in a further 58% with an overall success rate of 77%. The lower success rate with the MNS was ascribed to the limitations of the current generation of magnetically-enabled guide wires that have a 3-mm long stiff magnet at the tip, which reduced manoeuvrability within the occluded segment[70]. Improved magnetic guide wire technology, including more flexible tips with multiple magnets and a magnetically enabled radiofrequency ablation wire, has the potential to overcome current limitations.

The combination of MSCT-derived coronary roadmaps with imaging software integrated in the catheter laboratory, such as the MNS, also has the potential to revolutionize the way that PCI is performed. A small proof of concept study has introduced almost contrast-free PCI by the combination of MSCT-guided MNS and IVUS (Fig. 12.10)[71]. Patients who were referred for CA and PCI based on the results of MSCT obtained during the workup of chest pain symptoms were included. The MSCT roadmaps were coregistered with the patient anatomy based on the position of the guide catheter tip in the coronary ostium and without the use of contrast medium[71]. The guide wire was positioned distally in the target vessel, guided by centreline information extracted from the MSCT and using the MNS. IVUS was then performed to guide stent size and length selection. The optimal stent position was decided on IVUS and marked on the overhead display of the centreline at the point of the radiographic marker at the tip of the IVUS catheter (Fig. 12.10). The stent could be positioned under fluoroscopy guidance based on the marker on the overlay. Contrast was only used to verify optimal stent position before deployment and was minimal (Fig. 12.10). Although far removed from most current PCI practice, such procedures may ultimately change our concept of PCI.

Table 12.7 Indications and contraindications of CT CA using 64-slice CT scanner

Indications		Contraindications
Strong:	To exclude the presence of significant coronary stenosis in patients with low to intermediate pretest probability of CAD	Atrial fibrillation Severe calcifications Unable to cooperate during scanning
Good:	To evaluate the patency of bypass grafts To evaluate the patency of stents (excluding small <3mm stents) Informative prior to PCI CTO	

Conclusion

MSCT is now considered a useful non-invasive imaging modality to reliable rule out the presence of a significant coronary stenosis. It is less reliable in detecting coronary stenosis and frequently the stenosis severity is overestimated due to calcification of the lesion.

The indications and contraindications using current 64-slice CT scanners are listed in Table 12.7.

References

1. Achenbach S, Ulzheimer S, Baum U, *et al.* Noninvasive coronary angiography by retrospectively ECG-gated multislice spiral CT. *Circulation* 2000; **102**:2823–8.
2. Nieman K, Oudkerk M, Rensing BJ, *et al.* Coronary angiography with multi-slice computed tomography. *Lancet* 2001; **357**:599–603.
3. Achenbach S. Computed tomography coronary angiography. *J Am Coll Cardiol* 2006; **48**:1919–28.
4. De Feyter PJ, Meijboom WB, Weustink A, *et al.* Spiral multislice computed tomography coronary angiography: a current status report. *Clin. Cardiol* 2007; **30**:437–42.
5. Schoepf UJ, Zwerner PL, Savino G, *et al.* Coronary CT angiography. *Radiology* 2007; **244**:48–63.
6. Bluemke DA, Achenbach S, Budoff M, *et al.* Noninvasive coronary artery imaging magnetic resonance angiography and multidetector computed tomography angiography. A scientific statement from the American Heart Association Committee on Cardiovascular Imaging and Intervention of the Council on Cardiovascular Radiology and Intervention, and the Councils on Clinical Cardiology and

Cardiovascular Disease in the Young. *Circulation* 2008; **118**:586–606.

7. Schroeder S, Achenbach S, Bengel F, *et al.* Cardiac computed tomography: indications, applications, limitations, and training requirements. Report of a Writing Group deployed by the Working Group Nuclear Cardiology and Cardiac CT of the European Society of Cardiology and the European Council of Nuclear Cardiology. *Eur Heart J* 2008; **29**:531–56.
8. Roberts WT, Bax JJ, Davies LC. Cardiac CT and CT coronary angiography: technology and application. *Heart* 2008; **94**:781–92.
9. Lu B, Mao S, Zhuang N, *et al.* coronary artery motion during the cardiac cycle and optimal ECG triggering for coronary imaging. *Invest. Radiol* 2001; **36**:250–6.
10. Achenbach S, Ropers D, Holle J, Muschiol G, *et al.* In-plane coronary arterial motion velocity: measurement with electron-beam CT. *Radiology* 2000; **216**:457–63.
11. Hausleiter J, Meyer T, Hadamitzky M, *et al.* Radiation dose estimates from cardiac multislice computed tomography in daily practice impact of different scanning protocols on effective dose estimates. *Circulation* 2006; **113**:1305–10.
12. Earls JP, Berman EL, Urban AU, *et al.* Prospectively gated transverse coronary CT angiography versus retrospectively gated helical technique: improved image quality and reduced radiation dose. *Radiology* 2008; **246**:742–53.
13. Abdulla J, Abildstrom SZ, Gotzsche O, *et al.* 64-multislice detector computed tomography coronary angiography as potential alternative to conventional coronary angiography: a systematic review and meta-analysis. *Eur Heart J* 2007; **28**:3042–50.
14. Mowatt G, Cook JA, Hillis GS, *et al.* 64-slice computed tomography angiography in the diagnosis and assessment of coronary artery disease: systematic review and meta-analysis. *Heart* 2008; **94**:1386–93.
15. Stein PD, Yaekoub AY, Matta F, *et al.* 64-slice CT for diagnosis of coronary artery disease:a systematic review. *Am J Med* 2008; **121**:715–25.
16. Van Hoenacker PK, Decramer J, Bladt O, *et al.* Detection of non-ST-elevation myocardial infraction and unstable angina in the acute setting: a meta-analysis of diagnostic performance of MDCT-CA. *BMC Cardiovasc Disord* 2007; **7**:39.
17. Scheffel H, Alkadhi H, Plass A, *et al.* Accuracy of dual-source CT coronary angiography: first experience in a high pre-test probability population without heart rate control. *Eur Radiol* 2006; **16**:2739–47.
18. Weustink AC, Meijboom WB, Mollet NR, *et al.* Reliable high-speed coronary computed tomography in symptomatic patients. *J Am Coll Cardiol* 2007; **50**:786–94.
19. Leber AW, Johnson T, Becker A, *et al.* Diagnostic accuracy of dual-source multi-slice CT-coronary angiography in patients with an intermediate pretest likelihood for coronary artery disease. *Eur Heart J* 2007; **28**:2354–60.
20. Heuschmid M, Burgstahler C, Reimann A, *et al.* Usefulness of noninvasive cardiac imaging using dual-source computed tomography in an unselected population with high prevalence of coronary artery disease. *Am J Cardiol* 2007; **100**:587–92.
21. Ropers U, Ropers D, Pflederer T, *et al.* Influence of heart rate on the diagnostic accuracy of dual-source computed tomography coronary angiography. *J Am Coll Cardiol* 2007; **50**:2393–98.
22. Brodoefel H, Burgstahler C, Tsifikas I, *et al.* Dual-source CT: effect of heart rate, heart rate variability, and calcification on image quality and diagnostic accuracy. *Radiology* 2008; **247**:346–55.
23. Johnson TRC, Nikolaou K, Busch S, *et al.* Diagnostic accuracy of dual-source computed tomography in the diagnosis of coronary artery disease. *Invest Radiology* 2007; **42**:684–91.
24. Achenbach S, Ropers U, Kuettner A, *et al.* Randomized comparison of 64-slice single and dual-source computed tomography coronary angiography for the detection of coronary artery disease. *J Am Coll Cardiol Imaging* 2008; **1**:177–86.
25. Schuijf JD, Wijns W, Jukema JW, *et al.* Relationship between noninvasive coronary angiography with multislice computed tomography and myocardial perfusion imaging. *J Am Coll Cardiol* 2006; **48**:2508–14.
26. Meijboom WB, Van Mieghem CA, Van Pelt N, *et al.* Comprehensive assessment of coronary stenoses: computed tomography coronary angiography versus conventional coronary angiography and correlation with fractional flow reserve in patients with stable angina. *J Am Coll Cardiol* 2008; **52**:636–42.
27. Oncel D, Oncel G, Tastan A. Effectiveness of dual-source CT coronary angiography for the evaluation of coronary artery disease in patients with atrial fibrillation: initial experience. *Radiology* 2007; **245**:703–11.
28. Pache G, Saueressig U, Frydrychowicz A, *et al.* Initial experience with 64-slice cardiac CT: non-invasive visualization of coronary artery bypass grafts. *Eur Heart J* 2006; **27**:976–80.
29. Ropers D, Pohle FK, Kuettner A, *et al.* Diagnostic accuracy of noninvasive coronary angiography in patients after bypass surgery using 64-slice spiral computed tomography with 330-ms gantry rotation. *Circulation* 2006; **114**:2334–41.
30. Malagutti P, Nieman K, Meijboom WB, *et al.* Use of 64-slice CT in symptomatic patients after coronary bypass surgery: evaluation of grafts and coronary arteries. *Eur Heart J* 2007; **28**:1879–85.
31. Meyer TS, Martinoff S, Hadamitzky M, *et al.* Improved noninvasive assessment of coronary artery bypass grafts with 64-slice computed tomographic angiography in an unselected patient population. *J Am Coll Cardiol* 2007; **49**:946–50.
32. Onuma Y, Tanabe K, Chihara R, *et al.* Evaluation of coronary artery bypass grafts and native coronary arteries using 64-slice multidetector computed tomography. *Am Heart J* 2007; **154**:519–26.
33. Van Mieghem CAG, Cademartiri F, Mollet NR, *et al.* Multislice spiral computed tomography for the evaluation

of stent patency after main coronary artery stenting a comparison with conventional coronary angiography and intravascular ultrasound. *Circulation* 2006; **114**:645–53.

34. Oncel D, Oncel G, Karaca M. Coronary stent patency and in-stent restenosis: determination with 64-section multidetector ct coronary angiography-initial experience. *Radiology* 2007; **242**:403–9.
35. Rixe J, Achenbach S, Ropers D, *et al.* Assessment of coronary artery stent restenosis by 64-slice multi-detector computed tomography. *Eur Heart J* 2006; **27**:2567–72.
36. Ehara M, Kawai M, Surmely JF, *et al.* Diagnostic accuracy of coronary in-stent restenosis using 64-slice computed tomography comparison with invasive coronary angiography. *J Am Coll Cardiol* 2007; **49**:951–9.
37. Cademartiri F, Schuijf JD, Pugliese F, *et al.* Usefulness of 64-slice multislice computed tomography coronary angiography to assess in-stent restenosis. *J Am Coll Cardiol* 2007; **49**:2204–10.
38. Carbone I, Francone M, Algeri E, *et al.* Non-invasive evaluation of coronary artery stent patency with retrospectively ECG-gated 64-slice CT angiography. *Eur Radiol* 2008; **18**:234–43.
39. Pugliese F, Weustink AC, Van Mieghem C, *et al.* Dual source coronary computed tomography angiography for detecting in-stent restenosis. *Heart* 2008; **94**:848–54.
40. Rist C, Von Ziegler F, Nikolaou K, *et al.* Assessment of coronary artery stent patency and restenosis using 64-slice computed tomography. *Acad Radiol* 2008; **13**:1465–73.
41. Schmitt R, Froehner S, Brunn J, *et al.* Congenital anomalies of the coronary arteries: imaging with contrast-enhanced, multidetector computed tomography. *Eur Radiol* 2005; **15**:1110–21.
42. Topol EJ, Ellis SG, Fishman J, *et al.* Multicenter study of percutaneous transluminal angioplasty for right coronary artery ostial stenosis. *J Am Coll Cardiol* 1987; **9**: 1214–18.
43. Kereiakes DJ. Percutaneous transcatheter therapy of aorto-ostial stenoses. *Cathet Cardiovasc Diagn* 1996; **38**: 292–300.
44. Zampieri P, Colombo A, Almagor Y, *et al.* Results of coronary stenting of ostial lesions. *Am J Cardiol* 1994; **73**:901–3.
45. Horlitz M, Amin FR, Sigwart U, *et al.* Coronary stenting of aorto-ostial saphenous vein graft lesions. *J Invasive Cardiol* 2006; **68**:901–6.
46. Tierstein P, Stratienko AA, Schatz RA. Coronary stenting for ostial stenosis: Initial results and six-month follow-up. *Circulation* 1991; **84**(Suppl 2):II–250.
47. Kunadian B, Vijayalakshmi K, de Belder MA. Treatment of restenosis after bare-metal and drug-eluting stenting of an aorto-ostial lesion: challenges associated with excessive stent overhang. *J Cardiovasc Med* 2007; **8**(9):744–7.
48. Barlis P, Kaplan S, Dimopoulos K, *et al.* Comparison of bare-metal and sirolimus- or paclitaxel-eluting stents for aorto-ostial coronary disease. *Cardiology* 2008; **111**:270–6.
49. Roguin A, Abadi S, Engel A, *et al.* Novel method for real time hybrid cardiac ct andcoronary angiography image registration: visualising beyond luminology, proof-of-concept. *Eurointervention* 2009; **4**(5):648–53.
50. Louvard Y, Thomas M, Dzavik V, *et al.* Classification of coronary artery bifurcation lesions and treatments: time for a consensus! *Catheter Cardiovasc Interv* 2008; **71**(2):175–83.
51. Thuesen L, Kelbaek H, Kløvgaard L, *et al.* Comparison of sirolimus-eluting and bare metal stents in coronary bifurcation lesions: subgroup analysis of the Stenting Coronary Arteries in Non-Stress/Benestent Disease Trial (SCANDSTENT). *Am Heart J* 2006; **152**(6):1140–5.
52. Collins N, Seidelin PH, Daly P, *et al.* Long-term outcomes after percutaneous coronary intervention of bifurcation narrowings. *Am J Cardiol* 2008; **102**(4):404–10.
53. Adriaenssens T, Byrne RA, Dibra A, *et al.* Culotte stenting technique in coronary bifurcation disease: angiographic follow-up using dedicated quantitative coronary angiographic analysis and 12-month clinical outcomes. *Eur Heart J* 2008; **29**(23):2868–76.
54. Pflederer T, Ludwig J, Ropers D, *et al.* Measurement of coronary artery bifurcation angles by multidetector computed tomography. *Invest Radiol* 2006; **41**(11):793–8.
55. Van Mieghem CA, Thury A, Meijboom WB, *et al.* Detection and characterization of coronary bifurcation lesions with 64-slice computed tomography coronary angiography. *Eur Heart J* 2007; **28**(16):1968–76.
56. García-García H, Kukreja N, Daemen J, *et al.* Contemporary treatment of patients with chronic total occlusion: critical appraisal of different state-of-the-art techniques and devices. *EuroIntervention* 2007; **3**:188–96.
57. Mitsudo K, Yamashita T, Asakura Y, *et al.* Recanalization strategy for chronic total occlusions with tapered and stiff-tip guidewire. The results of CTO new techniQUE for STandard procedure (CONQUEST) trial. *J Invasive Cardiol* 2008; **20**(11):571–7.
58. Saito S. Different strategies of retrograde approach in coronary angioplasty for chronic total occlusion s. *Catheter Cardiovasc Interv* 2008; **71**(1):8–19.
59. Valenti R, Migliorini A, Signorini U, *et al.* Impact of complete revascularization with percutaneous coronary intervention on survival in patients with at least one chronic total occlusion. *Eur Heart J* 2008; **29**(19):2336–42.
60. Aziz S, Stables RH, Grayson AD, *et al.* Percutaneous coronary intervention for chronic total occlusions: improved survival for patients with successful revascularization compared to a failed procedure. *Catheter Cardiovasc Interv* 2007; **70**(1):15–20.
61. Hoye A, van Domburg RT, Sonnenschein K, *et al.* Percutaneous coronary intervention for chronic total occlusions: the Thoraxcenter experience 1992–2002. *Eur Heart J* 2005; **26**(24):2630–6.
62. Soon KH, Cox N, Wong A, *et al.* CT coronary angiography predicts the outcome of percutaneous coronary intervention of chronic total occlusion. *J Interv Cardiol* 2007; **20**(5):359–66.
63. Kaneda H, Saito S, Shiono T, *et al.* Sixty-four-slice computed tomography-facilitated percutaneous coronary

intervention for chronic total occlusion. *Int J Cardiol* 2007; **115**(1):130–2.
64. Mollet NR, Hoye A, Lemos PA, *et al.* Value of preprocedure multislice computed tomographic coronary angiography to predict the outcome of percutaneous recanalization of chronic total occlusions. *Am J Cardiol* 2005; **95**(2):240–3.
65. Yokoyama N, Yamamoto Y, Suzuki S, *et al.* Impact of 16-slice computed tomography in percutaneous coronary intervention of chronic total occlusions. *Catheter Cardiovasc Interv* 2006; **68**(1):1–7.
66. Tsuchida K, García-García HM, van der Giessen WJ, *et al.* Guidewire navigation in coronary artery stenoses using a novel magnetic navigation system: first clinical experience. *Catheter Cardiovasc Interv* 2006; **67**(3):356–63.
67. Ramcharitar S, Patterson MS, van Geuns RJ, *et al.* Technology insight: magnetic navigation in coronary interventions. *Nat Clin Pract Cardiovasc Med* 2008; **5**(3):148–56.
68. Ramcharitar S, Patterson MS, van Geuns RJ, *et al.* Magnetic navigation system used successfully to cross a crushed stent in a bifurcation that failed with conventional wires. *Catheter Cardiovasc Interv* 2007; **69**(6):852–5.
69. Ramcharitar S, van Geuns RJ, Patterson M, *et al.* A randomized comparison of the magnetic navigation system versus conventional percutaneous coronary intervention. *Catheter Cardiovasc Interv* 2008; **72**(6):761–70.
70. Ramcharitar S, van Geuns RJ, van der Giessen WJ, *et al.* Single centre experience of magnetic navigation in the management of chronically occluded vessels. In Ramcharitar S (ed) *Magnetic Navigation in Percutaneous Coronary and Non-coronary Interventions*, pp.187–202, PhD thesis 2009, Erasmus University, Rotterdam.
71. Ramcharitar S, Pugliese F, Schultz C, *et al.* Integration of multislice computer tomography with magnetic navigation facilitates percutaneous coronary interventions without contrast agents. *J Am Coll Cardiol* 2009; **53**:742–6.

CHAPTER 13

Cardiovascular magnetic resonance

Theodoros D. Karamitsos and
Stefan Neubauer

Introduction

Over the past decade, cardiovascular magnetic resonance (CMR) has undergone significant advancement in terms of imaging capabilities, ease of use, and speed of acquisition. A study of cardiac anatomy, function, and viability can now be completed in less than 30min with superb image quality and excellent reproducibility. This has led to widespread adoption of CMR in clinical practice. New CMR specialists and dedicated CMR units are rapidly emerging. The interventional cardiologist can now use CMR to find answers to many common clinical questions (e.g. inducible ischaemia, viability, coronary artery disease versus non-coronary causes of chest pain, etc.). Moreover, with the development of combined CMR-interventional units, interventional cardiologists are becoming an integral component of this evolving technology.

How CMR works

The fundamental principles of CMR imaging are briefly described here; greater detail can be found in more specialized texts[1]. For CMR imaging, a 1.5 Tesla magnetic field (approximately 30 000 times stronger than the earth's magnetic field) is most frequently used, although recently 3 Tesla magnets are increasingly being used. Hydrogen nuclei (protons), which are abundant in the human body, behave like small spinning magnets that have an alignment (magnetic moment) parallel to the direction of the external magnetic field and a rotation (*precession*) frequency proportional to the strength of the field. This frequency of precession is 63MHz for a field strength of 1.5 Tesla and is within the radiofrequency range. When the protons in a body region are intermittently excited by radiofrequency pulses at this resonant frequency, the magnetic moments in that region will be flipped out at an angle (flip angle) to the magnetic field (*excitation*). After this excitation, the net magnetization vector precesses around the direction of the main field, returning to its former position (*relaxation*). In magnetic resonance (MR) imaging, the contrast between tissues (e.g. heart muscle, fat, etc.) depends on the tissue density of hydrogen atoms (proton density), and on two distinct MR relaxation processes that affect the net magnetization; the longitudinal relaxation time (T1) and transverse relaxation time (T2). The differences in these parameters in distinct tissues are used to generate contrast in MR images. Image contrast can also be modified by modulating the way the radiofrequency pulses are played out (the MR sequence): For example, in so-called T1-weighted images, myocardial tissue is dark whereas fat is bright. On the other hand, T2-weighted images highlight unbound water in the myocardium and are used to demonstrate myocardial oedema due to inflammation or acute ischaemia[2].

A CMR *scanner* consists of a superconducting *magnet*, which produces a homogeneous and stable magnetic field, *gradient coils* within the bore of the magnet which generate the gradient fields, a *radiofrequency amplifier* to excite the spins with radiofrequency pulses, and a radiofrequency antenna (coil), which receives the radio signals coming from the patient. A *computer* and *specific software* are also needed to control the scanner and generate (reconstruct) the images.

A *CMR sequence* consists of a series of radiofrequency pulses, magnetic gradient field switches, and timed data acquisitions, all applied in a precise order to generate the CMR image. Most CMR images are acquired using two basic sequences known as spin echo and gradient echo. *Spin echo* sequences are mainly used for anatomic imaging and tissue characterization. *Gradient echo* sequences show fat and blood as white and can be used to acquire cine images. The so called *steady state free precession (SSFP)* sequences are now the standard cardiac MR sequences for imaging of cardiac function, as they provide the best contrast between chamber blood (white) and myocardium (dark). *Fat suppression* sequences allow signal from fat to be specifically suppressed with special pre-pulses. Other common prepulses are *inversion recovery*, which is used for infarct/viability imaging, and *saturation recovery*, which is used in perfusion imaging. Several other approaches exist, and CMR sequence development is a rapidly evolving field. However, a detailed description of this is beyond the scope of this chapter.

To prevent *artefacts* from cardiac motion, most CMR images are generated with ultrafast sequences gated to the R wave of the electrocardiogram. Respiratory motion, which is another factor that can produce artefacts, is eliminated by acquiring most CMR images in end-expiratory breath-hold. When acquisition is long and cannot be completed within one breath-hold, special free-breathing sequences that track the diaphragm's position (navigators) are used.

CMR safety

CMR scan subjects and operators are not exposed to ionizing radiation and there are no known detrimental biological side effects of MR imaging if safety guidelines are followed[(3)]. Claustrophobia may be a problem in a small percentage of patients, and mild sedation usually helps to overcome this. Only trained staff should have access to the magnet room, as the superconducting magnet is 'always on', and hence, any iron-based item with ferromagnetic properties can become a flying projectile, potentially causing serious injury to the patient or the operator and damage to the scanner. The presence of a pacemaker or defibrillator is considered a strong relative contraindication to routine MR examination, which is therefore discouraged[(4)]. This may change in the future with further technical development (specifically-designed CMR-compatible pacemakers etc). Some neurovascular clips continue to pose a problem, as do metallic objects in delicate positions, e.g. within the eye. Generally, most medical metallic implants including nearly all prosthetic cardiac valves, coronary and vascular stents, and orthopaedic implants may produce local image artefacts but pose no hazard at the field strength of 1.5 Tesla. However, whenever there is uncertainty regarding a particular device or implant, the CMR operator should consult a more detailed source of information, such as reference manuals, dedicated Internet sites (e.g. http://www.mrisafety.com), or the manufacturer's product information when available[(4)].

Cardiovascular anatomy

Using standard MR techniques, cardiovascular anatomy can be assessed with high spatial resolution in conventional orthogonal (e.g. transverse, sagittal, coronal) and in CMR-specific double-angulated (e.g. oblique sagittal) planes. CMR has been widely utilized to characterize changes in morphology and anatomy for various cardiovascular disorders including complex congenital abnormalities, and historically, this was the first widespread application of the method[(5)].

Cardiac function

The accurate and reproducible assessment of global and regional cardiac function is an essential part of the management and follow-up assessment of patients with cardiovascular disease. CMR has been shown to be an excellent technique for assessing left and right ventricular volumes and systolic function. Cine images are obtained using SSFP sequences, resulting in images with excellent delineation of the blood–myocardium interface[(6)]. For ventricular volume assessment, a set of contiguous short-axis slices parallel to the atrioventricular ring that encompasses both ventricles from base to apex is required (Fig. 13.1)[(7)]. Left and right ventricular volumes are calculated by summing the endocardial areas multiplied by the interslice distance. Thus, the functional information derived from a CMR study includes the entire ventricular volume without the need to make any geometrical assumptions and, hence, applies to ventricles of all sizes and shapes, even those which have been extensively remodelled. Importantly, the inherent three-dimensional (3D) nature of CMR makes it particularly well suited to study the right ventricle given its complex and variable (even in normal volunteers) morphology. Ventricular mass can also be determined from the end-diastolic images by multiplication of the myocardial volume by its specific weight of 1.05g/cm^3. An important feature of CMR is the excellent interstudy reproducibility of volume and mass measurements. This has allowed reductions of sample sizes of 80–97% to achieve the same statistical power

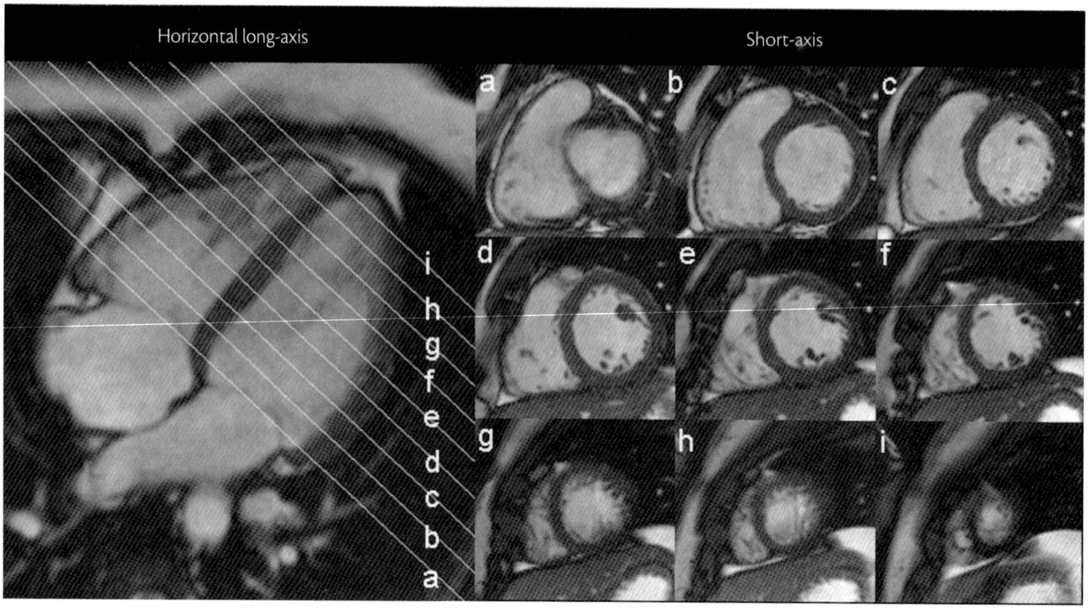

Fig. 13.1 End-diastolic still images from multiple contiguous short-axis SSFP cines (a-i) that encompass the left ventricle, from base to apex. Note the position of the short-axis slices marked on the still frame of an end-diastolic horizontal long axis cine image (left panel).

for demonstrating a given change in left ventricular (LV) volumes, ejection fraction, or cardiac mass[8].

CMR is also an excellent technique for visualizing regional wall motion abnormalities. It allows the identification of even subtle wall motion abnormalities at rest and during dobutamine stress. Quantification of regional wall motion is usually performed by visual inspection of cine images, although quantification of wall thickening is also possible but is usually reserved for research studies. Another technique for quantitative analysis of regional systolic and diastolic function is MR tagging. Selective saturation pre-pulses are used to superimpose a grid across the field of view. These grid lines are deformed by myocardial contraction, strain, and torsion, allowing direct quantification of myocardial deformation and strain[9]. Similar information can be derived by CMR tissue velocity mapping, a technique analogous to tissue Doppler echocardiography, which can provide measurements of 3D myocardial velocities, strains, and strain rates[10]. The clinical application of these techniques is currently limited by complex and time-consuming post-processing, but this is likely to be simplified in the future.

Blood flow

Phase contrast mapping of velocities through planes transecting blood flow in the main pulmonary artery and the ascending aorta can provide accurate measurements of cardiac output, shunt flow, aortic or pulmonary regurgitation, and, indirectly, of mitral and tricuspid regurgitation[11]. For stenotic jets, the peak velocity can be measured on *in-plane* or *through-plane* velocity-encoded images[12]. Peak pressure gradients can be estimated according to the modified Bernoulli's equation. Valve morphology can be assessed with the use of SSFP cine images, although valve structure is generally better assessed by echocardiography. For example, CMR is not the ideal technique to demonstrate valve calcification which appears as local signal loss, but valve area can be assessed with accuracy by direct planimetry using cross-sectional cine images[12]. Bicuspid aortic valves or fused valve leaflets can be readily identified. Valvular regurgitation is usually evident from the signal loss in the receiving chamber on cine images. However, this is not a reliable way to grade the severity of the disease. Instead, CMR provides a different way for excellent quantitative assessment of regurgitation. If a single valve is affected, the regurgitant volume can be measured from the difference in left and right ventricular stroke volumes. If both the mitral and tricuspid valves are affected, the regurgitant volumes can be calculated by subtracting the flow in main pulmonary artery and the ascending aorta, measured by CMR velocity mapping, from the left and right stroke volumes (measured by the volumetric method), respectively[13].

This technique compares favourably with measurements from catheterization and Doppler echocardiography techniques[14]. For pulmonary and aortic regurgitation, direct measurement of regurgitant volume is also possible using CMR velocity mapping[13]. These CMR techniques have high interstudy reproducibility and can be used for the longitudinal follow-up of patients with valve disease over time.

Apart from the evaluation of patients with valve pathologies, flow imaging by CMR is regularly used in assessing patients with congenital heart disease[11]. By measuring flow in the ascending aorta and main pulmonary artery with velocity-encoding CMR, the pulmonary-to-systemic flow ratio (Qp/Qs) can be determined[15]. This can also be estimated from the ventricular stroke volume comparison, if no significant valvular regurgitation exists. Importantly, pulmonary-to-systemic flow ratios measured by velocity-encoding CMR show excellent correlation with calculations obtained from oximetry during haemodynamic catheterization[15].

Ischaemia

In patients with stable angina, the interventional cardiologist should proceed to revascularization only when a given coronary artery stenosis results in significant stress-induced ischaemia[16,17]. The identification of myocardial ischaemia by CMR involves stressing the patient with either a vasodilator agent (adenosine or dipyridamole) to assess regional myocardial perfusion, or with an inotropic agent (dobutamine) to assess regional wall motion abnormalities. Perfusion defects are induced early in the ischaemic cascade (superior sensitivity), whereas regional wall motion abnormalities come on at a later stage (superior specificity). ECG changes and angina only occur later in the ischaemic cascade. CMR can visualize different stages of this continuum of events.

Perfusion

Perfusion imaging by CMR is an attractive method to assess myocardial ischaemia. It is radiation-free and can be performed as part of a comprehensive study in patients with acute or chronic ischaemic heart disease. Perfusion CMR was first introduced in 1990 but initially had limited application restricted to research studies[18]. However, perfusion imaging has undergone significant technical development with improvements in MR hardware, software (e.g. sequences), and analysis methods. Its validation included preclinical studies using microspheres in animal models and clinical studies in patients with suspected or documented CAD.

In first-pass perfusion CMR, the dynamic passage of a bolus of gadolinium-based contrast agent is followed through the cardiac chambers and the myocardium. For clinical application, most CMR centres prefer adenosine as the stressor agent because it is generally well tolerated and easily controlled[19]. After 3-4min of adenosine infusion at a rate of 140mcg/kg/min, an intravenous bolus of gadolinium is injected through a peripheral vein in the antecubital fossa, and a set of at least three short-axis slices (one basal, one equatorial, and one apical) is acquired every cardiac cycle during the first pass of the contrast[20]. Pharmacologic vasodilation induces a three- to fivefold increase of blood flow in myocardial areas subtended by normal coronary arteries, whereas no (or only minimal) change is found in areas subtended by stenotic coronary arteries. Such areas therefore show lower peak enhancement with delayed uptake of the contrast and, hence, appear hypointense (dark) compared to adjacent normal myocardium (Fig. 13.2). The same sequence is then repeated at rest. For routine clinical application, visual analysis of the perfusion images at stress and rest is adequate. More complex analysis for the measurement of myocardial perfusion reserve index based on the upslope of signal intensity versus time curves at stress and rest is time consuming and, hence, currently reserved only to research studies[21]. The same applies to absolute quantification of myocardial blood flow (in mL/min/g), which is perhaps the most exciting application of CMR perfusion imaging in clinical research.

There are several imaging sequences that can be used in perfusion imaging, but there are generally little differences amongst them, and what matters much more is the experience of the operator reviewing the images[22]. Occasionally, dark rim artefacts which resemble perfusion defects appear at the subendocardium, but with experience these can almost always be distinguished from true perfusion defects[23]. They appear early, together with the rapid increase in the signal from the blood pool, and are less persistent (last only up to 4–5 frames) than true perfusion defects (which last longer). The exact nature of these artefacts is still debated, but both susceptibility effects on the blood–subendocardium interface and other factors such as cardiac motion play a role[23]. With the improvement in spatial resolution, which is expected with the application of parallel imaging techniques and the higher field strength of 3 Tesla, these artefacts should become less of a problem for perfusion imaging.

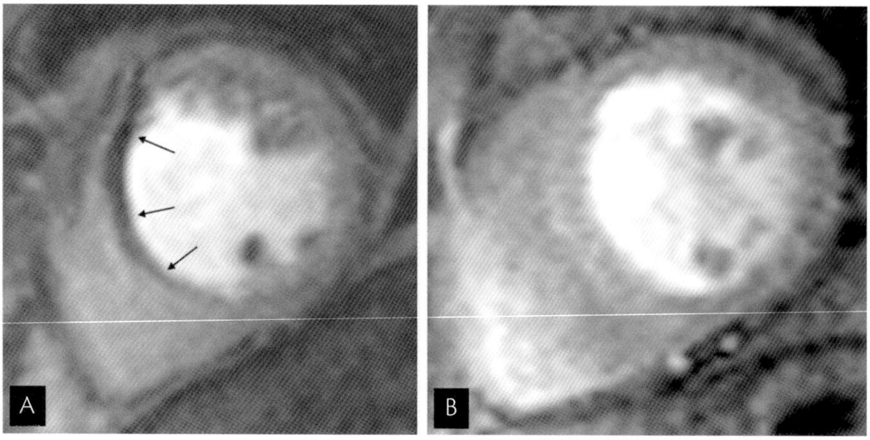

Fig. 13.2 Two representative examples of CMR perfusion scans during adenosine stress. (A) This patient had a significant stenosis of the left anterior descending coronary artery. Note the area of hypoenhancement in the anteroseptum (black arrows); this represents a perfusion defect. (B) Example of a young normal volunteer without cardiac risk factors. Note the homogeneous enhancement in all myocardial regions during the infusion of adenosine.

Compared to radionuclide techniques, perfusion CMR has many potential advantages. A typical voxel (3D) size for a perfusion CMR study measures 2.1× 2.4 × 8mm versus 6.5 × 6.5cm which is the pixel size of a single photon emission computed tomography (SPECT) study[24]. The difference in spatial resolution is almost an order of magnitude higher for CMR, allowing separate visualization of the subendocardial and subepicardial layers. Moreover, perfusion imaging is part of a comprehensive CMR examination, which typically lasts 45min and also includes imaging of cardiac function with cine CMR and viability assessment with the late gadolinium technique. This comprehensive assessment is feasible without exposure to ionizing radiation.

First-pass perfusion imaging with adenosine is a safe CMR technique and is generally well tolerated with only few well-described minor side effects (chest tightness, shortness of breath, flush, etc.) which usually resolve within a few minutes of stopping the infusion[25]. Adenosine has also been associated with various degrees of heart block. The incidence of advanced atrioventricular block (≥second-degree block) is 5–8%, and in most cases this is transient and terminates spontaneously without major haemodynamic effects. No deaths and only one case of acute myocardial infarction as a result of adenosine administration has been reported for SPECT studies involving more than 10 000 patients with suspected CAD[26]. The history of asthma and advanced atrioventricular block are contraindications for the administration of adenosine. A fully equipped crash trolley and medications including aminophylline, the adenosine antidote, must be available.

Stress-induced wall motion abnormalities: high-dose dobutamine CMR

High-dose dobutamine stress CMR (DSCMR) is now an established method for the assessment of stress-induced regional wall motion abnormalities[27]. Unlike echocardiography, DSCMR has no acoustic window limitations and high quality images for wall motion assessment can be acquired regardless of body habitus. In practice, the technique is performed in a manner analogous to dobutamine stress echo. To ensure an adequate heart rate response to dobutamine, beta-blockers are withheld for 24–48h prior to the CMR scan. Dobutamine is infused intravenously during 3-min stages at dosages of 10, 20, 30, and 40mcg/kg/min. If the target heart rate [(220 − age) × 0.85] is not reached, additional atropine doses are administered in 0.25mg/min increments up to the maximal dose of 1.0mg intravenously. At each stress level, three short-axis (basal, mid-equatorial, and apical) and three long axis (2-, 3-, 4-chamber view) cines are acquired. These are compared to the rest cine images (which were acquired before dobutamine) for evidence of new or worsened wall motion abnormalities. A pathologic response is characterized by stress-induced wall motion abnormalities (hypokinesis, akinesis, or dyskinesis) in at least one segment that was graded normal at rest. For standardized assessment and reporting, the use of the LV 17-segment model of the

American Heart Association is recommended[28]. The infusion is terminated if a new wall motion abnormality is noted, when peak heart rate is achieved and/or if serious side effects (e.g. deteriorating chest pain, infarction, sustained ventricular tachycardia, ventricular fibrillation) ensue. Due to the risk of severe side effects, patients have to be closely monitored (continuous monitoring of heart rhythm, blood pressure, and symptoms). The presence of trained personnel including at least one physician experienced in stress testing and particularly on-line wall motion analysis, is absolutely mandatory. Resuscitation equipment and medications must be available.

Previous studies with high-dose dobutamine stress echocardiography in patients with coronary artery disease (CAD) have shown that severe complications occur in 0.25–0.6% of patients including sustained ventricular tachycardia, myocardial infarction, ventricular fibrillation, and even death[29,30]. Significant arrhythmias have been reported to be more frequent in patients with a history of ventricular arrhythmias or LV dysfunction at rest[29]. Compared to dobutamine stress echocardiography, similar rates of severe complications have been reported for during DSCMR. However, there are additional difficulties[31]. During a CMR study, observation of the patient is hampered by confinement within the magnet, and ST-segment analysis is precluded by distortion caused by the magnetic field. Moreover, in case of an emergency, resuscitation involves rapid removal of the patient from the magnet room and transfer to a predetermined magnetically safe location, where full resuscitation efforts can be performed. For these reasons, the routine clinical use of DSCMR is currently limited, and instead, adenosine stress perfusion is much more commonly performed to assess myocardial ischaemia.

Myocardial injury

The visualization of irreversible injury using a T1-weighted segmented inversion-recovery gradient echo sequence has revolutionized the role of CMR in the evaluation of CAD patients. This method, which is commonly termed *late gadolinium enhancement* (LGE), provides high spatial resolution images of irreversible myocardial injury both in the acute and chronic setting. Importantly, this technique showed excellent correlation with histopathological specimens of infarcted and viable myocardium in large animal models. Kim and colleagues were the first to show in an experimental study of permanent coronary ligation that a near perfect correlation exists between LGE-CMR and histopathology-evidenced scar size in both the acute ($r = 0.99$, $p < 0.001$) and chronic ($r = 0.97$, $p < 0.001$) phases of infarction infarct[32]. Several other studies confirmed these findings and established CMR as a technique capable of distinguishing between reversible and irreversible myocardial injury independent of wall motion, infarct size, or reperfusion status[32–34].

The physiologic basis of LGE is an increase in its volume of distribution within areas of scarring or fibrosis and an abnormally prolonged wash-out related to decreased functional capillary density in the irreversibly injured myocardium[35–38]. In the setting of acute myocardial infarction, the loss of sarcolemmal membrane integrity provides a mechanism for extravasation of gadolinium[37]. In chronic infarction, the interstitial space is expanded because the loss of myocytes and increase in extracellular collagen content provide a greater volume of distribution for gadolinium[37]. Histopathological data support these proposed mechanisms in either acute or chronic myocardial infarction. The regional increase in extracellular volume of gadolinium distribution produces T1 shortening, which manifests as hyperenhancement (high signal) in areas of abnormality on so-called inversion-recovery LGE images: by nulling the normal myocardial signal, the area of myocardial injury appears with extremely high contrast relative to the black normal myocardium. This *in vivo* demonstration of the spatial extent of myocardial necrosis allows the identification of even small subendocardial infarcts previously undetectable by lower resolution techniques such as SPECT[34]. The LGE technique has also been used to characterize the pathological significance of Q-waves post myocardial infarction. The primary determinant of the presence of Q-waves on ECG is the total size of the underlying territorial infarction and not its transmural extent.

The use of LGE-CMR to predict functional recovery post-revascularization is another important application of CMR in daily clinical practice. An inverse relationship between the functional improvement after revascularization and the transmural extent of myocardial scarring before revascularization has been demonstrated (Fig. 13.3)[39,40]. In these studies, the relationship was even steeper for segments with severe dysfunction at baseline. These segments are the most difficult to assess with dobutamine echocardiography, as contractile reserve has reduced predictive accuracy if severe dysfunction is present at rest. For example, in akinetic segments, the sensitivity of dobutamine echocardiography for predicting functional improvement

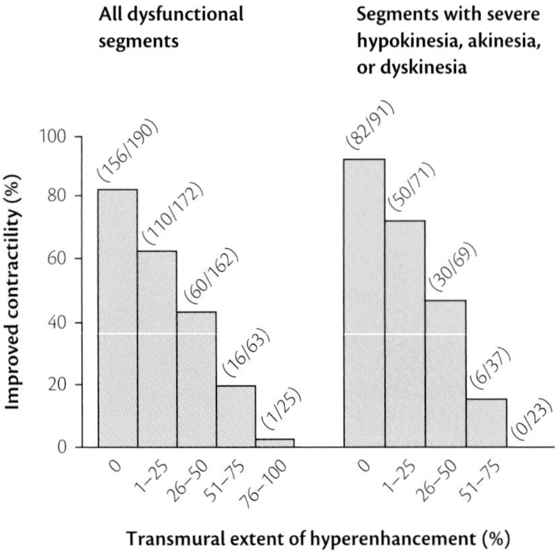

Fig. 13.3 Relationship between transmural extent of hyperenhancement before by-pass surgery and likelihood of increased contractility after revascularization in all dysfunctional segments (left) and in all segments with severe hypokinesia, akinesia, or dyskinesia. Reproduced with permission from Selvanayagam JB, Kardos A, Francis JM, *et al.* Value of delayed-enhancement cardiovascular magnetic resonance imaging in predicting myocardial viability after surgical revascularization. *Circulation* 2004; **110**(12):1535–41.

may be as low as 26%[41]. This is because any degree of inotropic stimulation may render these segments ischaemic, preventing enhanced contractility with inotropic stimulation. LGE-CMR, on the other hand, does not involve any form of stress and shows better predictive value if severe dysfunction is present at rest. This is, indeed, one of the strengths of LGE-CMR as it is safer, requires less intense monitoring, is easier to implement, and is faster to complete than the other non-invasive imaging methods for viability assessment. On the other hand, all studies using LGE-CMR highlight relatively lower specificity of the technique, which is mainly due to the variable functional recovery in myocardial segments with 25–75% hyperenhancement. A low-dose dobutamine study may be helpful in equivocal cases[42].

In the current era of modern stent technology and potent antiplatelet therapy, percutaneous coronary intervention (PCI) is performed in many patients with high-risk lesions/procedural characteristics. Side-branch occlusion or distal embolization of particulate matter during balloon inflation and stenting are two main responsible mechanisms of procedure-related myocardial injury. Our work showed that this can be identified by LGE-CMR in about 30% of patients undergoing complex PCI[43]. The extent of the procedure-related myocardial injury correlates well with the magnitude of troponin elevation.

LGE-CMR not only defines the location and extent of infarction, but also shows areas with poor tissue perfusion following revascularization, the so-called *no-reflow phenomenon*. This appears as a central black area within a larger region of hyper- enhancement and represents severe microcirculatory damage, myocyte necrosis and localized oedema that compresses intramural vessels (Fig. 13.4). Such microvascular obstruction detected by CMR has been linked to aggravated ventricular remodelling and adverse cardiovascular events post acute myocardial infarction[44].

LGE-CMR cannot differentiate between acute and chronic irreversible myocardial injury. Both patterns of injury exhibit hyperenhancement and result in regional wall motion abnormalities, and although wall thinning is a feature of chronic injury, this finding is not usually present in subendocardial infarcts. However, if LGE is combined with T2-weighted imaging (to detect regional increases in myocardial water content), then CMR can differentiate between acute and chronic injury. Chronic myocardial infarction is clearly depicted on LGE imaging, whereas T2-weighted images are unremarkable in this situation. On the other hand, in acute myocardial infarction, T2-weighted images reveal an area of high

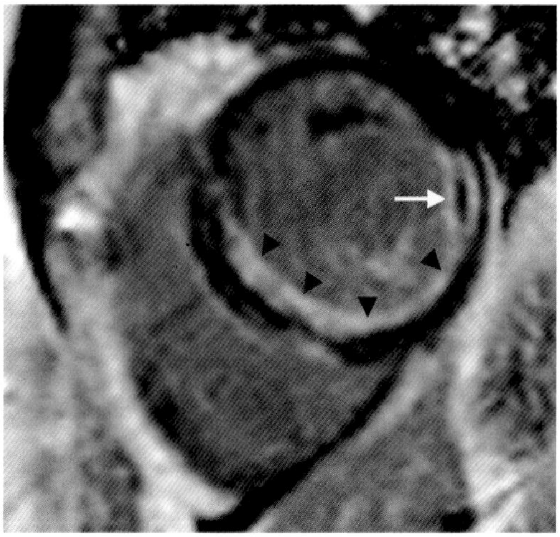

Fig. 13.4 Late gadolinium enhancement image showing two areas of infarction. A septal infarct involving 50–75% of wall thickness is marked with black arrowheads. There is also an inferior infarct which is predominantly subendocardial (0–25% transmural extent) but towards the inferolateral involves 50–75% of wall thickness and shows evidence of microvascular obstruction. Note the hypoenhanced (black) area in the inferolateral wall (white arrow) completely surrounded by hyper-enhanced regions.

signal ('area at risk') which exceeds that of irreversible injury[45]. The mechanisms underlying the development of myocardial oedema in acute myocardial infarction involve a disruption of the energy-regulated ionic transport mechanisms across the cell membrane after the ischaemic insult[46]. Moreover, in the setting of acutely reperfused infarction, the relation of myocardial oedema to irreversible myocardial injury provides additional information on the salvaged myocardium within the area at risk. Recently, this observation has been extended to the clinical setting. In patients with reperfused acute myocardial infarction CMR was able to visualize both reversible and irreversible injury, allowing the quantification of the salvaged area after revascularization (Fig. 13.5)[47]. Although oedema imaging needs further validation and improvement in terms of acquisition and quantitative analysis, it is a very promising CMR application which is expected to be of major use in the evaluation of new salvage strategies in primary PCI.

Viability assessment with low-dose dobutamine CMR

Low-dose DSCMR evaluates recruitment of inotropic reserve (i.e. improvement in contractility of viable but no improvement of non-viable segments), capitalizing on the excellent endocardial border definition, which enables accurate wall motion and wall thickening assessment. An improvement of regional contractile function with low-dose (5 or 10mcg/kg/min) dobutamine indicates the presence of viable myocardium. The standard cine views (2-, 3-, 4-chamber and basal, mid, and apical short-axis) are acquired at each level of stress. The images are projected side by side and graded for each stage of the protocol. As mentioned earlier, low-dose dobutamine CMR has been suggested as a method to improve viability assessment in patients with intermediate LGE (25–75% transmural extent); however, with the complexity of its implementation, it is rarely required in clinical practice[42,48].

Magnetic resonance coronary angiography

Invasive coronary angiography is still the gold standard technique for the diagnosis of CAD, and offers the potential for concurrent intervention. However, it is an invasive technique with a small risk of complications, and it exposes the patient and the operator to ionizing radiation. On the other hand, the number of patients who undergo invasive coronary angiography has increased dramatically over the past decade. In 2006 an estimated 1 115 000 in-patient diagnostic cardiac catheterizations where performed in the United States[49]. The search for an alternative non-invasive technique to image coronary arteries has triggered great interest, and multidetector computed tomography (MDCT) has made significant progress towards this goal. However, most MDCT exams currently involve 2–3 times more radiation exposure than conventional coronary angiography (though this is likely to be reduced with further technological development)[50]. CMR has the advantage of being radiation-free and offers high soft-tissue contrast for the visualization of coronary anatomy without the need to administer exogenous contrast (Fig. 13.6).

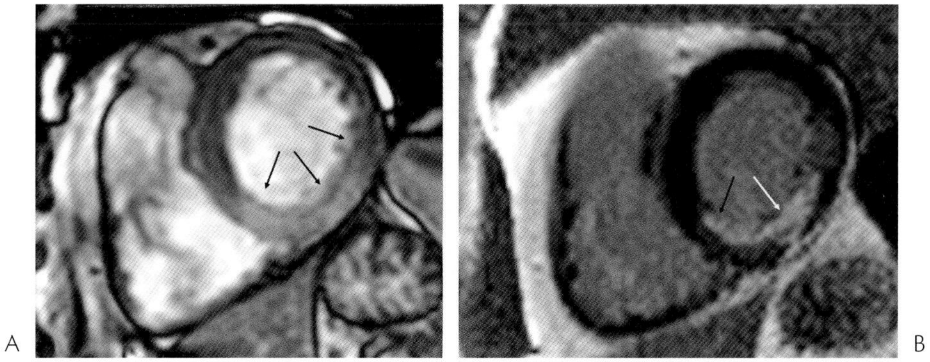

Fig. 13.5 A patient with acute inferior myocardial infarction. A) A T2-prepared SSFP image that shows an area of transmurally increased signal intensity involving the inferior septum and inferior wall; B) shows the corresponding late gadolinium enhancement image. Note that the spatial extent of myocardial injury in the oedema-sensitive T2 image is larger than that of the necrosis-sensitive late enhancement. Image courtesy of Dr. Erica Dall'Armellina, OCMR.

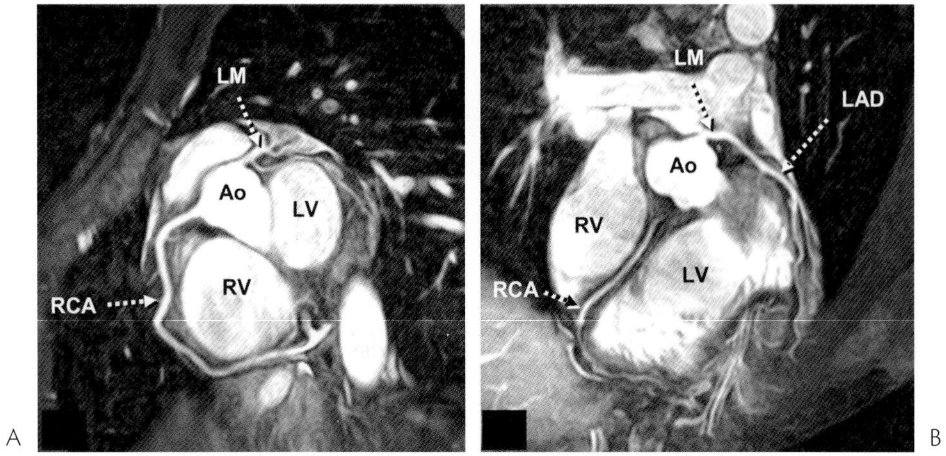

Fig. 13.6 SSFP coronary MRA of the right (A) and left (B) coronary systems of two healthy adult subjects, acquired using free-breathing and navigators. Ao, ascending aorta; LAD, left anterior descending; LV, left ventricle; RCA, right coronary artery; RV, right ventricle. Reproduced from Stuber M, Weiss RG. Coronary magnetic resonance angiography. *J Magn Reson Imaging* 2007; **26**(2):219–34. Reprinted with permission from John Wiley & Sons, Inc

However, the small size and tortuous course of the coronary arteries which move rapidly due to cardiac contraction and respiratory motion, makes magnetic resonance coronary angiography (MRCA) the most demanding of all CMR imaging techniques. To suppress the intrinsic cardiac motion, ECG gating is used and mid-diastole is the preferred time for image acquisition, because cardiac motion is minimized while coronary flow is high. A straightforward approach to suppress respiratory motion is to ask the patient to hold the breath during the acquisition. The disadvantage with this approach is that spatial and temporal image resolution is limited by the patient's breath-holding ability. Moreover, some patients may not be able to sustain adequate breath-holds, particularly when they last longer than a few seconds. Thus, at present, breath-hold strategies for MRCA have limited applicability. To overcome these limitations, navigator gating strategies have been used during free-breathing MRCA to track the position of the diaphragm during the scan. MRCA images are acquired only when the diaphragm is within 3–5mm of its end-expiratory position. Free-breathing navigator MRCA offers improved patient comfort as compared with breath-holding techniques and does not require significant patient effort[(50)]. However, this method prolongs the duration of acquisition (images can take up to 15min to acquire as image data are collected only when the end-expiratory position of the diaphragm coincides with the period of coronary artery diastasis. The spatial resolution of 3D MRCA imaging (0.7–0.8mm in-plane resolution and 1–3mm through-plane resolution) is still greatly inferior compared to that of X-ray coronary angiography (<0.3mm) or MDCT (~0.4mm)[(50)]. An important advantage of MRCA is that images are typically performed without the need for exogenous contrast agents. By applying special prepulses (e.g. fat-saturation prepulses, magnetization transfer contrast prepulses, or T2 preparatory pulses), the coronary lumen appears bright whereas the surrounding myocardium has reduced signal intensity[(51)]. Exogenous contrast enhancement with gadolinium-based contrast agents which quickly extravasate from the coronary lumen necessitates rapid first-pass imaging and breath-holding and, hence, images have reduced spatial resolution. Intravascular contrast agents, which typically remain in the vascular space for more than 1h, provide a prolonged time window for contrast-enhanced MRCA data acquisition, enabling the use of real-time navigator technology and 3D data collection with high spatial resolution. The use of SSFP sequences and parallel imaging techniques have substantially improved image quality of 3D MRCA encompassing the entire coronary arteries within a reasonably short imaging time[(51)]. However, at present, the method remains unreliable for the detection of stenosing CAD (see later section). In contrast, MRCA is a first-line investigation technique for the assessment of anomalous coronary arteries[(50)].

Atherosclerosis: vessel wall imaging

Vulnerable atherosclerotic plaque (plaque rupture) can lead to clinical events in the absence of significant stenosis. Therefore, a reliable non-invasive imaging tool able to detect early atherosclerotic disease and identify plaque composition is clinically desirable. High-resolution CMR has the potential to become the preferred non-invasive modality to study atherothrombotic disease in several vascular beds such as the aorta, the carotid arteries, and the coronary arteries. Several studies of the aorta, and particularly the carotid arteries(52), have demonstrated the ability of CMR to quantify atherosclerosis and its response to treatment (Fig. 13.7). Using a combination of inherent MR contrast, generated in T1-weighted, T2-weighted and proton-density-weighted images, it has been possible to characterize individual plaque components, including lipid-rich necrotic core, haemorrhage, and calcification(53). Although most CMR studies do not require exogenous contrast administration, gadolinium-based contrast agents can further improve delineation of individual plaque components such as the fibrous cap at submillimetre level(54). Thus, CMR differentiates plaque components on the basis of biophysical and biochemical parameters such as chemical composition, water content, physical state, molecular motion, or diffusion.

Importantly, as CMR provides imaging without ionizing radiation it can be repeated sequentially over time, enabling serial evaluation of the progression or regression of atherosclerosis over time. CMR findings have been extensively validated against pathology in *ex vivo* studies of carotid, aortic, and coronary artery specimen obtained at autopsy and using experimental models of atherosclerosis. The clinical implications of these capabilities were highlighted in a recent study of asymptomatic patients with moderate carotid stenosis (50–79% luminal narrowing) in which several high-risk features of plaques, observed by CMR, predicted subsequent cerebrovascular events(55). The foremost limitation of current CMR technology is the inability to reliably evaluate coronary artery walls due to limited spatial resolution, although initial promising attempts at this have been described(56,57). Furthermore, CMR is an attractive platform for molecular imaging studies of atherosclerosis using a large and expanding range of *in vivo* contrast agents that specifically target macrophages, platelets, and inflammatory cell adhesion molecules(53). Such methods can visualize molecular and cellular mechanisms that can give insights into the pathophysiology of atherosclerosis. Imaging of important molecular targets may in future transform clinical management by providing molecular specificity which would personalize drug selection tailored to an individual's proteome and genome(58).

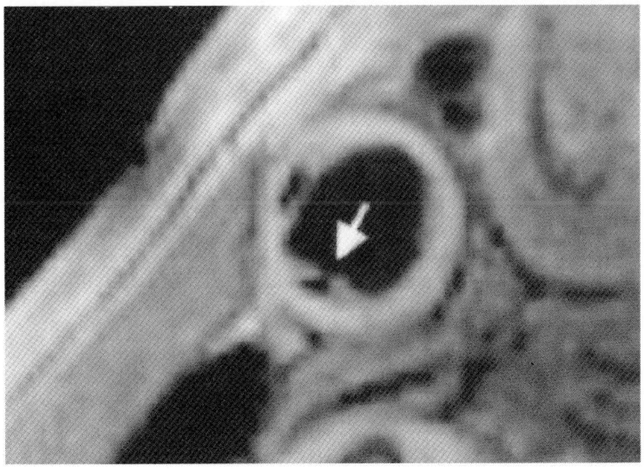

Fig. 13.7 Magnetic resonance T2-weighted turbo-spin-echo image in transverse orientation revealing increased wall thickness and two arteriosclerotic lesions in the right common carotid artery with dark lipid core and thin fibrous cap. One lesion is suggestive of a ruptured plaque showing discontinuity of the fibrous cap (white arrow). Reproduced with permission from Wiesmann F, Robson MD, Francis J, *et al.* Images in cardiovascular medicine. Visualization of the ruptured plaque by magnetic resonance imaging. *Circulation* 2003; **108**(20):2542.

Diagnosis of coronary artery disease

Acute coronary syndromes

The accurate triage of patients presenting with acute chest pain is a challenging problem in daily clinical practice. Only approximately 30% of patients with chest pain are clearly defined at presentation as having acute coronary syndromes based on history, ECG changes, and serial enzyme elevations(59). Because of the potential catastrophic consequences of the premature discharge of patients at risk for coronary events, the threshold to keep these patients in hospital is low, leading to many unnecessary admissions with major logistic and financial implications for healthcare providers. On the other hand, 2–4% of patients with chest pain discharged from emergency departments experience an acute coronary syndrome within 30 days(60). The application of a comprehensive CMR study in patients presenting with chest pain could potentially improve the efficiency of evaluation and reduce unnecessary admissions. To perform such examinations on patients with acute coronary syndromes in a timely and safe fashion, the MR scanner should be fully integrated with the emergency department. The safety and feasibility of a CMR approach for evaluation of patients presenting with chest pain to the emergency department has been demonstrated. A combination of cine, rest perfusion, and LGE imaging showed a sensitivity and specificity of approximately 85% for detecting acute coronary syndrome(61). Most of these patients had unstable angina because, by design, they had negative initial cardiac biomarkers and a negative ECG. One main limitation of this study was the difficulty in differentiating prior myocardial infarction from new acute coronary syndrome. However, as discussed earlier, the addition of T2-weighted imaging to cine and late enhancement CMR allows the differentiation between acute and chronic myocardial infarction. This new approach improved the overall accuracy of CMR to identify patients with acute coronary syndromes[(62)]. Inclusion of T2-weighted imaging improved specificity (from 84% to 96%), compared to the standard CMR protocol (cine, perfusion, and LGE) but sensitivity remained the same (85%). On the other hand, LV wall motion analysis at rest had poor specificity (10%) but excellent sensitivity (100%), which shows the complementary nature of information that can be derived from a comprehensive CMR study[(62)]. Another study determined the diagnostic value of adenosine CMR in 135 troponin-negative patients with chest pain[(63)]. The imaging protocol included regional and global function, adenosine stress perfusion, and infarct imaging within 72h of presentation to the emergency department. Adenosine CMR perfusion abnormalities had 100% sensitivity and 93% specificity for detection of significant coronary artery disease, and an abnormal CMR scan added significant prognostic value over that of clinical risk factors regarding prediction of a future diagnosis of CAD, myocardial infarction, or death.

CMR is effective in demonstrating the complications of acute myocardial infarction including ventricular aneurysm, pseudoaneurysm, ventricular septum rupture, and mitral regurgitation[(64)]. As echocardiography may yield a comparably high rate of false positive and false negative results regarding detection of LV thrombi post-infarction, the highly reliable CMR method is particularly useful in this setting (Fig. 13.8). The safety and diagnostic accuracy of stress CMR imaging early after ST- segment elevation myocardial infarction has been demonstrated[(65)]. Thirty-five patients admitted with first acute ST-segment elevation myocardial infarction underwent a comprehensive CMR protocol (rest cine, rest and stress perfusion, and LGE) and exercise tolerance testing before standard invasive coronary angiography. No complications occurred and all patients completed the CMR protocol. CMR was more sensitive (86% vs. 48%, $p = 0.007$) and specific (100% vs. 50%, $p < 0.001$) than exercise tolerance testing to detect significant coronary stenoses, and more sensitive (94% vs. 56%, $p = 0.04$) to predict the need for revascularization.

Acute myocarditis may present with acute chest pain masquerading as acute coronary syndrome. CMR imaging has an important role in establishing the diagnosis of this condition. Such patients may show areas of subepicardial/mid wall hyperenhancement with typical sparing of the subendocardium, and the septal and inferolateral walls are frequently involved[(66)]. T2-weighted images early after symptom onset may show regions of increased signal defining focal areas of myocardial oedema. Importantly, CMR provides information on the exact localization of myocardial damage caused by myocarditis which can be used to guide biopsy, enhancing sensitivity and specificity.

Aortic diseases and particularly aortic dissection should be ruled out in a patient presenting in the emergency department with abrupt onset chest pain. CMR has excellent diagnostic accuracy, combining high sensitivity and specificity for the detection of nearly all forms of aortic dissection[(67)]. However, rapid access to CMR imaging is limited in most centres, unstable patients are unsuitable for CMR, because patient monitoring/access during scanning is limited, and because a CMR study is much more time consuming than a MDCT scan. Therefore, CMR is typically only used in clinically/haemodynamically stable patients, and in chronic aortic dissections for follow-up imaging[(68)].

Assessment of stable coronary artery disease

In clinical practice, interventional cardiologists want to know whether a patient with stable chest pain has evidence of inducible ischaemia (and what the extent and locality of this is) and whether there is viable myocardium to justify revascularization. CMR can give reliable answers to all these questions. Both viability and ischaemia assessment are CMR techniques now firmly established in clinical practice. The relative technical ease of LGE imaging has enabled its widespread application and, currently, LGE forms a fundamental part of the scanning protocol for patients with CAD (see also Myocardial injury section)[(39,40)]. An example of the extent to which LGE has changed our perception of viability is in patients with significantly thinned (<6mm) myocardial segments, which would previously have been considered non-viable. Post revascularization, such segments can show improvement in contractile function and recovery of diastolic wall thickness[(69)] if they exhibit no or only subendocardial (1–25% transmural extent) scarring.

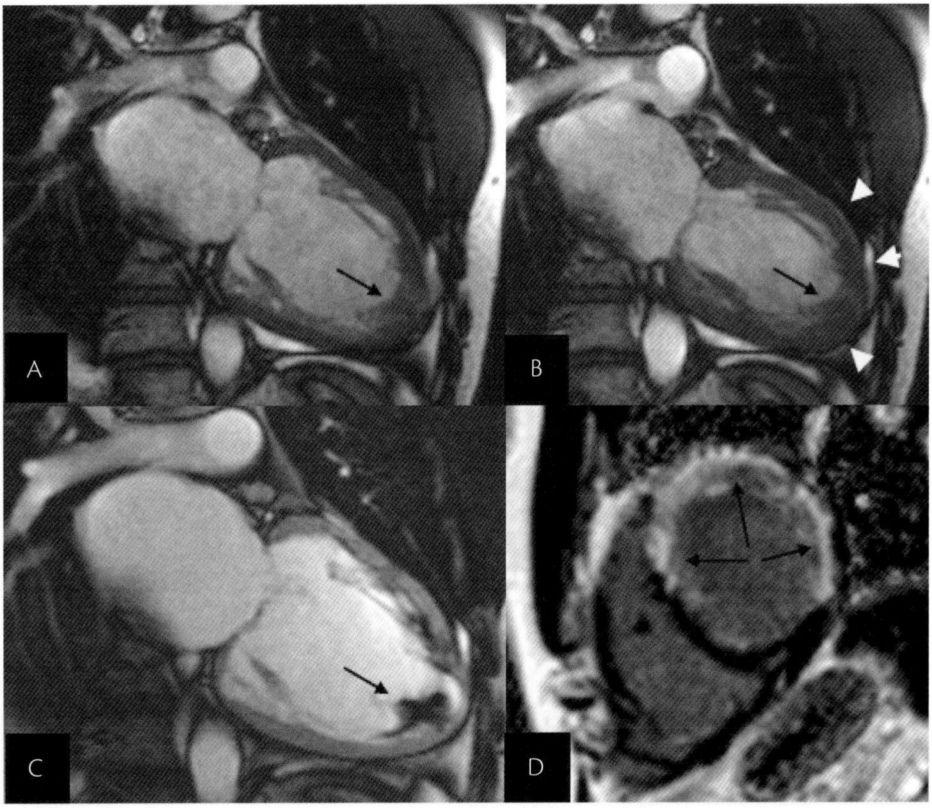

Fig. 13.8 A patient with extensive septal and anterolateral infarct. Panels (A) and (B) are still-frames from the vertical long-axis (2-chamber view) cine in end-diastole and end-systole respectively. Note the area of akinesis (white arrowheads) in the anterior wall, and the presence of a thrombus ((black arrow) at the akinetic apex. C) Image obtained early post-contrast with a segmented inversion recovery gradient echo sequence (long inversion time, 450ms) confirming the presence of thrombus at the apex (black arrow). Panel (D) is the late gadolinium enhancement (LGE) short-axis image which shows a near transmural infarct of the anterior septum, anterior and lateral walls. The inferior septum, which shows <25% of LGE and the inferior wall which has no LGE, are viable.

Multiple studies have proven the clinical feasibility, safety and high diagnostic accuracy of first-pass perfusion CMR with vasodilator stress for the detection of CAD (see also'Perfusion' section)[25,70–74]. A recent meta-analysis of 14 single-centre studies (1183 patients) demonstrated a pooled sensitivity of 91% and specificity of 81%, compared to conventional X-ray coronary angiography[70]. Recently, a multicentre-multivendor trial compared CMR perfusion with SPECT in 234 patients and showed at least equivalent diagnostic performance of CMR (area under the receiver operator characteristic curve 0.86 for CMR vs. 0.75 for SPECT, $p = 0.12$)[75]. Higher field strengths have the advantage of improved signal-to-noise ratio with theoretical advantages for perfusion imaging. Therefore, adenosine stress perfusion imaging at 3 Tesla has yielded improved diagnostic accuracy for the identification of single- and multivessel disease compared to 1.5 Tesla[71]. Recently, a multimodality approach incorporating elements of cine function, LGE, and stress perfusion imaging has been proposed to increase the accuracy of CAD detection (Fig. 13.9)[76]. With this approach, perfusion defects that have similar intensity and extent during both stress and rest ('fixed defects') without exhibiting LGE are considered to be artefacts, thereby improving the specificity of the test.

The efficacy of high-dose DSCMR (up to 40mcg/kg/min and atropine) for detecting CAD has clearly been shown (see also 'Stress-induced wall motion abnormalities: high-dose dobutamine CMR' section)[77]. Furthermore, the diagnostic performance of DSCMR has been compared with dobutamine stress echo in the

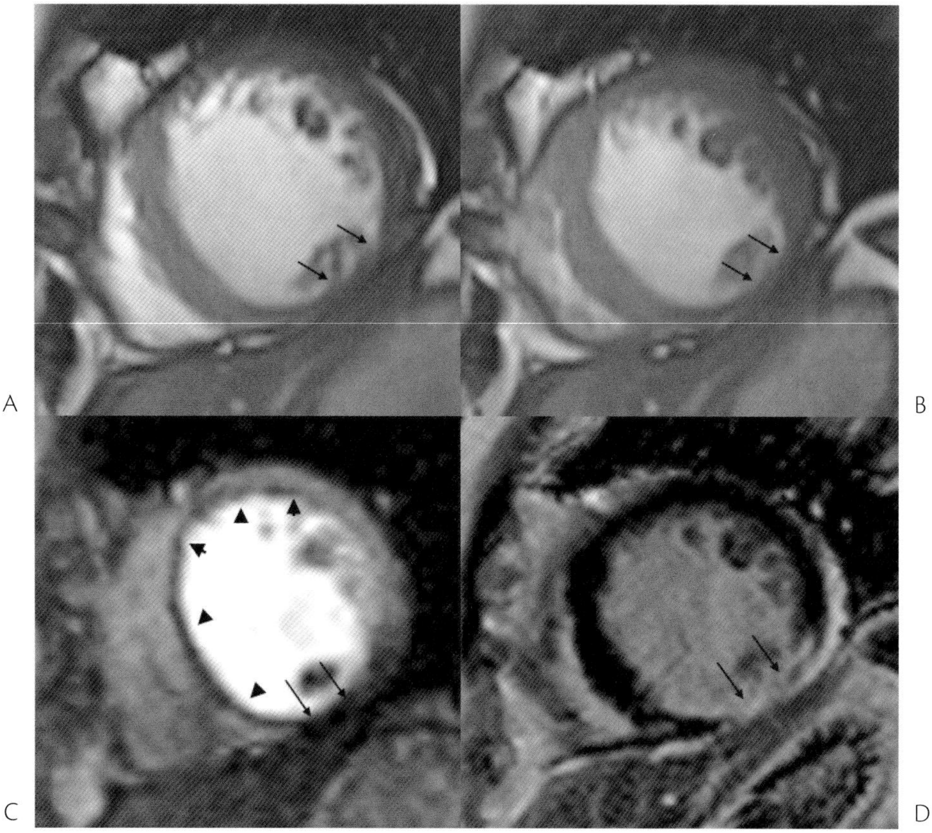

Fig. 13.9 A patient with previous inferior infarct and inducible ischaemia in 2-vessels. Panels (A) and (B) are still frames from the equatorial short-axis cine in end-diastole and end-systole respectively. Note the area of akinesis (black arrows) in the inferior wall. Panel (C) is a still frame from the stress perfusion cine (on the same slice position) showing an extensive subendocardial perfusion defect involving the anterior, septal and inferior walls (black arrow heads). Panel (D) is the corresponding LGE image showing a near transmural inferior infarct (black arrows). Thus, overall, this patient has evidence of two vessel disease (LAD and RCA) but the inferior wall is akinetic and non-viable whereas the anterior wall and the septum are fully viable.

same cohort of patients who underwent both procedures and found to have superior diagnostic accuracy (86% vs. 73%, p <0.05)[77]. The application of DSCMR is particularly advantageous in patients with poor acoustic windows[78]. Only one study has compared DSCMR with adenosine perfusion CMR in the same patient cohort. Adenosine perfusion CMR had slightly better sensitivity (91% vs. 89%), but worse specificity (62% vs. 80%) than DSCMR[79]. A recent meta-analysis of stress CMR studies showed that, overall, CMR perfusion imaging is more sensitive (91% vs. 85%) but less specific (81% vs. 86%) compared to imaging of stress-induced wall motion abnormalities[70]. In most CMR colleagues' clinical practice, adenosine perfusion CMR is the routine stress test and DSCMR is applied only when contraindications to adenosine such as asthma or atrioventricular block preclude its use.

In addition to ischaemia and viability imaging, CMR can provide some information on coronary anatomy, although luminal stenosis assessment is still challenging. In clinical practice, the main application of MRCA is the identification of anomalous origin and course of coronary arteries, and the assessment of Kawasaki disease and coronary artery aneurysms[50,80]. Reliable detection of CAD beyond the proximal coronary arteries requires further improvements in MR sequences (see also 'Magnetic resonance coronary angiography' section). The only multicentre but single-vendor study of 3D MRCA involved 109 patients and demonstrated 93% sensitivity, 58% specificity, and 81% negative predictive value for the identification of ≥50% diameter stenosis by invasive quantitative coronary angiography[81]. The sensitivity and negative predictive value for the identification of left-main or three-vessel disease were

100%, thereby demonstrating a role for MRCA for this subset. However, 16% of proximal and middle segments of coronary arteries were non-interpretable and were excluded from final analysis. Single-centre data obtained with free-breathing navigator-gated whole-heart MRCA suggest that the whole-heart approach (a technique for imaging the entire coronary tree in a single volume) provides faster acquisition (<15min) and superior accuracy, with sensitivities ranging between 80–90% and specificity of around 90%[50]. Two comparison studies of coronary MRA and 16-slice MDCT demonstrated similar accuracy when compared with free-breathing MRCA[82] and superior results for MDCT when compared with a combination of free-breathing and lower-resolution breath-hold coronary MRA[83]. Importantly, the studies discussed here were performed at research-oriented centres that have the expertise to perform high-quality MRCA. The utility of coronary MRCA in general practice has not been established, and multivendor trials have not been conducted yet.

CMR and prognosis in ischaemic heart disease

An important goal of any stress modality in cardiology is to not only distinguish the presence from the absence of functionally significant coronary artery stenoses but also to discriminate those patients at high risk for future cardiac events from those with a low cardiac event rate. A wealth of prognostication data from nuclear techniques is available from the last two decades. Although CMR, and particularly the LGE or first-pass perfusion techniques, are relatively new imaging tools, data on the prognostic role of CMR imaging in patients with CAD are rapidly emerging.

Recently, the utility of CMR adenosine perfusion imaging and of dobutamine wall motion imaging for predicting cardiac death and non-fatal myocardial infarction in a large patient population with known or suspected CAD has been demonstrated[84]. A patient with ischaemia detected by adenosine stress CMR has a 12-fold increased risk for experiencing a subsequent cardiac event over 3 years. The risk of major cardiac events is fivefold increased if wall motion abnormalities are detected by DSCMR. Similar data are also available for dipyridamole stress CMR[85].

Data on the rapidly expanding prognostic value of LGE-CMR are also available. The presence of LGE in patients with suspected CAD but no known history of myocardial infarction is the most important independent predictor of major cardiac adverse events over other clinical predictors, including ejection fraction[86]. Even patients with small amounts of scarring involving just 1.4% of LV mass experienced more than a sevenfold increased risk for major adverse cardiac events[86]. In diabetic patients without clinical evidence of myocardial infarction, the presence of LGE is strongly associated with major adverse cardiac events and mortality hazards[87]. Furthermore, the presence of extensive peri-infarct regions of intermediate hyperenhancement (defined as hyperenhancement with signal intensity two to three standard deviations above normal) is associated with increased mortality risk[88]. Increased infarct tissue heterogeneity identified by CMR augments the susceptibility to ventricular arrhythmias in patients with prior myocardial infarction and LV dysfunction[89]. These findings suggest that tissue characterization by CMR may serve as a novel tool for arrhythmia risk assessment after myocardial infarction and several studies are underway testing this hypothesis.

CMR to guide intervention

Standard X-ray fluoroscopy as used in the cardiac catheterization lab provides excellent spatial and temporal resolution, but soft tissues are virtually impossible to distinguish. On the other hand, CMR offers excellent soft tissue visualization in any plane without exposing patients and staff to ionizing radiation. As a result, interventional CMR has emerged as a complement to X-ray techniques for cardiovascular interventions (e.g. closure of septal defects or percutaneous placement of heart valves), and for peripheral vascular and cardiac electrophysiology applications. A combination of X-ray and CMR imaging (XMR) in a single suite has been designed for new interventional procedures. It should be borne in mind, however, that most commercially available diagnostic and guide catheters, balloon expandable stents, guide wires, and device delivery systems are not MR compatible and thus not suitable for interventional CMR. Therefore, specific MR compatible devices for visualization and minimal image distortion are being developed. Two approaches have been developed for tracking vascular intervention in the MR environment, *passive* and *active* catheter tracking [23,25]. Passive catheter tracking relies on material properties of the endovascular catheter allowing sufficient contrast with the blood pool on the MR images. This was achieved by coating the shaft or tip of the catheter with MR markers[26] or inflating a balloon with carbon dioxide at the tip of the catheter to cause signal loss[29]. Active catheter tracking[23,25] involves incorporating a radiofrequency coil into the catheter itself.

Early feasibility studies for interventional CMR targeted large peripheral vessels not subject to significant cardiac and respiratory motion. Carotid, renal, and iliac arteries have been successfully subjected to angiography and angioplasty solely under CMR control(90). More complex interventions have been performed under MR-guidance such as endovascular stenting of aortic aneurysms and dissections, as well as carotid, iliac, and renal arteries(90). One of the most compelling potential applications of interventional CMR is its use in the recanalization of chronic total occlusions. It is well known that X-ray angiography with contrast identifies the arteries up- and downstream of the occlusion, but the occluded segment itself remains invisible. Interventional CMR has been used in a swine model of peripheral artery chronic total occlusion to help operators traverse the occluded segment while keeping the equipment inside the walls of the target artery(91). Clinical-grade devices are currently under development to translate this experience into humans. Moreover, coronary angiography, angioplasty, and stent deployment in healthy swine have been described(92). Diagnostic catheterization in patients with congenital disease with the use of a hybrid XMR system has been reported(93).

CMR imaging has the potential to non-invasively measure the success of therapies such as intramyocardial injection of cells or of angiogenesis growth factors. Furthermore, the use of iron particles for labelling such cells allows the possibility to track the injection and distribution of injected cells in myocardium and other tissues. Real-time CMR has been used to deliver cells, by customized injection catheters, to the infarct border in a swine model(94). This study highlighted real-time infarct imaging, anatomically targeted endomyocardial injection, and verification of delivery with the use of an intracellular MR contrast agent.

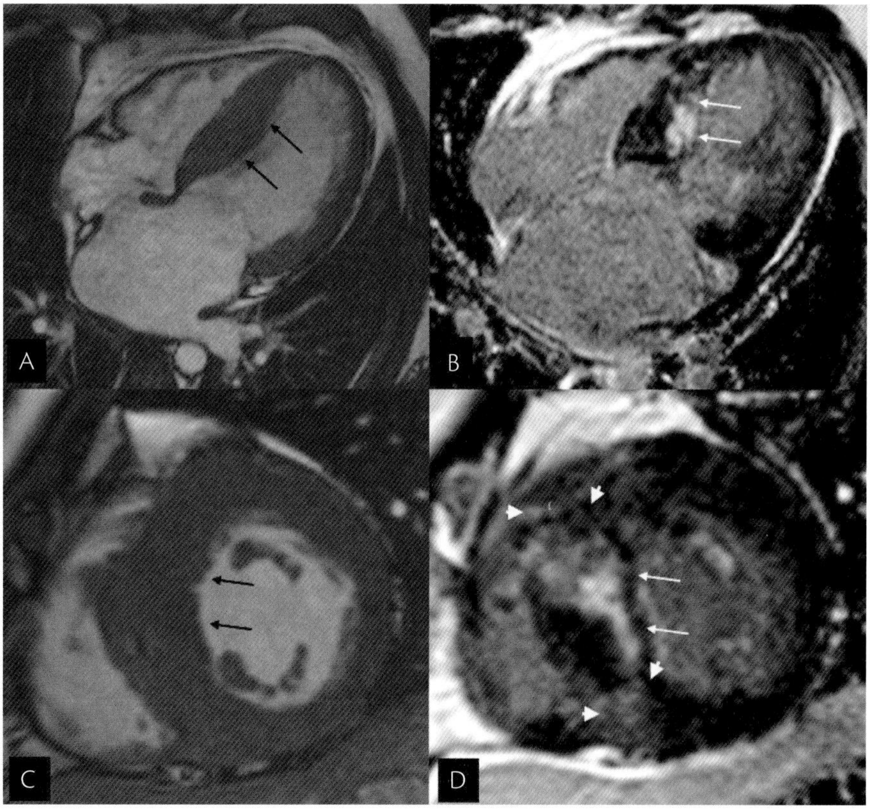

Fig. 13.10 A patient with hypertrophic cardiomyopathy. Still end-diastolic frames from SSFP cines—horizontal long axis (A) and short-axis at the mid-ventricular level (C) showing significant asymmetric septal hypertrophy (black arrows). Corresponding images using the late gadolinium enhancement (LGE) technique—(B) and (D) respectively. The pattern of mid-wall septal hyperenhancement is patchy, diffuse (white arrows), and typically involves both LV–RV junctions (white arrowheads). Note the differences from 'ischaemic' pattern of LGE which always involves the subendocardium (see Fig. 13.6 for comparison).

Interventional CMR might also afford surgical-style anatomic imaging guidance to electrophysiology procedures, in positioning and in depicting actual ablation lesions during procedures[(95)]. Recently, the first active-imaging MR catheters with appropriate filtering to acquire intracardiac electrograms during real-time CMR were described and first-in-man intracardiac electrograms in patients during CMR were obtained[(96)].

The future growth of endovascular MR-guided procedures depends on the safety and availability of MR-friendly devices and delivery systems. Clearly, interventional CMR has great potential and significant progress has been made in this area over the past few years. However, much work remains to be done towards the widespread clinical application of interventional CMR.

CMR for the diagnosis of non-ischaemic heart disease

CMR has found fertile ground in the field of non-ischaemic cardiomyopathies, mainly because of its intrinsic ability to provide information on myocardial tissue characterization. In hypertrophic cardiomyopathy, CMR can diagnose and determine the extent of hypertrophy more accurately than echocardiography. Moreover, diffuse areas of myocardial fibrosis can be identified with the use of LGE (Fig. 13.10)[(97)]. In patients with arrhythmogenic right ventricular cardiomyopathy, CMR can detect global right ventricular abnormalities, right ventricular aneurysms, or regional wall motion abnormalities. In advanced cases, fibrofatty myocardial infiltration might also be identified[(98)]. Myocardial and liver iron overload as a result of thalassaemia can be quantitatively assessed by measurement of myocardial $T2^*$[(99)]. This is useful to guide treatment and monitor response to iron chelating drug regimens[(100)]. CMR is also helpful in differentiating constrictive from restrictive cardiomyopathy. Thickened pericardium and abnormal motion of the septum due to increased interventricular dependence can be readily recognized in cases of constriction[(101)]. Systemic amyloidosis, sarcoidosis and other infiltrative diseases such as Fabry disease or endomyocardial fibroelastosis show characteristic abnormalities on LGE imaging[(102)].

Conclusions

CMR has enabled a new, advanced approach for assessing patients with ischaemic heart disease without exposure to ionizing radiation. CMR has become the gold standard imaging technique to assess myocardial anatomy, regional/global function and viability and also allows the assessment of perfusion and acute tissue injury (oedema and necrosis). The information derived from CMR can be used to guide management and stratify risk in patients with ischaemic heart disease. The high measurement accuracy of CMR makes it an ideal technique for monitoring of disease progression and of the effects of treatment. Interventional CMR is an area of active development and will be increasingly used to guide therapeutic procedures.

References

1. Fieno DS. Cardiac magnetic resonance: physics, pulse sequences, and clinical applications. *Rev Cardiovasc Med* 2008; **9**(3):174–86.
2. Abdel-Aty H, Simonetti O, Friedrich MG. T2-weighted cardiovascular magnetic resonance imaging. *J Magn Reson Imaging* 2007; **26**(3):452–9.
3. Shellock FG, Crues JV. MR procedures: biologic effects, safety, and patient care. *Radiology* 2004; **232**(3):635–52.
4. Levine GN, Gomes AS, Arai AE, *et al.* Safety of magnetic resonance imaging in patients with cardiovascular devices: an American Heart Association scientific statement from the Committee on Diagnostic and Interventional Cardiac Catheterization, Council on Clinical Cardiology, and the Council on Cardiovascular Radiology and Intervention: endorsed by the American College of Cardiology Foundation, the North American Society for Cardiac Imaging, and the Society for Cardiovascular Magnetic Resonance. *Circulation* 2007; **116**(24):2878–91.
5. Chung T. Assessment of cardiovascular anatomy in patients with congenital heart disease by magnetic resonance imaging. *Pediatr Cardiol* 2000; **21**(1):18–26.
6. Sarwar A, Shapiro MD, Abbara S, *et al.* Cardiac magnetic resonance imaging for the evaluation of ventricular function. *Semin Roentgenol* 2008; **43**(3):183–92.
7. Karamitsos TD, Hudsmith LE, Selvanayagam JB, *et al.* Operator induced variability in left ventricular measurements with cardiovascular magnetic resonance is improved after training. *J Cardiovasc Magn Reson* 2007; **9**(5):777–83.
8. Bellenger NG, Davies LC, Francis JM, *et al.* Reduction in sample size for studies of remodeling in heart failure by the use of cardiovascular magnetic resonance. *J Cardiovasc Magn Reson* 2000; **2**(4):271–8.
9. Reichek N. MRI myocardial tagging. *J Magn Reson Imaging* 1999; **10**(5):609–16.
10. Petersen SE, Jung BA, Wiesmann F, *et al.* Myocardial tissue phase mapping with cine phase-contrast MR imaging: regional wall motion analysis in healthy volunteers. *Radiology* 2006; **238**(3):816–26.
11. Kilner PJ, Gatehouse PD, Firmin DN. Flow measurement by magnetic resonance: a unique asset worth optimising. *J Cardiovasc Magn Reson* 2007; **9**(4):723–8.
12. Chai P, Mohiaddin R. How we perform cardiovascular magnetic resonance flow assessment using phase-contrast velocity mapping. *J Cardiovasc Magn Reson* 2005; **7**(4):705–16.

13. Gatehouse PD, Keegan J, Crowe LA, *et al.* Applications of phase-contrast flow and velocity imaging in cardiovascular MRI. *Eur Radiol* 2005; **15**(10):2172–84.
14. Kizilbash AM, Hundley WG, Willett DL, *et al.* Comparison of quantitative Doppler with magnetic resonance imaging for assessment of the severity of mitral regurgitation. *Am J Cardiol* 1998; **81**(6):792–5.
15. Beerbaum P, Korperich H, Barth P, *et al.* Noninvasive quantification of left-to-right shunt in pediatric patients:phase-contrast cine magnetic resonance imaging compared with invasive oximetry. *Circulation* 2001; **103**(20):2476–82.
16. King SB, 3rd, Smith SC, Jr, Hirshfeld JW, Jr, *et al.* 2007 focused update of the ACC/AHA/SCAI 2005 guideline update for percutaneous coronary intervention:a report of the American College of Cardiology/American Heart Association Task Force on Practice guidelines. *J Am Coll Cardiol* 2008; **51**(2):172–209.
17. Shaw LJ, Berman DS, Maron DJ, *et al.* Optimal medical therapy with or without percutaneous coronary intervention to reduce ischemic burden: results from the Clinical Outcomes Utilizing Revascularization and Aggressive Drug Evaluation (COURAGE) trial nuclear substudy. *Circulation* 2008; **117**(10):1283–91.
18. Atkinson DJ, Burstein D, Edelman RR. First-pass cardiac perfusion: evaluation with ultrafast MR imaging. *Radiology* 1990; **174**(3 Pt 1):757–62.
19. Pennell DJ. Cardiovascular magnetic resonance and the role of adenosine pharmacologic stress. *Am J Cardiol* 2004; **94**(2A): 26D–31D; discussion 1D–2D.
20. Gebker R, Schwitter J, Fleck E, *et al.* How we perform myocardial perfusion with cardiovascular magnetic resonance. *J Cardiovasc Magn Reson* 2007; **9**(3):539–47.
21. Jerosch-Herold M, Seethamraju RT, Swingen CM, *et al.* Analysis of myocardial perfusion MRI. *J Magn Reson Imaging* 2004; **19**(6):758–70.
22. Kellman P, Arai AE. Imaging sequences for first pass perfusion—a review. *J Cardiovasc Magn Reson* 2007; **9**(3):525–37.
23. Di Bella EV, Parker DL, Sinusas AJ. On the dark rim artifact in dynamic contrast-enhanced MRI myocardial perfusion studies. *Magn Reson Med* 2005; **54**(5):1295–9.
24. Sakuma H, Suzawa N, Ichikawa Y, *et al.* Diagnostic accuracy of stress first-pass contrast-enhanced myocardial perfusion MRI compared with stress myocardial perfusion scintigraphy. *AJR Am J Roentgenol* 2005; **185**(1):95–102.
25. Karamitsos TD, Arnold JR, Pegg TJ, *et al.* Tolerance and safety of adenosine stress perfusion cardiovascular magnetic resonance imaging in patients with severe coronary artery disease. *Int J Cardiovasc Imaging* 2009; **25**(3):277–83.
26. Cerqueira MD, Verani MS, Schwaiger M, *et al.* Safety profile of adenosine stress perfusion imaging: results from the Adenoscan Multicenter Trial Registry. *J Am Coll Cardiol* 1994; **23**(2):384–9.
27. Mandapaka S, Hundley WG. Dobutamine cardiovascular magnetic resonance: a review. *J Magn Reson Imaging* 2006; **24**(3):499–512.
28. Hundley WG, Bluemke D, Bogaert JG, *et al.* Society for Cardiovascular Magnetic Resonance guidelines for reporting cardiovascular magnetic resonance examinations. *J Cardiovasc Magn Reson* 2009; **11**(1):5.
29. Poldermans D, Fioretti PM, Boersma E, *et al.* Safety of dobutamine-atropine stress echocardiography in patients with suspected or proven coronary artery disease. *Am J Cardiol* 1994; **73**(7):456–9.
30. Lattanzi F, Picano E, Adamo E, *et al.* Dobutamine stress echocardiography: safety in diagnosing coronary artery disease. *Drug Saf* 2000; **22**(4):251–62.
31. Wahl A, Paetsch I, Gollesch A, *et al.* Safety and feasibility of high-dose dobutamine-atropine stress cardiovascular magnetic resonance for diagnosis of myocardial ischaemia: experience in 1000 consecutive cases. *Eur Heart J* 2004; **25**(14):1230–6.
32. Kim RJ, Fieno DS, Parrish TB, *et al.* Relationship of MRI delayed contrast enhancement to irreversible injury, infarct age, and contractile function. *Circulation* 1999; **100**(19):1992–2002.
33. Fieno DS, Kim RJ, Chen EL, *et al.* Contrast-enhanced magnetic resonance imaging of myocardium at risk: distinction between reversible and irreversible injury throughout infarct healing. *J Am Coll Cardiol* 2000; **36**(6):1985–91.
34. Wagner A, Mahrholdt H, Holly TA, *et al.* Contrast-enhanced MRI and routine single photon emission computed tomography (SPECT) perfusion imaging for detection of subendocardial myocardial infarcts: an imaging study. *Lancet* 2003; **361**(9355):374–9.
35. Schaefer S, Malloy CR, Katz J, *et al.* Gadolinium-DTPA-enhanced nuclear magnetic resonance imaging of reperfused myocardium: identification of the myocardial bed at risk. *J Am Coll Cardiol* 1988; **12**(4):1064–72.
36. Rehwald WG, Fieno DS, Chen EL, *et al.* Myocardial magnetic resonance imaging contrast agent concentrations after reversible and irreversible ischemic injury. *Circulation* 2002; **105**(2):224–9.
37. Mahrholdt H, Wagner A, Judd RM, *et al.* Delayed enhancement cardiovascular magnetic resonance assessment of non-ischaemic cardiomyopathies. *Eur Heart J* 2005; **26**(15):1461–74.
38. Kim RJ, Chen EL, Lima JA, *et al.* Myocardial Gd-DTPA kinetics determine MRI contrast enhancement and reflect the extent and severity of myocardial injury after acute reperfused infarction. *Circulation* 1996; **94**(12):3318–26.
39. Kim RJ, Wu E, Rafael A, *et al.* The use of contrast-enhanced magnetic resonance imaging to identify reversible myocardial dysfunction. *N Engl J Med* 2000; **343**(20):1445–53.
40. Selvanayagam JB, Kardos A, Francis JM, *et al.* Value of delayed-enhancement cardiovascular magnetic resonance imaging in predicting myocardial viability after surgical revascularization. *Circulation* 2004; **110**(12):1535–41.
41. Bonow RO. Identification of viable myocardium. *Circulation* 1996; **94**(11):2674–80.
42. Kaandorp TA, Bax JJ, Schuijf JD, *et al.* Head-to-head comparison between contrast-enhanced magnetic

resonance imaging and dobutamine magnetic resonance imaging in men with ischemic cardiomyopathy. *Am J Cardiol* 2004; **93**(12):1461–4.

43. Selvanayagam JB, Porto I, Channon K, *et al.* Troponin elevation after percutaneous coronary intervention directly represents the extent of irreversible myocardial injury: insights from cardiovascular magnetic resonance imaging. *Circulation* 2005; **111**(8):1027–32.
44. Wu KC, Zerhouni EA, Judd RM, *et al.* Prognostic significance of microvascular obstruction by magnetic resonance imaging in patients with acute myocardial infarction. *Circulation* 1998; **97**(8):765–72.
45. Aletras AH, Tilak GS, Natanzon A, *et al.* Retrospective determination of the area at risk for reperfused acute myocardial infarction with T2-weighted cardiac magnetic resonance imaging: histopathological and displacement encoding with stimulated echoes (DENSE) functional validations. *Circulation* 2006; **113**(15):1865–70.
46. Mukherjee A, Buja LM, Scales FE, *et al.* Abnormal myocardial fluid retention as an early manifestation of ischemic injury. *Recent Adv Stud Cardiac Struct Metab* 1976; **12**:245–52.
47. Friedrich MG, Abdel-Aty H, Taylor A, *et al.* The salvaged area at risk in reperfused acute myocardial infarction as visualized by cardiovascular magnetic resonance. *J Am Coll Cardiol* 2008; **51**(16):1581–7.
48. Wellnhofer E, Olariu A, Klein C, *et al.* Magnetic resonance low-dose dobutamine test is superior to SCAR quantification for the prediction of functional recovery. *Circulation* 2004; **109**(18):2172–4.
49. DeFrances CJ, Lucas CA, Buie VC, *et al.* 2006 National Hospital Discharge Survey. *Natl Health Stat Report* 2008; **5**:1–20.
50. Bluemke DA, Achenbach S, Budoff M, *et al.* Noninvasive coronary artery imaging: magnetic resonance angiography and multidetector computed tomography angiography: a scientific statement from the American Heart Association Committee on Cardiovascular Imaging and Intervention of The Council on Cardiovascular Radiology and Intervention, and the Councils on Clinical Cardiology and Cardiovascular Disease In The Young. *Circulation* 2008; **118**(5):586–606.
51. Stuber M, Weiss RG. Coronary magnetic resonance angiography. *J Magn Reson Imaging* 2007; **26**(2):219–34.
52. Wiesmann F, Robson MD, Francis J, *et al.* Images in cardiovascular medicine. Visualization of the ruptured plaque by magnetic resonance imaging. *Circulation* 2003; **108**(20):2542.
53. Lindsay AC, Choudhury RP. Form to function: current and future roles for atherosclerosis imaging in drug development. *Nat Rev Drug Discov* 2008; **7**(6):517–29.
54. Cai J, Hatsukami TS, Ferguson MS, *et al.* In vivo quantitative measurement of intact fibrous cap and lipid-rich necrotic core size in atherosclerotic carotid plaque: comparison of high-resolution, contrast-enhanced magnetic resonance imaging and histology. *Circulation* 2005; **112**(22):3437–44.
55. Takaya N, Yuan C, Chu B, *et al.* Association between carotid plaque characteristics and subsequent ischemic cerebrovascular events: a prospective assessment with MRI—initial results. *Stroke* 2006; **37**(3):818–23.
56. Botnar RM, Stuber M, Kissinger KV, *et al.* Noninvasive coronary vessel wall and plaque imaging with magnetic resonance imaging. *Circulation* 2000; **102**(21):2582–7.
57. Fayad ZA, Fuster V, Fallon JT, *et al.* Noninvasive in vivo human coronary artery lumen and wall imaging using black-blood magnetic resonance imaging. *Circulation* 2000; **102**(5):506–10.
58. Jaffer FA, Libby P, Weissleder R. Molecular imaging of cardiovascular disease. *Circulation* 2007; **116**(9):1052–61.
59. Pope JH, Ruthazer R, Beshansky JR, *et al.* Clinical Features of Emergency Department Patients Presenting with Symptoms Suggestive of Acute Cardiac Ischemia: A Multicenter Study. *J Thromb Thrombolysis* 1998; **6**(1): 63–74.
60. Pope JH, Aufderheide TP, Ruthazer R, *et al.* Missed diagnoses of acute cardiac ischemia in the emergency department. *N Engl J Med* 2000; **342**(16):1163–70.
61. Kwong RY, Schussheim AE, Rekhraj S, *et al.* Detecting acute coronary syndrome in the emergency department with cardiac magnetic resonance imaging. *Circulation* 2003; **107**(4):531–7.
62. Cury RC, Shash K, Nagurney JT, *et al.* Cardiac magnetic resonance with T2-weighted imaging improves detection of patients with acute coronary syndrome in the emergency department. *Circulation* 2008; **118**(8):837–44.
63. Ingkanisorn WP, Kwong RY, Bohme NS, *et al.* Prognosis of negative adenosine stress magnetic resonance in patients presenting to an emergency department with chest pain. *J Am Coll Cardiol* 2006; **47**(7):1427–32.
64. Shapiro MD, Guarraia DL, Moloo J, *et al.* Evaluation of acute coronary syndromes by cardiac magnetic resonance imaging. *Top Magn Reson Imaging* 2008; **19**(1):25–32.
65. Greenwood JP, Younger JF, Ridgway JP, *et al.* Safety and diagnostic accuracy of stress cardiac magnetic resonance imaging vs exercise tolerance testing early after acute ST elevation myocardial infarction. *Heart* 2007; **93**(11): 1363–8.
66. Mahrholdt H, Goedecke C, Wagner A, *et al.* Cardiovascular magnetic resonance assessment of human myocarditis: a comparison to histology and molecular pathology. *Circulation* 2004; **109**(10):1250–8.
67. Kersting-Sommerhoff BA, Higgins CB, White RD, *et al.* Aortic dissection: sensitivity and specificity of MR imaging. *Radiology* 1988; **166**(3):651–5.
68. Erbel R, Alfonso F, Boileau C, *et al.* Diagnosis and management of aortic dissection. *Eur Heart J* 2001; **22**(18):1642–81.
69. Kim RJ, Shah DJ. Fundamental concepts in myocardial viability assessment revisited: when knowing how much is "alive" is not enough. *Heart* 2004; **90**(2):137–40.
70. Nandalur KR, Dwamena BA, Choudhri AF, *et al.* Diagnostic performance of stress cardiac magnetic resonance imaging in the detection of coronary artery

disease: a meta-analysis. *J Am Coll Cardiol* 2007; **50**(14):1343–53.

71. Cheng AS, Pegg TJ, Karamitsos TD, *et al.* Cardiovascular magnetic resonance perfusion imaging at 3-tesla for the detection of coronary artery disease: a comparison with 1.5-tesla. *J Am Coll Cardiol* 2007; **49**(25):2440–9.
72. Nagel E, Klein C, Paetsch I, *et al.* Magnetic resonance perfusion measurements for the noninvasive detection of coronary artery disease. *Circulation* 2003; **108**(4):432–7.
73. Plein S, Radjenovic A, Ridgway JP, *et al.* Coronary artery disease: myocardial perfusion MR imaging with sensitivity encoding versus conventional angiography. *Radiology* 2005; **235**(2):423–30.
74. Cury RC, Cattani CA, Gabure LA, *et al.* Diagnostic performance of stress perfusion and delayed-enhancement MR imaging in patients with coronary artery disease. *Radiology* 2006; **240**(1):39–45.
75. Schwitter J, Wacker CM, van Rossum AC, *et al.* MR-IMPACT: comparison of perfusion-cardiac magnetic resonance with single-photon emission computed tomography for the detection of coronary artery disease in a multicentre, multivendor, randomized trial. *Eur Heart J* 2008; **29**(4):480–9.
76. Klem I, Heitner JF, Shah DJ, *et al.* Improved detection of coronary artery disease by stress perfusion cardiovascular magnetic resonance with the use of delayed enhancement infarction imaging. *J Am Coll Cardiol* 2006; **47**(8):1630–8.
77. Nagel E, Lehmkuhl HB, Bocksch W, *et al.* Noninvasive diagnosis of ischemia-induced wall motion abnormalities with the use of high-dose dobutamine stress MRI: comparison with dobutamine stress echocardiography. *Circulation* 1999; **99**(6):763–70.
78. Hundley WG, Hamilton CA, Thomas MS, *et al.* Utility of fast cine magnetic resonance imaging and display for the detection of myocardial ischemia in patients not well suited for second harmonic stress echocardiography. *Circulation* 1999; **100**(16):1697–702.
79. Paetsch I, Jahnke C, Wahl A, *et al.* Comparison of dobutamine stress magnetic resonance, adenosine stress magnetic resonance, and adenosine stress magnetic resonance perfusion. *Circulation* 2004; **110**(7):835–42.
80. Mavrogeni S, Papadopoulos G, Douskou M, *et al.* Magnetic resonance angiography is equivalent to X-ray coronary angiography for the evaluation of coronary arteries in Kawasaki disease. *J Am Coll Cardiol* 2004; **43**(4):649–52.
81. Kim WY, Danias PG, Stuber M, *et al.* Coronary magnetic resonance angiography for the detection of coronary stenoses. *N Engl J Med* 2001; **345**(26):1863–9.
82. Kefer J, Coche E, Legros G, *et al.* Head-to-head comparison of three-dimensional navigator-gated magnetic resonance imaging and 16-slice computed tomography to detect coronary artery stenosis in patients. *J Am Coll Cardiol* 2005; **46**(1):92–100.
83. Dewey M, Teige F, Schnapauff D, *et al.* Noninvasive detection of coronary artery stenoses with multislice computed tomography or magnetic resonance imaging. *Ann Intern Med* 2006; **145**(6):407–15.
84. Jahnke C, Nagel E, Gebker R, *et al.* Prognostic value of cardiac magnetic resonance stress tests: adenosine stress perfusion and dobutamine stress wall motion imaging. *Circulation* 2007; **115**(13):1769–76.
85. Bodi V, Sanchis J, Lopez-Lereu MP, *et al.* Prognostic value of dipyridamole stress cardiovascular magnetic resonance imaging in patients with known or suspected coronary artery disease. *J Am Coll Cardiol* 2007; **50**(12):1174–9.
86. Kwong RY, Chan AK, Brown KA, *et al.* Impact of unrecognized myocardial scar detected by cardiac magnetic resonance imaging on event-free survival in patients presenting with signs or symptoms of coronary artery disease. *Circulation* 2006; **113**(23):2733–43.
87. Kwong RY, Sattar H, Wu H, *et al.* Incidence and prognostic implication of unrecognized myocardial scar characterized by cardiac magnetic resonance in diabetic patients without clinical evidence of myocardial infarction. *Circulation* 2008; **118**(10):1011–20.
88. Yan AT, Shayne AJ, Brown KA, *et al.* Characterization of the peri-infarct zone by contrast-enhanced cardiac magnetic resonance imaging is a powerful predictor of post-myocardial infarction mortality. *Circulation* 2006; **114**(1):32–9.
89. Schmidt A, Azevedo CF, Cheng A, *et al.* Infarct tissue heterogeneity by magnetic resonance imaging identifies enhanced cardiac arrhythmia susceptibility in patients with left ventricular dysfunction. *Circulation* 2007; **115**(15):2006–14.
90. Raman VK, Lederman RJ. Interventional cardiovascular magnetic resonance imaging. *Trends Cardiovasc Med* 2007; **17**(6):196–202.
91. Raval AN, Karmarkar PV, Guttman MA, *et al.* Real-time magnetic resonance imaging-guided endovascular recanalization of chronic total arterial occlusion in a swine model. *Circulation* 2006; **113**(8):1101–7.
92. Spuentrup E, Ruebben A, Schaeffter T, *et al.* Magnetic resonance-guided coronary artery stent placement in a swine model. *Circulation* 2002; **105**(7):874–9.
93. Razavi R, Hill DL, Keevil SF, *et al.* Cardiac catheterisation guided by MRI in children and adults with congenital heart disease. *Lancet* 2003; **362**(9399):1877–82.
94. Dick AJ, Guttman MA, Raman VK, *et al.* Magnetic resonance fluoroscopy allows targeted delivery of mesenchymal stem cells to infarct borders in Swine. *Circulation* 2003; **108**(23):2899–904.
95. Peters DC, Wylie JV, Hauser TH, *et al.* Detection of pulmonary vein and left atrial scar after catheter ablation with three-dimensional navigator-gated delayed enhancement MR imaging: initial experience. *Radiology* 2007; **243**(3):690–5.
96. Nazarian S, Kolandaivelu A, Zviman MM, *et al.* Feasibility of real-time magnetic resonance imaging for catheter guidance in electrophysiology studies. *Circulation* 2008; **118**(3):223–9.

97. Moon JC, Reed E, Sheppard MN, *et al.* The histologic basis of late gadolinium enhancement cardiovascular magnetic resonance in hypertrophic cardiomyopathy. *J Am Coll Cardiol* 2004; **43**(12):2260–4.
98. Tandri H, Saranathan M, Rodriguez ER, *et al.* Noninvasive detection of myocardial fibrosis in arrhythmogenic right ventricular cardiomyopathy using delayed-enhancement magnetic resonance imaging. *J Am Coll Cardiol* 2005; **45**(1):98–103.
99. Anderson LJ, Holden S, Davis B, *et al.* Cardiovascular T2-star (T2*) magnetic resonance for the early diagnosis of myocardial iron overload. *Eur Heart J* 2001; **22**(23):2171–9.
100. Tanner MA, Galanello R, Dessi C, *et al.* A randomized, placebo-controlled, double-blind trial of the effect of combined therapy with deferoxamine and deferiprone on myocardial iron in thalassemia major using cardiovascular magnetic resonance. *Circulation* 2007; **115**(14):1876–84.
101. Francone M, Dymarkowski S, Kalantzi M, *et al.* Assessment of ventricular coupling with real-time cine MRI and its value to differentiate constrictive pericarditis from restrictive cardiomyopathy. *Eur Radiol* 2006; **16**(4):944–51.
102. Karamitsos TD, Francis JM, Myerson S, *et al.* The role of cardiovascular magnetic resonance imaging in heart failure. *J Am Coll Cardiol.* 2009; **54**(15):1407–24.

SECTION 3

Percutaneous coronary intervention by clinical syndrome

CHAPTER 14

Stable coronary artery disease: medical therapy versus percutaneous coronary intervention versus surgery

Scot Garg, Joanna J. Wykrzykowska, and Patrick W. Serruys

Introduction

Coronary artery disease (CAD) represents a wide spectrum of underlying anatomical disease ranging from near normal, minor single-vessel disease (SVD), to extensive triple-vessel disease. Its presentation is similarly variable, from a single episode of chest pain to acute coronary syndrome (ACS) or even death. The aim of treatment in CAD is to relieve symptoms and improve quality of life, reduce cardiovascular (CV) events, and prolong survival. There have been vast improvements in management over the years, following a greater understanding of the underlying pathophysiology, the identification and appropriate management of risk factors, development of new medication, and advances in revascularization techniques, both percutaneous and surgical. These developments have resulted in a move towards an anatomic treatment for CAD even though it is the minor lesion, so-called vulnerable plaque, which is suggested as the most likely culprit for mortality. Nevertheless, in those patients presenting with ACS or ST-elevation myocardial infarction the long-term benefits of percutaneous coronary intervention (PCI) have been confirmed in multiple randomized trials[(1)]; however, debate surrounds the ideal management of the majority of patients who have angina, and who have not experienced any previous CV events or had an interventional procedure, so-called stable CAD.

Medical therapy versus mechanical revascularization

Medical therapy which encompasses lifestyle modification, risk factor reduction, and pharmacological therapy (antiplatelet and antianginal) has a strong evidence base and clearly has a central role in the management of every patient with CAD. Intuitively it would seem apparent that PCI would be the ideal treatment for every patient, however the current evidence taken at face value would tend to suggest otherwise. The largest trial to date comparing PCI (and best medical therapy) with best medical therapy (BMT) was the COURAGE trial (Clinical Outcomes Utilizing Revascularization and Aggressive Drug Evaluation) whose publication has been well publicised and debated amongst general cardiologists, interventional cardiologists, and the general public. This trial, which recruited only 6.4% of the 35 539 patients who were assessed for entry, reported at median follow-up of 4.6 years no significant difference in the primary event rate (death or non fatal MI) with PCI compared with BMT (19.0% vs. 18.5%; 95% confidence interval [CI], 0.87–1.27; $p = 0.62$)[(2)]. This added to the evidence from earlier meta-analyses in 2000[(3)] and 2005[(4)] both of which concluded that PCI improved symptoms but did not reduce mortality or the incidence of CV events. There is no doubt that PCI helps relieve symptoms[(2,3,5)] but what is its true effect on mortality and morbidity, and can these general conclusions be applied to all groups of patients? The importance of this issue cannot be overstated given the vast resources that are spent on managing these patients who comprise 85% of the PCI workload in the United States[2]. Most importantly a recent meta-analysis which included the COURAGE data and comprised 7915 patients found a 20% reduction in all cause death amongst the PCI-treated patients compared with BMT (271 deaths vs. 335 deaths; odds ratio [OR], 0.80; 95% CI, 0.64–0.99; p = 0.263)[6].

It is essential to consider some of the limitations of the previous trials which have been performed comparing the two groups. They have all suffered from the low risk[7] of the population being studied, and have been under-powered to detect a significant mortality difference. In addition, mean follow-up time has been just under 4 years, which may be too short to detect morbidity in the BMT group, whilst those in the PCI group may experience peri-procedural events which will be detected on short-term follow-up. Importantly in the COURAGE trial the rate of spontaneous MI (not peri-procedural) in the BMT group was higher than in the PCI arm (119 vs. 108), but peri-procedural MIs were much higher in the PCI group (35 vs. 9). Peri-procedural MIs are not benign and do affect prognosis[8], some of these may occur through trying to achieve the 'perfect' angiographic appearance, when simpler less complicated procedures may produce the same symptomatic benefit, at a lower risk. The advantages of PCI are further reduced by high cross over rates, ranging from 6–44%, from BMT to PCI although this is a reality of the chronic nature of CAD rather than a 'fault' of the trials. The benefit of PCI has also been hampered by the trials being performed before the drug eluting stent (DES) era. It is well documented that restenosis, which is reduced significantly by DES compared with bare metal stent (BMS) or balloon angioplasty (POBA), is not a benign phenomenon and can present as an acute MI in between 9.5–19.4% of cases[9].

The presence of ischaemia affects clinical outcome but amongst the trials there is considerable variation in the objective evidence of ischaemia required for patient enrolment, with some simply relying on symptoms and angiographic evidence of stenosis. PCI is very effective at relieving the subjective symptoms of ischaemia. Evidence from the nuclear subset of the COURAGE trial which looked at 313 patients who had myocardial perfusion imaging before, and 6–18 months post randomization, would suggest that it is also more effective than BMT at relieving objective ischaemia. In this subset of patients those having PCI and BMT had a greater reduction in significant myocardial ischaemia than BMT controls (p = 0.004), and this translated clinically into a significantly lower rate of death and MI in these patients (13.4% vs. 24.7%, p = 0.037). Also of note were the zero rates of death and MI in those patients having no evidence of residual ischaemia at 6–18 months, compared with a rate of 39.3% in those with grater than 10% residual ischaemia. In summary, PCI with BMT has been shown to be better than BMT at relieving subjective and objective ischaemia, and this has translated into better clinical outcomes. The SWISS II study showed similar benefits in the presence of proven silent ischaemia[10]. Future trials need to ensure that the degree of myocardial ischaemia is accurately assessed to guarantee the validity of the conclusions reached.

In the 'real world' aggressive medical therapy is frequently difficult to implement because real-world patients experience side effects from therapy, and may subsequently be non-compliant with medication, or lifestyle advice. The COURAGE trial has shown what can be achieved in the ideal world with reductions in blood pressure, LDL cholesterol, smoking rates, and improvements in diet, and exercise; however, these require additional resources and the manpower which most healthcare providers are simply unable to deliver.

In summary, medical therapy plays an important part in the management of patients with CAD, and the role of revascularization should be considered to be complementary to BMT which is central to management. PCI should be considered if BMT fails to control symptoms in those patients who are deemed to be at a low risk of CV events, whilst in those who are at higher risk, revascularization with either PCI or coronary artery bypass grafting (CABG) and BMT must be considered early.

Risk stratification

From the previous discussion it is apparent that risk stratification plays a vital role in helping guide the management of patients with CAD. It also has an important role in providing patients, and their relatives, with answers to questions they may have about the likely course of their condition and their prognosis, and can also help inform other health professions planning other treatments and procedures.

Which patients are at high risk of events? The European Society of Cardiology defines those patients with an annual CV risk of >2% as high risk, <1% as low risk, and between 1–2% intermediate risk, and recommends that risk stratification takes into consideration:

1. Clinical evaluation of the patient

A clinical evaluation of the patient is essential in all cases and can provide information with regards prognosis, and the following factors—although by no means exhaustive—are all associated with an increased risk of adverse prognosis in those with stable CAD:

- History of diabetes mellitus, hypercholesterolaemia, hypertension, and renal impairment.
- Severity of angina presentation.
- Current smoking.
- Examination findings suggestive of peripheral vascular disease, or signs of left ventricular (LV) dysfunction.
- An abnormal ECG (previous MI, left bundle branch block, left anterior hemiblock, LV hypertrophy, atrial fibrillation, and second- or third-degree heart block).

2. Response to stress testing

Stress testing provides additional information regarding the patient's risk, and currently numerous different non-invasive stress tests are available, which are able to provide prognostic information obtained not only from the presence or absence of ischaemia, but also from the degree and severity of ischaemia, the exercise capacity, and the ischaemic threshold.

There are no randomized trials comparing individual stress tests, and issues other than the patient's physical and functional ability to exercise, or the presence of an abnormal ECG such as availability, local expertise, and preference of the referring physician do have an influence on which test is ultimately used. Table 14.1 lists the criteria on non-invasive stress testing which suggest a high risk of CV events and subsequently indicate the need for revascularization. Currently multisliced CT scanning provides an anatomical assessment of CAD, with limited data available on its correlation with inducible ischaemia; however, with further evaluation in progress this may change. Whichever test is used, a normal result doesn't exclude the presence of CAD or the risk of future events.

3. An assessment of left ventricular function

LV function is the most important marker of prognosis in those patients with CAD. Studies have shown that mortality is inversely proportional to LV function, and in those with an LV ejection fraction <35%, the annual risk of mortality is in excess of 3%[11].

Table 14.1 Prognostic variables and criteria indicating a high risk of cardiovascular events amongst various non-invasive stress tests

Modality	Prognostic variables	Criteria for high risk of CV events	Annual mean CV event rate in normal test
Echocardiography	LVEF at rest LVEF on exercise	LVEF <35% at rest LVEF <35% on exercise	
Stress echocardiography	Number of resting WMA Number of inducible WMA with stress	WMA (involving >2 segments) developing at: ◆ A low dose of dobutamine (≤10mg/kg/min) or ◆ At a low heart rate (<120bpm) Stress echocardiographic evidence of extensive ischaemia	<0.5%[11]
Exercise testing	Exercise-induced angina Exercise capacity BP response to exercise Changes in ST segment Exercise-induced ischaemia	High-risk Duke treadmill score (< −10)*	Low Duke score (>4) 0.25% (annual mortality)
Myocardial perfusion imaging	Large stress-induced perfusion defects Defects in multiple coronary arteries Transient post stress LV dilation Lung uptake with Tl-201	Stress-induced: ◆ Larger perfusion defect (particularly if anterior) ◆ Multiple perfusion defects of moderate size ◆ Moderate perfusion defect with LV dilation or increased lung uptake (Tl-201) Large, fixed perfusion defect with LV dilation or increased lung uptake (Tl-201)	0.7%[67]

* The Duke treadmill score equals the exercise time in minutes minus (5× the ST-segment deviation, during or after exercise, in millimetres) minus (4× the angina index, which has a value of '0' if there is no angina, '1' if angina occurs, and '2' if angina is the reason for stopping the test)[68].

BP, blood pressure; LVEF, left ventricular ejection fraction; Tl-201, thallium-201; WMA, wall motion abnormality.

4. An assessment of the coronary anatomy

Coronary anatomy provides valuable information in assessing the patient's risk of CV events, and in particular the extent, severity, and location of the disease are important factors which influence prognosis. A simple risk assessment can be based on the number of coronary arteries involved, which is supported by data from the CASS medical registry which showed that 12-year survival was 91%, 74%, 59%, and 50% in those with normal, single-, double-, or triple-vessel disease respectively[12], furthermore survival rates were poorer in those with a combination of two- or three-vessel disease and a left main stem (LMS) lesion. Early data has shown the poor prognosis in LMS lesions treated medically[13], and the improved survival with revascularization, which at the time of publication was predominantly CABG, in those with triple-vessel disease, two-vessel disease which includes the proximal left anterior descending artery (LAD), or two- or three-vessel disease and a positive exercise test[14].

It has been argued that coronary angiography is inappropriate in those patients who are deemed low risk after non-invasive testing in view of the risk of the procedure, and the small chance that repeat revascularization is required.

Once the patient has been risk stratified, and a decision reached to proceed with mechanical revascularization, the patient must be evaluated with respect to their suitability for PCI or CABG. This decision is often complex and requires a multidisciplinary team approach, with the cardiologist, interventional cardiologist, and cardiac surgeon all participating in the discussion. The last two decades have provided us with a large body of evidence to guide these complex decisions, and in the following section we will review the available data on stenting in multivessel disease (MVD) and CABG, including the most recent evidence from the SYNTAX, FAME, and CARDIA trials.

Mechanical revascularization: PCI versus CABG

After its introduction in the 1960s, CABG become the accepted treatment for MVD[15]; however, advances made in the percutaneous treatment of stable CAD from POBA to stenting with initially BMS[16] and now DES[17–19], have made PCI a progressively more attractive alternative (Fig. 14.1). All randomized clinical trials to date, whether performed in the early days with POBA or more recently with BMS or DES, show no mortality difference between PCI and CABG[20–22]. However the advantage of CABG over PCI in terms of restenosis rate and the need for re-intervention has progressively narrowed, especially in some patient subsets.

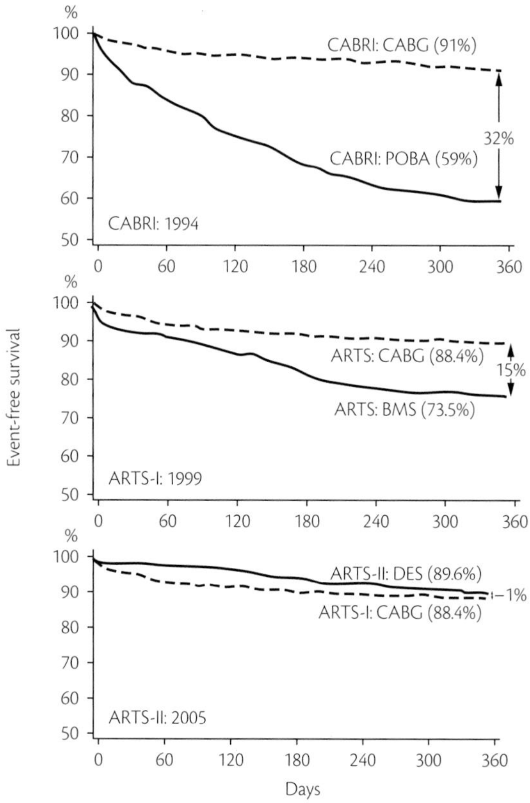

Fig. 14.1 Event-free survival at 1 year follow-up in the CABRI, ARTS-I, and ARTS-II studies showing a reduction in the difference in outcomes between CABG compared with balloon angioplasty, bare-metal stenting, and drug-eluting stents. Reproduced from Serruys, PW, ARTS I – the rapamycin eluting stent; ARTS II – the rosy prophecy. *Eur Heart J* 2002; **23**:757–9 by permission of Oxford University Press.

Pre-DES era: balloon angioplasty and bare metal stenting versus CABG

The six randomized trials comparing POBA to CABG are summarized in Table 14.2, together with the results at the longest published follow-up. In 1995, prior to the publication of the BARI trial, a 3-year meta-analysis was published of the other five trials which found no difference in the rates of death and non-fatal MI (CABG vs. POBA HR 1.03; 95% CI 0.81–1.32; $p = 0.81$)[20].

In view of the superior results with stenting compared with POBA (Fig. 14.2)[16], five subsequent randomized trials compared BMS to CABG in MVD. These five trials are summarized in Table 14.3 together with results at the longest published follow-up. The ARTS-I study was the largest of these trials and enrolled 1205 patients with

Table 14.2 Results at longest reported follow-up in the six randomized trials of balloon angioplasty versus coronary artery bypass surgery

Study	Year	No. of patients	Longest reported follow-up (years)	Death POBA vs. CABG	MI POBA vs. CABG	Re-intervention POBA vs. CABG
CABRI[69]	1994	1054	1	3.9% vs. 2.7% p = NS	p=NS	33.6% vs. 6.5% p <0.001
ERACI[70]	1993	127	3	4.7% vs. 9.5% p = 0.5	7.8% vs. 7.8% p = 0.8	37% vs. 6.3% p <0.001
RITA[71]	1993	1011	6.5	7.6% vs. 9.0% p = 0.51	10.8% vs. 7.4% p = 0.08	44.3% vs. 10.8%
EAST[72]	1994	392	8	20.7% vs. 17.3% p = 0.40	–	65.3% vs. 26.5% p <0.001
BARI[73]	1991	1829	10	71.0% vs. 73.5% p = 0.18	16.4% vs. 16.6% p = NS	76.8% vs. 20.3% p <0.001
GABI[74]	1994	359	13	25% vs. 21.9% p = 0.64	4.3% vs. 5.6% p = 0.6	82.9% vs. 58.8%

CABG, coronary artery bypass grafting; NS, not significant; POBA, balloon angioplasty; BARI, Bypass Angioplasty Revascularization Investigation; CABRI, Coronary Angioplasty versus Bypass Revascularization Investigation; EAST, Emory Angioplasty versus Surgery Trial; ERACI, Argentine Randomized Trial of Percutaneous Transluminal Coronary Angioplasty versus Coronary Artery Bypass Surgery in Multivessel Disease; GABI, German Angioplasty Bypass Surgery Investigation; RITA, Randomized Intervention Treatment of Angina.

MVD that had an equivalent baseline chance for complete revascularization. There was no difference between the two groups in either the prespecified primary endpoint of major adverse cardiac and cerebrovascular events (MACCE) at 1 year, or mortality at 5 years (8% vs. 7.6%; p = 0.83). However, when compared with CABG the rates of repeat revascularization were higher in the stenting group both at 1-year (16.8% vs. 3.5%) and 5-year (30.3% vs. 8.8%; p <0.001) follow-up[15,23].

A meta-analysis of all five trials showed similar MACCE rates and higher repeat revascularization rates in the PCI group at both 1- and 5-year follow-up[22,24,25]. The only study that has been at variance with these randomized trial results has been the New York Cardiac Registry[26] which looked retrospectively at risk-adjusted outcomes in 60 000 patients undergoing PCI or CABG. Risk adjusted survival was significantly higher in the CABG group (HR 0.64; 95% CI 0.56–0.74) with the difference being most pronounced in patients with three-vessel disease and proximal LAD disease. The criticism of this registry is that risk adjustment is likely to be impossible and that clinical judgement could not be adjusted for in this complex cohort of patients (J. Daemen, N. Kukreja, and P.W.J.C. Serruys, personal correspondence).

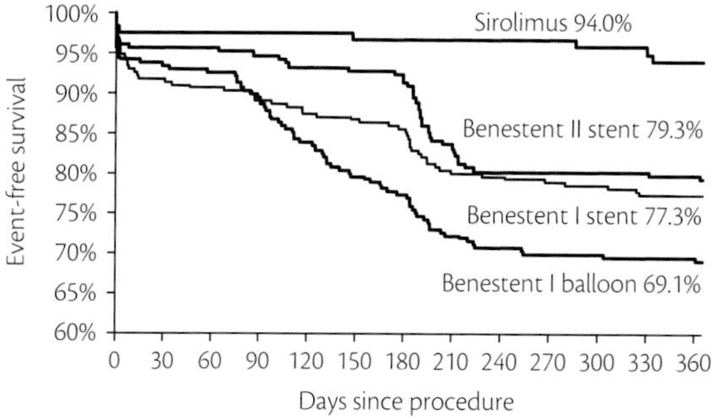

Fig. 14.2 The improved event-free survival in the Benestent I and II trials with the use of a bare-metal stent (Benestent I stent) or a heparin-coated stent (Benestent II) compared to only balloon angioplasty (Benestent balloon). The event-free survival, however, is much greater with a sirolimus-eluting stent.

The DES era—the game is getting closer

Randomized trials comparing DES and BMS have shown a reduction in the restenosis rates with DES. In addition, DES use has expanded to more complex patients and lesions including patients with MVD, which comprise close to 40% of PCI patients. The effectiveness of these devices has been shown in 'real world' registries such as RESEARCH and T-SEARCH[27]. ARTS-II was the first CABG-PCI registry/trial to evaluate the performance of DES specifically in MVD against CABG. It prospectively collected data on 607 patients with MVD treated with DES[28] who were then compared to historical CABG control from ARTS-I. One-year follow-up showed that PCI with DES was non-inferior to CABG with respect to MACCE rates. The rates of repeat revascularization, although lower than in the BMS arm of ARTS-I, were still significantly higher than in the historical CABG controls. These results were maintained at

Table 14.3 Results at longest reported follow-up in five randomized trials of bare metal stenting versus coronary artery bypass surgery

Study	Year	No. of patients	Longest reported follow-up (years)	Death PCI vs. CABG	MI PCI vs. CABG	Re-intervention PCI vs. CABG
AWESOME[75]	2000	142	3	24% vs. 27% p = NS	–	–
ARTS-I[23]	2001	1205	5	8.0% vs. 7.6% p = 0.83	9.5% vs. 6.4%	30.3% vs. 8.3% p <0.001
ERACI-II[76]	2001	450	5	7.1% vs. 11.5% p = 0.18	2.8% vs. 6.2% p = 0.13	28.4% vs. 7.2% p = 0.0002
MASS-II[77]	2003	611	5	15.5% vs. 12.8% p = NS	11.2% vs. 8.3%	32.2% vs. 3.5%
SOS[78]	1999	988	6	10.9% vs. 6.8% p = 0.022	–	–

CABG, coronary artery bypass grafting; NS, not significant; PCI, percutaneous coronary intervention; ARTS-I, Arterial Revascularization Therapy Study; AWESOME, Angina With Extremely Serious Operative Mortality Evaluation; ERACI-II, Argentine Randomized Study: Coronary Angioplasty with Stenting versus Coronary Bypass Surgery in Multivessel Disease; MASS-II, Medicine, Angioplasty or Surgery Study for multivessel coronary artery disease; SOS, Stent or Surgery

3-year follow-up with equivalent survival without MACCE (80.6% vs. 83.8%, p = 0.21) and lower freedom from repeat revascularization with PCI (85.5% vs. 93.4%, p <0.001). In ERACI-III which prospectively added a 205 patient cohort to the ERACI-II population, PCI with DES had a lower MACE rate than an historical CABG group (freedom from MACE was 88% vs. 80.5%; p = 0.038)[29]. One observational study in 1680 patients confirmed these findings with equivalent MACCE rates in a non-diabetic population with two-vessel disease[30]. However, again the New York registry of 17 400 patients appeared to contradict these results showing lower mortality rates for CABG at 18 months post procedure (adjusted survival of 96% vs. 94.6%; p = 0.003). Notably the difference was smaller than with a similar registry for BMS and the same concern regarding inability to adjust for all confounding risk factors remained.

SYNTAX, FAME, and CARDIA—results of the randomized trials: more answers but also more questions

Some of these earlier controversies in data interpretation are finally being partially resolved following the results of three major randomized trials presented in 2008 of DES versus CABG in patients with MVD. In addition, these trials also attempted to define more clearly which specific patient populations benefit from CABG or PCI.

Synergy between percutaneous coronary intervention with TAXus and cardiac surgery (SYNTAX) is a prospective, multicentre, multinational, randomized trial of all-comers design. It recruited 1800 patients with the goal to assess the best revascularization treatment for patients with de novo triple-vessel or LMS disease by randomizing them to either stenting with a paclitaxel-eluting Taxus® stent (Boston Scientific, Natick, USA) or CABG and also keeping a registry of those patients who were eligible for only PCI or only CABG[31]. The trial design was unique in that it employed the angiographic scoring system of lesion severity called the 'SYNTAX score'[32]. The patients recruited in SYNTAX are a unique study group in the PCI field, given their exceptionally complex anatomy and advanced disease. The average SYNTAX patient received 4.6 stents compared to the average 1.5 stents implanted in everyday practice. In addition, the patient profile included 33% with >100mm stented length, 84% with bi/trifurcations, 22% with chronic total occlusions, and 39% with LMS disease. Some of the sickest patients in the trial were not eligible for surgery and were treated with DES. The main results are summarized in Table 14.4. One of the most interesting results came from the SYNTAX score subgroup analysis which showed that PCI but not surgical outcomes were influenced by the angiographic SYNTAX score (lesion complexity). Analysis showed non-inferior results of PCI to CABG in patients with a SYNTAX score up to 32, whilst CABG was superior in those with a SYNTAX score above 32. Further analysis of the data will be required together with longer-term follow-up. The complexity of the patient population in this study certainly makes the data generalizable; however, one has to keep in mind that the surgery and

Table 14.4 12-month results from the SYNTAX study[31]

Events at 1 year	PCI N = 903 (%)	CABG N = 897 (%)	P-value
MACCE	160 (17.8)	109 (12.1)	0.002
Death/CVA/MI	69 (7.6)	69 (7.7)	0.98
All-cause death	39 (4.3)	31 (3.5)	0.37
MI	43 (4.8)	29 (3.2)	0.11
CVA	5 (0.6)	20 (2.2)	0.003
Repeat revascularization	124 (13.7)	53 (5.9)	<0.001

CVA, stroke; MACCE, major adverse cardiovascular and cerebrovascular events (all-cause death, CVA, MI, and repeat revascularization); MI, myocardial infarction.

complex PCI in this study was performed in highly selected centers of excellence in Europe and the United States who were used to high volumes of complex patients and cases.

The CARDIA (Coronary Artery Revascularisation in Diabetes) study randomized 510 diabetic patients with MVD or complex SVD to treatment with either CABG (n = 254) or PCI (n = 256; 71% DES). The primary outcome—death, MI and stroke—was comparable between CABG and PCI at 1 year (10.2% vs. 11.6%; p = 0.63), whilst repeat revascularization was significantly higher in the PCI group with a rate of 9.9% vs. 2.0% for CABG (p = 0.001). Similar results were seen in the DES subgroup analysis with no difference in the primary endpoint (CABG vs. DES PCI, p = 0.98) and higher repeat revascularization with DES compared to CABG group. Stroke, however, was more prevalent in the CABG group[33]. The results of the Future Revascularization Evaluation in patients with Diabetes Mellitus; Optimal Management of Multivessel Disease (FREEDOM) trial which is enrolling at least 2000 diabetic patients with MVD randomized to CABG versus multivessel stenting with DES are eagerly awaited.

Lastly, the Fractional flow reserve versus Angiography for Multivessel Evaluation (FAME) trial offers another approach to MVD treatment. It incorporates the idea of revascularizing the territory which has evidence of reversible ischaemia and uses the fractional flow reserve (FFR) measurement as a gold standard for the haemodynamic significance of the lesion. The premise of the study is based on the result that deferral of PCI based on the FFR cut-off point of 0.75 has been associated with favorable outcomes in patients with MVD[34] and that only lesions with inducible ischaemia benefit from invasive mechanical revascularization over medical therapy. FAME enrolled 1005 patients with at least two vessels with >50% lesions randomized to either angiographic guided, or FFR-guided stenting using an FFR cut off value of 0.8. The main results are shown in Fig. 14.3 There was a 35% reduction in overall MACE which was achieved without prolonging the procedure, (p = 0.51) and approximately one-third of angiographically significant lesions were found not to be haemodynamically significant by FFR. In addition the FFR-guided stenting strategy lead to a significant reduction in contrast use (272 ± 133mL vs. 302 ± 127; P <0.001) and a significant cost saving ($5332 vs. $6007, p <0.001) compared to the angiographic-guided stenting[35].

Lesion subsets

The previous section has been a general discussion comparing PCI and CABG. In the next section we have concentrated on six commonly encountered lesion subsets.

Single-vessel disease

Patients having revascularization have significantly lower 1-year mortality with SVD when compared with those having MVD; in fact the RITA trial showed this trend was maintained at 4.7 years follow-up (5.8% vs. 3.9%). In addition, those with SVD having revascularization have lower rates of MI and cardiac death compared to MVD, and also have better angina control at 1 and 3 years, compared to those with MVD having the same type of revascularization[21].

At present, approximately 4% of CABG is performed for SVD, however previously the rates were much

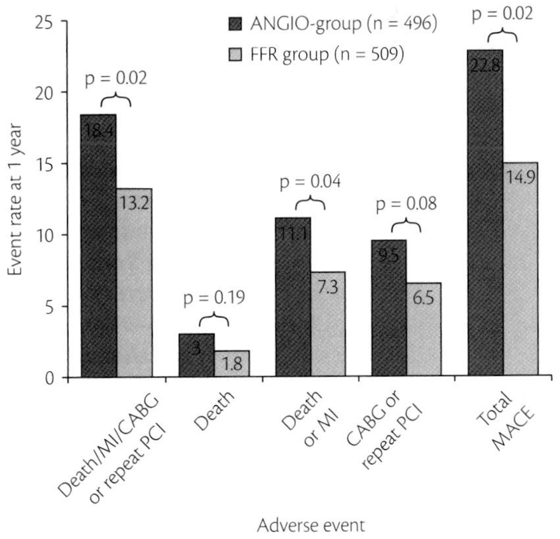

Fig. 14.3 The adverse event rates at one year from the 1005 patients in the FAME study showing improved outcomes with the use of an FFR-guided strategy[35].

higher, for example in the New York surgical registry of over 29 000 patients the rate of single-vessel CABG was 8.7%[36]. These initial high rates of surgical revascularization are the result of the early trials which showed a distinct advantage for CABG compared with medical therapy in patients with specific SVD—namely a significant proximal LAD lesion[37]; in fact in the previously mentioned New York registry 74.3% (n = 1917) of patients having single-vessel CABG, had proximal LAD disease. It is not surprising therefore that most data on the outcomes of revascularization in patients with SVD has concentrated on those with a significant proximal LAD lesion.

Two registries have concurred with the initial trials regarding surgical revascularization in those with significant proximal LAD disease; the New York registry was by far the larger containing 3-year outcome data on 23 808 patients (PCI = 21 231, CABG = 2577) with SVD. At follow-up those patients with SVD not including an LAD lesion had a much better survival with PCI than CABG (95.3% vs. 92.4%, p = 0.003); however, if there was a >70% LAD lesion, CABG conferred a significantly better prognosis. (96.6% vs. 95.2%, p = 0.01). Irrespective of the type of revascularization there was no significant difference between outcomes in those with SVD in the non-proximal LAD. In fact any patient with a proximal LAD lesion, whether with single-, double-, or triple-vessel disease did better with CABG. The Duke registry was much smaller, containing 9263 patients (medical therapy 2449; PCI 2924; CABG 3890), but concluded similar results at mean 5.3-year follow-up. Patients with SVD, including those with SVD and a mid/distal LAD lesion <75% severity, had better survival with PCI compared with CABG, whilst those with SVD due to a proximal LAD lesion >95% tended to do better with CABG.

It is, however, important to accept the limited clinical applicability of this data in the current era. Two main factors which may have influenced outcome were stent usage, which was only 11.8% in the New York registry, and usage of left internal mammary artery (LIMA) grafts. The Duke registry ran from 1984–1990 and the New York registry from 1993–1995, and although there is no comment on LIMA usage, in the 1980s studies reported rates of LIMA use of approximately 15%[37], whilst in the late 1990s rates of over 90% have been reported[38]. The relevance of low or even moderate use of the LIMA graft is the fact that they have significantly higher patency at follow-up, and confer a long term survival benefit when compared with saphenous vein grafts[39,40].

In recent years two meta-analyses have been published examining outcomes in patients with proximal LAD disease randomized to either PCI or surgical revascularization; Kapoor *et al.* concentrating on any surgical technique[41], whilst Aziz *et al.* examined specifically those having the minimally invasive direct coronary artery bypass (MIDCAB)[42]. In both studies patients tended to be young with a total mean age of 58.9 years, and with well-preserved ejection fractions (mean of 61.4%). The PCI technique varied in both, but of note the usage of DES was low, comprising of only 18.8% in Kapoor *et al.*'s study.

Kapoor *et al.* showed no differences in procedural stroke or MI, whilst Aziz *et al.* showed no difference in MI, and stroke at maximum follow-up. In both studies angina relief was significantly greater after CABG than after PCI, and following on from this, repeat revascularization was significantly less after CABG than after PCI; with results maintained to 5 years in Kapoor *et al.*'s study (7.3% vs. 33.5%, p <0.0001). Results from both studies showed that no significant difference in survival amongst patients assigned to either CABG or PCI, this extending out to 5 years in Kapoor *et al.*'s study. The excellent long-term prognosis of both treatments is further enhanced following the publication of Goy *et al.*'s randomized study comparing bare-metal stenting with LIMA grafting for proximal LAD lesions, which showed no mortality difference at 10-year follow-up (PCI 8% vs. CABG 4%; p = 0.4)[43].

So what can be concluded from the evidence presented? Many clinicians would have no hesitation for contemplating PCI for a single-vessel lesion (excluding proximal LAD) and registry data would support that in the current absence of randomized data—which is unlikely to ever be available. With regards proximal LAD lesions, data has shown no significant difference in mortality between PCI and CABG (up to 10 years) and the final decision should therefore be influenced by other factors such as patient preference, operator skill, and lesion characteristics.

Bifurcation lesions

Coronary artery bifurcations are at an increased risk for the development of coronary atherosclerosis because of turbulent flow and low shear stress, and have long posed a problem for interventional cardiologists. Despite advances in PCI they are associated with higher rates of MACE, restenosis, and a lower probability of success when compared to single-vessel intervention. Currently there is no randomized data comparing the treatment of patients with only bifurcation lesions between PCI and CABG; however, 1310 patients (657

CABG, 653 PCI), comprising 72.8% of the total cohort in the SYNTAX study had a bifurcation lesion.

Of the previous published studies most specified the number of vessels diseased, as opposed to the precise lesion type, and therefore did not include a separate subset of patients with bifurcation lesions, or report the percentage of lesions which were bifurcation lesions. The ARTS-II study did have a bifurcation subset which comprised approximately 34% of the total cohort; however the study compared PCI in these patients with PCI in non-bifurcation lesions. The results showed no significant difference in 1-year MACCE between PCI in the bifurcation and non-bifurcation lesions (13.3% vs. 11.0%, p = 0.46)[44]; which is comparable with the MACCE in the surgical arm of ARTS-I (12.2%), which included 188 (31%) patients who had bifurcation lesions[15].

There is a lack of randomized data at present to point to whether PCI or CABG is appropriate for non-LMS bifurcation lesions; however interventionalists are moving away from mandatory complex bifurcation stenting techniques towards the provisional T-stenting techniques[45] in view of recent studies showing similar outcomes between the two techniques, and only a low requirement of side-branch stenting in the single-stent strategy[46]. This is important as some would argue that bifurcation lesions should simply be regarded as high-risk single-vessel lesions, and treated accordingly, whilst being aware of the extent of the myocardium at risk, i.e. how large and important is the side branch? The ARTS-II data show similar MACCE in dealing with bifurcation lesions compared to a surgical cohort, and therefore the decision with regards revascularization technique should be based on the same arguments as previously discussed with SVD, namely patient preference, operator skill, lesion characteristic, and extent of myocardium at risk.

Chronic total occlusions

Chronic total occlusions remain the most challenging aspect of a complete revascularization strategy. They are present in up to 20% of patients but their procedural success rate has been the lowest of all interventional procedures, 60–70% (with conventional techniques), and reaches 98% on the second attempt only in most experienced hands[47]. Use of novel techniques such as retrograde technique[48], dedicated wires (Miracle series and Confienza), smaller balloons with very low crossing profiles (1mm in diameter) and other dedicated devices (Tornus, laser and blunt dissection devices) has improved acute procedural success, however, it has not reduced the likelihood of complications (such as perforation and dissection).

Multidetector CT has been very helpful in predicting interventional success as the assessment of lesion length and degree of calcification is more accurate than with angiography[49]. Even with better acute outcomes, long-term patency of chronic total occlusions remains low and has improved only somewhat with the use of DES[50–52]. In the PRISON II trial restenosis rates in chronic total occlusion lesions were 11% with sirolimus-eluting stents and 41% with BMS (p = 0.001)[50]. The ability to achieve complete revascularization in patients with a combination of MVD and chronic total occlusion whilst challenging is also of the utmost importance as it confers a long-term survival benefit[53–55].

Diabetes

Diabetic patients present a particular challenge for all revascularization strategies given the extent of their coronary disease, its aggressive nature, and other comorbidities. The long-term survival in diabetics after both PCI and CABG is lower than in non-diabetics[56,57]. Until recently, based on BARI trial experience where mortality was 19% with CABG and 35% with PCI in diabetics (HR 1.87; p = 0.00249), CABG has usually been advocated as the preferred revascularization strategy for diabetic patients. However, as BMS and DES were introduced the mortality difference between CABG and PCI has been eliminated, and now only the difference in the need for repeat revascularization has remained. In the ARTS-I trial amongst diabetics there was no mortality difference between PCI with BMS, and CABG (6.3 vs. 3.1%; p = 0.294); however, there was a 20% absolute difference in freedom from repeat revascularization in favour of CABG. The 3-year follow-up of the ARTS-II trial looking at outcomes in diabetic patients showed that this difference in freedom from MACCE and target-vessel revascularization has narrowed significantly since the introduction of DES, such that there was no significant difference between the MACCE in ARTS-II and the CABG arm of ARTS-I (p = 0.09). The incidence of death, CVA, and MI was significantly lower in ARTS-II than in ARTS-I PCI (adjusted OR, 0.67; 95% CI, 0.27–1.65) and was similar to that of ARTS-I CABG[25]. The analysis of this and other similar trials has been limited by the post hoc nature of the substudy.

The first dedicated trial of CABG versus PCI in diabetics using 70% DES was recently published[33]. As previously noted, there was no difference in the primary outcome of MACE at 1 year (Fig. 14.4). Overall repeat revascularization was higher in the stenting group (9.9% vs. 2%) and also in the DES subgroup compared to the CABG group, but the absolute difference has

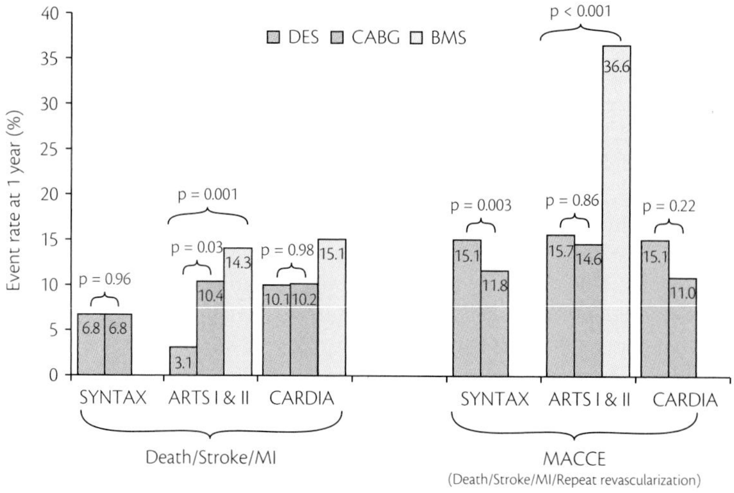

Fig. 14.4 The combined rates of death, stroke, and MI, and MACCE (death, stroke, MI, and repeat revascularization with either PCI or CABG) at 1 year amongst diabetic patients from ARTS-I, ARTS-II, CARDIA, and SYNTAX studies. From the limited data available there is an improvement in events with the use of drug-eluting stents, but repeat revascularization is still a prominent problem; however, matters appears to be improving.

narrowed to only 7% in favour of CABG. With further improvements in DES technology, this difference is likely to become even smaller, and the higher incidence of stroke in diabetic patients undergoing CABG may offset its benefit in terms of lower repeat revascularization rates.

Chronic renal insufficiency

Chronic renal insufficiency often complicates diabetes and is also a risk factor for accelerated CAD. In addition, patients with moderate renal insufficiency are at risk for worsening of disease both after contrast administration during complex PCI and during CABG. To our knowledge the only study to date that looked specifically at long-term outcomes of patients with moderate renal disease is ARTS-I[(58)]. At 5 years, there was no significant difference between the two groups in terms of mortality (14.5% vs. 12.3%, p = 0.81), or combined endpoint of death, cerebrovascular accident, or MI (30.4% in the stent group vs. 23.3% in the CABG group, p = 0.35). The rate of repeat revascularization was 18.8% in the stent group and 8.2% in the surgery group (p = 0.08). The event-free survival at 5 years was 50.7% in the stent group and 68.5% in the surgery group (p = 0.04). Larger prospective analysis of these patients with and without concomitant diabetes will be helpful in determining the relative risks of the two revascularization approaches.

Low and high body mass index (BMI) or the obesity paradox

Another group of patients that probably merits further investigation is the underweight and overweight group. In ARTS-I trial obese patients treated with bypass surgery had a significant advantage over low BMI patients in terms of freedom from MACE and repeat revascularization[(59)]. For patients who had been randomized to undergo CABG, there was a significant decrease in repeat revascularization procedures in obese patients (p = 0.03). Major adverse cardiac or cerebrovascular event rates were significantly lower for patients who were obese (11%) or overweight (16%) compared with patients who had a normal BMI (24%; p = 0.008). No such effect of BMI was observed on outcomes of treatment with stents. In the ARTS-II trial, BMI had no effect on outcomes of stenting with sirolimus-eluting stents[(60)]. These results contrast with findings of the BARI trial where obesity conferred significant increased risk in the surgical group[(61,62)]. On the other hand another found a U-shaped relationship with a BMI of 30 being optimal[(63)].

Risk–benefit and cost–benefit analysis of choosing between PCI and CABG

Whilst clinical trial evidence shows that both CABG and PCI increase health-related quality of life (HRQL), in the long term CABG has a greater HRQL, and lower repeat revascularization rate, especially compared to bare-metal stenting[(64)]. This deferred benefit, however, occurs at the expense of higher morbidity and delayed relief from pain in the time period immediately post procedure. Thus a decision regarding the procedure choice for a particular patient should be carefully weighed. Recently performed analysis based on ARTS study data using risk–benefit acceptability curve (RBAC), showed that the average patient has a risk of 0.7 for an additional revascularization procedure during the 3-year period after the index PCI procedure, in exchange for being pain free within 1 month of the initial treatment. Specifically, there is a risk of 0.96 clinical events at 3 years, including a risk of 0.57 for repeat PCIs and 0.33 for additional CABG events[65]. Similar analysis further stratified by other patient characteristics such as SYNTAX score will need to be performed in the current DES era. The SYNTAX trial may raise a further issue of the increased risk of stroke in CABG patients in exchange for the higher risk of repeat revascularization events with PCI[31].

Assuming the advantageous risk–benefit ratio, the issue of cost-effectiveness of the PCI versus CABG is an important one from a societal standpoint. In the BARI trial initial PCI costs were lower than CABG costs, however, at 5-year follow-up given the need for repeat procedures in the PCI group the cost difference has narrowed. At 10–12 years there was no economic advantage of one procedure over the other[66]. In the ARTS-I trial at 1 year PCI was less expensive, however, at 3 years whilst a cost saving was still present, it was significantly reduced in the stent arm due to repeat procedures[64]. Similar cost analysis will be needed in the SYNTAX and FREEDOM trials given the high costs of DES, and often wide spread use of glycoprotein IIb/IIIa inhibitors and novel antithrombin agents in the PCI arm.

Summary

A large proportion of patients with CAD have stable symptoms. Patients must undergo risk stratification using available resources and expertise to determine who requires additional revascularization. In those deemed low risk, symptoms can be appropriately controlled with medication with no detriment to long-term prognosis. Those patients who are high risk, or not controlled with medical therapy, should undergo revascularization, although the ideal form of revascularization is yet to be determined.

Whilst over the last decade we have accumulated a lot of evidence regarding outcomes of PCI versus CABG in the treatment of MVD, it is only recently that trials such as SYNTAX are starting to provide us with scores and tools in terms of anatomic and clinical patient characteristics that will allow us to better individualize the treatment choice for each patient. The SYNTAX score is one such tool that may facilitate better decision making in complex cases. This tool, however, still requires both retrospective and prospective validation in larger cohorts of patients.

References

1. Fox KA, Poole-Wilson P, Clayton TC, *et al.* 5-year outcome of an interventional strategy in non-ST-elevation acute coronary syndrome: the British Heart Foundation RITA 3 randomised trial. *Lancet* 2005; **366**(9489):914–20.
2. Boden WE, O'Rourke RA, Teo KK, *et al.* Optimal medical therapy with or without PCI for stable coronary disease. *N Engl J Med* 2007; **356**(15):1503–16.
3. Bucher HC, Hengstler P, Schindler C, *et al.* Percutaneous transluminal coronary angioplasty versus medical treatment for non-acute coronary heart disease: meta-analysis of randomised controlled trials. *BMJ* 2000; **321**(7253):73–7.
4. Katritsis DG, Ioannidis JP. Percutaneous coronary intervention versus conservative therapy in nonacute coronary artery disease: a meta-analysis. *Circulation* 2005; **111**(22):2906–12.
5. Henderson RA, Pocock SJ, Clayton TC, *et al.* Seven-year outcome in the RITA-2 trial: coronary angioplasty versus medical therapy. *J Am Coll Cardiol* 2003; **42**(7):1161–70.
6. Schomig A, Mehilli J, de Waha A, *et al.* A meta-analysis of 17 randomized trials of a percutaneous coronary intervention-based strategy in patients with stable coronary artery disease. *J Am Coll Cardiol* 2008; **52**(11):894–904.
7. Poole-Wilson PA, Voko Z, Kirwan B-A, *et al.* Clinical course of isolated stable angina due to coronary heart disease. *Eur Heart J* 2007; **28**(16):1928–35.
8. Ioannidis JP, Karvouni E, Katritsis DG. Mortality risk conferred by small elevations of creatine kinase-MB isoenzyme after percutaneous coronary intervention. *J Am Coll Cardiol* 2003; **42**(8):1406–11.
9. Lee MS, Pessegueiro A, Zimmer R, *et al.* Clinical presentation of patients with in-stent restenosis in the drug-eluting stent era. *J Invasive Cardiol* 2008; **20**(8):401–3.
10. Erne P, Schoenenberger AW, Burckhardt D, *et al.* Effects of percutaneous coronary interventions in silent ischemia after myocardial infarction: the SWISSI II randomized controlled trial. *JAMA* 2007; **297**(18):1985–91.
11. Fox K, Garcia MA, Ardissino D, *et al.* Guidelines on the management of stable angina pectoris: executive summary: The Task Force on the Management of Stable Angina Pectoris of the European Society of Cardiology. *Eur Heart J* 2006; **27**(11):1341–81.
12. Emond M, Mock MB, Davis KB, *et al.* Long-term survival of medically treated patients in the Coronary Artery Surgery Study (CASS) Registry. *Circulation* 1994; **90**(6):2645–57.
13. Coles JC, Goldbach MM, Ahmed SN, *et al.* Left main-stem coronary artery disease: surgical versus medical management. *Can J Surg* 1984; **27**(6):571–3.
14. Rahimtoola SH. A perspective on the three large multicenter randomized clinical trials of coronary bypass surgery for chronic stable angina. *Circulation* 1985; **72** (6 Pt 2):V123–35.

15. Serruys PW, Unger F, Sousa JE, *et al.* Comparison of coronary-artery bypass surgery and stenting for the treatment of multivessel disease. *N Engl J Med* 2001; **344**(15):1117–24.
16. Serruys PW, de Jaegere P, Kiemeneij F, *et al.* A comparison of balloon-expandable-stent implantation with balloon angioplasty in patients with coronary artery disease. Benestent Study Group. *N Engl J Med* 1994; **331**(8):489–95.
17. Daemen J, Ong AT, Stefanini GG, *et al.* Three-year clinical follow-up of the unrestricted use of sirolimus-eluting stents as part of the Rapamycin-Eluting Stent Evaluated at Rotterdam Cardiology Hospital (RESEARCH) registry. *Am J Cardiol* 2006; **98**(7):895–901.
18. Daemen J, Serruys PW. Optimal revascularization strategies for multivessel coronary artery disease. *Current Opin Cardiol* 2006; **21**(6):595–601.
19. Stone GW, Ellis SG, Cannon L, *et al.* Comparison of a polymer-based paclitaxel-eluting stent with a bare metal stent in patients with complex coronary artery disease: a randomized controlled trial. *JAMA* 2005; **294**(10): 1215–23.
20. Sim I, Gupta M, McDonald K, *et al.* A meta-analysis of randomized trials comparing coronary artery bypass grafting with percutaneous transluminal coronary angioplasty in multivessel coronary artery disease. *Am J Cardiol* 1995; **76**(14):1025–9.
21. Pocock SJ, Henderson RA, Rickards AF, *et al.* Meta-analysis of randomised trials comparing coronary angioplasty with bypass surgery. *Lancet* 1995; **346**(8984):1184–9.
22. Daemen J, Boersma E, Flather M, *et al.* Long-term safety and efficacy of percutaneous coronary intervention with stenting and coronary artery bypass surgery for multivessel coronary artery disease: a meta-analysis with 5-year patient-level data from the ARTS, ERACI-II, MASS-II, and SoS trials. *Circulation* 2008; **118**(11): 1146–54.
23. Serruys PW, Ong AT, van Herwerden LA, *et al.* Five-year outcomes after coronary stenting versus bypass surgery for the treatment of multivessel disease: the final analysis of the Arterial Revascularization Therapies Study (ARTS) randomized trial. *J Am Coll Cardiol* 2005; **46**(4):575–81.
24. Mercado N, Wijns W, Serruys PW, *et al.* One-year outcomes of coronary artery bypass graft surgery versus percutaneous coronary intervention with multiple stenting for multisystem disease: a meta-analysis of individual patient data from randomized clinical trials. *J Thorac Cardiovasc Surg* 2005; **130**(2):512–19.
25. Daemen J, Kuck KH, Macaya C, *et al.* Multivessel coronary revascularization in patients with and without diabetes mellitus 3-year follow-up of the ARTS-II (Arterial Revascularization Therapies Study-Part II) trial. *J Am Coll Cardiol* 2008; **52**(24):1957–67.
26. Hannan EL, Racz MJ, Walford G, *et al.* Long-term outcomes of coronary-artery bypass grafting versus stent implantation. *N Engl J Med* 2005; **352**(21):2174–83.
27. Daemen J, Serruys PW. Lessons from the unrestricted use of drug-eluting stents: Insights from the RESEARCH and T-SEARCH Registry. *Indian Heart J* 2006; **58**(1):10–14.
28. Serruys PW, Ong ATL, Morice MC, *et al.* Arterial Revascularisation Therapies Study Part II- Sirolimus-eluting stents for the treatment of patients with multivessel de novo coronary artery lesions. *EuroIntervention* 2005; **1**(2):147–56.
29. Rodriguez AE, Maree AO, Mieres J, *et al.* Late loss of early benefit from drug-eluting stents when compared with bare-metal stents and coronary artery bypass surgery: 3 years follow-up of the ERACI III registry. *Eur Heart J* 2007; **28**(17):2118–25.
30. Javaid A, Steinberg DH, Buch AN, *et al.* Outcomes of coronary artery bypass grafting versus percutaneous coronary intervention with drug-eluting stents for patients with multivessel coronary artery disease. *Circulation* 2007; **116**(11 Suppl):I200–6.
31. Serruys PW, Morice MC, Kappetein AP, *et al.* Percutaneous coronary intervention versus coronary-artery bypass grafting for severe coronary artery disease. *N Engl J Med* 2009; **360**(10):961–72.
32. Sianos G, Morel MA, Kappetein AP, *et al.* The SYNTAX score: an angiographic tool grading the complexity of coronary artery disease. *EuroIntervention* 2005; **1**:219–27.
33. Kapur A, Hall R, Malik I, *et al.* Randomized comparison of percutaneous coronary intervention with coronary artery bypass grafting in diabetic patients. *JACC* 2010; **55**(5):432–40.
34. Berger A, Botman KJ, MacCarthy PA, *et al.* Long-term clinical outcome after fractional flow reserve-guided percutaneous coronary intervention in patients with multivessel disease. *J Am Coll Cardiol* 2005; **46**(3):438–42.
35. Tonino PA, De Bruyne B, Pijls NH, *et al.* Fractional flow reserve versus angiography for guiding percutaneous coronary intervention. *N Engl J Med* 2009; **360**(3): 213–24.
36. Hannan EL, Racz MJ, McCallister BD, *et al.* A comparison of three-year survival after coronary artery bypass graft surgery and percutaneous transluminal coronary angioplasty. *J Am Coll Cardiol* 1999; **33**(1):63–72.
37. Chaitman BR, Ryan TJ, Kronmal RA, *et al.* Coronary Artery Surgery Study (CASS): comparability of 10 year survival in randomized and randomizable patients. *J Am Coll Cardiol* 1990; **16**(5):1071–8.
38. Karthik S, Fabri BM. Left internal mammary artery usage in coronary artery bypass grafting: a measure of quality control. *Ann R Coll Surg Engl* 2006; **88**(4):367–9.
39. Cameron A, Davis KB, Green G, *et al.* Coronary bypass surgery with internal-thoracic-artery grafts – effects on survival over a 15-year period. *N Engl J Med* 1996; **334**(4):216–19.
40. Loop FD, Lytle BW, Cosgrove DM, *et al.* Influence of the internal-mammary-artery graft on 10-year survival and other cardiac events. *N Engl J Med* 1986; **314**(1):1–6.
41. Kapoor JR, Gienger AL, Ardehali R, *et al.* Isolated disease of the proximal left anterior descending artery: comparing

the effectiveness of percutaneous coronary interventions and coronary artery bypass surgery. *J Am Coll Cardiol Intv* 2008; **1**(5):483–91.

42. Aziz O, Rao C, Panesar SS, *et al.* Meta-analysis of minimally invasive internal thoracic artery bypass versus percutaneous revascularisation for isolated lesions of the left anterior descending artery. *BMJ* 2007; **334**(7594):617.
43. Goy JJ, Kaufmann U, Hurni M, *et al.* 10-year follow-up of a prospective randomized trial comparing bare-metal stenting with internal mammary artery grafting for proximal, isolated de novo left anterior coronary artery stenosis: the SIMA (Stenting versus Internal Mammary Artery grafting) Trial. *J Am Coll Cardiol* 2008; **52**(10):815.
44. Tsuchida K, Colombo A, Lefevre T, *et al.* The clinical outcome of percutaneous treatment of bifurcation lesions in multivessel coronary artery disease with the sirolimus-eluting stent: insights from the Arterial Revascularization Therapies Study part II (ARTS II). *Eur Heart J* 2007; **28**(4):433–42.
45. Morice M-C. Bifurcation lesions: a never-ending challenge. *Eur Heart J* 2008; **29**(23):2831–2.
46. Steigen TK, Maeng M, Wiseth R, *et al.* Randomized Study on Simple Versus Complex Stenting of Coronary Artery Bifurcation Lesions: The Nordic Bifurcation Study. *Circulation* 2006; **114**(18):1955–61.
47. Hoye A, Onderwater E, Cummins P, *et al.* Improved recanalization of chronic total coronary occlusions using an optical coherence reflectometry-guided guidewire. *Catheter Cardiovasc Interv* 2004; **63**(2):158–63.
48. Kukreja N, Serruys PW, Sianos G. Retrograde recanalization of chronically occluded coronary arteries: illustration and description of the technique. *Catheter Cardiovasc Interv* 2007; **69**(6):833–41.
49. Mollet NR, Hoye A, Lemos PA, *et al.* Value of preprocedure multislice computed tomographic coronary angiography to predict the outcome of percutaneous recanalization of chronic total occlusions. *Am J Cardiol* 2005; **95**(2):240–3.
50. Suttorp MJ, Laarman GJ, Rahel BM, *et al.* Primary Stenting of Totally Occluded Native Coronary Arteries II (PRISON II): a randomized comparison of bare metal stent implantation with sirolimus-eluting stent implantation for the treatment of total coronary occlusions. *Circulation* 2006; **114**(9):921–8.
51. Ge L, Iakovou I, Cosgrave J, *et al.* Immediate and mid-term outcomes of sirolimus-eluting stent implantation for chronic total occlusions. *Eur Heart J* 2005; **26**(11):1056–62.
52. Lotan C, Almagor Y, Kuiper K, *et al.* Sirolimus-eluting stent in chronic total occlusion: the SICTO study. *J Interv Cardiol* 2006; **19**(4):307–12.
53. Valenti R, Migliorini A, Signorini U, *et al.* Impact of complete revascularization with percutaneous coronary intervention on survival in patients with at least one chronic total occlusion. *Eur Heart J* 2008; **29**(19):2336–42.
54. Suero JA, Marso SP, Jones PG, *et al.* Procedural outcomes and long-term survival among patients undergoing percutaneous coronary intervention of a chronic total occlusion in native coronary arteries: a 20-year experience. *J Am Coll Cardiol* 2001; **38**(2):409–14.
55. Aziz S, Stables RH, Grayson AD, *et al.* Percutaneous coronary intervention for chronic total occlusions: improved survival for patients with successful revascularization compared to a failed procedure. *Catheter Cardiovasc Interv* 2007; **70**(1):15–20.
56. Niles NW, McGrath PD, Malenka D, *et al.* Survival of patients with diabetes and multivessel coronary artery disease after surgical or percutaneous coronary revascularization: results of a large regional prospective study. Northern New England Cardiovascular Disease Study Group. *J Am Coll Cardiol* 2001; **37**(4):1008–15.
57. Detre KM, Guo P, Holubkov R, *et al.* Coronary revascularization in diabetic patients: a comparison of the randomized and observational components of the Aypass Angioplasty Revascularization Investigation (BARI). *Circulation* 1999; **99**(5):633–40.
58. Aoki J, Ong AT, Hoye A, *et al.* Five year clinical effect of coronary stenting and coronary artery bypass grafting in renal insufficient patients with multivessel coronary artery disease: insights from ARTS trial. *Eur Heart J* 2005; **26**(15):1488–93.
59. Gruberg L, Mercado N, Milo S, *et al.* Impact of body mass index on the outcome of patients with multivessel disease randomized to either coronary artery bypass grafting or stenting in the ARTS trial: The obesity paradox II? *Am J Cardiol* 2005; **95**(4):439–44.
60. Khattab AA, Daemen J, Richardt G, *et al.* Impact of body mass index on the one-year clinical outcome of patients undergoing multivessel revascularization with sirolimus-eluting stents (from the Arterial Revascularization Therapies Study Part II). *Am J Cardiol* 2008; **101**(11):1550–9.
61. Gurm HS, Brennan DM, Booth J, *et al.* Impact of body mass index on outcome after percutaneous coronary intervention (the obesity paradox). *Am J Cardiol* 2002; **90**(1):42–5.
62. Gurm HS, Whitlow PL, Kip KE. The impact of body mass index on short- and long-term outcomes inpatients undergoing coronary revascularization. Insights from the bypass angioplasty revascularization investigation (BARI). *J Am Coll Cardiol* 2002; **39**(5):834–40.
63. Wagner BD, Grunwald GK, Rumsfeld JS, *et al.* Relationship of body mass index with outcomes after coronary artery bypass graft surgery. *Ann Thorac Surg* 2007; **84**(1):10–16.
64. Legrand VM, Serruys PW, Unger F, *et al.* Three-year outcome after coronary stenting versus bypass surgery for the treatment of multivessel disease. *Circulation* 2004; **109**(9):1114–20.
65. Federspiel JJ, Stearns Sm Van Domburg R, *et al.* Risk-benefit trade offs in revascularisation choices. *Medical Decision Making*. In press.
66. Weintraub WS, Becker ER, Mauldin PD, *et al.* Costs of revascularization over eight years in the randomized and

eligible patients in the Emory Angioplasty versus Surgery Trial (EAST). *Am J Cardiol* 2000; **86**(7):747–52.

67. Underwood SR, Anagnostopoulos C, Cerqueira M, *et al.* Myocardial perfusion scintigraphy: the evidence. *Eur J Nucl Med Mol Imaging* 2004; **31**(2):261–91.
68. Mark DB, Hlatky MA, Harrell FE, Jr., *et al.* Exercise treadmill score for predicting prognosis in coronary artery disease. *Ann Intern Med* 1987; **106**(6):793–800.
69. First-year results of CABRI (Coronary Angioplasty versus Bypass Revascularisation Investigation). CABRI Trial Participants. *Lancet* 1995; **346**(8984):1179–84.
70. Rodriguez A, Mele E, Peyregne E, *et al.* Three-year follow-up of the Argentine Randomized Trial of Percutaneous Transluminal Coronary Angioplasty Versus Coronary Artery Bypass Surgery in Multivessel Disease (ERACI). *J Am Coll Cardiol* 1996; **27**(5): 1178–84.
71. Henderson RA, Pocock SJ, Sharp SJ, *et al.* Long-term results of RITA-1 trial: clinical and cost comparisons of coronary angioplasty and coronary-artery bypass grafting. *Lancet* 1998; 352(9138):1419–25.
72. King SB, III, Kosinski AS, Guyton RA, *et al.* Eight-year mortality in the Emory Angioplasty versus Surgery Trial (EAST). *J Am Coll Cardiol* 2000; 35(5):1116–21.
73. The final 10-year follow-up results from the BARI randomized trial. *J Am Coll Cardiol* 2007; **49**(15): 1600–6.
74. Kaehler J, Koester R, Billmann W, *et al.* 13-year follow-up of the German angioplasty bypass surgery investigation. *Eur Heart J* 2005; **26**(20):2148–53.
75. Morrison DA, Sethi G, Sacks J, *et al.* Percutaneous coronary intervention versus repeat bypass surgery for patients with medically refractory myocardial ischemia: AWESOME randomized trial and registry experience with post-CABG patients. *J Am Coll Cardiol* 2002; **40**(11):1951–4.
76. Rodriguez AE, Baldi J, Pereira CF, *et al.* Five-Year Follow-Up of the Argentine Randomized Trial of Coronary Angioplasty With Stenting Versus Coronary Bypass Surgery in Patients With Multiple Vessel Disease (ERACI II). *J Am Coll Cardiol* 2005; **46**(4):582–8.
77. Hueb W, Lopes NH, Gersh BJ, *et al.* Five-year follow-up of the Medicine, Angioplasty, or Surgery Study (MASS II): a randomized controlled clinical trial of 3 therapeutic strategies for multivessel coronary artery disease. *Circulation* 2007; **115**(9):1082–9.
78. Booth J, Clayton T, Pepper J, *et al.* Randomized, controlled trial of coronary artery bypass surgery versus percutaneous coronary intervention in patients with multivessel coronary artery disease: six-year follow-up from the Stent or Surgery Trial (SoS). *Circulation* 2008; **118**(4):381–8.

CHAPTER 15

Percutaneous coronary intervention in non-ST elevation acute coronary syndrome

Michael Mahmoudi and Nick Curzen

Pathophysiology

Ischaemic heart disease (IHD) accounts for 30% of all deaths in men and 25% of all deaths in women in England and Wales. IHD also remains the commonest cause of death in many industrialized countries. The current global impact of IHD is one of marked contrasts. Many countries with previously high rates of IHD, including the United Kingdom, United States, and Finland, are experiencing declines whereas the rates of IHD are rising in many countries such as central and eastern Europe where the rates were previously 'low'[1]. The annual incidence of non-ST elevation acute coronary syndrome (NSTEACS) has been estimated at approximately three per 1000 populations. Hospital mortality is greater than in those patients presenting with ST-elevation myocardial infarction (STEMI) (7% vs. 5%), although at 6 months, the mortality rates become similar[2].

Atherosclerosis is no longer considered a disorder purely of lipid accumulation, but a disease process characterized by the dynamic interaction between endothelial dysfunction, subendothelial inflammation, and the 'wound healing response' of vascular smooth muscle cells (VSMCs)[3]. The atherosclerotic lesion is defined by arterial intimal smooth muscle and inflammatory cell recruitment, lipid accumulation, and connective tissue deposition. The three main cellular components of the atherosclerotic plaque are VSMCs and lymphocytes, which dominate the fibrous cap, and macrophages, which are most abundant in the lipid-rich core. However, atherogenesis can be viewed as a dynamic continuum of several stages, involving accumulation of lipid, endothelial activation, inflammation, and VSMC repair.

Vascular endothelial cells orchestrate the dynamic balance between vasodilatation and vasoconstriction, the inhibition and stimulation of smooth muscle cell proliferation and migration, as well as thrombosis and fibrinolysis. Endothelial dysfunction is considered one of the earliest manifestations of a pathophysiological process that leads to atherosclerosis, and describes an imbalance between endothelium-dependent vasodilatation and endothelium-dependent contraction. It is characterized by loss of normal endothelium-dependent vasodilatation. Common causes of endothelial dysfunction include the conventional risk factors for atherosclerosis, such as hyperlipidaemia, diabetes mellitus, hypertension, and smoking, as well as infectious agents such as cytomegalovirus (CMV) and *Chlamydia pneumoniae.*

The pathophysiological process includes decreased bioavailability of nitric oxide (NO) and expression of endothelial cell surface receptors such as vascular cell adhesion molecule-1 (VCAM-1), intercellular adhesion molecule-1 (ICAM-1), and P selectin which bind platelets, monocytes, and T lymphocytes, thus initiating an inflammatory process which will lead to the formation of an atherosclerotic plaque. The plaque will ultimately consist of an acellular core of cholesterol esters covered by an endothelialized fibrous cap containing VSMCs, macrophages, T lymphocytes, and mast cells.

Fundamentally, there are two mechanisms by which atherosclerotic plaques can lead to symptoms. Firstly, if the lesion becomes sufficiently large to restrict blood flow, tissue ischaemia will occur as a result of mismatch between oxygen supply and demand leading to stable angina. By contrast, the second mechanism involves plaque rupture or erosion which will expose the highly thrombogenic acellular core to blood leading to platelet activation, aggregation, thrombosis, vessel occlusion, and ultimately to an acute coronary syndrome. Plaques containing a large lipid pool, a thin fibrous cap, high density of macrophages, and low density of VSMCs are more likely to rupture than those with a thick cap which is more able to resist local mechanical stresses. It is now clear that the most important determinant of plaque stability is the composition of the fibrous cap with a predominance of inflammatory cells and relative paucity of VSMCs favouring plaque rupture[4].

There are three potential mechanisms by which inflammatory cells may weaken the fibrous cap. Firstly, they produce matrix metalloproteinases that degrade matrix proteins, and proinflammatory cytokines such as interferon-γ, which inhibit VSMC proliferation and collagen synthesis thus affecting matrix protein turnover. Secondly, they produce a variety of other inflammatory cytokines such as interleukin-1β, and tumour necrosis factor-α, which synergistically cause VSMC apoptosis. Finally, activated macrophages have been shown to induce VSMC apoptosis by direct cellular contact. This is exacerbated by a reduction in the proliferative capacity and an increased susceptibility to apoptosis of plaque VSMCs[5–7].

In NSTEACS, plaque rupture or erosion leads to platelet activation and aggregation within the lipid core. As the thrombus begins to protrude into the lumen, the fibrin content of the clot increases and clumps of platelets may be swept downstream into the distal intramyocardial arteries leading to myocyte necrosis and subsequent release of cellular contents such as troponins. This is the pathological hallmark of non-STEMI (NSTEMI). The thrombus may grow to contain a loose network of fibrin and large numbers of entrapped red blood cells and ultimately occlude the artery. This is the pathological hallmark of STEMI. The persistence of the thrombotic process so that it neither progresses to occlude the vessel or heal is due to a balance between the prothrombotic and antithrombotic factors.

Clinical syndromes

The term acute coronary syndrome (ACS) embraces two conditions[8,9]:

1) STEMI or ST-elevation ACS (STEACS). This refers to patients presenting with cardiac-sounding chest pain or discomfort and ST-segment elevation on the electrocardiogram (ECG). The aim of therapy is to achieve immediate reperfusion either by thrombolysis or primary angioplasty.

2) NSTEACS. This refers to patients presenting with cardiac sounding chest pain or discomfort, and ECG changes such as ST-segment depression, T-wave inversion, T-wave flattening, pseudo-normalization of T waves, or, rarely, no ECG changes. The term NSTEMI refers to patients with elevated cardiac markers of necrosis, most frequently troponins. Patients with unstable angina do not exhibit elevated cardiac markers of necrosis.

Risk stratification

Patients with NSTEACS represent a heterogeneous population with varying risks of death and adverse cardiac events both in the short and long term. In these patients, risk stratification is important since the benefits of aggressive and costly revascularization strategies are proportional to individual risk scores. Three risk score tools are commonly used in routine clinical practice to facilitate management decisions:

1) Thrombolysis In Myocardial Infarction (TIMI) risk score[10] (Table 15.1)

2) Global Registry of Acute Coronary Events (GRACE) risk score[11] (Table 15.2)

3) Platelet glycoprotein IIb/IIIa in unstable angina: receptor suppression using integrilin (PURSUIT) risk score[12] (Table 15.3).

The TIMI risk score consists of seven risk indicators: age, coronary artery risk factors, known coronary artery stenosis, aspirin use in the preceding 7 days, recent severe angina, elevated cardiac markers, and ST-segment deviation. The composite endpoint of all-cause mortality, new or recurrent MI, or severe recurrent ischaemia has been shown to increase as the TIMI risk score increases. This has been validated in a number of large scale studies such as the Efficacy and Safety of Subcutaneous Enoxaparin in Unstable Angina and Non-Q wave Myocardial Infarction (ESSENCE) trial[13].

The GRACE risk score was developed from 11 389 unselected patients with ACS. It utilizes eight variables: age, heart rate, systolic blood pressure, creatinine, Killip class, cardiac arrest at presentation, and the presence of elevated cardiac markers. The total score is compared to a reference monogram to determine all-cause mortality from hospital discharge up to 6 months. The model has been validated in GRACE and GUSTO-2B trials[14].

Table 15.1 The TIMI risk score (0–7 points)

Factors	Points
Age (years)	
<65	0
≥65	1
CAD risk factors	
0–2	0
≥3	1
Known CAD (stenosis ≥50%)	
No	0
Yes	1
Aspirin use in the preceding 7 days	
No	0
Yes	1
Recent severe angina (<24h)	
No	0
Yes	1
Elevated cardiac markers	
No	0
Yes	1
ST-segment deviation ≥0.5mm	
No	0
Yes	1

Table 15.2 The GRACE risk score (0–258 points)

Factors	Points
Age (years)	
< 40	0
40–49	18
50–59	36
60–69	55
70–79	73
≥80	91
Heart rate (bpm)	
<70	0
70–89	7
90–109	13
110–149	23
150–199	36
>200	46
Systolic BP (mmHg)	
<80	63
80–99	58
100–119	47
120–139	37
140–159	26
160–199	11
>200	0
Creatinine (mg/dL)	
0.0–0.39	2
0.4–0.79	5
0.8–1.19	8
1.2–1.59	11
1.6–1.99	14
2.0–3.99	23
>4	31
Killip class	
Class I	0
Class II	21
Class III	43
Class IV	64
Cardiac arrest on presentation	
No	0
Yes	43
Elevated cardiac markers	
No	0
Yes	15

The PURSUIT risk score utilizes five variables: age, sex, CCS class in the preceding 6 weeks, signs of heart failure, and the presence of ST-segment depression in the presenting ECG. The 30-day incidence of death and the composite of death or MI increases with increasing PURSUIT risk score as has been shown in a number of registries.

Both the American College of Cardiology (ACC) and the European Society of Cardiology (ESC) guidelines for the diagnosis and treatment of NSTEACS have recommended that such risk scores should be utilized in both the initial and subsequent risk assessment of these patients[8,9].

Trials of medical/conservative therapy versus early invasive strategy

The management of patients with NSTEACS may be 'invasive' or 'conservative'. With the conservative approach, patients are commenced on optimal medical

Table 15.3 The PURSUIT risk score (0–18 points)

Factors	Points
Age (years)	
40–50	8
60	9
70	11
80	12
Sex	
Male	1
Female	0
CCS class in the previous 6 weeks	
I–II	0
III–IV	2
Signs of heart failure	
No	0
Yes	2
ST-segment depression in the presenting ECG	
No	0
Yes	1

therapy and angiography and revascularization only considered in those patients with either ongoing ischaemia clinically or with inducible ischaemia on non-invasive testing.

Both the ACC and ECS guidelines recommend an early invasive strategy in the following patients and circumstances:

- Elevated troponin levels
- Dynamic ST or T-wave changes
- Diabetes mellitus
- Impaired renal function (glomerular filtration rate <60mL/min/1.73m^2)
- Severe left ventricular systolic dysfunction (ejection fraction <40%)
- Post-MI angina
- Percutaneous coronary intervention (PCI) within the preceding 6 months
- Previous coronary artery bypass graft (CABG)
- Intermediate and high-risk patients according to risk score assessment.

The evidence for an early invasive strategy

Several randomized clinical trials have compared the routine early invasive strategy with a 'selective invasive strategy' in the treatment of patients with NSTEMI.

The Framingham and Fast Revascularization During Instability in Coronary Artery Disease (FRISC) II trial was the first randomized study to demonstrate that an early invasive strategy was associated with improved outcomes[15]. This randomized, prospective study enrolled 2457 ACS patients without ST-segment elevation to either an early invasive strategy or a non-invasive treatment strategy. All patients received aspirin and open-label dalteparin for at least 5 days. Randomization occurred within 72h and revascularization within 10 days. At 6 months, the early invasive strategy was associated with a significantly lower rate of the primary composite endpoint of death or MI in intermediate and high-risk patients (9.4% invasive vs. 12.1 conservative; p = 0.03). At 2 years, there was an absolute 4.2% reduction in the combined endpoint (12.1% vs. 16.3%). Hospital admissions were also significantly lower in the invasive arm (44.8% vs. 64.5%; p <0.001). The reduction in mortality seen in the invasive group did not reach statistical significance. At 5 years, the results remained consistent with a significantly lower rate of the primary endpoint (19.9% vs. 24.5%; p = 0.009). This was primarily driven by a reduction in MI (12.9% vs. 17.7%; p = 0.002). There was no difference in the rate of mortality between the two groups (9.7% vs. 10.1%; p = 0.69) (Fig. 15.1).

The benefits of an early invasive strategy have been confirmed in other studies. The TACTICS-TIMI 18 study randomized 2220 patients with NSTEACS to either an early invasive strategy, with routine catheterization

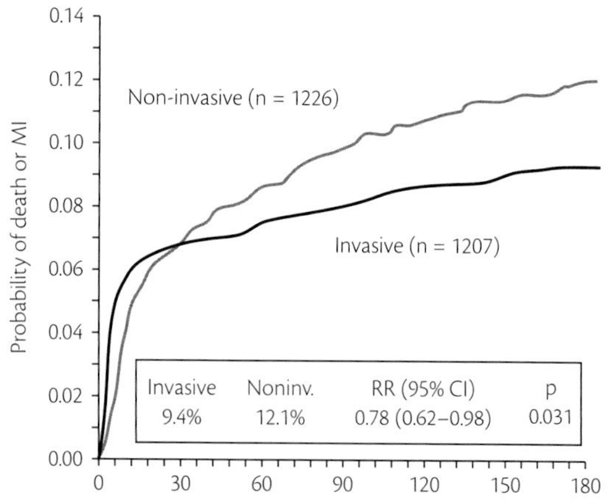

Fig. 15.1 The probability of death or MI in the FRISC II population. Reproduced from Long-term low-molecular-mass heparin in unstable coronary-artery disease: FRISC II prospective randomised multicentre study. *The Lancet* 1999; **354**:701–7, with permission of Elsevier.

within 4–48h and revascularization as appropriate or a conservative strategy[16]. All patients were treated with aspirin, heparin, and the glycoprotein IIb/IIIa inhibitor tirofiban. At 6 months, the early invasive strategy was associated with a significantly lower rate of the primary composite endpoint of death, non-fatal MI, and re-hospitalization for an ACS (15.9% vs. 19.4%; p = 0.03) (Fig. 15.2). The rate of death or non-fatal MI at 6 months was similarly reduced (7.3% vs. 9.5%; p <0.05). The greatest benefit from intervention was seen in high- or intermediate-risk patients (raised troponin, ST-depression on the ECG, diabetes mellitus, and the elderly). This constituted 75% of the study patients. In the 25% of patients that were classified as low risk, the outcomes were similar with the use of either strategy. A prospective analysis of the data demonstrated that in patients with an elevated troponin at baseline, an early invasive strategy reduced event rates to those of patients who did not have an elevated troponin.

The Randomized Intervention Trial of unstable Angina (RITA) 3 randomized 1810 NSTEACS patients to either routine early angiography and PCI (within 72h) or a conservative approach[17]. The cumulative risk of death, MI, or refractory angina was lower in the invasive arm at 4 months (9.6% vs. 14.5%; p = 0.001). This benefit was maintained at 1 year (13.6% vs. 18.4%; p = 0.003) (Fig. 15.3). At 5 years, there was a 22% relative reduction in the incidence of all cause death/MI (16.6% vs. 20%; p = 0.04), a 24% reduction in death (12.1% vs. 15.1%; p = 0.05), and a 26% reduction in the incidence of cardiovascular death/MI (12.2% vs. 15.9%; p = 0.03). Benefits were seen mainly in high-risk

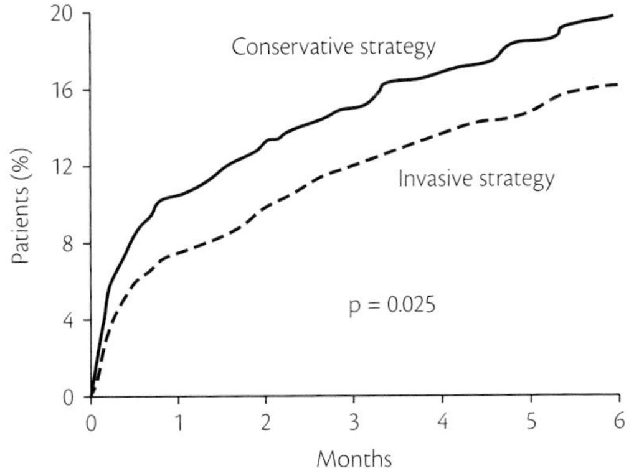

Fig. 15.2 Cumulative incidence of the primary endpoint of death, MI, or re-hospitalization for an ACS during the 6-month follow-up period. Reproduced from Cannon, CP *et al* TACTICS-TIMI 18 Comparison of early and conservative strategies in patients with unstable coronary syndromes treated with the glycoprotein IIb/IIIa inhibitor Tirofiban; *NEJM*, **344**: 1879–87. Copyright © 2001 Massachusetts Medical Society. All right reserved.

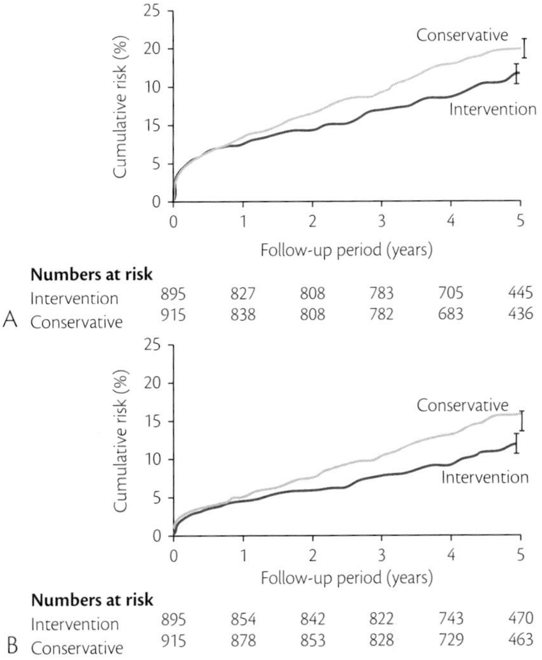

Fig. 15.3 The cumulative risk of death or MI in patients with NSTEACS (A) and the cumulative risk of death in patients with NSTEACS (B) in the RITA 3 patients. Interventional versus conservative treatment for patients with unstable angina or non-ST-elevation myocardial infarction: the British Heart Foundation RITA 3 randomised trial, *The Lancet*, **360**: 743–51.

patients, emphasizing the need for appropriate risk stratification.

FRISC II, TACTICS-TIMI 18, and RITA 3 all suggested that, in terms of clinical outcomes, an early invasive strategy was beneficial. However, none of these studies established the optimal timing of an 'invasive strategy'. This issue was subsequently addressed by two studies. The Intracoronary Stenting with Antithrombotic Regimen Cooling-Off Trial (ISAR-COOL) set out to determine the clinical efficacy of a 'cooling-off' period prior to PCI in patients with NSTEACS[18]. The study randomized 410 patients to either antithrombotic pre-treatment for 72–120h (cooling-off) followed by PCI or immediate PCI (mean 2.4h). The antithrombotic pre-treatment was similar in the two groups and consisted of aspirin (500-mg IV bolus followed by 100mg twice daily), clopidogrel (600-mg oral bolus followed by 75mg twice daily), tirofiban (10-mcg/kg bolus followed by 0.10mcg/kg/min), and heparin (60-U/kg bolus infusion). Peri-interventional treatment included tirofiban 0.15mcg/kg/min for 24h, heparin 60-U/kg bolus, aspirin 2 × 100mg, and clopidogrel 75mg twice daily for 5 days followed 75mg. Following PCI, tirofiban was continued for 24h, clopidogrel for 4 weeks, and aspirin indefinitely.

At 30 days, the early intervention group had a significantly lower rate of the primary composite endpoint of death, and non-fatal MI (5.9% vs. 11.6%; p = 0.04). This was primarily driven by a reduction in the rates of non-fatal MI. This study not only emphasized the importance of an early intervention strategy, but also suggested that a 'cooling-off' period may be disadvantageous in patients presenting with NSTEACS.

Further support for the benefit of an early invasive strategy in the management of NSTEACS has been provided by the Value of first day angiography/angioplasty in evolving non-ST segment elevation myocardial infarction (VINO) study[19]. This study randomized 131 patients with NSTEACS to either first day angiography and revascularization (mean randomization to angiography time 6.2h; N = 64) or an early conservative strategy (N = 67). At 6 months, the early invasive strategy was associated with a significantly lower rate of the primary endpoints of death and re-infarction (6.2% vs. 22.3%; p <0.001). Six-month mortality was significantly lower with the early invasive strategy (3.1% vs. 13.4%; p <0.03) as was the rate of non-fatal MI (3.1% vs. 14.9%; p <0.02). Interestingly, 40% of patients in the conservative group had undergone revascularization within 6 month of randomization. The study concluded that first day angiography and PCI whenever possible reduces mortality and re-infarction in patients presenting with NSTEACS.

Still further support for 'early' angiography and revascularization in the NSTEACS population has been provided by the Superior Yield of the New Strategy of Enoxoparin, Revascularization, and Glycoprotein IIb/IIIa inhibitors (SYNERGY) trial[20]. This trail demonstrated significantly lower rates of death or MI as the time from presentation to angiography was reduced, with an adjusted odds ratio of 0.56 when angiography was performed <6h compared to angiography undertaken at a later time point. This benefit persisted until angiography was performed at up to 30h (Fig. 15.4).

A recent meta-analysis of seven randomized trials incorporating 8375 patients has demonstrated a significant reduction in all-cause mortality at 2 years (4.9% vs. 6.5%; p = 0.001), non-fatal MI (7.6% vs. 9.1%; p = 0.01), as well as hospitalization RR = 0.69, 95% CI 0.65–0.74; p <0.0001) in those patients undergoing an early invasive strategy[21]. Furthermore, a review of contemporary randomized trials using the Cochrane Database has reached similar conclusions[22].

On the basis of the studies discussed here, it is apparent that an invasive strategy is superior to conservative management in patients with NSTEACS, particularly in troponin-positive patients. However, the Early Invasive versus Selectively Invasive Management for Acute Coronary Syndromes (ICTUS) trail has challenged this notion[23]. ICTUS randomized 1200 patients with NSTEMI to either an early invasive strategy or to a more conservative strategy. Patients received aspirin daily, enoxaparin for 48h, and abciximab at the time of PCI. The use of clopidogrel and intensive lipid-lowering therapy was recommended. At 12 months, there was no difference in the primary composite endpoint of death, non-fatal MI, or re-hospitalization for anginal symptoms within 1 year after randomization or MI in intermediate- and high-risk patients (22.7% vs. 21.2%; p = 0.33).

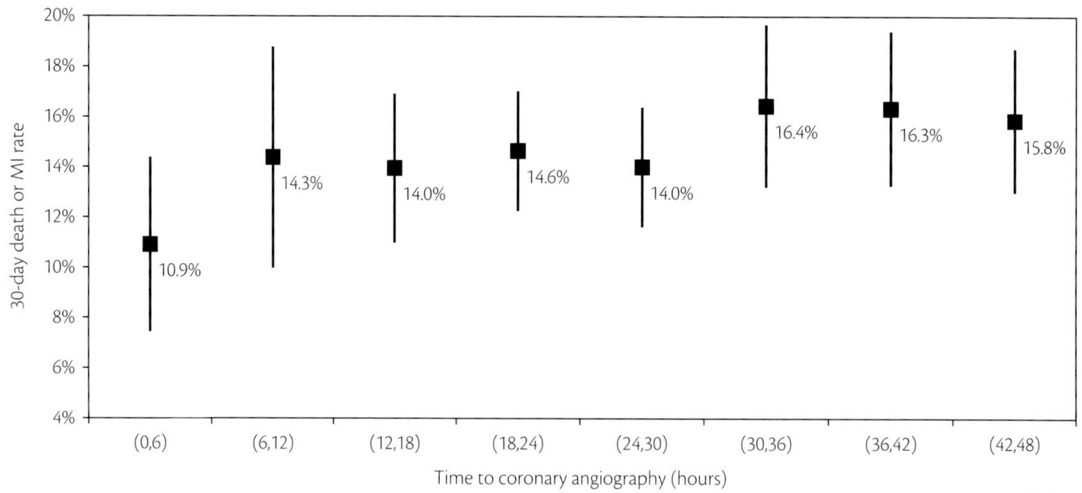

Fig. 15.4 Adjusted rates of death or MI through 30 days by time from hospitalization to coronary angiography. Reproduced with permission from SYNERGY Trial. Time to Coronary Angiography and Outcomes Among Patients With High-Risk Non-ST-Segment-Elevation Acute Coronary Syndromes. *Circulation* 2007; **116**: 2669–77.

The mortality rate was similar in the two groups (2.5%). MI was significantly more frequent in the early invasive arm of the study (15% vs. 10%; p = 0.005), but re-hospitalization was less frequent in this group (7.4% vs. 10.9%; p = 0.04). Another important finding of this study was that there was no difference in adverse clinical outcomes between patients who underwent early PCI (mean time of 23h) and those who underwent delayed PCI (mean time of 11.8 days) either during hospitalization or up to 1 year after randomization. The discrepant findings of ICTUS demand closer scrutiny. Firstly, recurrent MI was defined as any elevation in the CK-MB level above the upper limit of normal, irrespective of whether this elevation was spontaneous or peri-procedural. The excess MI rate observed in the invasive arm was thus driven largely by a relatively small rise in the CK-MB fraction (≥1× to ≤3× the upper limit of normal). This is compared to ≥1.5× used in FRISC II and ≥3× used in TACTICS-TIMI 18. It is therefore possible that the strict definition of MI used in this study may have disadvantaged the 'outcome' of patients designated to the invasive strategy. Secondly, ICTUS required troponin positivity for entry and it has been suggested that a combination of troponin and other markers of high risk should be used in the selection of the optimal management strategy. However, what ICTUS has demonstrated is that a conservative strategy may be an effective and appropriate management option in patients with NSTEACS and that further data is required regarding the optimal risk stratification and management of such patients.

Despite the wealth of evidence available for the management of NSTEACS, the optimal timing of an invasive strategy remains controversial. ISAR-COOL, VINO, and SYNERGY all advocate angiography and revascularization within a 6-h window although an average of 12h appears more realistic particularly for patients presenting out of working hours, weekends, and units that require patients to be transferred to regional centres with coronary revascularization capabilities. However, none of the international guidelines currently advocate a systematic approach of immediate angiography in patients with NSTEACS except those with refractory angina, clinical symptoms of heart failure or shock, and those with ventricular fibrillation or tachycardia.

Pharmacological therapy

Established treatments

Aspirin

Aspirin is as an inhibitor of platelet aggregation. It acts by inhibiting cyclo-oxygenase 1, thus preventing the production of thromboxane A2 within platelets. In patients with NSTEACS, aspirin therapy has been shown to reduce the risk of MI or death (RR 0.52; CI 0.37–0.72) and severe angina (RR 0.71; CI 0.56–0.91). The combined event rate of death or MI or referral for coronary angiography was reduced at 3 month (RR 0.44; CI 0.3–0.66) and 1 year (RR 0.65; CI 0.54–0.79)[24]. Similar findings were noted in a meta-analysis from the Antithrombotic Trialists' Collaboration[25]. Antiplatelet therapy, predominantly aspirin, was associated with a 30% reduction in vascular events at 1 month (10.4% vs. 14.2%; p <0.05). The ideal dose is unknown, but 75–150mg is effective. Higher doses have not been shown to provide any additional benefit. Aspirin should be commenced at a loading dose of 162–325mg as soon as the diagnosis of ACS is suspected to produce a rapid antithrombotic effect by immediate and complete inhibition of thromboxane A2 production. Aspirin at doses of 75–162mg should be continued indefinitely regardless of whether the patient proceeds to revascularization or not. The long-term benefits derived from aspirin is dose independent[24].

Clopidogrel

Clopidogrel is an adenosine diphosphate receptor (P2Y12) antagonist. Its antiplatelet effect is irreversible, but in the absence of a loading dose, its optimal effect takes several days to be established.

The benefit of clopidogrel in the management of NSTEACS was established in the Clopidogrel in Unstable angina to prevent Recurrent ischemic Events (CURE) trial[26]. The trail randomized 12 562 patients who had presented within 24h after the onset of a NSTEACS to clopidogrel, 300mg loading and 75mg maintenance, or placebo. All patients were given aspirin (75–320mg/day). At an average follow-up of 9 months, the combination of aspirin and clopidogrel was associated with a significant reduction in the composite of cardiovascular death, non-fatal MI, or stroke (9.3% vs. 11.4%; p <0.001) (Fig. 15.5). Clopidogrel was also associated with reduced in-hospital ischaemia, heart failure, and need for a revascularization procedure. Clopidogrel was associated with a significant increase in the risk of major bleeding (3.7% vs. 2.7%; p = 0.001) but not life-threatening bleeding or haemorrhagic stoke.

The PCI-CURE study was a substudy of the 2658 patients who underwent PCI. The patients were pre-treated with aspirin alone or aspirin and clopidogrel for a median of 6 days prior to intervention and combination therapy for 4 weeks post intervention. Clopidogrel reduced the composite of cardiovascular death, MI, or

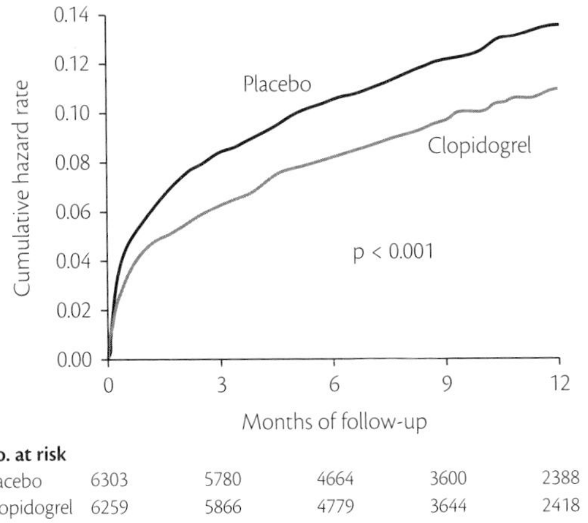

Fig. 15.5 Cumulative hazard rates for the first primary outcome (death from cardiovascular causes, non-fatal MI, or stroke) during the 12 months of the study. Reproduced from The clopidogrel in unstable angina to prevent recurrent events trial investigators, Effects of clopidogrel in addition to Asprin in patients with acute coronary syndromes without ST-segment elevation *NEJM* (2001) **1345**: 494–502. Copyright © 2001 Massachusetts Medical Society. All rights reserved.

urgent target vessel revascularization within 30 days and cardiovascular death or MI at 8 month (4.5% vs. 6.4%; p = 0.03). This benefit was seen in both the stented and non-stented patients.

The Clopidogrel for the Reduction of Events During Observation (CREDO) trial was designed to determine the optimal timing for initiating antiplatelet therapy in patients undergoing PCI[27]. The trial randomized 2116 patients to pre-treatment with clopidogrel 300mg and aspirin 325mg as a loading dose or placebo and aspirin 325mg as a loading dose 3–24h before PCI. Post procedure, all patients who underwent PCI and stenting received clopidogrel 75mg/day for 28 days. From day 28 to 1 year, patients that had been randomized to clopidogrel and aspirin pre-treatment were continued on clopidogrel 75mg/day, whilst patients that had been randomized to placebo continued with placebo. Approximately one-third of patients had an ACS, 89% were stented using a bare-metal stent, and 40% were treated with a glycoprotein IIb/IIIa inhibitor. At 12 months, the combination of aspirin and clopidogrel resulted in a significant reduction in the composite endpoint of death, MI, and stroke (11.5% vs. 8.5%; p = 0.02). This benefit was predominantly driven by fewer acute thrombotic complications and was independent of diabetes mellitus, ACS, or glycoprotein IIb/IIIa inhibitor. When analyzing the timing of clopidogrel loading, there was no difference in outcome between the two groups if pre-treatment was given less than 6h prior to PCI. However, a 39% reduction in the composite endpoint was observed when pre-loading was administered between 6–24h before PCI.

The optimal loading dose of clopidogrel remains controversial. In the Assessment of the Best Loading Dose of Clopidogrel to Blunt Platelet Activation, Inflammation and Ongoing Necrosis (ALBION) trial, 103 patients with NSTEMI were randomized to loading doses of 300mg, 600mg, and 900mg followed by 75mg maintenance. Whilst the 600-mg and 900-mg loading doses were associated with a more rapid and higher level of platelet activation and aggregation, there was no significant difference in major adverse cardiac events in the two groups[28].

The Antiplatelet Therapy for Reduction of Myocardial damage During Angioplasty (ARMYDA-2) study randomized 255 patients with NSTEACS or exertional angina and a positive stress test scheduled to undergo PCI to either 600-mg or 300-mg loading dose of clopidogrel 4–8h before diagnostic catheterization[29]. All patients were pre-treated with aspirin 100mg, a dose that was continued indefinitely as well as clopidogrel 75mg/day for up to 9 month. Baseline clinical and angiographic characteristics were similar in both groups, including the incidence of diabetes (30%) and ACS (25%). Drug eluting stents were used in 20% of cases and 13% of patients received GP IIb/IIIa inhibitors. At 30 days, the composite primary endpoint of MI, death, and target vessel revascularization was significantly greater in the 300-mg loading group (12% vs. 4%; p = 0.04) and was due entirely to peri-procedural MI. The 300-mg loading group also had a significantly higher elevations in CK-MB (26% vs. 14%; p = 0.036), troponin I (44% vs. 26%; p = 0.04), and myoglobin (46% vs. 30%; p = 0.015) concentrations. Multivariate analysis identified pre-treatment with 600-mg loading dose and statin therapy as independent predictors of decreased risk of peri-procedural MI (p = 0.44 and p = 0.02 respectively).

It has become increasingly apparent that there is a wide degree of heterogeneity in the response of individual patients to clopidogrel. Those patients with a relatively poor response have been shown to have adverse procedural and medium-term outcome after PCI[30]. Attempts to address the variability of response to clopidogrel and, specifically, to tailor clopidogrel dose to individual patient response have yielded important results. The RELOAD study (Reload with clopidogrel before coronary angioplasty in subjects treated long term with dual antiplatelet therapy) examined whether a dose–effect relationship could be seen across three loading regimens (300mg, 600mg, 900mg) in clopidogrel treated patients (75mg/day) as had previously been observed in clopidogrel naïve patients[31]. One hundred and sixty-six consecutive patients scheduled to undergo cardiac catheterization for NSTEACS or stable angina were serially allocated to clopidogrel 300mg, 600mg, and 900mg. Four hours after the first loading dose, a second loading dose of 600mg, 300mg, or 0mg was administered such that all patients received a total of 900mg loading. Thereafter, all patients continued on clopidogrel 75mg/day and aspirin ≤100mg/day. The three groups had similar baseline characteristics including the incidence of diabetes (32%) and previous MI (49%). Forty-eight per cent were admitted with NSTEACS and 52% with stable angina. Inhibition of residual platelet aggregation (IRPA) was measured at baseline, at 4h after the initial load and at 24h. At 4h following the first loading, the primary endpoint of inhibition of RIPA was significantly greater after 900mg versus 600mg (64% vs. 40.3%; p = 0.02) and 300mg (64% vs. 30.7%; p = 0.0008). After the first loading, patients that had been loaded with 900mg had lower intersubject variability compared to 600mg (0.13% vs. 0.29%; p = 0.006). The percentage IRPA was not significantly different at 24h when all patients had received 900mg. The incidence of suboptimal response, defined as IRPA <10%, were 23%, 20.4%, and 5.3% with 300mg, 600mg, and 900mg respectively (p = 0.02 for all). Although non-randomized, this study demonstrated that between one-third to one-fourth of patients on clopidogrel 75mg/day may have inadequate platelet inhibition. The study also demonstrated that a 900-mg loading dose is more effective than either 600mg or 300mg loading in inhibiting platelet activity within 4h, although at 24h, platelet inhibition was similar across the three groups.

Statins

Cholesterol is an important component of eukaryotic cell membranes and serves as the immediate precursor of steroid hormones.

The enzyme 3-hydroxy-3-methylglutaryl coenzyme A (HMG-CoA) reductase is the rate-limiting enzyme in the cholesterol biosynthetic pathway. Statins reversibly inhibit this enzyme leading to a reduction in the hepatic synthesis and secretion of lipoproteins, as well as upregulation of LDL receptors on hepatocytes, and apolipoprotein E and B- containing lipoproteins. In addition to reducing LDL, statins also reduce lipoprotein remnants including those of very low-density lipoprotein (VLDL) and intermediate-density lipoprotein (IDLP).

Statins also inhibit the synthesis of other intermediate metabolites such as farnesyl pyrophosphate (FPP) and geranylgeranyl pyrophosphate (GGPP). These intermediates are involved in the post-translational modification of a variety of proteins such as nuclear lamins and the GTP-binding proteins Ras and Rho. The inhibition of Rho geranylgeranylation and its downstream target, Rho kinase, has been postulated to mediate some of the pleiotropic effects of statins[32].

In addition to its lipid-lowering properties, statins have also recently been shown to be able to modify many of the steps involved in the evolution of the atherosclerotic plaque. Statins have been shown to increase endothelial NO synthase (eNOS) mRNA half-life, augment eNOS function, and attenuate endothelial cell apoptosis[33]. From a clinical perspective, brachial artery flow-mediated dilatation in elderly diabetic individuals has been shown to improve after 3 days of therapy with cerivastatin whilst improvements in the coronary endothelial function was seen 24h after a single oral dose of 40mg of pravastatin[34,35]. This is a predictable outcome for an agent that improves endothelial function.

After the discovery of the effects of statins on eNOS, other studies have demonstrated eNOS-independent anti-inflammatory actions for statins. For example, simvastatin has been shown to inhibit leucocyte–endothelial cell interactions independently of any lipid-lowering actions[36], atorvastatin was demonstrated to reduce neointimal inflammation and macrophage infiltration[37]. Statins have also been demonstrated to suppress the growth of macrophages expressing matrix metalloproteinases and tissue factor[38] thereby providing a mechanism for increasing plaque stability and decreasing thrombogenicity.

Statins have also been demonstrated to have other potentially important anti-inflammatory properties. The Pravastatin Inflammation/CRP Evaluation (PRINCE) study was conducted to determine whether pravastatin has anti-inflammatory effects as evidenced by a reduction in CRP. After 24 weeks, there was a decrease of 16.9% in the statin treated group, but no change in the CRP level of the placebo group. This effect was seen as early as 12 weeks and was present in all subgroups regardless of age, smoking, baseline lipid profile, presence of diabetes, and use of aspirin or hormone replacement therapy[39]. This trial demonstrated the anti-inflammatory action of statins independently of their lipid-lowering properties. Thus a variety of data puts statins in a position in which they may well be equipped to modify the inflammatory milieu seen in ACS.

The Myocardial ischemia reduction in Aggressive Cholesterol Lowering (MIRACL) study randomized 2402 individuals with NSTEACS to atorvastatin 80mg/day or placebo within 24–96h of admission for 16 weeks.

CRP, IL-6, and serum amyloid A (SAA) were measured at baseline and at 16 weeks[40]. Atorvastatin produced a 34% reduction in CRP and a 13% reduction in SAA after 16 weeks. There was no significant change in the levels of IL-6. This study demonstrated that statin therapy enhanced the resolution of the marked inflammatory response associated with ACS. At this dose, atorvastatin has also been shown to halt the progression of coronary plaque growth in the Reversal of Atherosclerosis with Aggressive Lipid Lowering (REVERSAL) trial[41].

In the Pravastatin or Atorvastatin Evaluation and Infection Therapy-Thrombolysis in Myocardial Infarction 22 (PROVE IT-TIMI 22) study, therapy with statins to achieve a target level of CRP less than 2mg/L was associated with a significant improvement in event-free survival in individuals with ACS independently of the serum LDL concentration (2.8 vs. 3.9 events per 100 person-years; p = 0.006)[42].

Heparin

The benefits of unfractionated heparin (UFH) and low molecular weight heparin (LMWH) in the management of ACS are well established. A meta-analysis of six trials comparing UFH versus placebo demonstrated a 33% risk reduction for death and MI (OR 0.67; 95% CI 0.45–0.99; p = 0.045). This was primarily driven by a reduction in the rate of MI[43].

The superiority of the LMWH enoxoparin to UFH has been demonstrated in a number of studies such as the TIMI 11B trial[44] and ESSENCE study[12]. TIMI 11B randomized 3910 patients with NSTEACS to UFH or enoxoparin 1mg/kg twice daily as their antithrombotic treatment. After 8 days, the primary endpoint of death, MI, or urgent revascularization was significantly lower in the enoxoparin group (12.4% vs. 14.5%; p = 0.048). After 43 days, the results were maintained (17.3% vs. 19.7%; p = 0.048).

ESSENCE randomized 3171 NSTEACS patients to UFH or enoxoparin 1mg/kg twice daily as their antithrombotic treatment. At 14 days, the primary endpoint of death, MI or recurrent angina was significantly lower in the enoxoparin group (16.6% vs. 19.8%; p = 0.019). This benefit was maintained at 30 days (19.8% vs. 23.3%; p = 0.016). Overall, bleeding complications occurred more commonly with enoxoparin (18.4% vs. 14.2%; p = 0.001), predominantly because of the development of bruising at the site of enoxoparin administration.

A meta-analysis of six trials comparing UFH with enoxoparin demonstrated no difference in mortality at 30 days between the two compounds. At 30 days, enoxoparin caused a reduction in the combined endpoint of death or MI compared to UFH (10.1% vs. 11%; OR 1; 95% CI 0.83–0.99). There was no difference in blood transfusions or major bleeding between the two groups [45].

Platelet glycoprotein IIb/IIIa receptor antagonists

Platelet activation is accompanied by conformational changes in their surface glycoprotein (GP) IIb/IIIa receptor leading to increased receptor affinity for fibrinogen and subsequent platelet aggregation. The IIb/IIIa receptors therefore represent a logical therapeutic target in the process of platelet aggregation, one of the key components of the vascular inflammatory response that mediates ACS.

There are currently three commercially available GP IIb/IIIa inhibitors:

1) Abciximab: a Fab fragment of a humanized murine antibody, with a plasma half-life of 10–30min. Platelet aggregation returns to baseline within 24–48h after discontinuation of the drug
2) Tirofiban: a non-peptide mimetic of the Arg–Gly–Asp sequence, with a plasma half-life of approximately 2h. Coagulation parameters return to baseline within 4–8h of discontinuing the drug
3) Eptifibatide: a cyclic heptapeptide containing the Lys–Gly–Asp sequence, with a plasma half-life of 2.5h. Platelet aggregation returns to baseline within 4h after discontinuation of the drug.

The evidence for the role of GP IIb/IIIa inhibitors in the management of NSTEACS can be considered under two headings:

1) Evidence for benefit in PCI in NSTEACS
2) Evidence for medical benefit in NSTEASC.

Evidence for benefit in PCI in NSTEACS

A number of clinical trials have provided support for the benefit of GP IIb/IIIa inhibitors in NSTEACS. The randomized placebo-controlled trial of abciximab before and during coronary intervention in refractory unstable angina trial (CAPTURE study) assessed whether abciximab could improve outcome in patients with refractory unstable angina who were undergoing percutaneous transluminal coronary angioplasty (PTCA)[46]. Patients were recruited within 24h of angiography and angioplasty was scheduled 18–24h after randomization. All patients received aspirin, intravenous GTN, β-blockers, and calcium channel antagonists. Heparin was given prior to randomization and continued for at least 1h after PTCA. At randomization, patients were given either abciximab 0.25mcg/kg bolus followed by 10mcg/kg infusion or a placebo.

The treatment was started within 2h of randomization and continued for the 18–24h before PTCA and for 1h after the procedure. The trial was discontinued after the third interim analysis of 1050 patients demonstrated the efficacy of abciximab, but the data for 1265 patients are presented here. At 30 days, the primary endpoint of death, MI, and target vessel revascularization was significantly lower in the abciximab group (11.3% vs. 15.9%; p = 0.012) which was mainly driven by a reduction in MI (4.1% vs. 8.2%); p = 0.002). The findings were consistent in all subgroups and were independent of age, sex, and the presence of diabetes mellitus, peripheral vascular disease, or renal impairment. Major bleeding was more frequent in the abciximab group (3.8% vs. 1.9%; p = 0.04). At 6-month follow-up, there was no significant difference in the primary endpoint between the two groups.

The benefit of abciximab in ischaemic complications was further evaluated by the EPIC trial (Evaluation of 7ES in Preventing Ischemic Complications)[47]. Four hundred and eighty-nine patients undergoing high-risk PTCA or directional atherectomy were randomized to placebo, abciximab 0.25mcg/kg bolus before the intervention, or abciximab 0.25mcg/kg bolus followed by 20-mcg/min infusion for 12h. All patients were given aspirin and bolus heparin to achieve an activated clotting time of 300–350s. At 30 days, there was a graded effect on the rate of the primary composite endpoint of death, MI, or urgent repeat revascularization with a 39% reduction among patients randomized to abciximab bolus versus placebo and a 62% reduction among patients randomized to abciximab bolus and infusion (12.5% vs. 7.8% vs. 4.8%; p = 0.01). By 6 months, cumulative death (1.8% vs. 6.6%; p = 0.02) and MI (2.4%% vs. 11.1%; p = 0.002) were further reduced by abciximab.

The Intracoronary Stenting and Antithrombotic Regimen Rapid Early Action for Coronary Treatment (ISAR-REACT 2) trial examined the effects of abciximab in 2022 patients with NSTEACS undergoing PCI[48]. All patients received clopidogrel 600mg, at least 2h before PCI, as well as oral or intravenous aspirin 500mg. Randomization was performed after the decision to perform PCI but before crossing the lesion with the guide wire. One thousand and twelve patients were randomized to the abciximab group (0.25mg/kg of body weight bolus followed by a 0.125-mcg/kg/min infusion for 12h) and heparin 70U/kg of body weight. The 1010 patients designated to the placebo group received a placebo bolus and infusion as well as heparin bolus of 140U/kg. Post procedure, all patients received aspirin 200mg indefinitely, clopidogrel 75mg twice daily until discharge but not for more than 3 days, followed by 75mg/day for at least 6 months, and other conventional secondary preventive medications. At 30 days, the primary endpoint of the combined cumulative incidence of death from any cause, MI, and urgent target vessel revascularization was significantly lower in the abciximab group (8.9% vs. 11.9%; p = 0.03). Most of the risk reduction was attributed to a reduction in the incidence of death and MI. There was no difference in the incidence of ischaemic events between the two groups in patients without an elevated troponin, whereas, by contrast, in those with an elevated troponin, the incidence of ischaemic events was lower in the abciximab group (13.1% vs. 18.3%; p = 0.02). There was no significant difference between the two groups regarding major or minor bleeding. Thrombocytopenia was significantly more common following an abciximab infusion (0.8% vs. 0%; p = 0.008).

The timing of GP IIb/IIIa inhibitor administration was studied in the Acute Catheterization and Urgent Intervention Triage Strategy (ACUITY) Timing trail[49]. The trail randomized 9207 patients due to undergo an invasive strategy to receive either GP IIb/IIIa inhibitor (tirofiban or eptifibatide at the investigator's preference) prior to angiography or during angiography as needed (abciximab or eptifibatide). Angiography was performed at a median of 19.6h. GP IIb/IIIa inhibitors were used in 98.3% of the upstream group and 55.7% of the deferred group and for a significantly longer duration (18.3h vs. 13.1h; p <0.001). In the upstream group, GP IIb/IIIa inhibitors were commenced at a median time of 35min after randomization and continued for a median of 4h before PCI. In the deferred group, GP IIb/IIIa inhibitors were commenced immediately prior to PCI, a delay of approximately 3.9h compared to the upstream group. At 30 days, the composite endpoint of death, MI, or revascularization was non-inferior in the two groups (11.7% in both groups; p <0.001 for non-inferiority). The triple ischaemic endpoint again did not meet the criteria for non-inferiority (7.1% vs. 7.9%; p >0.05). Major bleeding was significantly lower in the delayed group (4.9% vs. 6.1%; p = 0.009). There was no difference in mortality (1.3% for upstream vs. 1.5% for delayed) or MI (4.9% vs. 5.0%) but unplanned revascularization for ischaemia was lower in the upstream group (2.1% vs. 2.8%; p = 0.03 for superiority). In patients who received PCI (n = 5170), the composite ischaemic endpoint was significantly lower in the upstream therapy group (8.0% vs. 9.5%; p = 0.05).

GP IIb/IIIa inhibitors have been shown to be particularly beneficial in patients with diabetes mellitus and those with a previous history of CABG. In a meta-analysis of six randomized trial, which included 6458 diabetic patients, GP IIb/IIIa inhibitor therapy was associated with a lower 30-day mortality. Similarly, in the 12% of CABG patients that had been enrolled in the PURSUIT trial, eptifibatide was associated with a trend (although statistically non-significant) toward a lower 30-day rate of death or MI.

Evidence for medical benefit in NSTEASC

The use of tirofiban in NSTEACS has been studied in two major clinical trials. In the Platelet Receptor Inhibition in Ischemic Syndrome Management (PRISM) trial, 3232 patients with NSTEACS were randomized to receive tirofiban or heparin for 48h[50]. All patients received aspirin. PCI was undertaken in 1.9% of patients during this time. Tirofiban resulted in a 32% reduction in the composite endpoint of death, MI, or refractory ischaemia at 48h (3.8% vs. 5.6%; p = 0.01). At 30 days, there was no difference in the two treatment groups in the primary endpoint although mortality was lower in the tirofiban group (2.3% vs. 3.6%; p = 0.02). Major bleeding was similar in the two groups. Thrombocytopenia occurred more commonly with tirofiban (1.1% vs. 0.4%; p = 0.04). The study therefore concluded that tirofiban may have a role in the management of NSTEACS.

The Platelet Receptor Inhibition in Ischemic Syndrome Management in Patients Limited by Unstable Signs and Symptoms (PRISM-PLUS) trial randomized 1915 patients with NSTEACS to receive either tirofiban, heparin, or tirofiban and heparin[51]. Coronary angiography and PCI was performed when indicated after 48h. The tirofiban-only arm was terminated prematurely because of increased mortality trend at 7 days. The composite primary endpoint of death, MI, or refractory ischaemia within 7 days after randomization was lower in the tirofiban plus heparin group (12.9% vs. 17.9%; p = 0.004). This benefit was maintained at 30 days (18.5% vs. 22.3%; p = 0.03) and at 6 months (27.7% vs. 32.1%; p = 0.02). Death or non-fatal MI was also reduced at 7 days. This benefit was also similar whether the patients were treated medically or by PCI. Tirofiban, in combination with heparin, has therefore been approved in the treatment of patients with NSTEACS who are treated medically or with PCI.

The addition of eptifibatide therapy, for 72h, to standard medical therapy was investigated in the PURSUIT trial[52]—10 948 patients with NSTEACS were randomized to receive either eptifibatide or placebo for 72h or until hospital discharge, whichever occurred first. If PCI was performed towards the end of the 72-h infusion period, the infusion could be continued for an additional 24h. At 30 days, the composite endpoint of death or non-fatal MI was lower in the eptifibatide group (14.2% vs. 15.7%; p = 0.04). The benefit was apparent by 96h and persisted through 30 days. Event rate reduction was greater in patients who underwent PCI within 72h (11.6% vs. 16.7%; p = 0.01). The effect was consistent in most major subgroups except for women. Bleeding was more common with eptifibatide (10.6% vs. 9.1%; p = 0.02). Like tirofiban, eptifibatide has been approved in the treatment of patients with NSTEACS who are treated medically or with PCI.

In contrast to the above studies, the Global Use of Strategies to Open occluded Coronary Arteries (GUSTO) IV-ACS trial found no benefit in the use of abciximab as first-line medical therapy in patients with NSTEACS in whom early (less than 48h) revascularization was not intended[53]. The study randomized 7800 patients with NSTEACS to placebo, an abciximab bolus and 24h infusion, or abciximab bolus and 48h infusion. All patients received aspirin and either UFH or LMWH. Coronary angiography was not to be done within 60h after randomization unless the patient had recurrent ischaemia with ECS changes that was unresponsive to optimal medical therapy. At 30 days, the combined primary endpoint of death or MI was similar among the three treatment groups (8% vs. 8.2% vs. 9.1%; p = 0.2). At 48h, a significantly higher mortality rate was observed in patients receiving the 24-h (0.7%) or 48-h (0.9%) abciximab infusion than those receiving placebo (0.3%; p = 0.008). Death and MI were more common in patients with high-risk features such as advanced age, ST segment depression, elevated troponin, and diabetes mellitus. Abciximab was not shown to be of any benefit in any particular subgroup although an impaired outcome was seen in women. Bleeding rates and thrombocytopenia were also higher in the abciximab group. As a result, routine administration of abciximab as an upstream medical treatment of NSTEACS in its own right is not recommended.

Beta-blockers

Beta-blockers competitively inhibit the effect of catecholamines on the membrane receptors resulting in a decrease in the myocardial oxygen demand.

Two double-blind randomized trials have compared beta-blockers with placebo in NSTEACS. In the 'Trial of heparin versus atenolol in prevention of myocardial infarction in intermediate coronary syndrome', 214 patients were randomized to receive placebo, heparin, atenolol, or a combination of the two[54]. At 30 days,

MI had developed in 17% of the placebo group, 13% of the atenolol group, 2% of the heparin group, and 2% of the combined group (p = 0.024). This was maintained at 6-month follow up.

In the 'Efficacy of nifedipine and metoprolol in the early treatment of unstable angina in the coronary care unit' trial, 338 patients with NSTEASC who had not been previously on a beta-blocker were randomized to receive nifedipine, metoprolol, or their combination[55]. Nifedipine was also compared to placebo in 177 patients who were on a beta-blocker on admission. The main outcome of the study was MI or refractory ischaemia within 48h. Trial medication effect was expressed as event rates relative to placebo. In beta-blocker naïve patients, metoprolol was shown to have a beneficial effect on unstable angina, with the addition of nifedipine providing no additional benefit (rate ratio for nifedipine: 1.15, for metoprolol: 0.76 and for the combination: 0.80). However, the addition of nifedipine to patients who were already taking a beta-blocker on admission was also shown to be beneficial (rate ratio: 1.51).

Calcium channel antagonists

There are three classes of calcium channel antagonists: the dihydropyridines (e.g. nifedipine), benzothiazepines (e.g. diltiazem), and phenylalkylamines (e.g. verapamil). Although similar in their ability to produce coronary vasodilatation, they differ in their ability to produce peripheral arterial vasodilatation (greatest with nifedipine and amlodipine), decrease myocardial contractility, and suppress atrioventricular conduction.

The evidence base for benefit in NSTEACS is greatest for diltiazem. The effect of diltiazem on re-infarction after a non-Q-wave MI was studied in multicentre, randomized study of 576 patients[56]. Two hundred and eighty-seven patients were randomized to diltiazem 90mg four times daily within 24–72h after MI and continued for 14 days or placebo. At 14 days, the primary endpoint of re-infarction was significantly lower in the diltiazem group (5.2% vs. 9.3%; p = 0.03). Diltiazem also reduced the frequency of post-infarction angina by 49.7% (p = 0.03). Mortality was similar in both groups (3.8 % and 3.1%).

The ESC guidelines for the diagnosis and treatment of NSTEACS recommend that calcium channel blockers should be used for symptom relief in patients already receiving nitrates and beta-blockers. They are also recommended in patients intolerant of beta-blockers and those with vasospastic angina.

Nitrates

The use of nitrates in NSTEACS has been based on clinical experience as well as pathophysiological considerations. The vasodilatory effect of nitrates leads to a reduction in pre-load, and left ventricular end-diastolic volume with a resultant fall in myocardial oxygen consumption. They also increase flow through any pre-existing collaterals.

There are currently no randomized studies to confirm the beneficial effects of these agents in either relieving symptoms or improving prognosis. However, a number of small observational studies have demonstrated symptomatic benefit with intravenous nitrate in patients with unstable angina[57].

Newer agents

Prasugrel

Prasugrel is an ADP receptor inhibitor. The TRITON-TIMI 38 trial directly compared clopidogrel to prasugrel in 13 608 moderate- to high-risk patients with ACS undergoing PCI, including 10 074 patients with NSTEMI[58]. Patients were randomized to receive prasugrel (60mg loading and 10mg maintenance) or clopidogrel (300mg loading and 75mg maintenance) for 6–15 months. All patients received aspirin. The study medication was administered at any time between randomization and 1h after leaving the cardiac catheterization laboratory. The coronary anatomy had to be demonstrated to be suitable for PCI prior to randomization in all patients with NSTEACS. If the coronary anatomy had been previously documented or primary PCI was being undertaken for STEMI, pre-treatment with the study drug was permitted for up to 24h before PCI. At 15-month follow-up, the primary endpoint of cardiovascular death, non-fatal MI, or non-fatal stroke was lower in the prasugrel group (HR 0.81; p <0.001). This was primarily driven by a reduction in non-fatal MI (7.4% vs. 9.7%; p <0.001). The prasugrel group also had lower rates of target vessel revascularization (2.5% vs. 3.7%; p <0.001), and stent thrombosis (1.1% vs. 2.4%; p <0.001). However, patients receiving prasugrel had significantly higher rates of life-threatening bleeding (1.4% vs. 0.9%; p = 0.01) including fatal bleeding (0.4% vs. 0.1%; p = 0.002). Patients ≥75 years, ≤60kg in weight, and those with a previous history of stroke or transient ischaemic attack were identified to be at the greatest risk of bleeding and therefore the least to benefit from prasugrel. Although the absolute risk of bleeding was small, no excess in fatal bleeding has ever been reported in any of the dual antiplatelet therapy trials. The study also included a significant number of elderly patients as well as patients with moderate renal dysfunction, and this in part may explain the higher tendency for bleeding complications. However, like many antithrombotic trials, the study excluded patients that were perceived to be at high risk of bleeding, such that in a 'real-world' setting the bleeding complications with prasugrel could be potentially even higher. Based on enhanced platelet inhibition and endorsed by committee guidelines, clinicians are increasingly using high-dose clopidogrel loading, usually 600mg, prior to PCI. Prasugrel 60mg has been shown to achieve greater inhibition of platelet aggregation than clopidogrel 600mg in patients with chronic CAD[59]. The Prasugrel in Comparison to Clopidogrel for Inhibition of Platelet Activation and Aggregation (PRINCIPLE)-TIMI 44 trial demonstrated greater inhibition of platelet aggregation with prasugrel in the doses used in the TRITON-TIMI 38 trial compared to clopidogrel 600mg loading and 150mg maintenance[60]. However, the study was not powered to study clinical endpoints. Nevertheless, with careful patient selection, prasugrel can serves as an acceptable alternative to clopidogrel, particularly in patients at high risk of ischaemic events but at low risk of bleeding. The role of prasugrel in the treatment of NSTEACS is the subject of an appraisal by the National Institute of Health and Clinical Excellence (NICE) at the time of writing, and the FDA in the United States has recently recommended its use.

Fondaparinux

Fondaparinux binds specifically to antithrombin and therefore serves as a selective factor Xa inhibitor. It has no effect on the activated prothrombin time or the activated clotting time. It is administered subcutaneously at 2.5mg/day. It is excreted by the kidneys and is therefore contraindicated in patients with a creatinine clearance less than 30mL/min.

The safety and efficacy of fondaparinux compared to enoxaparin in patients with unstable angina (USA) and NSTEMI was investigated in the OASIS-5 study[61]. This randomized, double blind, multi-centre study randomized 20 078 patients to fondaparinux 2.5mg once daily or enoxoparin 1mg/kg twice daily for a maximum of 8 days. All patients were given aspirin, clopidogrel, and GP IIb/IIIa inhibitors. At 9 days, the combined endpoint of death, MI, and recurrent intervention was similar in the two groups, but the rate of major bleeding was less frequent in the fondaparinux group (2.2% vs. 4.1%; $p < 0.001$). At 30 days, the fondaparinux group had a significantly lower rate of death (3.5% vs. 3.9%; $p = 0.02$) and refractory ischaemia (2.3% vs. 2.2%; $p = 0.03$). At 6 months, the fondaparinux group had a significantly lower rate of death and MI (10.3% vs. 11.2%; $p = 0.04$), death (5.8% vs. 6.3%; $p = 0.04$), and stroke (1.3% vs. 1.8%; $p = 0.03$). Among 6238 patients undergoing PCI, fondaparinux was associated with similar rates of ischaemic complications at 9 days, a lower rate of major bleeding, but a higher rate of catheter thrombus formation, which for the interventional cardiologist is a major source of concern. Therefore, if fondaparinux is chosen as the anticoagulant therapy of choice, additional anticoagulant therapy must be used at the time of PCI.

Bivalirudin

Bivalirudin binds directly to thrombin and inhibits the conversion of fibrinogen to fibrin. Bivalirudin leads to prolongation of both the activated prothrombin time and the activated clotting time. It is administered intravenously and eliminated by both the kidneys and the liver.

In the setting of PCI, bivalirudin has been shown to reduce the rate of death, MI, or repeat revascularization as well as bleeding compared to UFH. Bivalirudin plus provisional GP IIb/IIIa inhibitors has been shown to be non-inferior to UFH and GP IIb/IIIa inhibitors in protecting against ischaemic events during PCI with a lower rate of major bleeding complications.

The ACUITY trial investigated the effectiveness of bivalirudin in moderate to high-risk patients with NSTEACS[62]. The trial compared UFH or enoxaparin and a GP IIb/IIIa inhibitor (the control group) versus bivalirudin and a GP IIb/IIIa inhibitor versus bivalirudin monotherapy in 13 819 patients undergoing early invasive management. Angiography was performed in all patients within 72h after randomization. All patients were given aspirin, 75–325mg/day indefinitely, and clopidogrel 75mg/day for 1 year. The following three primary 30-day endpoint were pre-specified: a composite ischaemia endpoint (death from any cause, MI, or unplanned revascularization for ischaemia), major bleeding, and a net clinical outcome endpoint (defined as the occurrence of the composite ischaemia endpoint or major bleeding). Bivalirudin plus GP IIb/IIIa inhibitors, as compared with heparin plus GP IIb/IIIa inhibitors, resulted in non-inferior 30-day rates of the composite ischaemia endpoint (7.7% vs. 7.3%; $p = 0.39$), major bleeding (5.3% vs. 5.7%; $p = 0.38$), and the net clinical outcome endpoint (11.8% vs. 11.7%; $p = 0.93$). Bivalirudin alone, as compared with heparin plus GP IIb/IIIa inhibitors, was associated with a non-inferior rate of the composite ischaemia endpoint (7.8% vs. 7.3%; $p = 0.32$), significantly reduced rate of major bleeding (3% vs. 5.7%; $p < 0.001$), and reduced rate of the net clinical outcome endpoint (10.1% vs. 11.7%; $p = 0.02$). Bivalirudin alone also reduced the rate of bleeding. Subgroup analysis showed no interaction between the primary study endpoints and various demographic and treatment variables. Among the 2472 patients who underwent angiography or intervention more than 24h after randomization (median 45h), bivalirudin monotherapy, as compared with heparin and GP IIb/IIIa inhibitors, resulted in a similar rate of the composite ischaemia endpoint (8.9% vs. 9.1%; p = 0.89), reduced rate of major bleeding (3.3% vs. 8.9%; p <0.001), and reduced rate of the net clinical outcome endpoint (11.4% vs. 16.4%; p = 0.003). It is notable with analysis of this complex trial design that there was no treatment arm representing heparin alone (Fig. 15.6).

Special subgroups

Gender and early invasive therapy: are women different?

On balance, the data support an early invasive strategy, with revascularization where appropriate in the NSTEACS population. However, important areas of uncertainty remain. For example, the original interesting observation that women with NSTEACS in some studies do not obtain prognostic benefit from early revascularization in contrast to their male counterpart has now become robust enough to raise concern. Thus the female cohort in FRISC II and RITA 3 showed no overall outcome benefit from an early invasive strategy[15–17]. This has been further demonstrated in a recent independent paper[63]. The difference in outcome that is apparently observed here is not explained. The consistency of the signal in relation to women with NSTEACS certainly demands further investigation, particularly since female patients are currently treated in exactly the same way.

Anaemia

Anaemia may be present in up to 15% of patients with MI, and in up to 43% of elderly patients with acute MI. Furthermore, many of the medical treatments used in the management of ACS can aggravate pre-existing anaemia. Anaemia has been shown to be associated with a higher mortality in a wide range of disorders such as heart failure, renal failure, malignancy, as well as the whole spectrum of ACS[64].

The adverse effects of anaemia upon the cardiovascular system include increased heart rate and cardiac output, compensatory left ventricular hypertrophy, and a mismatch between oxygen demand and delivery. Anaemia will also exacerbate any reduction in the delivery of oxygen to anywhere within the body as the oxygen delivery equation has haemoglobin in it. In the context of NSTEACS, compromised oxygen delivery to the ischaemic myocardium has the potential to increase infarct size, predispose to arrhythmias, and worsen prognosis.

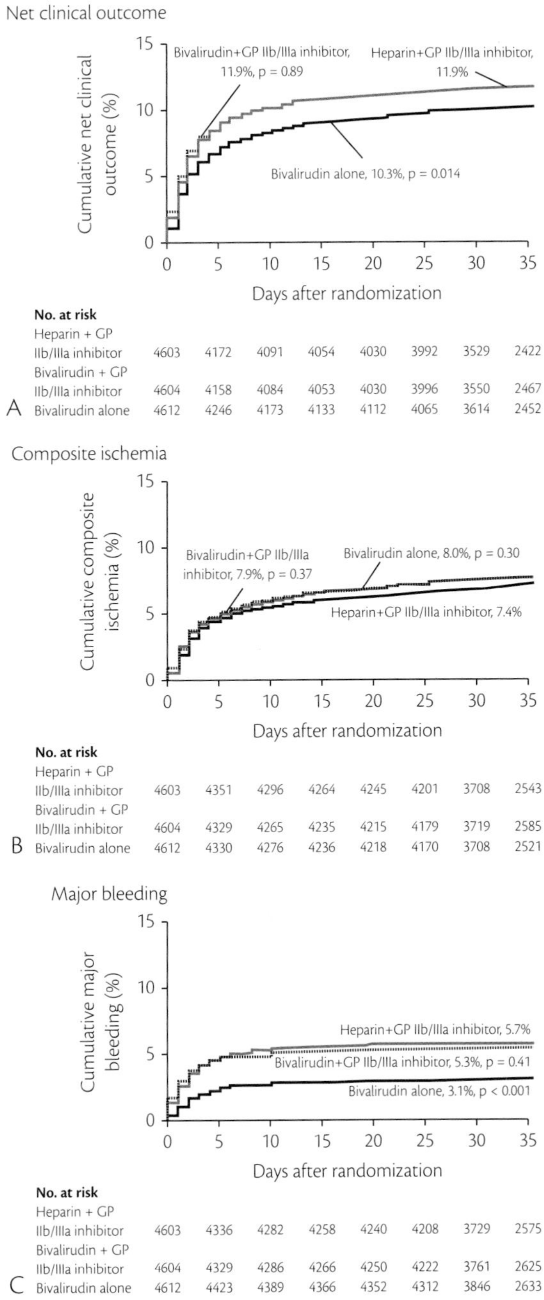

Fig. 15.6 Kaplan–Meier time-to-event curves for the endpoints of net clinical outcome (A), composite ischaemia (B), and major bleeding (C). Reproduced with permission from Stone G, *et al*, Bivalirudin for patients with acute coronary syndromes, *NEJM* 2006, **355**: 2203–16. Copyright © 2006 Massachusetts Medical Society. All rights reserved.

Using a baseline haemoglobin concentration of 15–16g/dL, a meta-analysis of nearly 40 000 patients across the whole spectrum of ACS demonstrated that those with lower baseline haemoglobin levels were more likely to be older, female, smokers, and have renal impairment. In the 14 503 patients with NSTACS, the risk of cardiovascular death, recurrent ischaemia, and the composite of death, ischaemia and recurrent MI increased as the haemoglobin concentration fell below 11g/dL with an adjusted OR of 1.45 (95% CI 1.33–1.58; p <0.001). Furthermore, there was a dose–response effect with lower survival rates in those patients with the greater degree of anaemia. Interestingly, the rate of adverse events also started to increase in those with very high haemoglobin levels (>16g/dL) with an OR of 1.31 (95% CI 1.03–1.66; p = 0.03). This has been attributed to increased blood viscosity leading to increased coronary vascular resistance and decreased coronary blood flow, which in turn predispose to thrombosis and increased cardiac workload[65].

It is therefore essential to place special attention to the baseline haemoglobin level when deciding upon the management strategy of patients presenting with NSTEMI and every effort taken to investigate and treat the underlying cause of anaemia.

Diabetes mellitus

As in CKD, diabetes mellitus (DM) is increasing in prevalence, and serves as an independent risk factor for the development and progression of cardiovascular disease. Diabetic patients are more commonly women, and have other comorbidities such as obesity, hypertension, CKD, stroke, heart failure, and general vascular disease.

In patients presenting with USA/NSTEMI, the prevalence of DM has been estimated at approximately 20–30%, most of whom have type II DM. Across the whole spectrum of ACS, DM is associated with a greater risk of 30-day and 1-year mortality after controlling for comorbidities. Diabetic patients with ACS are also at a greater risk of developing left ventricular failure than their non-diabetic counterparts[66,67].

The precise mechanism by which hyperglycaemia adversely affects the outcome of patients presenting with ACS is unknown. However, some of the proposed mechanisms include decreased collateral circulation leading to increased infarct size, microvascular dysfunction, higher incidence of no-reflow, higher free fatty acid concentration, insulin resistance, and impaired myocardial glucose utilization.

In the Diabetes mellitus, Insulin Glucose infusion in Acute Myocardial Infarction (DIGAMI) study, tight glycaemic control using intravenous insulin and glucose reduced 1-year mortality by 30% in patients with STEMI[68]. However, this benefit was not confirmed in the subsequent DIGAMI-2 study, although DIGAMI-2 ended up comparing differing strategies of insulin therapy rather than differing intensities of glucose control[69]. Nevertheless, this study demonstrated that glucose level is an independent predictor of mortality in type II diabetic patients presenting with MI, and tight glycaemic control remains an important part of the management of diabetic patients with ACS.

An early invasive strategy is recommended for diabetic patients with USA/NSTEMI. Both FRISC II and TACTICS-TIMI 18 demonstrated a significant reduction in death and non-fatal MI in the diabetic patients undergoing an invasive strategy. In those with multivessel disease, surgical revascularization remains the optimal treatment option. GP IIb/IIIa inhibitors should be commenced as part of the initial medical management and continued through the completion of PCI. As many diabetic patients may also have CKD, care must be taken to minimize the risk of CIN. The use of metformin should be prohibited for at least 24h before coronary angiography/PCI, and recommenced 48h later in the absence of renal failure developing.

Conclusion

The management of NSTEACS has undergone rapid evolution over the past 20 years as result of giant leaps made in the understanding of molecular mechanisms contributing to plaque development, plaque rupture, and atherothrombosis. The next 20 years is likely to see a further revolution with regard to development of more effective antiplatelet and antithrombotic agents and developments in stent technology. The current strategy of optimal medical therapy and early invasive investigation and revascularization is well established. However, clarification of ongoing uncertainty in various areas is required. These include:

- The apparent lack of benefit for this aggressive strategy in women
- Optimal timing of invasive management
- Optimal adjuvant antithrombotic and antiplatelet therapy
- The role for novel disease modification.

References

1. British Heart Foundation. *Coronary Heart Disease Statistics*. London: British Heart Foundation, 1998.
2. Volmink JA, Newton JN, Hicks NR, *et al*. Coronary event and case fatality rates in an English population: results of the Oxford myocardial infarction incidence study. *Heart* 1998; **80**:40–4.
3. Mahmoudi M, Curzen N, Gallagher PJ. *et al*. Atherogenesis: the role of inflammation and infection. *Histopathology* 2007; **50**:535–46.
4. Davies M. Stability and instability. The Paul-Dudley-White lecture 1995. *Circulation* 1996; **94**:2013–20.
5. Ross R. Atherosclerosis–an inflammatory disease. *NEJM* 1999; **340**:115–26.
6. Bennett MR, Evan GI, Schwartz SM. Apoptosis of human vascular smooth muscle cells derived from normal vessels and coronary atherosclerotic plaques. *J Clin Invest* 1995; **95**:2266–74.
7. Hansson G. Inflammation, atherosclerosis and coronary artery disease. *NEJM* 2005; **352**:1685–1695.
8. Anderson JL, Adamas CD, Antman EM, *et al*. ACC/AHA 2007 guidelines for the management of patients with unstable angina/non-ST-elevation myocardial infarction: Executive summary. *Circulation* 2007; **116**:e148–e304.
9. Bassand JP, Hamm CW, Ardissino D, *et al*. Guidelines for the diagnosis and treatment of non-ST-segment elevation acute coronary syndromes. *Eur Heart J* 2007; **28**: 1598–660.
10. Antman EM, Cohen M, Bernink PJ, *et al*. The TIMI risk score for unstable angina/non-ST elevation MI: a method for prognostication and therapeutic decision making. *JAMA* 2000; **284**:835–42.
11. Fox KA, Goodman SG, Klein W, *et al*. Management of acute coronary syndromes.Variation in practice and outcome; findings from the Global Registry of Acute Coronary Events (GRACE). *Eur Heart J* 2002; **23**:1177–89.
12. Boersma E, Pieper KS, Steyerberg EW, *et al*. Predictors of outcome in patients with acute coronary syndromes without persistent ST-segment elevation. Results from an international trial of 9461 patients. *Circulation* 2000; **101**:2557–67.
13. Cohen, M, Demers C, Gurfinkel EP, *et al*. A comparison of low-molecular-weight heparin with unfractionated heparin for unstable coronary artery disease. *NEJM* 1997; **337**:447–52.
14. Metz BK, White HD, Granger CB, *et al*. Randomized comparison of direct thrombin inhibition versus heparin in conjunction with fibrinolytic therapy for acute myocardial infarction: results from the GUSTO-IIb trial. *J Am Coll Cardiol* 1998; **31**:1493–8.
15. FRagmin Fast Revascularisation during In Stability in Coronary artery disease (FRISC II) Investigators. Long-term low-molecular-mass heparin in unstable coronary artery disease: FRISC II prospective randomised multicentre study. *Lancet* 1999; **354**:701–7.
16. Cannon CP, Weintraub WS, Demopoulos LA, *et al*. Comparison of early invasive and conservative strategies in patients with unstable coronary syndromes treated with the glycoprotein IIb/IIIa inhibitor tirofiban. *NEJM* 2001; **344**:1879–87.
17. Fox KA, Poole-Wilson PA, Henderson RA, *et al*. Interventional versus conservative treatment for patients with unstable angina or non-ST-elevation myocardial infarction: the British Heart Foundation RITA 3 randomized trial. *Lancet* 2002; **360**:743–51.
18. Neumann FJ, Kastrati A, Pogatsa-Murray G, *et al*. Evaluation of prolonged antithrombotic pretreatment(Cooling-Off strategy) before intervention in patients with unstable coronary syndromes. *JAMA* 2003; **290**:1593–9.
19. Spacek R, Widimský P, Straka Z, *et al*. Value of first day angiography/angioplasty in evolving non-ST segment elevation myocardialinfarction: an open multicenter randomized trial.The VINO study. *Eur Heart J* 2002; **23**:230–8.
20. Tricoci, P, Lokhnygina Y, Berdan LG, *et al*. Time to coronary angiography and outcomes among patients with high risk non-ST-segment elevation acute coronary syndromes. *Circulation* 2007; **116**:2669–77.
21. Bavry AA, Kumbhani DJ, Rassi AN, *et al*. Benefit of early invasive therapy in acute coronary syndromes: a meta-analysis of contemporary randomized clinical trials. *J Am Coll Cardiol* 2006; **48**:1319–25.
22. Hoenig M, Doust J, Aroney CN, *et al*. Early invasive versus conservative strategies for unstable angina and non-ST elevation myocardial infarction in the stent era. *Cochrane Database Syst Rev* 2006; **3**:CD004815.
23. de Winter R, Windhausen F, Cornel JH, *et al*. Early invasive versus selectively invasive management for acute coronary syndromes. *NEJM* 2005; **353**:1095–104.
24. Wallentin L. Aspirin (75mg/day) after an episode of unstable coronary artery disease: long term effects on the risk of myocardial infarction, occurrence of severe angina and the need for revascularization. *J Am Coll Cardiol* 1991; **18**:1587–93.
25. Antithrombotic Trialists' Collaboration. Collaborative meta-analysis of randomized trials of antiplatelet therapy for prevention of death, myocardial infarction, and stroke in high risk patients. *BMJ* 2002; **324**:71–86.
26. Yusuf S, Zhao F, Mehta SR, *et al*. Effects of clopidogrel in addition to aspirin in patients with acute coronary syndromes without ST-segment elevation. *NEJM* 2001; **345**:494–502.
27. Steinhubl S, Berger P, Mann JT 3rd, *et al*. Early and sustained dual oral antiplatelet therapy following percutaneous coronary intervention: a randomized controlled trial. *JAMA* 2002; **288**:2411–20.
28. Montalescot G, Sideris G, Meuleman C, *et al*. A randomized comparison of high clopidogrel loading doses in patients with non-ST-segment elevation acute coronary syndromes: the ALBION (Assessment of the Best

Loading Dose of Clopidogrel to Blunt Platelet Activation, Inflammation and Ongoing Necrosis) trial. *J Am Coll Cardiol* 2006; **48**:931–8.

29. Patti G, Colonna G, Pasceri V, *et al.* Randomized trial of high loading dose of clopidogrel for reduction of periprocedural myocardial infarction in patients undergoing coronary intervention. *Circulation* 2005; **111**:2099–106.
30. Hobson A, Curzen N. Improving outcome with antiplatelet therapy in percutaneous coronary intervention and stenting. *Thromb Haemost* 2009; **101**: 23–30.
31. Collet JP, Silvain J, Landivier A, *et al.* Dose effects of clopidogrel reloading in patients already on 75-mg maintenance dose. *Circulation* 2008; **118**:1225–33.
32. Takemoto M, Sun J, Hiroki J, *et al.* Rho-kinase mediates hypoxia-induced down-regulation of endothelial nitric oxide synthase. *Circulation* 2002; **106**:57–62.
33. Laufs U, Liao J. Post transcriptional regulation of endothelial nitric oxide synthase mRNA stability by Rho GTPase. *J Biol Chem* 1998; **273**:24266–71.
34. Tsunekawa T, Hayashi T, Kano H, *et al.* Cerivastatin, an HMG-CoA reductase inhibitor, improves endothelial function in elderly diabetic patients within 3 days. *Circulation* 2001; **104**:376–9.
35. Wassmann S, Faul A, Hennen B, *et al.* Rapid effects of HMG-CoA reductase inhibition on coronary endothelial function. *Circ Res* 2003; **93**:98–103.
36. Pruefer D, Scalia R, Lefer AM, *et al.* Simvastatin inhibits leukocyte-endothelial cell interaction and protects against inflammatory processes in normo-cholesterolemic rats. *ATVB* 1999; **19**:2894–900.
37. Bustos C, Hernandez-Presa MA, Ortego M, *et al.* HMG-CoA reductase inhibition by atorvastatin reduces neointimal inflammation in a rabbit model of atherosclerosis. *Am J Cardiol* 1998; **32**:2027–34.
38. Aikawa M, Rabkin E, Sugiyama S, *et al.* The HMG-CoA reductase inhibitor cerivastatin suppresses growth of macrophages expressing matrix metalloproteinases and tissue factor in vivo and in vitro. *Circulation* 2001; **103**:276–83.
39. Albert M, Danielson E, Rifai N, *et al.* Effect of statin therapy on CRP levels: the Pravastatin Inflammation/CRP Evaluation (PRINCE). *JAMA* 2001; **286**:64–70.
40. Kinlay S, Schwartz GG, Olsson AG, *et al.* High dose atorvastatin enhances the decline in inflammatory markers in patients with acute coronary syndrome in the MIRACL study. *Circulation* 2003; **108**:1560–6.
41. Nissen SE, Tuzcu EM, Schoenhagen P, *et al.* Statin therapy, LDL cholesterol, CRP, and coronary artery disease. *NEJM* 2005; **352**:29–38.
42. Ridker PM, Cannon CP, Morrow D, *et al.* C-reactive protein levels and outcomes after statin therapy. *NEJM* 2005; **352**:20–8.
43. Eikelboom JW, Anand SS, Malmberg K, *et al.* Unfractionated heparin and low-molecular-weight heparin in acute coronary syndrome without ST elevation: a meta-analysis. *Lancet* 2000; **355**:1936–42.
44. Antman EM, McCabe CH, Gurfinkel EP, *et al.* Enoxaparin prevents death and cardiac ischemic events in unstable angina/non-Q-wave myocardial infarction. *Circulation* 1999; **100**:1593–601.
45. Petersen JL, Mahaffey KW, Hasselblad V, *et al.* Efficacy and bleeding complications among patients randomized to enoxaparin or unfractionated heparin for antithrombin therapy in non-ST-segment elevation acute coronary syndromes: a systematic overview. *JAMA* 2004; **292**:89–96.
46. The CAPTURE Investigators. Randomised placebo-controlled trial of abciximab before and during coronary intervention in refractory unstable angina: the CAPTURE Study. *Lancet* 1997; **349**:1429–35.
47. Lincoff AM, Califf RM, Anderson KM, *et al.* Evidence for prevention of death and myocardial infarction with platelet membrane glycoprotein IIb/IIIa receptor blockade by abciximab among patients with unstable angina undergoing percutaneous coronary revascularization. *J Am Coll Cardiol* 1997; **330**:149–56.
48. Kastrati A, Mehilli J, Neumann FJ, *et al.* Abciximab in patients with acute coronary syndromes undergoing percutaneous coronary intervention after clopidogrel pretreatment. *JAMA* 2006; **295**:1531–8.
49. Stone GW, Bertrand ME, Moses JW, *et al.* Routine upstream initiation vs. deferred selective use of glycoprotein IIb/IIIa inhibitors in acute coronary syndromes. *JAMA* 2007; **297**:591–602.
50. The Platelet Receptor Inhibition in Ischemic Syndrome Management (PRISM) Study Investigators. A comparison of aspirin plus tirofiban with aspirin plus heparin for unstable angina. *NEJM* 1998; **338**:1498–505.
51. The Platelet Receptor Inhibition in Ischemic Syndrome Management in Patients Limited by Unstable Signs and Symptoms (PRISM-PLUS) Study Investigators. Inhibition of the platelet glycoprotein IIb/IIIa receptor with tirofiban in unstable angina and non-Q-wave myocardial infarction. *NEJM* 1998; **338**:1488–97.
52. The PURSUIT Trial Investigators. Inhibition of platelet glycoprotein IIb/IIIa with eptifibatide in patients with acute coronary syndromes. *NEJM* 1998; **339**:436–43.
53. Simoons ML; GUSTO IV-ACS Investigators. Effect of glycoprotein IIb/IIIa receptor blocker abciximab on outcome in patients with acute coronary syndromes without early coronary revascularization: the GUSTO IV-ACS randomized trial. *Lancet* 2001; **357**:1915–24.
54. Telford A, Wilson C. Trial of heparin versus atenolol in prevention of myocardial infarction in intermediate coronary syndrome. *Lancet* 1981; **1**:1225–8.
55. Lubsen J, Tijssen J. Efficacy of nifedipine and metoprolol in the early treatment of unstable angina in the coronary care unit: findings from the Holland Interuniversity Nifedipine/metoprolol Trial (HINT). *Am J Cardiol* 1987; **60**:18A–25A.
56. Gibson RS, Boden WE, Theroux P, *et al.* Diltiazem and reinfarction in patients with non-Q-wave myocardial

infarction. Results of a double-blind, randomized, multicenter trial. *NEJM* 1986; **315**:423–9.
57. Kaplan K, Davison R, Parker M, *et al.* Intravenous nitroglycerine for the treatment of angina at rest unresponsive to standard nitrate therapy. *Am J Cardiol* 1983; **51**:694–8.
58. Wiviott SD, Braunwald E, McCabe CH, *et al.* Prasugrel versus clopidogrel in patients with acute coronary syndromes. *NEJM* 2001; **357**:2001–15.
59. Wallentin L, Varenhorst C, *et al.* Prasugrel acheives greater and faster P2Y12 receptor-mediated platelet inhibition than clopidogrel due to more efficient generation of its active metabolitein aspirin treated patients with coronary artery disease. *Eur Heart J* 2008; **29**:21–30.
60. Wiviott SD, Trenk D, Frelinger AL, *et al.* Prasugrel compared to high loading- and maintenance-dose clopidogrel in patients with planned percutaneous coronary intervention: the PRINCIPLE-TIMI 44 trial. *Circulation* 2006; **116**:2923–32.
61. Yusuf S, Mehta S, *et al.* Efficacy and safety of fondaparinux compared to enoxaparin in acute coronary syndromes. *NEJM* 2006; **354**:1464–76.
62. Stone GW, McLaurin BT, Cox DA, *et al.* Bivalirudin for patients with acute coronary syndromes. *NEJM* 2006; **355**:2203–16.
63. Swahn E, Alfredsson J, Afzal R, *et al.* Early invasive compared with a selective invasive strategy in women with non-ST elevation acute coronary syndromes: a substudy of the OASIS 5 trial and a meta-analysis of previous randomized trials. *Eur Heart J* [Epub Feb 2009].
64. Nikolsky E, Stone GW, *et al.* Gastrointestinal bleeding in patients with acute coronary syndrome: incidence, predictors and clinical implications: Analysis from the ACUITY trial. *J Am Coll Cardiol.* 2009; **54**:293–302.
65. Sabatine MS, Morrow DA, Giugliano RP, *et al.* Association of hemoglobin levels with clinical outcomes in acute coronary syndromes. *Circulation* 2005; **111**:2042–9.
66. Beckman JA, Creager MA, Libby P. Diabetes and atherosclerosis: epidemiology, pathophysiology, and management. *JAMA* 2002; **287**:2570–81.
67. Franklin K, Goldberg RJ, Spencer F, *et al.* Implications of diabetes in patients with acute coronary syndromes. *Arch Intern Med* 2004; **164**:1457–63.
68. Malmberg K, Rydén L, Efendic S, *et al.* Randomized trial of insulin-glucose infusion followed by subcutaneous insulin treatment in diabetic patients with acute myocardial infarction. *J Am Coll Cardiol* 1995; **26**:57–65.
69. Malmberg K, Rydén L, Wedel H, *et al.* Intense metabolic control by means of insulin in patients with diabetes mellitus and acute myocardial infarction (DIGAMI 2): effects on mortality and morbidity. *Eur Heart J* 2005; **26**:650–61.

CHAPTER 16

Primary percutaneous coronary intervention for ST elevation myocardial infarction

Zulfiquar Adam and Mark A. de Belder

Introduction

One of the first reports on the use of intravenous thrombolysis in the treatment of acute myocardial infarction (AMI) was published 50 years ago when Fletcher and colleagues described the use of intravenous streptokinase to restore the patency of arteries occluded by thrombus[(1)]. However, it was not until the early 1980s that the real impetus towards the 'open artery' concept was realised when an angiographic study defined the high prevalence of total coronary occlusion in the early hours of AMI[(2)]. By this time, the era of interventional cardiology had begun and in 1978 there had already been pilot studies of mechanically opening the infarct-related artery (IRA) as well as selective use of intracoronary streptokinase[(3,4)]. In 1983, Hartzler and colleagues reported a small case series on the feasibility of percutaneous transluminal coronary angioplasty (PTCA) during AMI in patients treated with and without prior thrombolysis[(5)]. The use of angioplasty as the main means of opening an occluded vessel (i.e. instead of thrombolysis) was termed 'primary angioplasty' but now, in the era of intracoronary stents and other devices, is referred to as primary percutaneous coronary intervention (PPCI).

During the early 1980s, interventional cardiology was in its infancy and with the lack of suitably trained operators and interventional facilities there was limited development of PPCI. Instead, a number of trials published in the mid-1980s demonstrated a significant benefit from intravenous thrombolytic therapy. A meta-analysis of nine trials with 58 600 patients showed a reduction in mortality at 35 days from 11.5% in control subjects to 9.6%[(6)]. Although thrombolysis became a mainstream treatment, its limitations also became apparent and with the development of interventional techniques there was renewed interest in primary angioplasty. The simultaneous publication of the Primary Angioplasty in Myocardial Infarction (PAMI), Zwolle, and Mayo clinic trials in 1993 paved the way for PPCI as the preferred therapy for the treatment of ST elevation myocardial infarction (STEMI)[(7–9)].

Limitations of thrombolysis and potential benefits of PPCI

- The studies of thrombolysis showed that its efficacy diminished with time following the onset of symptoms. The Fibrinolytic Therapy Trialists' (FTT) collaborative group showed that within 6h of symptom onset there was an absolute mortality reduction of 30 per 1000 patients treated, diminishing to 20 per 1000 patients treated between 6–12h. Beyond 12h, the benefit was not statistically significant from placebo[(6)]. In 2002, a meta-analysis comparing thrombolysis with PPCI showed a similar relationship with time but the decay in benefit is not as steep as with thrombolysis[(10)]. Patients were assigned to three groups according to symptom onset: early (<2h), intermediate (2–4h), and late (>4h). For PPCI, 30-day mortality was 3.9%, 4.1%, and 4.7%

respectively, compared with 5.0%, 6.3%, and 12% respectively in the thrombolysis-treated patients. Another important point highlighted by this study was that the majority of patients (approximately 70% for both groups) were intermediate or late presenters in whom most benefit is derived from PPCI

- The early restoration of normal (Thrombolysis in Myocardial Infarction [TIMI] grade 3) flow in the IRA following the use of various thrombolytic regimens ranges from 40–60%[11], which is in contrast to that seen with PPCI where TIMI 3 flow rates have been reported in over 90% of patients[12]
- One of the most significant complications of thrombolytic therapy is major haemorrhage, in particular intracerebral haemorrhage that occurs in 1% of all patients treated[6]
- It is estimated that up to 25% of patients have contraindications to thrombolysis
- Of the patients treated with thrombolysis about 10% will already be undergoing clot resolution (either spontaneously or due to the effects of aspirin) and thus will have been subjected to the risks of thrombolytic therapy unnecessarily. The use of angiography leading to PPCI allows direct visualization of the coronary anatomy and coronary flow and thus avoids treatment where it is not necessary. Moreover, it enables alternate diagnoses such as myocarditis to be sought if angiographic findings do not correlate with electrocardiogram (ECG) findings
- Up to 10% of patients presenting with STEMI may require CABG on the basis of multi-vessel or LMS disease and these patients can be identified sooner with a PPCI programme.

In addition, early invasive therapy has been shown to be superior to medical therapy in cardiogenic shock. Although not specifically a trial of primary angioplasty, the Should We Emergently Revascularise Occluded Coronaries in Cardiogenic Shock? (SHOCK) trial showed that early revascularization by PCI or CABG was superior to medical therapy at 6 months and 1 year in patients with AMI complicated by cardiogenic shock. One-year survival was 46.7% for patients in the early revascularization group compared with 33.6% in the medical therapy group (absolute difference in survival, 13.2%; 95% CI 2.2–24.1%; p <0.03; relative risk for death, 0.72; 95% CI 0.54–0.95). Of the 10 pre-specified subgroup analyses, only age (<75 vs. ≥75 years) interacted significantly (p <0.03), in that treatment benefit was apparent only for patients younger than 75 years (51.6% survival vs. 33.3% in the medical therapy group)[13,14].

Evidence for PPCI

As mentioned earlier, one of the landmark trials in favour of PPCI was the PAMI trial (n = 395), in which in-hospital mortality was 2.6% for those treated with PPCI versus 6.0% in patients treated with tissue plasminogen activator (t-PA) (p = 0.06) and the combined endpoint of death and non-fatal reinfarction was 10% vsersus 24%. The benefit of PPCI over thrombolysis was maintained on long-term follow-up. At 2 years, patients undergoing primary angioplasty had less recurrent ischaemia (36.4% vs. 48% for t-PA, p = 0.026), lower reintervention rates (27.2% vs. 46.5%, p <0.0001), and reduced hospital readmission rates (58.5% vs. 69.0%, p = 0.035). The combined endpoint of death or reinfarction was 14.9% for angioplasty versus 23% for t-PA, p = 0.034. Multivariate analysis found angioplasty to be independently predictive of a reduction in death, reinfarction, or target vessel revascularization (p = 0.0001)[15].

A number of trials comparing the two strategies were performed following the original series and in 1997, a systematic review combining the results of 10 randomized trials (n = 2606) showed mortality at 30 days or less was 4.4% for the 1290 patients treated with primary angioplasty compared with 6.5% for the 1316 patients treated with thrombolysis (34% reduction; OR, 0.66; 95% CI 0.46–0.94; p = 0.02). The rates of death or non-fatal reinfarction were 7.2% for angioplasty and 11.9% for thrombolytic therapy (OR, 0.58; 95% CI 0.44–0.76; p <0.001). Angioplasty was associated with a significant reduction in total stroke (0.7% vs. 2.0%; p = 0.007) and haemorrhagic stroke (0.1% vs. 1.1%; p<0.001)[16].

In 2003, Keeley and colleagues combined the results of the original 10 trials and a further 13 trials including the use of stents and glycoprotein (GP) IIb/IIIa inhibitors (n = 7739). They showed that short-term mortality was 7% for PPCI versus 9% with thrombolysis (p = 0.0002), stroke occurred in 1% compared to 2% (p = 0.0004) respectively, and non-fatal reinfarction occurred in 3% versus 7% (p <0.0001) respectively. The combined endpoint of these three outcomes was also significantly lower in the PPCI group—8% compared to 14% in the thrombolysis group (p <0.0001) (Fig. 16.1)[17].

The superiority of PPCI over hospital-administered thrombolysis seen in this analysis influenced the current European Society for Cardiology (ESC) guidelines that recommend PPCI as the preferred strategy for

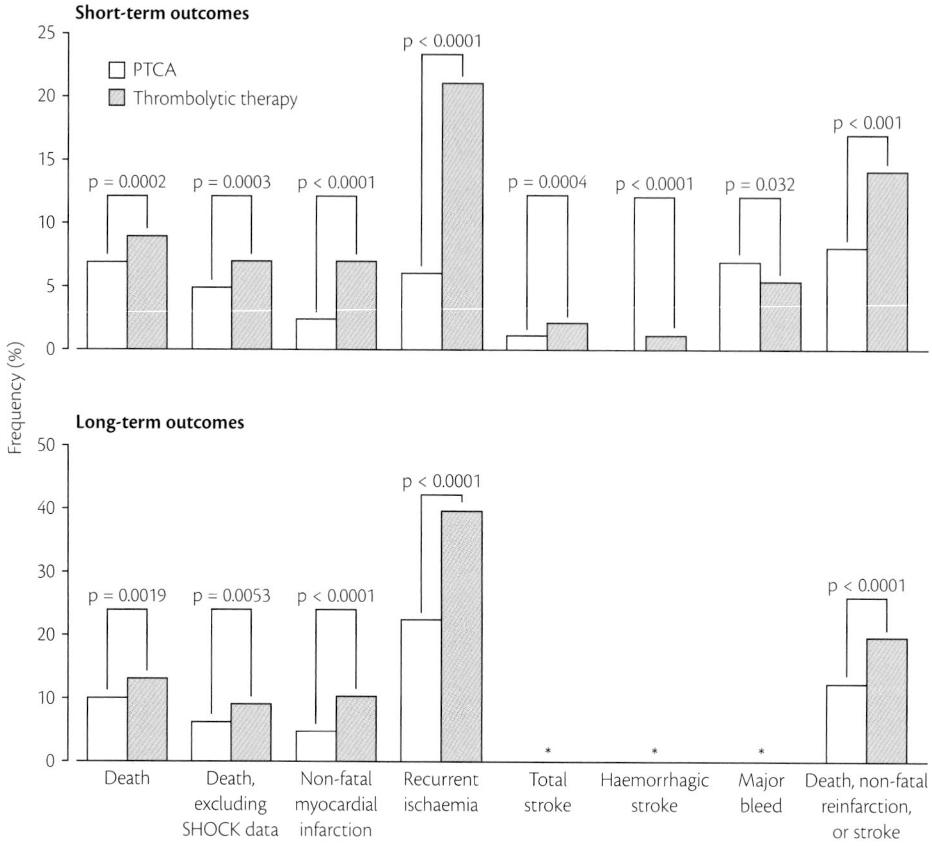

Fig. 16.1 Short-term and long-term clinical outcomes following PTCA versus thrombolysis. Reproduced from Keeley EC, Boura JA, Grines CL. Primary angioplasty versus intravenous thrombolytic therapy for acute myocardial infarction: a quantitative review of 23 randomised trials. *Lancet* 2003; **361**:13–20. Copyright ©2003, with permission from Elsevier.

reperfusion for STEMI, but the recommendation is dependent on how soon PPCI can be performed after first medical contact (FMC) (recommendation level of evidence Class 1, level A)[(18)].

There are a number of factors that require consideration with regards to PPCI:

1) Whereas thrombolytic therapy is easy to give and can even be administered in ambulances, PPCI has to be delivered by specialized teams and requires transportation of the patients to a cardiac catheterization laboratory;
2) Previously, the majority of patients have either not presented or been delivered to hospitals with PPCI capabilities;
3) Transportation of patients takes time, and for some the time taken may negate the potential advantages of PPCI; and
4) Before considering the widespread uptake of PPCI, the cost-effectiveness of this strategy also has to be considered, taking into account the importance of time and issues with respect to transportation.

Optimal timing for PPCI versus thrombolysis

Although the time versus muscle conservation relationship differs between PPCI and thrombolysis, probably because PPCI offers successful early opening of the artery and restoration of good flow in significantly more patients, a number of time factors need to be considered. First, there is a delay before the patient seeks FMC and, in spite of a number of public education programmes, this remains longer than is desirable. This is important, as the PRAGUE-2 trial in particular demonstrated that PPCI was superior to thrombolysis in terms of lives saved when the delay to randomization was 3h or more from symptom onset (vide infra)[19]. This fact has been reinforced in ESC guidelines on the use of PPCI, which recommend that all patients presenting late should be considered for PPCI rather than thrombolysis[18].

Although trials summarize the overall outcomes of patients, this can hide the fact that patients with STEMI vary from those presenting with a 'big bang' (when significant myocardial damage occurs very early and for whom very early reperfusion therapy may be crucial) to those with 'stuttering infarction' when myocardium may be relatively preserved in spite of considerable delays to presentation (possibly because of collateral vessel formation and a number of adaptive physiological responses to ischaemia). When transportation of a patient for PPCI is very long, say >3h, there may be cases where so much myocardial damage occurs prior to successful PPCI that relatively small amounts of myocardium can be salvaged. This has led to the study of the impact of PPCI-related delay on outcomes, i.e. is there a time between when thrombolysis could be started and PPCI can be performed when the advantages of PPCI are lost?

Ideally, one would want to compare the time taken to successful reperfusion with these two treatments. However, it is not possible to accurately analyse the time to successful reperfusion with thrombolysis for a number of reasons: 1) because of a lack of consensus on how to identify successful reperfusion with thrombolysis on clinical and electrocardiographic criteria; 2) because the time to certain pre-defined ECG changes has not been routinely recorded in these trials; and 3) because thrombolysis does not achieve successful and/or timely reperfusion in a significant number of patients. Instead, one can record the time of onset of the major symptoms heralding the infarct (not always easy to be precise about), the time of call of the patient for help or the time of FMC, the time of arrival at the hospital, and/or the time of the start of the thrombolytic treatment (the 'needle' time). From these, one can measure symptom-to-needle, call-to-needle, FMC-to-needle, or door-to-needle times—i.e. the relevant times to the *start* of treatment.

With PPCI, a number of other times can be recorded, e.g. the time of arrival on the catheter laboratory table, the time when local anaesthetic was first administered, the time when the first balloon is inflated (or nowadays the first device used, especially as this might be a thrombus-removing device), or the time when angiographic TIMI-3 flow is restored. However, because TIMI-3 flow may not always be restored and because of intra-observer variability in defining angiographic flow patterns, it is has become conventional to utilize the first balloon (device) time to calculate symptom-to-balloon, call-to-balloon, FMC-to-balloon, or door-to-balloon (DTB) times. If patients are transferred from one non-PCI hospital to another centre with PCI capabilities, one also has to record the arrival times at each hospital (door 1 and door 2 times). Unlike thrombolysis, the time of onset of the procedure to successful reperfusion is usually short, and is much more reflective of the time to *successful therapy*. In general, PCI centre DTB times reflect the efficiency of that centre, whereas the call-to-balloon times reflect an overview of the whole system of care, from identifying the patient with a STEMI to the start of PCI. In considering the issues of PCI-related delay, a number of important observations have been made, as discussed in the following sections.

Time from symptom onset to thrombolysis versus balloon inflation

In the landmark 'reappraisal of the golden hour' study, Boersma and colleagues found that treatment within an hour after onset of symptoms with thrombolysis results in a 6.5% absolute reduction in mortality compared with placebo; this benefit falls quickly with time to 3.7% at 1–2h, 2.6% at 2–3h, 2.9% at 3–6h, 1.8% at 6–12h, and 0.9% at 12–24h[20].

For PPCI, however, there has been somewhat conflicting evidence concerning the relationship between symptom-to-balloon time and outcome. A prospective observational study from the Second National Registry of Myocardial infarction (NRMI-2) of 27 080 patients at 661 community and tertiary care hospitals who underwent PPCI showed that there was no correlation between in-hospital mortality and the symptom-to-balloon time[21], whereas, in a study of 1791 patients, the Zwolle group showed that presentation more than 4h after symptom onset was an independent predictor of mortality. On further analysis of these data, a continuous relationship was found such that for every 30-min delay in balloon inflation from symptom onset, mortality increased by 1.075 times[22].

Time from first medical contact to thrombolysis ('door-to-needle' time) versus balloon inflation ('door-to-balloon' time)

One of the most-quoted analyses addressing this issue was performed by Nallamothu and Bates (n = 7419). They extracted the 4–6-week mortality, incidence of reinfarction and stroke, and the PCI-related time delay defined as the mean (or median) DTB time minus the door-to-needle time data from the Keeley meta-analysis (excluding data from two trials—one had missing data on time to treatment and the other involved patients in cardiogenic shock). In what some consider to be a flawed analysis, their principal finding was that at 62-min delay, PCI loses its potential to save more lives (there is 'equipoise' as regards survival) (Fig. 16.2)[23].

An extended analysis performed by the same authors showed that the acceptable PCI-related delay appears to be shorter for thrombin-specific thrombolytic agents than with streptokinase. In 13 thrombin-specific trials, the absolute mortality reduction favouring PPCI decreased significantly as PPCI-related delay increased (1.1% decrease for every additional 10-min delay, $p = 0.044$). In contrast, the impact of PPCI-related delay on mortality was not significant in the streptokinase studies (absolute 0.3% decrease for every 10-min delay, $p = 0.78$). The time to equipoise between the two reperfusion strategies was >170min in the seven streptokinase studies, 62min in the 13 thrombin-specific studies, and 88min for all 20 trials (absolute 0.5% decrease for every 10-min delay, $p = 0.22$)[24].

It is worth pointing out that the Nallamothu and Bates analysis used the differences between mean or median times to start of treatment, not absolute times for individual patients and also they did not take account of the time delay between symptom onset and presentation. Another criticism of these analyses relates to the use of a weighted meta-regression providing an

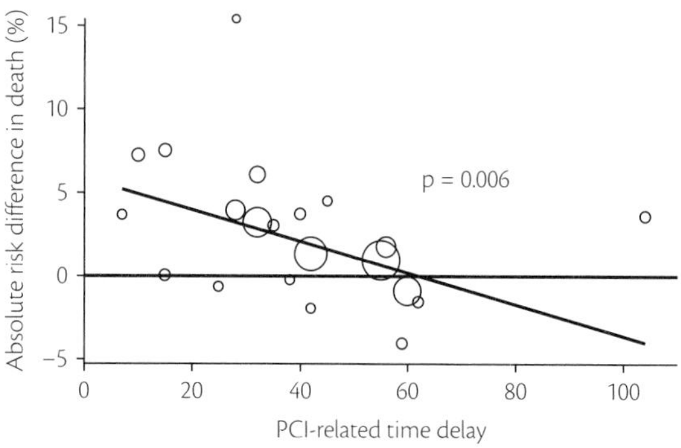

Fig. 16.2 Absolute risk reduction in 4- to 6-week mortality rates with primary PCI as a function of PCI-related time delay. *Circle* sizes reflect the sample size of the individual study. Values >0 represent benefit and values <0 represent harm. *Solid line*, weighted meta-regression. Reproduced from Nallamothu BK, Bates ER. Percutaneous coronary intervention versus fibrinolytic therapy in acute myocardial infarction: is timing (almost) everything? *Am J Cardiol* 2003; **92**:824–6. Copyright ©2003, with permission from Elsevier.

'absolute' cut-off, in spite of the fact that there are virtually no data points beyond 60min. Asseburg and colleagues repeated this analysis with a different statistical approach and, with more complete data from the trials, demonstrated that although one can derive a time for equipoise for mortality outcomes, there is considerable uncertainty about these results. In contrast to Nallamothu and Bates, they determined that for mortality, angioplasty is better than thrombolysis, on average, at time delays up to 90min. Moreover, they demonstrated that PPCI was highly likely to be superior to thrombolysis as regards the development of reinfarction or stroke, regardless of time delay (Fig. 16.3)[25].

Boersma performed a different analysis of the same data but was able to obtain patient-specific data from most of the trials. In this study combining the results of 22 trials ($n = 6763$), both the influences of presentation delay and PCI-related delay were assessed. Overall 30-day mortality was less in the PPCI group (5.3% vs. 7.9% $p < 0.001$) and the negative influence of presentation delay on mortality in both groups was also apparent (Table 16.1). An important point to make from this analysis is that for patients presenting very early, PPCI appeared to be superior to thrombolysis[26].

The results for the effect of PCI-related delay showed that PPCI was superior to thrombolysis overall but particularly in patients with a PCI-related delay of less than 35min. The negative impact of longer time to treatment was also clearly highlighted (Table 16.2)[26].

The NRMI registry data ($n = 192\,409$) provided insights into this debate using prospective non-randomized data more likely to be reflective of real-world practice. In this analysis, a PCI-related delay of 114min represented the 'equipoise' point for mortality between the two treatment strategies. Subgroup analyses suggested that time may be more important for different groups of patients[27]. For example, for patients aged less than 65 years with anterior location of infarct, the equipoise point was at only 40min (Fig. 16.4). This study had its limitations due to its observational design. Selection bias could well have been an important factor, as PPCI was more likely to be performed in patients with cardiogenic shock. In addition, the majority of thrombolysis treated patients received thrombin-specific agents with a median door-to-needle time of approximately 40min (i.e. almost ideal) whereas PPCI was mainly performed at low-volume centres and the majority of patients had DTB times greater than 90min (i.e. not ideal).

These studies highlight the uncertainties with relation to the effect of the acceptable limits of PCI-related delay. The Nallamothu and Bates, Asseburg, and Boersma

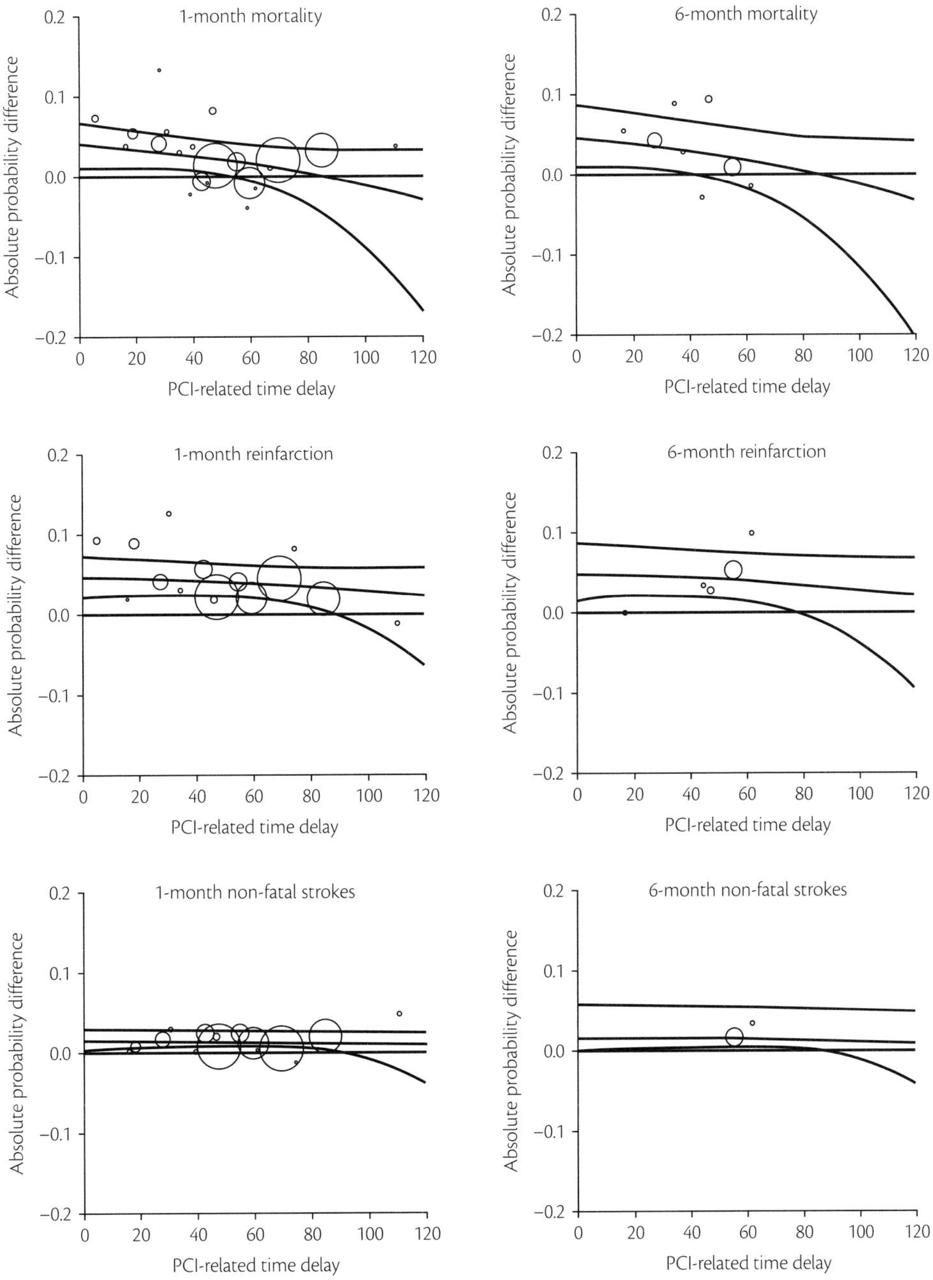

Fig. 16.3 Treatment effect of primary angioplasty relative to thrombolytic treatment, shown as the absolute probability differences for each key outcome (death, non-fatal reinfarctions, non-fatal strokes) and point of follow-up (1 month, 6 months). The graphs show means and 95% credibility intervals plotted against the additional time delay to initiating primary angioplasty. Values above the 0.0 horizontal line indicate that angioplasty results in fewer clinical events. Each point represents a trial and their size is proportional to the trial sample size. Reproduced from Asseburg C, Vergel YB, Palmer S, *et al.* Assessing the effectiveness of primary angioplasty compared with thrombolysis and its relationship to time delay: a Bayesian evidence synthesis. *Heart* 2007; **93**:1244–50, with permission from BMJ Publishing Group Ltd.

Table 16.1 Mortality according to presentation delay

	Overall	Presentation delay				
		0–1h	>1–2h	>2–3h	>3–6h	>6h
Thrombolysis (n)	3383	368	997	818	876	324
Mortality (%)	7.9	6.0	6.2	7.3	9.5	12.7
PPCI (n)	3380	379	1003	894	764	340
Mortality (%)	5.3	4.7	4.2	5.1	5.6	8.5

Data from Boersma E. Does time matter? A pooled analysis of randomized clinical trials comparing primary percutaneous coronary intervention and in-hospital fibrinolysis in acute myocardial infarction patients. *Eur Heart J* 2006; **27**:779–88.

Table 16.2 Mortality according to PCI-related delay

PCI-related delay (min)	Number of patients	30-day mortality (%)	
		Thrombolysis	PPCI
0–35	1417	8.2	2.8
>35–50	1292	6.8	5.4
>50–62	1425	5.4	4.8
>62–79	1280	9.5	6.9
>79–120	1349	9.6	6.6
All patients	6763	7.9	5.3

Data from Boersma E. Does time matter? A pooled analysis of randomized clinical trials comparing primary percutaneous coronary intervention and in-hospital fibrinolysis in acute myocardial infarction patients. *Eur Heart J* 2006; **27**:779–88.

analyses all used a similar dataset but had different results using different statistical techniques. However, the earlier reperfusion therapy is delivered, the better the results regardless of strategy and a consistent theme is that, in general, PPCI is superior to thrombolysis. However, caution is required in interpreting these analyses and it would appear that, based on the Boersma analysis, a PCI related delay of up to 120min may be acceptable.

Current ESC guidelines recommend that for PPCI, time from FMC should be less than 2h in any case or less than 90min in those presenting early (symptom onset less than 2h) with a large infarct and low bleeding risk (Class 1, level B) (Fig. 16.5)[18].

Regional transfers

Despite the evidence for benefit of PPCI over thrombolysis, there are still those that believe that the latter should remain the treatment of choice for many patients with STEMI. This is mainly based on the additional

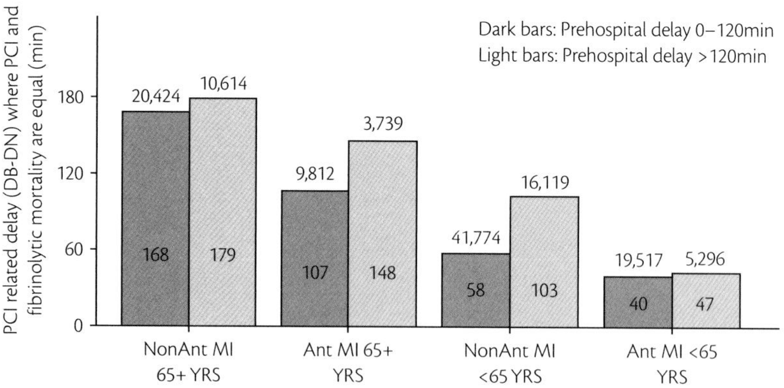

Fig. 16.4 Adjusted analysis illustrating significant heterogeneity in the PCI-related delay for which the mortality rates with PPCI and thrombolysis were comparable after the study population was stratified by pre-hospital delay, location of infarct, and age. PCI-related time at which the mortality benefit was lost was based on multivariate models. Data from Pinto DS, Kirtane AJ, Nallamothu BK, *et al.* Hospital delays in reperfusion for ST-elevation myocardial infarction: implications when selecting a reperfusion strategy. *Circulation* 2006; **114**:2019–25.

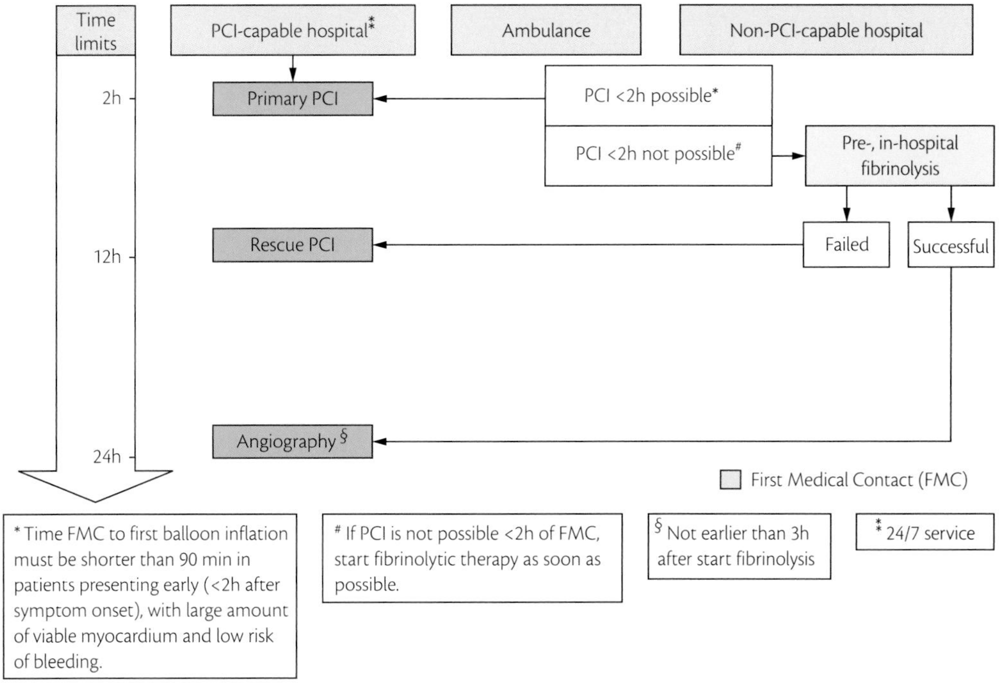

Fig. 16.5 Flow chart demonstrating current ESC guidelines regarding reperfusion treatment for STEMI. Reproduced from Van de Werf F, Bax J, Betriu A, *et al.* Management of acute myocardial infarction in patients presenting with persistent ST-segment elevation: the Task Force on the Management of ST-Segment Elevation Acute Myocardial Infarction of the European Society of Cardiology. *Eur Heart J* 2008; **29**:2909–45.

time and resource required for PPCI and is one of the main sources of ongoing debate as the majority of patients have traditionally presented to non-PCI capable hospitals.

This question was addressed mainly by two large trials, the PRAGUE-2 study in 2002 (n = 850)[19] and the Danish Multicenter Randomized Study on Fibrinolytic Therapy versus Acute Coronary Angioplasty in Acute Myocardial Infarction (DANAMI-2) study in 2003 (n = 1572)[28]. In both studies, patients presenting with an STEMI with symptom duration less than 12h were randomized to either thrombolysis (streptokinase in PRAGUE-2, alteplase in DANAMI-2) or transfer to a PCI-capable hospital. Patients presenting directly to the PCI-capable hospitals were also included in DANAMI-2.

Patients were transported distances up to 120km in the PRAGUE-2 study. The primary outcome was 30-day mortality, which was lower in the PPCI group compared to the thrombolysis group (6.8% vs. 10%; p = 0.12). For patients presenting less than 3h since onset of symptoms, mortality was similar in both groups (7.3% vs. 7.4% respectively). For those presenting 3–12h since onset, PPCI was associated with lower mortality (6% vs. 15.3% respectively). The combined clinical endpoint of death, disabling stroke, and reinfarction was significantly lower in the PPCI group (8.4% vs. 15.2% respectively; p <0.003).

In the DANAMI-2 trial, the combined endpoint of death, reinfarction, and disabling stroke was significantly lower in the PPCI group (8.5% vs. 14.2%; p = 0.002) for patients attending referral hospitals. This was mainly accounted for by the reduction in reinfarction (1.9% vs. 6.2%; p <0.001) although there was no significant difference in mortality (6.5% vs. 8.5%; p = 0.20). The median distance that patients were transported was 50km (range 3–150km).

These and five other smaller trials were analysed separately in the meta-analysis performed by Keeley and colleagues and the results favoured PPCI (Fig. 16.6)[17].

The trials also demonstrated that transport of these patients was safe. In the DANAMI-2 trial, eight of 559 (1.4%) patients transferred from their local hospital for PCI had a VF arrest. No patients died en route (median distance transported was 50km). Of 425 patients transferred in PRAGUE-2, three (0.71%) were successfully resuscitated from VF and two died en route (0.47%).

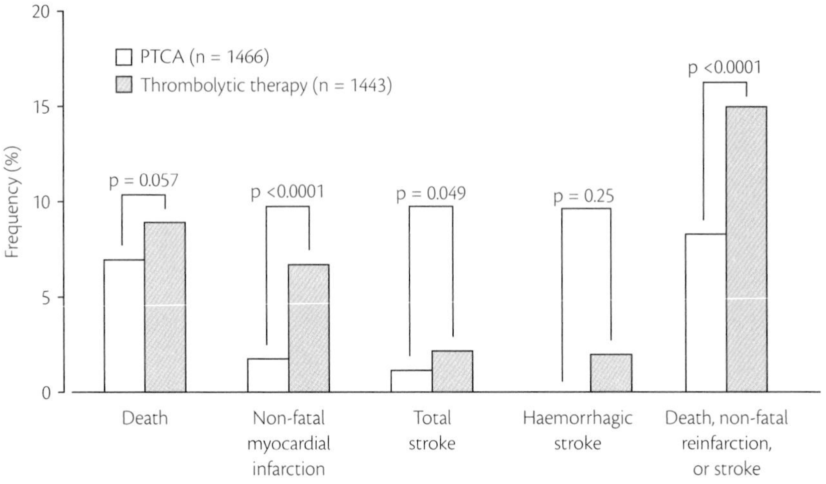

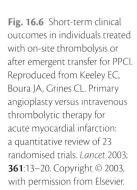

Fig. 16.6 Short-term clinical outcomes in individuals treated with on-site thrombolysis or after emergent transfer for PPCI. Reproduced from Keeley EC, Boura JA, Grines CL. Primary angioplasty versus intravenous thrombolytic therapy for acute myocardial infarction: a quantitative review of 23 randomised trials. *Lancet* 2003; **361**:13–20. Copyright © 2003, with permission from Elsevier.

It is of note that these favourable results for PPCI were seen even when the patient had presented first to the non-PCI hospital, been randomized, and then transferred. It is also of note that, although the transfer took time, the PCI centre angioplasty teams were activated whilst the patient was en route, such that the PCI centre DTB times were favourable in these studies.

Pre-hospital thrombolysis, facilitated PCI, and routine early PCI

Pre-hospital thrombolysis

One criticism of these trials is that PPCI was compared against delivery of thrombolysis once the patient had arrived in hospital. However, efforts to expedite thrombolysis have included delivering it pre-hospital, usually in the ambulance. In the United Kingdom (UK), the targets of delivering thrombolytic therapy are within 60min of calling for help and 30min of arrival in hospital for STEMI. A protocol for the initiation of pre-hospital thrombolysis (PHT) has also been introduced mainly for the benefit of those patients where the journey time to the nearest hospital is greater than 45min. PHT has been shown to reduce mortality compared with in-hospital thrombolysis (IHT)[29].

In the UK, however, PHT is only administered to a proportion of patients. This relates to the Joint Royal Colleges Liaison Committee (JRCALC) guidelines for the administration of thrombolysis by paramedics, which state that treatment can only be started for patients under 80 years, with symptom duration less than 6h and in the absence of haemodynamic compromise (heart rate 40–140bpm, systolic blood pressure [BP] 80–180mmHg, diastolic BP <110mmHg)[30]. In 2007/8, 3176 patients (2972 in England and 204 in Wales) received pre-hospital thrombolytic treatment compared with 2942 patients in 2006/7, an increase of 8.0%, but this represented only 22% of all patients receiving thrombolysis[31].

In 2002, the Comparison of Angioplasty and Pre-hospital Thrombolysis in Acute Myocardial Infarction (CAPTIM) study group randomized patients presenting within 6h of symptom onset of AMI in the ambulance. This trial was limited by funding and enrolment issues and so only 840 patients of the required 1200 patients were recruited. No statistically significant differences were seen in the primary endpoint between the two therapies. The composite endpoint of death, reinfarction, and stroke at 30 days was numerically lower in the PPCI group (6.2% vs. 8.2%; p = 0.29). Some trends in the secondary endpoints are worthy of mention, with lower rates of recurrent ischaemia in the PPCI group (4.0% vs. 7.2%; p = 0.09) but, interestingly, less occurrence of cardiogenic shock in the PHT group (2.5% vs. 4.0%; p = 0.09). This latter finding provided part of the impetus for exploration of the role of facilitated PCI (discussed below)[32]. Moreover, in a non pre-specified subgroup analysis, the 30-day death rates for patients presenting within 2h of the onset of pain were 2.2% in the PHT group compared to 5.7% in the PPCI group (p = 0.058)[33]. It should be noted though that 30–40% of patients receiving PHT underwent immediate rescue angioplasty and about 70% had undergone PCI prior to discharge. In other words, this was a study of PHT associated with liberal use of rescue and early PCI versus PPCI.

These and results from other studies have stimulated the ongoing Strategic Reperfusion Early After Myocardial Infarction (STREAM) trial in which a larger cohort of high-risk patients who present within 3h of symptoms are being randomized between these strategies.

The CAPTIM trial subgroup results differ from those found in a large Swedish registry from 2006. In this prospective observational cohort study (n = 26 205), the adjusted 30-day mortality was lower with PPCI than PHT (4.9% vs. 7.6%; HR 0.70; 95% CI 0.58–0.85) and similarly at 1 year (7.6% vs. 10.3%; HR 0.81; 95% CI 0.69–0.94). Beyond 2-h treatment delay, the observed mortality reductions with PHT tended to decrease while the benefits with PPCI seemed to remain regardless of time delay (Table 16.3). PPCI was also associated with shorter hospital stay and less reinfarction than either PHT or IHT[34].

For patients presenting early, PHT may be an attractive option for reperfusion therapy but, in the UK at least, its use is restricted, as most ambulance services do not have emergency physicians available. Moreover, a strategy of PHT appears to get best results when linked to the use of rescue or early PCI and so such a strategy ideally requires that patients receiving PHT be taken immediately to a hospital with PCI capabilities. In addition, for those not receiving PHT, then a system of immediate transfer to a PCI-capable hospital is desirable. Either way, apart from those patients who self-present to hospital, the use of PHT actually started to influence the thinking behind 'heart attack centres', i.e. those hospitals with PCI capability, and the strategy of ambulances bypassing non-PCI capable centres.

In the UK, the investment in PHT has been extremely useful for PPCI. The training of paramedic crews in pre-hospital assessment of AMI, including ECG interpretation, means that more efficient triage and transfer of these patients to PCI centres can occur.

Table 16.3 Comparison of mortality between in hospital thrombolysis (IHT), pre-hospital thrombolysis (PHT), and primary percutaneous coronary intervention (PPCI) amongst ST elevation MI patients*

	IHT	PHT	PPCI
Mortality at 30 days (%):			
<2h to reperfusion	8.6	5.6	3.8
≥2h to reperfusion	11.4	8.9	4.5
Mortality at 1 year (%):			
<2h to reperfusion	11.9	8.0	6.7
≥2h to reperfusion	16.3	11.8	7.3

*Data from Stenestrand *et al.*[34].

Facilitated PCI

The difficulties in transferring patients in a timely manner for PPCI led to another strategy, that of facilitated PCI. The idea behind this is that patients who are unlikely to be transferred for PPCI within the recommended time limits are pre-treated with pharmacological therapy which can involve thrombolysis, platelet GP IIb/IIIa inhibitors or a combination of the two (half-dose lytic therapy + GP IIb/IIIa inhibitor) and subsequently transferred for coronary angiography with a view to revascularization with PCI. The potential benefits would be earlier reperfusion and possibly less occurrence of slow flow or the no-reflow phenomenon, (discussed in a later section). These trials were stimulated by a number of studies that demonstrated that the lowest mortality appeared to be for patients with TIMI-3 flow prior to PCI as well as TIMI-3 flow post PCI[35,36]. However, there is clearly a potential for worse outcomes in other patients—thrombolysis may lead to haemorrhagic transformation of an infarcted zone, may predispose to cardiac rupture and stimulates platelet aggregation through activation by fibrin degradation products[37]. Randomized trials were needed to evaluate the risk:benefit ratio of a facilitated approach.

The Combined Angioplasty and Pharmacological Intervention Versus Thrombolysis Alone in Acute Myocardial Infarction (CAPITAL AMI) study investigated 170 high-risk STEMI patients (two or more of anterior location, extensive non-anterior location, Killip class 3 or systolic BP <100mmHg). The patients were randomly assigned to tenecteplase followed by immediate transfer for PCI or tenecteplase alone. The composite primary endpoint at 6 months (death, recurrent MI, recurrent unstable ischaemia, or stroke) was found less often in patients who received facilitated PCI (11.6% vs. 24.4%, p = 0.04), being driven by a significant reduction in recurrent unstable ischaemia (8.1% vs. 20.7%, p = 0.03) and trend towards reduction in reinfarction (5.8% vs. 14.6 %, p = 0.07). There were no significant differences in mortality (3.5% vs. 3.7%, p = 1.0) or stroke (1.2% vs. 1.2%, p = 1.0)[38].

The Assessment of the Safety and Efficacy of a New Treatment Strategy with Percutaneous Coronary Intervention (ASSENT-4 PCI) investigators planned to enrol 4000 patients with acute STEMI of less than 6h duration who were scheduled to undergo primary PCI with an anticipated delay of 1–3h and were to be randomly assigned to tenecteplase or placebo prior to angioplasty. The primary endpoint was the composite of death, heart failure, or shock within 90 days. The data and safety monitoring board recommended early cessation of enrolment after 1667 patients because of a significant increase in mortality in the tenecteplase group (6% vs. 3% p = 0.01). Among the patients who were randomized, facilitated PCI with tenecteplase was associated with significant increases in the primary endpoint (19% vs. 13%, relative risk 1.39, 95% CI 1.11–1.74) and in the rate of in-hospital stroke (1.8 vs. 0%; 8 of 13 classified strokes were due to intracranial haemorrhage) and, at 90 days, reinfarction (6% vs. 4%), and target vessel revascularization (7% vs. 3%)[39].

A comprehensive meta-analysis (n = 4504) performed in 2006 involving 17 trials did not show any benefit for this approach when compared to PPCI[40]. Although the initial TIMI 3 flow rates were better in the facilitated PCI group (37% vs. 15%, OR 3·18; 95% CI 2·22–4·55; p = 0·0001), there was no significant difference between the final TIMI-3 flow rates (89% vs. 88%; OR 1·19, 95% CI 0·86–1·64; p = 0.30). The primary endpoints of short-term (up to 42day) mortality (5% vs. 3%; OR 1·38, 95% CI 1·01–1·87), non-fatal reinfarction (3% vs. 2%; OR 1·71, 95% CI 1·16–2·51), urgent target vessel revascularization (4% vs. 1%; OR 2.39, 95% CI 1.23–4.66), and major bleeding (7% vs. 5%; OR 1.51, 95% CI 1.10–2.08) all favoured the PPCI group. The facilitated PCI group also had increased rates of both haemorrhagic (0.7% vs. 0.1%, p = 0.0014) and total stroke (1.1% vs. 0.3%, p = 0.0008). These findings were mainly as a result of the regimens that used up-front thrombolytic therapy. When analysed separately, the facilitated regimens that only involved platelet GP IIb/IIIa inhibitors did not show an increase in major adverse clinical outcomes.

This latter finding was replicated in the FINESSE study (n = 2452) in 2008[41]. In this study, patients within 6h of onset of STEMI were randomized to abciximab alone pre-PCI, half-dose reteplase + abciximab pre-PCI, or PPCI with abciximab therapy during the procedure. There were no significant differences in the primary composite endpoint of death, ventricular fibrillation occurring more than 48h after randomization, cardiogenic shock, and congestive heart failure requiring rehospitalization or an emergency room visit through 90 days (9.8%, 10.5%, and 10.7 % respectively). From a safety perspective, patients receiving thrombolytic therapy had significantly more bleeding (combination of TIMI major and minor) complications than the PPCI group (14.5% vs. 6.9%, p <0.001). Haemorrhagic stroke was also higher in this group compared to PPCI (0.6% vs. 0.1%). The abciximab group findings were in keeping with the previous meta-analysis.

The conclusions that can be drawn from these results are that, within the time windows in these trials (up to 4h delay), facilitated PCI with thrombolytic therapy should be avoided, and facilitated PCI with platelet GP IIb/IIIa inhibitors cannot be recommended because of the lack of benefit. This is reflected in current ESC guidelines[18]. Whether facilitated PCI has a role for specific subgroups of patients (e.g. high-risk patients with very long transfer times) requires further study.

Routine early PCI

With the lack of evidence for a facilitated approach, another strategy for dealing with those patients who present to non-PCI capable hospitals involves the use of routine early PCI where coronary angiography is performed within hours of thrombolysis rather than immediately. Given the short half-life of most fibrin-specific thrombolytic agents, the rationale here is that delayed PCI might confer some benefit but without the early hazards that can occur when PCI is performed early.

This was investigated by the Grupo de Análisis de la Cardiopatía Isquémica Aguda (GRACIA) collaborators. In GRACIA-1 (n = 500), patients were randomized to thrombolysis with either transfer to a PCI centre for angiography and PCI if indicated within 24h of thrombolysis or an ischaemia-driven approach to coronary angiography ± PCI. There was a significant reduction in the primary endpoint of death, non-fatal reinfarction, or revascularization by 1 year (9% vs. 21%, p = 0.0008) in favour of the early transfer group[42].

The GRACIA-2 study (n = 212) was a trial designed to show non-inferiority of a routine early PCI strategy compared to PPCI. In this trial, patients were randomized to PPCI alone or PCI 3–12h following thrombolysis. The investigators used surrogate markers as their primary endpoint. There was a significant benefit in favour of the routine early PCI group in terms of degree of epicardial and myocardial reperfusion after PCI (defined as TIMI 3 epicardial flow, TIMI 3 myocardial perfusion, and ≥70% resolution of the initial sum of ST-segment elevation). Infarct size was similar between the two groups determined by area under the curve for troponin and creatine kinase–MB levels, and left ventricular function assessment by echocardiography. There were no significant differences in major cardiovascular events or bleeding complications[43].

The Combined Abciximab Reteplase Stent Study in Acute Myocardial Infarction (CARESS-in-AMI) evaluated the optimum reperfusion strategy in 600 STEMI patients with one or more high-risk features (extensive ST-segment elevation, new left bundle branch block, prior MI, Killip class >2, or left ventricular ejection fraction ≤35%) who were initially admitted to hospitals without PCI capability. Patients were treated with half-dose reteplase and abciximab and then randomly assigned to either immediate transfer to the nearest interventional centre for PCI or to continued medical therapy with transfer only in case of persistent ST-segment elevation or clinical deterioration. The mean time between thrombolysis and angiography in the early intervention group was 125min. The primary composite endpoint (death, reinfarction, or refractory ischaemia at 30 days) occurred significantly less often in the immediate PCI group compared with the standard care/rescue group (4.4% vs. 10.7%, p = 0.004). This result was driven primarily by a reduction in refractory ischaemia (0.3% vs. 4.0% for standard care, p = 0.003). There were no significant differences in death (3.0% vs. 4.7% for standard care, p = 0.40) or reinfarction (1.3% vs. 2.0% for standard care, p = 0.75)[(44)]. A noteworthy point about this trial is that the combination of half-dose lytic and GP IIb/IIIa inhibitor has not been recommended as a reperfusion strategy (even with additional rescue or selective angiography ± PCI).

In the Trial of Routine Angioplasty and Stenting after Fibrinolysis to Enhance Reperfusion in Acute Myocardial Infarction (TRANSFER-AMI), 1059 STEMI patients who presented to a non-PCI hospital were given thrombolytic therapy (tenecteplase) within 2h of the onset of chest pain[(45)]. They were then randomly assigned to either urgent transfer for cardiac catheterization within 6h or to standard care, which was defined as transfer for rescue and/or urgent PCI with elective routine catheterization encouraged for successfully reperfused patients after 24h. The median time to catheterization after randomization was 2.8h in the urgent transfer group and 32.5h in the standard care group. At 30 days, the primary composite endpoint (death, reinfarction, heart failure, severe recurrent ischaemia, or shock) occurred significantly less often in the urgent transfer group (11.0% vs. 17.2%, p = 0.004). This was mainly accounted for by a reduction in reinfarction (3.4% vs. 5.7%, p = 0.06) and recurrent ischaemia (0.2% vs. 2.1%, p = 0.003) in the pharmacoinvasive group. Mortality was not significantly different (4.5% vs. 3.4% for standard care, p = 0.39). The bleeding rates were similar in the two groups.

The latter two trials suggest that giving thrombolysis or a combination of lytic and GP IIb/IIIa inhibitors and then sending for early care is better than selective transfer for rescue or 'standard care'. The obvious difficulty in interpreting these results is that they did not compare the routine early strategy with PPCI. In the ASSENT-4PCI trial, the 90-day mortality was 5% compared to a 30-day mortality of 4.5% in TRANSFER AMI. Although these are different trials with different populations, there is no convincing evidence that routine early angiography following thrombolysis is likely to be better than PPCI. Moreover, these trials look at selected subsets of patients and so lead to the potential for complex algorithms for care rather than a simple one for PPCI. Increasing complexity in treatment algorithms may jeopardize feasibility and currently there is no evidence that this would lead to better overall outcomes. Further research is needed but currently ESC guidelines recommend routine early angiography ± PCI for patients with evidence of successful reperfusion within 3–24h post thrombolysis for STEMI (Class IIa, level A)[(18)].

Systems of care: factors related to PCI hospitals

Door-to-balloon time

The effect of DTB time on mortality has been studied extensively. One of the largest studies was the observational NRMI registry analysis (n = 29 222). In patients who underwent PPCI for STEMI at 395 hospitals in the United States, longer DTB times were associated with higher mortality (3.0%, 4.2%, 5.7%, and 7.4% for DTB time of ≤90min, 91–120min, 121–150min, and >150min, respectively)[(46)].

After adjusting for patient characteristics, this relationship remained significant (OR 1.42; 95% CI 1.24–1.62) (Fig. 16.7).

Another important study highlighted the importance of DTB times in high-risk patients. In this study (n = 2322), patients were prospectively followed up for 7 years. A longer DTB time (>2h) was associated with greater long-term mortality in high-risk patients (defined as one or more of Killip class III or IV heart failure, age >70 years, or anterior MI), 32.5% compared to 21.5% for DTB ≤2h, p = 0.0002). In lower-risk patients, though, there was no significant difference (10.8% vs. 9.2%, p = 0.53)[(47)]. There was also a significant increase in 7-year mortality in patients presenting ≤3h from symptom onset (24.7% for DTB time >2h vs. 15.0% for DTB time ≤2h) but not in patients presenting after 3h (21.1% for DTB time >2h vs. 18.5% for DTB time ≤2h). In other words, short DTB times are especially important for high-risk patients and those presenting within 3h of symptom onset. This analysis does not

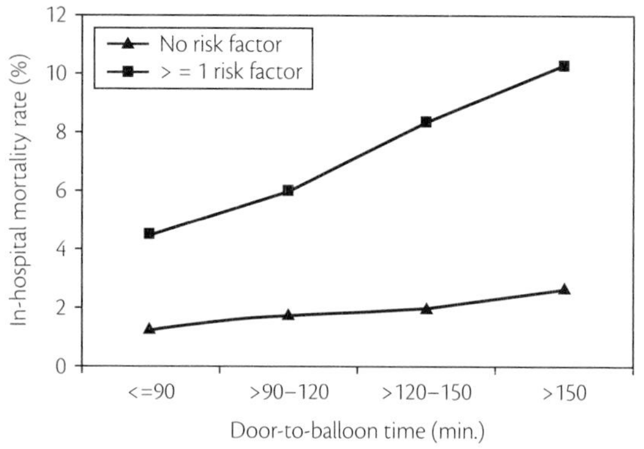

Fig. 16.7 In-hospital mortality and door-to-balloon time in patients stratified by risk factor status; p for trend <0.001 for each line. Risk factors include anterior/septal location, diabetes mellitus, heart rate >100 beats/min, systolic blood pressure <100mm Hg. Reproduced from McNamara RL, Wang Y, Herrin J, *et al.* Effect of door-to-balloon time on mortality in patients with ST-segment elevation myocardial infarction. *J Am Coll Cardiol* 2006; **47**:2180–6. Copyright © 2006, with permission from Elsevier.

justify delaying treatment in the lower-risk patients, as it was not an analysis of any randomized comparison.

The Nallamothu and Bates analysis mentioned previously also highlighted the importance of DTB times(23). They showed that for every additional 10-min delay in PCI compared to the administration of thrombolysis, the absolute mortality benefit favouring PPCI decreased by 0.94% (p = 0.006). There was an absolute decrease in benefit of 1.17% (p = 0.016) for a combined endpoint of death, stroke, and reinfarction for every 10-min delay in PCI over thrombolysis.

In conclusion, DTB times are an important determinant of outcome in patients treated with PPCI for STEMI and hospitals delivering a PPCI service should have systems in place to minimize delays.

Strategies to improve DTB times

In recent times, there has been considerable focus on methods to reduce DTB times. A survey of 365 hospitals in the United States highlighted six important strategies that were associated with a faster DTB time(48). Using multivariate analysis, these strategies (and the time saved) included:

- Having emergency medicine physicians activate the catheterization laboratory (mean reduction in DTB time, 8.2min)
- Having a single call to a central page operator activate the laboratory (13.8min)
- Having the emergency department activate the catheterization laboratory while the patient is en route to the hospital (15.4min)
- Expecting staff to arrive in the catheterization laboratory within 20min after being paged (vs. >30min) (19.3min)
- Having an attending cardiologist always on site (14.6min)
- Having staff in the emergency department and the catheterization laboratory use real-time data feedback (8.6min).

A useful way of using real-time data feedback is through the use of statistical process control charts (Fig. 16.8)(49). They not only allow the effects of various interventions on the service delivery to be seen but as importantly, also highlight outliers so that these cases can be investigated individually.

DTB time is an important measure that is easily audited and can help to monitor individual hospital performance. The recent National Infarct Angioplasty Project (NIAP) report in the UK has suggested that monitoring the percentage of patients with a DTB <90min and call-to-balloon time of <120min may aid quality improvements in the system of care(50).

Hospital and operator experience in PPCI

It is logical to expect that experience and familiarity with a particular process or technique would lead to better outcomes. This has already been shown with regards to the management of STEMI. In a large cohort of Canadian patients, there was lower mortality in hospitals where physicians treated more than 24 AMI cases annually compared to those who treated five or fewer AMI cases per year (11.8% vs. 15.3% respectively, p <0.001)(51). With regards to PCI alone, numerous studies have shown a significant relationship between hospital and operator volumes and outcome(52–58).

For PPCI, there have only been a few analyses to date. Registry PCI data from the greater Paris area showed that, in high volume centres (defined as >400 procedures per year based on French guidelines), the difference in in-hospital mortality rates was significant in the subgroup of emergency procedures performed in patients presenting with AMI, cardiogenic shock, or out-of-hospital cardiac arrest (6.75% vs. 8.54% in low-volume centres, p = 0.028)(59). A German study has also highlighted that the volume-outcome relationship applies most to the highest-risk patients,

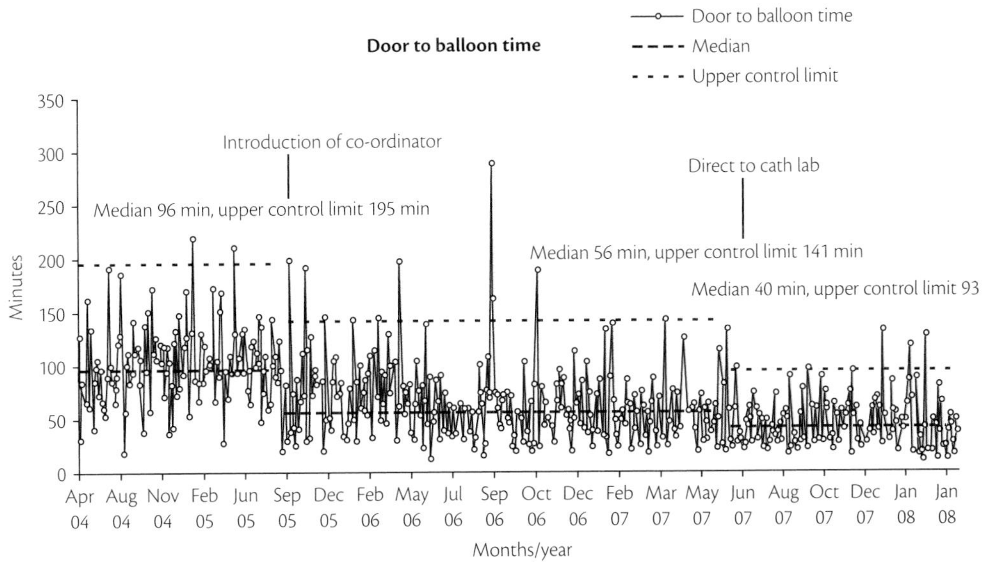

Fig. 16.8 Example of a statistical process control chart from a tertiary regional cardiac centre in northeast England demonstrating effects of (A) introducing a single coordinator to receive calls from the ambulance services and emergency departments and (B) organizing transfer of the patient direct to the cath lab in order to reduce DTB times. There were significant falls in DTB times with changes to the system of care.

including those being treated for non-STEMI and STEMI[(60)].

An interesting analysis using NRMI data showed that for hospitals with high (≥49 procedures) and intermediate annual PPCI volumes (17–48 procedures), there was a mortality benefit of PPCI compared to thrombolysis similar to that found in the randomized trials (3.4% vs. 5.4%, $p < 0.001$; 4.5% vs. 5.9%, $p < 0.001$ respectively) but in low-volume centres (≤16 procedures), there was no significant benefit (6.2% vs. 5.9%, $p = 0.58$)[(61)].

Analyses based on New York state observational data have investigated the effect of operator volume on the relationship between hospital volume and mortality during PPCI. In an earlier analysis using data from 1995, in-hospital mortality was reduced by 57% among patients who underwent primary angioplasty by high-volume (≥11 cases per year) as opposed to low-volume operators (<11 cases per year) (adjusted relative risk 0.43; 95% CI 0.21–0.83). In high-volume hospitals (≥57 cases per year) rather than low-volume institutions (<57 cases per year), the relative risk reduction for in-hospital mortality was 44% (adjusted relative risk 0.56; 95% CI 0.29–1.1). Compared with patients treated at low-volume hospitals by low-volume operators, patients treated at high-volume hospitals by high-volume operators had a 49% reduction in the risk of in hospital mortality (adjusted relative risk 0.51; 95% CI 0.26–0.99)[(62)]. A more recent analysis using data from 2001–2002 PPCI by high-volume hospitals (>50 cases per year) and high-volume physicians (>10 cases per year) was associated with significantly lower unadjusted in hospital mortality (3.2% vs. 6.7%, $p = 0.03$) and a trend to lower adjusted in hospital mortality (3.8% vs. 8.4%, $p = 0.09$) compared to low-volume hospitals (≤50 cases per year) and low-volume operators (≤10 cases per year). When the analysis was performed using operator volume of >20 cases versus ≤20 cases, the results for both adjusted and unadjusted in-hospital mortality were statistically significant. The authors also assessed the relationship between low-volume operators and high-volume operators in low-volume hospitals and showed that although there was a lower average risk-adjusted mortality rate, the result was not statistically significant (8.4% vs. 4.8% for high-volume physicians; OR 1.44, 95% CI 0.68–3.03). However, in high-volume hospitals, a statistically significant result was seen. The risk-adjusted mortality rate for high-volume physicians was 3.8% versus 6.5% for low-volume physicians (OR 0.58; 95% CI 0.39–0.86)[(63)].

Although there appears to be evidence for a relationship between hospital volume and/or operator volume and outcomes in PPCI, further research is required. Currently, it is difficult to make a specific recommendation about minimum volume of activity, but it is likely that better outcomes will be seen in units performing a large number of PPCIs. The trade-off in this context is with the time of access to PPCI, and each region has to balance these two factors in determining which PCI centres should be designated a heart attack centre. Similar to DTB times, PPCI volumes can therefore also be easily monitored and thus can be used in assessing service delivery and safety on both an individual operator level and hospital level.

Need for on-site surgical support?

The developments in interventional cardiology over the last two decades have meant that complications, in particular the need for emergency CABG, have decreased. In 1991, 2.6% of patients required emergency CABG following PCI compared to only 0.29% in 2003 in the UK(64). The Atlantic Cardiovascular Patient Outcomes Research Team (C-PORT) trial (n = 451) randomized patients to PPCI or thrombolysis (accelerated tPA) in 11 hospitals without on-site surgical cover. There was a significant benefit in the combined primary endpoint of death, recurrent MI, and stroke (10.7% vs. 17.7%, p = 0.03) in favour of the PPCI group. None of the patients in the PPCI group required transport for emergency CABG(65). The study was limited by funding issues and so the required number of patients was not recruited. Important additional points to note about this study are that no comparison was made with transfer to a high-volume tertiary centre for PPCI and most patients (62%) presented between 8am and 4pm. The latter is particularly relevant as 'off hours' presentation has been shown to be associated with longer times to treatment for PCI during STEMI(66).

Although the Atlantic C-PORT trial demonstrated the feasibility of PPCI in community hospitals without on-site cardiac surgical back up, there are still issues regarding its widespread applicability. By considering all of the hospital-related factors as discussed previously, it is important that when developing and maintaining a PPCI programme certain principles are upheld: 1) it should have sufficient experience to maintain expertise; 2) the centre should ideally be performing over 400 PCI cases per annum; and 3) it should be able to deal with the sickest patients (e.g. cardiogenic shock) and have appropriate support staff and available intensive care beds. Current ESC guidelines recommend that centres performing PPCI should provide the service at all hours(18).

Technical aspects of delivering PPCI

Triage and telemetry

There should be rapid triage and preparation for patients presenting with STEMI, using pre-hospital ECGs to activate the catheter lab and thereby reduce DTB times (67). This can be done by transmission of ECGs by telemed systems to a central CCU coordinator. Trained paramedics have been shown to have similar accuracy in interpreting 12-lead ECGs to identify STEMI as physician reviewers(68) and, therefore can activate catheter labs directly. Although many units have found telemed systems to be extremely useful, others rely only on a telephonic call from the paramedic or emergency team and accept patients without the use of ECG transmission systems.

Clinical evaluation

For patients who meet the criteria for PPCI, a targeted history and physical examination should be performed. In addition to eliciting the relevant symptoms, particular attention should be paid to the presence of allergies, bleeding risk, current use of anticoagulant therapy, history of renal disease, and functional status. Examination should focus on haemodynamic status, signs of heart failure, or mechanical complications of MI (e.g. ventricular septal defect or acute mitral regurgitation). Time should be taken for echocardiographic evaluation if such problems are suspected but routine echocardiography prior to angiography is not needed. The duration of dual antiplatelet therapy following stenting may become an important issue and so a history of dyspeptic problems should also be sought and patients asked whether they are scheduled for any planned surgery. For patients in shock or in pulmonary oedema, a cardiothoracic anaesthetic team should be called to assist with the case.

Oral antiplatelet therapy

The patients should be given 300mg of aspirin (usually administered by the paramedics in the UK). In addition, morphine and a suitable antiemetic should be given intravenously for the relief of chest pain. Either before or immediately after PPCI, a loading dose of clopidogrel is recommended. Although the licensed loading dose is 300mg, in this context many centres use 600mg (see later section). Some units do not like to give dual antiplatelet therapy prior to angiography, in case cardiac surgery is needed, but the need for immediate surgery is rare, and a single loading dose of clopidogrel is unlikely to be associated with major life-threatening bleeding should surgery be required.

Arterial access

Traditionally, the femoral route of access has been preferred for PPCI. Operators are accustomed to this approach, it allows easy use of an intra-aortic balloon pump (IABP) if required, and larger guide catheters can be used (which can facilitate the use of some thrombus removal devices). However, radial access has been shown to be a safe and effective alternative with fewer occurrences of local bleeding complications and reduced hospital stay(69). The radial or femoral site should therefore be prepared depending on operator preference and clinical factors and angiography performed in accordance with standard techniques. Insertion of a femoral venous sheath may be needed for placement of a temporary pacing wire in some cases, but is usually avoided as it can increase bleeding risks. Some operators perform the diagnostic angiography with an appropriately selected guide catheter to try and save some time; others prefer to use routine diagnostic catheters first as the findings then help aid the selection of the most appropriate guide catheter.

Intra-aortic balloon pump

The role of prophylactic insertion of an IABP was investigated in the PAMI-2 trial in which cardiac catheterization was performed in 1100 patients within 12h of onset of an acute STEMI. Four hundred and thirty-seven patients with one or more high-risk characteristics (age >70, left ventricular ejection fraction <45%, suboptimal PTCA result, malignant arrhythmias, three-vessel coronary disease, saphenous vein graft occlusion, or failed PTCA) were randomly assigned to 36–48h of IABP or traditional care. There was no difference in the primary combined endpoint of death, reinfarction, infarct-related artery reocclusion, stroke or new-onset heart failure, or sustained hypotension between the two groups (28.9% vs. 29.2%, p = 0.95). The IABP was associated with a modest reduction in recurrent ischaemia and the need for repeat catheterization compared to traditional care, but a higher incidence of stroke(70). Other studies have failed to demonstrate a convincing role for routine use of an IABP and most operators use them selectively in patients with poor haemodynamic status either during or immediately after PPCI. For patients with cardiogenic shock, however, the use of IABP is believed to be beneficial and is recommended by current ESC guidelines (Class1, Level C)(18).

Platelet glycoprotein IIb/IIIa inhibitors

The role of platelet GP IIb/IIIa inhibitors in PPCI, of which abciximab has been most extensively studied, has been evaluated in major randomized clinical trials and a meta-analysis (n = 27 115, 11 trials) showed that abciximab therapy was associated with a significant reduction in mortality at 30 days (2.4% vs. 3.4% with placebo, p = 0.047) and at 6–12 months (4.4% vs. 6.2%, p = 0.01) and in reinfarction at 30 days (1.0% vs. 1.9%, p = 0.03). There was no increase in bleeding (4.7% vs. 4.0% for placebo, p = 0.36)(71).

The Controlled Abciximab and Device Investigation to Lower Late Angioplasty Complications (CADILLAC) trial was included in the meta-analysis but deserves separate mention. This trial (n = 2082) was designed to address the hypothesis that stenting was superior to angioplasty with or without abciximab. Patients were randomized to angioplasty alone, angioplasty plus abciximab, stenting alone, or stenting plus angioplasty. The group that had the greatest benefit from abciximab therapy was the patients treated with angioplasty alone whilst the best results were seen in the stenting group regardless of whether they had been treated with abciximab(12).

The CADILLAC and other trials in the meta-analysis were, however, performed prior to the use of 600-mg loading doses of clopidogrel. In the Bavarian Reperfusion Alternatives Evaluation 3 (BRAVE-3 trial), patients were treated with aspirin, intravenous heparin, and a loading dose of 600mg of clopidogrel and randomized to either abciximab or placebo. There were no significant differences in mortality (3.2% vs. 2.5% for placebo, p = 0.53) or the combined endpoint of death, recurrent MI, urgent revascularization, and stroke (5% vs. 3.9%, p = 0.39)(72). Further studies are needed to verify whether high loading doses of oral dual antiplatelet therapy blunt the previously recognized advantages of giving abciximab.

The timing of platelet GP IIb/IIIa inhibitor therapy in relation to PPCI has also been investigated. The FINESSE study (discussed previously) did not show a significant clinical benefit of early (i.e. prior to the catheter lab) abciximab therapy(41). A meta-analysis in 2004 of six trials (three involving the use of abciximab and three involving the use of tirofiban, n = 931) similarly showed no significant impact of early platelet GP IIb/IIIa inhibitor therapy on reducing mortality rates (3.4% vs. 4.7%, p = 0.42). There was, however, a significantly higher rate of TIMI 3 flow prior to PCI in the IRA in the early group (20.3% vs. 12.2, p <0.001)(73). The Ongoing

Tirofiban In Myocardial infarction Evaluation (On-TIME) 2 study group assessed the use of early pre-hospital initiation of high dose bolus of tirofiban versus placebo with bailout use of tirofiban in the catheter lab whilst using a 600-mg loading dose of clopidogrel. The primary endpoint was mean residual ST segment deviation. There was significantly greater ST segment resolution in the patients that received pre-hospital tirofiban. There was also significant benefit in the combined secondary endpoint of death, recurrent MI, urgent target vessel revascularization, or thrombotic bailout (26.0% vs.32.9% for placebo, p = 0.02), which was mainly accounted for by greater use of 'thrombotic bailout', i.e tirofiban use for <TIMI 3 flow, complications during PCI or prolonged ischaemia in the placebo group[74]. Of note, there was no significant difference in TIMI flow pre and post PCI and there was no comparison made between pre-hospital and catheter lab use of tirofiban. Early use of GP IIb/IIIa inhibitors has therefore been shown to result in improved angiographic and surrogate markers of reperfusion but not clinical endpoints. Upstream use of these drugs is therefore not currently recommended.

Antithrombotic therapy

Current ESC guidelines recommend intravenous unfractionated heparin as the anticoagulant therapy of choice for use during PPCI[18]. A bolus dose of 100U/kg weight (60U/kg weight if a platelet GP IIb/IIIa inhibitor is used) is recommended and subsequently further doses may be required to maintain an activated clotting time of 250–350s (200–250s if a GP IIb/IIIa inhibitor is used). At present, low-molecular-weight heparins have been insufficiently studied in PPCI and are therefore not used routinely.

Alternate anticoagulants have been studied. The Harmonizing Outcomes with Revascularisation and Stents in Acute Myocardial Infarction (HORIZONS-AMI) trial (n = 3602) randomized patients to bivalirudin, a direct thrombin inhibitor, with bailout GP IIb/IIIa inhibitor or intravenous heparin plus routine GP IIb/IIIa inhibitor. There was a net clinical benefit in favour of bivalirudin treatment (9.2% vs. 12.1%, p = 0.005) due to a reduction mainly in major bleeding rate at 30 days. Mortality at 30 days was significantly less in the bivalirudin group when all patients were included on an intention-to-treat analysis (2.1% vs. 3.1%, p = 0.047) but when the outcomes for only the PPCI population were assessed, there was only a trend towards lower mortality (2.0% vs. 2.9%, p = 0.067). Important additional points to note about this study were that the authors did not document the use of the radial route, there were higher rates of acute stent thrombosis in the bivalirudin arm (1.3% vs. 0.3%, p <0.001), and approximately 60% of the patients had received a bolus of heparin prior to randomization. At 30 days, however, there was no statistically significant difference in subacute stent thrombosis[75]. Bivalirudin with the option of bailout usage of a GP IIb/IIIa inhibitor is therefore a suitable alternative to unfractionated heparin with routine use of a GP IIb/IIIa inhibitor.

Thrombus removal devices

Once the guide wire has been introduced, consideration can be given to the use of a thrombus removal device. Although previous studies had shown benefits as regards surrogate end-points, previous meta-analyses had failed to show any meaningful clinical benefits. Most recently, in the Thrombus Aspiration during Percutaneous coronary intervention in Acute myocardial infarction (TAPAS) study (n = 1071), patients were randomized to thrombus aspiration with a 6-French Export® Aspiration Catheter (Medtronic) or conventional PCI. Thrombus aspiration resulted in improved myocardial reperfusion as shown by an improvement in myocardial blush grade and resolution of ST elevation. This was associated with a trend to reducing death in the aspiration group at 30 days (2.1% vs. 4.0%, p = 0.07)[76]. At 1 year, there was a clear survival advantage in the arm where a thrombus removal device was used (cardiac death at 1 year was 3.6% in the thrombus aspiration group and 6.7% in the conventional PCI group; p = 0.020)[77]. Further studies are needed to verify this finding (especially as the trial was not powered for this endpoint).

Stenting versus balloon angioplasty

One of the limitations of angioplasty in the setting of STEMI is the risk of reocclusion as well as restenosis. In this context, stenting was first compared with balloon angioplasty in the Stent-PAMI (n = 900) trial. This showed an overall benefit of stenting over angioplasty that was entirely due to a reduction in the need for target vessel revascularization (TVR). Interestingly, TIMI 3 flow post stenting was seen in slightly fewer patients in the stenting group (89.4% vs. 92.7%, p = 0.1) and there was also a numerically higher mortality rate (4.2% vs. 2.7%, p = 0.27), although this was not statistically significant[78]. Abciximab was used in only 5% of patients. The CADILLAC trial, mentioned earlier, showed a clear benefit of stenting over angioplasty (MACE 10.5% vs. 18.0% for angioplasty, p <0.001) but again this was solely due to a reduction in TVR (6.8% vs. 14.7%, p <0.001)[12].

A systematic Cochrane review in 2005 (n = 4433, nine trials) subsequently showed that stenting was associated with significant reductions in reinfarction (OR 0.52; 95% CI 0.31–0.87 at 30 days, and OR 0.67; 95% CI 0.45–0.98 at 1 year) and TVR (OR 0.45; 95% CI 0.34–0.60 at 30 days, and OR 0.47; 95% CI 0.38–0.57 at 1 year). There was no significant difference in mortality (OR 1.06; 95% CI 0.77–1.45 at 1 year)[79].

There were conflicting results from a large randomized trial (n = 1683) from the Netherlands. In this study, there was no significant difference in the primary endpoint of death or reinfarction between stenting and angioplasty (12.4% v 11.3%) and, although angiographically there was less restenosis in the stenting group, TVR was also not significantly different[80]. Despite these conflicting results, primary stenting of the IRA has become the standard therapy for STEMI.

Drug eluting stents versus bare metal stents

Drug eluting stents (DES) are more effective at reducing the need for repeat vascularization than bare-metal stents (BMS) in the setting of elective PCI. Whether they would have the same impact during PPCI required specific study. In addition, given the concern regarding the occurrence of late stent thrombosis with DES, there have been particular questions whether stent thrombosis would limit their use in the context of an acutely thrombotic artery. The simultaneous publication of two of the largest trials comparing DES with BMS provided some of the answers. The Trial to Assess the Use of the Cypher® Stent in Acute Myocardial Infarction Treated with Balloon Angioplasty (TYPHOON) study (n = 712) randomized patients to either sirolimus-eluting stents or BMS and showed that the occurrence of the primary endpoint of target vessel failure at 1 year was significantly lower in the DES group (7.3% vs. 14.3%, p = 0.004) and this was driven almost entirely by a lower need for TVR. The rates of mortality (2.3% and 2.2%, respectively; p = 1.00), recurrent myocardial infarction (1.1% and 1.4%, respectively; p = 1.00), or in-stent thrombosis (3.4% and 3.6%, respectively; P = 1.00) were virtually the same[81].

The Paclitaxel-Eluting Stent versus Conventional Stent in Myocardial Infarction with ST-Segment Elevation (PASSION) study (n = 619) investigated the difference between paclitaxel-eluting stents and BMS and found that the primary combined endpoint of death, ischaemia-driven TVR, and reinfarction at 1 year was lower in the DES group although the result did not reach statistical significance (8.8% vs. 12.8%, p = 0.12). Surprisingly, the rates of TVR were also similar (5.3% vs. 7.8% respectively, p = 0.23)[82].

These trials accounted for almost 50% of the patients in a meta-analysis (n = 2786, eight trials) comparing the different stents published in 2007. The mean length of follow-up was 12–24 months. DES significantly reduced the risk of reintervention (hazard ratio (HR) 0.38; 95% CI 0.29–0.50; p <0.001). The overall risk of stent thrombosis (HR 0.80; 95% CI 0.46–1.39; p = 0.43); death (HR 0.76; 95% CI 0.53–1.10; p = 0.14); and recurrent myocardial infarction (HR 0.72; 95% CI 0.48 1.08; p = 0.11) was not significantly different for patients receiving DES compared to BMS[83].

The largest randomized trial to date on this subject, Harmonizing Outcomes with Revascularization and Stents in Acute Myocardial Infarction (HORIZONS-AMI), included 3602 patients from multiple centers randomizing 2257 patients to paclitaxel eluting stents compared to 749 patients to bare metal stents in a 3 to 1 fashion. There was no difference in the composite primary safety endpoint (8.1% for DES vs. 8.0%; p = 0.92) or any of its components of death, stroke, reinfarction or stent thrombosis at 1 year but patients treated with DES had significantly lower 12-month rates of ischaemia-driven target lesion revascularization (4.5% vs. 7.5%; p = 0.002) and target-vessel revascularization (5.8% vs. 8.7%; p = 0.006)[84].

Currently, there remains uncertainty whether DES are superior to BMS in the context of PPCI. Given that the need for TVR following PPCI has not been as large as that seen in trials in other settings, there is uncertainty about the cost-effectiveness of routine use of DES. Although none of these randomized trials have shown an increase in stent thrombosis with DES, the longer-term effects are not yet known. Most operators use them selectively in patients deemed to be at especially high risk of restenosis.

Suboptimal reperfusion after PPCI

The main aim of therapy in STEMI is normal myocardial reperfusion in the territory of the IRA. Although it has its limitations, one of the most widely used measures of reperfusion therapy is the Thrombolysis In Myocardial Infarction (TIMI) angiographic flow grading system (Table 16.4)[85].

In many studies, TIMI 3 flow has been reported in over 90% of patients with PPCI as shown by the PAMI investigators (other studies using core labs tend to show a slightly lower rate). Of 3362 patients who underwent PPCI in the various PAMI trials, only 232 (6.9%) had less than TIMI 3 flow. Multivariate analysis identified

Table 16.4 Thrombolysis in myocardial infarction (TIMI) flow grading system

Grade 0	Complete occlusion of the infarct-related artery
Grade 1	Some penetration of contrast material beyond the point of obstruction but without perfusion of the distal coronary bed
Grade 2	Perfusion of the entire infarct vessel into the distal bed but with delayed flow compared with a normal artery
Grade 3	Full perfusion of the infarct vessel with normal flow

Table 16.5 Reasons for not attaining TIMI 3 flow post PPCI

Persistent pathological process	Complications of PCI	Other
Persistent stenosis/ thrombosis	Coronary dissection	No-reflow phenomenon
Coronary spasm	Acute stent thrombosis	Cell oedema
	Branch occlusion	Reperfusion injury
	Failed stent deployment	
	Intramural haematoma	
	Distal macro-/ microembolism	

age >70, diabetes, symptom to presentation, left ventricular ejection fraction < 50%, and initial TIMI flow ≤1 as independent predictors in these patients. They also showed that achieving TIMI 3 flow in the IRA post PPCI was associated with better outcomes at 1 year (Fig. 16.9)[86].

Most of the causes of failure to attain TIMI 3 flow post PCI are a result of persisting pathological process or mechanical complications during PCI (Table 16.5). Of the other causes, the no-reflow phenomenon and reperfusion injury are thought to be multifactorial. No-reflow is defined as the reduction in coronary blood flow (TIMI flow ≤2) despite vessel patency at the site of PCI.

Changes at a microscopic level such as distal microembolization of plaque or thrombus with platelet or fibrin plugging, endothelial cell and myocyte injury with accompanying oedema, oxygen free radical formation and release from trapped leucocytes, and vasoconstriction are all thought to be implicated [87,88].

No-reflow has been described in up to 15% of cases of AMI. Angiographic predictors include:

- Cut-off pattern of occlusion in the IRA (52.4% vs. 10.3%, p <0.001)
- Accumulated thrombus (>5mm) proximal to the occlusion (37.5% vs. 3.4%, p <0.001)
- Presence of floating thrombus (66.7% vs. 12.7%, p <0.001)
- Persistent dye stasis distal to the obstruction (51.9% vs. 13.8%, p <0.001)
- Reference lumen diameter (RLD) of the IRA ≥4mm (46.3% vs. 9.6%, p <0.001)

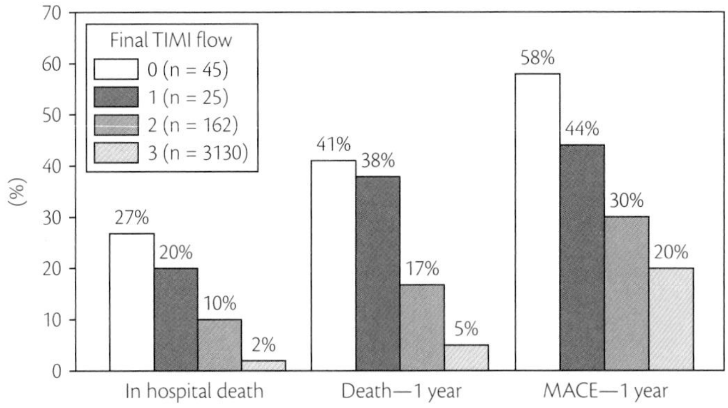

Fig. 16.9 Relationship of final TIMI flow grades after primary percutaneous coronary intervention with in-hospital and 1-year mortality and major adverse cardiovascular events (MACE). p for trend <0.0001 for all three outcomes. Reproduced from Mehta RH, Harjai KJ, Cox D, *et al.* Clinical and angiographic correlates and outcomes of suboptimal coronary flow in patients with acute myocardial infarction undergoing primary percutaneous coronary intervention. *J Am Coll Cardiol* 2003; **42**:1739–46. Copyright © 2003, with permission from Elsevier.

- Incomplete obstruction with presence of accumulated thrombus with a linear dimension more than three times the RLD of the IRA (51.7% vs. 3.9, p <0.0001)[89].

No-reflow remains a difficult problem in the treatment of STEMI with PPCI and has been correlated with increased mortality and thus represents a challenge in a minority of patients. Avoiding it in the first place may be a better strategy. Thrombus removal devices are useful in this context and encouraging early results in the TAPAS trial have been seen as discussed earlier. Other strategies include:

- The use of platelet GP IIb/IIIa inhibitors, which have been shown to improve epicardial flow in patients receiving them prior to angiography in AMI. This has already been discussed with regards to facilitated PCI. Whether they confer clinical benefit in the setting of no-flow is not known
- Distal protection devices aimed at preventing distal embolization. However, they have little effect on outcome except in the treatment of saphenous vein graft lesions[90]. The disappointing results may relate, in part, to embolization during delivery of the devices
- Direct stenting of the IRA. This has been evaluated in a randomized trial of 206 patients with an AMI undergoing primary stenting with or without pre-dilation. Although the incidence of TIMI grade 3 flow and the corrected TIMI frame count were not significantly different with both approaches, the incidence of the composite angiographic endpoint (slow and no-reflow or distal embolization) was significantly lower with direct stenting (11.7% vs. 26.9% with pre-dilation before stenting, p = 0.01). ST-segment resolution was also significantly improved after direct stenting (no ST-segment resolution in 20.2% vs. 38.1% with pre-dilation, p = 0.01)[91]
- The use of arteriolar vasodilators such as adenosine. In the Acute Myocardial Infarction Study of Adenosine (AMISTAD I), in patients (n = 236) treated with thrombolysis for STEMI, there was a 33% reduction in infarct size in patients treated with adenosine compared to placebo. This effect was seen in anterior infarcts only[92]. In the subsequent AMISTAD II trial, only patients (n = 2118) with anterior infarcts treated by thrombolysis or PPCI were investigated. There was no benefit with adenosine compared to placebo in the primary endpoint of congestive heart failure or death within 6 months but there was a trend towards smaller infarct size in the adenosine group (17% vs. 27% for placebo, p = 0.074), which became significant when only the high-dose adenosine group was compared to placebo (11% vs. 27% for placebo, p = 0.023)[93]. Although the effect of other vasodilators such as verapamil and nicorandil on angiographic parameters of reperfusion has been studied, no studies have yet shown convincing evidence of clinical benefits.

Post-PPCI care and rehabilitation

Following reperfusion therapy for STEMI, patients should be routinely offered cardiac rehabilitation (which should start in the index hospitalization) and secondary preventive therapies[18]. This is particularly important following PPCI, because the shorter hospital stay potentially jeopardizes what a patient might be offered, and may influence a patient's perception of the diagnosis[49]. Lifelong aspirin, beta-blocker, statin, and ACE-inhibitor therapy should be prescribed routinely, and measures taken to ensure appropriate up-titration of doses. Clopidogrel should be prescribed for at least 6 months and many centres now routinely use dual antiplatelet therapy for the first year. Patients should be evaluated with echocardiography or other imaging modalities, and consideration made for delayed investigation with ambulatory ECG recordings to identify those who should be offered implantable cardioverter-defibrillator (ICD) therapy. Appropriate follow-up should be arranged and communication with primary care services is essential.

Conclusion

Over the course of the past 15 years, one of the most important developments in cardiology has been the improvement in hospital outcomes following treatment for STEMI. Although reperfusion therapy per se has been highly important, the widespread introduction of primary PCI has represented a step-change in the management of these patients. Several countries now offer PPCI as the major means of reperfusion therapy, but the geographical considerations in larger countries have been associated with a poorer uptake. However, most industrialized nations are now taking strides to improve access to PPCI. System redesigns remain a challenge but lessons learned in countries that have led the way should make it easier for other countries to follow. In areas where PCI facilities are few and far between, some hospitals not currently undertaking PPCI should be encouraged to set up a programme and supported to enable greater access to this form of reperfusion therapy. In the UK, PPCI has been shown not only to be effective but also cost-effective as long as it is delivered in a timely fashion[49,94].

Several key questions remain regarding the choice of therapy. Further research is needed on those patients who live a long way (>3h) from a PPCI centre and high-risk patients who present early. Further work is needed to determine the best pharmacological approaches during PPCI, trying to optimize reperfusion but at the same time minimize bleeding risks. Research continues on new methods to improve the immediate outcomes following PPCI—these include the use of core temperature cooling and the use of conditioning techniques that may help in preservation of ischaemic myocardium. Where clinicians continue to use thrombolysis (for whatever reason) as the primary treatment for an individual patient, the patient should immediately be transferred to a centre with PCI capability.

The concept of 'heart attack centres' is here to stay, but although the aim of these centres is to optimize early reperfusion following STEMI, the best results will only be obtained where these early efforts feed into a system of care that provides routine cardiac rehabilitation and optimal use of secondary preventive therapies. Regional networks of care should work to overcome the logistical barriers to a full service.

References

1. Fletcher AP, Sherry S, Alkjaersig N, *et al.* The maintenance of a sustained thrombolytic state in man. II. Clinical observations on patients with myocardial infarction and other thromboembolic disorders. *J Clin Invest* 1959; **38**(7):1111–19.
2. DeWood MA, Spores J, Notske R, *et al.* Prevalence of total coronary occlusion during the early hours of transmural myocardial infarction. *N Engl J Med* 1980; **303**(16): 897–902.
3. Rentrop KP, Blanke H, Karsch KR, *et al.* Initial experience with transluminal recanalization of the recently occluded infarct-related coronary artery in acute myocardial infarction – comparison with conventionally treated patients. *Clin Cardiol* 1979; **2**(2):92–105.
4. Rentrop KP, Blanke H, Karsch KR, *et al.* Acute myocardial infarction: intracoronary application of nitroglycerin and streptokinase. *Clin Cardiol* 1979; **2**(5):354–63.
5. Hartzler GO, Rutherford BD, McConahay DR, *et al.* Percutaneous transluminal coronary angioplasty with and without thrombolytic therapy for treatment of acute myocardial infarction. *Am Heart J* 1983; **106**(5 Pt 1): 965–73.
6. Fibrinolytic Therapy Trialists' (FTT) Collaborative Group. Indications for fibrinolytic therapy in suspected acute myocardial infarction: collaborative overview of early mortality and major morbidity results from all randomised trials of more than 1000 patients. *Lancet* 1994; **343**(8893):311–22.
7. Grines CL, Browne KF, Marco J, *et al.* A comparison of immediate angioplasty with thrombolytic therapy for acute myocardial infarction. The Primary Angioplasty in Myocardial Infarction Study Group. *N Engl J Med* 1993; **328**(10):673–9.
8. Zijlstra F, de Boer MJ, Hoorntje JC, *et al.* A comparison of immediate coronary angioplasty with intravenous streptokinase in acute myocardial infarction. *N Engl J Med* 1993; **328**(10):680–4.
9. Gibbons RJ, Holmes DR, Reeder GS, *et al.* Immediate angioplasty compared with the administration of a thrombolytic agent followed by conservative treatment for myocardial infarction. The Mayo Coronary Care Unit and Catheterization Laboratory Groups. *N Engl J Med* 1993; **328**(10):685–91.
10. Zijlstra F, Patel A, Jones M, *et al.* Clinical characteristics and outcome of patients with early (<2h), intermediate (2–4h) and late (>4h) presentation treated by primary coronary angioplasty or thrombolytic therapy for acute myocardial infarction. *Eur Heart J* 2002; **23**(7):550–7.
11. The GUSTO Angiographic Investigators. The effects of tissue plasminogen activator, streptokinase, or both on coronary-artery patency, ventricular function, and survival after acute myocardial infarction. *N Engl J Med* 1993; **329**(22):1615–22.
12. Stone GW, Grines CL, Cox DA, *et al.* Comparison of angioplasty with stenting, with or without abciximab, in acute myocardial infarction. *N Engl J Med* 2002; **346**(13):957–66.
13. Hochman JS, Sleeper LA, Webb JG, *et al.* Early revascularization in acute myocardial infarction complicated by cardiogenic shock. SHOCK Investigators. Should We Emergently Revascularize Occluded Coronaries for Cardiogenic Shock. *N Engl J Med* 1999; **341**(9):625–34.
14. Hochman JS, Sleeper LA, White HD, *et al.* One-year survival following early revascularization for cardiogenic shock. *JAMA* 2001; **285**(2):190–2.
15. Nunn CM, O'Neill WW, Rothbaum D, *et al.* Long-term outcome after primary angioplasty: report from the primary angioplasty in myocardial infarction (PAMI-I) trial. *J Am Coll Cardiol* 1999; **33**(3):640–6.
16. Weaver WD, Simes RJ, Betriu A, *et al.* Comparison of primary coronary angioplasty and intravenous thrombolytic therapy for acute myocardial infarction: a quantitative review. *JAMA* 1997; **278**(23):2093–8.
17. Keeley EC, Boura JA, Grines CL. Primary angioplasty versus intravenous thrombolytic therapy for acute myocardial infarction: a quantitative review of 23 randomised trials. *Lancet* 2003; **361**(9351):13–20.
18. Van de Werf F, Bax J, Betriu A, *et al.* Management of acute myocardial infarction in patients presenting with persistent ST-segment elevation: the Task Force on the Management of ST-Segment Elevation Acute Myocardial Infarction of the European Society of Cardiology. *Eur Heart J* 2008; **29**(23):2909–45.

19. Widimsky P, Budesinsky T, Vorac D, *et al.* Long distance transport for primary angioplasty vs immediate thrombolysis in acute myocardial infarction. Final results of the randomized national multicentre trial – PRAGUE-2. *Eur Heart J* 2003; **24**(1):94–104.
20. Boersma E, Maas AC, Deckers JW, *et al.* Early thrombolytic treatment in acute myocardial infarction: reappraisal of the golden hour. *Lancet* 1996; **348**(9030):771–5.
21. Cannon CP, Gibson CM, Lambrew CT, *et al.* Relationship of symptom-onset-to-balloon time and door-to-balloon time with mortality in patients undergoing angioplasty for acute myocardial infarction. *JAMA* 2000; **283**(22):2941–7.
22. De Luca G, Suryapranata H, Ottervanger JP, *et al.* Time delay to treatment and mortality in primary angioplasty for acute myocardial infarction: every minute of delay counts. *Circulation* 2004; **109**(10):1223–5.
23. Nallamothu BK, Bates ER. Percutaneous coronary intervention versus fibrinolytic therapy in acute myocardial infarction: is timing (almost) everything? *Am J Cardiol* 2003; **92**(7):824–6.
24. Nallamothu BK, Antman EM, Bates ER. Primary percutaneous coronary intervention versus fibrinolytic therapy in acute myocardial infarction: does the choice of fibrinolytic agent impact on the importance of time-to-treatment? *Am J Cardiol* 2004; **94**(6):772–4.
25. Asseburg C, Vergel YB, Palmer S, *et al.* Assessing the effectiveness of primary angioplasty compared with thrombolysis and its relationship to time delay: a Bayesian evidence synthesis. *Heart* 2007; **93**(10):1244–50.
26. Boersma E. Does time matter? A pooled analysis of randomized clinical trials comparing primary percutaneous coronary intervention and in-hospital fibrinolysis in acute myocardial infarction patients. *Eur Heart J* 2006; **27**(7):779–88.
27. Pinto DS, Kirtane AJ, Nallamothu BK, *et al.* Hospital delays in reperfusion for ST-elevation myocardial infarction: implications when selecting a reperfusion strategy. *Circulation* 2006 Nov 7; **114**(19):2019–25.
28. Andersen HR, Nielsen TT, Rasmussen K, *et al.* A comparison of coronary angioplasty with fibrinolytic therapy in acute myocardial infarction. *N Engl J Med* 2003; **349**(8):733–42.
29. Morrison LJ, Verbeek PR, McDonald AC, *et al.* Mortality and prehospital thrombolysis for acute myocardial infarction: A meta-analysis. *JAMA* 2000; **283**(20):2686–92.
30. UK Ambulance Service Clinical Practice Guidelines (2006). 2006; Available from: http://www2.warwick.ac.uk/fac/med/research/hsri/emergencycare/prehospitalcare/jrcalcstakeholderwebsite/guidelines.
31. Myocardial Ischaemia National Audit Project (MINAP) How the NHS manages heart attacks Seventh Public Report 2008. Royal College of Physicians UK, 2008; Available from: http://www.rcplondon.ac.uk/clinical-standards/organisation/partnership/Documents/Minap%202008.pdf.
32. Bonnefoy E, Lapostolle F, Leizorovicz A, *et al.* Primary angioplasty versus prehospital fibrinolysis in acute myocardial infarction: a randomised study. *Lancet* 2002; **360**(9336):825–9.
33. Steg PG, Bonnefoy E, Chabaud S, *et al.* Impact of time to treatment on mortality after prehospital fibrinolysis or primary angioplasty: data from the CAPTIM randomized clinical trial. *Circulation* 2003; **108**(23):2851–6.
34. Stenestrand U, Lindback J, Wallentin L. Long-term outcome of primary percutaneous coronary intervention vs prehospital and in-hospital thrombolysis for patients with ST-elevation myocardial infarction. *JAMA* 2006; **296**(14):1749–56.
35. Ross AM, Coyne KS, Reiner JS, *et al.* A randomized trial comparing primary angioplasty with a strategy of short-acting thrombolysis and immediate planned rescue angioplasty in acute myocardial infarction: the PACT trial. PACT investigators. Plasminogen-activator Angioplasty Compatibility Trial. *J Am Coll Cardiol* 1999; **34**(7):1954–62.
36. Stone GW, Cox D, Garcia E, *et al.* Normal flow (TIMI-3) before mechanical reperfusion therapy is an independent determinant of survival in acute myocardial infarction: analysis from the primary angioplasty in myocardial infarction trials. *Circulation* 2001; **104**(6):636–41.
37. Weitz JI, Califf RM, Ginsberg JS, *et al.* New antithrombotics. *Chest* 1995; **108**(4 Suppl):471S–85S.
38. Le May MR, Wells GA, Labinaz M, *et al.* Combined angioplasty and pharmacological intervention versus thrombolysis alone in acute myocardial infarction (CAPITAL AMI study). *J Am Coll Cardiol.* 2005; **46**(3):417–24.
39. Assessment of the Safety and Efficacy of a New Treatment Strategy with Percutaneous Coronary Intervention (ASSENT-4 PCI) Investigators. Primary versus tenecteplase-facilitated percutaneous coronary intervention in patients with ST-segment elevation acute myocardial infarction (ASSENT-4 PCI): randomised trial. *Lancet* 2006; **367**(9510):569–78.
40. Keeley EC, Boura JA, Grines CL. Comparison of primary and facilitated percutaneous coronary interventions for ST-elevation myocardial infarction: quantitative review of randomised trials. *Lancet* 2006; **367**(9510):579–88.
41. Ellis SG, Tendera M, de Belder MA, *et al.* Facilitated PCI in patients with ST-elevation myocardial infarction. *N Engl J Med* 2008; **358**(21):2205–17.
42. Fernandez-Aviles F, Alonso JJ, Castro-Beiras A, *et al.* Routine invasive strategy within 24 hours of thrombolysis versus ischaemia-guided conservative approach for acute myocardial infarction with ST-segment elevation (GRACIA-1): a randomised controlled trial. *Lancet* 2004; **364**(9439):1045–53.
43. Fernandez-Aviles F, Alonso JJ, Pena G, *et al.* Primary angioplasty vs. early routine post-fibrinolysis angioplasty for acute myocardial infarction with ST-segment elevation: the GRACIA-2 non-inferiority, randomized, controlled trial. *Eur Heart J* 2007; **28**(8):949–60.
44. Di Mario C, Dudek D, Piscione F, *et al.* Immediate angioplasty versus standard therapy with rescue angioplasty after thrombolysis in the Combined Abciximab REteplase Stent Study in Acute Myocardial Infarction (CARESS-in-AMI): an open, prospective,

randomised, multicentre trial. *Lancet* 2008; **371**(9612):559–68.
45. Cantor WJ, Fitchett D, Borgundvaag B, *et al.* for the TRANSFER-AMI Trial Investigators. *N Engl J Med* 2009; **360**(26):2705–18.
46. McNamara RL, Wang Y, Herrin J, *et al.* for the NRMI Investigators. *J Am Coll Cardiol* 2006; **47**:2180–6.
47. Brodie BR, Hansen C, Stuckey TD, *et al.* Door-to-balloon time with primary percutaneous coronary intervention for acute myocardial infarction impacts late cardiac mortality in high-risk patients and patients presenting early after the onset of symptoms. *J Am Coll Cardiol* 2006; **47**(2):289–95.
48. Bradley EH, Herrin J, Wang Y, *et al.* Strategies for reducing the door-to-balloon time in acute myocardial infarction. *N Engl J Med* 2006; **355**(22):2308–20.
49. Benneyan JC, Lloyd RC, Plsek PE. Statistical process control as a tool for research and healthcare improvement. *Qual Saf Health Care* 2003; **12**(6):458–64.
50. Treatment of Heart Attack: National Guidance Final Report of the National Infarct Angioplasty Project (NIAP) British Cardiovascular. Department of Health, 2008; Available from: http://www.bcis.org.uk/resources/documents/NIAP%20Final%20Report.pdf.
51. Tu JV, Austin PC, Chan BT. Relationship between annual volume of patients treated by admitting physician and mortality after acute myocardial infarction. *JAMA* 2001; **285**(24):3116–22.
52. Ellis SG, Weintraub W, Holmes D, *et al.* Relation of operator volume and experience to procedural outcome of percutaneous coronary revascularization at hospitals with high interventional volumes. *Circulation* 1997; **95**(11):2479–84.
53. Jollis JG, Peterson ED, Nelson CL, *et al.* Relationship between physician and hospital coronary angioplasty volume and outcome in elderly patients. *Circulation* 1997; **95**(11):2485–91.
54. Hannan EL, Racz M, Ryan TJ, *et al.* Coronary angioplasty volume-outcome relationships for hospitals and cardiologists. *JAMA* 1997; **277**(11):892–8.
55. Zahn R, Vogt A, Seidl K, *et al.* [Balloon dilatation in acute myocardial infarct in routine clinical practice: results of the register of the Working Society of Leading Cardiologic Hospital Physicians in 4,625 patients]. *Z Kardiol* 1997; **86**(9):712–21.
56. McGrath PD, Wennberg DE, Malenka DJ, *et al.* Operator volume and outcomes in 12,998 percutaneous coronary interventions. Northern New England Cardiovascular Disease Study Group. *J Am Coll Cardiol* 1998; **31**(3): 570–6.
57. Malenka DJ, McGrath PD, Wennberg DE, *et al.* The relationship between operator volume and outcomes after percutaneous coronary interventions in high volume hospitals in 1994-1996: the northern New England experience. Northern New England Cardiovascular Disease Study Group. *J Am Coll Cardiol* 1999; **34**(5): 1471–80.
58. Canto JG, Every NR, Magid DJ, *et al.* The volume of primary angioplasty procedures and survival after acute myocardial infarction. National Registry of Myocardial Infarction 2 Investigators. *N Engl J Med* 2000; **342**(21):1573–80.
59. Spaulding C, Morice MC, Lancelin B, *et al.* Is the volume-outcome relation still an issue in the era of PCI with systematic stenting? Results of the greater Paris area PCI registry. *Eur Heart J* 2006; **27**(9):1054–60.
60. Zahn R, Gottwik M, Hochadel M, *et al.* Volume-outcome relation for contemporary percutaneous coronary interventions (PCI) in daily clinical practice: is it limited to high-risk patients? Results from the Registry of Percutaneous Coronary Interventions of the Arbeitsgemeinschaft Leitende Kardiologische Krankenhausärtze (ALKK). *Heart* 2008; **94**:329–35.
61. Magid DJ, Calonge BN, Rumsfeld JS, *et al.* Relation between hospital primary angioplasty volume and mortality for patients with acute MI treated with primary angioplasty vs thrombolytic therapy. *JAMA* 2000; **284**(24):3131–8.
62. Vakili BA, Kaplan R, Brown DL. Volume-outcome relation for physicians and hospitals performing angioplasty for acute myocardial infarction in New York state. *Circulation* 2001; **104**(18):2171–6.
63. Srinivas VS, Hailpern SM, Koss E, *et al.* Effect of physician volume on the relationship between hospital volume and mortality during primary angioplasty. *J Am Coll Cardiol* 2009; **53**(7):574–9.
64. Dawkins KD, Gershlick T, de Belder M, *et al.* Percutaneous coronary intervention: recommendations for good practice and training. *Heart* 2005; **91**(Suppl 6): vi1–27.
65. Aversano T, Aversano LT, Passamani E, *et al.* Thrombolytic therapy vs primary percutaneous coronary intervention for myocardial infarction in patients presenting to hospitals without on-site cardiac surgery: a randomized controlled trial. *JAMA* 2002; **287**(15): 1943–51.
66. Magid DJ, Wang Y, Herrin J, *et al.* Relationship between time of day, day of week, timeliness of reperfusion, and in-hospital mortality for patients with acute ST-segment elevation myocardial infarction. *JAMA* 2005; **294**(7): 803–12.
67. Brown JP, Mahmud E, Dunford JV, *et al.* Effect of prehospital 12-lead electrocardiogram on activation of the cardiac catheterization laboratory and door-to-balloon time in ST-segment elevation acute myocardial infarction. *Am J Cardiol* 2008; **101**(2):158–61.
68. Feldman JA, Brinsfield K, Bernard S, *et al.* Real-time paramedic compared with blinded physician identification of ST-segment elevation myocardial infarction: results of an observational study. *Am J Emerg Med* 2005; **23**(4): 443–8.
69. Philippe F, Larrazet F, Meziane T, *et al.* Comparison of transradial vs. transfemoral approach in the treatment of

acute myocardial infarction with primary angioplasty and abciximab. *Catheter Cardiovasc Interv* 2004; **61**(1):67–73.

70. Stone GW, Marsalese D, Brodie BR, *et al.* A prospective, randomized evaluation of prophylactic intraaortic balloon counterpulsation in high risk patients with acute myocardial infarction treated with primary angioplasty. Second Primary Angioplasty in Myocardial Infarction (PAMI-II) Trial Investigators. *J Am Coll Cardiol* 1997; **29**(7):1459–67.
71. De Luca G, Suryapranata H, Stone GW, *et al.* Abciximab as adjunctive therapy to reperfusion in acute ST-segment elevation myocardial infarction: a meta-analysis of randomized trials. *JAMA* 2005; **293**(14):1759–65.
72. Mehilli J, Kastrati A, Schulz S, *et al.* for the Bavarian Reperfusion Alternatives Evaluation-3 (BRAVE-3) Study Investigators. Abciximab in patients with acute ST elevation myocardial infarction undergoing primary percutaneous coronary intervention after clopidogrel loading. A randomized double-blind trial. *Circulation* 2009; **119**(14):1933–40.
73. Montalescot G, Borentain M, Payot L, *et al.* Early vs late administration of glycoprotein IIb/IIIa inhibitors in primary percutaneous coronary intervention of acute ST-segment elevation myocardial infarction: a meta-analysis. *JAMA* 2004; **292**(3):362–6.
74. Van't Hof AW, Ten Berg J, Heestermans T, *et al.* Prehospital initiation of tirofiban in patients with ST-elevation myocardial infarction undergoing primary angioplasty (On-TIME 2): a multicentre, double-blind, randomised controlled trial. *Lancet* 2008; **372**(9638): 537–46.
75. Stone GW, Witzenbichler B, Guagliumi G, *et al.* Bivalirudin during primary PCI in acute myocardial infarction. *N Engl J Med* 2008; **358**(21):2218–30.
76. Svilaas T, Vlaar PJ, van der Horst IC, *et al.* Thrombus aspiration during primary percutaneous coronary intervention. *N Engl J Med* 2008; **358**(6):557–67.
77. Vlaar PJ, Svilaas T, van der Horst IC, *et al.* Cardiac death and reinfarction after 1 year in the Thrombus Aspiration during Percutaneous coronary intervention in Acute myocardial infarction Study (TAPAS): a 1-year follow-up study. *Lancet* 2008; **371**(9628):1915–20.
78. Grines CL, Cox DA, Stone GW, *et al.* Coronary angioplasty with or without stent implantation for acute myocardial infarction. Stent Primary Angioplasty in Myocardial Infarction Study Group. *N Engl J Med* 1999; **341**(26):1949–56.
79. Nordmann AJ, Bucher H, Hengstler P, *et al.* Primary stenting versus primary balloon angioplasty for treating acute myocardial infarction. *Cochrane Database Syst Rev* 2005; **2**:CD005313.
80. Suryapranata H, De Luca G, van 't Hof AW, *et al.* Is routine stenting for acute myocardial infarction superior to balloon angioplasty? A randomised comparison in a large cohort of unselected patients. *Heart* 2005; **91**(5):641–5.
81. Spaulding C, Henry P, Teiger E, *et al.* Sirolimus-eluting versus uncoated stents in acute myocardial infarction. *N Engl J Med* 2006; **355**(11):1093–104.
82. Laarman GJ, Suttorp MJ, Dirksen MT, *et al.* Paclitaxel-eluting versus uncoated stents in primary percutaneous coronary intervention. *N Engl J Med* 2006; **355**(11): 1105–13.
83. Kastrati A, Dibra A, Spaulding C, *et al.* Meta-analysis of randomized trials on drug-eluting stents vs. bare-metal stents in patients with acute myocardial infarction. *Eur Heart J* 2007; **28**(22):2706–13.
84. Stone GW, Lansky AJ, Pocock SJ, *et al.* Paclitaxel-Eluting Stents versus Bare-Metal Stents in Acute Myocardial Infarction. *N Engl J Med* 2009; **360**(19):1946–59.
85. The Thrombolysis in Myocardial Infarction (TIMI) trial. Phase I findings. TIMI Study Group. *N Engl J Med* 1985; **312**(14):932–6.
86. Mehta RH, Harjai KJ, Cox D, *et al.* Clinical and angiographic correlates and outcomes of suboptimal coronary flow inpatients with acute myocardial infarction undergoing primary percutaneous coronary intervention. *J Am Coll Cardiol* 2003; **42**(10):1739–46.
87. Kloner RA. Does reperfusion injury exist in humans? *J Am Coll Cardiol* 1993; **21**(2):537–45.
88. Rezkalla SH, Kloner RA. No-reflow phenomenon. *Circulation* 2002; **105**(5):656–62.
89. Yip HK, Chen MC, Chang HW, *et al.* Angiographic morphologic features of infarct-related arteries and timely reperfusion in acute myocardial infarction: predictors of slow-flow and no-reflow phenomenon. *Chest* 2002; **122**(4):1322–32.
90. Mamas MA, Fraser D, Fath-Ordoubadi F. The role of thrombectomy and distal protection devices during percutaneous coronary interventions. *EuroIntervention* 2008; **4**(1):115–23.
91. Loubeyre C, Morice MC, Lefevre T, *et al.* A randomized comparison of direct stenting with conventional stent implantation in selected patients with acute myocardial infarction. *J Am Coll Cardiol* 2002; **39**(1):15–21.
92. Mahaffey KW, Puma JA, Barbagelata NA, *et al.* Adenosine as an adjunct to thrombolytic therapy for acute myocardial infarction: results of a multicenter, randomized, placebo-controlled trial: the Acute Myocardial Infarction STudy of ADenosine (AMISTAD) trial. *J Am Coll Cardiol* 1999; **34**(6):1711–20.
93. Ross AM, Gibbons RJ, Stone GW, *et al.* A randomized, double-blinded, placebo-controlled multicenter trial of adenosine as an adjunct to reperfusion in the treatment of acute myocardial infarction (AMISTAD-II). *J Am Coll Cardiol* 2005; **45**(11):1775–80.
94. Bravo Vergel Y, Palmer S, Asseburg C, *et al.* Is primary angioplasty cost-effective in the UK? Results of a comprehensive decision analysis. *Heart* 2007; **93**: 1238–43.

CHAPTER 17

Percutaneous coronary intervention in patients with impaired left ventricular function

Divaka Perera and Simon Redwood

Impact of left ventricular function on outcome after percutaneous coronary intervention

Changes in left ventricular (LV) function are an early manifestation of the ischaemic cascade and often precede the well recognized markers of ischaemia, such as ST segment changes or chest pain. Decreased ventricular compliance, diminished regional and global contractility, and elevated end-diastolic pressure occur within a few seconds of interruption of coronary blood flow by balloon occlusion, whereas recovery of these parameters can lag several minutes behind balloon deflation, restoration of blood flow, and resolution of electrocardiogram (ECG) changes[1]. Prolonged post-ischaemic myocardial dysfunction, or stunning, can occur following recurrent ischaemia, which may persist for several hours or days even when blood flow is restored[2]. The impact of transient or repetitive coronary occlusion on LV function is rarely of clinical consequence when percutaneous coronary intervention (PCI) is performed in patients with preserved ventricular function, but is potentially hazardous in those who have LV impairment at the outset, particularly when there is a large amount of myocardium at risk. These patients have attenuated haemodynamic reserve and may recover incompletely from post-ischaemic stunning, which increases the risk of entering a deteriorating spiral of decreasing cardiac output and worsening ischaemia that could culminate in cardiogenic shock or ventricular arrhythmias. Furthermore, patients with impaired LV function tend to be older and have more advanced comorbidities, which are independently associated with an adverse outcome following any form of revascularization.

The theoretical risks of PCI in the presence of impaired LV function have been borne out in several registries. A report from the NHLBI Dynamic Registry involving 1158 patients undergoing (predominantly elective) PCI between 1997 and 1998 showed that LV ejection fraction was a strong predictor of in-hospital death, with mortality rates of 3% in those with LV ejection fraction (LVEF) <30% compared to 0.1% when LVEF >50%[3]. Similarly, a recent analysis of nearly 56 000 patients who underwent elective PCI in the State of New York between 1998 and 1999 has shown that an EF <45% is associated with significantly decreased chances of survival to hospital discharge, compared to patients with a LVEF ≥55%. After multivariate adjustment, the odds ratio for in-hospital death was 2.2 if EF 25–35% and 3.9 if EF ≤25%[4]. More than a quarter of patients in this cohort had an LVEF <45%, confirming that PCI is commonly performed in this group of patients, despite the adverse outcome associated with depressed LV function. Considerable technological advances have occurred in PCI during the last decade, which are generally assumed to have translated to improved clinical outcomes, particularly in patients who have been traditionally deemed to be at high risk of complications. Nevertheless, contemporary registries confirm the continued adverse impact of LV dysfunction on mortality following PCI[5,6]. These observational series demonstrate higher in-hospital mortality when LV function is impaired (due to a greater risk of procedural events) as well as reduced mid-term survival, which reflects the adverse prognosis in this group of patients, regardless of the mode of revascularization[7]. Non-fatal complications are also more common in patients with poor LV function, although the relationship is less clear cut than observed with mortality, given the varied determinants of adverse cardiac and cerebrovascular events in this group (see Fig. 17.1).

The degree of risk associated with PCI varies with the extent of LV impairment; while severely depressed function is consistently linked to poor outcomes, even moderate degrees of LV dysfunction have been shown to affect prognosis following PCI[4]. The Mayo Risk Score incorporates actual LVEF, rather than a dichotomous classification of function as 'good' or 'poor', and seeks to grade the procedural risk associated with even modest changes in LV systolic function[5]. As such, quantitative (or semi-quantitative) assessment of LV function should be an integral process in guiding management and risk stratification of every patient scheduled to undergo PCI. This principle is equally pertinent to ad hoc PCI, when assessment of LV function is often omitted in the interests of expediency or limiting contrast volume. Identification of significant LV impairment in advance allows selection of adjunctive therapies to optimize outcome following PCI and to counsel these patients about the increased risk of major adverse events.

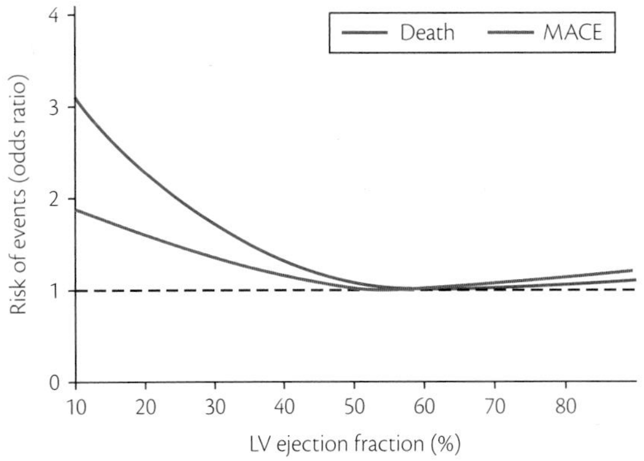

Fig. 17.1 Impact of baseline left ventricular ejection fraction on the relative risk of in-hospital death (red line) or major adverse cardiovascular events (blue line) following PCI. Data from Singh M, Rihal CS, Lennon RJ, *et al.* Bedside estimation of risk from percutaneous coronary intervention: the new Mayo Clinic risk scores. *Mayo Clin Proc* 2007; **82**:701–8.

Optimizing PCI when left ventricular function is impaired

Major advances have been made in the medical treatment of heart failure in the past two decades, resulting in appreciable prognostic benefits in these patients. Strategies such as medical therapy with ACE inhibitors/angiotensin receptor antagonists, beta-blockers, aldosterone antagonists and diuretics, or cardiac resynchronization should be employed (in accordance with current heart failure management guidelines) to improve LV function prior to PCI, when LV dysfunction is identified beforehand. When urgent PCI is indicated by an acute presentation, limiting the opportunity to optimize haemodynamic conditions before the procedure, such therapies should be instituted very early following PCI to maximize outcome following revascularization.

Distinguishing hypovolaemia from incipient cardiogenic shock is important, should hypotension occur during PCI in a patient with depressed LV function. Indeed, many of these patients will have received diuretic therapy beforehand and may have relative intravascular volume depletion, predisposing them to hypotension, particularly if nitrates or other vasodilators are administered. In these situations, assessment of pulmonary artery pressure (PAP) (and pulmonary capillary wedge pressure, PCWP) can be helpful, as a low diastolic PAP (or PCWP <12mmHg) effectively excludes shock. Significant myocardial ischaemia causes elevation of diastolic pressure[1], which in turn causes elevation of PAP and PCWP and as such, PAP monitoring can provide an additional early warning of potential haemodynamic compromise. However, changes in PAP do not reliably detect ischaemia[8] and continuous PAP monitoring would only be recommended for patients with poor LV function and borderline haemodynamics.

It is well recognized that myonecrosis is a frequent undesirable by-product of PCI, the impact of which depends on the extent of peri-procedural infarction, as well as the degree of baseline LV impairment. As such, every effort needs to be made to avoid procedural complications, such as side-branch occlusion or distal embolization, which are recognized as the major causes of peri-procedural myonecrosis[9]. This is turn requires judicious patient selection and a lower threshold for using adjunctive treatments such as thrombus aspiration, embolic protection devices, and powerful platelet inhibition. Even transient episodes of ischaemia can result in stunning[1], which is poorly tolerated by a bad ventricle; the length of ischaemia during PCI should be minimized in such cases.

In addition to these general measures, invasive support of the circulation could be considered, as an adjunct to high-risk PCI, in patients with severely depressed LV function.

Intra-aortic balloon counterpulsation

Principles of counterpulsation

Fifty years ago, the Harvard surgeon Dwight Harken demonstrated that the failing heart could be supported by removing blood from the femoral artery in systole and replacing this volume in diastole[10]. The principle of diastolic augmentation led to the development of the intra-aortic balloon pump (IABP) in the 1960s. Counterpulsation is carried out by placing a balloon catheter in the descending aorta, which is inflated in diastole and deflated just prior to the onset of systole; balloon inflation and deflation are synchronized with the cardiac cycle by monitoring the aortic pressure waveform and ECG respectively. Augmentation of aortic diastolic pressure increases the aorto-coronary pressure gradient, with consequent increase in coronary flow[11], while rapid deflation of the balloon just prior to the beginning of systole causes a void in the aorta, leading to a drop in end-diastolic pressure and subsequent systolic wall tension[12]. The simultaneous increase in coronary perfusion and decrease in oxygen demand is a unique feature of balloon counterpulsation and contrasts with the action of pharmacological inotropic agents, which increase cardiac output at the expense of increased myocardial oxygen demand. The IABP was introduced into clinical practice as a means of supporting patients undergoing surgical revascularization but technological developments in catheter design, coupled with improved understanding of the physiological effects of counterpulsation, have led to increasing use of the IABP as an adjunct to PCI in cardiogenic shock or when haemodynamic decompensation is imminent.

IABP to support PCI for shock

Owing to its emergent nature, to date, there have been no randomized controlled trials that have specifically evaluated the use of IABP in cardiogenic shock. Notwithstanding the selection bias inherent in observational data involving critically ill patients, there is reasonable non-randomized evidence supporting the use of balloon counterpulsation during the treatment of AMI complicated by shock. Most of these data are derived from the thrombolysis era. While the advent of thrombolysis led to impressive reduction in infarct size and improved survival, the magnitude of benefit is attenuated in the presence of cardiogenic shock, in part due to decreased coronary perfusion[13]. IABP therapy appears to have a synergistic effect with thrombolysis, which may be via augmentation of coronary flow[14]. The largest of these registries is NRMI-2, which included 5681 patients with shock who were treated with thrombolysis, nearly 40% of whom also received IABP therapy[15]. Mortality in the IABP group was significantly lower than in those receiving thrombolysis alone (49% vs. 77%) and these results were reproduced in a meta-analysis, which also included six other cohort studies[16] (see Fig. 17.2). Interestingly, this synergy is not seen in shock patients treated with PCI and IABP support, with even a suggestion of increased mortality in this group, compared to those who have PCI without counterpulsation. However, these are retrospective, non-randomized data which need to be interpreted cautiously. Firstly, the available information does not allow distinction between elective and bail-out IABP use, the latter indicating sicker patients, whose haemodynamics either deteriorate or fail to improve following revascularization. If counterpulsation was primarily used to rescue haemodynamic compromise in these series, the increased mortality observed in the IABP group may merely be a reflection of a higher risk cohort. In contrast, patients receiving thrombolysis and IABP therapy tended to be younger, included a greater frequency of men, and were more likely to receive subsequent revascularization, all of which are independent predictors of improved outcome, and may explain the lower mortality seen in this group. Despite the gaps in the evidence base, the role of IABP therapy in supporting PCI for shock has virtually become dogma; the current ACC/AHA guidelines describe IABP therapy as a Class I indication for treatment of shock complicating AMI, without distinguishing between modes of reperfusion[17].

IABP use during high-risk PCI

Patients who are haemodynamically stable but have poor LV function are another group who are at increased risk of death or major cardiovascular complications; the use of elective IABP support to ameliorate this risk is controversial at present. In a registry of approximately 1500 consecutive patients undergoing PCI for AMI, Brodie and colleagues found that the use of IABP before intervention was a significant independent predictor of freedom from adverse events during the procedure (odds ratio, 0.5)[18]. The beneficial effect was most significant in those with cardiogenic shock but

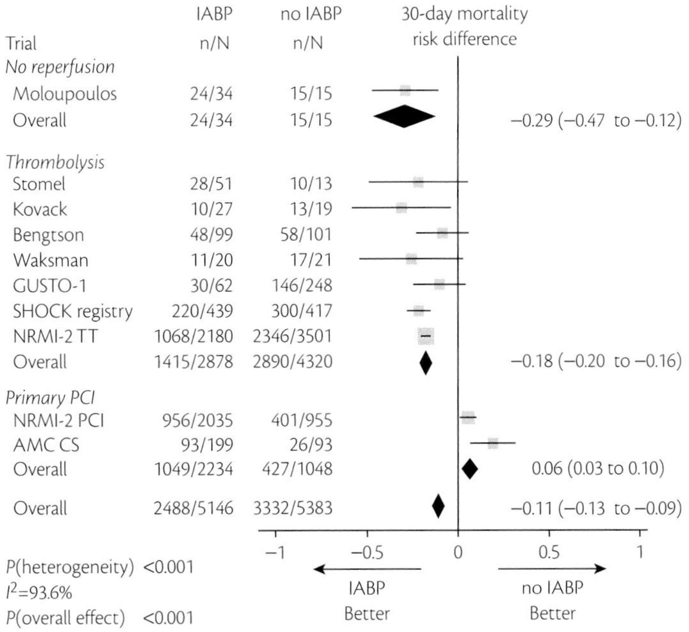
IABP
no IABP
30-day mortality risk difference
Trial
n/N
n/N
No reperfusion
Moloupoulos 24/34 15/15
Overall 24/34 15/15 −0.29 (−0.47 to −0.12)
Thrombolysis
Stomel 28/51 10/13
Kovack 10/27 13/19
Bengtson 48/99 58/101
Waksman 11/20 17/21
GUSTO-1 30/62 146/248
SHOCK registry 220/439 300/417
NRMI-2 TT 1068/2180 2346/3501
Overall 1415/2878 2890/4320 −0.18 (−0.20 to −0.16)
Primary PCI
NRMI-2 PCI 956/2035 401/955
AMC CS 93/199 26/93
Overall 1049/2234 427/1048 0.06 (0.03 to 0.10)
Overall 2488/5146 3332/5383 −0.11 (−0.13 to −0.09)
−1
−0.5
0
0.5
1
P(heterogeneity) <0.001
I²=93.6%
P(overall effect) <0.001
IABP Better
no IABP Better

Fig. 17.2 Comparison of 30-day mortality in patients receiving IABP therapy with those who did not, for treatment of acute MI complicated by shock. The width of each square represents the weight of each study in the meta-analysis. NRMI-2 TT denotes cohort from NRMI-2 study of patients treated with thrombolysis, and NRMI-2 PCI denotes cohort from NRMI-2 study of patients treated with primary PCI. Reproduced with permission from Sjauw KD, Engstrom AE, Vis MM, *et al.* A systematic review and meta-analysis of intra-aortic balloon pump therapy in ST-elevation myocardial infarction: should we change the guidelines? *Eur Heart J* 2009; **30**:459–68.

there was a clear trend toward fewer events with prophylactic IABP insertion even in the high-risk patients who were haemodynamically stable at the outset. Brigouri and colleagues reported similar findings in a retrospective study of IABP use during PCI in 133 clinically stable patients with significantly impaired LV function (EF <30%)[19]. Compared to conventional treatment (including bail-out IABP insertion if required), elective IABP use was associated with significantly fewer cardiac and cerebral events during the procedure and a strong trend to a lower in-hospital MACE rate. The combination of LV impairment and a large area of myocardium at risk augured a particularly adverse outcome in this study; a high jeopardy score conferred a 5.4-fold risk of major cardiovascular events. It has also been demonstrated that insertion of an IABP before high-risk PCI is associated with better in-hospital and 6-month survival than when it is used to rescue haemodynamic compromise during the procedure[20].

Albeit persuasive, given the observational nature of this data, there are no formal recommendations for counterpulsation in this setting. The current AHA/ACC guidelines suggest that 'IABP support during PCI should be reserved only for patients at the extreme end of the spectrum of haemodynamic compromise'[21]. However, the real-world utilization of IABP is at variance with these guidelines, and more than 20% of all IABP insertions are in the context of high-risk PCI or angiography in patients who are not in shock[22]. The Balloon pump assisted Coronary Intervention Study (BCIS-1) is the first randomized controlled trial of IABP use in this setting. BCIS-1 randomized 300 patients with poor LV function (EF <30%) and a large amount of myocardium at risk (BCIS-1 Jeopardy Score ≥8/12) to receive elective IABP support or have conventional treatment (including bail-out IABP), with a primary outcome measure of major adverse cardiac or cerebrovascular events to hospital discharge[23]. Secondary outcome measures included procedural complications (hypotension, VT/VF or cardiorespiratory arrest) and 6 month mortality.

BCIS-1 showed that elective IABP insertion does not reduce in-hospital MACCE compared to a strategy of no planned IABP support in these high-risk patients (14.6% vs. 15.3% respectively, p=0.35[24]). However, approximately 1 in 8 cases carried out without planned IABP support suffered intra-procedural complications such as hypotension or vessel closure, requiring bailout IABP insertion during the PCI procedure (see Fig. 17.3). Despite bail-out IABP use, the latter group suffered a higher rate of peri-procedural myocardial infarction than those receiving elective IABP support (22% vs. 11.3%). Hence it is likely that there may be a "very high-risk" cohort within this group, perhaps characterized by complex lesion morphology as well as high coronary jeopardy and severely impaired LV function. Where it

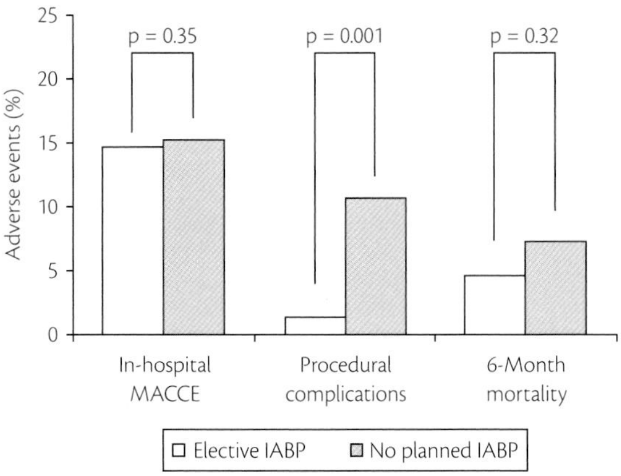

Fig. 17.3 Primary and secondary Outcomes in elective IABP group (open bars) and No Planned IABP group (filled bars) in BCIS-1. Elective IABP insertion failed to reduce in-hospital MACCE in a high-risk cohort, characterized by poor LV function and high coronary jeopardy scores. However, intra-procedural complications occurred more frequently when an IABP was not inserted electively. 6-month mortality was not significantly different in the two groups[24]. Reprinted with permission from Sjauw KD, Engstrom AE, Vis MM, *et al.* A systematic review and meta-analysis of intra-aortic balloon pump therapy in ST-elevation myocardial infarction: should we change the guidelines? *Eur Heart J* 2009; **30**:459–68.

is possible to prospectively identify such patients, elective IABP support would be expected to reduce the incidence of intraprocedural complications.

An alternative to elective IABP support is a 'standby' strategy, whereby preparation of the patient and catheter laboratory team in advance can facilitate swift and uncomplicated bail-out IABP insertion if required. Typically, contralateral femoral arterial access is obtained with a small calibre sheath, the balloon pump console turned on, and the ECG inputs required for IABP function secured at the start of the procedure. In addition to minimizing delay in obtaining IABP support if required emergently, this strategy also serves to highlight the high-risk nature of the intervention to the entire team.

Left ventricular assist devices

Left ventricular assist devices (LVAD) can provide invaluable support to a failing ventricle and have traditionally been large devices requiring surgical implantation, as a bridge to cardiac transplantation. However, impressive technological developments in recent years have allowed progressive miniaturization of these devices, which can now be inserted in the cardiac catheterization laboratory. Two main types of percutaneous LVAD are in clinical use at present, the Impella® (Abiomed Inc., Massachusetts, USA) and TandemHeart® (CardiacAssist, Pittsburgh, USA) devices.

The Impella® system is based on a microaxial pump, mounted on a pigtail catheter, which is advanced retrogradely via the femoral artery into the ventricle across the aortic valve (see Fig. 17.4). The pump continually aspirates blood from the ventricular cavity, which is delivered directly to the ascending aorta, and can augment cardiac output by up to 2.5L/min with a device requiring 12F femoral access. By unloading the ventricle, the Impella® reduces end-diastolic pressure[25], which may translate to decreased wall tension and myocardial oxygen demand. There is also evidence that it has a beneficial effect on coronary perfusion[26], which theoretically achieves a similar net effect as the IABP, although systematic comparison of the two treatments is yet to be carried out. Hypothetically, the Impella® may be a preferable means of supporting the circulation when intrinsic cardiac output is severely depressed, as in cardiogenic shock. A small randomized comparison of the two devices, ISAR-SHOCK, has shown better cardiac output parameters when the Impella® device (rather than the IABP) was used as an adjunct to PCI for treatment of cardiogenic shock, although a similar clinical outcome was observed in both groups[27]. Preliminary data also suggest that the Impella® constitutes a safe means of supporting high-risk PCI in patients with impaired LV function who are haemodynamically stable[28], but adequately powered studies of efficacy in this setting are awaited.

The TandemHeart® system involves drawing oxygenated blood from the left atrium (via a 21F trans-septal cannula inserted through the femoral vein), which is returned to the systemic circulation via a 12–15F femoral artery cannula. The extracorporeal circulation is powered by a centrifugal pump. More invasive than the Impella® system, the TandemHeart® device is reported to provide up to 4.5L/min of additional circulatory support and has been used as an adjunct to high-risk PCI in patients with poor ventricular function[29]. However, there is a significant increase in the rate of bleeding and vascular complications with the use of these devices, which need to be balanced against any potential benefits of circulatory support.

PCI to improve left ventricular function

The concept of viable but dysfunctional myocardium emerged approximately three decades ago, when it was observed that patients undergoing coronary artery

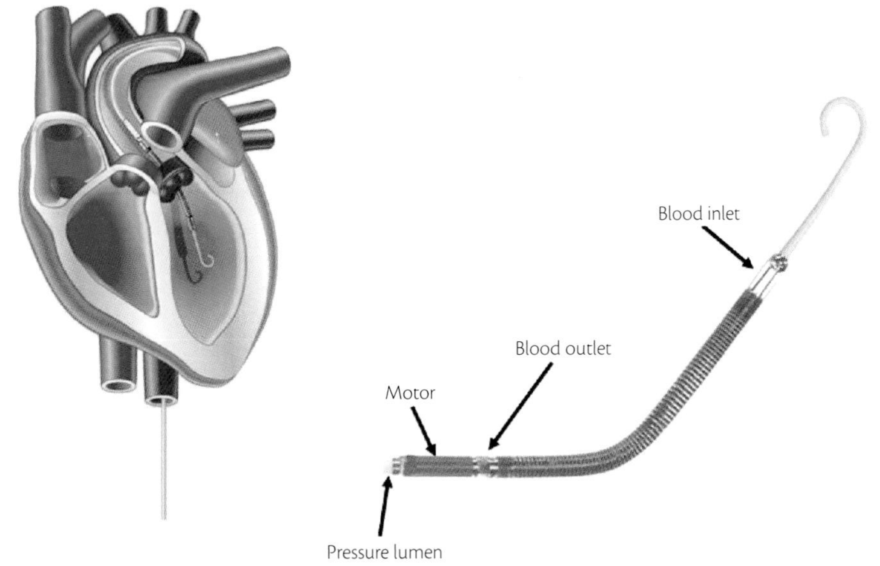

Fig. 17.4 The Impella 2.5 left ventricular assist device is inserted percutaneously via the femoral artery and can augment cardiac output by a maximum of 2.5L/min. Adapted from Allman KC, Shaw LJ, Hachamovitch R, Udelson JE. Myocardial viability testing and impact of revascularization on prognosis in patients with coronary artery disease and left ventricular dysfunction: a meta-analysis. *J Am Coll.Cardiol.* 2002; **39**:1151–8. Copyright © 2002 American College of Cardiology Foundation. Published by Elsevier Science Inc.

bypass graft (CABG) surgery for chronic stable angina had improvement or normalization of LV function following revascularization[30]. The energy utilized during myocyte contraction far exceeds the requirement for sustaining viability and as such, myocardial tissue may survive in a hypocontractile state in the presence of reduced coronary blood flow or decreased coronary flow reserve, known as hibernation[31]. Improvement of blood flow by revascularization of hibernating myocardium can lead to restoration of regional and global LV function and reversal of adverse remodelling[32–34], provided this is achieved before the onset of irreversible cellular and ultrastructural alterations[35]. The importance of diagnosing and treating hibernation is underscored by epidemiological studies and registries that have demonstrated that coronary artery disease is now the predominant cause of heart failure in the western world[36,37]. A meta-analysis of 24 major heart failure trials reported in the past 20 years has shown that coronary disease was the underlying cause of heart failure in 65% of cases[38], although this may have been an underestimation, given that few of these studies mandated systematic exploration of aetiology.

Viability testing

Potentially reversible, dysfunctional myocardium is characterized by preserved cellular integrity and a degree of contractile reserve, whereas scarring and absence of inducible contraction tend to reflect irreversible myocardial damage. Each of these distinguishing features can be used to predict myocardial viability or the likelihood of functional recovery following revascularization. Single-photon emission computed tomography (SPECT) and positron emission tomography (PET) are used to delineate viable tissue, based on the uptake and retention of tracers (which require intact cell membranes and mitochondrial function) or myocardial glucose metabolism respectively. Metabolism-perfusion mismatch (reduced perfusion but normal metabolism) on PET has high negative and positive predictive value in predicting functional recovery[39]. In contrast, magnetic resonance imaging (MRI) is used to image scar, which appears bright due to chelation of gadolinium within collagenous scar; the transmural extent of scarring has a strong inverse correlation with myocardial viability[39]. Contractile reserve is assessed by measuring the augmentation of function of hypocontractile myocardium in response to inotropic stimulation. The most commonly used agent is dobutamine (at doses up to 20mcg/kg/min) while the change in regional and global contractility could be imaged by echocardiography (dobutamine stress echocardiography, DSE) or cine-MRI. In practice, the modality chosen to assess viability depends on the individual patient as well as the expertise within each centre and may involve more than one technique in a given case. A MRI protocol incorporating scar-imaging and dobutamine contractile reserve may well emerge as the gold-standard viability test but at present this modality has restricted availability and further prognostic data are awaited.

Despite variation in the sensitivity and specificity of these techniques, patients found to have viable myocardium (by any modality) have been shown to have a strong survival advantage following revascularization compared to medical therapy alone. A meta-analysis of more than 3000 patients in 24 randomized studies (in which viability was assessed by SPECT, PET, or DSE) showed an impressive 80% relative reduction (and 12.8% absolute reduction) in mortality with revascularization compared to medical therapy in patients found to have significant viable myocardium[33]. In contrast, no survival benefit was seen in the absence of viability and even a trend to worse outcome with revascularization (Fig. 17.5). These data also argue against a strategy of revascularizing all patients with heart failure and coronary disease, regardless of viability; mortality following revascularization (predominantly CABG surgery) in patients without viability was more than double that observed in those who did have viable myocardium. It has traditionally been held that completeness of revascularization (in relation to the angiographic findings) is a major determinant of outcome in ischaemic

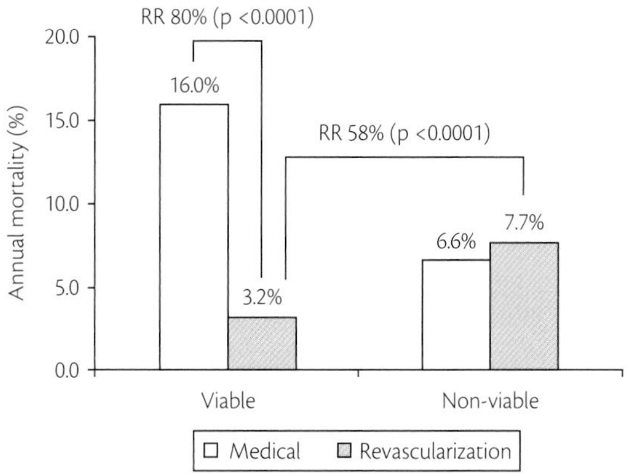

Fig. 17.5 Annual mortality rates in patients with LV dysfunction following revascularisation (filled bars) or treated medical therapy alone (open bars). Patients with viable myocardium had 80% reduction in mortality rate when revascularised, whereas this benefit was not seen when there was no viability. Patients undergoing revascularisation had a significantly higher survival rate if they had viable myocardium at baseline. Reprinted with permission from Chareonthaitawee P, Gersh BJ, Araoz PA, Gibbons RJ. Revascularization in severe left ventricular dysfunction: the role of viability testing. *J Am Coll. Cardiol.* 2005; **46**:567–74. Copyright © 2005 American College of Cardiology Foundation Published by Elsevier Inc.

cardiomyopathy[41]; whether regional viability can be used to guide the extent (and hence the mode) of revascularization in a given patient, remains untested to date.

Notwithstanding the powerful prognostic utility of viability testing suggested by these studies, translation of these results to clinical practice can sometimes be difficult. While the extremes of the spectrum of viability can be reliably detected by most modalities, a large proportion of patients lie within the 'grey-zone' (for example, 30–70% transmurality of scar on late gadolinium MRI). In these cases, a second viability test may help but often will rest on the clinical judgement of a multidisciplinary team (MDT). Furthermore, the critical mass of viable myocardium required to justify intervention is unclear, which may in turn depend on the perceived risks of the chosen modality of coronary intervention.

Surgical revascularization for ischaemic cardiomyopathy

To date, there have been no randomized controlled comparisons of any form of coronary revascularization with medical therapy for treatment of LV dysfunction in patients who do not have angina. As such, current recommendations for CABG surgery in patients with ischaemic cardiomyopathy are based on data from registries and cohort studies that were carried out more than 20 years ago, before the routine use of medical therapies that have been shown to improve survival and symptoms in this group of patients. The two largest observational cohorts are the CASS and Duke Registries. The CASS registry included 651 (of a total of approximately 20 000) patients who had a LVEF <50%, 231 of whom received CABG surgery. CABG provided a mortality benefit over medical therapy only in the subgroup of patients with severe LV dysfunction (EF <25%), where angina was the predominant symptom, rather than heart failure[7]. The Duke registry of 1391 patients with ischaemic cardiomyopathy (EF <40%), treated over a period of 25 years, demonstrated a sustained survival benefit in the group receiving CABG surgery (339 patients) compared to those treated with medical therapy alone[42]. Despite the paucity of randomized data, the available evidence (summarized in Fig. 17.6) [43] has been considered sufficiently convincing for the AHA/ACC to classify CABG as a class I indication for treatment of impaired LV function in the presence of significant proximal coronary disease, regardless of the whether the patient has angina[44].

However, revascularization of ischaemic cardiomyopathy embodies a paradox often encountered by

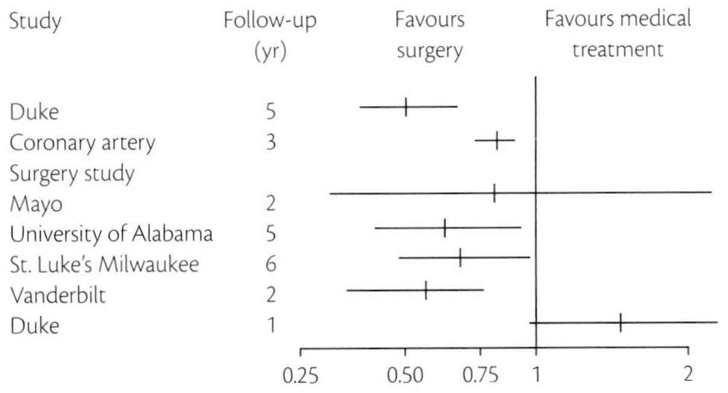

Fig. 17.6 Relative risk of mortality for CABG compared to medical therapy in moderate-to-severe LV systolic dysfunction, ranked in order of study quality. Studies were observational, most patients had limiting angina, and preoperative viability testing was not routinely performed. Reprinted with permission from the Journal of the American College of Cardiology[43]. Copyright 2005, The American College of Cardiology Foundation.

cardiologists and cardiothoracic surgeons; patients who are most likely to benefit from treatment (namely those with severely impaired LV function) are also at highest risk of mortality and morbidity from the procedure. Perioperative mortality rates in patients with LV dysfunction can vary between 5–30%, the risk increasing with age, comorbidities, and degree of LV impairment[(45)]. The relative risk of early death following CABG surgery in patients with severe LV function is 3- to 4-fold higher than in those with mild dysfunction or preserved systolic function[(46,47)]. Given the increasing scrutiny of individual and institutional outcome data following CABG surgery, this paradox can often lead to a reluctance of surgeons to take on the highest risk cases with severe LV dysfunction. The increased perception of risk, coupled with technological advancements in PCI has led to the latter emerging as an alternative treatment for ischaemic cardiomyopathy. It should be noted that either form of revascularization is associated with more major complications in this group than in those with preserved LV function; careful selection (including assessment of viability) is central to optimizing the risk–benefit balance in these patients.

PCI for ischaemic cardiomyopathy

Numerous comparisons have been made between PCI and CABG surgery for patients with symptomatic coronary disease or evidence of significant reversible ischaemia, but most of the large randomized trials excluded patients with impaired LV function (EF <30%)[(48–50)]. Less than 2% of all patients included in the largest and most recent randomized controlled trial, SYNTAX, had significant LV impairment (EF <30%) at baseline[(51)]. A meta-analysis of 10 such trials has found similar 5-year survival following surgery or PCI in the combined cohort, as well as in the subgroup (17% of all patients) who had modest LV dysfunction[(52)].

There have been a few non-randomized comparisons of the two modalities in patients with poor LV function. In the pre-stent era, observational studies suggested better early outcomes but less complete revascularization and more mid-term repeat revascularization procedures following balloon angioplasty than surgery, with similar long-term survival following either treatment[(41,53)]. The AWESOME (Angina With Extremely Serious Operative Mortality Evaluation) investigators combined the data from randomized and registry cohorts in a pre-specified subgroup analysis and demonstrated equivalent 3-year survival following surgery or bare-metal stent PCI[(54)]. The advent of drug-eluting stents has vastly reduced the incidence of restenosis and has facilitated a greater degree of revascularization with PCI, which are particularly pertinent factors in the treatment of ischaemic cardiomyopathy[(55)]. A recent observational study has confirmed these theoretical benefits by demonstrating comparable mortality at 15 months following drug-eluting stent PCI or CABG surgery, although there was a greater improvement in New York Heart Association (NYHA) functional class with surgery, possibly due to more complete revascularization[(56)]. However, these studies were relatively underpowered, retrospective analyses that included patients who had significant angina and were not balanced in terms of baseline characteristics or completeness of revascularization. At present, although conceptually appealing, there is no clear evidence supporting the use of PCI for patients with ischaemic cardiomyopathy and predominant symptoms of heart failure rather than angina.

In the absence of explicit guidelines, CABG and PCI should be considered complementary techniques for treating patients with ischaemic cardiomyopathy and significant viable myocardium, with the management strategy tailored to the individual by a MDT, including imaging physicians, cardiologists and cardiac surgeons, in discussion with the patients themselves. The presence of multiple comorbidities, advanced age, or a history of previous cardiac surgery may favour PCI while complex coronary anatomy (including chronic occlusions and diffuse disease), the need for concomitant mitral valve surgery and distal vessels suitable for grafting may mean CABG is most appropriate. The ability to carry out surgical ventricular reconstruction has also been traditionally considered an indication for CABG surgery rather than PCI, but the recently concluded STICH (Surgical Treatment for Ischemic Heart Failure) trial suggests that ventricular restoration does not offer survival or functional benefit over revascularization alone[57].

There is a convincing body of evidence supporting coronary angiography and subsequent revascularization in patients with symptoms and signs of heart failure who also have angina, which is a class I indication in the AHA/ACC guidelines. The guidance on management of patients with heart failure who do not have angina or have atypical chest pain is less distinct and coronary angiography has a class IIa recommendation in this group[58]. However, it is the authors' view that coronary angiography is extremely valuable in defining the aetiology of heart failure as well as determining anatomical suitability for revascularization and should be considered in all individuals who are sufficiently robust to undergo PCI or CABG surgery. In addition to selection of patients who would benefit from revascularization, knowledge of coronary anatomy often allows optimization of medical therapy in such patients, leading to a greater use of agents such as aspirin and statins, which in turn are associated with improved outcomes[59]. A suggested algorithm for revascularizing patients without angina who have heart failure and coronary disease is contained in Fig. 17.7. It should be emphasized that medical therapy (including ACE inhibitors/angiotensin receptor blockers, beta-blockers, aldosterone antagonists, and any other novel therapies) should be offered to all patients with heart failure, as soon as this diagnosis is established. The optimal timing of revascularization in relation to initiation and titration of medical therapy has not been formally studied but observational studies suggest that delay in revascularization is associated with increased mortality in patients with hibernating myocardium[35,60,61]. Until randomized trial data are available, early assessment of viability and consideration of revascularization is recommended, rather than restriction of this option to those who fail a trial of medical therapy.

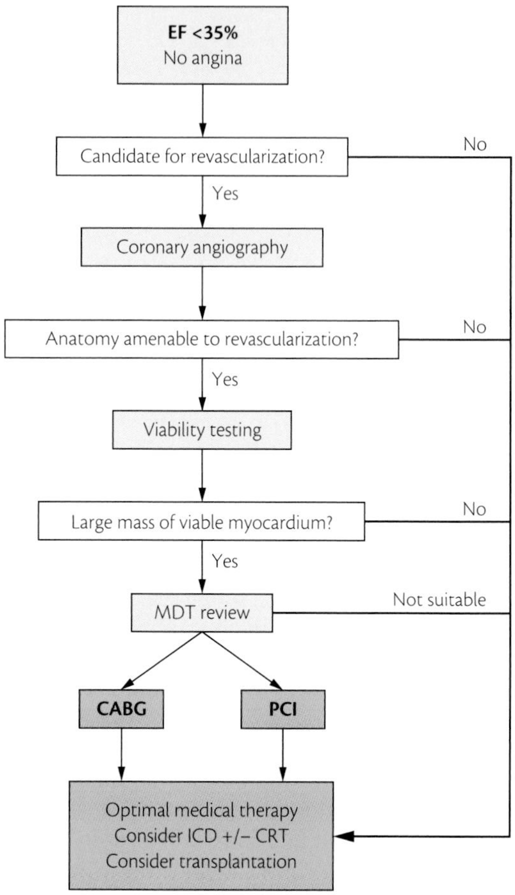

Fig. 17.7 Algorithm for revascularizing patients without angina who have heart failure and coronary disease.

References

1. Nesto RW, Kowalchuk GJ. The ischemic cascade: temporal sequence of hemodynamic, electrocardiographic and symptomatic expressions of ischemia. *Am J Cardiol* 1987; **59**:23C–30C.
2. Braunwald E,.Kloner RA. The stunned myocardium: prolonged, postischemic ventricular dysfunction. *Circulation* 1982; **66**:1146–9.
3. Keelan PC, Johnston JM, Koru-Sengul T, *et al.* Comparison of in-hospital and one-year outcomes in patients with left ventricular ejection fractions <or=40%, 41% to 49%, and >or=50% having percutaneous coronary revascularization. *Am J Cardiol* 2003; **91**:1168–72.
4. Wallace TW, Berger JS, Wang A, *et al.* Impact of left ventricular dysfunction on hospital mortality among patients undergoing elective percutaneous coronary intervention. *Am J Cardiol* 2009; **103**:355–60.

5. Singh M, Rihal CS, Lennon RJ, *et al.* Bedside estimation of risk from percutaneous coronary intervention: the new Mayo Clinic risk scores. *Mayo ClinProc* 2007; **82**:701–8.
6. Chowdhary S, Ivanov J, Mackie K, *et al.* The Toronto score for in-hospital mortality after percutaneous coronary interventions. *Am Heart J* 2009; **157**:156–63.
7. Alderman EL, Fisher LD, Litwin P, *et al.* Results of coronary artery surgery in patients with poor left ventricular function (CASS). *Circulation* 1983; **68**:785–95.
8. van Daele ME, Sutherland GR, Mitchell MM, *et al.* Do changes in pulmonary capillary wedge pressure adequately reflect myocardial ischemia during anesthesia? A correlative preoperative hemodynamic, electrocardiographic, and transesophageal echocardiographic study. *Circulation* 1990; **81**:865–71.
9. Porto I, Selvanayagam JB, Van Gaal WJ, *et al.* Plaque volume and occurrence and location of periprocedural myocardial necrosis after percutaneous coronary intervention: insights from delayed-enhancement magnetic resonance imaging, thrombolysis in myocardial infarction myocardial perfusion grade analysis, and intravascular ultrasound. *Circulation* 2006; **114**:662–9.
10. Harken DE. Presentation at the International College of Cardiology, Brussels, Belgium 1958.
11. Kern MJ, Aguirre F, Bach R, *et al.* Augmentation of coronary blood flow by intra-aortic balloon pumping in patients after coronary angioplasty. *Circulation* 1993; **87**:500–11.
12. Williams DO, Korr KS, Gewirtz H, *et al.* The effect of intraaortic balloon counterpulsation on regional myocardial blood flow and oxygen consumption in the presence of coronary artery stenosis in patients with unstable angina. *Circulation* 1982; **66**:593–7.
13. Bates ER, Topol EJ. Limitations of thrombolytic therapy for acute myocardial infarction complicated by congestive heart failure and cardiogenic shock. *J Am Coll Cardiol* 1991; **18**:1077–84.
14. Sanborn TA, Sleeper LA, Bates ER, *et al.* Impact of thrombolysis, intra-aortic balloon pump counterpulsation, and their combination in cardiogenic shock complicating acute myocardial infarction: a report from the SHOCK Trial Registry. SHould we emergently revascularize Occluded Coronaries for cardiogenic shocK? *J Am Coll Cardiol* 2000; **36**:1123–9.
15. Barron HV, Every NR, Parsons LS, *et al.* The use of intra-aortic balloon counterpulsation in patients with cardiogenic shock complicating acute myocardial infarction: data from the National Registry of Myocardial Infarction 2. *Am Heart J* 2001; **141**:933–9.
16. Sjauw KD, Engstrom AE, Vis MM, *et al.* A systematic review and meta-analysis of intra-aortic balloon pump therapy in ST-elevation myocardial infarction: should we change the guidelines? *Eur Heart J* 2009; **30**:459–68.
17. Antman EM, Anbe DT, Armstrong PW, *et al.* ACC/AHA guidelines for the management of patients with ST-elevation myocardial infarction: a report of the American College of Cardiology/American Heart Association Task Force on Practice Guidelines (Committee to Revise the 1999 Guidelines for the Management of Patients with Acute Myocardial Infarction). *Circulation* 2004; **110**:e82–292.
18. Brodie BR, Stuckey TD, Hansen C, *et al.* Intra-aortic balloon counterpulsation before primary percutaneous transluminal coronary angioplasty reduces catheterization laboratory events in high-risk patients with acute myocardial infarction. *Am J Cardiol* 1999; **84**:18–23.
19. Briguori C, Sarais C, Pagnotta P, *et al.* Elective versus provisional intra-aortic balloon pumping in high-risk percutaneous transluminal coronary angioplasty. *Am Heart J* 2003; **145**:700–7.
20. Mishra S, Chu WW, Torguson R, *et al.* Role of prophylactic intra-aortic balloon pump in high-risk patients undergoing percutaneous coronary intervention. *Am J Cardiol* 2006; **98**:608–12.
21. Smith SC, Jr, Feldman TE, Hirshfeld JW, Jr, *et al.* ACC/AHA/SCAI 2005 guideline update for percutaneous coronary intervention: a report of the American College of Cardiology/American Heart Association Task Force on Practice Guidelines (ACC/AHA/SCAI Writing Committee to Update the 2001 Guidelines for Percutaneous Coronary Intervention). *J Am Coll Cardiol* 2006; **47**:e1–121.
22. Ferguson JJ, III, Cohen M, Freedman RJ, Jr, *et al.* The current practice of intra-aortic balloon counterpulsation: results from the Benchmark Registry. *J Am Coll Cardiol* 2001; **38**:1456–62.
23. Perera D, Stables RH, Booth J, Thomas M, Redwood S. The Balloon pump-assisted Coronary Intervention Study (BCIS-1): Rationale and Design. *Am Heart J* 2009; **158**:910–16.
24. Redwood S. Balloon pump assisted Coronary Intervention Study (BCIS-1). *Presentation at Transcatheter Cardiovascular Therapeutics Conference, San Francisco* 2009.
25. Valgimigli M, Steendijk P, Sianos G, *et al.* Left ventricular unloading and concomitant total cardiac output increase by the use of percutaneous Impella Recover LP 2.5 assist device during high-risk coronary intervention. *Catheter Cardiovasc Interv* 2005; **65**:263–7.
26. Remmelink M, Sjauw KD, Henriques JP, *et al.* Effects of left ventricular unloading by Impella recover LP2.5 on coronary hemodynamics. *Catheter Cardiovasc Interv* 2007; **70**:532–7.
27. Seyfarth M, Sibbing D, Bauer I, *et al.* A randomized clinical trial to evaluate the safety and efficacy of a percutaneous left ventricular assist device versus intra-aortic balloon pumping for treatment of cardiogenic shock caused by myocardial infarction. *J Am Coll Cardiol* 2008; **52**:1584–8.
28. Dixon SR, Henriques JP, Mauri L, *et al.* A prospective feasibility trial investigating the use of the Impella 2.5 system in patients undergoing high-risk percutaneous coronary intervention (The PROTECT I Trial): initial U.S. experience. *JACC Cardiovasc Interv* 2009; **2**:91–6.

29. Vranckx P, Schultz CJ, Valgimigli M, *et al.* Assisted circulation using the TandemHeart® during very high-risk PCI of the unprotected left main coronary artery in patients declined for CABG. *Catheter Cardiovasc Interv* 2009; **74**(2):302–10.
30. Rahimtoola SH. Coronary bypass surgery for chronic angina –1981. A perspective. *Circulation* 1982; **65**:225–41.
31. Rahimtoola SH. The hibernating myocardium. *Am Heart J* 1989; **117**:211–21.
32. Bax JJ, Visser FC, Poldermans D, *et al.* Time course of functional recovery of stunned and hibernating segments after surgical revascularization. *Circulation* 2001; **104**:I314–I318.
33. Allman KC, Shaw LJ, Hachamovitch R, *et al.* Myocardial viability testing and impact of revascularization on prognosis in patients with coronary artery disease and left ventricular dysfunction: a meta-analysis. *J Am Coll Cardiol* 2002; **39**:1151–8.
34. Carluccio E, Biagioli P, Alunni G, *et al.* Patients with hibernating myocardium show altered left ventricular volumes and shape, which revert after revascularization: evidence that dyssynergy might directly induce cardiac remodeling. *J Am Coll Cardiol* 2006; **47**:969–77.
35. Dispersyn GD, Borgers M, Flameng W. Apoptosis in chronic hibernating myocardium: sleeping to death? *Cardiovasc Res* 2000; **45**:696–703.
36. Lloyd-Jones DM, Larson MG, Leip EP, *et al.* Lifetime risk for developing congestive heart failure: the Framingham Heart Study. *Circulation* 2002; **106**:3068–72.
37. Adams KF, Jr, Fonarow GC, Emerman CL, *et al.* Characteristics and outcomes of patients hospitalized for heart failure in the United States: rationale, design, and preliminary observations from the first 100,000 cases in the Acute Decompensated Heart Failure National Registry (ADHERE). *Am Heart J* 2005; **149**:209–16.
38. Gheorghiade M, Sopko G, De Luca L, *et al.* Navigating the crossroads of coronary artery disease and heart failure. *Circulation* 2006; **114**:1202–13.
39. Knuuti J, Schelbert HR, Bax JJ. The need for standardisation of cardiac FDG PET imaging in the evaluation of myocardial viability in patients with chronic ischaemic left ventricular dysfunction. *Eur J Nucl Med Mol Imaging* 2002; **29**:1257–66.
40. Knuesel PR, Nanz D, Wyss C, *et al.* Characterization of dysfunctional myocardium by positron emission tomography and magnetic resonance: relation to functional outcome after revascularization. *Circulation* 2003; **108**:1095–100.
41. Toda K, Mackenzie K, Mehra MR, *et al.* Revascularization in severe ventricular dysfunction (15% < OR = LVEF < OR = 30%): a comparison of bypass grafting and percutaneous intervention. *Ann Thorac Surg* 2002; **74**:2082–7.
42. O'Connor CM, Velazquez EJ, Gardner LH, *et al.* Comparison of coronary artery bypass grafting versus medical therapy on long-term outcome in patients with ischemic cardiomyopathy (a 25-year experience from the Duke Cardiovascular Disease Databank). *Am J Cardiol* 2002; **90**:101–7.
43. Chareonthaitawee P, Gersh BJ, Araoz PA, *et al.* Revascularization in severe left ventricular dysfunction: the role of viability testing. *J Am Coll Cardiol* 2005; **46**:567–74.
44. Eagle KA, Guyton RA, Davidoff R, *et al.* ACC/AHA 2004 guideline update for coronary artery bypass graft surgery: a report of the American College of Cardiology/American Heart Association Task Force on Practice Guidelines (Committee to Update the 1999 Guidelines for Coronary Artery Bypass Graft Surgery). *Circulation* 2004; **110**: e340–e437.
45. Baker DW, Jones R, Hodges J, *et al.* Management of heart failure. III. The role of revascularization in the treatment of patients with moderate or severe left ventricular systolic dysfunction. *JAMA* 1994; **272**:1528–34.
46. Kennedy JW, Kaiser GC, Fisher LD, *et al.* Clinical and angiographic predictors of operative mortality from the collaborative study in coronary artery surgery (CASS). *Circulation* 1981; **63**:793–802.
47. Stahle E, Bergstrom R, Edlund B, *et al.* Influence of left ventricular function on survival after coronary artery bypass grafting. *Ann Thorac Surg* 1997; **64**:437–44.
48. Serruys PW, Unger F, Sousa JE, *et al.* Comparison of coronary-artery bypass surgery and stenting for the treatment of multivessel disease. *N Engl J Med* 2001; **344**:1117–24.
49. Rodriguez A, Bernardi V, Navia J, *et al.* Argentine Randomized Study: Coronary Angioplasty with Stenting versus Coronary Bypass Surgery in patients with Multiple-Vessel Disease (ERACI II): 30-day and one-year follow-up results. ERACI II Investigators. *J Am Coll Cardiol* 2001; **37**:51–8.
50. Hueb W, Soares PR, Gersh BJ, *et al.* The medicine, angioplasty, or surgery study (MASS-II): a randomized, controlled clinical trial of three therapeutic strategies for multivessel coronary artery disease: one-year results. *J Am Coll Cardiol* 2004; **43**:1743–51.
51. Serruys PW, Morice MC, Kappetein AP, *et al.* Percutaneous coronary intervention versus coronary-artery bypass grafting for severe coronary artery disease. *N Engl J Med* 2009; **360**:961–72.
52. Hlatky MA, Boothroyd DB, Bravata DM, *et al.* Coronary artery bypass surgery compared with percutaneous coronary interventions for multivessel disease: a collaborative analysis of individual patient data from ten randomised trials. *Lancet* 2009; **373**:1190–7.
53. O'Keefe JH, Jr, Allan JJ, McCallister BD, *et al.* Angioplasty versus bypass surgery for multivessel coronary artery disease with left ventricular ejection fraction < or = 40%. *Am J Cardiol* 1993; **71**:897–901.
54. Sedlis SP, Ramanathan KB, Morrison DA, *et al.* Outcome of percutaneous coronary intervention versus coronary bypass grafting for patients with low left ventricular ejection fractions, unstable angina pectoris, and risk factors for adverse outcomes with bypass (the AWESOME

Randomized Trial and Registry). *Am J Cardiol* 2004; **94**:118–20.

55. Gioia G, Matthai W, Benassi A, *et al.* Improved survival with drug-eluting stent implantation in comparison with bare metal stent in patients with severe left ventricular dysfunction. *Catheter Cardiovasc Interv* 2006; **68**:392–8.
56. Gioia G, Matthai W, Gillin K, *et al.* Revascularization in severe left ventricular dysfunction: outcome comparison of drug-eluting stent implantation versus coronary artery by-pass grafting. *Catheter Cardiovasc Interv* 2007; **70**: 26–33.
57. Jones RH, Velazquez EJ, Michler RE, *et al.* Coronary bypass surgery with or without surgical ventricular reconstruction. *N Engl J Med* 2009; **360**:1705–17.
58. Hunt SA, Abraham WT, Chin MH, *et al.* 2009 Focused update incorporated into the ACC/AHA 2005 Guidelines for the Diagnosis and Management of Heart Failure in Adults A Report of the American College of Cardiology Foundation/American Heart Association Task Force on Practice Guidelines Developed in Collaboration With the International Society for Heart and Lung Transplantation. *J Am Coll Cardiol* 2009; **53**:e1–e90.
59. Flaherty JD, Rossi JS, Fonarow GC, *et al.* Influence of coronary angiography on the utilization of therapies in patients with acute heart failure syndromes: findings from Organized Program to Initiate Lifesaving Treatment in Hospitalized Patients with Heart Failure (OPTIMIZE-HF). *Am Heart J* 2009; **157**:1018–25.
60. Beanlands RS, Hendry PJ, Masters RG, *et al.* Delay in revascularization is associated with increased mortality rate in patients with severe left ventricular dysfunction and viable myocardium on fluorine 18-fluorodeoxyglucose positron emission tomography imaging. *Circulation* 1998; **98**:II51–II56.
61. Bax JJ, Schinkel AF, Boersma E, *et al.* Early versus delayed revascularization in patients with ischemic cardiomyopathy and substantial viability: impact on outcome. *Circulation* 2003; **108**(Suppl 1):II39–II42.

SECTION 4

Percutaneous coronary intervention by lesion and patient subsets

CHAPTER 18

Coronary bifurcation stenting: state of the art

Yves Louvard and Thierry Lefèvre

Background

The difference between a coronary bifurcation lesion and an ordinary lesion lies in the presence of a side branch (SB). Such branches are particularly instrumental in the development of atheroma because of local blood flow patterns and are also a predictive factor of peri-procedural myocardial infarction (MI) when percutaneous coronary angioplasty (PCI) is performed.

The clinical importance of a SB depends on its diameter which is strongly correlated with its flow and the muscular mass that it vascularizes; the diameter of the SB, main branch (MB), and of proximal segment of the MB are indeed interdependent as evidenced by Murray's law. Therefore, a coronary bifurcation should be divided into three segments, each with its own reference diameter.

Before the advent of coronary stenting, and later with bare-metal stents (BMS), PCI of coronary bifurcation lesions was associated with a lower success rate, a higher risk of complications, and a higher restenosis rate compared to non-bifurcation lesions. Although the use of drug-eluting stents (DES) has resulted in reduced restenosis rates and reintervention, coronary bifurcation lesions remain a higher risk setting especially when the bifurcation is proximal.

Over the past few years, the subject of many debates has been the identification of optimal BMS or DES strategies for improving angiographic success, reducing the risk of peri-procedural complications, and decreasing the rate of restenosis and reintervention. The vast majority of registry studies (BMS and DES) and randomized studies (DES) have demonstrated that the systematic stenting of both branches is not superior to the strategy of 'provisional side-branch stenting'. Indications for systematic double stenting as well as the type of strategy to be implemented are still being debated because of heterogeneous studies with respect to lesion type, and of the multiplicity of inadequately described or applied techniques.

Adapting the technique to the lesion, as reported by several recent randomized studies, is complicated by the emergence of a new prognostic factor, namely the angle or angles of the bifurcation, which are still very difficult to measure precisely.

Various types of 'dedicated' stents specifically designed for bifurcation lesions have been included in debates about the adaptation of the technique (or stent) to the type of bifurcation lesion to be treated.

Finally, stenting of bifurcation lesions has been shown to be a risk factor of acute, late, or very late stent thrombosis and the influence of the technique or its imperfect implementation, has not been adequately assessed.

The purpose of the present chapter is to provide an overview of coronary bifurcation lesions and their current treatment and address the fundamental as well as practical issues inherent in this setting.

Fundamental aspects

Coronary trees, as well as other arborescences (tree-like patterns) in humans, trees, rivers, and in the natural world in general, are objects of fractal geometry, with a self replicating asymmetric branching[1–3]. Coronary trees are constructed according to the hypothesis of minimum energy cost[4–5]. The cumulated cross sectional area and the velocity are constant in this 'distributive' part of the vessel. There is a linear relationship between vessel diameter and flow in all segments, and between vessel diameter in a given segment and the vascular volume of its distribution area (crown). There is also a linear relationship between the diameter of a vessel and the muscular mass vascularized by this vessel, which allows the definition of an infarction index for each branch in relation to its diameter[6,7]. In practical terms, this means that the diameter and length of a vessel may be used to determine its physiological, physiopathological, and clinical importance and to identify the main distal segment of a bifurcation and the SB.

For each asymmetric branching, the diameter (D) of the proximal segment and both distal segments are defined by Murray's law: D prox. main^3 = D dist. main^3 + D side branch^3[4]. This formula has been simplified after an IVUS study in humans by Finet and colleagues as follows: D prox. main = (D dist. main + D side branch) × 0.678[8]. The practical consequences of this branching law are the following:

- A bifurcation has no MB or SB but is comprised of three segments
- The diameter of a coronary artery tapers towards the distal end due to its branching nature. The diameter is constant between two bifurcations. Consequently, there is no continuous linear reference function in the MB. Each segment has its own reference function
- Conventional QCA computer programs are not suitable for coronary bifurcations because they underestimate the reference diameter of the main proximal segment and overestimate the reference diameter of the main distal segment. The ostium of the side branch may be over- or underestimated according to the method used[9]
- In practice, a stent selected for the main vessel on the basis of the distal segment diameter is too small for the proximal segment and vice versa.

In a coronary bifurcation the flow is pulsatile (anterograde during diastole and inverted during systole) and no longer linear, with a parabolic transversal speed profile. The flow remains linear and rapid on each side of the carena (flow divider), but it is turbulent and slow along the walls opposite the carena[10]. Endothelial shear stress (ESS) is low or oscillatory in areas with low velocity turbulent flow. A negative correlation was found between intimal thickness and ESS[11]. A low ESS is a major stimulus of atherogenesis, the lower it is, the more likely it is to generate high-risk plaque, thinning of the fibrous plaque, fragmentation of the inner elastic layer, inflammation, and remodelling which may create new areas of low ESS[11].

The distribution of low ESS values in the coronary tree is in accordance with the frequent localization of atherosclerosis lesions[11]. Atherosclerosis occurs predominantly in the vicinity of bifurcations. Different types of involvement of coronary bifurcations by atherosclerosis have been described (Fig. 18.1). Carinal involvement is extremely unusual[12]. As a consequence, it is very unlikely that the deterioration of the SB ostium subsequent to the stenting of the MB across the SB is a result of the often reported plaque shifting or snow-plough phenomenon. It should rather be attributed to the shifting of the carena towards the SB caused by the stent[13,14].

How shall we define, designate, measure, and classify coronary bifurcation lesions and treatments?

Numerous definitions of coronary bifurcation lesions have been proposed. The European Bifurcation Club (EBC)[15] has suggested the following definition: 'a bifurcation lesion is a coronary artery narrowing occurring adjacent to, and/or involving the origin of a significant SB'. 'A significant SB is a branch that you do not want to lose in the global context of a particular patient (symptoms, location of ischaemia, branch responsible for symptoms of ischaemia, viability, collateralizing vessel, left ventricular function…)'. Post PCI myonecrosis, defined as three times the maximal normal value of CK-MB according to the European Society of Cardiology (ESC) and American College of Cardiology (ACC) guidelines[16] is an established factor of late mortality, especially in the presence of moderate (>5×) to significant (>8–10×) elevation. One of the established causes of myonecrosis is the occlusion of the SB. In the NIRVANA study[20], MI is reported in 40% of SB occlusion instances.

The elevation of biomarkers after PCI has been shown to be associated with documented necrosis by MRI assessment[21] and more recently it has been demonstrated that troponin elevation without CK-MB elevation is a predictive factor of long-term mortality[21]. Given the linear relationship between the vascularized muscular mass and the artery diameter in each vessel, we should be able to improve the definition of coronary bifurcation lesions by determining the diameter of arteries in which occlusion would have long-term clinical consequences.

The classification of bifurcation lesions is indispensable for several reasons

Some lesion morphologies carry a reduced clinical risk. Certain operators advocate the selection of a particular stenting technique adapted to a given morphology.

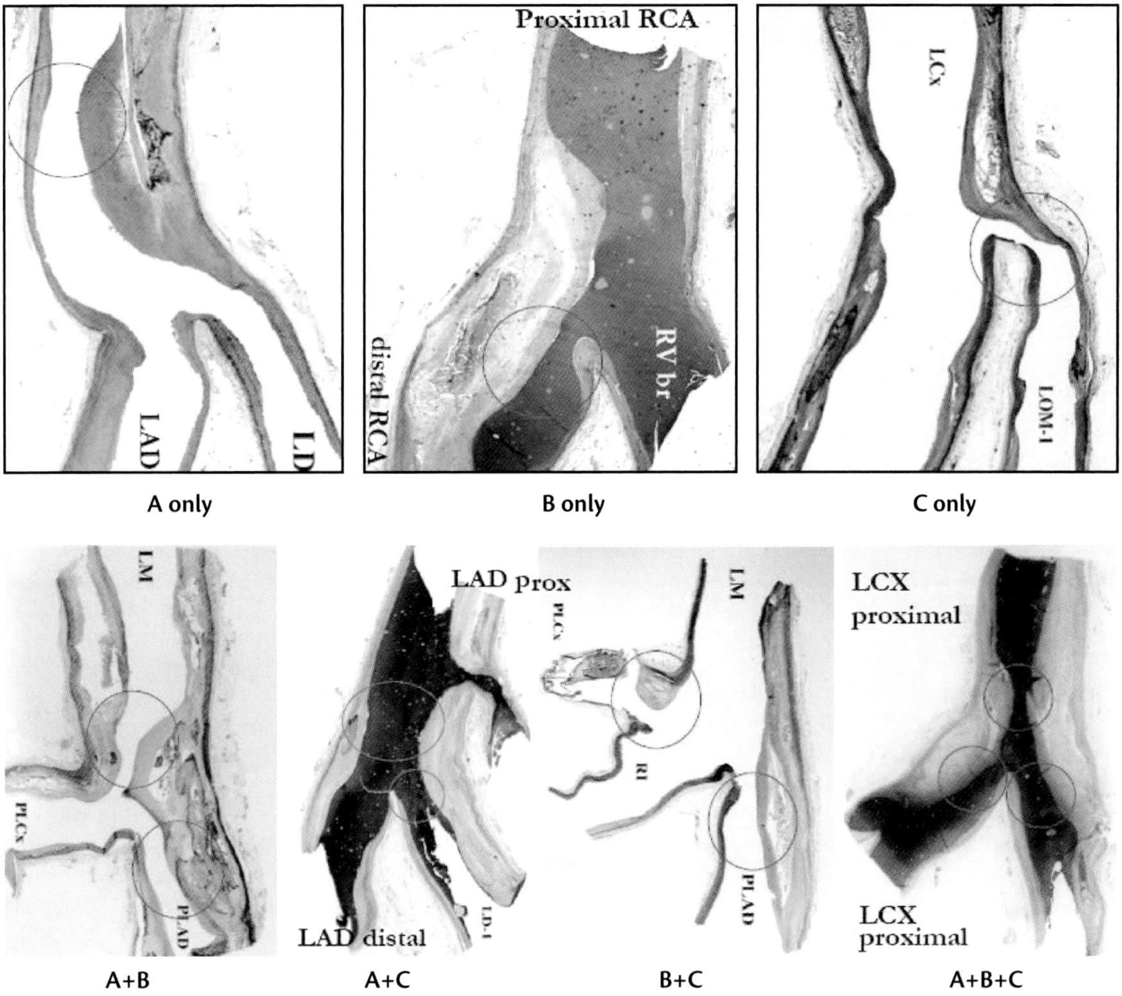

Fig. 18.1 Anatomopathologic types of involvement of coronary bifurcations by atherosclerosis presented by Renu Virmani (European Bifurcation Club, Rome, September 2006, http://www.bifurc.net). Types are remarkably similar to the Medina angiographic classification without significant carena disease. Adapted from R. Virmani.

The pattern of clinical and angiographic follow-up varies according to the lesion. To date, numerous classifications of coronary bifurcation lesions have been proposed(23–31). In 2005, the EBC recommended the adoption of the Medina classification (Fig. 18.2)(32), which does not need to be memorized, provided it is used on the basis of quantitative coronary angiography (QCA). Attempts at improving this definition, by including the potential presence of calcifications, the length of the SB lesion, or even the angle between two distal branches, have been discontinued in order to keep the original classification simple. Furthermore, this would have transformed numerically continuous data into symbols based on mere visual assessment. In the presence of trifurcations, one more comma and a digit can be added by order of importance of the vessels.

Why and how should a bifurcation lesion be 'named'(15)

In addition to localizing a lesion in the coronary tree, it is necessary to determine which distal branch is the main branch in order to establish the Medina classification and describe the technique used adequately. A nosological classification is inappropriate because although diagonal

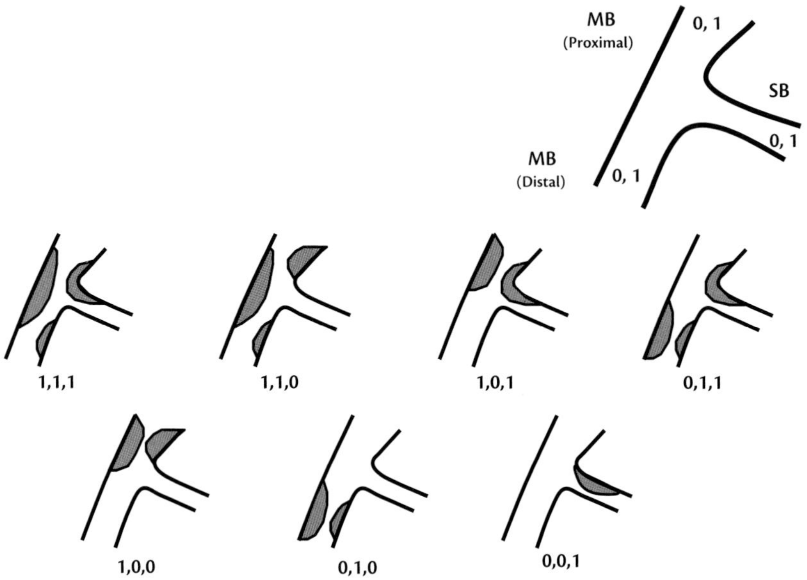

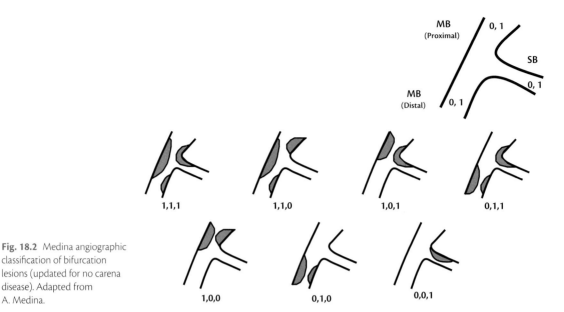

Fig. 18.2 Medina angiographic classification of bifurcation lesions (updated for no carena disease). Adapted from A. Medina.

and septal branches are usually secondary branches, this is not always the case for marginal branches and the posterolateral branch (PLA) of the distal right coronary artery. In theory, the distal MB is the largest/longest segment. However, the operator may run counter to this rule in patients with a history of MI, coronary artery bypass grafting (CABG), or coronary artery collateralization.

The EBC has suggested the designation of bifurcations using the same notation as the Medina classification: abbreviated name of the proximal main branch, comma, abbreviated name of the distal main branch, comma, abbreviated name of the side branch. In order to describe a trifurcation, a name and a comma may be added as in the Medina classification (Fig. 18.3).

Classification of coronary bifurcation treatment techniques

A widely adopted classification may facilitate the description and understanding of complex techniques; such an undertaking, however, represents a considerable challenge. Several classifications have been proposed. The MADS classification[(15)] suggested by the EBC in 2007 is based on the strategy of stent deployment and final placement (Fig. 18.4). All techniques included in the classification have been reported or presented, but the classification remains open. Inverted techniques[(15)] consist of stenting the bifurcation whilst considering the SB (the smallest branch) as the distal MB (Fig. 18.5). The chronological classification of sequential stent placement is not sufficient to define a technique adequately. The preparation of the lesion, guide wire protection of the branch, and successive final kissing inflations may have a considerable impact on acute as well as longer-term outcome[(33)]. It would be possible to design an e-CRF in which all procedural manoeuvres would be chronologically recorded in order to constitute a posteriori homogeneous group[(15)]. Nevertheless, the MADS classification allows the recording of the operator's intended strategy at the beginning of the procedure and of the actual strategy used upon completion of the procedure.

Angiographic analysis of bifurcations

The angiographic analysis is both the source of the Medina classification and its indispensable complement. New computer programs[(34,35)] allow the construction of reference diameters for the three segments of the bifurcation according to Murray's law. This enables the operator to perform an accurate analysis of the degree of stenosis before and after the stenting procedure and during the follow-up period. The construction of the SB reference function is not continuous to the proximal MB. Consequently, the SB is not constructed from its ostium, thus eliminating a potential underestimation of the SB lesion attributable to an increasing reference function. This analysis can be performed on-line and may greatly assist the operator in the selection of stents suitable for certain technical

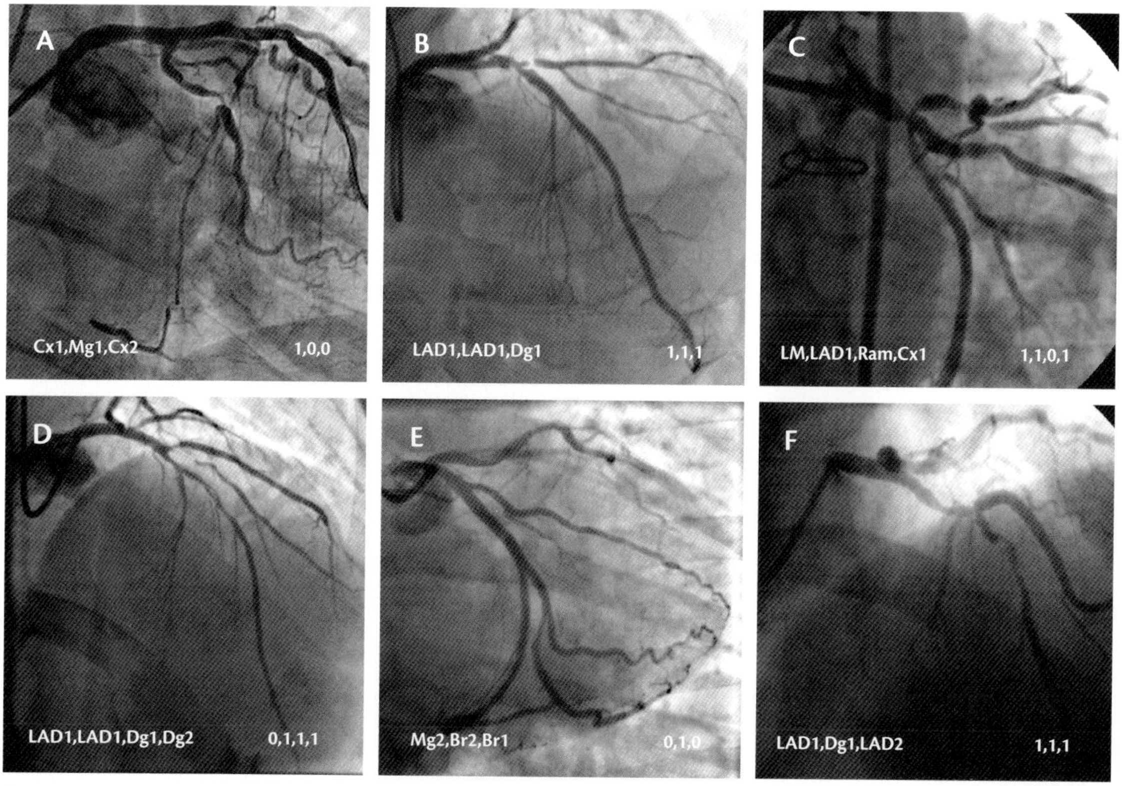

Fig. 18.3 How to name a bifurcation lesion? Names adapted from medina classification: A) the mid circumflex artery is very small but fills the RCA, this lesion is, therefore, a bifurcation lesion, marginal branch is clearly the main distal vessel. B) Both main proximal and main distal vessels are LAD 1, 1st diagonal is the SB. C) Name of a LM trifurcation: LM is the proximal main vessel, the distal vessels are in decreasing order of importance, note that the Ramus is not stenosed. D) Two diagonal branches are involved in this proximal-mid LAD, even if this is not a real bifurcation, they are listed in decreasing order of importance. E) This bifurcation is situated on the second marginal branch. F) In this case the large diagonal branch was considered more important than the distal LAD, hence the name.

strategies. These computer programs allow the measurement of the lesion length (MB and SB). They also permit analysis and multi-segment reporting as recommended by the EBC[36]. In addition to in-stent analysis, this includes the analysis of the edges in each of the three bifurcation segments as well as the accurate analysis of areas specific to bifurcation such as the ostia of the two distal branches (gap or overlapping), the overlapping or crush areas of stents (Fig. 18.6). The influence of bifurcation angles on the short- and mid-term outcome of certain stenting techniques has given rise to a new quantitative angiographic analysis method[37]. This method allows reliable measurement of the bifurcation angles as well as assessment of their potential modification after stent placement. Angle A (access) is the angle between the proximal MB and the SB and defines the difficulty of accessing the SB. Angle B (between) is the angle between the two distal branches, its acuteness is commensurate with the risk of SB occlusion during stent placement across the MB due to the carena displacement phenomenon[13,14].

Bench testing

The simulated deployment of stents in bench tests provided very valuable information for stenting in patients. The first bench tests consisted of silicon elements with bifurcations of variable angles regardless of the rules of branching. Stent deployment, guide wire manoeuvres, or balloon inflations carried out during bench test evaluation were filmed or photographed.

The data collected were only of a qualitative nature[38], namely, distortion of the MB stent during balloon inflation towards the SB[39,40] and feasibility of stenting both branches (MB and SB ostium) using only the MB stent.

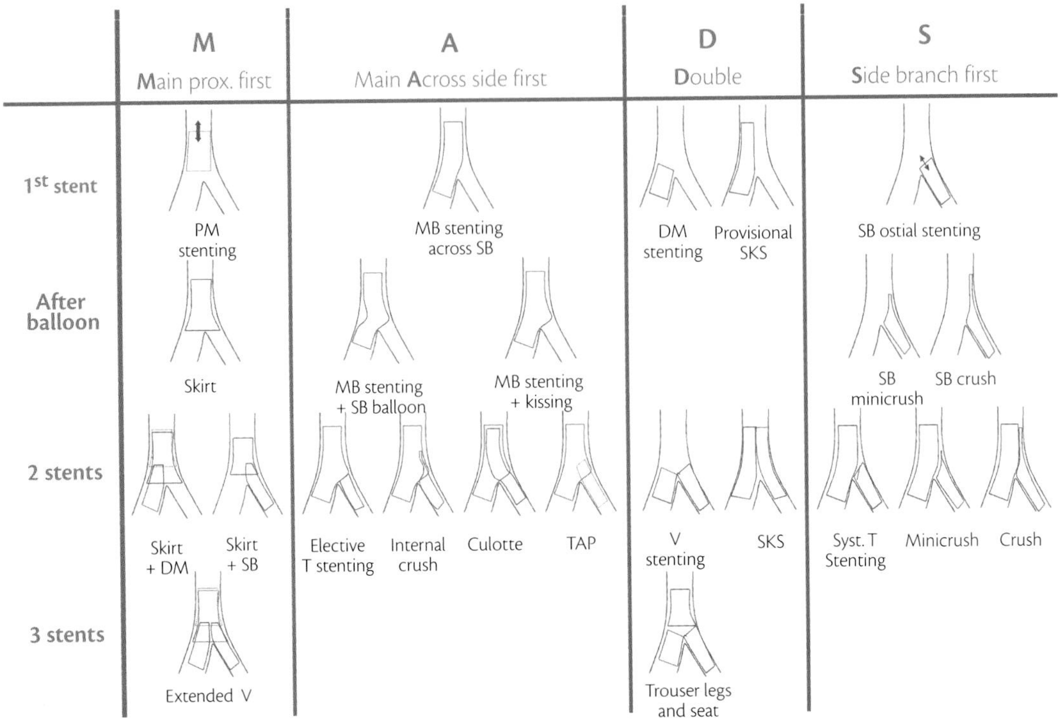

Fig. 18.4 MADS classification of stenting techniques for bifurcation lesions. All these techniques have been published or reported. New names are proposed to avoid confusion. The classification is based on strategy, especially on implantation of the first stent, and on final stent positions. This is not an exhaustive description of all the techniques which include also the use of wires, single balloon inflation, and kissing balloon techniques.

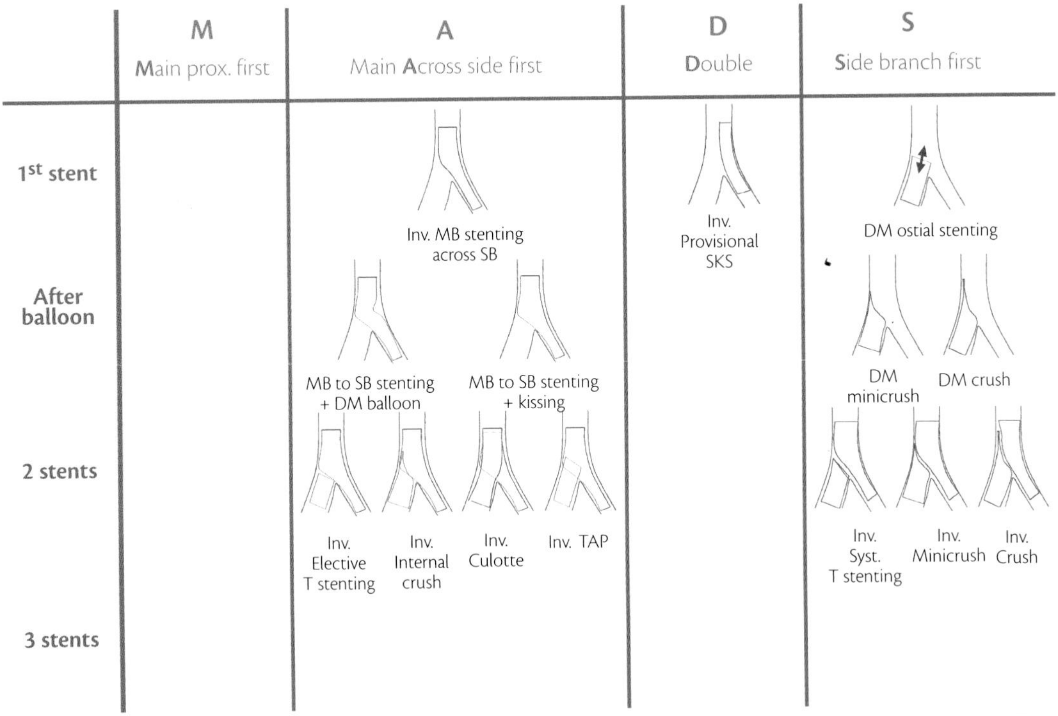

Fig. 18.5 MADS classification of inverted techniques.

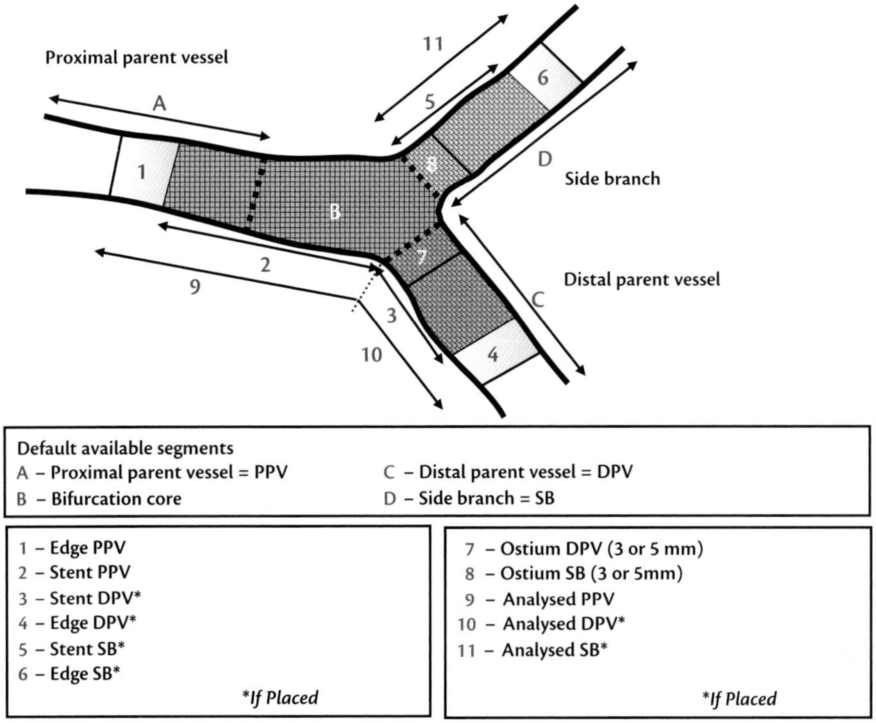

Fig. 18.6 Bifurcation QCA edge segment analysis with the new definition of 3 segments (from A. Lansky).

Bench testing has gradually become more sophisticated, following the fractal nature of bifurcations, and sometimes tri-dimensional(41). Their configuration can be digitalized following micro CT imaging(41). Today, the images obtained may be viewed under various angles or fragmented. Stent deployment and stent cell area may be measured. These bench studies can be used as a valuable learning and teaching tool and for comparison with the difficulties encountered and the results obtained in patients.

Virtual reality software may also provide coronary tree(42) and stent deployment(43) models and enable the measurement of cell size in various situations. Technical strategies can also be taught by means of virtual procedures.

Bifurcation stenting techniques and results

Historical aspects

Balloon angioplasty of bifurcation lesions was attempted in the 1980s with a low success rate and a high complication and restenosis rate despite early introduction of the kissing balloon technique. The use of directional or rotational atherectomy slightly improved the success rate without reducing the complication and restenosis rates. The advent of the initial bare stents, at first hand crimped(44) and then pre-mounted on a balloon, was soon followed by the description of numerous deployment techniques(45–51) which were indexed and classified(52,53). The most commonly implemented strategies were the implantation of a stent first in the SB and then in the MB across the SB (the so called planned T-stenting technique)(46), stenting of the two distal branches with overlapping stents into the proximal branch (culotte)(50), or simultaneous stent placement in the ostium of the two distal branches by applying the V-stenting technique(45). An alternative T-stenting strategy was the implantation of a stent in the MB across the SB followed by the placement of a second stent in the ostium of the SB.

The opening of a cell of the MB stent towards the SB to allow SB stenting led to the new concept that SB stenting could be provisional(54). Conversely, ostial restenosis of the SB was often associated with a gap; this gave rise to the modified T-stenting technique(55), and later the crush technique(56). In parallel, *in vitro* stent deployment experiments showed that the opening of a cell stent was likely to cause severe stent distortion(57), warranting the systematic simultaneous inflation of two balloons (kissing balloon inflation)(53) in order to correct stent deformation. The question as to whether or not we should perform systematic final kissing balloon inflation is still being debated. The Nordic IV will probably provide an answer to this question.

The use of BMS was associated with acute results inferior to those achieved in non-bifurcated lesions and with high restenosis and reintervention rates, especially with 'metallic' strategies such as the culotte technique(59,60). Technical comparisons involved exclusively single versus double stenting in various lesion types with heterogeneous and often inadequately described techniques in non-randomized, retrospective studies without or with incomplete angiographic follow-up. None of these studies has demonstrated the benefit of using a systematic double stenting technique(61–64).

The advent of DES was associated with a clear reduction of the restenosis rate in bifurcation lesions, which encouraged the operators to carry out extensive bifurcation stenting and implement new technical strategies such as crush, extended V stenting, simultaneous kissing stent. . .(56,66,67), thus refuelling the debate of single versus double stenting. The randomized studies performed in heterogeneous lesion subsets, mainly with the Cypher® stent, have confirmed the non-superiority of the systematic double stenting strategy over provisional(68–75) SB stenting. Specific angiographic settings where double stenting may provide superior results are currently being examined in randomized studies using the new classification of bifurcation lesions(32) and carrying out intention-to treat analysis of head-to-head comparison of well described techniques with a single stent.

The strategy of stenting the distal left main followed a similar path, though a little later. Although no randomized studies were performed, the accumulation of registry data has shown that systematic double stenting does not provide superior results over simple procedures.

Over the past few years, 'dedicated' stents have been specifically designed for bifurcation lesions in order to allow the simple and rapid implementation of provisional SB stenting with permanent access to the SB. However, the technical difficulties have not been overcome and the benefit of these dedicated stents has not been established. Only one randomized study has been conducted with BMS(71). A few new-generation dedicated stents have been implanted using new strategies with interesting preliminary results but randomized studies are needed.

Stenting of the main branch only or stenting of both branches with BMS?

There have been a number of comparative, non-randomized studies of BMS implanted with simple or complex techniques, as well as registries involving a specific technique or strategy. Complex techniques are essentially T stenting, modified T stenting, or culotte. Comparisons including angiographic and clinical follow-up (Fig. 18.7) have not shown any benefit in terms of acute events for the complex two-stent techniques, and have often shown a higher rate of restenosis in the SB. A higher in-hospital MACE rate was associated with the double stenting strategy. It has been suggested that this event rate was related to the fact that most of the time these comparative registries were not assessed by intent-to-treat analysis.

This means that certain patients received a stent in the SB because of suboptimal results or complications, and others did not receive a stent in the SB because of technical procedural failure. In complex settings, the impact of the technique used was evidenced in several series. In the study by Al Suwaidi, the use of the culotte technique in a few complex cases seems to account for the poor results associated with the double stenting strategy(62). Two important registries have confirmed the poor mid-term outcome of the culotte technique with BMS(60,72).

Stenting of the main branch only or stenting of both branches with DES

Since the advent of DES, a number of registries and non-randomized comparative studies have been carried out in addition to randomized studies comparing simple with complex strategies. Most of these studies have flaws; indeed they were conducted in non-selected populations of patients with simple and complex coronary bifurcation disease, without intent-to-treat analysis (the

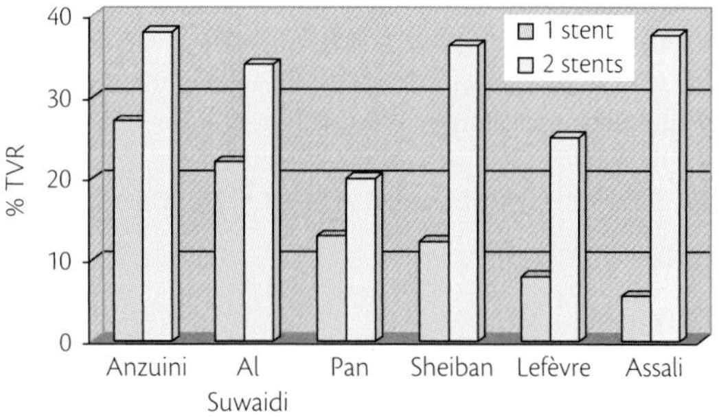

Fig. 18.7 Two BMS are not better than one: TVR rates after bifurcation stenting with BMS in the literature.

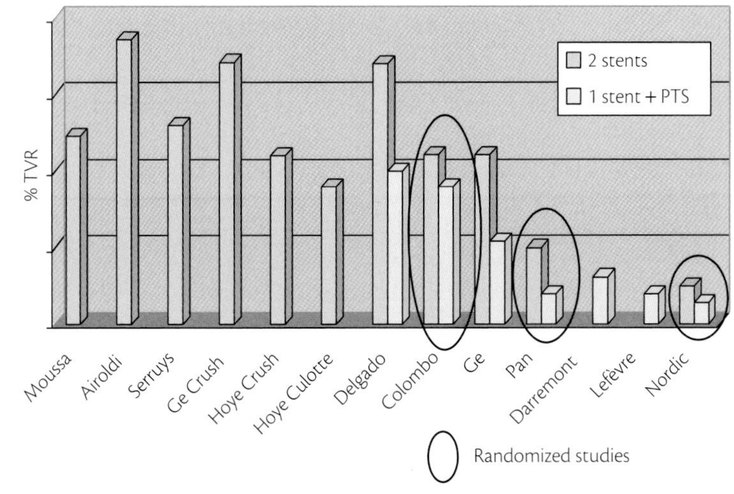

Fig. 18.8 Two DES are not better than one (clinical follow up): TVR rates after bifurcation stenting with DES in the literature.

technical failure rate was not reported). Certain randomized studies had very small patient samples[73] or an unacceptable percentage of crossover[74]. Overall, the benefit of systematic stent placement in the SB was not demonstrated (Figs. 18.8 and 18.9). These results corroborate the provisional SB stenting strategy starting with stent implantation in the MB and potentially followed by stenting of the SB if required.

The outcome of two large randomized studies has reinforced this strategy. One of these studies, the Nordic study, has already been published[68] and the other has been reported at the TCT meeting in 2008 (BBC ONE). In the Nordic study, 413 patients presenting with unspecified bifurcation lesions were randomized to receive either a Cypher Select® stent in the MB across the SB with possible crossover to SB stenting in cases of TIMI 0 flow after balloon inflation (in order to achieve TIMI >2), or to systematic double stenting treatment by means of the crush, culotte, or any other technique used at the operator's discretion. In instances when SB stenting was performed, final kissing balloon inflation was recommended. Six-month clinical outcome did not show any differences in terms of overall or cardiac mortality, MI, target vessel revascularization (TVR), or stent thrombosis. QCA showed a paradoxical result in the SB ostium, i.e. a higher late loss in recipients of DES compared to patients treated with balloon angioplasty alone, which corroborated the results reported in SIRIUS bifurcation[74]. The acute results showed, however, that the two-stent technique was associated with a significantly

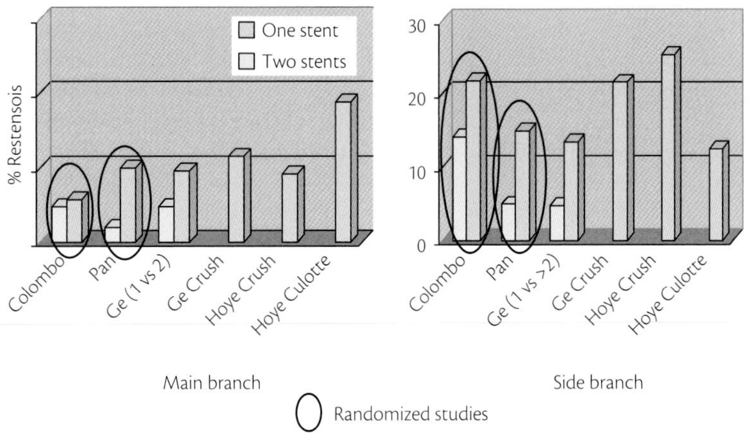

Fig. 18.9 Two DES are not better than one (angiographic follow-up): restenosis rates on main branch and side branch in the literature.

higher rate of myonecrosis biomarker elevation, longer procedural time, increased contrast volume, and X-ray exposure. In the BBC ONE study, 500 patients were randomized to a simple strategy as in the Nordic study with a potential crossover to T stenting in cases of SB TIMI flow <3, dissection > grade A, severe ostial pinching (>70%), or threatened SB closure (n = 7) or a two-stent technique (crush in 169 or culotte in 75 patients) at the operator's discretion. Contrary to the Nordic study, the Medina classification was performed and true bifurcation lesions were observed in 83% of cases. The composite endpoint at 9 months (death, target vessel failure, and MI) was 8% in the single-stent technique versus 15.2% in the two-stent technique (p <0.009). Peri-procedural MACE (death, MI, CABG), 2.0 versus 7.6% (p = 0.003), procedure duration, X-ray exposure, volume of contrast, and equipment used were higher in the two-stent group. As in the Nordic study, there was a significant elevation of peri-procedural biomarkers of myonecrosis in the two-stent group.

Consequently, the consensus in 2009 is that there is no benefit in performing systematically a complex procedure with two stents rather than a provisional SB stenting approach as evidenced by a higher frequency of AMI at the acute phase unrelated to the occurrence of a complication, and an unchanged risk of reintervention during the follow-up period. Nevertheless, the adverse outcome associated with complex procedures could be attributable to one of the techniques used in these heterogeneous groups. The recommendation of the EBC is that more accurate studies should be conducted with the purpose of comparing only two technical strategies using the same stents in 'true' bifurcation lesions.

Matching technique to lesion?

Given that the efficiency of the provisional SB stenting strategy has been demonstrated in all global studies, thus invalidating the concept of treatments indexed to lesions, it remains to be established which particular settings require the use of complex strategies. Do 'true' bifurcation lesions require complete coverage and which technique should be applied? These issues have been addressed in recent randomized studies. The BBK study[70] randomly compared two techniques using the Cypher® stent only: a simple technique (101 patients), the provisional SB strategy with authorized crossover only in instances of SB stenosis >60% or flow-limiting dissection versus the T-stenting technique (101 patients), but starting with the MB, with systematic stenting of the SB. The percentage of final kissing balloon inflation was 100% in both groups. However, the percentage of 'true' bifurcation lesions was only 68%. The primary endpoint (in-segment per cent diameter stenosis of the SB at angiographic follow-up) was again in favour of the simple approach (crossover = 18.8%) compared to complex procedures (crossover = 3%), p = 0.07. No clinical differences were observed during the 2-year follow-up period. The NORDIC II study examined the results of the Cypher® stent in a head-to-head comparison of the crush and culotte techniques in groups of 160 and 164 patients respectively, presenting with 78% and 85% of 'true' bifurcation lesions. The primary endpoint was the rate of cardiac death, AMI, TVR, or stent thrombosis. The 6-month clinical follow-up did not show any differences albeit a higher in-stent restenosis rate at the SB ostium associated with the crush technique (with less kissing balloon inflation). The CACTUS study[75] compared the strategy of provisional SB stenting with the crush technique using the Cypher® stent in a population of 350 patients with 'true' bifurcation lesions in 92% of cases. The 6-month follow-up analysis showed no clinical, angiographic, or stent thrombosis differences. Final kissing balloon inflation in the overall study population led to a reduction in the restenosis rate (MB and SB), AMI, and stent thrombosis rate.

The implementation of a simple strategy seems, therefore, appropriate in the setting of 'true' bifurcation lesions. A number of operators, however, still advocate the use of complex strategies in 'true' bifurcation lesions in the presence of a long lesion in the SB, a subject which calls for additional randomized studies.

Other data have shed some light on the question of the indexation of treatments to lesions. These data have been provided by studies on the efficacy of the crush technique in relation to the angle between the two distal branches[76]. When the angle was greater than 50°, the reported 2-year MACE-free survival rate was significantly decreased from 90% to 75%. The absence of kissing balloon inflation resulted in a reduction of the survival rate down to approximately 45%, whereas this did not have any impact when the angle was inferior to 50°.

Isolated ostial lesions of the LAD (0,0,1) and sometimes of the circumflex coronary artery (0,0,1) pose specific problems. Some operators are reluctant to use conventional techniques of bifurcation stenting with coverage of the left main, even the less 'metallic' ones (provisional SB stenting strategy), quoting the established fact that the angle between the two branches of the left main is more open than in other bifurcations[77] and suggesting that the ostium should be stented with or without protection or balloon inflation in the other branch. Very few studies have been devoted to this issue except for a reported series of provisional SB stenting procedures with good results[78].

Ostial stenosis of the SB (0,0,1) is an even more specific situation. Though stenosis of the SB ostium may account for symptoms or document ischaemia, the degree of angiographic stenosis may be difficult to assess (phenomenon of slow flow opposite to the carena) or to measure (inadequate QCA software). Stent implantation in this type of lesion is difficult and may carry the risk of incomplete lesion coverage or involvement of the MB. Several techniques have been proposed: the stenting of the SB ostium using a stent delivery balloon inflated at a very low pressure ('dog bone technique') and then pulled to the contact of a balloon inflated in the MB before complete deployment, which is a compromise between ensuring ostium coverage and avoiding stent protrusion (proposed by Zehtgruber); the inverted provisional T technique (proposed by Brunel), with the stent delivered at low pressure from the proximal MB towards the SB followed by kissing balloon inflation; the SB crush or mini crush (proposed by Ormiston) with the stent delivered in the SB while protruding in the MB where it is crushed with a balloon before final kissing balloon inflation. Selection of the appropriate technique depends on the angle between the two branches and is still a matter of debate.

Which DES should be used in bifurcation lesions?

There is only one randomized study comparing two DES, the Cypher® and the Taxus® stent (n = 102 vs. 103). Patients with bifurcation lesions treated by SES showed a significantly lower rate of late loss, restenosis, and target lesion revascularization[79] than patients treated with PES. This needs to be confirmed in other studies.

Bifurcation lesions and stent thrombosis

There is absolutely no doubt that stent implantation in a coronary bifurcation lesion is a predictive factor of stent thrombosis. Several major studies have reported stenting as an independent factor of stent thrombosis with a risk ratio between 3–10 times that associated with stent placement in a non-bifurcated lesion[80–83]. The impact of double stenting as a factor of stent thrombosis is still being debated. Analysis of the literature shows a higher rate of stent thrombosis in reported series of complex treatment procedures (Fig. 18.10). The influence of double stenting is documented as a predictive factor in the substantial J-Cypher® Registry which included 5015 patients with a risk ratio of 2. This increased risk of stent thrombosis associated with double stenting was not reported in the NORDIC study where stent thrombosis remained a rare occurrence, or in the BBK study. However, a trend was observed in the BBC ONE study (2 vs. 0.4% at 9 months). In the CACTUS study, absence of final kissing balloon inflation in the overall population (crush or provisional SB stenting) was a predictive factor of stent thrombosis[75].

Stenting of coronary bifurcations: the step by step techniques

The different techniques are described according to the MADS classification which is now established as a reference and covers all types of treatment available to date (see Figs. 18.4 and 18.5).

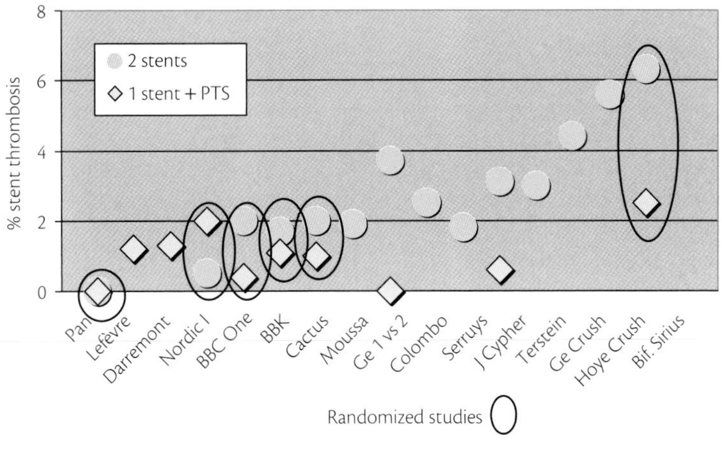

Fig. 18.10 Bifurcation stenting techniques with DES and stent thrombosis: thrombosis rates after provisional SB stenting or systematic side branch stenting in the literature.

The MADS classification: the 'M' strategy ('main')

This strategy involves the stenting of the proximal main vessel first, not by manually crimping a stent onto two balloons as with the SKIRT technique, but by placing a stent as close as possible to the carena. The first stent may prove sufficient in certain lesion types (1,0,0). This is the strategy used with a dedicated DES, the Axxess stent (Devax) stent, a conical, self-expandable stent coated with biolimus[84]. The stent is advanced on a single wire, preferably along the most angulated distal branch. Once the sheath has been removed, the distal part, the widest part of the cone, is deployed at the level of carena in the ostium of both branches. After placement of the first stent, the distal branches may also be stented separately or by simultaneous implantation of two stents side by side with slight internal protrusion in the proximal stent, the so-called extended V technique[85]. The Devax stent combined with other DES was assessed in relatively substantial series and was associated with good immediate and mid-term results. It was not, however, compared with standard treatment techniques. The drawbacks associated with these techniques are the fact that both branches of the bifurcation must be pre-dilated, the number of stents required, the overlapping areas, the cost, and the technical expertise required for implantation of the Devax stent.

The MADS classification: the 'A' strategy ('across')

This is the provisional SB stenting strategy. Here are the successive steps:

1) *Insertion of two guide wires* into each distal branch starts generally with the most difficult branch to access, the one where guide rotation is expected to be the widest, in order to avoid wire wrap. The second wire is then inserted into the easiest branch by limiting the rotation manoeuvre (no more than a wrist rotation). Keeping the wires separate and well identified outside the patient helps prevent wire wrap. The wire inserted in the SB are metallic in preference to hydrophilic polymeric wires because the coating can be peeled off or the wire broken (Choice PT® wires) during removal of the jailed wire. Systematic placement of a protection guide wire in the SB in the initial phase of the procedure facilitates the opening of angle A (access) which further facilitates access to the SB during guide wire exchange[86]. Another advantage of this technique is that it preserves the patency of the SB during stent placement across the MB[86] and if an occlusion occurs, the guide serves as a marker in order to find the SB lumen. When using this approach, it is very important to prepare the distal tip of the MB wire in order to access the SB through the MB stent strut by pulling back the wire orientated toward the SB.

   The insertion of a simple protection wire in the SB, which is removed if the flow remains normal, is a simplified version of this very flexible strategy. When guide wire insertion in both branches proves difficult, placement of a hydrophilic wire (later exchanged by means of a microcatheter), use of an orientable microcatheter (Venture® catheter, St Jude Medical)[87] or even rotational or directional atherectomy may be useful.

2) *Pre-dilatation of the MB* is left to the operator's discretion, but in patients with acute coronary syndromes, direct stenting should be preferred (lower risk of distal embolization, slow flow or no-reflow).

3) *Pre-dilatation of the SB* is still controversial, but after 14 years of bifurcation stenting in our institution, we came to the conclusion that it was preferable not to pre-dilate the SB in the majority of cases. During the ESC meeting in September 2008, Remo Albiero explained why we should not pre-dilate the SB (Fig. 18.11). Pre-dilatation increases the lumen toward the SB and supposedly the chance of engaging the SB through the MB stent. But at the same time it creates a dissection. After MB stenting, strut crossing may be more difficult because of dissection.

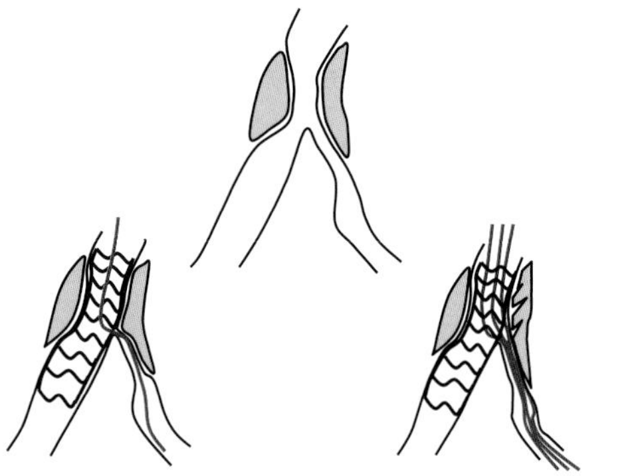

Fig. 18.11 Why not pre-dilate the SB?: after pre-dilatation of the side branch there are more stent cells available for crossing and sometimes a dissection. When no pre-dilatation is performed there is frequently only one cell available for crossing, the one close to carena free of atheroma (distal or 'carinal cell'), allowing projection of struts in the ostium of the SB.

Moreover, the chances of traversing a distal strut (carenal strut) are decreased. In some instances (severe calcifications), it seems advisable to pre-dilate with a small balloon. Pan suggested a variant of this strategy as follows: pre-dilatation of the SB followed by stent deployment in the MB across the SB with no further manoeuvre if no SB complication occurs.

4) *A stent is then implanted in the MB across the SB.* Selection of the stent is an important decision. Preference should be given to a tubular stent with good longitudinal stability. The cell area must be homogeneous and well adapted to the SB ostium, the surface of which varies according to angle A. The more open the angle, the wider the SB ostium area. Mortier created a model of stent deployment in order to perform stent cell measurements and determine the compatibility of a stent with the bifurcation type according to stent expansibility, stent cell area, SB reference diameter, and angle A[(88)]. The stent diameter should be selected according to the diameter of the distal MB rather than that of the proximal MB in order to avoid excessive carena shifting and to keep to the rules of coronary artery branching. Inevitably, and especially in bifurcation lesions with large SB, the proximal segment of the stent is inadequately deployed in the proximal MB, which may pose technical problems during guide wire exchange (mainly SB access). Darremont[(89)] has proposed the use of the POT technique (proximal optimization technique): prior to guide wire exchange, in order to optimize stent deployment proximal to the bifurcation, post dilatation is performed with a short 0.5mm bigger balloon. As a result, the diameter of the proximal stent segment is optimal and the stent struts facing the SB are larger, which facilitates SB guide wire insertion, particularly in the most distal cell. Albiero[(90)] has suggested that this technique should be implemented with a spherical balloon of large diameter.

5) *The next step is optional: the guide-wires are exchanged* starting with the removal of the guide wire from the distal MB in order to insert it into the SB, followed by the release of the SB jailed wire which is subsequently placed in the distal MB. But the procedure may be completed at the operator's discretion if the SB has been dilated, or if the result is acceptable. In the presence of a large SB, we systematically open the stent cell towards the SB. In order to do this, we carefully remove the wire from the MB and manoeuvre it towards the SB in order to enter the most distal cell during removal (carena cell). Prior to the procedure, the guide wire must be made into the appropriate distal angle. As the SB has not been pre-dilated, the only accessible strut is that situated in front of the lesion-free carena[(92)] and because we select the stent diameter according to Murray's law, the risk of SB occlusion due to carena shifting is very low. The jailed wire, pre-shaped in a short configuration, is withdrawn proximal to the stent, (care must be taken that the guiding catheter does not engage the coronary artery abruptly) and then advanced into the distal MB branch. Shaping the wire into a U form or a loop can be useful to avoid crossing outside the stent. When insertion of a free wire into the SB proves difficult, the use of a hydrophilic wire or of the Venture® catheter, as well as the optimized deployment of the proximal MB stent segment (POT technique) may help solve this problem.

   In vitro experiments have shown that the opening of a stent strut causes complex stent distortion[(38)]. When a proximal cell is opened toward the SB, there is no SB scaffolding and no significant stent deformation opposite the SB. When a distal cell is opened, a piece of crescent-shaped metal is projected into the side branch ostium (Fig. 18.12). On the opposite wall of the stent, struts are attracted towards the middle of the MB. These two phenomena are interrelated. Stent strut attraction is commensurate with the amount of metal pushed into the SB (opening of a distal strut) as well as the size of the SB and MB. It is inversely related to the expansibility of the stent. Stent projection in the proximal SB allows the placement of a stent in the SB in a T shape configuration without any gap even in Y shape angulations. In vitro stent deformation also occurs in vivo as revealed by the stent boost technique[(93)]. Untoward stent deformation may be corrected by kissing balloon inflation.

6) *Kissing balloon inflation* is performed immediately upon guide wire exchange. The diameter of the two balloons is selected according to the diameter of the two distal vessels. Short balloons are used to avoid the occurrence of 'geographical miss' in the MB and to ensure that only one strut is opened towards the SB in order to reposition the carena appropriately. Only one small, randomized study was conducted on the benefit of kissing balloon inflation associated with this strategy and it showed good acute results[(58)]. The inflation of two kissing balloons

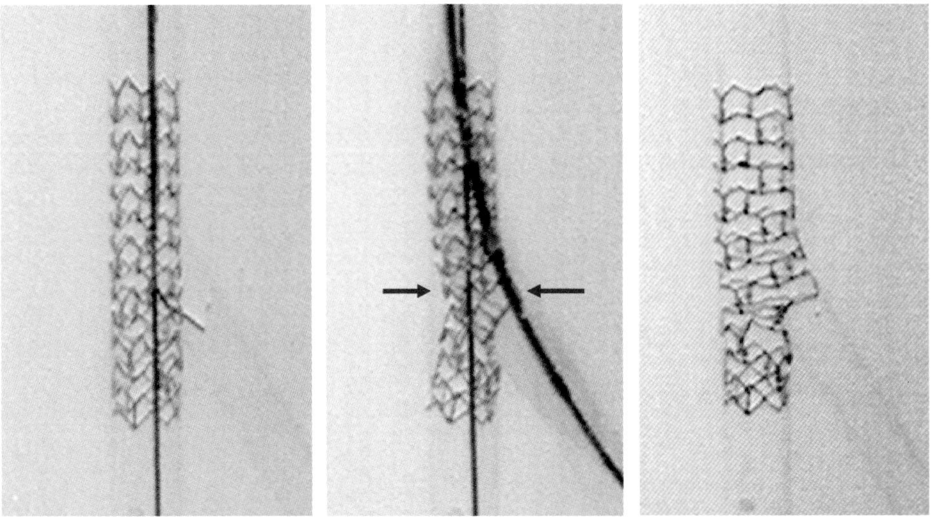

Fig. 18.12 Typical distortion of a tubular stent after SB cell opening (proximal versus distal cross) and after kissing balloon inflation as presented by Ormiston *et al*. An optimal result is obtained after distal cross and SB balloon inflation with some metal pushed in the ostium of the SB (the good) whereas opposite the SB, the stent is attracted in the middle of the main branch (the bad). Correction of the distortion is obtained after kissing balloon inflation.

completes the procedure in the vast majority of cases, especially in 'false' bifurcations (–,–,0). The need for a second stent in the SB is assessed according to the results of the procedure.

Although implantation of a stent in the SB is warranted in cases of flow-limiting complications, the presence of residual stenosis is a more complex issue. Indeed, there is an inconsistency between the percentage of residual stenosis in the SB ostium after MB stenting and FFR assessment. In instances where the residual stenosis in the SB is <75%, FFR is always >0.75 (normal), but it is also the case in 38% of cases when stenosis is >75%[94] which may lead one to consider that residual stenosis <75% by QCA is an acceptable result for the SB. The suggested reasons for this discrepancy are an inadequate contrast filling in the SB or a suboptimal assessment of the result in the SB due to a poor angiographic view, the stenosis pattern being no longer symmetrical but oval- or slit-shaped (carena shift).

The decision to stent the SB depends upon several factors: size of the branch, flow, presence of chest pain, or EKG documented ischaemia and quality of the result, bearing in mind that late loss is higher after stenting compared to balloon angioplasty alone. The beauty of the provisional SB stenting approach is that it is fully open to a large variety of techniques when SB stenting is needed. Stent placement in the SB is usually easy provided that deployment of the proximal MB stent has been adequately achieved. Following insertion of a second stent, the procedure is completed by repeat kissing balloon inflation.

The stent may be placed at the ostium (elective T stenting)[15] without protrusion in at least two angiographic views (only the proximal marker of the stent protrudes into the main branch stent, but stent/markers relationships may vary according to the different types of stent).

A slight systematic protrusion into the MB may be achieved using the TAP technique (T and Protrusion)[95]. The stent may be deployed using the internal crush technique[96] with protrusion into the MB followed by balloon crushing of the proximal stent segment with subsequent guide wire re-insertion into the SB prior to kissing balloon inflation. The procedure may be also completed by the culotte technique with wide deployment of the SB stent in the MB and subsequent re-insertion of the MB guide wire next to the carena prior to final kissing inflation[15,97].

Provisional SB strategy with dedicated stents: this strategy is used with a number of dedicated non-coated stents[98,99] and very acceptable mid-term data. The first human use of the Taxus Petal® paclitaxel-eluting bifurcation stent was associated with excellent 6-month angiographic and clinical follow-up results[100].

The advantage of the procedure is that it provides permanent access to both branches. The main issue with this type of dedicated stent is that of 'wire wrap' which results in the impossibility of 'pushing' the stent at the right level. This can be avoided by taking adequate measures in order to, first, prevent wire wrap (wire the most difficult branch first, no more than a wrist rotation with the second wire, no wire wrap on the table), second, identify wire wrap (sometimes visible on the screen when using an optimal view), which causes some resistance to be felt when advancing the device. Third, solve the problem by withdrawing one of the two wires and re-advance it without criss-crossing. A randomized study has been published comparing Frontier® stent and standard bifurcation stenting with no differences in clinical follow-up outcome except for a reduction in X-ray exposure time and contrast medium volume[71]. In the future, this kind of study will be very important to validate the potential benefit of dedicated devices. The main difficulty will be to find the optimal procedural endpoint.

The MADS classification: the 'D' strategy ('distal' or 'double')

This heterogeneous class involves the simultaneous treatment of both distal branches with two stents (and sometimes one stent and one balloon). This is not recommended in false bifurcation lesions. Historically, the first technique used was V stenting (touching stent)[40], mainly used in the Medina 0,1,1 anatomic type. For treatment of stenosis in the proximal MB, this technique evolved into the simultaneous kissing stent (SKS) strategy using DES[101], which implies the creation of a double lumen in a gun barrel configuration over a segment of variable length in the proximal MB. Bench studies have shown that these two lumens rarely form an ideal configuration and that they often interlace, especially when the angle between the proximal MB and the SB is wide. In areas where two stents are joined, the circular nature of balloons results in stent malapposition (turbulence, no biological effect). The outcome of this technique, as reported in the literature, varies from acceptable[102–104] to very poor. Certain studies have shown a high rate of stent thrombosis. A membrane growth on the neo-carina complicates the treatment of restenosis as well as any new intervention. In the absence of relevant data, it seems reasonable to limit the length of the neo-carina. Both these techniques, V stenting and SKS, require an adequate preparation of the bifurcation by balloon pre-dilatation. The treatment of a proximal dissection and restenosis in the follow-up period is very complex.

The MADS classification: the 'S' strategy ('side')

This class involves the majority of complex procedures starting with the stenting of the SB. An S strategy should not be used in 'false bifurcation lesions' because there is no disease in the SB and, therefore, no need for systematic SB stenting. Historically, the first technique applied was conventional T stenting[41], which was apparently an ideal strategy in T-shape bifurcations (a rare occurrence) although carrying the risk of creating a gap in lesions with a sharp B angle.

In order to solve the gap issue, the SB stent may be implanted so as to protrude into the MB. In such cases, however, the stent prevents the passage of a wire, balloon, or second stent. This technique evolved into the 'modified T stenting' strategy proposed by Colombo[50] as follows: implantation of the stent in the SB with a slight protrusion into the MB; the MB stent already in place is subsequently deployed after withdrawal of the SB balloon and wire. The frequent occurrence of ostial restenosis in the SB was attributed to incomplete coverage of the SB ostium and a new approach was developed by Colombo, the crush technique[51].

For the original crush technique, in order to facilitate guide wire re-insertion into the distal MB, two guide wires should be positioned at the beginning of the procedure with subsequent pre-dilation of both branches of the bifurcation. A stent is placed in the SB with variable protrusion into the proximal MB. The balloon and SB guide wire are removed before deployment of the MB stent positioned at the beginning of the procedure. After re-insertion of a guide wire into the SB, kissing balloon inflation is performed. It has been shown that final kissing divides the rate of repeat intervention by three[104]. There are several drawbacks to the crush technique, namely, the need for an 8F guiding catheter, the presence of three layers of stent in a segment of the proximal MB which may prevent or delay endothelialization, result in fracture[105], and is associated with turbulence, the non-apposition of the stent on the carina[106], difficult re-insertion of the wire into the SB with resulting high failure rate of kissing balloon inflation[107], and non-alignment between the arterial lumen and the two layers of stent[106]. Several improvements to the crush technique have been proposed in order to solve these issues: crushing the SB stent with a balloon rather than a stent (balloon crush or step crush technique compatible with 6F catheters)[108]; reinsertion of the guide wire into the SB through the most proximal strut and not next to the carina where the stent is often inadequately applied (risk of SB stent crush)[106,109]; high-pressure non-compliant balloon inflation in the SB before final kissing inflation for cell alignment[106] or two kissing inflations after stent implantation in the SB and balloon crush (double kissing or DK crush has proven superior to conventional crush)[110]; final kissing balloon inflation with adequately sized balloons in order to reduce the risk of local turbulence[106]. In order to prevent the occurrence of delayed endothelialization, the length of the crushed stent should be limited. The minicrush technique[111] was developed for this reason. However, it is hard to differentiate from the modified T-stenting technique. In the crush technique, the guide wire is reinserted into the SB through the SB stent cell whereas in the modified T technique, the wire is inserted in the SB through the SB stent lumen. Such a distinction may be made in a test bench but may prove very difficult *in vivo*.

Consequently, it seems that the crush technique is mostly efficient in bifurcations with a sharp angle[76], that the crushed segment must be as short as possible, and that double kissing balloon inflation or the double step approach must be carried out in order to improve the alignment of the stents cells on the SB ostium.

Another option is the culotte inverted technique which involves the stenting of the proximal MB towards the SB, followed by distal cell opening toward the MB, MB stent implantation, and final kissing balloon inflation (see Fig. 18.5). The main limitation is the significant difference in diameter between the proximal MB and the SB.

Distal left main stenosis: just another bifurcation?

The left main coronary artery vascularizes a large myocardial territory, which accounts for the severity of any lesion involving the left main itself and its two main branches, and for the higher frequency of ischaemia and symptoms. In at least 70% of cases, left main stenoses involve the distal bifurcation[112]. The left main coronary artery is a large-diameter vessel which is seldom <4mm as documented by IVUS. Its diameter as well as that of its branches is governed by the rules previously described; this is particularly important in the setting of diffuse stenosis of the left main where the diameter of the largest vessel should not be considered as the actual diameter of the left main trunk. In the absence of a proximal reference diameter, Finet's formula may be used to calculate the proximal MB reference diameter. Compared to other bifurcation sites, the angle between the left main and the circumflex artery is smaller and the angle between the distal branches is wider. These angle characteristics worsen with time and may be affected by other factors such as hypertension or left ventricular enlargement.

Left main stenting: historical perspective

Left main stenting: BMS or DES?

Even though acceptable results of left main stenting with BMS have been reported in the setting of patients not eligible for surgery, a small-size randomized study has shown that the use of DES under ultrasound guidance is associated with a reduction in binary stenosis at 6 months (22% vs. 6%, $p = 0.021$)[113].

Left main stenting: which DES?

Another randomized study compared SES ($n = 305$) vs. PES ($n = 302$) implantation in the left main coronary artery, with only 63% of distal left main segments. Half of the patients received a single stent, whereas the other half were treated by means of the culotte technique. No clinical difference was evidenced at 30 days and 2 years, even in diabetic patients, and the rates of binary stenosis and stent thrombosis were also similar[114].

Left main stenting: which technique?

Numerous technical strategies have been implemented in the left main coronary artery: crush[115], culotte, SKS[102,103], T stenting, provisional SB stenting[116], or more simply, stenting the MB across the SB (normally the circumflex artery) without protection, or any other manoeuvre[117]. No randomized study has been conducted so far to compare the efficiency of the available techniques (single, basic stenting across the SB or provisional SB stenting strategy vs. double stenting) in the distal left main coronary artery. Nevertheless, the analysis of several published or reported studies has shown that a better outcome was associated with simple techniques compared to complex strategies as in other bifurcation sites[117,118]. In the recently published SYNTAX study[119], it has been shown for the first time that distal LM had similar 1-year clinical outcomes compared to non-distal left main treated with PCI. Furthermore, in the presence of LM disease, the 1-year outcome after stenting was comparable to surgery. Furthermore, it has been clearly shown that the best clinical results in patients with distal left main lesions were observed when a single stent was used (compared to two stents), and when a provisional SB stenting approach was performed (compared to other techniques). These are, of course, not randomized data, but a similar trend was observed in the French pilot registry, where the use of two stents was shown to be a predictor of death at 2-year follow-up[116].

Left main stenting: IVUS guidance

In the Korean registry (Main Compare) including 2311 left main coronary arteries[120], renal and cardiac failure, chronic obstructive pulmonary disease, and the absence of IVUS guidance were identified as independent predictive factors of mortality after left main stenting. Therefore, IVUS should be strongly recommended when treating left main disease with PCI, at least in the learning phase.

Conclusion

Stenting of coronary bifurcation lesions using DES is still associated, as were BMS, with higher procedural complexity and in-hospital complications and poorer angiographic and clinical outcomes compared to non-bifurcation lesions. However, DES have dramatically improved angiographic and clinical outcomes compared to BMS.

In bifurcation lesions not involving the left main, the majority of acute clinical events are associated with the SB, whereas the infrequent occurrence of mid-term clinical events is often related to MB restenosis, the SB being too small to trigger symptoms.

Whether using BMS or DES, systematic SB stenting is not associated with better outcome compared to MB stenting with provisional SB treatment and may be associated with a higher rate of peri-procedural MI and stent thrombosis. Consequently, it is better to think twice before stenting the SB and, when in doubt, physiological assessment of the degree of residual SB stenosis may be useful.

In the absence of dedicated randomized trials, one cannot rule out the possibility that in certain instances, such as the presence of a long lesion in the SB, complete coverage of the bifurcation may be required. When and how is still a subject of debate.

Finally, the main objectives of the interventionalist when treating a bifurcation lesion should be to prevent the occurrence of peri-procedural MI which is most frequently observed when strategies that are either too simple (SB sacrificed) or too complex are implemented, and to focus on MB treatment by taking into account the respective diameters of the three bifurcation segments and by avoiding stent overlapping or mal apposition likely to result in flow turbulence, stent thrombosis, and restenosis.

References

1. Kassab GS. Scaling laws of vascular trees: of form and function. *Am J Physiol Heart Circ Physiol* 2006; **290**(2):H894–903.
2. Kassab GS. Functional hierarchy of coronary circulation: direct evidence of a structure-function relation. *Am J Physiol Heart Circ Physiol* 2005; **289**(6):H2559–65.
3. Kalsho G, Kassab GS. Bifurcation asymmetry of the porcine coronary vasculature and its implications on coronary flow heterogeneity. *Am J Physiol Heart Circ Physiol* 2004; **287**(6):H2493–500.
4. Murray CD. The physiological principle of minimum work: I. The vascular system and the cost of blood volume. *Proc Natl Acad Sci USA* 1926; **12**:207–14.
5. Kassab GS. Design of coronary circulation: the minimum energy hypothesis. *Comput Methods Appl Mech Engrg* 2007; **196**:3033–42.
6. Kamiya A, Takahashi T. Quantitative assessments of morphological and functional properties of biological trees based on their fractal nature. *J Appl Physiol* 2007; **102**(6):2315–23.
7. Choy JS, Kassab GS. Scaling of myocardial mass to flow and morphometry of coronary arteries. *J Appl Physiol* 2008; **104**(5):1259.
8. Finet G, Gilard M, Perrenot B, *et al.* Frcatla geometry of cornary bifurcations : a quantitative coronary angiography and intravascular ultrasoubnd analysis. *EuroIntervention* 2008; **3**:490–98.
9. Lansky A, Tuinenburg J, Costa M, *et al.* European Bifurcation Angiographic Sub-Committee.Quantitative angiographic methods for bifurcation lesions: a consensus statement from the European. *Catheter Cardiovasc Interv* 2009; **73**(2):258–66.
10. Asakura T, Karino T. Flow patterns and spatial distribution of atherosclerotic lesions in human coronary arteries. *Circ Res* 1990; **66**(4):1045–66.
11. Chatzizisis YS, Jonas M, Coskun AU, *et al.* Prediction of the localization of high-risk coronary atherosclerotic plaques on the basis of low endothelial shear stress: an intravascular ultrasound and histopathology natural history study. *Circulation* 2008; **117**(8):993–1002.
12. Shimada Y, Courtney BK, Nakamura M, *et al.* Intravascular ultrasonic analysis of atherosclerotic vessel remodeling and plaque distribution of stenotic left anterior descending coronary arterial bifurcation lesions upstream and downstream of the side branch. *Am J Cardiol* 2006; **98**(2):193–6.
13. Louvard Y, Sashikand G, Lefèvre T, *et al.* Angiographic predictors of side branch occlusion during the treatment of bifurcation lesions. *Cath Cardiovasc Interv* 2005 (Abstr. Supp.).
14. Vassilev D, Gil R. Clinical verification of a theory for predicting side branch stenosis after main vessel stenting in coronary bifurcation lesions. *J Interv Cardiol* 2008; **21**(6):493–503.

15. Louvard Y, Thomas M, Dzavik V, *et al.* Classification of coronary artery bifurcation lesions and treatments: time for a consensus! *Catheter Cardiovasc Interv* 2008; **71**(2):175–83.
16. Thygesen K, Alpert JS, White HD. Universal definition of myocardial infarction. *J Am Coll Cardiol* 2007; **50**:2173.
17. Califf RM, Abdelmeguid AE, Kuntz RE, *et al.* Myonecrosis after revascularization procedures. *J Am Coll Cardiol* 1998; **31**:241–51.
18. Jang JS, Hong MK, Park DW, *et al.* Impact of periprocedural myonecrosis on clinical events after implantation of drug-eluting stents. *Int J Cardiol* 2008; **129**:368–72.
19. Kini AS, Lee P, Marmur JD, *et al.* Correlation of postpercutaneous coronary intervention creatine kinase-MB and troponin I elevation in predicting mid-term mortality. *Am J Cardiol* 2004; **93**:18–23.
20. Bhargava B, Waksman R, Lansky AJ, *et al.* Clinical outcomes of compromised side branch [stent jail] after coronary stenting with the NIR stent. *Catheter Cardiovasc Interv* 2001; **54**:295–300.
21. Prasad A, Singh M, Lerman A, *et al.* Isolated elevation in troponin T after percutaneous coronary intervention is associated with higher long-term mortality. *J Am Coll Cardiol* 2006; **48**:1765–1770.
22. Ricciardi MJ, Wu E, Davidson CJ, *et al.* Visualization of discrete microinfarction after percutaneous coronary intervention associated with mild creatine kinase-MB elevation. *Circulation* 2001; **103**(23):2780–3.
23. George BS, Myler RK, Stertzer SH, *et al.* Balloon angioplasty of coronary bifurcation lesions: the kissing balloon technique. *Cathet Cardiovasc Diagn* 1986; **12**: 124–38.
24. Popma J, Bashore T. Qualitative and quantitative angiography –Bifurcation lesions. In Topol E (ed) *Textbook of Interventional Cardiology*, pp.1055–8. Philadelphia, PA: W.B. Saunders, 1994.
25. Spokojny AM, Sanborn TM. The bifurcation lesion. In Ellis SG, Holmes DR (eds) *Strategic Approaches in Coronary Intervention*, p.288. Baltimore, MD: Williams and Wilkins, 1996.
26. Safian RD. Bifurcation lesions. In Safian RD, Freed MS (eds) *The Manual of Interventional Cardiology*, p.222. Royal Oak, MI: Physician's Press, 2001.
27. Lefevre T, Louvard Y, Morice MC, *et al.* Stenting of bifurcation lesions: classification, treatments, and results. *Catheter Cardiovasc Interv* 2000; **49**:274–83.
28. Iakovou I, Ge L, Colombo A. Contemporary stent treatment of coronary bifurcations. *J Am Coll Cardiol* 2005; **46**(8):1446–55.
29. Tsuchida K, Colombo A, Lefevre T, *et al.* The clinical outcome of percutaneous treatment of bifurcation lesions in multivessel coronary artery disease with the sirolimus-eluting stent: insights from the Arterial Revascularization Therapies Study part II (ARTS II). *Eur Heart J* 2007; **28**:433–42.
30. Chen J-L, Gao R-L, Yang Y-J, *et al.* Short and long-term outcomes of two drug eluting stents in bifurcation lesions. *Chin Med J* 2007; **120**(3):183–86.
31. Movahed MR, Kern K, Thai H, *et al.* Coronary artery bifurcation lesions: a review and update on classification and interventional techniques. *Cardiovasc Revasc Med* 2008; 9:263–8.
32. Medina A, Suarez de Lezo J, Pan M. A new classification of coronary bifurcation lesions. *Rev Esp Cardiol* 2006; **59**:183.
33. Ge L, Airoldi F, Iakovou I, *et al.* Clinical and angiographic outcome after implantation of drug-eluting stents in bifurcation lesions with the crush stent technique: importance of final kissing balloon post-dilation. *J Am Coll Cardiol* 2005; **46**(4):613–20.
34. Goktekin O, Kaplan S, Dimopoulos K, *et al.* A new quantitative analysis system for the evaluation of coronary bifurcation lesions: comparison with current conventional methods. *Catheter Cardiovasc Interv* 2007; **69**(2):172–80.
35. Ramcharitar S, Onuma Y, Aben JP, *et al.* A novel dedicated quantitative coronary analysis methodology for bifurcation analysis. *EuroIntervention* 2008; **3**: 553–7.
36. Lansky A, Tuinenburg J, Costa M, *et al.*; European Bifurcation Angiographic Sub-Committee. Quantitative angiographic methods for bifurcation lesions: a consensus statement from the European Bifurcation Group. *Catheter Cardiovasc Interv* 2009; **73**(2):258–66.
37. Ramcharitar S, Daeman J, Patterson M, *et al.* First direct in vivo comparison of two commercially available three-dimensional quantitative coronary angiography systems. *Catheter Cardiovasc Interv* 2008; **71**(1):44–50.
38. Ormiston JA, Currie E, Panther MJ, *et al.* The driver stent for coronary bifurcations: a clinical case and bench testing of provisional "culotte" side-branch stenting. *J Invasive Cardiol* 2004; **16**(2):1–3.
39. Pomerantz RM, Ling FS. Distortion of Palmaz–Schatz stent geometry following side- branch balloon dilation through the stent in a rabbit model. *Cathet Cardiovasc Diagn* 1997; **40**:422–6.
40. Ormiston JA, Webster MW, Ruygrok PN, *et al.* Stent deformation following simulated side-branch dilatation: a comparison of five stent designs. *Catheter Cardiovasc Interv* 1999; **47**(2):258–64.
41. Murasato Y, Horiuchi M, Otsuji Y. Three-dimensional modeling of double-stent techniques at the left main coronary artery bifurcation using micro-focus X-ray computed tomography. *Catheter Cardiovasc Interv* 2007; **70**(2):211–20.
42. Mittal N, Zhou Y, Ung S, *et al.* A computer reconstruction of the entire coronary arterial tree based on detailed morphometric data. *Ann Biomed Eng* 2005; **33**(8):1015–26.
43. Mortier P, De Beule M, Van Loo D, *et al.* Finite element analysis of side branch access during bifurcation stenting. *Med Eng Phys* 2009; **31**:434–40.
44. Kobayashi Y, Colombo A, Adamian M, *et al.* The skirt technique: A stenting technique to treat a lesion immediately proximal to the bifurcation

(pseudobifurcation). *Catheter Cardiovasc Interv* 2000; **51**(3):347–51.

45. Colombo A, Gaglione A, Nakamura S, *et al.* “Kissing” stents for bifurcation coronary lesion. *Cathet Cardiovasc Diagn* 1993; **30**:327–30.
46. Carrie D, Karouny E, Chouairi S, *et al.* “T”-shaped stent placement: a technique for the treatment of dissected bifurcation lesions. *Cathet Cardiovasc Diagn* 1996; **37**:311–3.
47. Fort S, Lazzam C, Schwartz L. Coronary ‘Y’ stenting: a technique for angioplasty of bifurcation stenoses. *Can J Cardiol* 1996; **12**:678–82.
48. Khoja A, Ozbek C, Bay W, *et al.* Trouser-like stenting: a new technique for bifurcation lesions. *Cathet Cardiovasc Diagn* 1997; **41**:192–6.
49. Carrie D, Elbaz M, Dambrin G, *et al.* Coronary stenting of bifurcation lesions using “T” or “reverse Y” configuration with Wiktor stent. *Am J Cardiol* 1998; **82**:1418–21, A8.
50. Chevalier B, Glatt B, Royer T, *et al.* Placement of coronary stents in bifurcation lesions by the “culotte” technique. *Am J Cardiol* 1998; **82**:943–9.
51. Morice M-C, Mansour S, Louvard Y, *et al.* Provisional versus systematic T stenting: insights from a large prospective single-center database. *J Am Coll Cardiol* 2004; 43(5), Supplement A.
52. Lefèvre T, Louvard Y, Morice MC, *et al.* Stenting of bifurcation lesions: classification, treatments, and results. *Catheter Cardiovasc Interv* 2000; **49**:274–83.
53. Louvard Y, Lefèvre T, Morice M-C. Percutaneous coronary intervention for bifurcation coronary disease. *Heart* 2004; **90**:713–722.
54. Lefèvre T, Louvard Y, Morice MC, *et al.* Stenting of bifurcation lesions: a rational approach. *J Interv Cardiol* 2001; **14**:573–85.
55. Kobayashi Y, Colombo A, Akiyama T, *et al.* Modified “T” stenting: a technique for kissing stents in bifurcational coronary lesion. *Cathet Cardiovasc Diagn* 1998; **43**:323–6.
56. Colombo A, Stankovic G, Orlic D, *et al.* Modified T-stenting technique with crushing for bifurcation lesions: immediate results and 30-day outcome. *Catheter Cardiovasc Interv* 2003; **60**(2):145–51.
57. Ormiston JA, Webster MW, Ruygrok PN, *et al.* Stent deformation following simulated side-branch dilatation: a comparison of five stent designs. *Catheter Cardiovasc Interv* 1999; **47**:258–64.
58. Brueck M, Scheinert D, Flachskampf FA, *et al.* Sequential vs. kissing balloon angioplasty for stenting of bifurcation coronary lesions. *Catheter Cardiovasc Interv* 2002; **55**(4):461–6.
59. Garot P, Lefèvre T, Savage M, *et al.* Nine-month outcome of patients treated by percutaneous coronary interventions for bifurcation lesions in the recent era: a report from the Prevention of Restenosis with Tranilast and its Outcomes (PRESTO) trial. *J Am Coll Cardiol* 2005; **46**(4):606–12.
60. Carlier SG, Colombo A, de Scheerder I, *et al.* Stenting of bifurcational coronary lesions: results of the multicentric European culottes registry. *Eur Heart J* 2001; **22**(Abst. suppl):348.
61. Pan M, Suárez de Lezo J, Medina A, *et al.* Simple and complex stent strategies for bifurcated coronary arterial stenosis involving the side branch origin. *Am J Cardiol* 1999; **83**(9):1320–5.
62. Al Suwaidi J, Berger PB, Rihal CS, *et al.* Immediate and long-term outcome of intracoronary stent implantation for true bifurcation lesions. *J Am Coll Cardiol* 2000; **35**(4):929–36.
63. Anzuini A, Briguori C, Rosanio S, *et al.* Immediate and long-term clinical and angiographic results from Wiktor stent treatment for true bifurcation narrowings. *Am J Cardiol* 2001; **88**(11):1246–50.
64. Assali AR, Teplitsky I, Hasdai D, *et al.* Coronary bifurcation lesions: to stent one branch or both? *J Invasive Cardiol* 2004; **16**(9):447–50.
65. Thuesen L, Kelbaek H, Kløvgaard L, *et al.*; SCANDSTENT Investigators. Comparison of sirolimus-eluting and bare metal stents in coronary bifurcation lesions: subgroup analysis of the Stenting Coronary Arteries in Non-Stress/Benestent Disease Trial (SCANDSTENT). *Am Heart J* 2006; **152**(6):1140–5.
66. Sharma SK, Choudhury A, Lee J, *et al.* Simultaneous kissing stents (SKS) technique for treating bifurcation lesions in medium-to-large arteries. *Am J Cardiol* 2004; **94**(7):913–7.
67. Helqvist S, Jørgensen E, Kelbaek H, *et al.* Percutaneous treatment of coronary bifurcation lesions: a novel “extended Y” technique with complete lesion stent coverage. *Heart* 2006; **92**(7):981–2.
68. Steigen TK, Maeng M, Wiseth R, *et al.* Randomized study on simple versus complex stenting of coronary artery bifurcation lesions: the Nordic bifurcation study. Nordic PCI Study Group. *Circulation* 2006; **114**(18):1955–61.
69. Pan M, de Lezo JS, Medina A, *et al.* Rapamycin-eluting stents for the treatment of bifurcated coronary lesions: a randomized comparison of a simple versus complex strategy. *Am Heart J* 2004; **148**(5):857–64.
70. Ferenc M, Gick M, Kienzle RP, *et al.* Randomized trial on routine vs. provisional T-stenting in the treatment of de novo coronary bifurcation lesions. *Eur Heart J* 2008; **29**(23):2859–67.
71. Cervinka P, Bystron M, Spacek R, *et al.* Treatment of bifurcation lesions using dedicated bifurcation stents versus classic bare-metal stents. Randomized, controlled trial with 12-month angiographic follow up. *J Invasive Cardiol* 2008; **20**(10):516–20.
72. Lefèvre T, Morice M-C, Sengottuvel G, *et al.* Influence of technical strategies on the outcome of coronary bifurcation stenting. *EuroIntervention* 2005; **1**:31–37.
73. Pan M, de Lezo JS, Medina A, *et al.* Rapamycin-eluting stents for the treatment of bifurcated coronary lesions: a randomized comparison of a simple versus complex strategy. *Am Heart J* 2004; **148**(5):857–64.
74. Colombo A, Moses JW, Morice MC, *et al.* Randomized study to evaluate sirolimus-eluting stents implanted

at coronary bifurcation lesions. *Circulation* 2004; **109**(10):1244–9.
75. Colombo A, Bramucci E, Saccà S, *et al.* Randomized study of the crush technique versus provisional side-branch stenting in true coronary bifurcations: the CACTUS (Coronary Bifurcations: Application of the Crushing Technique Using Sirolimus-Eluting Stents) Study. *Circulation* 2009; **119**(1):71–8.
76. Dzavik V, Kharbanda R, Ivanov J, *et al.* Predictors of long-term outcome after crush stenting of coronary bifurcation lesions: importance of the bifurcation angle. *Am Heart J* 2006; **152**(4):762–9.
77. Kawasaki T, Koga H, Serikawa T, *et al.* The bifurcation study using 64 multislice computed tomography. *Catheter Cardiovasc Interv* 2009; **73**(5):653–8.
78. Cubeddu RJ, Wood FO, Saylors EK, *et al.* Isolated disease of the ostium left anterior descending or circumflex artery: management using a left main stenting technique. Clinical outcome at 2 years. *J Invasive Cardiol* 2007; **19**(11):457–61.
79. Pan M, Suárez de Lezo J, Medina A, *et al.* Drug-eluting stents for the treatment of bifurcation lesions: a randomized comparison between paclitaxel and sirolimus stents. *Am Heart J* 2007; **153**(1):15.e1–7.
80. Iakovou I, Schmidt T, Bonizzoni E, *et al.* Incidence, predictors, and outcome of thrombosis after successful implantation of drug-eluting stents. *JAMA* 2005; **293**(17):2126–30.
81. Ong AT, McFadden EP, Regar E, *et al.* Late angiographic stent thrombosis (LAST) events with drug-eluting stents. *J Am Coll Cardiol* 2005; **45**(12):2088–92.
82. Kuchulakanti PK, Chu WW, Torguson R, *et al.* Correlates and long-term outcomes of angiographically proven stent thrombosis with sirolimus- and paclitaxel-eluting stents. *Circulation* 2006; **113**(8):1108–13.
83. Daemen J, Wenaweser P, Tsuchida K, *et al.* Early and late coronary stent thrombosis of sirolimus-eluting and paclitaxel-eluting stents in routine clinical practice: data from a large two-institutional cohort study. *Lancet* 2007; **369**(9562):667–78.
84. Grube E, Buellesfeld L, Neumann FJ, *et al.* Six-month clinical and angiographic results of a dedicated drug-eluting stent for the treatment of coronary bifurcation narrowings. *Am J Cardiol* 2007; **99**(12):1691–7.
85. Helqvist S, Jørgensen E, Kelbaek H, *et al.* Percutaneous treatment of coronary bifurcation lesions: a novel "extended Y" technique with complete lesion stent coverage. *Heart* 2006; **92**(7):981–2.
86. Terkamp C, Gaede A, Werner PC, *et al.* Combining stenting with the double wire technique effectively prevents side branch occlusion. *Z Kardiol* 2002; **91**(11):899–904.
87. Lilli A, Vecchio S, Giuliani G, *et al.* Venture wire control catheter in percutaneous treatment of complex coronary bifurcation. A case report. *Minerva Cardioangiol* 2008; **56**(2):255–8.
88. Mortier P, Van Loo D, De Beule M, *et al.* Comparison of drug-eluting stent cell size using micro-CT: important data for bifurcation stent selection. *EuroIntervention* 2008; **4**(3):391–6.
89. Darremont O. The POT technique. Personal communication European bifurcation club. *Valencia*, September 2007. http://www.bifurc.net
90. Albiero R. Spherical balloon. Personal communication European bifurcation club, Valencia. *Roma* 2006. http://www.bifurc.net
91. Pan M, de Lezo JS, Medina A, *et al.* Rapamycin-eluting stents for the treatment of bifurcated coronary lesions: a randomized comparison of a simple versus complex strategy. *Am Heart J* 2004; **148**(5):857–64.
92. Albiero R. Why we should not predilate the side branch? Personal communication. *European Society of Cardiology*, September 2008.
93. Agostoni P, Verheye S. Bifurcation stenting with a dedicated biolimus-eluting stent: X-ray visual enhancement of the final angiographic result with "StentBoost Subtract". *Catheter Cardiovasc Interv* 2007; **70**(2):233–6.
94. Koo BK, Kang HJ, Youn TJ, *et al.* Physiologic assessment of jailed side branch lesions using fractional flow reserve. *J Am Coll Cardiol* 2005; **46**(4):633–7.
95. Burzotta F, Gwon HC, Hahn JY, *et al.* Modified T-stenting with intentional protrusion of the side-branch stent within the main vessel stent to ensure ostial coverage and facilitate final kissing balloon: the T-stenting and small protrusion technique (TAP-stenting). Report of bench testing and first clinical Italian-Korean two-centre experience. *Catheter Cardiovasc Interv* 2007; **70**(1):75–82.
96. Ormiston JA, Webster MW, El Jack S, *et al.* Drug-eluting stents for coronary bifurcations: bench testing of provisional side-branch strategies. *Catheter Cardiovasc Interv* 2006; **67**(1):49–55.
97. Adriaenssens T, Byrne RA, Dibra A, *et al.* Culotte stenting technique in coronary bifurcation disease: angiographic follow-up using dedicated quantitative coronary angiographic analysis and 12-month clinical outcomes. *Eur Heart J* 2008; **29**(23):2868–76.
98. Lefèvre T, Ormiston J, Guagliumi G, *et al.* The Frontier stent registry: safety and feasibility of a novel dedicated stent for the treatment of bifurcation coronary artery lesions. *J Am Coll Cardiol* 2005; **46**(4):592–8.
99. Ormiston J, Webster M, El-Jack S, *et al.* The AST petal dedicated bifurcation stent: first-in-human experience. *Catheter Cardiovasc Interv* 2007; **70**(3):335–40.
100. Ormiston JA, Lefèvre T, Grube E, *et al.* First human use of the taxus petal paclitaxel-eluting bifurcation stent. *J Am Coll Cardiol* 2009; **59**:A79.
101. Sharma SK, Choudhury A, Lee J, *et al.* Simultaneous kissing stents (SKS) technique for treating bifurcation lesions in medium-to-large arteries. *Am J Cardiol* 2004; **94**(7):913–17.

102. Price MJ, Cristea E, Sawhney N, *et al.* Serial angiographic follow-up of sirolimus-eluting stents for unprotected left main coronary artery revascularization. *J Am Coll Cardiol* 2006; **47**(4):871–7.
103. Morton AC, Siotia A, Arnold ND, *et al.* Simultaneous kissing stent technique to treat left main stem bifurcation disease. *Catheter Cardiovasc Interv* 2007; **69**(2):209–15.
104. Ge L, Airoldi F, Iakovou I, *et al.* Clinical and angiographic outcome after implantation of drug-eluting stents in bifurcation lesions with the crush stent technique: importance of final kissing balloon post-dilation. *J Am Coll Cardiol* 2005; **46**:613–20.
105. Surmely JF, Kinoshita Y, Dash D, *et al.* Stent strut fracture-induced restenosis in a bifurcation lesion treated with the crush stenting technique. *Circ J* 2006; **70**(7): 936–8.
106. Ormiston JA, Currie E, Webster MW, *et al.* Drug-eluting stents for coronary bifurcations: insights into the crush technique. *Catheter Cardiovasc Interv* 2004; **63**(3):332–6.
107. Gunnes P, Niemela M, Kervinen K, *et al.* For the Nordic-Baltic PCI Study Group. Eight months angiographic follow-up in patients randomised to crush or culotte stenting of coronary artery bifurcation lesions. The Nordic Bifurcation Stent Technique study. Paper presented at ACC 2008 Late Breaking Trials; April 1, 2008; Chicago, IL.
108. Lim PO, Dzavík V. Balloon crush: treatment of bifurcation lesions using the crush stenting technique as adapted for transradial approach of percutaneous coronary intervention. *Catheter Cardiovasc Interv* 2004; **63**(4):412–6.
109. Murasato Y, Suzuka H, Suzuki Y. Incomplete stent apposition in a left main bifurcated lesion after kissing stent implantation. *J Invasive Cardiol* 2006; **18**(11): E279–84.
110. Chen SL, Zhang JJ, Ye F, *et al.* Study comparing the double kissing (DK) crush with classical crush for the treatment of coronary bifurcation lesions: the DKCRUSH-1 Bifurcation Study with drug-eluting stents. *Eur J Clin Invest* 2008; **38**(6):361–71.
111. Galassi AR, Colombo A, Buchbinder M, *et al.* Long-term outcomes of bifurcation lesions after implantation of drug-eluting stents with the "mini-crush technique". *Catheter Cardiovasc Interv* 2007; **69**(7):976–83.
112. Biondi-Zoccai GG, Lotrionte M, Moretti C, *et al.* A collaborative systematic review and meta-analysis on 1278 patients undergoing percutaneous drug-eluting stenting for unprotected left main coronary artery disease. *Am Heart J* 2008;**155**:274–83.
113. Erglis A, Narbute I, Kumsars I, *et al.* A randomized comparison of paclitaxel-eluting stents versus bare-metal stents for treatment of unprotected left main coronary artery stenosis. *J Am Coll Cardiol* 2007; **50**(6):491–7.
114. Mehilli J, Kastrati A, Byrne RA, *et al.* Paclitaxel- Versus Sirolimus-Eluting Stents for Unprotected Left Main Coronary Artery Disease. *J Am Coll Cardiol* 2009; **53**(19):1760–8.
115. Jim MH, Chow WH, Ho HH. Stenting of unprotected distal left main coronary artery bifurcation stenoses using modified crush technique with double kissing balloon inflation (sleeve technique): immediate procedure result and early clinical outcome. *J Interv Cardiol* 2007; **20**(1):17–22.
116. Vaquerizo B, Lefèvre T, Darremont O, et al. Unprotected left main stenting in the real world: Two-year outcomes of the french left main taxus registry. *Circulation* 2009 (in press).
117. Kim YH, Park SW, Hong MK, *et al.* Comparison of simple and complex stenting techniques in the treatment of unprotected left main coronary artery bifurcation stenosis. *Am J Cardiol* 2006; **97**(11):1597–601.
118. Park SJ. Which is the most appropriate stenting technique with drug-eluting stent for unprotected left main bifurcation stenosis? *Catheter Cardiovasc Interv* 2008; **71**(2):173–4.
119. Serruys PW, Morice MC, Kappetein AP, *et al.* Percutaneous Coronary Intervention versus Coronary-Artery Bypass Grafting for Severe Coronary Disease. *N Engl J Med* 2009; **360**:961–72.
120. Seung KB, Park DW, Kim YH, *et al.* Stents versus coronary-artery bypass grafting for left main coronary artery disease. *N Engl J Med* 2008; **358**:1781–92.

CHAPTER 19

Percutaneous coronary intervention for unprotected and protected left main stem disease

Christine Hughes, Bruno Farah, and Jean Fajadet

Introduction: to stent or not to stent the left main—why is that the question?

Significant unprotected left main coronary artery (ULMCA) disease occurs in 5–7% of patients undergoing coronary angiography[1,2] and patients with ULMCA disease treated medically have a 3-year mortality rate of 50%[3,4]. Several studies have shown a significant benefit following treatment of left main (LM) stenosis with coronary bypass grafting compared with medical treatment[5–8]. Until recently coronary bypass grafting has been the gold standard therapy for LM disease. However, advances in percutaneous intervention techniques and stent technology have allowed re-evaluation of the role of percutaneous coronary intervention (PCI) for LM disease. Recent studies have focused on the safety and efficacy of stenting the left main coronary artery (LMCA) to determine if it does provide a true alternative to coronary artery bypass grafting (CABG). So should we stent the LM?

CABG versus PCI

Because of concern about procedural risk and long-term durability, PCI has usually been restricted to patients who are poor candidates for surgery or have LMCA disease that is 'protected' by a patent bypass graft to the left anterior descending or circumflex artery. The European guidelines for PCIs stated that 'stenting for unprotected LMCA disease should only be considered in the absence of other revascularization options' (Class II_{B3})[9]. Likewise, the American guidelines writing committee considered coronary artery bypass grafting as the gold standard for revascularization of lesions in the LMCA in patients eligible for CABG given the proven benefit in the long-term (Class III indication)[10].

However, some cardiac interventionalists feel that these guidelines do not take into account the advances in stent technology and the development of antiplatelet regimens which have minimized the incidence of acute and subacute stent thrombosis and restenosis[11]. It is necessary, therefore, to examine the evidence for LMCA stenting.

Initial reviews of angioplasty and stenting in the LM showed that while the procedure was in general technically successful and safe, there was a high incidence of early mortality in the few months after the procedure. Many of these patients had been turned down for surgery due to high surgical risk and patients were not routinely treated with dual antiplatelets. These were undoubtedly contributing factors although the actual 'causes of death' for the high mortality rate were unproven. There was also a very high rate of restenosis in patients followed-up with coronary angiography[12]. However, more recent studies investigating the use of bare-metal stents in LM stenting have had more favourable results and development of drug-eluting stents have led to

Table 19.1 In-hospital and long-term mortality after CABG for LMCA disease

Author (year)	Year of surgery	N	Mortality			
			Hospital	30-day	1-year	2-years
Jonsson (2006)	1970–1999	1888	2.7	–	–	–
Lu *et al.* (2006) (2005)	1997–2003	1197	2.8	3	5	6
Keogh and Kinsman (2003)	2003	5003	3	–	–	–
Dewey *et al.* (2006) (2001)	1998–1999	728	–	4.2	–	–
Yeatman *et al.* (2006) (2001)	1996–2000	387	2.4	–	–	5
Ellis *et al.* (2006) (1998)	1990–1995	1585	2.3	–	–	–
Weighted average	–	10 788	2.8	–	–	–

Reproduced from Taggart, DP, Kaul, S, Boden, WE *et al.* Revascularization for unprotected left main stem coronary artery stenosis: stenting or surgery. *J Am Coll Cardiol* 2008; **51**:885–92 © 2008, with permission from Elsevier.

renewed questions about the role of stenting and CABG in LM disease.

So what does the evidence show?

Results of CABG in patients with LM stenosis

Coronary artery bypass surgery is a well established technique, with excellent proven results for the treatment of coronary artery disease, dating back to the early 1970s. The Coronary Artery Surgery Study (CASS) registry reported on 1477 patients with LM disease(3). Of these, 53 (3.6%) were asymptomatic. The survival rate 5 years after surgery for treatment of LMCA stenosis was 84% for the symptomatic patients and 88% for the asymptomatic patients. Medical management of LMCA disease produced a 5-year survival rate of 57% for asymptomatic patients and 58% for symptomatic patients.

A more recent review by Taggart and colleagues published in 2008 reported on a series of studies, all of which had an in-hospital mortality of between 2–3% after CABG for LM stenosis and, although there was a less data on long-term follow-up, those studies which did report on long-term outcomes had results showing 5–6% mortality at 5 years (Table 19.1)(13).

Some studies had suggested that patients with LM disease had poorer outcomes after surgery than patients with coronary artery disease that did not involve the LM. Using data from the Karolinska registry, Jönsson and colleagues(14), however, showed that although patients with LM disease operated on between 1985–1994 did appear to have a higher mortality at 30 days and 5 years, compared to patients who had CABG for coronary artery disease not involving the LM, this finding was not reproduced in data on patients operated on between 1995–1999. They found that patients with LM stenosis operated on between 1995–1999 had a 2% 30-day mortality and 7% 5-year mortality, compared to 2.2% and 6.6% respectively for patients with non-LM disease (Table 19.2). Therefore, it would appear that with current surgical practice, CABG is as safe and as effective for patients who have LM stenosis as for those with non-LM disease.

In their review of the Cleveland Clinic experience of CABG for patients with LM stenosis, Sabik and colleagues(15) report a 20-year follow-up of all patients operated on between 1971–1998. They have shown that for the 3803 patients with LM stenosis, 30-day survival is 97.6%, with 93.6% at 1 year and 83% at 5 years. Ten-year survival rate is 64%. Importantly, rates of freedom from coronary reintervention are 99.7% at 30 days, 98.9% at 1 year, and 89% at 5 years. At 10 years, 76% of

Table 19.2 Results from the Karolinska registry

	CABG with LM	CABG without LM
N	1888	8759
30-day mortality (%)		
1985–1994	2.6	2.2
1995–1999	2.0	2,2
5-year mortality (%)		
1985–1994	12.4	9.2
1995–1999	7.0	6.6

Reproduced from Jönsson A, Hammar N, Nordquist T, *et al.* Left main coronary artery stenosis no longer a risk factor for early and late death after coronary artery bypass surgery – an experience covering three decades. *Eur J Cardiothorac Surg* 2006; **30**:311–17 © 2006 with permission from Elsevier.

surviving patients remain free from re-intervention and 61% at 20 years.

These studies represent the benchmark against which other treatments of the LM stem (LMS) must be compared.

Results of PCI with bare-metal stents in LM stenosis

The first reported balloon angioplasty of the LMS was performed in 1979 by Dr Gruentzig as one of five angioplasties that he performed(16). After the first series of 129 patients, reported by O'Keefe and colleagues in 1989(17), showed a 10% in-hospital mortality and 64% 3-year mortality, the practice was quickly abandoned due to poor outcomes and better surgical results. The development of stenting techniques and dual antiplatelet regimens, however, allowed PCI to be considered as a treatment again by the mid 1990s. Partly driven by case reports of successful emergency PCI to the LMS and partly by the poor survival of patients with LM stenosis who were turned down for surgery and treated only with medical management, several studies and registries reported their experiences of LM stenting in the era of the bare metal stent. There was also a drive to establish this technique in Eastern countries where CABG is culturally undesirable(18).

Silvestri and colleagues(19) published their review of a single-centre experience of LM PCI from 1993–1998. During this time they performed 140 LM PCI procedures. They reported 100% procedural success. Short-term results were also encouraging, with 9% mortality in high-risk patients and 0% mortality in low-risk cases at 1 month and 89% versus 97% survival respectively at 1 year. There was a restenosis rate of 23% and TLR in 17%.

These results were similar to those published by Park and colleagues in 1998, from their small group of 42 patients(18). Park and colleagues subsequently published a longer-term follow-up of 270 patients treated with ULM stenting(20). In a multicentre study of patients with LM stenting and normal left ventricular (LV) function they reported 98.9% procedural success. Three-year outcomes demonstrated a restenosis rate of 21%, with 17% TLR and 12% new lesion revascularization. Event-free survival was 81.9%, 78.4%, and 77.7% at 1, 2, and 3 years respectively (Fig. 19.1).

Tagaki and colleagues(21) also reported a 91% 3-year survival in their study of 62 patients following LM stenting. They identified poor LV function and increased Parsonnet score as predictors of increased cardiac mortality rate. Patients with a Parsonnet score >15 had a 21% cardiac mortality rate compared with 4% in the lower-risk group (Parsonnet score ≤15). Both Park and Tagaki reported reference vessel size as a significant factor in the development of restenosis and adverse events including repeat revascularization.

Black and colleagues also found a significant difference in mortality in patients with a high surgical risk score in their study of 92 consecutive patients who underwent unprotected LMCA stenting between March 1994 and December 1998(22). Initially angioplasty was performed only when surgical revascularization was contraindicated (Group I, 39 patients); however, the remaining 53 patients (group II) also included patients

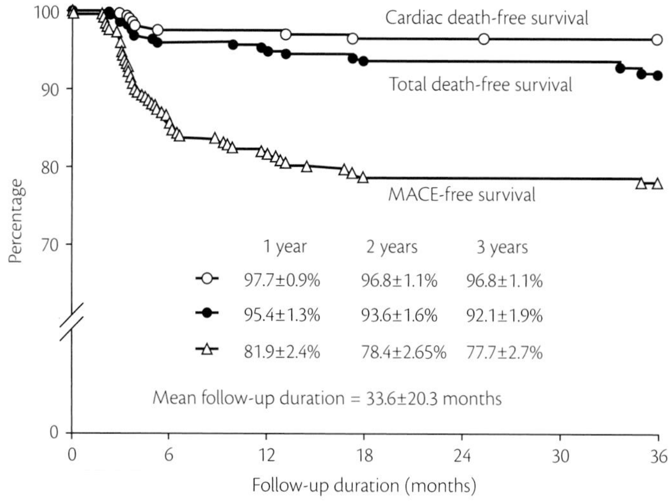

Fig. 19.1 Cumulative probability of survival free from cardiac death, total death, and MACE. Reproduced from Park S-J, Park S-W, Hong MK, *et al.* Long-term (three-year) outcomes after stenting of unprotected left main coronary artery stenosis in patients with normal left ventricular function *Am J Cardiol* 2003; **91**:12–16, © 2003 with permission from Elsevier.

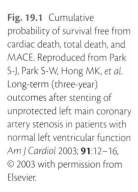

in whom surgery was feasible. Patients were followed for 7.3 ± 5.8 months. Group II patients had higher LV ejection fraction and lower surgical risk score. The procedural success rate was 100%. In-hospital mortality was 4%. During follow-up there were six deaths, 13 patients required repeat PCI, and two required CABG surgery. Survival rates were 89% at 500 days and 85% at 1000 days post stenting. Overall mortality was 3.8% in group II and 20.5% in group I.

The ULTIMA registry was a multicentre registry established in to evaluate outcome after unprotected LM coronary stenting in 25 PCI centres between 1993–1998. Their early findings raised concern over a high rate of early death in patients after LM stenting (10.6% at 6 months). However, 46% of the 279 patients enrolled were deemed to be inoperable or high surgical risk. Longer-term follow-up showed a 24% mortality at 1 year, however subset analysis of high- and low-risk groups showed only a 3.4 % mortality in the low risk group at 1 year[23]. Low-risk patients were those aged less than 65 years with LV function greater than 30% and absence of cardiogenic shock. Severe LV impairment (ejection fraction <30%), significant mitral regurgitation, renal impairment, and cardiogenic shock were identified as predictors of adverse outcome. Lesion calcification was also associated with poorer long-term results (Table 19.3).

In summary:

- Stenting the LMS with bare-metal stents is technically feasible and initial procedural success rates are reported between 98–100%
- Overall mortality is between 10–20 % at 1 year
- In low-risk patients, however, mortality rates are reported as <5% at 3 years
- Risk factors for cardiac mortality are increasing age, impaired LV function, significant mitral regurgitation, and renal impairment
- Restenosis remains a major issue with approximately 20% restenosis and 17–20 % TLR at 3 years.

Results of PCI with drug-eluting stents for LM stenosis

The evolution of drug-eluting stents has been a major breakthrough in PCI. In view of the high incidence of restenosis in the LM population, this has been of particular importance. Safety concerns arose, however, regarding the incidence of acute and late stent thrombosis and the consequences this would have for a patient with a stent *in situ* in the LMS. Despite these concerns, a recent survey suggests that as many as 30% of patients in Europe and 20% of patients in the UK now undergo PCI with stents for LMCA stenosis[24].

Studies investigating the efficacy and safety of drug-eluting stents in the LMCA have, however, had promising results. Chieffo and colleagues[25] have reported favourable long-term results from a multicentre registry of patients who have had drug-eluting stents implanted in ostial and 'body' lesions in the unprotected LMS. These patients were unsuitable for surgery due to either a high EuroSCORE or Parsonnet score or had had previous CABG with failed conduits. The 147 patients were

Table 19.3 One-year actuarial outcomes in the entire population and selected subgroups*

Population	Death† (%)	Cardiac death† (%)	MI (%)	CABG (%)	Repeat PCI (%)	Death/MI/CABG (%)
All (n = 278)	24.2	20.2	9.8	9.4	24.2	34.6
High-risk LVEF ≤30% (n = 26)	78.7	73.7	40.1	0.0	67.7	83.7
MR grade 3 or 4 (n = 10)	80.0	80.0	0.0	46.7	0.0	90.0
Cardiogenic shock (n = 37)	67.6	65.3	0.0	45.8	14.1	78.4
Creatinine ≥2mg/dL (n = 16)	68.4	68.4	22.1	0.0	52.8	68.4
Severe calcification (n = 21)	56.2	56.2	8.3	10.1	46.0	57.2
Intermediate risk (n = 118)	24.4	20.4	14.2	7.8	27.1	33.9
Low risk (n = 89) (<65 years, LVEF >30%, and not in cardiogenic shock)	3.4	3.4	2.3	11.4	20.4	16.9

* Includes in-hospital outcomes.

† All deaths considered cardiac unless clearly from other causes, e.g. cancer.

LVEF, left ventricular ejection fraction; MI, myocardial infarction.

Reproduced from Tan WA, Tamai H, Park, S-J, *et al.* Long-term clinical outcomes after unprotected left main trunk percutaneous revascularization in 279 patients. *Circulation* 2001; **104**:1609–14.

treated with either sirolimus-eluting or paxitaxel-eluting stents and followed for 886 ± 308 days. They achieved 99% procedural success. Angiographic follow-up in 106 (72%) of patients showed only −0.01mm late loss and only one patient (0.9%) had restenosis. Seven patients had target vessel revascularization, and only one of these was a TLR. They found a major adverse event rate of 7.4% and there was one death in the patient group, due to a respiratory infection.

Pavei and colleagues[26] have reported on a single-centre experience (Clinique Pasteur, France) of stenting de novo ULMCA lesions, in patients unsuitable or unwilling for CABG, with drug-eluting stents. Between 2002–2006, LM PCI was performed on 148 patients, 94 (63.5%) of whom had distal LMCA stenosis. There was a 99.3% procedural success rate and the intra-procedural complication rate was 1.4% (two patients) with one death. Patients were followed up for 874 ± 382 days and 78 patients had control angiograms between 6–8 months after the index procedure. There was a 4.7% mortality rate at 1 year and 10% at 874 days. The MACE rate was 20.3%. The rate of restenosis was 10.8% and 13 patients (8.8%) had TLR. Patients with TLR had a higher prevalence of distal stenosis. There was only 1 case of ostial lesion restenosis, the majority (9 cases) of the 16 cases of restenosis occurred at the ostium of the side branch (LCx) and 3 were in the bifurcation. A further 3 cases involved mid-shaft lesions. They showed that patients with low ejection fraction (EF) and distal stenosis were more likely to have suffered an adverse event.

These results are similar to those published by Park and colleagues[27] who evaluated a group of 784 patients undergoing drug-eluting stent implantation between 2003–2006. They report 91% survival at 3 years, with an 11.5% MACE rate and a 9.3% rate of TLR.

Valgimigli and colleagues[28] have shown that the long-term outcome of ULMCA PCI is significantly worse in patients with distal disease of the LMS compared to those with non-bifurcational lesions. They reported a significantly higher MACE rate in patients with distal LM disease (30%) compared to non-distal LM disease (11%) in their study of 130 patients. All patients were stented with either rapamycin-eluting or Taxus® stents and were followed up for approximately 590 days. Results at 30 days were similar between the two groups, however at long-term follow-up the group with distal LM disease (DLMD) had a much higher incidence of TLR and a composite endpoint of death and non-fatal myocardial infarction was twice as likely in the DLMD group (17% vs. 8%).

The recently published date from the FRIEND registry[29], however, showed excellent results when stenting the LMS despite having 66% of patients with DLMD. In a prospective multicentre study of LM stenting with paclitaxel stents, 151 patients were stented, 100 with DLMD. In the DLMD group they opted for an approach of 'provisional T' stenting where possible and 72% of the DLMD patients had only one stent inserted. At median follow-up of over 450 days they reported a mortality rate of 2% and major adverse cardiac and cerebrovascular event (MACCE) rate of 10.6% despite the inclusion of a high proportion of patients with DLMD.

In a systematic review and meta-analysis of 1278 patients, Biondi-Zoccai and colleagues[30] have shown that treating ULMCA lesions with drug-eluting stents is associated with a 5.5% (3.3–7.7%) risk of death, a 16.5% (11.7–21.3%) MACE rate, and a TLR rate of 6.5% (3.7–9.2%). DLMD is a predictor of MACE and TLR, however, it is the presence of high risk features that predicts death. The review also shows that most series have reported low rates of stent thrombosis (0–2%) apart from the Price *et al.*[31] group (4%).

In summary:

- Most of the available data regarding drug-eluting stent use in the LMS is taken from registries and non-randomized trials
- Most of these report experience in small numbers of patients, almost all less than 150 patients and follow-up is rarely greater than 2–3 years
- There is also often a lack of complete angiographic follow-up to accurately assess restenosis rates
- However, in a cohort of patients including many with high-risk features and multiple comorbidities, current stenting practice is associated with high procedural and short-term success
- There is a 5–10% risk of death over a 2–3-year-follow-up in a population of patients, many of whom have a high EuroSCORE or Parsonnet score and who were high surgical risk candidates
- Restenosis rates are usually <5% but are higher in patients with distal bifurcation lesions (10%). Rates of TLR are <10%.

Comparison between CABG and PCI with drug-eluting stents

Despite the many trials reporting outcomes of LM treatment there have been very few comparative studies looking at CABG versus PCI. In 2006 Chieffo and colleagues[25] reported on registry data from their centre on all patients treated for LMCA disease between 2002–2004. During this period they treated 249 patients,

142 with CABG and 109 with PCI with drug-eluting stents. Treatment strategy for each patient was based on physician and patient preference. The aim in each case was to provide complete revascularization. In the PCI group, 87 patients (81%) had distal LMS disease and two branches were stented in 74% of cases. Although the PCI group were younger, and had a lower incidence of hypertension and renal impairment, there was no significant difference in LV function or EuroSCORE values between the two patient cohorts. At 1-year follow-up there were no significant differences in primary endpoints of death, myocardial infarction, and revascularization. There was however a significantly lower mortality rate in the PCI group (2.8%) compared to the CABG group (6.4%). The PCI group did have a significantly higher rate of TLR (15.8%) and TVR (19.6%) than the CABG group (3.6% for each).

Lee and colleagues[32] reported similar findings from their single-centre study evaluating 173 patients who underwent CABG or PCI for ULMCA disease after 2003. All of the 50 patients in the PCI group received drug-eluting stents. In the CABG group 46% were considered high risk (Parsonnet score >15) compared with 64% in the PCI group. However, although there was a significantly higher rate of MACE in the CABG group (17% vs. 2%) at 30 days, there was no difference in MACE rates between the groups at 6 and 12 months.

The MAIN-COMPARE registry[33] is a Korean multicentre registry that compared long-term outcomes in a matched cohort of 1102 patients with unprotected LMCA disease who underwent stent implantation and 1138 patients who underwent CABG in Korea between January 2000 and June 2006. In the group of 318 patients stented between January 2000 and May 2003, coronary stenting was performed exclusively with bare-metal stents, whereas from May 2003 until June 2006, exclusively drug-eluting stents were used in the remaining 784 patients (71%). Patients treated with bare-metal stents were prescribed clopidogrel or ticlopidine for at least 1 month, and patients treated with drug-eluting stents were prescribed clopidogrel for at least 6 months. Patients were matched into 542 paired PCI and CABG groups (396 drug-eluting stents with 60% in each having DLMD). This large observational study showed that the risk of death and myocardial infarction or stroke were not significantly different between the matched PCI and the CABG groups. These results were consistent when bare-metal stents or drug-eluting stents were compared with CABG. They also reported that the rate of target-vessel revascularization was significantly lower in the CABG group than in the PCI group.

These registry data suggested that randomized trials were needed to truly compare the treatment strategies.

The first randomized trial, the LEMANS study was published in 2008[34]. In this small multicentre study, 105 patients with ULMCA stenosis were randomized to PCI (52 patients) or CABG (53 patients). The primary endpoint was change in LV function. PCI patients had significantly lower MACCE at 1 month. There was no significant difference between the groups at 12 months for MACCE, however, there was a significantly improved ejection fraction in the PCI group.

Initial results from the large, multicentre SYNTAX study were also presented at the European Society of Cardiology congress in 2008[35]. Patients who were eligible for treatment by both PCI and CABG were randomized to receive either PCI and stenting with a Taxus® drug-eluting stent, or CABG. Individuals deemed better candidates for one approach or the other were sent for the appropriate procedure and then entered into SYNTAX PCI or CABG registries. The decision on patients' suitability is made jointly by a cardiothoracic surgeon and an interventional cardiologist. Patients are to be followed-up for 5 years.

The 1-year follow-up presented in 2008 reported that of the 1800 patients randomized to PCI (903 patients) or CABG (897 patients), 705 had LM disease. Most of the patients (87%) with LM disease also had significant lesions in at least one other vessel. In the LM subset, the composite MACCE rate between the two treatment strategies at 1 year was comparable (13.7% for CABG vs. 15.8% for PCI). There was, however, a significantly higher risk of stroke in the CABG group, while PCI patients had a higher risk of reintervention. They also noted that the need for repeat procedures increased in patients with LM and multivessel disease compared to isolated LM or LM +1 vessel disease. This was supported using analysis by SYNTAX score which demonstrated that while there were no significant differences in risk of

Table 19.4 SYNTAX trial endpoints in left main subset

Endpoint	CABG (%)	Taxus (%)	p
Death	4.4	4.2	0.88
Stroke	2.7	0.3	0.009
Myocardial infarction (MI)	4.1	4.3	0.97
Revascularization	6.7	12.0	0.02
Death/stroke/MI	9.1	7.0	0.29
MACCE	13.6	15.8	0.44

Reproduced with permission from Serruys P. TCT 2008; October 14, 2008; Washington, DC.

MACCE between the treatment strategies for patients with low or intermediate SYNTAX scores, patients with the highest scores (33 or higher) had significantly lower MACCE rates if treated by CABG.

In summary:

- Patients undergoing PCI for LMS stenosis have a mortality rate which is comparable to CABG in the short and medium term
- PCI is, however, associated with significantly higher rates of reintervention
- The presence of multi-vessel disease may be a greater indicator of reintervention than the presence of LM stenosis
- The long-term follow-up of recent trials may provide further information.

What is important about LM stenosis?

The LMCA is of particular importance as it supplies approximately two-thirds of the blood to the heart and almost 100% of the blood flow to the left ventricle. The LM is a large artery and therefore tends to have a high plaque volume in order to cause a significant lesion. LM lesions are also prone to calcification, with over 50% having significant calcification on angiogram. Plaque shift and incomplete stent expansion are therefore important technical considerations when thinking about stenting the LM.

The distal LM, by definition, always ends in a bifurcation, or even trifurcation, giving rise to the left anterior descending (LAD) and left circumflex (LCx) arteries, and possibly an intermediate artery. Seventy per cent of significant LM lesions involve the distal LM and its branches. Compromise of these 'branches' would obviously cause important procedural and clinical effects for the patients.

LM disease is often associated with lesions in the other coronary arteries, giving a pattern of complex multi-vessel disease. The treatment of these lesions needs to be considered when deciding on the treatment strategy of the LM and the feasibility of a complete revascularization approach.

Finally, the LM is the artery of guide catheter intubation which may also give rise to some technical issues, especially with ostial and very proximal lesions.

Ostial and mid-vessel lesions of the LM

These lesions are very amenable to stenting and have good procedural and long-term results[25]. The techniques are straightforward and should involve a single-stent strategy. Mid-vessel lesions can be treated as with stenosis in any other vessel, taking into account considerations such as plaque shift and vessel calcification. Ostial lesions are also very amenable to stenting; however, the position of the guide catheter during balloon and stent placement requires careful consideration. The guide catheter may also have a significant occlusive effect on left coronary artery blood flow if there is an ostial lesion, therefore careful assessment of the patient and ECG for signs of ischaemia are mandatory. Ostial LM lesions, like all ostial lesions, require careful stent deployment and post dilatation at the aorto-arterial junction to minimize the risk of subsequent restenosis (Fig. 19.2).

Distal LMS lesions

The distal LM is a much more challenging target for stenting and as discussed is more prone to restenosis and subsequent target vessel revascularization. Distal LM lesions are by definition bifurcation lesions, at least, and a number of stenting techniques can be considered. These will be discussed in detail in the section on stenting techniques.

Protected LM stenosis

LM disease occurs when one or both of the two main branches are 'protected' by a patent graft, especially an internal mammary graft, can usually be safely treated if required by PCI at very low risk to the patient. The stenting strategy depends on the pattern of disease and the distribution of vessels 'protected' by patent grafts.

Patient selection

The first step in safely performing PCI to the LMS is careful patient selection. There are two important areas to consider when selecting patients for LMS PCI. The first is the clinical characteristics of the patient and the second is the angiographic characteristics. A through assessment of these factors should be used to determine which patients should be selected for PCI and which should be sent for surgery. These discussions should usually involve both the cardiology and surgical team.

Clinical characteristics

Clinical characteristics to consider are:

- Age
- Diabetes
- Renal function
- Functional class

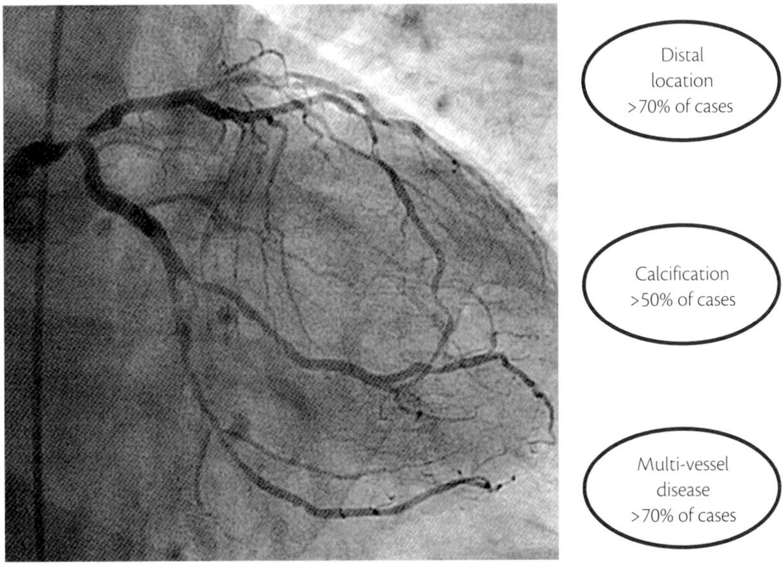

Fig. 19.2 Distal LM stenosis with multi-vessel disease.

- Cognitive status
- Valvular disease
- Carotid disease
- Previous cardiac intervention
- Other comorbidities.

The presence of other comorbidities and increasing age are important considerations when assessing the risks involved in PCI and the feasibility of safely performing the procedure. Increasing age and worsening renal function may contribute to a higher procedural risk but they may also, however, have a higher impact on the surgical risk associated with an individual patient and weight the overall assessment in favour of PCI.

The presence of other comorbidities and impaired cognitive status may also mean that the long-term benefits of surgery and concerns over restenosis may not be particularly applicable to every patient.

The EuroSCORE gives us a useful method of assessing the patient's surgical risk based on these clinical characteristics.

Angiographic characteristics

The important angiographic features to consider are:

- LV function
- Distal or no distal LM
- LM anatomy (trifurcation)
- Length of LM lesion
- Calcification
- Diffuse disease
- Multi-vessel disease
- RCA occlusion
- Additional complex lesions (bifurcation, chronic total occlusion) on the other vessels
- Quality of the distal vessels.

The development of the SYNTAX score has provided a numerical assessment tool for grading the complexity of the angiographic anatomy.

After analysis of the clinical and angiographic features, patients can be divided into one of three treatment groups. These are:

1) Favourable for stenting:
   - Low-risk patients, with good LV function, non distal and non-calcified LM stenosis
   - Ostial LM lesions
   - Mid-shaft LM lesions.

These patients have been shown to have excellent outcomes following LM stenting as shown in Table 19.5.

2) Technically difficult and controversial:
   Patients with preserved LV function and non-calcified distal LM bifurcation lesion involving the ostium of LAD and LCx.

Table 19.5 Mortality after LM stenting

	In Hospital	Follow-Up (886±308 Days)
Cardiac death, n (%)	0	4 (2.7)
Cardiac death in 60 high-risk patients, n (%)	0	4 (6.6)
Cardiac death in 87 low-risk patients, n (%)	0	0
Total death, n (%)	1 (0.7)	5 (3.4)

Reproduced with permission from Chieffo A, Park SJ, Valgimigli M, *et al.* Favorable long-term outcome after drug-eluting stent implantation in nonbifurcation lesions that involve unprotected left main coronary artery. a multicenter registry. *Circulation* 2007; **116**:158–62.

PCI could be considered when:

- Elderly (octogenarians)
- Small LCx
- No complex additional lesions
- Non diabetic
- Poor surgical candidate:
  - distal coronary disease unfavourable to CABG
  - high surgical risk (EuroSCORE)
  - comorbidity (chronic obstructive lung disease)
  - emergency clinical situation i.e. acute LM occlusion

3) Surgery preferred:

- Heavy calcified LM disease
- Reduced LV function
- Diabetic patients
- Multi-vessel disease suitable for CABG:
  - with distal bifurcation lesion and reduced LV function
  - with distal bifurcation lesion and occluded RCA
  - with additional complex lesions on the other vessels (high SYNTAX score).

Risk stratification tools

The EuroSCORE is an assessment tool which looks at clinical characteristics of the patient, including age, sex, presence of comorbidities such as renal failure and recent acute coronary event, and gives these a 'weighting score'. The additive EuroSCORE has been shown to be an accurate reflection of the surgical mortality risk at 30 days. A EuroSCORE ≥6 is considered high risk. The logistic EuroSCORE has subsequently been shown to have greater predictive power[36,37].

The Parsonnet surgical risk score[38] has also been used in some studies to assess patient characteristics prior to LM stenting. This score was developed in the USA in the 1980s and also uses clinical characteristics, comorbidities, and type of surgery to estimate surgical risk. It has largely been overtaken by the EuroSCORE in recent practice. A Parsonnet score of ≥15 was considered high risk.

A criticism of the previous two scores was that neither took account of the number of vessels and lesions involved and the complexity of these for either the surgeon or the interventionalist. In response the SYNTAX score[39] was recently developed and piloted during the multicentre SYNTAX study. This angiographic score calculates a total based on cumulative scores for each vessel and each lesion, assessing tortuosity, calcification, lesion length, and the presence of side branches as well as the location of the lesion within the vessel and the overall vessel calibre. The SYNTAX study results at 1 year suggest that a raw score of <22 is low risk, an intermediate group has a SYNTAX score of 22–32, and ≥33 is high risk. These scores will, however, be weighted when the results of the long-term follow-up (5 years) are known.

Summary

- Patient selection is crucial
- Global appraisal of the patient (clinical and angiographic characteristics)—use the EuroSCORE and SYNTAX score
- Based on medical-surgical consultation and ethics of information
- Stenting can be performed with good results in selected patients
- Long-term careful follow-up is needed to evaluate safety and efficacy of our procedures
- Feasibility does not mean indication!

Equipment for stenting the LMCA

Do we need special equipment when stenting the LM? No. Most LM stenting does not require any different equipment; however, the key issue is to be well prepared. It is important to consider the equipment that will be required and have this immediately available.

The equipment that may be required is:

- IABP—in general this should be on standby for all LM stenting. The placement of a 5F sheath in the contralateral femoral at the beginning of the procedure allows rapid intra-aorta balloon pump (IABP) insertion if required and should be considered, especially for all patients with impaired LV function. Consider elective placement of an IABP at the start of the procedure for very high-risk patients
- Temporary pacing wire—not routinely required
- Guide catheters—usually requires 6F or 7F for complex distal LM lesions or for adjuvant strategies, e.g. rotablation. Complex stenting strategies may occasionally require an 8F catheter. The EBU, XB, and Amplatz guides generally provide good support during stenting. The EBU (or JFL) can also be used from the radial route. The Amplatz guides should not be used in ostial lesions
- Short tipped catheter may also be useful in severe ostial lesions
- Intravascular ultrasound (IVUS)—should be used to assist in correct stent sizing and ensure adequate stent deployment
- Rotablator—remember the LM often has significant calcification.

Stenting techniques

Ostial and mid vessel lesions

These lesions should be stented with a single-stent strategy (Fig. 19.3).

Mid vessel lesions can essentially be treated as in any other vessel. It is possible to successfully direct stent the mid vessel but careful assessment should be made of the vessel diameter, lesion length, and degree of calcification. The potential for plaque shift should also be considered. If any doubt then pre-dilate in the same manner as with any discrete lesion in any vessel. It is common practice to wire both main distal branches before stenting.

There are some important techniques required when stenting ostial lesions:

- Ostial lesions are often pre-dilated
- Careful imaging must be performed to ensure adequate visualization of the ostium and adjacent aorta. Appropriate working views should be selected before commencing any interventional practice (usually from AP–cranial to LAO–cranial)
- If the stenosis is severe, the guide catheter may be occlusive. After the angioplasty wire is in position in the distal vessel, the guide can be carefully disengaged slightly from the ostium by pushing gently on the wire. This will help to minimize coronary ischaemia. The guide can then be gently moved towards the ostium, by slight traction on the wire, to allow contrast injections and imaging
- A short-tip 6F or 7F catheter with side holes is also available for severe ostial lesions
- The stent needs to be placed carefully with 1–2mm protruding into the aorta
- The guide then needs to be completely removed from the LM before the stent is deployed to avoid being trapped by the stent. Keep the guide close to the ostium to allow contrast injection into the LM. Ensure that the stent position is not altered by guide catheter manipulation
- After deploying the stent, the balloon should be withdrawn slightly into the ascending aorta. Post dilate the proximal part of the stent to 'flare it' and ensure good stent apposition at the ostium. This is also useful in facilitating catheter engagement if further angiography is required
- Be aware that excessive or aggressive dilatation at the ostium can cause dissection of the ascending aorta
- Use IVUS to ensure a satisfactory result.

Distal LM lesions

Distal LM lesions are in most cases treated as true bifurcation lesions. The exception to this is when one branch is recessive (usually the LCx) and of very small calibre, when one branch is chronically occluded or if protected by a good quality graft. In these circumstances the distal lesion may be stented with a single-stent technique, stenting across the ostium of the other vessel, and treating essentially a single distal vessel.

True distal bifurcation lesions may be treated by either a single-stent or by a two-stent strategy. Choice of strategy is based on vessel and lesion characteristics but also on operator experience and expertise. The provisional T stenting is a single-stent strategy, although it allows the placement of a second stent if required. More complex lesions may require T stenting, crush, culotte or V-stenting, depending on the pattern of disease at the bifurcation, the diameter of the branches, and the angle between them. Data from several registries (RESEARCH and T-SEARCH) have not shown a significant benefit of

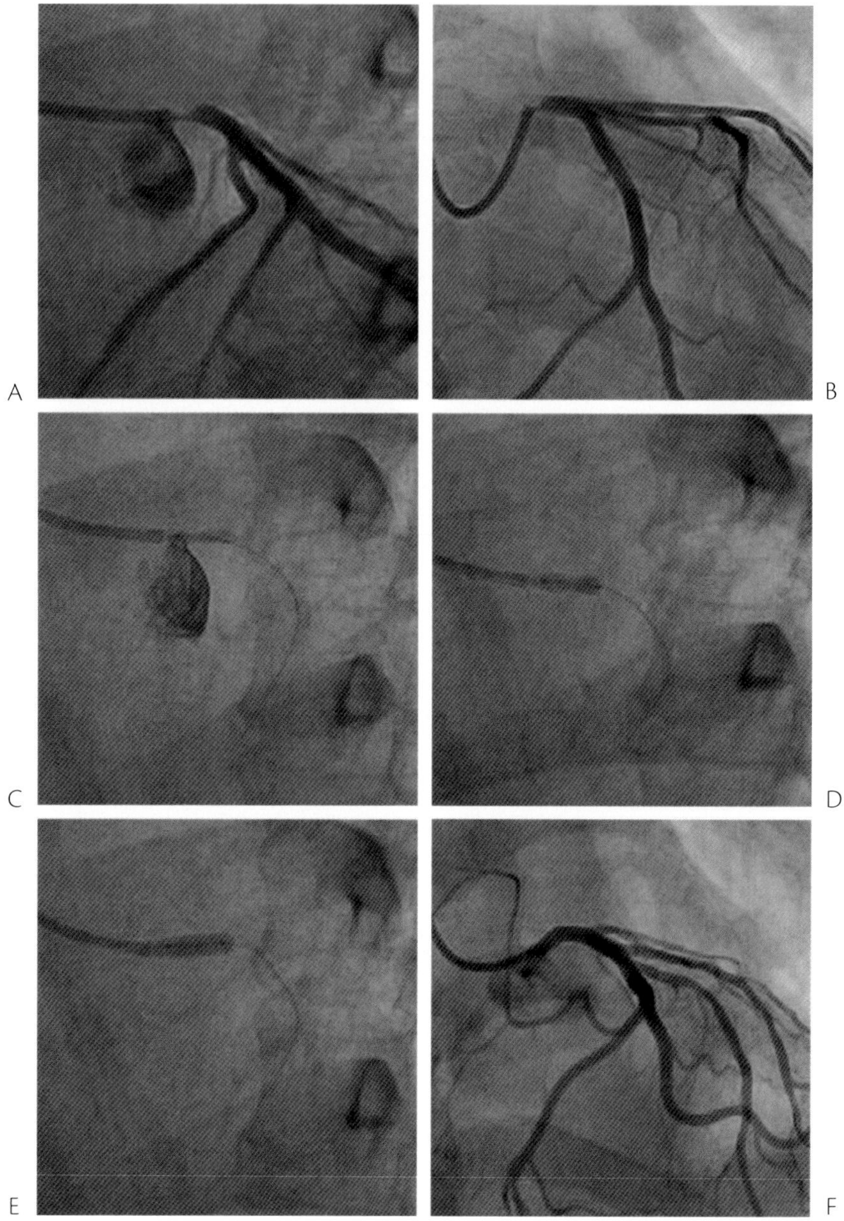

Fig. 19.3 Ostial LM stenting. A and B). Initial appearance. C) Positioning stent with guide disengaged. D) Stent deployment with proximal stent protruding into aorta. E) High pressure post dilatation. F) Final appearance.

any one technique and MACE and restenosis rates were similar for one- and two-stent techniques. Others studies have suggested that stenting the side branch or using the crush technique may be associated with higher rates of restenosis. The different methods will be discussed in detail.

In deciding which strategy to use the important thing to consider is the anatomy of the side branch, which is almost always the LCx.

The LCx is one of the key elements for indication of LM PCI due to:

- Size
- Area of jeopardized myocardium
- Ostial location of atheroma plaque
- Bifurcation angle.

The LCx is a major issue because:

- Frequently involved
- Often calcified
- Influences treatment strategy
- Influences PCI technique
- Problem of restenosis.

The size of the LCx and the anatomy of the ostium are the two important features (Fig. 19.4).

By this strategy, if there is an occluded or very small circumflex then the main vessel, the LAD, is treated exclusively. A wire placed in a small LCx may help to maintain flow after a single stent is placed across the ostium. Due to the small diameter of the vessel, however, it is not considered suitable for further intervention (Fig. 19.5)

Single-stent strategy

The provisional T stent

This is a single-stent strategy but allows the positioning of a second stent if required. The main vessel (almost always the LAD) is wired. The decision to place a second wire is made using the pathways as described. The stent is deployed in the LM–LAD and post dilated as required.

The appearance of the ostial LCx is assessed, again using the pathways as described. The LCx may be left untouched or a wire may be passed through the stent into the LCx and a kissing inflation performed. Again, the angiographic appearances are assessed and if necessary a second stent may be passed into the ostial LCx and deployed if required. Post dilatation of the main vessel stent is mandatory after stenting of the LCx. A kissing inflation completes the procedure if two stents have been used (Fig. 19.6).

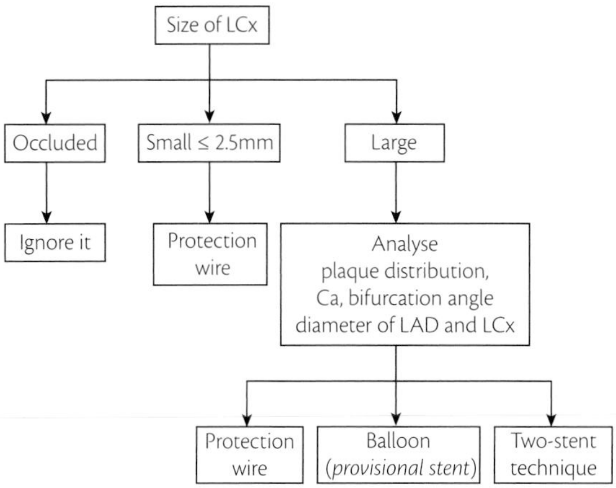

Fig. 19.4 Factors relevant in deciding strategy for managing the side branch (LCx).

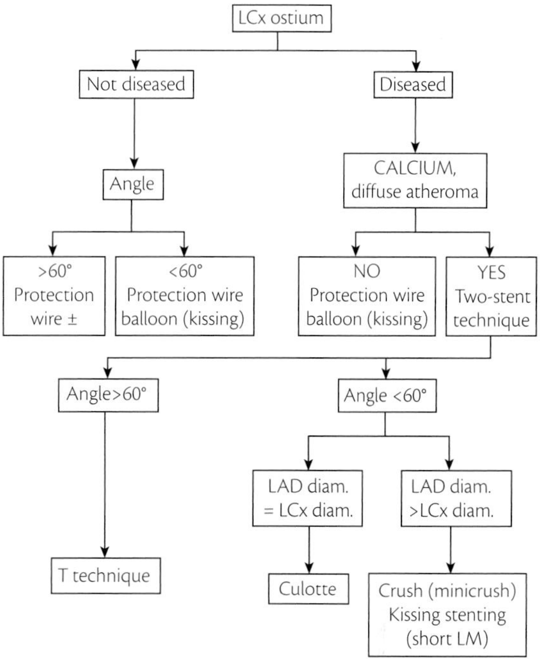

Fig. 19.5 Factors important in choosing which bifurcation stenting technique.

Double-stent strategies

The culotte stent

This is a strategy suitable for lesions where the ostium of the LCx is diseased, the angulation between the vessels is <60° (higher risk of plaque shift) and the two vessels are of similar diameter. Both vessels are wired. The main vessel, usually the LM–LAD, is stented. The side vessel is rewired and the side branch ostium pre-dilated to open the stent struts. A second stent is then passed through the struts of the first into the side vessel, leaving an overlap of both stents in the LM. The jailed and LAD wires are removed prior to the deployment of the second stent. The LM–LCx stent is deployed. A wire is passes back into the LAD and the procedure is completed with a 'kissing balloon' inflation (Fig. 19.7).

The T stent

The T stent is used when a two-stent strategy is required but the angulation between the two vessels approached 90°. The two vessels are wired. A stent is deployed in the side vessel, making sure to cover the ostium with only minimal protrusion into the LAD. The LM–LAD lesion is then stented. A wire is recrossed into the LCx side branch. Post dilatation of the LCx ostium and a 'kissing balloon' inflation are performed (Fig. 19.8).

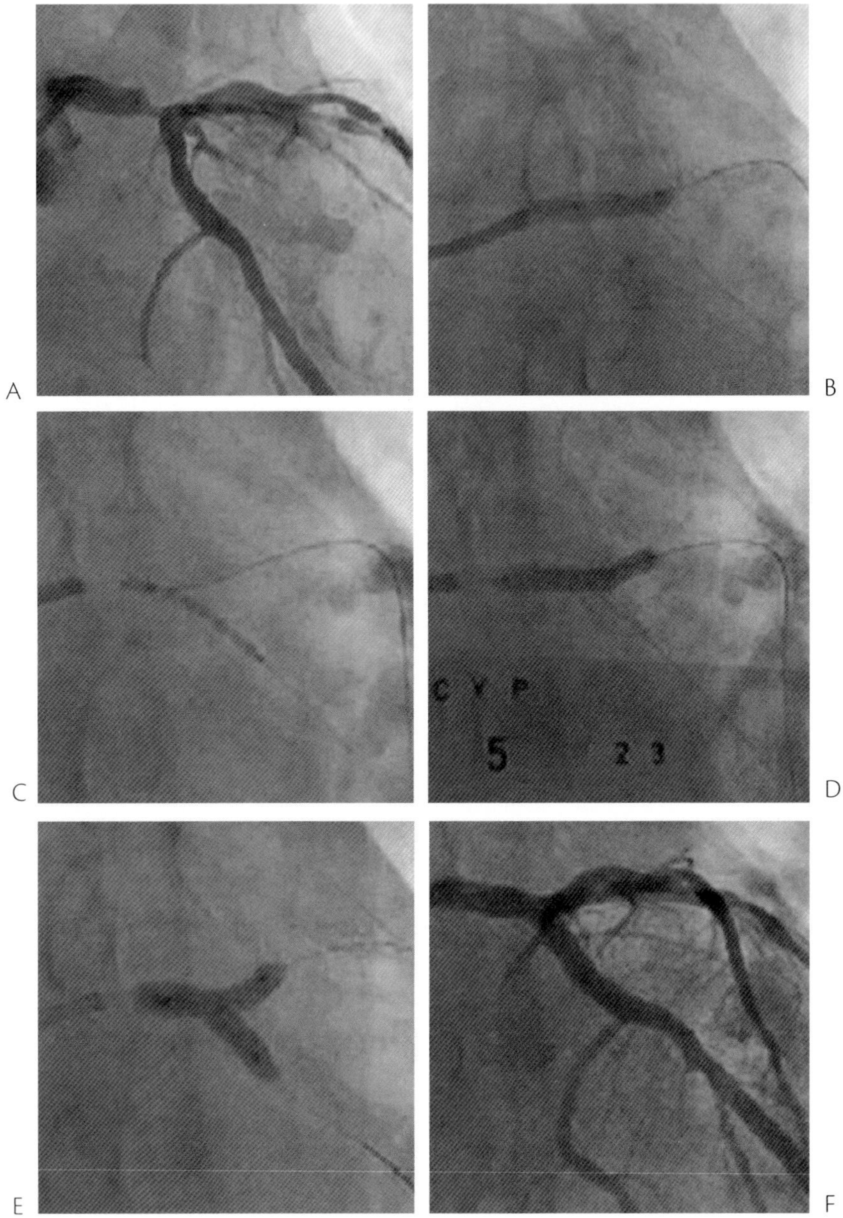

Fig. 19.6 The culotte technique. A) Initial appearance. B) Predilatation of the LAD. C) First stent deployed in the LCx. D) Second stent deployed in the LAD after recrossing with wire and predilatation. E) Kissing balloon post dilatation. F) Final result.

The crush stent

The crush technique can be used when the diameter of the main vessel is greater than the side branch and the angulation is favourable (approximately ≤60%). Both vessels are wired. The side branch is stented first, positioning the stent to allow 1–2mm (minicrush) to protrude into the LM. After deployment the wire is removed from the side branch. A prepositioned balloon in the main vessel is then inflated. This crushes the proximal side branch stent against the LM wall. The main vessel is then stented. The main vessel stent is positioned to ensure that the side vessel stent is completely covered within the LM. Deployment of the main vessel stent crushes the proximal side branch

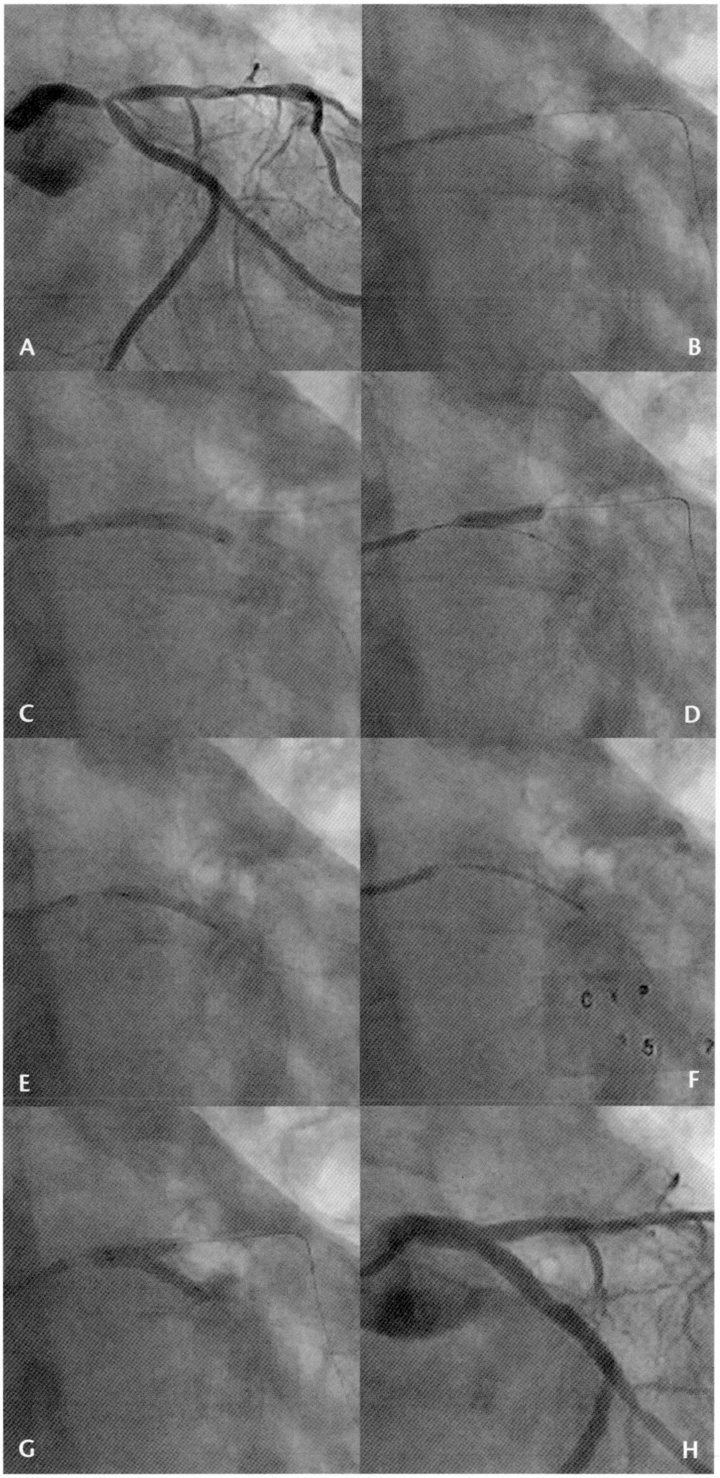

Fig. 19.7 The crush technique for left main stenting. A) Initial appearance. B) Pre dilatation of LAD. C) Pre dilatation of LCx. D) Stent to LAD ('side branch' due to large dominant LCx. E) Remove side branch wire and balloon to dilate main vessel (LCx) and 'crush' side vessel stent. F) Deploy main vessel. G) Rewire side branch and 'kissing balloon' post dilate. H) Final appearance.

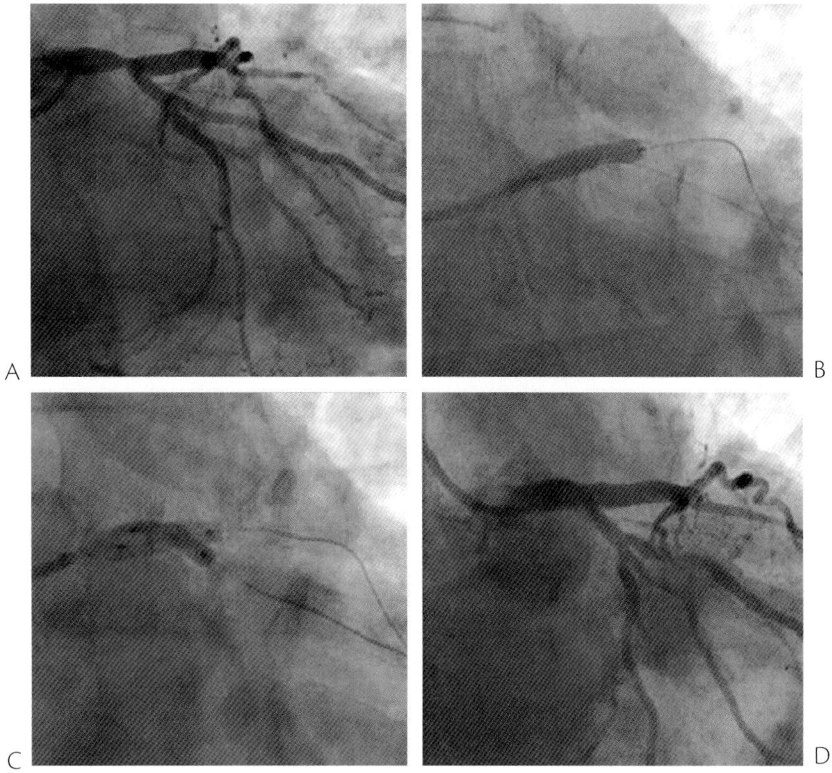

Fig. 19.8 Provisional T stenting of the LM. A) Initial appearance. B) Stent to LM–LAD. C) Kissing balloons post-stent deployment. D) Final result.

stent against the LM wall. It is necessary to rewire the LCx, through the stent struts of both the LAD and crushed LCx stent to perform a final post dilatation of the side branch ostium and a final 'kissing balloon' inflation. It is sometimes difficult to recross the crushed stent segment but it is very important to perform the final kissing inflation to achieve a satisfactory outcome (Fig. 19.9).

The V stent

The V stent technique (or 'kissing stent' technique) is suitable in similar situations to the crush technique. However it is important to have a large diameter LM with large but relatively smaller LAD and LCx. The two vessels are wired. The lesions are pre-dilated sequentially, if required. The two stents are placed into the LM and respective arteries. It is important that the proximal edges of both stents are placed together in the LM, while the distal ends are distal to the bifurcation. The stents are then deployed by simultaneous inflation of the stent balloons to equal pressures. Post dilatation, if required, can be performed by a 'kissing balloon' inflation (Fig. 19.10).

Special considerations during LM stenting

Technical tips

- Think carefully before you embark—is this an appropriate procedure?
- Anticipate potential problems
- Have a clear strategy at the outset—and a backup plan in the event of a less than desirable result
- Ensure all equipment is checked and ready if required. In the event of a complication the response must be rapid
- Ensure you have good guide support and clear views
- Keep inflations short—the balloon inflated in the LM is obstructing blood flow to almost all of the left ventricle

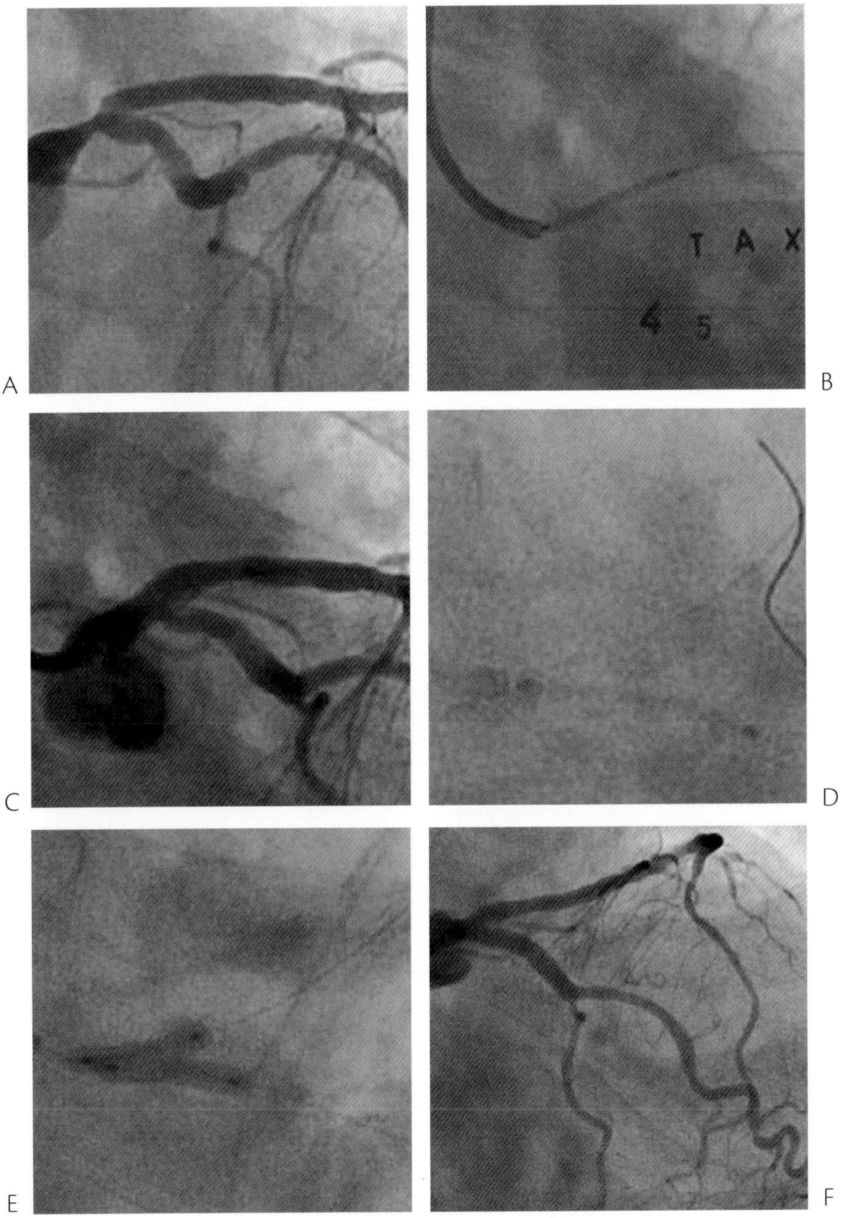

Fig. 19.9 Planned T stenting of the LM. A) Initial appearance. B) Stent to LM–LAD. C) Dissection of ostial LCx. D) Stent to LCx. E) Kissing balloons. F) Final result.

- Use IVUS to ensure appropriate stent selection and deployment
- Keep it simple.

Antiplatelet therapy

In elective LM stenting all patients should be pretreated with dual antiplatelet therapy or have a loading dose of aspirin 300mg and clopidogrel 300–600mg at least 24h prior to the procedure.

All patients should be anticoagulated with heparin 70–100unit/kg during the procedure.

Aspirin should be continued lifelong.

Clopidogrel 75mg should be continued for at least a year following deployment of drug-eluting stents in the LM. There is currently no evidence for longer regimens in LM stenting and studies suggest the probability of stent thrombosis is small. The use of longer regimens or tests for non-responders may become advisable for

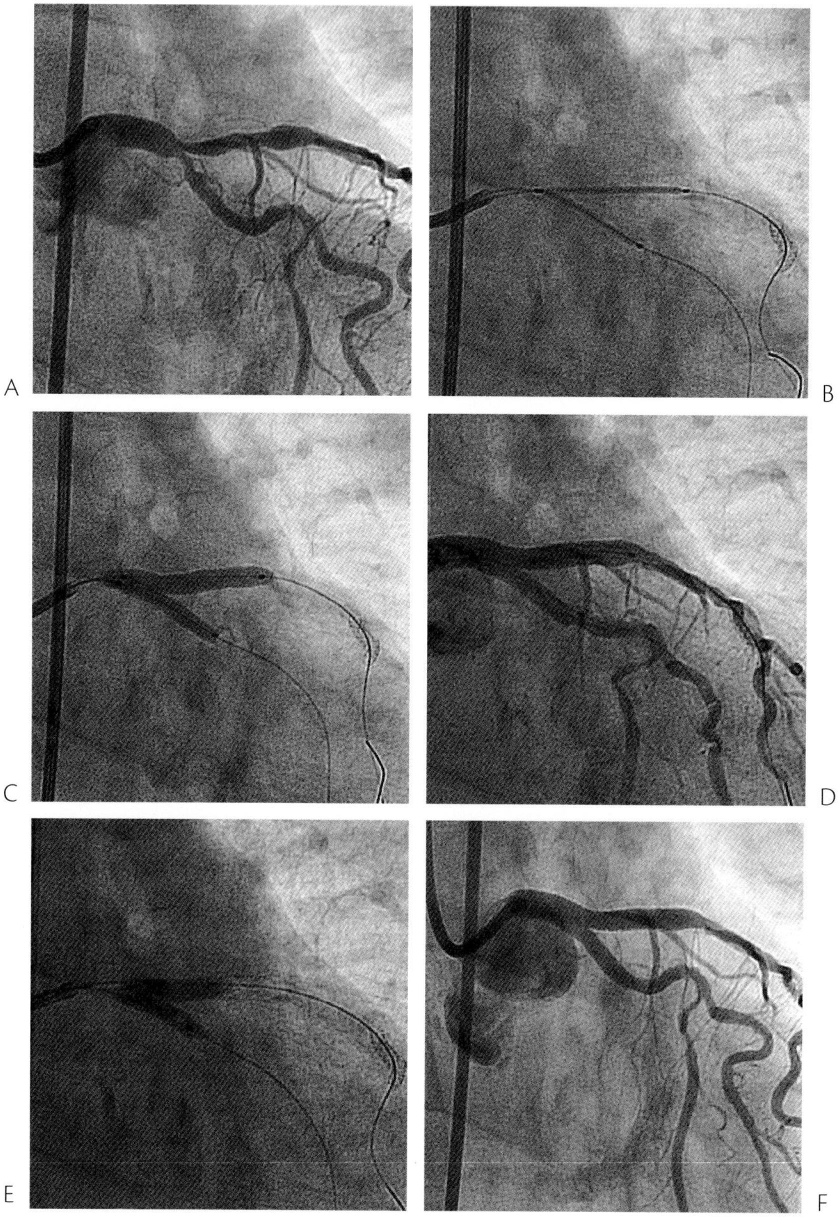

Fig. 19.10 V stenting of the LM. A) Initial appearance. B) Positioning of the two stents. C) Deploying the two stents. D) Post stenting. E) Kissing balloon post dilatation. F) Final result.

these patients, especially with complex reconstruction of the distal LM, which may predispose to higher risk of stent thrombosis.

In patients with bare-metal stents, the presence of other comorbidities is often important in the choice of stent and safely of long-term dual anticoagulation; however, 6–12 months is suggested where possible.

The use of glycoprotein IIb/IIIa in LM stenting is left to the operator's discretion and is likely to depend on the clinical scenario and the presence of acute ischaemia and thrombus.

Follow-up strategies

All patients should have regular clinical follow-up.

The practice of the authors is to routinely perform stress echocardiography or myocardial perfusion imaging at 3 months followed by multislice cardiac computed tomography (or angiography) at 6–9 months.

Recurrence of symptoms, however, should be an indication for urgent angiographic assessment.

Conclusion

- CABG remains the gold standard of care for patients with LM stenosis
- LM stenting is feasible and is generally technically safe although there are some special considerations during the stenting process
- Results of non-distal LM stenting are good
- Distal LM disease presents a true challenge but the use of current stenting techniques have allowed this to be performed with acceptable short- and long-term results
- A high EuroSCORE is an adverse predictor of mortality in these high-risk patients. Poor LV function is particularly associated with a high mortality rate
- The presence of multi-vessel disease and a high SYNTAX score is indicative of a high risk of MACCE and repeat intervention
- The use of drug-eluting stents has significantly reduced the risk of restenosis and there does not appear to be a significant risk on stent thrombosis
- The use of IVUS should be considered for all LM stenting. The need for adjunctive equipment and IABP must be carefully considered
- LM stenting provides an alternative for patients at high surgical risk or who find CABG unacceptable but it is important to consider CABG for all patients as long-term data is not yet available and the rate of reintervention remains high for many patients
- Think before you embark—feasibility does not mean indication!

References

1. Stone P, Goldschlager N. Left main coronary artery disease: review and appraisal. *Cardiovasc Med* 1979; **4**:165–77.
2. DeMots H, Rosch J, McAnulty J. Left main coronary artery disease. *Cardiovasc Clin* 1977; **8**:201–11.
3. Taylor H, Deumite N, Chaitman B, *et al.* Asymptomatic left main coronary artery disease in the Coronary Artery Surgery Study (CASS) registry. *Circulation* 1989; **79**: 1171–9.
4. Cohen M, Gorlin R. Main left coronary artery disease: clinical experience from 1964-1974. *Circulation* 1975; **52**:275–85.
5. Yusuf S, Zucker D, Peduzzi P, *et al.* Effect of coronary artery bypass graft surgery on survival: overview of 10-year results from randomised trials by the Coronary Artery Bypass Graft Surgery Trialists' Collaboration. *Lancet* 1994; **344**:1446.
6. Chaitman BR, Fisher LD, Bourassa MG, *et al.* Effect of coronary bypass surgery on survival patterns in subsets of patients with left main coronary artery disease: report of the Collaborative Study in Coronary Artery Surgery (CASS). *Am J Cardiol* 1981; **48**:765–77.
7. Takaro T, Peduzzi P, Detre KM, *et al.* Survival in subgroups of patients with left main coronary artery disease: Veterans Administration Cooperative Study of Surgery for Coronary Arterial Occlusive Disease. *Circulation* 1982; **66**:14–22.
8. Caracciolo EA, Davis KB, Sopko G, *et al.* Comparison of surgical and medical group survival in patients with left main equivalent coronary artery disease: longterm CASS experience. *Circulation* 1995; **91**:2335–44.
9. Silber S, Albertsson P, Aviles FF, *et al.* Guidelines for percutaneous coronary interventions. The Task Force for Percutaneous Coronary Interventions of the European Society of Cardiology. *Eur Heart J* 2005; **26**:804–47.
10. Smith SC Jr, Feldman TE, Hirshfeld JW Jr, *et al.* ACC/AHA/SCAI 2005 Guideline Update for Percutaneous Coronary Intervention—summary article: a report of the American College of Cardiology/American Heart Association Task Force on Practice Guidelines (ACC/AHA/SCAI Writing Committee to Update the 2001 Guidelines for Percutaneous Coronary Intervention). *Circulation* 2006; **113**:156–75.
11. Bottner RK, Klein LW. Do the current ACC/AHA guidelines correctly reflect the attitudes and utilization of PCI in patients with unprotected left main coronary artery stenosis? *Catheter Cardiovasc Interv* 2005; **64**:402–5.
12. Ellis SG, Tamai H, Nobuyoshi M, *et al.* Contemporary percutaneous treatment of unprotected left main coronary stenoses. Initial results from a multicenter registry analysis. 1994–1996 *Circulation* 1997; **96**:3867–72.
13. Taggart DP, Kaul S, Boden WE, *et al.* Revascularisation for unprotected left main stem coronary artery stenosis: stenting or surgery. *J Am Coll Cardiol* 2008; **51**:885–92.
14. Jönsson A, Hammar N, Nordquist T, *et al.* Left main coronary artery stenosis no longer a risk factor for early and late death after coronary artery bypass surgery – an experience covering three decades. *Eur J Cardiothorac Surgery* 2006; **30**:311–17.
15. Sabik JF, Blackstone EH, Firstenberg M, *et al.* A benchmark for evaluating innovative treatment of left main coronary disease. *Circulation.* 2007; **116**(Suppl I):I-232–I-239.
16. Gruntzig AR, Senning A, Siegenthaler WE. Nonoperative dilatation of coronary-artery stenosis: percutaneous transluminal coronary angioplasty. *N Engl J Med* 1979; **301**: 61–8.
17. O'Keefe JH Jr, Hartzler GO, Rutherford BD, *et al.* Left main coronary angioplasty: early and late results of

127 acute and elective procedures. *Am J Cardiol* 1989; **64**(3):144–7.
18. Park SJ, Park SW, Hong MK, *et al.* Stenting of unprotected left main coronary artery stenoses: immediate and late outcomes. *J Am Coll Cardiol* 1998; **31**:3–42.
19. Silvestri M, Barragan P, Sainsous J, *et al.* Unprotected left main coronary artery stenting: immediate and medium-term outcomes of 140 elective procedures. *J Am Coll Cardiol* 2000; **35**:1543–50.
20. Park SJ, Park SW, Hong MK, *et al.* Long-term (three-year) outcomes after stenting of unprotected left main coronary artery stenosis in patients with normal left ventricular function. *Am J Cardiol* 2003; **91**:12–16.
21. Takagi T, Stankovic G, Finci L, *et al.* Results and long-term predictors of adverse clinical events after elective percutaneous interventions on unprotected left main coronary artery. *Circulation* 2002; **106**:698–702.
22. Black A, Cortina R, Bossi I, *et al.* Unprotected left main coronary artery stenting: correlates of midterm survival and impact of patient selection. *J Am Coll Cardiol* 2001; **37**:832–8.
23. Tan WA, Tamai H, Park SJ, *et al.* Long-term clinical outcomes after unprotected left main trunk percutaneous revascularization in 279 patients. *Circulation* 2001; **104**:1609–14.
24. Kappetein AP, Dawkins KD, Mohr FW, *et al.* Current percutaneous coronary intervention and coronary artery bypass grafting practices for three-vessel and left main coronary artery disease. Insights from the SYNTAX run-in phase. *Eur J Cardiothorac Surg* 2006; **29**:486–91.
25. Chieffo A, Morici N, Maisano F, *et al.* Percutaneous Treatment With Drug-Eluting Stent Implantation Versus Bypass Surgery for Unprotected Left Main Stenosis: A Single-Center Experience. *Circulation* 2006; **113**:2542–47.
26. Pavei A, Oreglia J, Martin G, *et al.* Long-term follow-up of percutaneous coronary intervention of unprotected left main lesions with drug eluting stents: Predictors of clinical outcome. *EuroIntervention* 2009; **4**:457–63.
27. Park SJ, Kim YH, Lee BK, *et al.* Sirolimus-eluting stent implantation for unprotected left main coronary artery stenosis: comparison with bare metal stent implantation. *J Am Coll Cardiol* 2005; **45**:351–6.
28. Valgimigli M, van Mieghem CA, Ong AT, *et al.* Short- and long-term clinical outcome after drug-eluting stent implantation for the percutaneous treatment of left main coronary artery disease: insights from the Rapamycin-Eluting and Taxus Stent Evaluated At Rotterdam Cardiology Hospital registries (RESEARCH and T-SEARCH). *Circulation* 2005; **111**:1383–9.
29. Carrié D, Eltchaninoff H, Lefèvre T, *et al.* Twelve month clinical and angiographic outcome after stenting of unprotected left main coronary artery stenosis with paclitaxel-eluting stents – results of the multicentre FRIEND registry. *EuroIntervention* 2009; **4**:449–56.
30. Biondi-Zoccai GLG, Lotrionte M, Moretti C, *et al.* A collaborative systematic review and meta-analysis on 1278 patients undergoing percutaneous drug-eluting stenting for unprotected left main coronary artery disease. *Am Heart J* 2008; **155**:274–83.
31. Price MJ, Cristea E, Sawhney N, *et al.* Serial angiographic follow-up of sirolimus-eluting stents for unprotected left main coronary artery revascularization. *J Am Coll Cardiol* 2006; **47**:871–7.
32. Lee MS, Kapoor N, Jamal F, *et al.* Comparison of coronary artery bypass surgery with percutaneous coronary intervention with drug-eluting stents for unprotected left main coronary artery disease. *J Am Coll Cardiol* 2006; **47**:864–70.
33. Seung KB, Park DW, Kim YH, *et al.* Stents versus coronary-artery bypass grafting for left main coronary artery disease. *N Engl J Med* 2008; **358**:1781–92.
34. Buszman PE, Kiesz SR, Bochenek A, *et al.* Acute and late outcomes of unprotected left main stenting in comparison with surgical revascularization. *J Am Coll Cardiol* 2008; **51**:538–45.
35. Serruys PW, Morice MC, Kappetein AP, *et al.* Percutaneous coronary intervention versus coronary-artery bypass grafting for severe coronary artery disease. *N Engl J Med* 2009; **360**:961–72.
36. Nashef SA, Roques F, Michel P, *et al.* European system for cardiac operative risk evaluation (EuroSCORE). *Eur J Cardiothorac Surg* 1999; **16**:9–13.
37. Nashef SA, Roques F, Hammill BG, *et al.* Validation of European System for Cardiac Operative Risk Evaluation (EuroSCORE) in North American cardiac surgery. *Eur J Cardiothorac Surg* 2002; **22**:101–5.
38. Parsonnet V, Dean D, Bernstein AD. A method of uniform stratification of risk for evaluating the results of surgery in acquired adult heart disease. *Circulation* 1989; 79(Suppl I):3–12.
39. Sianos G, Morel MA, Kappetein AP, *et al.* The SYNTAX Score: an angiographic tool grading the complexity of coronary artery disease. *EuroIntervention* 2005; **1**: 219–27.

CHAPTER 20

Chronic total occlusions

Neville Kukreja, Pawel Tyczynski, and Carlo di Mario

Introduction

Chronic total occlusions (CTOs) remain the most technically challenging and time-consuming subset of coronary artery lesions to treat with percutaneous intervention (PCI). Particular difficulties may be encountered in crossing and dilating the lesion, whilst the rates of restenosis are higher than other lesions even after successful PCI. The presence of a CTO frequently prevents complete percutaneous revascularization, and may therefore provide justification for either revascularizing patients by means of coronary artery bypass grafting (CABG) or denying revascularization in favour of a more conservative approach. CTOs can cause severe disabling angina and lead to an impairment of regional and global left ventricular function. This explains why opening CTOs may provide a benefit exceeding the recognized ability of PCI to improve symptoms, and favourably impact upon long-term prognosis. This chapter aims to provide a comprehensive review of the literature on indications and results of CTO treatment as well as providing a modern practical technical guide to planning and executing CTO revascularization.

Definition

The presence of an occluded artery can only be determined by conventional selective coronary angiography. Computed tomography has advantages for the measurement of the occlusion length and to assess the severity of calcification, but is unable to distinguish subocclusive and occlusive stenoses and to detect the direction of the filling of the distal artery. European and Japanese operators define occlusions as complete interruption of anterograde blood flow (Thrombolysis in Myocardial Infarction [TIMI] grade 0 flow)[1] with no possibility to visualize a continuous residual lumen in the occluded segment. American operators also include lesions with minimal penetration of contrast material beyond the point of obstruction but without perfusion of the distal coronary bed (TIMI grade 1 flow)[2]. The inclusion of functional subocclusive lesions in the CTO group has implications in the assessment of the success rate, close to 100% in the first group but much lower for true TIMI 0 occlusions. We must recognize, however, that there is an element of subjectivity in the evaluation of the filling pattern and multiple views with a well-engaged catheter and optimal opacification are required to distinguish the direction of filling. A classical mistake of inexperienced operators is to confuse perivascular collaterals for the true lumen. The second element defining a chronic occlusion is its duration, ideally assessed based on a previous angiogram but more frequently estimated based on an acute coronary event such as a Q-wave myocardial infarction (MI) in the territory of distribution of the occluded artery. The published literature has used varying definitions and recent articles accept 1 month as cut-off criterion. The consensus view is that occlusions of more than 3 months' duration are chronic[1,2] but, when it is not possible to accurately determine the duration of occlusion[3], occlusions with TIMI 0 flow and distal filling via collaterals are also defined as chronic.

Prevalence

Without screening the entire population (including asymptomatic individuals), the true prevalence of CTOs is unknown. All available data comes from details of patients attending for diagnostic coronary angiography for clinical indications. In a registry analysis of 8004 consecutive patients presenting for diagnostic catheterization at a single institution from 1990–2000, after excluding patients with previous CABG or recent myocardial infarction (MI), a CTO was found in 24% of all patients and in 52% of those with significant (>70% diameter stenosis) coronary artery disease[4]. The territory supplied by the left anterior descending (LAD) artery was involved in 444 patients (28%), the left circumflex (LCx) artery in 560 patients (35%), and the right coronary artery (RCA) in 1027 patients (64%). In a multivariate analysis, CTO was the strongest predictor against the selection of PCI as a treatment strategy. A further, smaller registry found a CTO in 38% of patients undergoing angiography[5]. CABG was performed in 31% of patients with a CTO compared with 18% of non-CTO patients, whilst medical therapy without revascularization was the treatment of choice for 22% versus 9%. For this reason the percentage of CTO in patients treated with angioplasty is much lower than its prevalence in the general population with angiographically-determined significant coronary stenoses.

The American College of Cardiology–National Cardiovascular Data Registry (ACC–NCDR) analysed results of 100 292 PCIs performed between 1998–2000, and found that 12% of PCIs involved treatment of total occlusions[6]. However, analysis of the National Heart, Lung and Blood Institute (NHLBI) dynamic registry of four waves of patients (wave 1: July 1997 to February 1998; wave 2: February to June 1999; wave 3: October 2001 to March 2002; wave 4: February 2004 to May 2004) found a decrease in the percentage of patients treated for a CTO from 9.6% in wave 1 to 5.7% in wave 4[7]. This registry also highlighted the discrepancy in success rates for CTO treatment (71.4% to 79.7%) compared to other lesions (96% to 97%). The 2007 database from the British Cardiovascular Interventional Society (BCIS) included 77 093 patients treated with angioplasty and found that CTOs constituted 6.6% of all PCIs with a success rate of 67.5% (http://www.bcis.org.uk/resources/audit/audit2007). The absence of data verification via an independent angiographic core laboratory and the variability of definitions both in terms of timing and filling pattern suggest that the number of true CTOs treated and its average success rate is probably much lower.

Pathological findings

Histopathological examination of CTOs has provided us with valuable insights into the difficulties frequently encountered with PCI as well as providing clues as to potential treatment strategies. In an autopsy study of 96 CTOs, the majority (78%) of angiographic CTOs were actually found to be <99% occluded by histopathologic assessment, with extensive lumen recanalization in 59% of all CTOs, irrespective of age of the occlusion[8]. Furthermore, intimal plaque neovascular channels were observed in 85% of CTOs >1 year old as compared with 74% of CTOs <1 year old. Neovascular channels were also frequently found in the media and adventitia. A significant increase in the frequency of predominantly fibrocalcific lesions was evident with increasing CTO age, whereas younger lesions were more often cholesterol-laden. The proximal cap of the CTO in particular contains dense fibrous tissue and explains the tendency of PCI guide wires to take the path of least resistance with wires deflecting towards side branches or subintimal space rather than engaging the true lumen of the occluded vessel[9].

Benefits of treatment

Relief of angina

PCI is widely accepted as a valuable treatment option for the improvement of symptoms in patients with stable angina and flow-limiting coronary artery disease. The same holds for patients with CTOs, where approximately 70% of patients reported either a significant reduction or complete resolution of anginal symptoms[10].

Improvement in left ventricular function

Additionally, many patients with CTOs have regional abnormalities in left ventricular function, which may improve following successful revascularization provided that the myocardium is viable. An evaluation of 95 patients following successful PCI for a CTO found that when assessed by left ventriculography, the left ventricular ejection fraction (LVEF) for the whole cohort increased from 62 ± 13% before PCI to 67 ± 12% at 6-month follow-up ($p < 0.001$): this increase was found in patients with an open artery 62 ± 13% to 67 ± 11%, $p < 0.001$), whereas the eight patients with re-occlusion had no change in LVEF (63 ± 11% to 64 ± 13%, p = ns)[11]. An increase in LVEF was found in 65 of the 95 patients (68%). The Total Occlusion Study of Canada (TOSCA) also found an improvement in LVEF in the entire group of 410 patients (59% ± 11% to 61% ± 11%, $p = 0.003$)[12]. However, this study included patients with relatively recent occlusions (40% had an occlusion duration of ≤6 weeks) and multivariate analysis revealed baseline LVEF <60%, duration of occlusion ≤6 weeks, and Canadian Cardiology Society (CCS) angina class I or II to be independent predictors of improvement in LVEF. A study of 290 patients with paired echocardiographic data available before and after successful CTO recanalization found that the LVEF at 6 months was significantly increased after treatment when compared with the baseline value (46.5 ± 11.3 vs. 42.2 ± 12.1%; p <0.001)[13]. Dobutamine stress echocardiography (DSE) can help to predict recovery of left ventricular (LV) function: in a study of 40 patients with coronary artery disease and LV dysfunction (68% with a CTO), functional recovery occurred in 27 of the 34 segments (79%) with a biphasic response to DSE (defined as improvement at low dose and worsening at high dose dobutamine)[14]. The sensitivity, specificity, and accuracy of low-dose DSE for prediction of regional functional recovery were 71%, 90%, and 86%, respectively. Magnetic resonance imaging (MRI) can identify viable myocardium supplied by a CTO with the use of gadolinium and the assessment of late hyperenhancement which identifies the presence and transmural extent of fibrosis. In a study of 21 patients, following successful PCI, improved systolic wall thickening was identified in 55% of previously dysfunctional segments, particularly in those with a transmural extent of infarction (TEI) <25%, but also to a lesser extent in those with a TEI between 25–75%[15]. Overall, significant decreases in mean end-diastolic and mean end-systolic volume indexes were observed 3 years after recanalization, whilst mean LVEF tended to improve (60 ± 9% to 63 ± 11%; p = 0.11).

Improvement in survival

Theoretically, successful percutaneous treatment of a CTO might improve survival due to beneficial effects on LV function. Furthermore, the reduction in ischaemic burden (which can be confirmed by non-invasive perfusion imaging) may reduce the likelihood of further ischaemic events and may result in electrical stabilization with a reduction in life-threatening arrhythmias. Additionally, successful percutaneous CTO treatment may prevent patients being exposed to the small but definite mortality risk associated with CABG.

Several studies have suggested an improvement in survival following successful treatment for a CTO. A summary of these is shown in Table 20.1. A report of balloon angioplasty from Emory University found that at 4 years, freedom from CABG was 87% in the clinically successful group and 64% in the clinical failures[16]. The largest patient number and longest follow-up period from the mid-America Heart institute found a significant increase in survival with successful CTO treatment, although this population included some patients with relatively recent occlusions (minimum occlusion duration 7 days) and infrequent use of stent implantation[17]. A study from the Thoraxcenter in Rotterdam found lower survival in patients with unsuccessful CTO recanalization with a hazard ratio (HR) for death of 1.86 (95% confidence interval [CI] 1.12–3.10), whilst successful PCI was an independent predictor against death (adjusted HR 0.58; 95% CI 0.34–0.98)[18]. Although the difference in mortality rates did not reach statistical significance in the TOAST-GISE study, rates of cardiac death (0.4% vs. 3.6%, p = 0.04), CABG (2.5% vs. 15.7%, p <0.0001) and any major adverse cardiovascular event (MACE: 12.2% vs. 25.3%, p = 0.005) were all lower in the group with successful CTO treatment at 1 year follow-up[19]. A more recent study from Liverpool found that the crude HR for death with CTO failure was 3.92 (95% CI 1.56–10.07; p = 0.004)[20]. The rates of subsequent CABG were 3.2% vs. 21.7% (p <0.001) for the CTO success and CTO failure patients, respectively. The authors also propensity matched 157 CTO success to CTO failure patients and found the associated

Table 20.1 Survival benefit following successful percutaneous CTO treatment

Author (reference)	Years of enrolment	No. of patients	Procedural success rate	Stent use	DES use	Follow-up duration (years)	Mortality in successful patients	Mortality in unsuccessful patients	P
Ivanhoe[16]	1980–1988	480	66%	–	–	4	1%	4%	0.006
Suero[17]	1980–1999	2007	70%	7%	–	10	26.5%	34.9%	0.001
Hoye[18]	1992–2002	874	65%	81%	–	Median 4.48 (IQR 2.72–6.64)	6.5%	12%	0.02
Olivari[19]	1999–2000	376	73%	90%	–	1	1.1%	3.6%	0.13
Aziz[20]	2000–2004	543	69%	98%	17%	Mean 1.7 ± 0.5	2.5%	7.3%	0.004
Valenti[13]	2003–2006	486	71%	100%	100%	Median 2.0 (IQR 1.1–2.8)	8.4%	12.6%	0.025

DES, drug-eluting stent; IQR, interquartile range.

HR for death with CTO failure to be 4.63 (95% CI 1.01–12.61; p = 0.049). Multivariate analysis also showed that CTO failure was an independent predictor of death. In another large series of 1262 patients treated at the Mayo Clinic (United States) between 1979 and 2005, patients with technical success had improved long-term survival, although this was not apparent until 6 years after the procedure and technical success was not an independent predictor of mortality (adjusted HR 1.16, 95% CI 0.90–1.5, p = 0.25)[21].

Impact of complete revascularization

There is some evidence that the improvement in survival found with successful recanalization of a CTO may be related to the completeness of revascularization. The Coronary Angioplasty versus Bypass Revascularisation Investigation (CABRI) randomized 1054 patients with multivessel coronary disease to CABG or to coronary angioplasty: 223 of the patients had chronic occlusion of a major vessel[22]. Unsuccessful revascularization of the chronic occlusion (either by CABG or PCI) was associated with increased rates of death or Q-wave MI (HR 2.5; 95% CI 1.0–6.1; p <0.05). Completeness of revascularization was an independent predictor of lower rates of death or MI (HR 0.26; 95% CI 0.09—0.76; p = 0.01). The group in Florence (Italy) recently found that although successful treatment of a CTO was not associated with improved mortality and LVEF, the completeness of revascularization was independently related to the risk of death (HR 0.44; 95% CI 0.22–0.87; p = 0.02)[13].

Treatment of chronic occlusions

As with any patient with coronary artery disease, optimal medical therapy should be pursued in terms of treatment with antiplatelet agents, lipid-lowering therapy, and angiotensin-converting enzyme inhibitors. Beta-blockers should be prescribed if possible to patients with a previous MI, whilst attempts should be made to control angina symptoms with appropriate pharmacotherapy. Nevertheless, given the evidence in favour of revascularization, the presence of a CTO should not serve to deny patients appropriate revascularization. A non-invasive assessment of myocardial viability is essential before exposing patients to lengthy and expensive procedures, whilst an understanding of predictors of success (see Table 20.2), will help determine whether PCI is an appropriate treatment strategy. Joint cardiothoracic-surgical multidisciplinary team meetings are invaluable in 'grey' cases and patient preference should of course be taken into consideration, providing the risks and benefits of each treatment strategy have been fully discussed with the patient.

Percutaneous treatment of chronic occlusions

PCI of CTOs carries lower success rates than for any other lesion subtype (Table 20.1). The combination of a tough fibrous proximal cap, followed by fibrocalcific plaque and neovascular channels create unique difficulties requiring a frequent change in strategy and in the types of equipment required to successfully traverse the lesion. Unsurprisingly, this results in long procedure times, high radiation doses, and amount of contrast which can easily exceed 300–400mL[23]. Further specific potential complications include periprocedural MI due to compromise of collateral vessels, vessel perforation or rupture, and damage to the proximal vessel due to aggressive guiding catheter manipulation. Despite these issues, percutaneous treatment of CTOs can be undertaken safely in experienced hands: the European CTO

Table 20.2 Predictors of simple (high success rate) versus complex percutaneous CTO intervention*

	Simple	Complex
Vessel diameter (mm)	≥3.0	<3.0
Occlusion length (mm)	≤20	<20
Calcification of occluded segment	None–moderate	Severe
Tortuosity of occluded segment	Minimal–moderate	Severe
Occlusion stump	Tapered	Blunt or absent
Distal vessel opacification	Good–excellent	Poor
Distal vessel disease	Absent or moderate	Severe
Tandem/multiple occlusions	No	Yes
Tortuosity proximal to occlusion	Minimal–moderate	Severe
Disease of the proximal segment	Absent or moderate	Severe
Expected guiding catheter support	Good	Poor
Ostial location	No	Yes
Previous attempts	No	Yes
Renal insufficiency	No	Yes
Expected patient tolerance	Good	Poor

*Adapted from Di Mario *et al.*[1]

club analysis of 3403 patients undergoing CTO PCI in 2006 found acceptably low adverse events rates (death 0.12%, Q-wave MI 0.14%, any MI 1.96%, emergency CABG 0.27%, and tamponade 0.64%)[1]. A consensus view on parameters associated with high success rates are shown in Table 20.2. The degree of calcification, presence of a blunt stump, and occlusion length are features backed up by most of the current literature[24], but with progress in technique and especially the diffusion of retrograde recanalization factors previously associated with failure are no longer predictive. Favourable lesion and patient characteristics are expected to be associated with success rates of 90% or more in experienced hands, whilst unfavourable cases may have success rates of <60–70%[1].

Contralateral injection

Visualization of the distal lumen is essential to guide progression of the stiff dedicated wires used for CTO recanalization. If collaterals mainly originate from the contralateral artery as is almost the rule for RCA and LAD occlusions, a simultaneous injection of the occluded vessel and the donor artery is essential to plan the procedure, measure the length and direction of the occluded segment, and study the most appropriate entry site if the stump is not evident. Guidance of the crossing of the distal cap must be done with frequent assessment in multiple views of the orientation of the wire and the distal true lumen.

Guiding catheter support

It is imperative to have optimal guiding catheter support to assist with successful CTO crossing. The first step is in the selection of guiding catheter size and shape. The majority of other lesion subtypes and simple CTOs may be tacked with 6F guiding catheters, but a 7F or even 8F guiding catheter may be necessary for adequate support, delivery of bulky specialist equipment, use of two over-the-wire (OTW) catheters and intravascular ultrasound (IVUS)-guided techniques[1,23]. A supportive guiding catheter shape is also essential, for example, in the treatment of the right coronary artery, an Amplatz left catheter might be appropriate. A shorter length guiding catheter (85–90cm compared to the standard 100cm) may also be required for a retrograde case. Beyond the choice of guiding catheter, stenting the proximal segment of the coronary artery when it is also diseased may facilitate deep engagement of the guiding catheter. Advancing a guide wire into a non-target vessel, may also serve to increase guiding catheter support, e.g. inserting a guide wire into the LCx may stabilize the guiding catheter to allow treatment of a CTO in the LAD. Other techniques to improve support include the anchoring technique, consisting of inflating a balloon at low pressure in a non-target side branch[25] (Fig. 20.1). The child in Mother catheter technique (or five-in-six system) where a 5F guiding catheter is inserted into a 6F or 7F guiding catheter to increase backup support[26]. Usually, the 5F guiding catheter is 120cm and the 6F 100cm long (Fig. 20.2). The 5F must have a soft tip to negotiate any tortuosity it might encounter with the least possible damage.

Guide wire selection

This is generally a matter of personal preference, although the choice falls between hydrophilic floppy

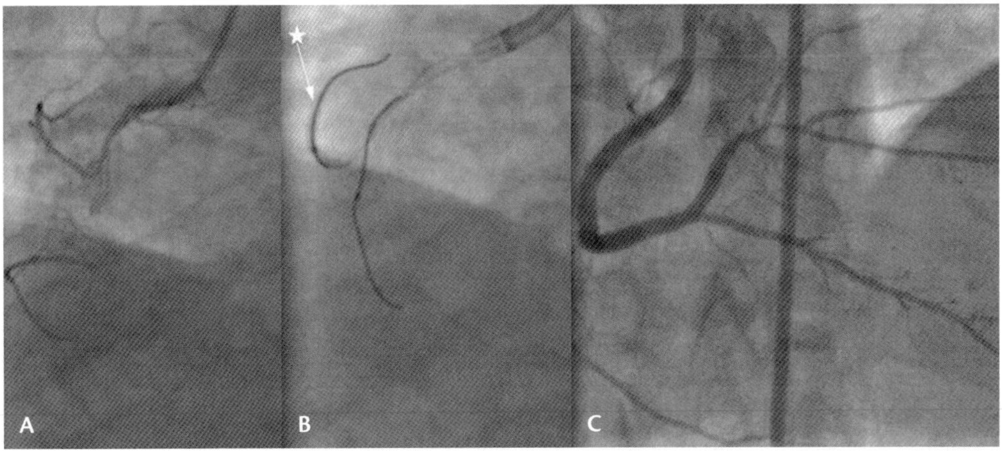

Fig. 20.1 A) Chronic total occlusion of the right coronary artery; B) anchor balloon (*) inflated at low pressure (6 atmospheres) in a branch originating from the proximal segment of the right coronary artery; C) final angiographic result.

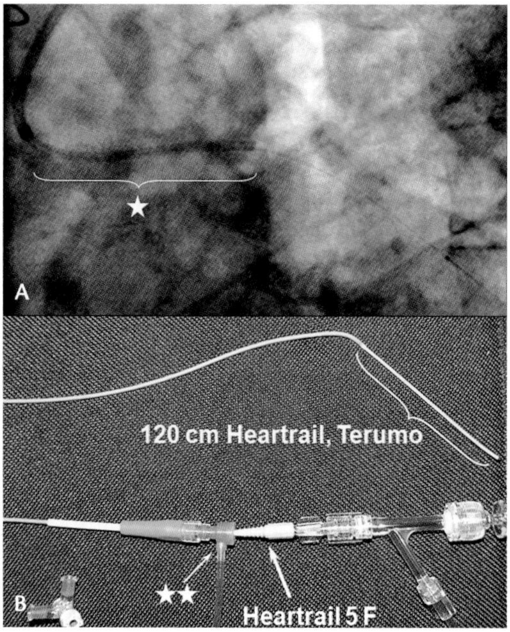

Fig. 20.2 'Mother and Child' guiding catheter technique. A) Angiographic appearance of a Terumo Heartrail® 5F catheter (*) protruding from a 7F guide catheter; B) *In vivo* image of the manifold of the 120cm Terumo Heartrail® 5F catheter within a conventional 100cm 7F guiding catheter ('mother catheter'), which is inserted via a short Luer-lock pressure valve (**).

wires which might traverse neovascular channels, and stiffer wires which might penetrate the fibrocalcific plaque. A regular floppy wire may be advisable to negotiate the vessel proximal to the occlusion: this can then be exchanged using an OTW balloon or microcatheter for a dedicated CTO wire[1]. Table 20.3 lists some of the guide wires commonly used for CTO treatment. Most operators employ a 'step-up' approach, sequentially using wires of increasing stiffness until the wire can be advanced. Appropriate shaping of the wire tip is also essential—a small (1.0–1.5mm length, 30–45° angulation) distal primary curve is suitable for engaging the proximal cap[27].

Over-the-wire balloon or microcatheter

While unsupported wire crossing and monorail balloons are standard for non-CTO lesions, only OTW balloons or microcatheters (Finecross®, Terumo, Japan; Transit®, Cordis, Miami, USA; Excelsior®, BSC, Natick, MS, USA etc.) should be used to support the guide wire for a CTO attempt. This allows negotiation of the proximal vessel with soft guide wires followed by safely switching to stiff wires only in front of the lesion, with the possibility to reshape the wire and exchange it for a stiffer and tapered wire or for a polymer coated wire at various stages in the procedure. Additionally once the

Table 20.3 Commonly-used guide wires for CTO treatment*

Manufacturer	Wire	Tip diameter	Stiffness	Coating
Abbott Vascular	Whisper® LS, MS	0.014 inch	1g	Polymer coated
	Pilot® 50, 150, 200	0.014 inch	2–5g	Polymer coated
	Cross-It® 100, 200, 300, 400	0.014–0.010 inch (tapered tip)	2–4g	Hydrophilic with moderate lubricity
Medtronic	Persuader®	0.014 inch	3–9g	Hydrophilic
Asahi	Fielder®	0.014 inch	1g	Polymer coated
	Fielder XT®	0.0014–0.009 inch (tapered tip)	1g	Polymer coated
	Miracle® 3, 4.5, 6, 12	0.014 inch	3–12g	Non-hydrophilic
	Conquest®/Confianza®	0.0014–0.009 inch (tapered tip)	9g	Non-hydrophilic
	Conquest®/Confianza Pro® 9, 12	0.0014–0.009 inch (tapered tip)	9–12g	Hydrophilic except tip with non-lubricious shaft
	Conquest/Confianza Pro® 8–20	0.0014–0.008 inch (tapered tip)	20g	Hydrophilic except tip with non-lubricious shaft
Cordis J&J	Shinobi®	0.01 inch	2g	Polymer coated
	Shinobi Plus®	0.014 inch	4g	Polymer coated
Terumo	Runthrough NS®	0.014 inch	1–3g	Hydrophilic
	Crosswire NT®	0.014 inch	12g	Polymer coated

*Adapted from Di Mario *et al.*[1]

wire has crossed the occlusion, the OTW catheter can be used to exchange the aggressive wires used for the initial crossing for safer workhorse wires. This can be facilitated by using 300-cm length guide wires, by attaching an extension wire or by using the Nanto technique (removal of the balloon or microcatheter attached to an indeflator maintained at a pressure of 14–16 atmospheres to hold the guide wire in place)[23,28]. Another use of an OTW catheter is in the common situation where there is uncertainty whether the guide wire is in the true lumen. The operator can carefully advance the OTW balloon up to the tip of the guide wire or as far as possible; once the guide wire is removed, an injection of 1 or 2cc of contrast media through the lumen of the OTW is performed, allowing visualization of the distal vessel thereby discerning whether the guide wire is in the true lumen. This technique offers useful confirmation that the wire has engaged the main distal vessel rather than diagonals or other smaller branches but should be used with caution once it is expected that the wire is in a false lumen because it may enlarge the subintimal space and compress the true lumen. Microcatheters tend to have more flexible tips and a single distal radiopaque marker facilitating identification of the distal tip; balloons on the other hand often have a single central radiopaque marker, but obviously have the advantage of being used for dilating the lesion.

Parallel wire technique

If the guide wire has entered a false channel, then the parallel wire technique can be employed. The wire which enters the subintimal space should be left in place since it occludes the false channel and provides an excellent landmark to point the second wire in the right direction, allowing easier engagement of the distal fibrous cap and penetration of the distal vessel[1,23,27] (Fig. 20.3). If the second wire also enters a subintimal position, then the first wire can be withdrawn and advanced again (the 'seesaw' technique).

Subintimal tracking and re-entry (STAR)

This technique was originally employed for peripheral arterial revascularization but has since been used for coronary CTOs. Briefly, if the wire enters the subintimal and does not reach the distal true lumen, using OTW support, a polymer-coated wire with a loop at the distal end is advanced along the subintimal plane until it re-enters the true lumen distal to the occlusion[29]. The subintimal track is then dilated and the entire segment stented. Although this technique can be successfully used, particularly in the RCA, there are several concerns regarding its use: side branches arising from the true lumen may become occluded, which may explain the peri-procedural MI rate of 16.1%. Furthermore, the risk of vessel perforation seems high (9.7% in the initial

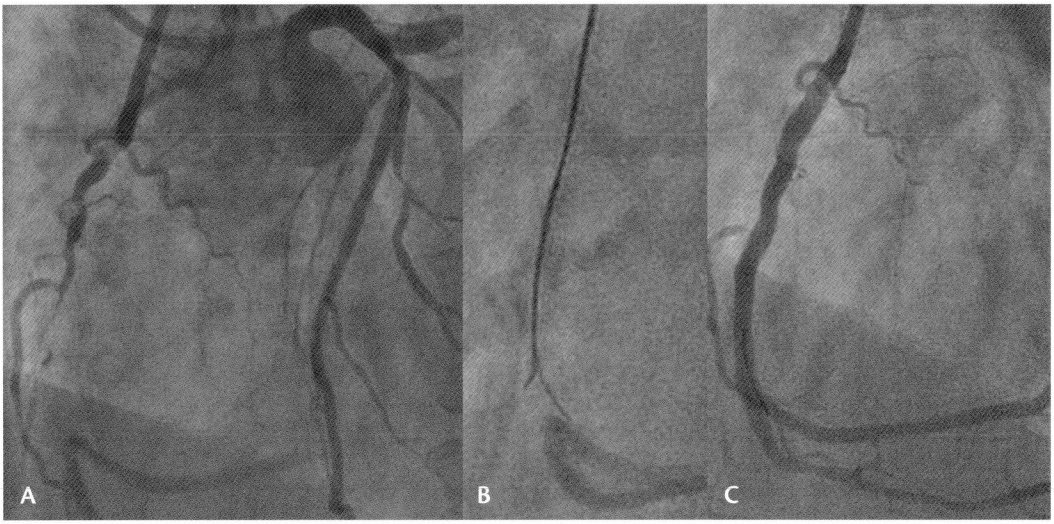

Fig. 20.3 A) Chronic total occlusion of right coronary artery. Simultaneous injection from the left and the right coronary artery; B) parallel wires negotiating the occlusion of the right coronary artery; C) final angiographic result.

series). Using contrast injections through the OTW to identify microchannels may facilitate the technique, but the rates of restenosis (target lesion revascularization [TLR] rate 29.4% even with drug-eluting stents) seems high[30].

Intravascular ultrasound-guided recanalization

IVUS can help to identify an occlusion site, in cases with a blunt stump where the occlusion site is situated next to a side branch and cannot be accurately identified angiographically (Fig. 20.4). Intravascular imaging from the side branch can assist in identifying the occlusion site as well as monitoring initial wire progress[31]. Additionally, as an alternative to the STAR technique to avoid too long dissections, an IVUS catheter can be advanced along the subintimal plane to assist re-entry into the true lumen[1]. The progression of a second wire is monitored from the proximal occlusion to identify the direction of the true lumen and orientate the wire appropriately. In peripheral vessels, an ultrasound-guided system with an integrated needle is used successfully to guide re-entry. In the coronaries, a flat balloon with two exit points (StingRay®, Bridgepoint Medical, Plymouth, MN, USA) has been designed to orientate the wire in the direction of the true distal lumen but the system only uses ultrasound guidance.

Retrograde recanalization

Since crossing the tough proximal cap is often the most challenging aspect of CTO recanalization, experienced Japanese operators pioneered the concept of crossing

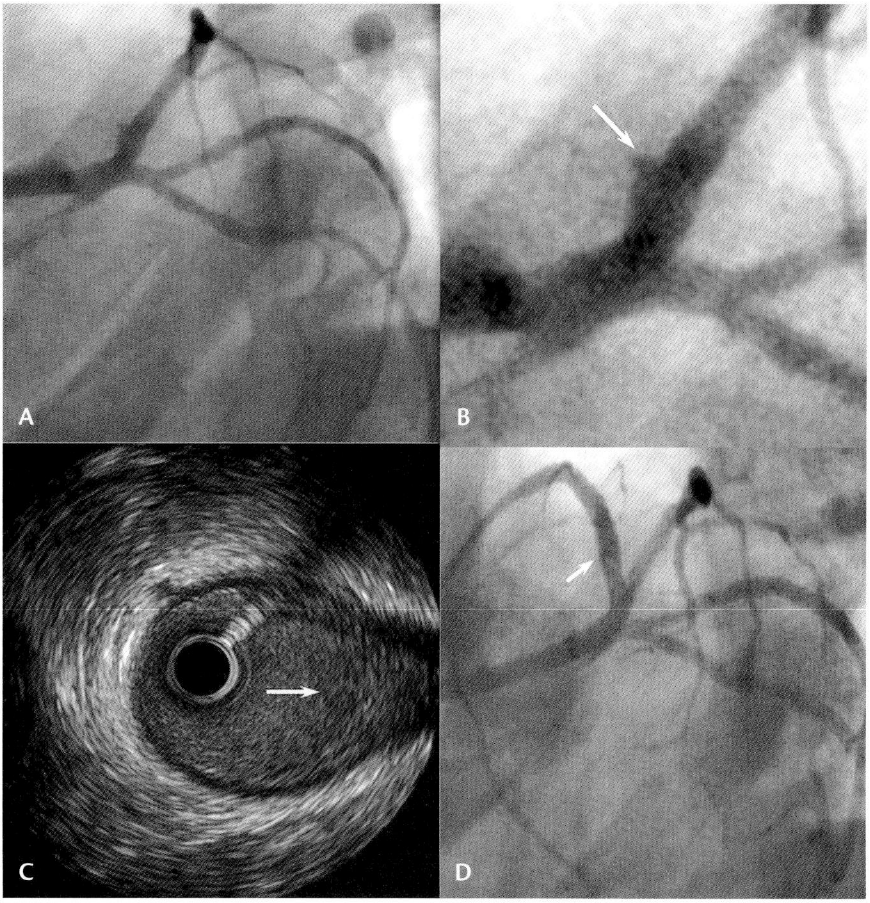

Fig. 20.4 A) Ostial occlusion of the left anterior descending artery; B) magnified image showing the site of chronic total occlusion (arrow); C) corresponding intravascular ultrasound image clearly showing the entry point of the occlusion (arrow); D) final angiographic result with recanalization of the left anterior descending artery (arrow).

the occlusion retrogradely by advancing a guide wire through collateral vessels to the distal cap and thence through the occlusion[32]. There are three possible routes to reach the distal cap: 1) via arterial or venous grafts anastomosed to the native vessel distal to the site of occlusion in patients who have previously undergone CABG; 2) via epicardial collaterals mainly between RCA and LCx through posterior atrial branches or between distal RCA and LAD over the apex; and C) septal collaterals between the distal RCA and LAD (Fig. 20.5)[33,34]. Bilateral arterial access is required for any route of retrograde approach. A soft-tipped polymer coated wire, such as a Whisper® (Abbott Vascular, Santa Clara, USA) or Fielder® (Asahi Intec, Japan) is used to access suitable collaterals with OTW catheter support. Supersoft® (Fielder FC) or tapered (Fielder XT®) polymer coated wires have been specifically designed for the most difficult tortuous collaterals. Injection of contrast through the OTW catheter can help the operator to identify if the chosen collateral does indeed directly communicate with the target vessel distal to the occlusion (Figs. 20.5 and 20.6). Please note that it is not rare that the wire can penetrate angiographically invisible (<100μm) collaterals and reach the distal vessel. Once the soft guide wire has reached the distal cap, it can be exchanged through the microcatheter for a stiffer dedicated CTO

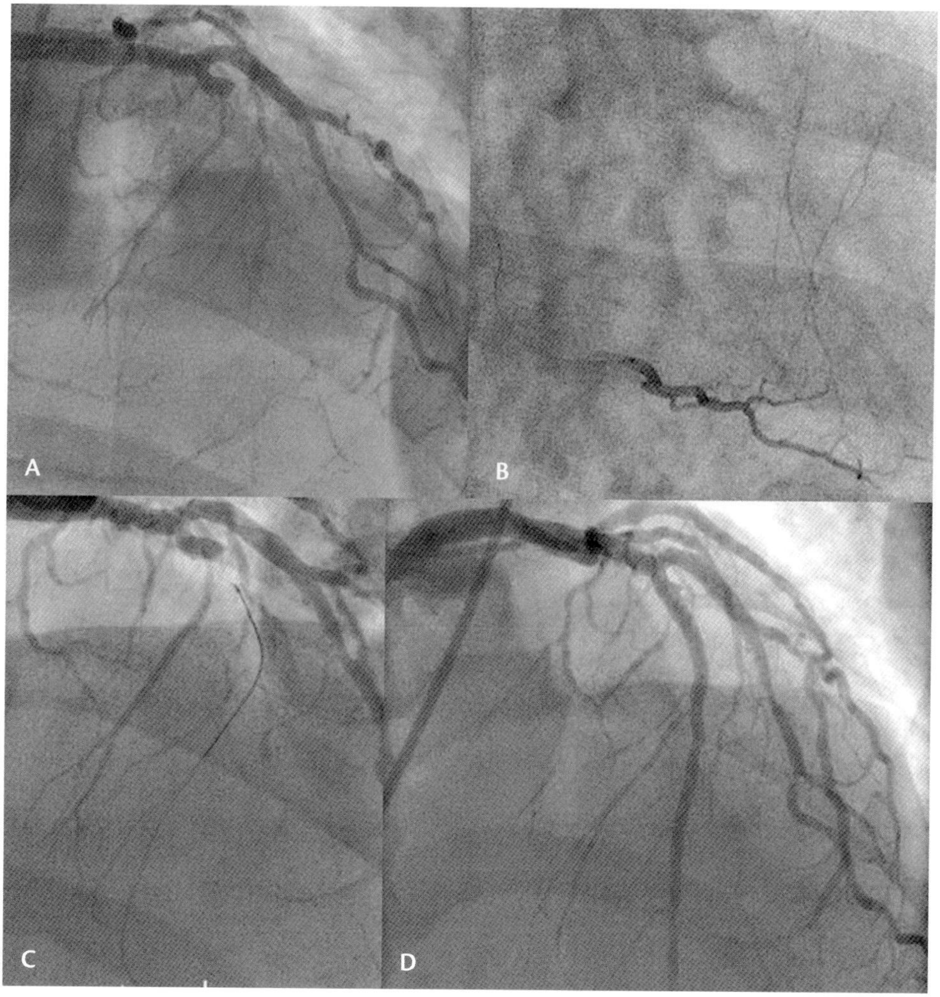

Fig. 20.5 A) Chronic total occlusion of the left anterior descending artery; B) sub-selective contrast injection of the septal collaterals via a micro-catheter (Finecross®) from the right coronary artery; C) retrograde approach to the occlusion of the left anterior descending artery via a septal collateral; D) final angiographic result.

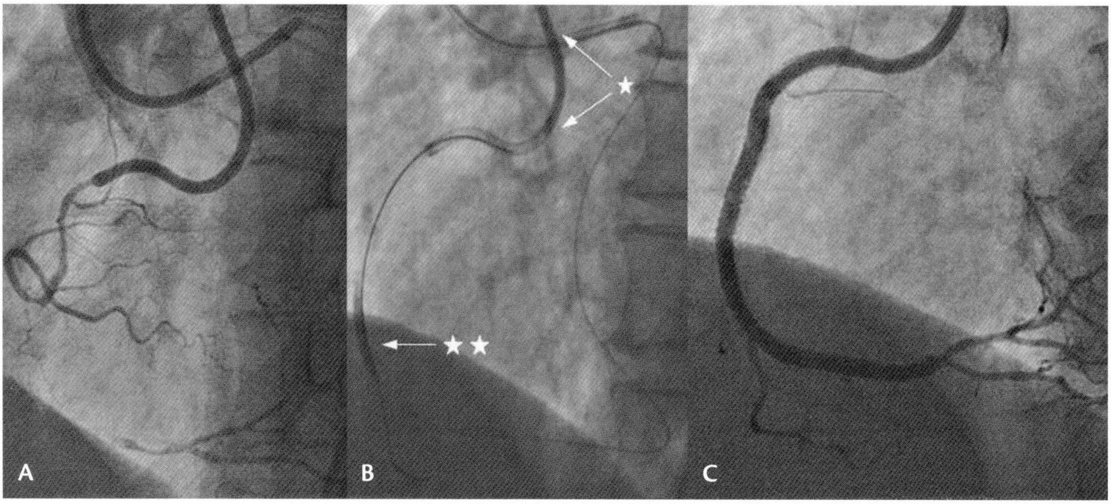

Fig. 20.6 A) Chronic total occlusion of the right coronary artery; B) retrograde and anterograde approach to open the occlusion. Retrograde guidewire jailed by an inflated balloon (*) within the RCA guiding catheter in order to facilitate crossing of balloon via occlusion of the right coronary artery (**); C) final angiographic result.

wire, such as a Miracle® or Confianza® (both Asahi Intec, Japan) to cross the lesion.

Since the tortuosity of the collateral vessel is often so extreme that balloons or microcatheters cannot be advanced, a dedicated braided metallic catheter with smooth lubricious coating has been developed (Corsair®, Asahi, Japan). This catheter is advanced with bilateral rotation of the proximal hub to force progression, and, when in place, allows easier manipulation of the retrograde wire and retrograde crossing. If the retrograde attempt allows advancement of the retrograde wire into the guiding catheter at the ostium of the occluded vessel, the wire can be trapped inside the anterograde guiding catheter and a balloon advanced retrogradely to open the occluded segment and allow progression of an anterograde wire (Fig. 20.6). If this is not successful, the retrograde wire can be externalized through the anterograde guiding catheter, often using a soft 300cm RotaWire® (Boston Scientific, Natick, MS, USA), and the balloon can be advanced anterogradely. If retrograde recanalization is not directly successful, this approach can be used in conjunction with an anterograde attempt, using the retrograde wire as a marker of the distal true lumen. A subintimal anterograde wire can then be manipulated to join the retrograde wire in the distal true lumen but this almost always requires a controlled anterograde and retrograde tracking (CART) technique[32], i.e. a dilatation of the anterograde or retrograde balloon in the subintimal space, creating a controlled dissection where the other wire can follow during advancement (Fig. 20.7). A report from the European CTO club of 175 patients undergoing retrograde recanalization of a CTO found an overall success rate of 83.4%[35]. Similar success rates have been reported by colleagues from Japan[36]. In the European series, the rate of collateral vessel perforation was 6.9%, whilst 1.1% of patients suffered dissection of the donor artery. There were no cases of tamponade. The rates of clinical adverse events were low—4.0% of patients suffered a peri-procedural MI (all non Q-wave), but there were no in-hospital deaths and no requirement for emergency CABG[35].

Atherectomy

Following successful guide wire crossing it may not always be possible to advance a balloon into the lesion. In these cases either dedicated CTO devices (see next section) or rotational atherectomy are possible strategies. For rotational atherectomy, the RotaWire® can be advanced though an OTW catheter to allow rotablation[1].

Dedicated chronic occlusion devices

A number of dedicated devices aimed at facilitating CTO treatment have been used over the years. Although some may have a role in specific situations, none have been proven to significantly improve overall procedural success rates when compared to advanced wire techniques[23].

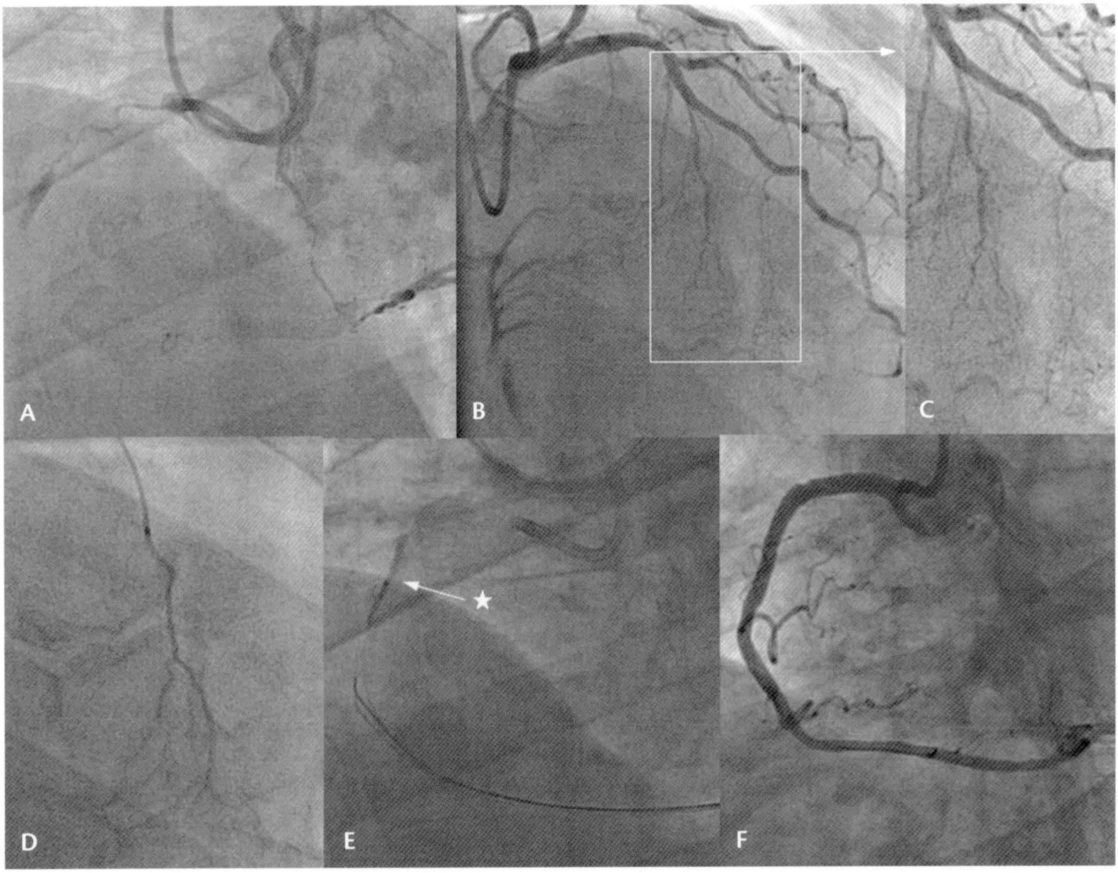

Fig. 20.7 A) Chronic total occlusion of the right coronary artery; B) the left anterior descending artery; C) septal collaterals; D) super-selective contrast injection to visualize the anatomy of a septal collateral; E) inflation of a small-diameter anterograde balloon (*) to create subintimal space in order to facilitate passage of the retrograde wire into the true vessel lumen; F) final angiographic result.

The Tornus® catheter (Asahi Intec, Japan) is a braided 2.1F or 2.6F support catheter, which can be advanced along the guide wire and through the occlusion using an anti-clockwise screwing motion. The benefit of this device in cases where a balloon or conventional micro-catheter was unable to cross has been demonstrated[37]. Crossing with the Tornus® creates a lumen of sufficient diameter to allow passage of a conventional balloon for further dilatation on the lesion (Fig. 20.8)[38].

Laser: the laser guide wire (Spectranetics®, Colorado Springs, CO, USA) consists of a 0.018-inch shapeable guide wire containing 12 silica fibres with a 45-micron diameter. The guide wire was designed to function as an exchange guide wire. The fluence typically used during a laser guide wire procedure is 60mJ/mm^2, with a pulse repetition rate of 25Hz[23]. A randomized trial comparing the laser wire against conventional guide wires for crossing CTOs found no difference in overall success rates (63% vs. 66%, $p = 0.6$)[39] so that this approach has been abandoned. A laser catheter (Spectranetics®) is also available (either 0.9mm or 0.7mm) and can be used to dilate lesions following guide wire passage, if no other device can cross or dilate the lesion[23]. Unfortunately this approach is only successful if the occlusion is fibrotic, since the laser is unable to penetrate thick calcium.

The CROSSER® CTO Recanalization System (FlowCardia Inc, CA) is vibrational angioplasty CTO device. It uses piezoelectric crystals to convert electrical energy into high-frequency vibrational energy (21 000 cycles per second), which provides mechanical impact and cavitational effects which may facilitate lesion crossing[40]. The catheter is monorail, hydrophilic, and 0.014-inch guide wire and 6F guiding catheter compatible. It can be used for primary crossing of the lesion,

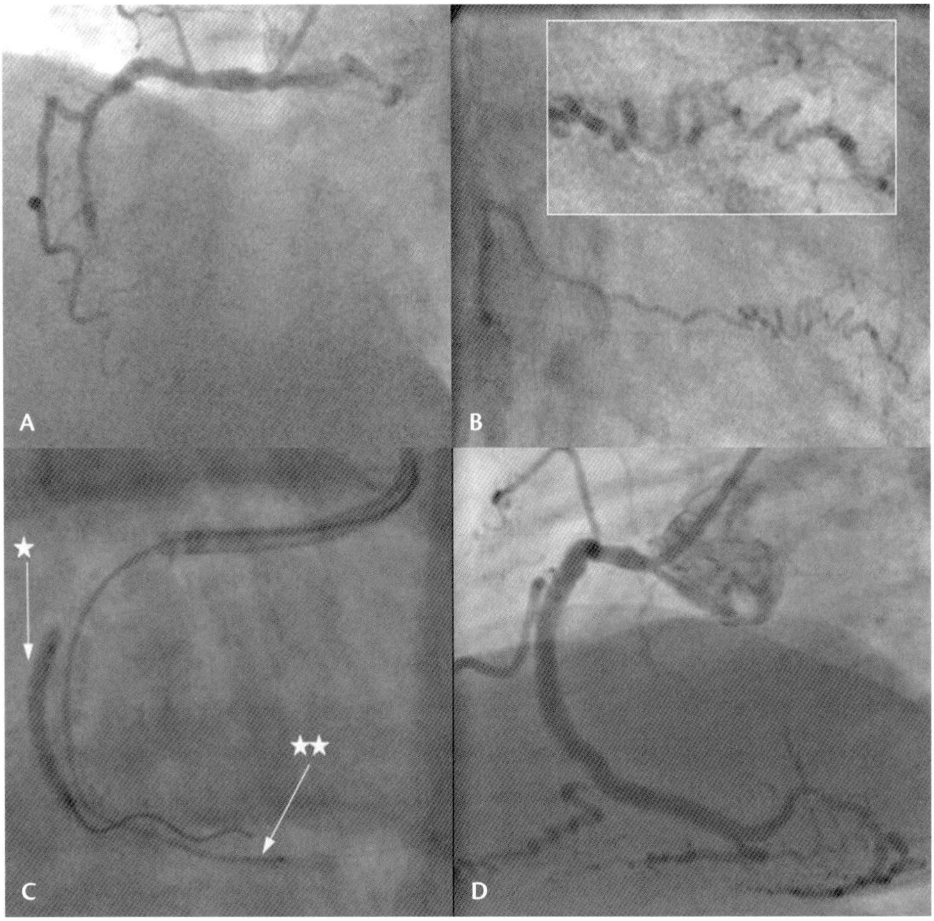

Fig. 20.8 A) Heavily calcified chronic total occlusion of the right coronary artery; B) super-selective contrast injection to septal collateral showing extremely tortuous anatomy, unsuitable for crossing with a guidewire; C) anchor balloon (*) dilated at low pressure (6 atmospheres) in a branch from the right coronary artery for additional catheter support during negotiating the occlusion with the Tornus® catheter (**); D) final angiographic result.

but can also help when the lesion is undilatable. The largest registry of the CROSSER® found a procedural success rates of 60%, with total major adverse event rates of 8.8% (perforation in 1.6%, and MI in 4.8%)[41].

More recently, the RVT CTO Guidewire Device® (ReVascular Therapeutics, Sunnyvale, CA, USA) has been described[42]. This device is designed to provide enhanced penetration and control and consists of a 0.014-inch guide wire with a mechanically active distal end, a handle attached proximally to the guide wire, with an adjustable torquer, and a non-disposable, battery-operated, control unit, that provides activation control and audio feedback during the CTO crossing procedure. The distal 4cm is radiopaque. The distal wire tip is shapeable and has 12g tip stiffness. When activated, the driveshaft tip rotates at 12 000rpm and changes rotation direction (oscillation). The adjustable torquer provides torque control in its passive mode, allowing fine movement and precise positioning of the guide wire distal tip, before the activation mode is switched on. The success rate of this device is reported at 62.5% with no adverse complications so far.

The Frontrunner® catheter (LuMend Inc.) is a blunt microdissection device. It consists of a blunt articulated distal tip which can be activated by a proximal control knob[43]. Opening the jaws of the device will fracture or separate the plaque to facilitate advancement of a guide wire. Although an initial report of three patients was promising, a further report of 50 patients found a significant learning curve and overall an angiographic success rate of only 50% with high rates of perforation (18%) and tamponade (4%)[44].

The SafeCross System® (Intraluminal Therapeutics, Carlsbad, CA, USA) is comprised of the Intraluminal guide wire, which is plugged directly into a console. The wire itself is 0.014inch in diameter and notably has a blunt tip; the distal 10mm is radiopaque. The system uses optical coherence reflectometry to enable accurate guidance of the wire and to reduce the risk of wire perforation. In addition, the system is forward-looking with a very high resolution of up to 15 microns. The Intraluminal guide wire has the capability of radiofrequency ablation with short-duration bursts (100-msec pulses) of low-frequency energy (250–500kHz) delivered at the tip to enhance forward wire passage[23]. A registry of 116 patients found success rates of 54%, with perforation in 2.6%[45].

Magnetic navigation system

The use of a magnetic navigation system (MNS) is a new option that may facilitate navigation in complex coronary anatomy[46]. In brief, the Stereotaxis Niobe® MNS consists of two permanent magnets positioned on either side of the fluoroscopic table. The MNS generates a composite magnetic field of 0.8 Tesla that is uniform in a 15-cm^3 volume within the chest of the patient. This creates a magnetic field vector that can be rotated, translated, and tilted in 360° in each plane, which allows fine control of the orientation of the tip of a magnetically-enabled guide wire. Coregistration of images from multislice CT angiography, allowing delineation of the direction of the occluded segment, is an important step allowed by the system software. Although a study of 350 consecutive patients undergoing complex PCI found that the success rate of MNS guide wire crossing was 93%, the majority (25 out of 35) of the failures were in CTOs[46]. Unfortunately, the ideal wires designed for the final crossing, able to emit radiofrequency at the tip and with a fragmented magnet to allow fine angulation of the tip, are not yet available for clinical applications.

Stent use

Following successful CTO recanalization, most operators would nowadays implant drug-eluting stents (DES): CTO lesions are associated with high rates of restenosis following balloon angioplasty only or bare-metal stent (BMS) implantation and there are several registries demonstrating the efficacy of DES in this setting; Table 20.4 summarizes the various registries evaluating the effect of DES. Additionally, a subgroup analysis of the Stenting Coronary Arteries in Non-Stress/Benestent Disease (SCANDSTENT) Trial randomizing patients to sirolimus-eluting stents (SES) or BMS has been reported[47]. The 127 patients (64 SES, 63 BMS) were well matched in demographic and angiographic baseline characteristics. At 6-month follow-up, patients who received SES had a minimal lumen diameter of 2.49mm compared with 1.46mm in those who received BMS ($p = 0.015$), 0% versus 38% developed restenosis ($p < 0.001$), and the target vessel failure rate 5% with SES versus 35% with BMS ($p < 0.001$). The Primary Stenting of Totally Occluded Native Coronary Arteries (PRISON) II study randomized 200 patients with a CTO to either SES or BMS[48]. After 3 years, TLR was 7% in the SES group vs. 27% in the BMS group ($p < 0.001$); and target vessel revascularization (TVR) was seen in 11% in the SES group vs. 30% in the BMS group ($p = 0.002$). Major adverse cardiac events were noted in 10% of the SES group vs. 34% in the BMS group ($p < 0.001$). There were no statistically significant

Table 20.4 Registry data evaluating the use of drug-eluting stents in chronic occlusions

Author (reference)	Years of enrolment	No. of BMS patients	No. of DES patients	Follow-up duration (months)	TVR BMS	TVR DES	p	MACE BMS	MACE DES	p
Garcia-Garcia[49]	2001–2003	71	76 SES	36	12.7%	9.2%	0.5	18.3%	15.8%	0.7
Ge[50]	2000–2004	259	122 SES	6	29%	9%	<0.001	35.1%	16.4%	<0.001
Migliorini[51]	2002–2004	26	92 SES or PES	6	23%	7.6%	0.03	23%	9.8%	0.07
Nakamura[52]	2002–2003	120	60 SES	12	30%	3%	0.001	42%	3%	0.001
Werner[53]	1999–2004	148	82 PES	12	53.4%	10%	<0.001	56.7%	13.3%	<0.001

BMS, bare metal stent; DES, drug-eluting stent; PES, paclitaxel-eluting stent; SES, sirolimus-eluting stent.

differences in death, MI, and stent thrombosis according to the Academic Research Consortium criteria between the two groups.

Conclusions

Despite the mounting evidence of the benefits, many patients with CTOs are still not offered percutaneous revascularization. Although a number of dedicated CTO devices have failed to improve success rates, the use of contemporary wires and techniques including retrograde recanalization in experienced hands reaches success rates to consistently greater than 80%, which becomes more than 95% if the retrograde wire successfully reaches the distal vessel and can be used as indicated to help recanalization. There is clear evidence that DES can reduce rates of restenosis and re-occlusion after successful CTO treatment to acceptably low levels. With high success rates in suitable patients, coupled to the benefits in morbidity and mortality, it seems logical that more patients with CTOs should be offered percutaneous revascularization. While the simplest occlusion should be carefully approached by any experienced PCI operator, concentration of the most difficult cases or of cases after initial failure in CTO centres appears the safest and most effective approach.

References

1. Di Mario C, Werner GS, Sianos G, *et al.* European perspective in the recanalisation of chronic total occlusions (CTO): consensus document from the EuroCTO Club. *EuroInterv* 2007; **3**: 30–43.
2. Stone GW, Kandzari DE, Mehran R, *et al.* Percutaneous recanalization of chronically occluded coronary arteries: a consensus document: part i. *Circulation* 2005; **112**(15): 2364–72.
3. Barlis, P, Kaplan S, Dimopoulos K, *et al.* An indeterminate occlusion duration predicts procedural failure in the recanalization of coronary chronic total occlusions. *Catheter Cardiovasc Interv* 2008; **71**(5): 621–8.
4. Christofferson RD, Lehmann KG, Martin GV, *et al.* Effect of chronic total coronary occlusion on treatment strategy. *Am J Cardiol* 2005; **95**(9): 1088–91.
5. Delacretaz E, Meier B. Therapeutic strategy with total coronary artery occlusions. *Am J Cardiol* 1997; **79**(2): 185–7.
6. Anderson HV, Shaw RE, Brindis RG, *et al.* A contemporary overview of percutaneous coronary interventions. The American College of Cardiology-National Cardiovascular Data Registry (ACC-NCDR). *J Am Coll Cardiol* 2002; **39**(7):1096–103.
7. Abbott, JD, Kip KE, Vlachos HA, *et al.* Recent trends in the percutaneous treatment of chronic total coronary occlusions. *Am J Cardiol* 2006; **97**(12):1691–6.
8. Srivatsa SS, Edwards WD, Boos CM, *et al.* Histologic correlates of angiographic chronic total coronary artery occlusions: influence of occlusion duration on neovascular channel patterns and intimal plaque composition. *J Am Coll Cardiol* 1997; **29**(5):955–63.
9. Hoye A. The how and why of. chronic total occlusions – part two: Why we treat CTOs the way we do. *EuroIntervention* 2006; **2**:382–8.
10. Puma JA, Sketch MH Jr, Tcheng JE, *et al.* Percutaneous revascularization of chronic coronary occlusions: an overview. *J Am Coll Cardiol* 1995; **26**(1):1–11.
11. Sirnes PA, Myreng Y, Mølstad P, *et al.* Improvement in left ventricular ejection fraction and wall motion after successful recanalization of chronic coronary occlusions. *Eur Heart J* 1998; **19**(2):273–81.
12. Dzavik V, Carere RG, Mancini GB, *et al.* Predictors of improvement in left ventricular function after percutaneous revascularization of occluded coronary arteries: a report from the Total Occlusion Study of Canada (TOSCA). *Am Heart J* 2001; **142**(2):301–8.
13. Valenti R, Migliorini A, Signorini U, *et al.* Impact of complete revascularization with percutaneous coronary intervention on survival in patients with at least one chronic total occlusion. *Eur Heart J* 2008; **29**(19): 2336–42.
14. Elhendy A, Cornel JH, Roelandt JR, *et al.* Impact of severity of coronary artery stenosis and the collateral circulation on the functional outcome of dyssynergic myocardium after revascularization in patients with healed myocardial infarction and chronic left ventricular dysfunction. *Am J Cardiol* 1997; **79**(7):883–8.
15. Kirschbaum SW, Baks T, van den Ent M, *et al.* Evaluation of left ventricular function three years after percutaneous recanalization of chronic total coronary occlusions. *Am J Cardiol* 2008; **101**(2):179–85.
16. Ivanhoe R.J, Weintraub WS, Douglas JS Jr, *et al.* Percutaneous transluminal coronary angioplasty of chronic total occlusions. Primary success, restenosis, and long-term clinical follow-up. *Circulation* 1992; **85**(1): 106–15.
17. Suero JA, Marso SP, Jones PG, *et al.* Procedural outcomes and long-term survival among patients undergoing percutaneous coronary intervention of a chronic total occlusion in native coronary arteries: a 20-year experience. *J Am Coll Cardiol* 2001; **38**(2):409–14.
18. Hoye A, van Domburg RT, Sonnenschein K, *et al.* Percutaneous coronary intervention for chronic total occlusions: the Thoraxcenter experience 1992–2002; *Eur Heart J* 2005; **26**(24):2630–6.
19. Olivari Z, Rubartelli P, Piscione F, *et al.* Immediate results and one-year clinical outcome after percutaneous coronary interventions in chronic total occlusions: data from a multicenter, prospective, observational study (TOAST-GISE). *J Am Coll Cardiol* 2003; **41**(10):1672–8.
20. Aziz S, Stables RH, Grayson AD, *et al.* Percutaneous coronary intervention for chronic total occlusions: improved survival for patients with successful

revascularization compared to a failed procedure. *Catheter Cardiovasc Interv* 2007; **70**(1):15–20.

21. Prasad A, Rihal CS, Lennon RJ, *et al.* Trends in outcomes after percutaneous coronary intervention for chronic total occlusions: a 25-year experience from the Mayo Clinic. *J Am Coll Cardiol* 2007; **49**(15):1611–18.
22. Martuscelli E, Clementi F, Gallagher MM, *et al.* Revascularization strategy in patients with multivessel disease and a major vessel chronically occluded; data from the CABRI trial. *Eur J Cardiothorac Surg* 2008; **33**(1):4–8.
23. Garcia-Garcia HM, Kukreja N, Daemen J, *et al.* Contemporary treatment of patients with chronic total occlusion: critical appraisal of different techniques and devices. *EuroIntervention* 2007; **3**:188–96.
24. Mollet NR, Hoye A, Lemos PA, *et al.* Value of preprocedure multislice computed tomographic coronary angiography to predict the outcome of percutaneous recanalization of chronic total occlusions. *Am J Cardiol* 2005; **95**(2):240–3.
25. Hirokami M, Saito S, Muto H. Anchoring technique to improve guiding catheter support in coronary angioplasty of chronic total occlusions. *Catheter Cardiovasc Interv* 2006; **67**(3):366–71.
26. Takahashi S, Saito S, Tanaka S, *et al.* New method to increase a backup support of a 6 French guiding coronary catheter. *Catheter Cardiovasc Interv* 2004; **63**(4):452–6.
27. Mitsudo K, The how and why of. Chronic Total Occlusions. Part One: How to treat CTOs. *EuroIntervention* 2006; **2**:375–81.
28. Nanto S, Ohara T, Shimonagata T, *et al.* A technique for changing a PTCA balloon catheter over a regular-length guidewire. *Cathet Cardiovasc Diagn* 1994; **32**(3):274–7.
29. Colombo A, Mikhail GW, Michev I, *et al.* Treating chronic total occlusions using subintimal tracking and reentry: the STAR technique. *Catheter Cardiovasc Interv* 2005; **64**(4):407–11; discussion 412.
30. Carlino M, Godino C, Latib A, *et al.* Subintimal tracking and re-entry technique with contrast guidance: a safer approach. *Catheter Cardiovasc Interv* 2008; **72**(6):790–6.
31. Furuichi S, Airoldi F, Colombo A. Intravascular ultrasound-guided wiring for chronic total occlusion. *Catheter Cardiovasc Interv* 2007; **70**(6):856–9.
32. Surmely JF, Tsuchikane E, Katoh O, *et al.* New concept for CTO recanalization using controlled antegrade and retrograde subintimal tracking: the CART technique. *J Invasive Cardiol* 2006; **18**(7):334–8.
33. Kukreja N, Serruys PW, Sianos G. Retrograde recanalization of chronically occluded coronary arteries: illustration and description of the technique. *Catheter Cardiovasc Interv* 2007; **69**(6):833–41.
34. Surmely JF, Katoh O, Tsuchikane E, *et al.* Coronary septal collaterals as an access for the retrograde approach in the percutaneous treatment of coronary chronic total occlusions. *Catheter Cardiovasc Interv* 2007; **69**(6):826–32.
35. Sianos G, Barlis P, Di Mario C, *et al.* European experience with the retrograde approach for the recanalisation of coronary artery chronic total occlusions. A report on behalf of the EuroCTO club. *EuroIntervention* 2008; **4**: 84–92.
36. Saito S. Different strategies of retrograde approach in coronary angioplasty for chronic total occlusion. *Catheter Cardiovasc Interv* 2008; **71**(1):8–19.
37. Tsuchikane E, Katoh O, Shimogami M, *et al.* First clinical experience of a novel penetration catheter for patients with severe coronary artery stenosis. *Catheter Cardiovasc Interv* 2005; **65**(3):368–73.
38. Reifart N, Enayat D, Giokoglu K. A novel penetration catheter (Tornus) as bail-out device after balloon failure to recanalise long, old calcified chronic occlusions. *EuroIntervention* 2008; **3**:617–21.
39. Serruys PW, Hamburger JN, Koolen JJ, *et al.* Total occlusion trial with angioplasty by using laser guidewire. The TOTAL trial. *Eur Heart J* 2000; **21**(21):1797–805.
40. Melzi G, Cosgrave J, Biondi-Zoccai GL, *et al.* A novel approach to chronic total occlusions: the crosser system. *Catheter Cardiovasc Interv* 2006; **68**(1):29–35.
41. Tiroch K, Cannon L, Reisman M, *et al.* High-frequency vibration for the recanalization of guidewire refractory chronic total coronary occlusions. *Catheter Cardiovasc Interv* 2008; **72**(6):771–80.
42. Chamié D, Abizaid A, Costa JR Jr, *et al.* The revascular active percutaneous interventional device for coronary total occlusions study. *Catheter Cardiovasc Interv* 2008; **72**(2):156–63.
43. Whitbourn RJ, Cincotta M, Mossop P, *et al.* Intraluminal blunt microdissection for angioplasty of coronary chronic total occlusions. *Catheter Cardiovasc Interv* 2003; **58**(2):194–8.
44. Orlic D, Stankovic G, Sangiorgi G, *et al.* Preliminary experience with the Frontrunner coronary catheter: novel device dedicated to mechanical revascularization of chronic total occlusions. *Catheter Cardiovasc Interv* 2005; **64**(2):146–52.
45. Baim DS, Braden G, Heuser R, *et al.* Utility of the Safe-Cross-guided radiofrequency total occlusion crossing system in chronic coronary total occlusions (results from the Guided Radio Frequency Energy Ablation of Total Occlusions Registry Study). *Am J Cardiol* 2004; **94**(7):853–8.
46. Kiemeneij F, Patterson MS, Amoroso G, *et al.* Use of the Stereotaxis Niobe magnetic navigation system for percutaneous coronary intervention: results from 350 consecutive patients. *Catheter Cardiovasc Interv* 2008; **71**(4):510–16.
47. Kelbaek H, Helqvist S, Thuesen L, *et al.* Sirolimus versus bare metal stent implantation in patients with total coronary occlusions: subgroup analysis of the Stenting Coronary Arteries in Non-Stress/Benestent Disease (SCANDSTENT) trial. *Am Heart J* 2006; **152**(5):882–6.
48. Rahel BM, Laarman GJ, Kelder JC, *et al.* Three-year clinical outcome after primary stenting of totally occluded native coronary arteries: a randomized comparison of bare-metal stent implantation with sirolimus-eluting stent implantation for the treatment of total coronary

occlusions (Primary Stenting of Totally Occluded Native Coronary Arteries [PRISON] II study). *Am Heart J* 2009; **157**(1):149–55.

49. García-García HM, Daemen J, Kukreja N, *et al.* Three-year clinical outcomes after coronary stenting of chronic total occlusion using sirolimus-eluting stents: Insights from the rapamycin-eluting stent evaluated at Rotterdam cardiology hospital-(RESEARCH) registry. *Catheter Cardiovasc Interv* 2007; **70**(5):635–9.
50. Ge L, Iakovou I, Cosgrave J, *et al.* Immediate and mid-term outcomes of sirolimus-eluting stent implantation for chronic total occlusions. *Eur Heart J* 2005; **26**(11): 1056–62.
51. Migliorini A, Moschi G, Vergara R, *et al.* Drug-eluting stent-supported percutaneous coronary intervention for chronic total coronary occlusion. *Catheter Cardiovasc Interv* 2006; **67**(3):344–8.
52. Nakamura S, Muthusamy TS, Bae JH, *et al.* Impact of sirolimus-eluting stent on the outcome of patients with chronic total occlusions. *Am J Cardiol* 2005; **95**(2):161–6.
53. Werner GS, Schwarz G, Prochnau D, *et al.* Paclitaxel-eluting stents for the treatment of chronic total coronary occlusions: A strategy of extensive lesion coverage with drug-eluting stents. *Catheter Cardiovasc Interv* 2006; **67**(1):1–9.

CHAPTER 21

Revascularization in diabetes mellitus

Akhil Kapur and Ayesha Qureshi

Introduction

Diabetes is occurring in epidemic proportions. In the general population in the developed world, approximately 8% of adults have diabetes[1,2]. The prevalence of diabetes will double over the next 15 years or so to an estimated 300 million people by the year 2025[3]. This is due almost totally to an increase in type 2 diabetes mellitus (T2DM). These figures are likely to understate the size of the problem as it has been estimated that up to one-half of affected patients in the general population remain undiagnosed[4–6]. In addition up to double the number of patients who have diabetes have insulin resistance syndrome with a heightened risk of developing T2DM[7]. This increase will be due mainly to an increasing prevalence of obesity, decreasing rates of physical activity, an increasing consumption of high calorie diets, and an ageing population[8].

In patients with T2DM, manifestations of atherosclerosis are often already present by the time of diagnosis suggesting that the pre-diabetic period is an important risk factor for plaque development. The cause of most deaths and a great deal of the morbidity in patients with diabetes is dominated by coronary heart disease (CHD), accompanied by increased rates of stroke and peripheral vascular disease, together defined as macrovascular disease[9–13]. Cardiovascular complications remain the leading cause of mortality among patients with T2DM accounting for up to 80% of deaths. While the overall age-adjusted mortality rate associated with CHD has declined over the past 20 years this trend has not been reflected in a decline of age-adjusted mortality rates in patients with T2DM[14–16]. Men with T2DM have a threefold higher absolute risk of cardiovascular death than non-diabetic men even after controlling for age, race, income, cholesterol levels, blood pressure, and smoking[13]. The higher mortality risk in diabetic patients with CHD occurs in all aspects of the manifestation and treatment of their CHD.

Diabetes trebles the risk of developing CHD and once CHD has developed, diabetes doubles the risk for acute coronary syndromes (ACS) with an additional doubling of the clinical risk once the event has occurred[17–20]. This risk of a first cardiovascular event is higher than in the population, and may be as high as in patients who have had a previous myocardial infarction (MI)[21]. The Framingham study showed that even after adjusting for other factors, patients with diabetes not only had a higher mortality, they also had a higher incidence of reinfarction and heart failure in the acute and post-infarction period[22].

This higher risk of mortality in patients with diabetes is true whether they are treated with fibrinolysis or with primary angioplasty[23,24]. One-year mortality of diabetic patients post MI is twofold compared to non-diabetic patients and this was consistent in all age groups[25]. Over 20% of patients diagnosed with ACS are known to have diabetes[19]. Furthermore among patients who have an acute MI and are subsequently found to be diabetic, approximately 50% are undiagnosed[26]. Just under 20% of patients undergoing cardiac catheterization[6] are also known to have diabetes, with diabetic patients accounting for over 20% of all revascularization procedures in many of the more recent randomized trials in this area[27–29]. This percentage is rising as the incidence of T2DM increases. It is projected that over 30% of all revascularizations for coronary artery disease by 2015 will be in patients with diabetes. Yet the outcomes following percutaneous coronary intervention (PCI) and coronary artery bypass grafting (CABG) remain worse in patients with diabetes[30–36].

Patients with diabetes have a greater need for further revascularization after their index procedure. In addition to the increased risk associated with diabetes itself, the manifestations of coronary heart disease are more severe in diabetic patients with more extensive and diffuse coronary artery disease(37). An analysis of baseline characteristics in the Bypass Angioplasty Revascularization Investigation (BARI) trial of diabetic versus non-diabetic patients showed that diabetic patients had a higher incidence of triple vessel disease (46% vs. 40%, respectively, $p < 0.05$) and left ventricular (LV) dysfunction, defined as an ejection fraction (EF) below 50% (20% vs. 31%, $p < 0.001$)(38). This translated into a significantly lower 5-year survival.

Likewise, in the angioplasty sub study of the Global Use of Strategies to Open Occluded arteries in acute coronary syndromes (GUSTO IIb), the incidence of multi-vessel disease was much higher in diabetic patients, compared to those without diabetes (45.3% vs 32.4%, $p = 0.006$), and the mean EF was lower (48% vs. 51%, $p = 0.003$)(24). In the same study diabetes was associated with a poorer outcome (death or reinfarction), both at 30 days (13.1% vs 8.5%, $p = 0.0001$) and at 6 months (18.8% vs. 11.4%, $p = 0.0001$)(18).

These differences in clinical features of coronary artery disease (CAD) are reflected in angiographic findings. Typically, diabetic patients have more diffuse, multi-vessel and distal coronary disease, smaller reference vessels (i.e. even the undiseased vessel is of smaller calibre than in a non-diabetic patient), poorer coronary collateral circulation, and more frequent left main stem disease (Fig. 21.1)(23,39–41). In an autopsy study, lesion morphological characteristics differed between unstable patients with and without diabetes with more plaque ulceration and intracoronary thrombus observed in diabetic patients(42).

Why is diabetes different?

Several biological mechanisms exist that can explain the premature development of atherosclerosis and the higher risk of CAD in patients with diabetes mellitus.

These increased risks are related not only to a higher frequency of general vascular risk factors in diabetic patients including hypertension and hyperlipidaemia(43) but to specific risks resulting from the triad of insulin resistance, hyperinsulinaemia, and hyperglycaemia(44) detailed further in Table 21.1 and summarized below.

Hyperglycaemia and chronic vascular complications characterize diabetes mellitus. While it is clear that improvements in glycaemic control can slow the development and progression of microvascular complications there is also evidence that macrovascular disease can be controlled by tighter glycaemic control, although probably less so(45). Various mechanisms may explain the translation of poor glycaemic control into vascular disorders including protein glycosylation, the formation of advanced glycation end products (AGEs), changes in haemostasis, specific lipid profile abnormalities, oxidative stress, and inflammation.

The biological mechanisms which contribute to the increased risk of coronary disease in patients with diabetes can be divided into biochemical abnormalities which include dyslipidaemia and AGEs, coagulation abnormalities including platelet hyperactivity and haemostatic abnormalities, and those that affect the arterial

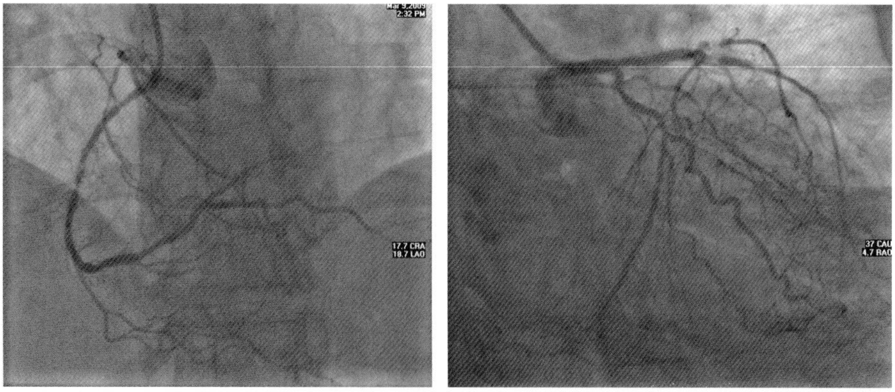

Fig. 21.1 Coronary angiograms demonstrating typical images of diabetic coronary disease. Note the small-calibre vessels with diffuse, distal disease.

Table 21.1 Features of diabetes which increase risk of CHD

Factor	Effect
Dyslipidaemia	Increased LDL and trigylceride-rich VLDL Reduced HDL
Endothelial dysfunction	Increased expression of cellular adhesion molecules Impaired vasomotor activity due to decreased availability of nitric oxide
Oxidative stress	Increased concentrations of markers such as oxidized LDLs and F2-isoprostanes
Inflammation	Increased expression of markers such as fibrinogen and CRP
Abnormalities of coagulation and fibrinolysis	Overproduction of fibrinogen, Expression of PAI-1 Reduced tPA
Glycation of proteins	Formation of proatherogenic advanced end products (AGE) in LDL and collagen within the arterial wall

HDL, high-density lipoprotein; LDH, low-density lipoprotein; VLDL, very low-density lipoprotein. tPA, tissue plasminogen activator; PAI-1, plasminogen activator inhibitor-1

wall including adverse arterial remodelling, endothelial dysfunction, and cellular proliferation and restenosis.

Dyslipidaemia

Patients with diabetes have a characteristic but abnormal lipid profile, probably as a result of insulin resistance and a failure of insulin activity in general. The result is an increase in the release of free fatty acids from adipose tissue, increased delivery of free fatty acids to the liver, and increased synthesis of very low-density lipoproteins (VLDL)[46,47]. The resulting abnormal lipid profile is characterized by increased concentrations of small dense LDLs, triglyceride-rich VLDLs, and low concentrations of high-density lipoproteins (HDLs), and is associated with a markedly increased cardiovascular risk[48,49]. Whilst triglyceride levels are directly related to the degree of glucose intolerance and glucose control[50] these appear to have less effect on HDL and LDL levels.

Endothelial dysfunction

It is well established that severe arteriopathy occurs during the pre-diabetic state. The earliest measurable feature of this is endothelial dysfunction which is also thought to be an early marker for the development of atherosclerosis. Early endothelial injury occurs probably through hyperglycaemia, hypertension, diabetic dyslipidaemia, and insulin resistance, and the resulting endothelial dysfunction is a manifestation of the development of both microvascular and macrovascular complications[51–53]. In support of the fact that there is a risk of macrovascular disease before the development of overt T2DM is that these patients have an increased concentration of markers of endothelial dysfunction including soluble vascular cell adhesion molecule (sVCAM), soluble intercellular adhesion molecule (sICAM), endothelin (ET)-1, and vWF(54).

Although it is accepted that there is clustering of cardiovascular risk factors before the development of T2DM it seems that the insulin resistance syndrome or the pre-diabetic state contribute to vascular risk over and above that of traditional risk factors. The protein kinase C (PKC) pathway is activated by hyperglycaemia and is associated with many abnormal cellular functions, including increased vascular contractility and endothelial dysfunction.

It is likely that endothelial dysfunction is linked to inflammatory cytokines and both IL-6 and C-reactive protein (CRP) have been linked to the development of both diabetes mellitus and central adiposity[55–57]. Further studies have shown that the use of pharmacological agents or visceral fat reduction results in a reduction in the circulating levels of cytokines, soluble markers of endothelial cell activation, and an improvement in endothelial function[58].

Other risk factors include oxidative stress (increased concentrations of markers such as oxidized LDLs and F2-isoprostanes) and glycation of proteins (resulting in the formation of AGEs in LDL and collagen within the arterial wall, which have a variety of proatherogenic effects). Prolonged exposure to hyperglycaemia causes endothelial and platelet dysfunction impairing vasodilatation and accelerating the atherosclerotic process[59].

Platelet hyperactivity

Increased platelet activity in diabetes contributes to the increased thrombogenic potential in diabetes and is a productive target for pharmacological intervention. Platelets of patients with diabetes are larger and have an increased number of glycoprotein (GP) IIb/IIIa receptors[60]. They aggregate more easily to known agonists *in vitro* than platelets from non-diabetic patients[61]. Hyperglycaemia may be the cause for the greater percentage of diabetic platelets, circulating in an activated state, possibly due to increased production of F2-isoprostane[59]. Hyperglycaemia may also promote platelet-mediated thrombosis. Serum glucose levels have been shown to be a key multivariate predictor of platelet dependent thrombosis[62].

Endothelial dysfunction results in reduction of prostacyclin and NO. Both these agents have potent antiplatelet aggregating properties and are released by intact endothelium. In patients with diabetes and insulin resistance the synthesis of agents, which have proaggregating properties such as adenosine diphosphate (ADP) and thromboxane, is up regulated. The combination of the action of these compounds may well be key in resulting in a propensity for platelet-mediated atherothrombosis in diabetes[63].

This is the basis for the marked clinical benefit that diabetic patients derive from antiplatelet therapies including aspirin[64–66], thienopyridine derivatives such as clopidogrel[67], and GP IIb/IIIa inhibitors[68].

The action of the GP IIb/IIIa receptor, which exists on the platelet surface, is to bind fibrinogen. When activated these receptors function as adhesion molecules, resulting in platelet cross-linking, an essential element of platelet aggregation. GP IIb/IIIa receptor inhibitors hinder platelet aggregation by binding to these receptors thus blocking the final common pathway[69]. In patients with diabetes mellitus who present with an ACS and/or who undergo PCI, the use of GP IIb/IIIa inhibitors results in increased short- and long-term event-free survival[70,71].

Haemostatic abnormalities

Several haemostatic abnormalities are associated with diabetes. These include increased levels of von Willebrand factor (vWF), factors VII, VIII, and X, and fibrinogen[72–75] resulting in an increased propensity for coagulation. Reductions of levels of protein C and antithrombin which are inhibitors of coagulation add to this propensity for coagulation[76].

Elevations of PAI-1 concentrations reflect profound suppression of the fibrinolytic pathway in patients with diabetes in association with insulin resistance[77]. There is a strong relationship between features of the metabolic syndrome and elevated PAI-1 levels with the correlation with triglyceride concentrations being particularly strong[77]. In patients with type 1 diabetes mellitus (T1DM) there is no consistent defect in fibrinolysis, in fact studies suggest that these patients have an increase in fibrinolytic activity and tPA concentrations, with either normal or reduced levels of PAI-1[78,79].

Adverse arterial remodelling

It is well known that patients with diabetes exhibit aggressive atherosclerosis and restenosis. During the early stages of atherosclerosis there is a tendency for negative arterial remodelling, a lack of collateral vessel formation, and a heightened risk of late vessel occlusion following conventional balloon angioplasty although this is no longer the case with intracoronary stenting.

As opposed to having an adaptive arterial response to atherosclerosis, patients with diabetes tend to respond with vessel contracture which in effect means that less plaque burden can cause a significant stenosis in patients with diabetes than in non-diabetic patients[80]. As a result, patients with diabetes tend to have smaller arteries with lesions of longer lengths and diffuse disease, all of which can add to medium- and long-term problems following revascularization.

Even though patients with diabetes have a tendency to have both earlier onset and more aggressive atherosclerosis they seem to be less able to collateralize occluded arteries. It has been shown that there is decreased gene expression of vascular endothelial growth factor (VEGF) in human diabetic myocardial samples as well as a decrease in expression of the VEGF receptor. This was increased in non-diabetic patients with CHD compared to controls[41].

Accelerated atherosclerosis

Endothelial dysfunction and the pro-thrombotic state play major roles in the accelerated atherosclerotic process. Hyperglycaemia, through a series of chemical reactions, results in the formation of AGEs. Engagement of RAGE, the cell surface receptor for AGEs, can activate inflammatory functions of endothelial cells, smooth muscle cells, and macrophages, cell types intimately involved in atherogenesis and compound the inflammatory stimuli encountered by the arterial wall in patients with diabetes. RAGE is therefore involved in the progression of atheroma and plaque vulnerability in uncontrolled diabetic patients[81–83]. Loredana and colleagues reported that the administration of soluble RAGE can inhibit the progression of already established atheroma, reducing the size of lesions and changing the characteristics of plaques that indicate reduced inflammation and increased stability[84]. Blockade of RAGE may be a novel strategy to stabilize atherosclerosis and vascular inflammation in established diabetes.

Haemoglobin A1c measures a protein (haemoglobin) that has undergone non-enzymatic glycation, and correlates with AGE levels. Thus, given the link between glycaemic control and ligands for RAGE, one might logically presume that strict glycaemic control would protect against vascular complications in diabetic patients. In terms of the lipid abnormalities in diabetes, it is the complex pattern of dyslipidaemia that may promote plaque inflammation and hence atherogenesis.

The multifactorial complexity of diabetic vascular disease suggests the need for aggressive treatment including strict glycaemic control and global risk factor modification for all diabetic patients including those undergoing coronary intervention. Aggressive reduction of such risk factors has been shown to improve the outcome after PCI and to reduce the incidence of subsequent MI and the need for repeat revascularization[85].

Cellular proliferation and restenosis

Several studies have shown that diabetes is an independent risk factor for restenosis after balloon angioplasty, with a reported restenosis rate ranging from 35–71%[86,87]. Following balloon dilatation it occurs as a result of three factors: abrupt vessel closure, adverse arterial modelling, and neointimal proliferation. Arterial remodelling and acute recoil of balloon-injured vessels contribute significantly to the restenosis process following balloon angioplasty, with neointimal proliferation playing a secondary role[88,89]. In diabetic patients, collagen-rich sclerotic content is increased in restenotic lesions undergoing remodelling and elastic recoil, suggesting an accelerated fibrotic rather than a proliferative response in diabetic lesions in post-angioplasty restenosis[90].

Late vessel occlusion is the other frequent mode of restenosis following balloon angioplasty associated with a significant decrease in ejection fraction[91], and was reported to be a major determinant of long-term mortality in diabetic patients[92]. Intravascular ultrasound data suggest that intimal hyperplasia is the main reason for increased restenosis in both stented and non-stented lesions in diabetic patients[93]. Since the advent of stenting, restenosis has been reduced in both diabetic and non-diabetic patients. This has been caused mainly by the elimination of abrupt vessel closure and vessel remodelling following PCI. Stenting has also significantly reduced the rate of occlusive restenosis in diabetic patients closer to the level of non-diabetic patients[94]. It follows therefore that restenosis following stenting is a direct result of neointimal proliferation. Patients with diabetes still have higher rates of restenosis following stenting than those who are non-diabetic[95].

Insulin and glucose have been suggested as key drivers of neointimal proliferation in patients with diabetes. In terms of restenosis itself it is unlikely that hyperglycaemia is the only factor and no direct link exists between glucose control and restenosis. Insulin itself is a weak growth factor but the coexpression of insulin like growth factor-1 and platelet derived growth factors have powerful mitogenic effects and may also play a role as one of the factors in restenosis[96].

Microalbuminuria

The presence of microalbuminuria is one of the major determinants of adverse outcome in diabetic patients[97]. When diabetic nephropathy develops, the prevalence of CHD increases dramatically[98]. In patients with T2DM, microalbuminuria is an independent predictor of increased cardiovascular mortality [99,100], increasing the risk for fatal CHD by a factor of two to four. One of the possible explanations for poor outcomes in diabetic patients with nephropathy is the accentuation of the atherogenic mechanisms present in diabetes. The early stages of diabetic nephropathy are associated with coexistence of multiple cardiovascular risk factors including hypertension, lipid abnormalities, and a hypercoagulable state[101].

Hypertension is frequently present in diabetic nephropathy, even when the creatinine concentrations remain normal, and can intensify coronary disease in diabetic patients. Microalbuminuria is associated with an atherogenic lipoprotein profile that includes elevated LDL and chylomicron remnants levels, decreased HDL levels, and elevated LpA levels[102–104]. In addition, PAI-1 activity, factor VII, and plasma fibrinogen are significantly higher in patients with T1DM and microalbuminuria[105,106]. Finally, nephropathy results in accelerated accumulation of AGEs in the circulation and tissue that parallels the severity of renal impairment.

Medical therapy versus revascularization in patients with diabetes

Acute coronary syndromes

At least eight trials have compared an invasive versus conservative strategy in the management of non-ST elevation MI (NSTEMI). The invasive strategy used rapid diagnostic coronary angiography and revascularization where necessary and the conservative strategy medical therapy with selective invasive therapy in patients with recurrent or inducible ischaemia[107,108]. In the setting of NSTEMI ACS diabetes mellitus has been identified as an independent predictor of long-term mortality[19], related to the proinflammatory and prothrombotic states present in diabetes[109]. Since no study has specifically addressed the value of an early invasive strategy in diabetic patients with ACS, we are left with subgroup analyses of the major trials. In FRISC II (Fragmin and Fast Revascularisation during InStability in Coronary artery disease Investigators) there was a strong trend to benefit in terms of 1-year death or MI in the patients with diabetes (n = 299), both in relative risk reduction (RRR, 39%) and absolute risk reduction (ARR, 9.3%)[(110)]. Among individuals without diabetes, the efficacy was less pronounced (RRR, 28%; ARR, 3.1%). However, because of the smaller sample size, the benefit observed did not reach statistical significance in patients with diabetes (p = 0.07), even though it was significant in patients without diabetes (p = 0.02). In the TACTICS TIMI-18 (Treat Angina with aggrastat and determine Cost of Therapy with Invasive or Conservative Strategy – Thrombolysis In Myocardial Infarction) trial all patients received platelet GP IIb/IIIa receptor inhibitors in contrast to FRISC II. Again, patients with diabetes derived a greater benefit from the early invasive strategy than those without diabetes, in terms of both RRR (27% and 13%, respectively) and ARR (7.6% and 1.8%, respectively). The benefit reached statistical significance in diabetes (n = 613), but not in patients without diabetes (n = 1607)[(111)].

The European Society of Cardiology (ESC) guidelines recommend that patients with diabetes and ACS benefit from an early invasive strategy[(112,113)]. The only randomized data that compare PCI and CABG in this setting are derived from the AWESOME (Percutaneous Coronary Intervention Versus Coronary Artery Bypass Graft Surgery for Patients with Medically Refractory Myocardial Ischemia and Risk Factors for Adverse Outcomes with Bypass) trial[(114)] which compared the two revascularization strategies in diabetic patients with medically refractory unstable angina who were at high risk for CABG. Patients had at least one of five risk factors for adverse outcomes after bypass (prior CABG, MI within 7 days, LV ejection fraction <35%, age >70 years, or an intra-aortic balloon being required to stabilize)[(114)]. Among 2431 patients identified, 454 were considered acceptable for both PCI and CABG; 1650 patients were deemed not to be candidates for either therapy and entered a physician-directed registry; and 327 who were considered candidates for both treatments but refused randomization entered a patient-choice registry. The respective CABG and PCI 3-year survival rates for patients with diabetes were 72% and 81% for randomized patients (n = 144), 85% and 89% for those who entered the patient-choice registry (n = 89), and 73% and 71% for the physician-directed registry patients (n = 525). None of the differences between patient groups was statistically significant. These results have to be interpreted with caution as the left internal mammary artery (LIMA) was used as an arterial conduit in 70% of cases and stents were used in only 54% of cases, with GP IIb/IIIa antagonists administered in 11% of patients.

Stable coronary disease

The controversy over the benefit of revascularization, particularly PCI, compared to medical therapy alone continues. This is despite the recent publication of the COURAGE (Clinical Outcomes Utilizing Revascularization and Aggressive Drug Evaluation) trial[(115)]. Between 1999–2004, the COURAGE trial enrolled and randomized 2287 patients either to PCI plus optimal medical therapy or to optimal medical therapy alone with no difference seen in all-cause deaths or non-fatal MIs (the primary outcome of COURAGE) Over the median 4.6 years of follow-up, more medical therapy patients than PCI treated patients underwent subsequent revascularization, usually due to refractive angina or objective, non-invasive evidence of worsening ischaemia. The only statistically significant difference between the two treatment strategies was reduced prevalence of angina, which was greater in the PCI group at 1 and 3 years but not at 5 years which was in part a reflection of subsequent revascularization in the medical therapy group as one-third of medically managed patients underwent PCI or CABG during the follow-up period. A subanalysis for the 766 patients with diabetes did not show a benefit for PCI in this subset either (OR 0.99; 95% CI 0.73–1.32) ([115]). It has been argued that these results are not unexpected in view of the earlier findings of the 1018 patient RITA (Randomised Intervention Treatment of Angina) 2 trial[(116)]. Seven year results showed that death or MI was no different between PCI patients (14.5%) and medical patients (12.3%) (p = 0.21). There were 43 deaths in both groups, 41% of which were cardiac. In the PCI group 12.7% subsequently had CABG, and 14.5% required additional non-randomized PCI. Most of these reinterventions occurred within a year of randomization, and after two years the reintervention rate was 2.3% per annum. In the medical group, 35.4% required myocardial revascularization: 15.0% in the first year and an annual rate of 3.6% after 2 years. An initial policy of PCI was associated with improved anginal symptoms and exercise times. These treatment differences narrowed over time, mainly because of coronary interventions in medical patients with severe symptoms. It should be noted that there were only 90 patients with diabetes recruited into this study.

A meta-analysis[(117)] purporting to summarize the data available to date was recently published and included 17 randomized trials comparing a PCI-based invasive treatment strategy with medical treatment in 7513 patients with symptoms or signs of myocardial ischemia but no ACS. The primary endpoint was all-cause death.

Follow-up was a median of 51 months. There was a 20% reduction in all-cause death in the PCI group (OR 0.80; 95% CI 0.64–0.99; p = 0.263 for heterogeneity across the trials). It has been argued that these findings suggest that a PCI-based invasive strategy may improve long-term survival compared with a medical treatment only strategy in patients with stable coronary artery disease. No separate subset analysis of patients with diabetes was reported.

Thus it is still not clear whether revascularization procedures are associated with an improvement in mortality among diabetic subjects, as compared with a more conservative medical treatment. In MASS II (Medicine, Angioplasty, or Surgery Study), 611 patients with stable multi-vessel coronary disease were randomly assigned to medical treatment, surgery, or angioplasty[118]. Of these, 190 patients had diabetes (75 medical, 56 angioplasty, 59 surgery). Mortality rates were analysed for the entire 5 years of follow-up. Separate analyses were also performed for mortality at two time intervals: during the first year and after the first year of follow-up. A calculation for the probability of death conditional on surviving to the start of the interval analysed was done. The cumulative 5-year mortality as well as the mortality during the first year of follow-up was not significantly different among treatment groups, both for diabetic and for non-diabetic subjects. Also, during years 2–5, the mortality of the three treatment groups was not different for non-diabetic subjects. Diabetic patients who underwent any form of revascularization had a significantly lower mortality between years 2–5 than those allocated to medical treatment (p = 0.039).

The BARI 2D (Bypass Angioplasty Revascularization Investigation 2 in Diabetes) Trial[119] is a 2 × 2 factorial trial which attempted to answer this question of which more is discussed later.

PCI versus surgery

There are two main types of study design, which have been used to compare angioplasty and surgery. In general terms they are prospective randomized studies and observational or registry studies which can be prospective or retrospective.

The relative merits of these two forms of studies came to light with the results of the BARI (Bypass Angioplasty Revascularization Investigation) study where both a randomized controlled trial and a registry of refusing patients were important elements of the investigation. A difference in demographics was noted between the randomized and registry elements[87]. The population in the randomized trial were less educated and contained a higher percentage from ethnic minorities than those in the registry. There was also more three-vessel disease in the PCI randomized patients than in the PCI registry patients who were allocated according to physician preference. The subset of diabetic patients in the randomized study who received PCI (Fig. 21.2) did significantly worse than those in the registry who received PCI (see Table 21.2).

However, the results of the subset of randomized patients in BARI have not been replicated in other studies which has produced conflicting results, possibly because the subsets in these were even smaller. In the absence of additional prospective randomized trial data, analyses of diabetic cohorts within large registry databases can add to the body of evidence. Patients who might otherwise not enter a randomized trial because of patient or physician refusal can be represented in such studies. While data from randomized trials can be difficult to generalize, the limitation of data from a registry or observational study is that selection bias cannot be overcome.

Randomized trials

Revascularization with PCI and CABG in diabetic patients has been under investigation for several years, but almost always comprises substudies of trials that are designed to compare PCI and CABG in the general population (diabetic and non-diabetic patients).

The randomized interventional studies comparing PCI with CABG occurred in three waves. The first recruited between 1986–1992 and the use of stents in the PCI arms of these studies was either non-existent or severely limited. These studies will be described as from the prestent era. The second wave comprised three main trials, which recruited patients between 1996–999, and were specifically designed to compare stenting with surgery and are described as those from the stent era. The third wave of studies compared drug-eluting stents (DES) and surgery recruiting from 2002 onwards.

Several trials have compared an initial treatment strategy of PCI with an initial treatment strategy of CABG[120–131]. Although these trials differed in design, they all enrolled patients who were clinically and angiographically suitable for randomization to either procedure. A meta-analysis of the earlier trials suggests no difference between the two strategies in terms of mortality, non-fatal MI, and CVA although the rates of further revascularization were much higher in the PCI groups[132].A more recent meta-analysis

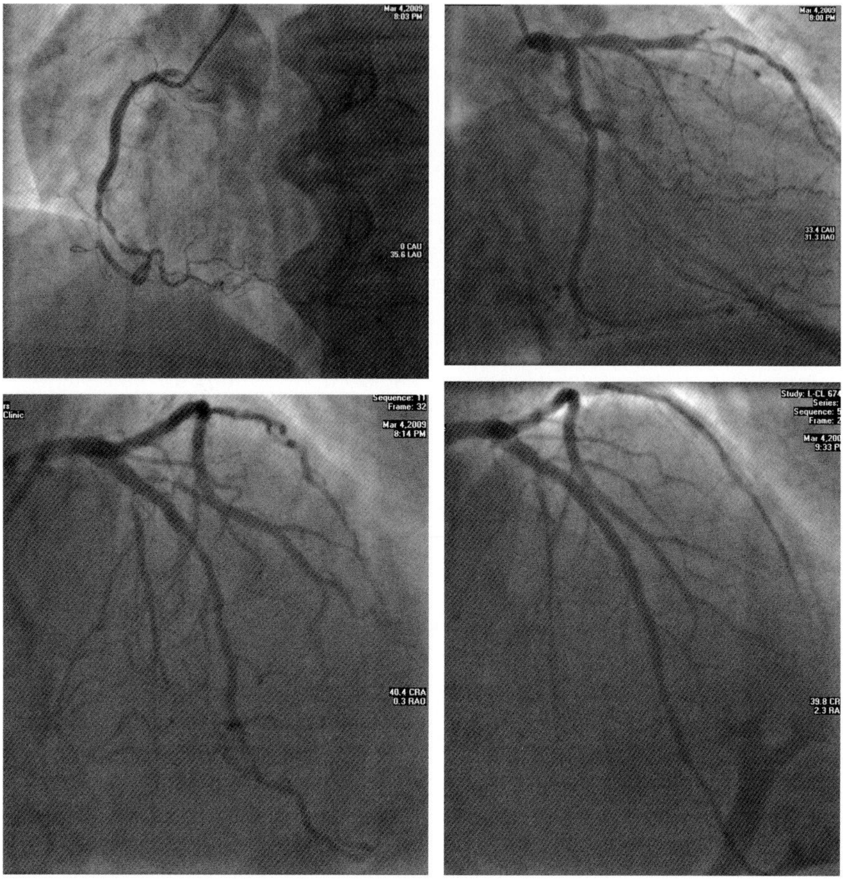

Fig. 21.2 Diagnostic coronary angiogram (A–C) of a diabetic patient showing a significant lesion in the mid LAD (B, C). The patient underwent PCI with an excellent result (D).

confirmed no difference in death or non-fatal MI but did confirm a lower rate of CVA in the PCI groups (0.6% vs. 1.2%, $p = 0.002$) as well as higher rates of repeat revascularization[(133)].

It has been suggested that there might be a difference in outcome between the two groups in the subset of patients with diabetes mellitus. The BARI trial showed that a diabetic subgroup of patients treated by an initial policy of PCI were at a higher risk of death, compared to patients treated by an initial policy of CABG (44% vs. 23.6% at 7 years, $p = 0.0011$)[(134)]. The importance of this finding has been debated since this subgroup was not pre-specified and the study was not designed to specifically look at patients with diabetes. The outcome of diabetic patients in the registry did not suggest a dramatic advantage of CABG over PCI (see Table 21.3)[(87)]. A similar but statistically non-significant difference in favour of CABG was also reported in 125 patients with diabetes in the CABRI (Coronary Artery Bypass Revascularization Investigation) trial[(121,135)]. Numerous studies have shown that diabetes increases the risk of restenosis after successful PCI and that insulin-requiring patients have an even worse outcome[(136,137)]. Until now there has been a trend amongst clinicians to favour

Table 21.2 BARI 5-year mortality randomized PCI versus CABG and registry PCI versus CABG

	5-year mortality (%)
Randomized PCI	34.5
Randomized CABG	19.4
Registry PCI	14.4
Registry CABG	14.9

Table 21.3 Size of diabetic subsets in the major interventional trials

Trial	Total number of patients	Number of diabetic patients	Recruitment period	CABG superior to PCI in diabetics at primary endpoint	Primary endpoint
BARI	1829	353	1988–1991	Yes	All-cause death at 5 years
CABRI	1054	125	1988–1992	No*	Death and angina status at 5 years
EAST	392	59	1987–1990	No	Death or MI or large ischaemic defect on perfusion scan at 3 years
RITA	1011	62	1988–1991	No*	Death or MI at 5 years
ERACI	127	13	1988–1990	No*	Death or MI at 3 years
GABI	359	43	1986–1991	No*	Freedom from angina at 1 year
ARTS	1205	208	1996–1997	Yes	Death or MI or CVA or repeat revascularization at 1 year
SoS	988	142	1996–1998	No*	Death or MI at 2 years
ERACI II	450	77	1996–1998	No	Death, MI, CVA, or repeat revascularization at 30 days
CARDia	510	510	2002–2007	No	Death, MI, CVA at 1 year
SYNTAX	1800	452	2005–2007	No	Death, MI, CVA and repeat revascularization at 1 year

*diabetic subset too small.

surgery, as a result of the BARI trial in particular. Both techniques have made advances in recent years, although in routine practice this may be more so for coronary angioplasty. Coronary stents reduce the risk of restenosis and the subsequent clinical event rate(138,139) with more marked benefits in diabetic patients(94,136). New pharmacological interventions appear to be improving the acute and the long-term results of PCI. Several trials have now shown that abciximab and other GPIIb/IIIa inhibitors improve acute outcome and that benefit may be sustained in the long term(140–142). These drugs seem to lower the risk of non-surgical revascularization in diabetic patients in particular(71), especially with the combination of stents and GPIIb/IIIa inhibitors(143). In addition, while the effects of lipid lowering are known to improve clinical outcome in patients with coronary artery disease(144) and those who undergo PCI(145) it was not known until recently whether the effect is the same with CABG(146,147). These advances have limited the relevance of the original trials of PCI versus CABG to current clinical practice. Data from the ARTS (Arterial Revascularisation Therapies Study) trial(130,148) suggested that multi-vessel stenting produces similar results in terms of clinical outcome to CABG in the overall population of patients but with a much lower repeat revascularization rate than was experienced in the original PCI versus CABG trials. However, the diabetic subset in this study was even smaller than that in BARI but again diabetes was an independent risk factor for PCI and not CABG(148).

The major randomized trials that compared PCI to CABG in both the pre stent and the stent era are listed in Table 21.3. This highlights the paucity of data that existed in these patients before the CARDia and SYNTAX trials. None of these randomized studies were specifically dedicated to patients with diabetes but some have undertaken substudy analyses in these patients. Whether any conclusions could be gleaned from these subsets and what these conclusions were will be discussed. Any data particularly relevant to diabetic patients is detailed at the end of the summary of each trial.

The registry studies

However, as already indicated, the results of the BARI trial have not been replicated in other randomized studies. When differing findings occur in randomized trials, this is often due to population differences. This is further magnified when the subsets being considered, in this case patients with diabetes, are small. Patients who might otherwise not enter a randomized trial because of patient or physician refusal can often be represented in these studies.

Several of these studies have been undertaken. As well as the BARI registry of randomizable but non-randomized patients(87) there are data from at least four other databases. Three of these are single institution databases: Duke(149), Emory(150), and the Mid America Heart

Institute (MAHI)[151]. The other was a large regional database comprising data from institutions in Northern New England[152].

In all of these studies patients, similar to the population with diabetes in BARI, were selected, and multivariate adjustment techniques were used to control for confounding factors.

Duke

In the Duke analysis[149], 3220 patients with multivessel disease of whom 24% were diabetic were studied between 1984–1990. Exclusions were similar to those that precluded entry to the BARI study and included significant left main stem stenosis, a history of prior revascularization, a history of valvular disease, and MI within 24h of catheterization. Survival at 5 years in the surgical group was 74% in diabetic and 86% in non-diabetic patients and was respectively 76% and 88% in the angioplasty group. After adjustment for baseline characteristics diabetes was associated with a worse outcome regardless of revascularization strategy ($p < 0.0001$). The outcomes in diabetes with PCI were no different to those of CABG however ($p = 0.91$).

MAHI

The MAHI analysis[151] was a retrospective study of diabetic patients with multi-vessel disease revascularized between 1987–1990. It had a similar patient population to the BARI randomized study and to the Duke registry and there was a strong, although non-significant trend for survival in favour of CABG versus PCI ($p = 0.08$) although there was significantly more three-vessel disease in the CABG group than in the PCI group. Incomplete revascularization occurred significantly more often in the PCI group than in the CABG group (58% vs. 21%, $p < 0.001$) and it was this, not mode of revascularization that was a predictor of late mortality. The inference was that the inability of angioplasty to provide complete revascularization, at least at the time of the study, contributed to poorer outcomes.

Emory

The Emory analysis studied 2639 diabetic patients with multi-vessel disease who received revascularization between 1981–1994[150]. The surgical group were on the whole higher risk with more three-vessel disease, more frequent history of MI, and lower ejection fractions. Once these baseline differences had been accounted for there was no statistical difference between the two groups but there was a strong trend to survival advantage in the surgical group at 5 years. However, multivariate analysis in a subset of 889 insulin-requiring patients revealed that they were worse off with angioplasty than surgery, in terms of survival, revealing a HR of 1.35 (95% CI 1.01–1.79).

The Northern New England Group

The Northern New England database group[152] examined the 5-year outcomes of 2766 patients, similar to those randomized in the BARI study and who were revascularized between 1992–1996. PCI was the initial treatment strategy in 736 patients and CABG in 2030. Patients who underwent PCI were younger, had higher ejection fractions, and less extensive coronary disease. After adjusting for baseline differences, patients with diabetes treated with PCI had significantly greater mortality than those undergoing CABG ($HR = 1.49$; 95% CI 1.02–2.17; $p = 0.037$). Mortality risk was greater among the 1251 who had three-vessel disease ($HR = 2.02$; 95% CI 1.04–3.91, $p = 0.038$) than the 1515 patients with two-vessel disease ($HR = 1.33$; 95% CI 0.84–2.1, $p = 0.21$). This study did not involve a significant usage of stenting (<5% of total patient years of follow-up). The results demonstrated a clear difference in survival with an initial CABG HR of 1.49 approaching that seen in the BARI randomized trial of 1.78.

In summary, it can be observed that there is at least a trend to benefit, if not a significant benefit, in favour of CABG over PCI in patients with diabetes in all of these studies.

Using the results of both randomized and registry studies to identify factors for optimal revascularization in diabetes

A study of the combined results of the BARI registry and randomized studies reveals that if diabetic patients with multi-vessel disease are assigned according to physician choice to either PCI or CABG they do significantly better than if they are randomly assigned to one or other treatment[87]. It did suggest that physicians were able to select those patients who benefited most from PCI. On further analysis there was a strong tendency to refer those with more extensive disease i.e. those with three-vessel disease rather than two-vessel disease to CABG (Fig. 21.3) This practice is supported by the Emory PTCA database[30], which showed that survival with PCI in a general population of patients undergoing revascularization is more favourable with less extensive disease. The results of the Northern New England database study in diabetic patients[152] supports this as among patients with three-vessel disease

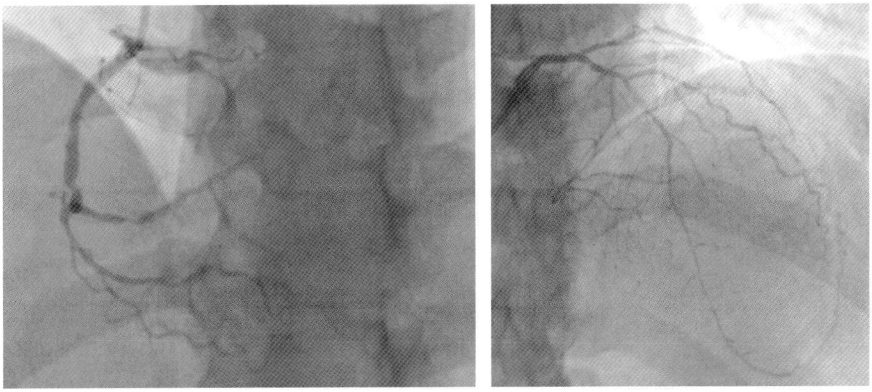

Fig. 21.3 Severe diffuse multi-vessel coronary artery disease in a patient with diabetes mellitus. Note that the RCA is occluded distally and the extensive collaterals from the RCA cross to the distal LAD. The patient was referred for a surgical opinion although the small calibre of the vessels and severity of the distal disease make them difficult to graft.

the HR was 2.02 favouring surgery. However in patients with two-vessel disease PCI is not significantly different to CABG in the short to long term. When abciximab is added to stenting during the revascularization of patients with diabetes, particularly with MVD, the absolute benefit seems to be over and above that seen with non-diabetic patients. In fact an eightfold reduction in mortality was achieved using this regimen according to the meta analysis of the EPISTENT (Evaluation of platelet IIb/IIIa inhibitor for stenting), EPILOG (Evaluation in PTCA to Improve Long-Term Outcome with Abciximab GP IIb/IIIa Blockade) and EPIC (Evaluation of 7E3 for the Prevention of Ischemic Complications) trials, albeit with only 173 patients in this subgroup(71).

Long-term survival may also be affected by completeness of revascularization. It has been suggested that complete revascularization in diabetic patients is more easily achieved with CABG than with PCI(150). It has also been shown that when incomplete revascularization is adjusted for, the mode of revascularization in patients with diabetes does not correlate with late mortality(30).

While the optimal strategy for single-vessel disease has not been specifically studied it is generally accepted that a reasonable approach would be to undertake PCI initially if technically feasible. It seems sensible, based on the randomized and registry trials to date, that patient allocation to one revascularization strategy versus the other should involve the consideration of several factors. More extensive disease, a great number of lesions, diffuse disease but good distal targets, chronic occlusions, multiple complex disease such as bifurcations or ostial disease, may all favour CABG while discreet lesions in the context of relatively limited disease where complete revascularization is possible would allow PCI to be considered. However the field of revascularization generally, and therefore in patients with diabetes and multi-vessel disease is continually changing with the advent of new techniques and adjunctive therapies many of which have not been tested in trials comparing PCI and CABG. The SYNTAX score which has recently been introduced can also help with this decision making process (see SYNTAX trial, page 366).

Have advances in coronary surgery improved outcomes in patients with diabetes?

Off-pump coronary surgery

Cardiopulmonary bypass with cardiac arrest (on-pump) provides a surgical field free of motion and blood, allowing safe anastamoses of grafts. Cardiopulmonary bypass has been found to be a major determinant of perioperative morbidity(153,154) and costs, partly through prolonged stay(155). The availability of cardiac stabilizers has allowed the reintroduction of cardiopulmonary bypass (off-pump)(156). It was hoped that off-pump bypass surgery may reduce perioperative morbidity and costs related to surgery, but it is not clear whether the outcome is similar to that involving the use of cardiopulmonary bypass (on-pump). One study(157) compared on-pump and off-pump coronary bypass surgery in low-risk patients and found no difference in cardiac outcome at 1 year. In this study of 282 patients with predominantly single- or double-vessel disease, 17% of patients in the on-pump group and 9% in the off-pump group were diabetic and so it is difficult to draw conclusions about the value of off-pump surgery in diabetic patients generally. An analysis of all randomized trials comparing on-pump and off-pump concluded that there was no evidence that off-pump reduced mortality, MI, repeat revascularization, or even stroke. However, there was convincing evidence that atrial fibrillation is reduced if off-pump surgery is used(158). In diabetic patients undergoing off-pump bypass surgery comparative operative mortality and perioperative MI rates have been demonstrated versus non-diabetic patients although an increased rate of renal insufficiency and infections were seen. Outcome was worse than in non-diabetic patients which is consistent with on-pump surgery and may similarly be due to more preoperative comorbidities and a lower use of multiple internal thoracic artery grafts(136). It has been shown that in diabetic patients undergoing off-pump bypass harvesting bilateral internal thoracic arteries (BITA) is a risk factor for wound infection(159).

Total arterial revascularization

The use of LIMA grafts has been clearly demonstrated to be beneficial in terms of cardiac event-free survival and long-term patency rates compared to saphenous vein grafts (SVG) in patients in general(160–163) and in diabetic patients(38). This has led to an interest in arterial coronary revascularization techniques generally.

The very early experience of radial artery grafting was disappointing(164) but interest has renewed after the experience of Acar *et al.*(165). Results since have been encouraging with several groups reporting short-term and mid-term clinical and angiographic results(166–169). However, while the use of a right internal mammary artery (RIMA), when used in addition to a LIMA, has been shown to reduce the risk of death, re-operation, and PCI when compared to single LIMA strategy(170–172), use of this technique is limited because of increased operative time, potentially increased morbidity rate, and technical difficulty of the operation with contradictory reports with respect to survival outcomes(173,174). A meta-analysis of bilateral versus single internal thoracic artery (SITA) graft survival, together with the two largest series in this field, show that a reduction in mortality of about 20% is achieved using this technique(171,172,175). The most recent data are from 1152 propensity matched patients from the Cleveland Clinic followed for a mean of 16.5 years with 50 patients followed for more than 20 years. The survival of BITA (bilateral internal thoracic artery) versus SITA (single internal thoracic artery) increased progressively over these 20 years. Subset analysis suggested that this difference persisted in several high-risk subgroups although no specific information has been reported in diabetic patients. The 3000 patient Arterial Revascularisation Trial (ART) randomizes patients to BITA and SITA and the endpoints are a 5% reduction in mortality from 25% to 20%, a 90% power, and a 5% alpha. This trial is ongoing and will follow patients for 5–10 years.

One study, which compared radial to RIMA when used as a second graft, showed that early and mid-term results are better with the radial rather than the RIMA assuming that the first graft is the LIMA(176). However, it is difficult to draw conclusions in patients with diabetes as only 6.3% of the 336 in the RIMA arm and 18.2% of the 325 radials had diabetes.

Buxton and colleagues compared radial artery revascularization to both RIMA and SVG over a 10-year period(177). Two groups were studied. Patients under 70 years underwent radial versus RIMA grafting and those over 70 years underwent radial versus saphenous vein grafting. In this study these grafts were anastamosed to the largest conduit remaining once the LIMA had been used. There was no evidence that the radial artery was associated with increased vessel patency or a decreased event rate. Another randomized comparison of radial artery and saphenous vein grafting showed at 1 year that the number of occlusions in the radial artery group was 8.2% and 13.6% which resulted in the authors concluding that the radial artery graft was superior. However 7% of the radial artery patients and 0.9% of the saphenous graft patients had a string sign which demonstrates internal functional occlusion. If this was added to the occlusion rate then the results were nearly identical(178). There are several studies ongoing in this area which may further answer this question including the RAPS (Radial Artery Patency Study) (179).

The current consensus is that the use of BITA is the preferred mode of revascularization and the addition of free arterial grafts to LIMAs is likely to be inferior to a second internal thoracic artery. Furthermore free arterial grafts have not been proven yet to be superior to SVGs.

In patients with diabetes caution should be exercised because it is recognized that SITA and BITA increase the likelihood of sternal wound infection(180,181). Many surgeons have hesitated to adopt the use of BITA routinely because of this perception of sternal wound infection, particularly in patients with diabetes.

Stents

Several studies have shown by multivariate analysis that diabetes is an independent risk factor for restenosis after balloon angioplasty, with a reported restenosis rate ranging from 35–71% in the pre drug-eluting stent era[86,87].

The STRESS (Stent Restenosis Study) and Benestent (BElgian NEtherlands STENT) trials demonstrated that in selected patients coronary stents reduce the risk of restenosis and subsequent clinical events[138,139] a reduction most marked in diabetic patients[136]. In one study in diabetic patients, coronary stenting was associated with a better 6-month angiographic outcome and 4-year clinical event rate compared to balloon angioplasty alone[94,136]. In the balloon group, the restenosis rate was almost twice as high in those patients with diabetes than those without (63% vs. 36%, $p = 0.0002$) due to the effects of both higher rates of late loss (0.79 vs. 0.41 mm, respectively, $p < 0.0001$) and a higher rate of late vessel occlusion (14% vs. 3% respectively, $p < 0.001$). In the stent group, however, diabetic and non-diabetic patients had similar restenosis rates (25% vs. 27% respectively) and late vessel occlusion rates (2% vs. 1% respectively). The balloon angioplasty patients experienced a significant reduction in ejection fraction at 6 months (2.4 ± 10.9%, $p < 0.02$), while, during the same period, no change was observed in the stent group. At 4 years, a significant reduction in the combined clinical endpoint of cardiac death and non-fatal MI was observed in the stent group (14.8% vs. 26.0%; $p < 0.02$), attributed to a lower rate of occlusive restenosis and preservation of LV function in the stent group. The requirement for repeat revascularization was 52.1% vs. 35.4% ($p < 0.001$) in the balloon and stent group respectively. Another study demonstrated that, even though restenosis rates have improved with stenting, diabetic patients still had a less favourable clinical outcome at 1 year compared to non-diabetic patients[95]. MI-free survival was significantly reduced in the diabetic group (89.9% vs. 94.4%; $p < 0.001$) and the incidence of both restenosis (37.5% vs. 28.3%; $p < 0.001$) and stent vessel occlusion (5.3% vs. 3.4%; $p = 0.037$) was still higher in diabetic patients.

The heterogeneity of diabetes was demonstrated by Abizaid and colleagues who investigated the clinical outcome following coronary stent implantation in insulin-requiring (IR) diabetic patients, non-insulin requiring (non-IR) diabetic patients, and non-diabetic patients[137].Patients with IR were at a significantly higher risk for subsequent target lesion revascularization (TLR) (28%) compared with non-IR patients (18%) and non-diabetic patients (16%), ($p < 0.05$). Late cardiac event-free survival was significantly lower ($p = 0.0004$) in IR patients (60%) compared with non-IR patients (70%) and non-diabetic patients (76%). Multivariate analysis showed that insulin requirement in diabetes was an independent predictor for 1 year MACE (OR 2.05; $p = 0.0002$).

Small reference vessel diameter is also of importance in patients with diabetes resulting in a rate of in-stent restenosis ranging from 40–70%[182,183]. In the series of Süselbeck *et al.*[182] a comparison of diabetic and non-diabetic patients according to vessel size revealed double the rate of in-stent restenosis in small vessels <3mm (44% vs. 23%, $p = 0.002$), whereas in vessels >3.0 mm the rate of in-stent restenosis was not significantly different between the two groups (18% vs. 15%). Lau *et al.*[183] found comparable results in a smaller group of 197 diabetic patients, demonstrating that diabetes and the diameter of the stent were strong predictors for the occurrence of in-stent restenosis. In this study, diabetic patients with stents <2.7 mm had the highest rate of in-stent restenosis (71%), whereas in non-diabetic patients the incidence of in-stent restenosis was only 24% ($p = 0.0028$). In stents >2.7 mm the difference was smaller (31% vs. 23%, $p = 0.006$). Therefore, both studies confirmed diabetes as a risk factor for the occurrence of in-stent restenosis in small vessels.

Antiplatelet therapy

Pharmacological interventions, such as GP IIb/IIIa inhibitors and clopidogrel, improve the outcomes of PCI[145,184,185]. Several trials have shown that abciximab and other GP IIb/IIIa inhibitors improve acute outcome and that this benefit may be sustained in the long term[140,142,186]. In particular, the combination of stents and GP IIb/IIIa inhibitors appears to be most effective[184].

The role of adjunctive peri-procedural pharmacotherapy has been examined in several randomized trials, including the EPIC[142,184,187], EPILOG, and EPISTENT trials, which all used a GP IIb/IIIa inhibitor, abciximab, as adjunctive therapy in PCI. Kleiman and colleagues compared the outcomes of 638 diabetic patients enrolled in the EPILOG trial to non-diabetic patients[187]. Diabetic patients had more baseline comorbid conditions. During hospitalization, a composite of death, MI, or urgent revascularization occurred in 7.1% of diabetic and 7.5% of non-diabetic patients. At 6 months, the composite of death or MI was 8.8% for diabetic and 7.4% for non-diabetic patients. Abciximab treatment significantly reduced the composite endpoint of death or MI among both diabetic and non-diabetic patients (HR 0.28 and 0.47 at 30 days, and 0.36 and 0.60 at 6 months for diabetics and non-diabetic patients respectively).

In the more recent EPISTENT study, the composite of death, MI, or TVR at 6 months was reduced by 48% (25% vs. 13%, p = 0.005) in 491 patients with diabetes treated with abciximab and stenting versus stenting alone[(68)]. Abciximab, regardless of whether patients underwent balloon or stent angioplasty, resulted in a significant decrease in the 6-month death or MI rate: 12.7% for stent-placebo, 7.8% for balloon angioplasty-abciximab, and 6.2% for the stent-abciximab group (p = 0.029). A pooled analysis of three abciximab trials (EPIC, EPILOG, and EPISTENT) also showed that abciximab decreased the 1-year mortality in patients with diabetes from 4.5% to 2.5% (p = 0.031) and in non-diabetic patients from 2.6% to 1.9% (p = 0.1)[(71)].

In the only head-to-head comparison of GP IIb/IIIa antagonists, the TARGET trial (Do Tirofiban and ReoPro Give similar Efficacy Trial) randomized 5308 patients to tirofiban or abciximab before PCI with the intent to perform stenting[(188,189)]. Abciximab was superior to tirofiban at reducing the 30-day primary endpoint of composite death, MI, or TVR (6.0% vs. 7.6%; p = 0.038). Both tirofiban and abciximab offered similar protection against death, MI, or TVR at 6 months (14.8% vs. 14.3%, p = NS). Among diabetic patients randomized to tirofiban (n = 560) and abciximab (n = 557), the incidence of death, MI, or TVR at 30 days was 6.2% vs. 5.4% respectively (p = 0.54). Both tirofiban and abciximab were associated with comparable event rates, including similar rates of 6-month TVR (9.5% vs. 11.1%, p = 0.366) and 1-year mortality (2.1% vs. 2.9%, p=0.436). The results of the ESPRIT (Enhanced Suppression of the Platelet IIb/IIIa Receptor with Integrilin Therapy) trial revealed that eptifibatide reduced death, MI, and urgent TVR at 2 days and 30 days in patients undergoing coronary stenting[(140)]. The 1-year results showed a significant reduction in MI and a non-significant reduction in death with a similar benefit in reducing cumulative events in diabetic and non-diabetic patients treated with eptifibatide[(190)].

In the management of ACS, a meta-analysis of the diabetic populations (n = 6458) enrolled in six trials looked at GP IIb/IIIa inhibitor use. It detected a 26% mortality reduction (from 6.2% to 4.6%; p = 0.007) associated with GP IIb/IIIa inhibitor use at 30 days when compared with placebo[(70)]. These findings were reinforced by a statistically significant interaction between treatment and diabetic status. The benefit among patients with diabetes undergoing PCI, corresponding to a 70% 30-day mortality reduction (from 4.0% to 1.2%, p = 0.002).

In summary, the combined use of GP IIb/IIIa inhibitors and stents in diabetic patients, at least with abciximab and tirofiban, appears to reduce the level of risk that diabetic patients undergoing PCI have to that of non-diabetic patients. Whether the results achievable with this regimen are comparable to those achieved with modern coronary artery bypass grafting can only be answered by prospective randomized trials. Two such trials have been designed to look at this question. CARDia reported its primary endpoint recently[(191)] and FREEDOM is ongoing.

The advent of the thienopyridine, clopidogrel, resulted in improved outcomes for patients following both acute coronary syndromes and PCI although patients continued to have atherothrombotic events despite dual antiplatelet therapy following PCI[(192,193)]. Subset analysis did not suggest additional benefit with clopidogrel in diabetic patients over and above that achieved in non-diabetic patients. CURE (Clopidogrel in Unstable Angina to Prevent Recurrent Events) demonstrated that the point estimate of benefit for the diabetic subgroup with clopidogrel was only 15% compared with 20% overall[(192)].

In patients being treated for stable coronary disease a subset analysis undertaken in the CAPRIE trial[(194,195)] suggested that most of the benefit demonstrated in this study was because of the benefit in patients with diabetes. As a result the National Institute for Health and Clinical Excellence (NICE) considered whether clopidogrel should be recommended in addition to aspirin in all patients with diabetes and coronary disease but rejected this. Data from ISAR Sweet (Intracoronary Stenting and Antithrombotic Regimen: Is Abciximab a Superior Way to Eliminate Elevated Thrombotic Risk in Diabetics) suggested that the use of clopidogrel might negate the need for GPIIb/IIIa inhibitors during PCI in patients with diabetes in some circumstances, especially in those patients undergoing elective and relatively low-risk procedures[(196)].

There are limitations to such therapy with marked interpatient variability[(197)] and delayed onset of action[(185)]. In the Optimising Antiplatelet Therapy in Diabetes Mellitus (OPTIMUS) trial it was demonstrated that two-thirds of the patients with stable coronary artery disease were hyporesponders to a standard dose of aspirin and clopidogrel[(198)]. When the hyporesponders were assigned to continue on standard dose clopidogrel or 150mg clopidogrel, a significant reduction in maximal platelet aggregation after ADP stimuli was seen with the higher dose of clopidogrel. The dose related clopidogrel effects are currently in the process of being replicated with outcomes in clinical trials.

Diabetes is a proinflammatory and prothrombotic state[199] and associated with increased oxidative stress and impaired endothelial function. In the insulin resistant state an upregulation of platelet membrane proteins including the $P2Y_{12}$ receptor pathway occurs[200]. Hence insulin treatment may identify a subset of individuals particularly likely to have a poor response to antiplatelet agents.

Prasugrel, a relatively new agent, is a thienopyridine pro-drug which like clopidogrel requires conversion to an active metabolite in the liver before binding to the platelet $P2Y_{12}$ receptor resulting in an antiplatelet effect. A 60-mg loading dose, followed by maintenance dosing with 10mg has demonstrated a more rapid, more consistent, and greater adenosine diphosphate-induced platelet inhibition than either standard or higher doses of clopidogrel in healthy volunteers[201], coronary artery disease[202,203], and following elective PCI[204].

TRITON-TIMI 38 (Trial to Assess Improvement in Therapeutic Outcomes by Optimizing Platelet Inhibition with Prasugrel-Thrombolysis In Myocardial Infarction) demonstrated that prasugrel (n = 6813) was associated with lower rates of ischaemic events in patients with acute coronary syndromes than occurred with conventional dual antiplatelet (n = 6795) therapy[205]. There was a significant reduction in the prasugrel group for MI (9.7% for clopidogrel vs. 7.4% for prasugrel, p <0.001), urgent TVR (3.7% vs. 2.5%, p <0.001), and stent thrombosis (2.4% vs 1.1%, p <0.001). However, this greater antiplatelet effect came at a price, with an increased risk of major bleeding with prasugrel (1.8% vs. 2.4%, p = 0.03), a significantly higher rate of life-threatening bleeding (0.9% vs. 1.4%, p = 0.01), and fatal bleeding (0.1% vs. 0.4%, p = 0.002).

The results for the diabetes mellitus subset of TRITON-TIMI 38 have been reported recently[206]. This involved 3146 patients of whom 776 were receiving insulin. The primary endpoint was a composite of cardiovascular death, non-fatal MI, non-fatal CVA, and was reduced significantly among subjects on prasugrel without diabetes (9.2% vs. 10.6%; HR = 0.86; p = 0.02), and with diabetes (12.2% vs. 17%; HR = 0.70; p <0.001). A benefit for prasugrel was observed among diabetic patients on insulin (14.3% vs. 22%; HR = 0.63; p = 0.009) and diabetic patients not on insulin (11.5% vs. 15.3%; HR = 0.74; p = 0.009). MI was reduced with prasugrel by 18% among patients without diabetes mellitus (7.2% vs. 8.7%; HR = 0.82; p = 0.006) and by 40% in those with diabetes (8.2% vs. 13.2%; HR = 0.6; p <0.001). Whilst TIMI (Thrombolysis In Myocardial Infarction) major haemorrhage was increased among subjects without diabetes on prasugrel (1.6% vs 2.4%, HR = 1.43, p = 0.02), rates were similar for patients with diabetes for clopidogrel and prasugrel (2.6% vs 2.5%; HR = 1.06; p = 0.81). Net clinical benefit with prasugrel was greater for patients with diabetes (14.6% vs. 19.2%; HR = 0.74; p = 0.001) than for those without diabetes (11.5% vs. 12.3%; HR 0.92; p = 0.16).

The findings from this study validate the concept that for diabetic patients, the degree of platelet inhibition may be an important marker of outcome. An absolute reduction in ischaemic events of approximately 8% was achieved in those diabetic patients treated with insulin, which would suggest that prasugrel has durable action across the whole spectrum of diabetes mellitus. The difference in ischaemic events was driven by a marked reduction in MI. Whilst the diabetic subgroup did experience a higher rate of TIMI major bleeding (2.6% vs. 2.0%) than the non-diabetic cohort, no difference was demonstrated in excess bleeding between the clopidogrel and prasugrel groups[199]. This has identified clearly that diabetic patients have a greater clinical benefit from a more intensive antiplatelet regimen. Further studies with larger cohorts of diabetic patients will be necessary to further assess the bleeding risk. Variability of response among diabetic patients will need to be assessed as will the role of GP IIb/IIIa inhibitors. Over 50% of the patients in this study also received these agents and it is possible that a better safety profile might have been identified without their routine use. The effectiveness of antiplatelet therapy may also be influenced by the extent of chronic glycaemic control and this will need to be studied further.

Drug-eluting stents

A major limitation of PCI has always been in-stent restenosis and a subsequent requirement for further revascularization procedures, reducing the overall impact of its initial success as a treatment strategy, when compared with CABG. That restenosis may become a thing of the past was first intimated by the RAVEL (Randomised Study with the Sirolimus-Coated Bx Velocity Balloon-Expandable Stent in the Treatment of Patients with de Novo Native Coronary Artery Lesions) trial suggesting that the use of sirolimus-coated stents during PCI can reduce or even prevent restenosis[207].

Data from the multicentre, randomized, double-blind SIRIUS (SIRolImUS-coated Bx Velocity stent in the treatment of patients with de novo coronary artery lesions) study were subsequently published[208]. The inclusion criteria were more liberal than RAVEL and allowed multi-lesion stenting, which occurred in a quarter of patients. The primary endpoint was target vessel failure, which included cardiac death, MI, or TVR at 9 months' follow-up. After 9 months, 8.6% of the patients receiving the Cypher (sirolimus-eluting) stent reached the primary endpoint of target vessel failure, compared with 21.0% in the control group. In the Cypher® group, in-stent restenosis was 2.0%, and in-lesion restenosis was 9.1%, these results confirming the potent anti-restenotic effects of Cypher® stents. In the diabetic subset, which comprised 279 out of 1058 patients 12.2% of the patients receiving the Cypher® stent reached the primary endpoint, compared to 27.1% in the control group, demonstrating a comparable benefit for diabetic patients also. Thus the relative reduction in recurrent events seen with sirolimus versus control remained constant but the absolute values for restenosis, TLR, and other indices were higher in both groups for diabetic patients and diabetes remained an independent predictor for restenosis and TLR.

These results were replicated in the TAXUS IV study. The TLR rate at 1 year was reduced from 15.1% in the control group to 4.4% ($p < 0.001$) in the Taxus® group in the study as a whole[209], and from 20.9% to 7.4% ($p = 0.0008$) in the patients with diabetes. This suggested that the benefit was as great with IR diabetic patients as with non-insulin dependent diabetics, a benefit not demonstrated in the SIRIUS trial, although in both studies the numbers in the subset of insulin-treated patients is very small so it is difficult to draw firm conclusions[28].

It is now apparent that DES represent a major advance for the prevention of restenosis and repeat revascularization after PCI in diabetic patients[27,28,208,210]. However, as in the SIRIUS study[27], diabetes was an independent predictor of TLR (OR 1.54; 95% CI 1.04–2.27) in the paclitaxel-eluting TAXUS IV stud[28]. As patients with diabetes were not prespecified for sub-analysis in either of these studies, the true value of DES in diabetic patients was initially questioned[211]. The comparison with thick strut BMS used in the control group of these trials may have increased the differential restenosis rate resulting in a relatively high BMS TLR rate thus enhancing the apparent anti-restenotic effects of DES. The use of angiographic follow-up in these studies can positively influence TLR, which might be higher than in studies with clinical follow-up only. This potential for bias might be particularly relevant for diabetic patients in whom restenosis might not be apparent, owing to silent ischaemia.

The 160 patient DIABETES (Diabetes and Sirolimus-Eluting Stent) trial specifically assessed the effects in diabetes of a sirolimus-eluting stent (SES) [210] randomized versus a bare-metal stent (BMS). The primary endpoint of the trial was in segment late lumen loss as assessed by quantitative coronary angiography at 9-month follow up. In segment late lumen loss was reduced from 0.47 ± 0.5 mm for standard stents to 0.06 ± 0.4 mm for sirolimus stents ($p < 0.001$). TLR and MACE were significantly lower in the sirolimus group (31.3% vs. 7.3% and 36.3% vs. 11.3%, respectively; both $p < 0.001$). Non-insulin and insulin requiring patients demonstrated similar reductions in angiographic and clinical parameters of restenosis after sirolimus eluting stent implantation. In the SIRTAX (SIRolimus- versus pacliTAXel-eluting stents) trial[210], the HR for major cardiovascular or cerebrovascular event rate (MACCE) was less in SES-treated patients compared with in paclitaxel eluting stents (PES)-treated patients and this difference was more pronounced in diabetes. In the ISAR (In-Stent Angiographic Restenosis)-DIABETES trial[213], in-segment restenosis was identified on follow-up angiography in 16.5 % of the patients in the PES group and 6.9 % of the patients in the SES group ($p = 0.03$). TLR was performed in 12.0 % of the patients in the PES group and 6.4 % of the patients in the SES group ($p = 0.13$). PCI with SES resulted in less in-segment restenosis in insulin treated ($p = 0.02$) and non-insulin treated ($p = 0.03$) diabetic patients.

In the last 2 years there have been concerns that first generation stents (Cypher® and Taxus®) increased the occurrence of major adverse events including death and MI.[214] This was because DES were felt to have a higher rate of stent thrombosis (including late stent thrombosis) than BMS, (which is a major cause of short-term mortality)[215]. Of particular concern were the results of a pooled analysis of four randomized trials which showed that although when comparing SES with BMS there was no overall increase in mortality with DES, in the diabetic subset there was a significant increase in mortality with DES[215]. A pooled analysis specifically in patients with diabetes of five trials of PES versus BMS trials showed no difference[217]. A recent meta-analysis appears to have clarified this issue further[218]. In patients with diabetes who receive dual antiplatelet therapy, i.e. aspirin and clopidogrel for less than 6 months, there is an increased mortality associated with DES. However, if they receive longer-term dual antiplatelet therapy, i.e. at least 6 months, there is no associated increased mortality. It is interesting to note that the only trials where dual antiplatelet therapy was given for less than 6 months were those involving SES.

Interventional trials in the DES era

ARTS 2

The Arterial Revascularisation Therapies Study 2 was a 45-centre single-arm study which used Cypher® stents for the revascularization of patients with multi-vessel disease[219]. Outcomes are now at 3 years and have been compared to the original ARTS study which randomized PCI with BMS and CABG. The inclusion and exclusion criteria were the same and they used the same definitions for MACCE. Patients were stratified by centre so that at least one-third of patients had three-vessel disease in order to achieve the same number of lesions as in ARTS 1. Stent thrombosis was readjudicated using the Academic Research Consortium (ARC) definitions[220]. In fact in ARTS 2, 46.6% of patients had three-vessel treatment as opposed to 18% in the PCI arm of ARTS 1. In ARTS 2, diabetes was present in 26.2% of patients as opposed to 17.3% in ARTS 1. In ARTS 2, 3.7 stents per patient were implanted resulting in a mean stent length of 72.5mm as opposed to 2.8 and 47.6mm in ARTS 1. The 3-year survival rate was 97.0% in ARTS 2 comparable to the 95.6% and 96.0% survival rates of the historical surgical and PCI cohorts from ARTS 1. The death/MI/CVA survival rate in ARTS 2 was 91.7% versus 89.1% ($p = 0.1$) and 87.2% ($p = 0.007$) in ARTS 1 surgical and PCI cohorts, respectively. Revascularization rates were 14.5% in ARTS 2, which is lower than ARTS 1 CABG 6.6% ($p < 0.001$) but higher than ARTS 1 PCI 26.3% ($p < 0.001$)[221]. At 3 years, in the diabetes subset the death rates were 5.0% in ARTS 2, 5.2% in the ARTS 1 CABG group, and 7.1% in the ARTS 1 PCI group, stroke rates were 2.5%, 5.2%, and 4.5% respectively, repeat revascularization was 18.3%, 4.2%, and 28.6%[222]. What is of particular note is that repeat revascularization rates have been progressively decreasing through the various eras with PCI, from the days of balloon angioplasty in BARI to stenting in ARTS and now DES use in ARTS 2 including in patients with diabetes.

CARDia

Adjunctive antiplatelet therapies, as described earlier, have improved outcome and reduced the need for early reintervention following PCI in diabetic patients. The rate of restenosis after an initial PCI has also been reduced following the advent of DES. The current wave of interventional studies comparing CABG and PCI involve comparisons addressing this question and employ these adjunctive therapies in the PCI arms.

In the United Kingdom, the CARDia Trial[191] reported its 1-year primary endpoint results at the European Society of Cardiology in 2008. It is an investigator-initiated study and is the first prospective study designed specifically to address the hypothesis that optimal PCI with stenting and abciximab is not inferior to up-to-date CABG as a revascularization strategy for diabetic patients with multi-vessel or complex single-vessel coronary disease. The primary outcome was a composite of death, MI, or stroke, and the study had a non-inferiority design. Between 2002–2007, 24 centres in the United Kingdom and Ireland randomized 510 diabetic patients with multi-vessel or complex single-vessel coronary disease to PCI plus stenting (and routine abciximab) versus CABG. BMS were used initially but a switch to Cypher® (sirolimus-drug eluting) stents was made when these became available.

At 1 year, the composite rate of death, MI, and stroke was 10.5% in the CABG group vs. 13.0%, in the PCI group (HR 1.25; 95% CI 0.75–2.09; $p = 0.39$). The non-inferiority margin was not met. All-cause mortality was 3.2% versus 3.2%, and rates of repeat revascularization 2.0% versus 11.8%, ($p < 0.001$) in the CABG and PCI groups respectively. When the subset of patients who received DES (69% of patients) was compared to those receiving CABG the composite outcome of death, MI, and stroke was 12.4% vs. 11.6% respectively.

FREEDOM

The FREEDOM (Future Revascularisation Evaluation in Patients with Diabetes Mellitus: Optimal Management of Multivessel Disease) study[223] in the United States started after CARDia and at the time of writing is 50% recruited. It is a larger head-to-head study comparing surgery with DES in patients with diabetes although use of a GPIIb/IIIa inhibitor is not mandatory in the PCI arm.

BARI 2D

The 1800-patient BARI 2D is a 2×2 comparison of firstly revascularization by either strategy versus aggressive medical therapy for coronary disease, and secondly of an insulin-providing regimen versus an insulin-sensitizing regimen. The SYNTAX score developed as a result of this trial has been a useful aid to assessing which revascularization patients should receive. In general terms it has been concluded that patients in the low risk or intermediate tercile can have PCI or CABG (SYNTAX score <33) and those in the high risk tercile should have CABG (SYNTAX score > or = 33) whether they have diabetes or not.

SYNTAX

The 1800-patient SYNTAX (Synergy between Percutaneous Coronary Intervention with TAXUS and Cardiac Surgery) trial, although not specifically in patients with diabetes (diabetic subset n = 452), is a non-inferiority randomized controlled trial which compares CABG with PCI in patients with three-vessel and/or left main stem disease and reported its main primary endpoint results at the ESC in the same session as CARDia. This trial was an 'all comers' design in which patients had to be deemed suitable for either PCI or CABG by consensus between an interventional cardiologist and a cardiac surgeon. If considered suitable only for one mode of intervention then they were allocated to either the PCI or CABG registry within the trial as appropriate. The primary endpoint was the MACCE at 1 year defined as all cause death, CVA, documented MI (using the ARC definition[220]), or any repeat revascularization. There was no significant difference at 1 year in all-cause death (3.5% in the CABG arm versus 4.3% in the PCI arm, $p = 0.37$) or MI (4.8% vs 3.2%, $p = 0.11$). There was a significantly higher rate of stroke with CABG at 1 year (2.2% vs 0.6%, $p = 0.003$). The rate of repeat revascularization was significantly higher with PCI at 1 year (5.9% vs 13.7%, $p <0.0001$). Finally the rate of MACCE at 1 year was significantly lower with CABG (12.1% vs 17.8%, $p = 0.0015$). In the diabetes subgroup there was no significant difference in all-cause death, MI, or CVA between CABG and PCI at 1 year (10.3% vs 10.1%, $p = 0.9558$)[224]. This showed that there was no significant difference in the rates of death and major cardiovascular events between those undergoing revascularization and those undergoing medical therapy or between strategies of insulin sensitization and insulin provision. This was a study of low risk patients, many of whom had single vessel disease. It is already known that such low risk patients have less prognostic benefit from revascularization. There was no stratification between PCI and CABG. Those who were assigned to receive CABG had more coronary disease and were therefore higher risk. This explains why there was prognostic benefit in this group for revascularization and why in the lower risk PCI patients this was not observed [119]. It should be noted that the non-inferiority parameters for the trial as a whole were not met.

Practical considerations

Percutaneous revascularization of patients with diabetes presents a number of unique challenges. These are anatomical (smaller vessels, more extensive and diffuse disease) on both a macro and microvascular level, metabolic (endothelial dysfunction, platelets increased in size, number, adhesiveness, and activation), and in the coagulation pathways. The average restenosis rate in a diabetic patient in the BMS era was 58%[91], furthermore occlusive restenosis was recognized as being a particular problem in these patients[92]. From the literature it is apparent that there is underuse of both pharmacotherapy and revascularization in these patients post AMI[225].

In order to optimize outcome following PCI it is important that these patients receive pre-procedure aspirin and clopidogrel[192]. A GP IIb IIIa inhibitor (preferably abciximab) should be considered in all complex or ACS cases[71]. The operator should have a lower threshold for consideration of pre-procedure hydration and renal protection than in non-diabetic patients[226–228]. Careful choice of guide catheter due to the higher potential for tortuous coronary anatomy is recommended. Pre-dilatation of lesions should be considered as tortuous anatomy, diffuse disease, and calcified lesions may make optimization of stent deployment more difficult in diabetic patients, all the more important given the potential increased risk of stent thrombosis. Preparation of lesions can be aided by rotational atherectomy in calcified lesions.

To enhance the outcomes following revascularization in general the following targets, which have been shown to be cost-effective, should be aimed for (HbA1c <7%, LDL <2.0 and BP <130/80)[229]. Strict blood glucose control with intensive insulin therapy improves mortality and morbidity of adult critically ill patients as well as of adult cardiac surgery patients. These guidelines also recommend screening for impaired glucose tolerance and diabetes mellitus in all patients with established cardiovascular disease by means of an oral glucose tolerance test. Lifestyle counselling (including regular exercise, smoking cessation, and weight loss) is the cornerstone of prevention of cardiovascular complications. Patients with diabetes mellitus should be offered early angiography and mechanical revascularization—either PCI or surgery. Where PCI is the mode of revascularization, DES should be used. Tailored risk assessment of patients with diabetes should be performed including investigation of autonomic dysfunction, heart failure, arrhythmias, hypotension, and peripheral vascular disease. The joint approach of cardiologists and diabetologists is essential for the sake of the millions of patients with diabetes, pre-diabetes, and cardiovascular disease, and in light of this, the first time joint effort of the European Association for the Study of Diabetes (EASD) and the European Society of Cardiology (ESC) is highly appropriate[229].

Conclusion

Revascularization in patients with diabetes and multi-vessel disease has traditionally been a high-risk area. Although it has long been thought that surgery is superior to angioplasty in these patients, this has been based on limited data. Despite the data from BARI and other studies large numbers of patients with diabetes and multi-vessel disease are receiving PCI. In the United Kingdom in 2007 an estimated 3800 patients with diabetes and multi-vessel disease underwent PCI (*British Cardiovascular Intervention Society-Central Cardiac Audit Database BCIS-CCAD, with analysis by Peter Ludman on behalf of BCIS*) indicating the importance of the data available for this complex group. Arguably, the gap between PCI and CABG has narrowed. This is certainly true for the rates of repeat revascularization, although this is still significantly higher with PCI. Conversely CABG remains a more traumatic procedure for patients requiring longer rehabilitation. There is a higher rate of stroke with surgery. It is also true that PCI has improved dramatically relative to CABG since the days of the BARI trial due to the advent of BMS, antiplatelet therapy, and DES. In terms of the composite of the 'hard' endpoints of death, non-fatal MI, and non-fatal CVA, the gap between PCI and CABG has been narrowed. However, the story of revascularization in diabetic patients is not over yet. Advances in both forms of revascularization, including robotic and minimally invasive surgery, as well as biodegradable stents and more effective adjunctive therapy, such as prasugrel, for PCI can only be good news for these high-risk patients.

References

1. Harris MI, Flegal KM, Cowie CC, *et al.* Prevalence of diabetes, impaired fasting glucose, and impaired glucose tolerance in U.S. adults. The Third National Health and Nutrition Examination Survey, 1988–1994. *Diabetes Care* 1998; **21**(4):518–24.
2. Kenny SJ, Aubert RE, Geiss LS. Prevalence and incidence of insulin-dependent diabetes. In Harris MI, Cowie CC (eds) *Diabetes in America*, 2nd edn, pp. 47–68 . Bethseda: National Diabetes Data Group, National Institute of Health, 1995.
3. King H, Aubert RE, Herman WH. Global burden of diabetes, 1995–2025: prevalence, numerical estimates, and projections. *Diabetes Care* 1998; **21**(9):1414–31.
4. Harris MI, Hadden WC, Knowler WC, *et al* Prevalence of diabetes and impaired glucose tolerance and plasma glucose levels in U.S. population aged 20–74 yr. *Diabetes* 1987; **36**(4):523–34.
5. Saydah SH, Loria CM, Eberhardt MS, *et al.* Subclinical states of glucose intolerance and risk of death in the U.S. *Diabetes Care* 2001; **24**(3):447–53.
6. Taubert G, Winkelmann BR, Schleiffer T, *et al.* Prevalence, predictors, and consequences of unrecognized diabetes mellitus in 3266 patients scheduled for coronary angiography. *Am Heart J* 2003; **145**(2):285–91.
7. Ford ES, Giles WH, Dietz WH. Prevalence of the metabolic syndrome among US adults: findings from the third National Health and Nutrition Examination Survey. *JAMA* 2002; **287**(3):356–9.
8. Popkin BM, Horton S, Kim S, *et al.* Trends in diet, nutritional status, and diet-related noncommunicable diseases in China and India: the economic costs of the nutrition transition. *Nutr Rev* 2001; **59**(12):379–90.
9. Role of cardiovascular risk factors in prevention and treatment of macrovascular disease in diabetes. American Diabetes Association. *Diabetes Care* 1989; **12**(8):573–9.
10. Kannel WB, McGee DL. Diabetes and cardiovascular disease. The Framingham study. *JAMA* 1979; **241**(19):2035–8.
11. Wingard DL, Barrett-Connor E. Heart disease and diabetes. In Harris MI, Cowie CC (eds) *Diabetes in America*, 2nd edn, pp. 429–48. Bethseda: National Diabetes Data Group, National Institute of Health, 1995.
12. Geiss LS, Herman WH, Smith PJ. Mortality in non-insulin-dependent diabetes. In Harris MI, Cowie CC (eds) *Diabetes in America*, 2nd edn, pp. 233–59. Bethseda: National Diabetes Data Group, National Institute of Health, 1995.
13. Stamler J, Vaccaro O, Neaton JD, *et al.* Diabetes, other risk factors, and 12-yr cardiovascular mortality for men screened in the Multiple Risk Factor Intervention Trial. *Diabetes Care* 1993; **16**(2):434–44.
14. McKinlay J, Marceau L. US public health and the 21st century: diabetes mellitus. *Lancet* 2000; **356**(9231):757–61.
15. Gu K, Cowie CC, Harris MI. Diabetes and decline in heart disease mortality in US adults. *JAMA* 1999; **281**(14):1291–7.
16. Norhammar A, Lindback J, Ryden L, *et al.* Improved but still high short- and long-term mortality rates after myocardial infarction in patients with diabetes mellitus: a time-trend report from the Swedish Register of Information and Knowledge about Swedish Heart Intensive Care Admission. *Heart* 2007; **93**(12):1577–83.
17. Aronson D, Rayfield EJ, Chesebro JH. Mechanisms determining course and outcome of diabetic patients who have had acute myocardial infarction. *Ann Intern Med* 1997; **126**(4):296–306.
18. McGuire DK, Emanuelsson H, Granger CB, *et al.* Influence of diabetes mellitus on clinical outcomes across the spectrum of acute coronary syndromes. Findings from the GUSTO-IIb study. GUSTO IIb Investigators. *Eur Heart J* 2000; **21**(21):1750–8.
19. Malmberg K, Yusuf S, Gerstein HC, *et al.* Impact of diabetes on long-term prognosis in patients with unstable angina and non-Q-wave myocardial infarction: results of the OASIS(Organization to Assess Strategies for Ischemic Syndromes) Registry. *Circulation* 2000; **102**(9):101–19.
20. Donahoe SM, Stewart GC, McCabe CH, *et al.* Diabetes and mortality following acute coronary syndromes. *JAMA* 2007; **298**(7):765–75.

21. Haffner SM, Lehto S, Ronnemaa T, *et al.* Mortality from coronary heart disease in subjects with type 2 diabetes and in nondiabetic subjects with and without prior myocardial infarction. *N Engl J Med* 1998; **339**(4):229–34.
22. Abbott RD, Donahue RP, Kannel WB, *et al.* The impact of diabetes on survival following myocardial infarction in men vs women. The Framingham Study. *JAMA* 1988; **260**(23):3456–60.
23. Mak KH, Moliterno DJ, Granger CB, *et al.* Influence of diabetes mellitus on clinical outcome in the thrombolytic era of acute myocardial infarction. GUSTO-I Investigators. Global Utilization of Streptokinase and Tissue Plasminogen Activator for Occluded Coronary Arteries. *J Am Coll Cardiol* 1997; **30**(1):171–9.
24. Hasdai D, Granger CB, Srivatsa SS, *et al.* Diabetes mellitus and outcome after primary coronary angioplasty for acute myocardial infarction: lessons from the GUSTO-IIb Angioplasty Substudy. Global Use of Strategies to Open Occluded Arteries in Acute Coronary Syndromes. *J Am Coll Cardiol* 2000; **35**(6):1502–12.
25. Malmberg K, Ryden L. Myocardial infarction in patients with diabetes mellitus. *Eur Heart J* 1988; **9**(3):259–64.
26. Norhammar A, Tenerz A, Nilsson G, *et al.* Glucose metabolism in patients with acute myocardial infarction and no previous diagnosis of diabetes mellitus: a prospective study. *Lancet* 2002; **359**(9324):2140–4.
27. Moussa I, Leon MB, Baim DS, *et al.* Impact of sirolimus-eluting stents on outcome in diabetic patients: a SIRIUS(SIRolImUS-coated Bx Velocity balloon-expandable stent in the treatment of patients with de novo coronary artery lesions) substudy. *Circulation* 2004; **109**(19):2273–8.
28. Hermiller JB, Raizner A, Cannon L, *et al.* Outcomes with the polymer-based paclitaxel-eluting TAXUS stent in patients with diabetes mellitus: the TAXUS-IV trial. *J Am Coll Cardiol* 2005; **45**(8):1172–9.
29. Serruys PW, Ong AT, Morice MC, *et al.* Arterial Revascularisation Therapies Study Part II:Sirolimus eluting stents for the treatment of patients with multivessel de novo coronary artery lesions. *EuroIntervention* 2005; **1**:147–56.
30. Stein B, Weintraub WS, Gebhart SP, *et al.* Influence of diabetes mellitus on early and late outcome after percutaneous transluminal coronary angioplasty. *Circulation* 1995; **91**(4):979–89.
31. Kip KE, Faxon DP, Detre KM, *et al.* Coronary angioplasty in diabetic patients. The National Heart, Lung, and Blood Institute Percutaneous Transluminal Coronary Angioplasty Registry. *Circulation* 1996; **94**(8):1818–25.
32. Alderman EL, Corley SD, Fisher LD, *et al.* Five-year angiographic follow-up of factors associated with progression of coronary artery disease in the Coronary Artery Surgery Study(CASS). CASS Participating Investigators and Staff. *J Am Coll Cardiol* 1993; **22**(4):1141–54.
33. Thourani VH, Weintraub WS, Stein B, *et al.* Influence of diabetes mellitus on early and late outcome after coronary artery bypass grafting. *Ann Thorac Surg* 1999; **67**(4):1045–52.
34. Flaherty JD, Davidson CJ. Diabetes and coronary revascularization. *JAMA* 2005; **293**(12):1501–8.
35. Abizaid A, Costa MA, Centemero M, *et al.* Clinical and economic impact of diabetes mellitus on percutaneous and surgical treatment of multivessel coronary disease patients: insights from the Arterial Revascularization Therapy Study(ARTS) trial. *Circulation* 2001; **104**(5): 533–8.
36. Marcheix B, Vanden EF, Demers P, *et al.* Influence of diabetes mellitus on long-term survival in systematic off-pump coronary artery bypass surgery. *Ann Thorac Surg* 2008; **86**(4):1181–8.
37. Nicholls SJ, Tuzcu EM, Kalidindi S, *et al.* Effect of diabetes on progression of coronary atherosclerosis and arterial remodeling: a pooled analysis of 5 intravascular ultrasound trials. *J Am Coll Cardiol* 2008; **52**(4):255–62.
38. Influence of diabetes on 5-year mortality and morbidity in a randomized trial comparing CABG and PTCA in patients with multivessel disease: the Bypass Angioplasty Revascularization Investigation (BARI). *Circulation* 1997; **96**(6):1761–9.
39. Morris JJ, Smith LR, Jones RH, *et al.* Influence of diabetes and mammary artery grafting on survival after coronary bypass. *Circulation* 1991; **84**(5 Suppl):III275–III284.
40. Moussa I Moses J, Wang X. Why do coronary vessels in diabetics appear to be angiographically small? *J Am Coll Cardiol* 1999; **33**(Suppl.1):78A.
41. Abaci A, Oguzhan A, Kahraman S, *et al.* Effect of diabetes mellitus on formation of coronary collateral vessels. *Circulation* 1999; **99**(17):2239–42.
42. Silva JA, Escobar A, Collins TJ, *et al.* Unstable angina. A comparison of angioscopic findings between diabetic and nondiabetic patients. *Circulation* 1995; **92**(7): 1731–6.
43. Claudi T, Midthjell K, Holmen J, *et al.* Cardiovascular disease and risk factors in persons with type 2 diabetes diagnosed in a large population screening: the Nord-Trondelag Diabetes Study, Norway. *J Intern Med* 2000; **248**(6):492–500.
44. Hayden JM, Reaven PD. Cardiovascular disease in diabetes mellitus type 2: a potential role for novel cardiovascular risk factors. *Curr Opin Lipidol* 2000; **11**(5):519–28.
45. Stratton IM, Adler AI, Neil HA, *et al.* Association of glycaemia with macrovascular and microvascular complications of type 2 diabetes (UKPDS 35): prospective observational study. *BMJ* 2000; **321**(7258):405–12.
46. Reaven GM, Hollenbeck C, Jeng CY, *et al.* Measurement of plasma glucose, free fatty acid, lactate, and insulin for 24 h in patients with NIDDM. *Diabetes* 1988; **37**(8): 1020–4.
47. Bierman EL. George Lyman Duff Memorial Lecture. Atherogenesis in diabetes. *Arterioscler Thromb* 1992; **12**(6):647–56.
48. Stampfer MJ, Krauss RM, Ma J, *et al.* A prospective study of triglyceride level, low-density lipoprotein particle diameter, and risk of myocardial infarction. *JAMA* 1996; **276**(11):882–8.

49. Lamarche B, Tchernof A, Moorjani S, *et al.* Small, dense low-density lipoprotein particles as a predictor of the risk of ischemic heart disease in men. Prospective results from the Quebec Cardiovascular Study. *Circulation* 1997; **95**(1):69–75.
50. Cowie CC, Harris MI. Physical and metabolic characteristics of persons with diabetes. In Harris MI, Cowie CC (eds) *Diabetes in America*, 2nd edn, pp.117–64. Bethseda: National Diabetes Data Group, National Institute of Health, 1995.
51. Williams SB, Cusco JA, Roddy MA, Johnstone MT, Creager MA. Impaired nitric oxide-mediated vasodilation in patients with non-insulin-dependent diabetes mellitus. *J Am Coll Cardiol* 1996; **27**(3):567–74.
52. McVeigh GE, Brennan GM, Johnston GD, *et al.* Impaired endothelium-dependent and independent vasodilation in patients with type 2 (non-insulin-dependent) diabetes mellitus. *Diabetologia* 1992; **35**(8):771–6.
53. Morris SJ, Shore AC, Tooke JE. Responses of the skin microcirculation to acetylcholine and sodium nitroprusside in patients with NIDDM. *Diabetologia* 1995; **38**(11):1337–44.
54. Lim SC, Caballero AE, Smakowski P, *et al.* Soluble intercellular adhesion molecule, vascular cell adhesion molecule, and impaired microvascular reactivity are early markers of vasculopathy in type 2 diabetic individuals without microalbuminuria. *Diabetes Care* 1999; **22**(11):1865–70.
55. Tomai F, Crea F, Gaspardone A, *et al.* Unstable angina and elevated c-reactive protein levels predict enhanced vasoreactivity of the culprit lesion. *Circulation* 2001; **104**(13):1471–6.
56. Pradhan AD, Manson JE, Rifai N, *et al.* C-reactive protein, interleukin 6, and risk of developing type 2 diabetes mellitus. *JAMA* 2001; **286**(3):327–34.
57. Festa A, D'Agostino R, Jr., Howard G, *et al.* Chronic subclinical inflammation as part of the insulin resistance syndrome: the Insulin Resistance Atherosclerosis Study (IRAS). *Circulation* 2000; **102**(1):42–7.
58. Fichtlscherer S, Rosenberger G, Walter DH, *et al.* Elevated C-reactive protein levels and impaired endothelial vasoreactivity in patients with coronary artery disease. *Circulation* 2000; **102**(9):1000–6.
59. Davi G, Ciabattoni G, Consoli A, *et al.* In vivo formation of 8-iso-prostaglandin f2alpha and platelet activation in diabetes mellitus: effects of improved metabolic control and vitamin E supplementation. *Circulation* 1999; **99**(2):224–9.
60. Tschoepe D, Roesen P, Kaufmann L, *et al.* Evidence for abnormal platelet glycoprotein expression in diabetes mellitus. *Eur J Clin Invest* 1990; **20**(2):166–70.
61. Aronson D, Bloomgarden Z, Rayfield EJ. Potential mechanisms promoting restenosis in diabetic patients. *J Am Coll Cardiol* 1996; **27**(3):528–35.
62. Shechter M, Merz CN, Paul-Labrador MJ, *et al.* Blood glucose and platelet-dependent thrombosis in patients with coronary artery disease. *J Am Coll Cardiol* 2000; **35**(2):300–7.
63. Vinik AI, Erbas T, Park TS, *et al.* Platelet dysfunction in type 2 diabetes. *Diabetes Care* 2001; **24**(8):1476–85.
64. Collaborative overview of randomised trials of antiplatelet therapy – I: Prevention of death, myocardial infarction, and stroke by prolonged antiplatelet therapy in various categories of patients. Antiplatelet Trialists' Collaboration. *BMJ* 1994; **308**(6921):81–106.
65. Physician's health study: aspirin and primary prevention of coronary heart disease. *N Engl J Med* 1989; **321**(26):1825–8.
66. Aspirin effects on mortality and morbidity in patients with diabetes mellitus. Early Treatment Diabetic Retinopathy Study report 14. ETDRS Investigators. *JAMA* 1992; **268**(10):1292–300.
67. Bhatt DL, Hirsch AT, Ringleb PA, *et al.* Reduction in the need for hospitalization for recurrent ischemic events and bleeding with clopidogrel instead of aspirin. CAPRIE investigators. *Am Heart J* 2000; **140**(1):67–73.
68. Marso SP, Lincoff AM, Ellis SG, *et al.* Optimizing the percutaneous interventional outcomes for patients with diabetes mellitus: results of the EPISTENT (Evaluation of platelet IIb/IIIa inhibitor for stenting trial) diabetic substudy. *Circulation* 1999; **100**(25):2477–84.
69. Bhatt DL, Topol EJ. Current role of platelet glycoprotein IIb/IIIa inhibitors in acute coronary syndromes. *JAMA* 2000; **284**(12):1549–58.
70. Roffi M, Chew DP, Mukherjee D, *et al.* Platelet glycoprotein IIb/IIIa inhibitors reduce mortality in diabetic patients with non-ST-segment-elevation acute coronary syndromes. *Circulation* 2001; **104**(23):2767–71.
71. Bhatt DL, Marso SP, Lincoff AM, *et al.* Abciximab reduces mortality in diabetics following percutaneous coronary intervention. *J Am Coll Cardiol* 2000; **35**(4): 922–8.
72. Conlan MG, Folsom AR, Finch A, *et al.* Associations of factor VIII and von Willebrand factor with age, race, sex, and risk factors for atherosclerosis. The Atherosclerosis Risk in Communities (ARIC) Study. *Thromb Haemost* 1993; **70**(3):380–5.
73. Fuller JH, Keen H, Jarrett RJ, *et al.* Haemostatic variables associated with diabetes and its complications. *BMJ* 1979; **2**(6196):964–6.
74. el Khawand C, Jamart J, Donckier J, *et al.* Hemostasis variables in type I diabetic patients without demonstrable vascular complications. *Diabetes Care* 1993; **16**(8): 1137–45.
75. Juhan-Vague I, Alessi MC, Vague P. Thrombogenic and fibrinolytic factors and cardiovascular risk in non-insulin-dependent diabetes mellitus. *Ann Med* 1996; **28**(4): 371–80.
76. Kwaan HC. Changes in blood coagulation, platelet function, and plasminogen-plasmin system in diabetes. *Diabetes* 1992; **41**(Suppl 2):32–5.
77. Juhan-Vague I, Alessi MC, Vague P. Increased plasma plasminogen activator inhibitor 1 levels. A possible link between insulin resistance and atherothrombosis. *Diabetologia* 1991; **34**(7):457–62.
78. Gough SC, Grant PJ. The fibrinolytic system in diabetes mellitus. *Diabet Med* 1991; **8**(10):898–905.

79. Walmsley D, Hampton KK, Grant PJ. Contrasting fibrinolytic responses in type 1 (insulin-dependent) and type 2 (non-insulin-dependent) diabetes. *Diabet Med* 1991; **8**(10):954–9.
80. Kornowski R, Mintz GS, Lansky AJ, *et al.* Paradoxic decreases in atherosclerotic plaque mass in insulin-treated diabetic patients. *Am J Cardiol* 1998; **81**(11): 1298–304.
81. Schmidt AM, Yan SD, Wautier JL, *et al.* Activation of receptor for advanced glycation end products: a mechanism for chronic vascular dysfunction in diabetic vasculopathy and atherosclerosis. *Circ Res* 1999; **84**(5):489–97.
82. Vlassara H. Recent progress in advanced glycation end products and diabetic complications. *Diabetes* 1997; **46**(Suppl 2):S19–S25.
83. Libby P, Plutzky J. Diabetic macrovascular disease: the glucose paradox? *Circulation* 2002; **106**(22):2760–3.
84. Bucciarelli LG, Wendt T, Qu W, *et al.* RAGE blockade stabilizes established atherosclerosis in diabetic apolipoprotein E-null mice. *Circulation* 2002; **106**(22):2827–35.
85. Smith SC, Jr., Blair SN, Criqui MH, *et al.* Preventing heart attack and death in patients with coronary disease. *Circulation* 1995; **92**(1):2–4.
86. Rozenman Y, Sapoznikov D, Mosseri M, *et al.* Long-term angiographic follow-up of coronary balloon angioplasty in patients with diabetes mellitus: a clue to the explanation of the results of the BARI study. Balloon Angioplasty Revascularization Investigation. *J Am Coll Cardiol* 1997; **30**(6):1420–5.
87. Detre KM, Guo P, Holubkov R, *et al.* Coronary revascularization in diabetic patients: a comparison of the randomized and observational components of the Aypass Angioplasty Revascularization Investigation (BARI). *Circulation* 1999; **99**(5):633–40.
88. Kimura T, Tamura T, Yokoi H, *et al.* Long-term clinical and angiographic follow-up after placement of Palmaz-Schatz coronary stent: a single center experience. *J Interv Cardiol* 1994; **7**(2):129–39.
89. Mehran R, Mintz GS, Satler LF, *et al.* Treatment of in-stent restenosis with excimer laser coronary angioplasty: mechanisms and results compared with PTCA alone. *Circulation* 1997; **96**(7):2183–9.
90. Moreno PR, Fallon JT, Murcia AM, *et al.* Tissue characteristics of restenosis after percutaneous transluminal coronary angioplasty in diabetic patients. *J Am Coll Cardiol* 1999; **34**(4):1045–9.
91. Van BE, Abolmaali K, Bauters C, *et al.* Restenosis, late vessel occlusion and left ventricular function six months after balloon angioplasty in diabetic patients. *J Am Coll Cardiol* 1999; **34**(2):476–85.
92. Van BE, Ketelers R, Bauters C, *et al.* Patency of percutaneous transluminal coronary angioplasty sites at 6-month angiographic follow-up: A key determinant of survival in diabetics after coronary balloon angioplasty. *Circulation* 2001; **103**(9):1218–24.
93. Kornowski R, Mintz GS, Kent KM, *et al.* Increased restenosis in diabetes mellitus after coronary interventions is due to exaggerated intimal hyperplasia. A serial intravascular ultrasound study. *Circulation* 1997; **95**(6):1366–9.
94. Van BE, Perie M, Braune D, *et al.* Effects of coronary stenting on vessel patency and long-term clinical outcome after percutaneous coronary revascularization in diabetic patients. *J Am Coll Cardiol* 2002; **40**(3):410–7.
95. Elezi S, Kastrati A, Pache J, *et al.* Diabetes mellitus and the clinical and angiographic outcome after coronary stent placement. *J Am Coll Cardiol* 1998; **32**(7):1866–73.
96. Bornfeldt KE, Raines EW, Nakano T, *et al.* Insulin-like growth factor-I and platelet-derived growth factor-BB induce directed migration of human arterial smooth muscle cells via signaling pathways that are distinct from those of proliferation. *J Clin Invest* 1994; **93**(3):1266–74.
97. Marso SP, Ellis SG, Tuzcu M, *et al.* The importance of proteinuria as a determinant of mortality following percutaneous coronary revascularization in diabetics. *J Am Coll Cardiol* 1999; 33(5):1269–77.
98. Krolewski AS, Kosinski EJ, Warram JH, *et al.* Magnitude and determinants of coronary artery disease in juvenile-onset, insulin-dependent diabetes mellitus. *Am J Cardiol* 1987; **59**(8):750–5.
99. Mattock MB, Morrish NJ, Viberti G, *et al.* Prospective study of microalbuminuria as predictor of mortality in NIDDM. *Diabetes* 1992; **41**(6):736–41.
100. Neil A, Hawkins M, Potok M, *et al.* A prospective population-based study of microalbuminuria as a predictor of mortality in NIDDM. *Diabetes Care* 1993; **16**(7):996–1003.
101. Deckert T, Kofoed-Enevoldsen A, Norgaard K, *et al.* Microalbuminuria. Implications for micro- and macrovascular disease. *Diabetes Care* 1992; **15**(9): 1181–91.
102. Jensen T, Stender S, Deckert T. Abnormalities in plasmas concentrations of lipoproteins and fibrinogen in type 1 (insulin-dependent) diabetic patients with increased urinary albumin excretion. *Diabetologia* 1988; **31**(3):142–5.
103. Jones SL, Close CF, Mattock MB, *et al.* Plasma lipid and coagulation factor concentrations in insulin dependent diabetics with microalbuminuria. *BMJ* 1989; **298**(6672):487–90.
104. Winocour PH, Durrington PN, Bhatnagar D, *et al.* Influence of early diabetic nephropathy on very low density lipoprotein (VLDL), intermediate density lipoprotein (IDL), and low density lipoprotein (LDL) composition. *Atherosclerosis* 1991; **89**(1): 49–57.
105. Gruden G, Cavallo-Perin P, Bazzan M, *et al.* PAI-1 and factor VII activity are higher in IDDM patients with microalbuminuria. *Diabetes* 1994; **43**(3):426–9.
106. Stehouwer CD, Nauta JJ, Zeldenrust GC, *et al.* Urinary albumin excretion, cardiovascular disease, and endothelial dysfunction in non-insulin-dependent diabetes mellitus. *Lancet* 1992; **340**(8815):319–23.

107. Mehta SR, Cannon CP, Fox KA, *et al.* Routine vs selective invasive strategies in patients with acute coronary syndromes: a collaborative meta-analysis of randomized trials. *JAMA* 2005; **293**(23):2908–17.
108. de Winter RJ, Windhausen F, Cornel JH, *et al.* Early invasive versus selectively invasive management for acute coronary syndromes. *N Engl J Med* 2005; **353**(11):1095–104.
109. Biondi-Zoccai GG, Abbate A, Liuzzo G, *et al.* Atherothrombosis, inflammation, and diabetes. *J Am Coll Cardiol* 2003; **41**(7):1071–7.
110. Norhammar A, Malmberg K, Diderholm E, *et al.* Diabetes mellitus: the major risk factor in unstable coronary artery disease even after consideration of the extent of coronary artery disease and benefits of revascularization. *J Am Coll Cardiol* 2004; **43**(4):585–91.
111. Cannon CP, Weintraub WS, Demopoulos LA, *et al.* Comparison of early invasive and conservative strategies in patients with unstable coronary syndromes treated with the glycoprotein IIb/IIIa inhibitor tirofiban. *N Engl J Med* 2001; **344**(25):1879–87.
112. Bertrand ME, Simoons ML, Fox KA, v Management of acute coronary syndromes in patients presenting without persistent ST-segment elevation. *Eur Heart J* 2002; **23**(23):1809–40.
113. Bassand JP, Hamm CW, Ardissino D, *et al.* Guidelines for the diagnosis and treatment of non-ST-segment elevation acute coronary syndromes. *Eur Heart J* 2007; **28**(13):1598–660.
114. Sedlis SP, Morrison DA, Lorin JD, *et al.* Percutaneous coronary intervention versus coronary bypass graft surgery for diabetic patients with unstable angina and risk factors for adverse outcomes with bypass: outcome of diabetic patients in the AWESOME randomized trial and registry. *J Am Coll Cardiol* 2002; **40**(9):1555–66.
115. Boden WE, O'Rourke RA, Teo KK, *et al.* Optimal medical therapy with or without PCI for stable coronary disease. *N Engl J Med* 2007; **356**(15):1503–16.
116. Henderson RA, Pocock SJ, Clayton TC, *et al.* Seven-year outcome in the RITA-2 trial: coronary angioplasty versus medical therapy. *J Am Coll Cardiol* 2003; **42**(7):1161–70.
117. Schömig A, Mehilli J, de Waha A, *et al.* A meta-analysis of 17 randomized trials of a percutaneous coronary intervention-based strategy in patients with stable coronary artery disease. *J Am Coll Cardiol* 2008; **52**(11):894–904.
118. Soares PR, Hueb WA, Lemos PA, *et al.* Coronary revascularization (surgical or percutaneous) decreases mortality after the first year in diabetic subjects but not in nondiabetic subjects with multivessel disease: an analysis from the Medicine, Angioplasty, or Surgery Study (MASS II). *Circulation* 2006; **114**(1 Suppl):I420–I424.
119. Sobel BE, Frye R, Detre KM. Burgeoning dilemmas in the management of diabetes and cardiovascular disease: rationale for the Bypass Angioplasty Revascularization Investigation 2 Diabetes (BARI 2D) Trial. *Circulation* 2003; **107**(4):636–42.
120. Coronary angioplasty versus coronary artery bypass surgery: the Randomized Intervention Treatment of Angina (RITA) trial. *Lancet* 1993; **341**(8845):573–80.
121. First-year results of CABRI (Coronary Angioplasty versus Bypass Revascularisation Investigation). CABRI Trial Participants. *Lancet* 1995; **346**(8984):1179–84.
122. Comparison of coronary bypass surgery with angioplasty in patients with multivessel disease. The Bypass Angioplasty Revascularization Investigation (BARI) Investigators. *N Engl J Med* 1996; **335**(4):217–25.
123. Carrie D, Elbaz M, Puel J, *et al.* Five-year outcome after coronary angioplasty versus bypass surgery in multivessel coronary artery disease: results from the French Monocentric Study. *Circulation* 1997; **96**(9 Suppl):II–6.
124. Goy JJ, Eeckhout E, Burnand B, *et al.* Coronary angioplasty versus left internal mammary artery grafting for isolated proximal left anterior descending artery stenosis. *Lancet* 1994; **343**(8911):1449–53.
125. Hamm CW, Reimers J, Ischinger T, *et al.* A randomized study of coronary angioplasty compared with bypass surgery in patients with symptomatic multivessel coronary disease. German Angioplasty Bypass Surgery Investigation (GABI). *N Engl J Med* 1994; **331**(16): 1037–43.
126. Hueb WA, Bellotti G, de Oliveira SA, *et al.* The Medicine, Angioplasty or Surgery Study (MASS): a prospective, randomized trial of medical therapy, balloon angioplasty or bypass surgery for single proximal left anterior descending artery stenoses. *J Am Coll Cardiol* 1995; **26**(7):1600–5.
127. King SB, III, Lembo NJ, Weintraub WS, *et al.* Emory Angioplasty Versus Surgery Trial (EAST): design, recruitment, and baseline description of patients. *Am J Cardiol* 1995; **75**(9):42C–59C.
128. Rodriguez A, Boullon F, Perez-Balino N, *et al.* Argentine randomized trial of percutaneous transluminal coronary angioplasty versus coronary artery bypass surgery in multivessel disease (ERACI): in-hospital results and 1-year follow-up. ERACI Group. *J Am Coll Cardiol* 1993; **22**(4):1060–7.
129. Rodriguez A, Bernardi V, Navia J, *et al.* Argentine Randomized Study: Coronary Angioplasty with Stenting versus Coronary Bypass Surgery in patients with Multiple-Vessel Disease (ERACI II): 30-day and one-year follow-up results. ERACI II Investigators. *J Am Coll Cardiol* 2001; **37**(1):51–8.
130. Serruys PW, Unger F, Sousa JE, *et al.* Comparison of coronary-artery bypass surgery and stenting for the treatment of multivessel disease. *N Engl J Med* 2001; **344**(15):1117–24.
131. Coronary artery bypass surgery versus percutaneous coronary intervention with stent implantation in patients with multivessel coronary artery disease (the Stent or Surgery trial): a randomised controlled trial. *Lancet* 2002; **360**(9338):965–70.
132. Sim I, Gupta M, McDonald K, *et al.* A meta-analysis of randomized trials comparing coronary artery bypass

grafting with percutaneous transluminal coronary angioplasty in multivessel coronary artery disease. *Am J Cardiol* 1995; **76**(14):1025–9.

133. Bravata DM, Gienger AL, McDonald KM, *et al.* Systematic review: the comparative effectiveness of percutaneous coronary interventions and coronary artery bypass graft surgery. *Ann Intern Med* 2007; **147**(10): 703–16.
134. Seven-year outcome in the Bypass Angioplasty Revascularization Investigation (BARI) by treatment and diabetic status. *J Am Coll Cardiol* 2000; **35**(5):1122–9.
135. Kurbaan AS, Bowker TJ, Ilsley CD, *et al.* Difference in the mortality of the CABRI diabetic and nondiabetic populations and its relation to coronary artery disease and the revascularization mode. *Am J Cardiol* 2001; **87**(8):947–50.
136. Van BE, Bauters C, Hubert E, *et al.* Restenosis rates in diabetic patients: a comparison of coronary stenting and balloon angioplasty in native coronary vessels. *Circulation* 1997; **96**(5):1454–60.
137. Abizaid A, Kornowski R, Mintz GS, *et al.* The influence of diabetes mellitus on acute and late clinical outcomes following coronary stent implantation. *J Am Coll Cardiol* 1998; **32**(3):584–9.
138. George CJ, Baim DS, Brinker JA, *et al.* One-year follow-up of the Stent Restenosis (STRESS I) Study. *Am J Cardiol* 1998; **81**(7):860–5.
139. Serruys PW, de Jaegere P, Kiemeneij F, *et al.* A comparison of balloon-expandable-stent implantation with balloon angioplasty in patients with coronary artery disease. Benestent Study Group. *N Engl J Med* 1994; **331**(8):489–95.
140. Novel dosing regimen of eptifibatide in planned coronary stent implantation (ESPRIT): a randomised, placebo-controlled trial. *Lancet* 2000; **356**(9247): 2037–44.
141. Adgey AA. An overview of the results of clinical trials with glycoprotein IIb/IIIa inhibitors. *Eur Heart J* 1998; **19**(Suppl D):D10–D21.
142. Use of a monoclonal antibody directed against the platelet glycoprotein IIb/IIIa receptor in high-risk coronary angioplasty. The EPIC Investigation. *N Engl J Med* 1994; **330**(14):956–61.
143. Topol EJ, Mark DB, Lincoff AM, *et al.* Outcomes at 1 year and economic implications of platelet glycoprotein IIb/IIIa blockade in patients undergoing coronary stenting: results from a multicentre randomised trial. EPISTENT Investigators. Evaluation of Platelet IIb/IIIa Inhibitor for Stenting. *Lancet* 1999; **354**(9195):2019–24.
144. MRC/BHF Heart Protection Study of cholesterol lowering with simvastatin in 20,536 high-risk individuals: a randomised placebo-controlled trial. *Lancet* 2002; **360**(9326):7–22.
145. Serruys PW, de Feyter P, Macaya C, *et al.* Fluvastatin for prevention of cardiac events following successful first percutaneous coronary intervention: a randomized controlled trial. *JAMA* 2002; **287**(24):3215–22.
146. Powell BD, Bybee KA, Valeti U, *et al.* Influence of preoperative lipid-lowering therapy on postoperative outcome in patients undergoing coronary artery bypass grafting. *Am J Cardiol* 2007; **99**(6):785–9.
147. Paraskevas KI. Applications of statins in cardiothoracic surgery: more than just lipid-lowering. *Eur J Cardiothorac Surg* 2008; **33**(3):377–90.
148. Legrand VM, Serruys PW, Unger F, *et al.* Three-year outcome after coronary stenting versus bypass surgery for the treatment of multivessel disease. *Circulation* 2004; **109**(9):1114–20.
149. Barsness GW, Peterson ED, Ohman EM, *et al.* Relationship between diabetes mellitus and long-term survival after coronary bypass and angioplasty. *Circulation* 1997; **96**(8):2551–6.
150. Weintraub WS, Stein B, Kosinski A, *et al.* Outcome of coronary bypass surgery versus coronary angioplasty in diabetic patients with multivessel coronary artery disease. *J Am Coll Cardiol* 1998; **31**(1):10–19.
151. Gum PA, O'Keefe JH, Jr, Borkon AM, *et al.* Bypass surgery versus coronary angioplasty for revascularization of treated diabetic patients. *Circulation* 1997; **96**(9 Suppl): II-10.
152. Niles NW, McGrath PD, Malenka D, *et al.* Survival of patients with diabetes and multivessel coronary artery disease after surgical or percutaneous coronary revascularization: results of a large regional prospective study. Northern New England Cardiovascular Disease Study Group. *J Am Coll Cardiol* 2001; **37**(4):1008–15.
153. Edmunds LH, Jr. Why cardiopulmonary bypass makes patients sick: strategies to control the blood-synthetic surface interface. *Adv Card Surg* 1995; **6**:131–67.
154. Roach GW, Kanchuger M, Mangano CM, *et al.* Adverse cerebral outcomes after coronary bypass surgery. Multicenter Study of Perioperative Ischemia Research Group and the Ischemia Research and Education Foundation Investigators. *N Engl J Med* 1996; **335**(25):1857–63.
155. Arom KV, Emery RW, Flavin TF, *et al.* Cost-effectiveness of minimally invasive coronary artery bypass surgery. *Ann Thorac Surg* 1999; **68**(4):1562–6.
156. Pavie A, Lima L, Bonnet N, *et al.* Perioperative management in minimally invasive coronary surgery. *Eur J Cardiothorac Surg* 1999; **16**(Suppl 2):S53–S57.
157. Nathoe HM, van Dijk D, Jansen EW, *et al.* A comparison of on-pump and off-pump coronary bypass surgery in low-risk patients. *N Engl J Med* 2003; **348**(5): 394–402.
158. Møller CH, Penninga L, Wetterslev J, *et al.* Clinical outcomes in randomized trials of off- vs. on-pump coronary artery bypass surgery: systematic review with meta-analyses and trial sequential analyses. *Eur Heart J* 2008; **29**(21):2601–16.
159. Nakano J, Okabayashi H, Hanyu M, *et al.* Risk factors for wound infection after off-pump coronary artery bypass grafting: should bilateral internal thoracic arteries be harvested in patients with diabetes? *J Thorac Cardiovasc Surg* 2008; **135**(3):540–5.

160. Loop FD, Lytle BW, Cosgrove DM, *et al.* Influence of the internal-mammary-artery graft on 10-year survival and other cardiac events. *N Engl J Med* 1986; **314**(1):1–6.
161. Cameron A, Davis KB, Green G, *et al.* Coronary bypass surgery with internal-thoracic-artery grafts – effects on survival over a 15-year period. *N Engl J Med* 1996; **334**(4):216–19.
162. Zeff RH, Kongtahworn C, Iannone LA, *et al.* Internal mammary artery versus saphenous vein graft to the left anterior descending coronary artery: prospective randomized study with 10-year follow-up. *Ann Thorac Surg* 1988; **45**(5):533–6.
163. Grondin CM, Campeau L, Lesperance J, *et* al. Comparison of late changes in internal mammary artery and saphenous vein grafts in two consecutive series of patients 10 years after operation. *Circulation* 1984; **70**(3 Pt 2):I208–I212.
164. Carpentier A, Guermonprez JL, Deloche A, *et al.* The aorta-to-coronary radial artery bypass graft. A technique avoiding pathological changes in grafts. *Ann Thorac Surg* 1973; **16**(2):111-21.
165. Acar C, Jebara VA, Portoghese M, *et al.* Revival of the radial artery for coronary artery bypass grafting. *Ann Thorac Surg* 1992; **54**(4):652–9.
166. Acar C, Ramsheyi A, Pagny JY, *et al.* The radial artery for coronary artery bypass grafting: clinical and angiographic results at five years. *J Thorac Cardiovasc Surg* 1998; **116**(6):981–9.
167. Possati G, Gaudino M, Alessandrini F, *et al.* Midterm clinical and angiographic results of radial artery grafts used for myocardial revascularization. *J Thorac Cardiovasc Surg* 1998; **116**(6):1015–21.
168. Chen AH, Nakao T, Brodman RF, *et al.* Early postoperative angiographic assessment of radial grafts used for coronary artery bypass grafting. *J Thorac Cardiovasc Surg* 1996; **111**(6):1208–12.
169. Weinschelbaum EE, Gabe ED, Macchia A, *et al.* Total myocardial revascularization with arterial conduits: radial artery combined with internal thoracic arteries. *J Thorac Cardiovasc Surg* 1997; **114**(6):911–16.
170. Calafiore AM, Teodori G, Di Giammarco G, *et al.* Multiple arterial conduits without cardiopulmonary bypass: early angiographic results. *Ann Thorac Surg* 1999; **67**(2):450-6.
171. Lytle BW, Blackstone EH, Loop FD, *et al.* Two internal thoracic artery grafts are better than one. *J Thorac Cardiovasc Surg* 1999; **117**(5):855–72.
172. Taggart DP, D'Amico R, Altman DG. Effect of arterial revascularisation on survival: a systematic review of studies comparing bilateral and single internal mammary arteries. *Lancet* 2001; **358**(9285):870–5.
173. Sergeant PT, Blackstone EH, Meyns BP. Does arterial revascularization decrease the risk of infarction after coronary artery bypass grafting? *Ann Thorac Surg* 1998; **66**(1):1–10.
174. Leavitt BJ, Olmstead EM, Plume SK, *et al.* Use of the internal mammary artery graft in Northern New England. Northern New England Cardiovascular Disease Study Group. *Circulation* 1997; **96**(9 Suppl): II-6.
175. Buxton BF, Komeda M, Fuller JA, Gordon I. Bilateral internal thoracic artery grafting may improve outcome of coronary artery surgery. Risk-adjusted survival. *Circulation* 1998; **98**(19 Suppl):II1–II6.
176. Caputo M, Reeves B, Marchetto G, *et al.* Radial versus right internal thoracic artery as a second arterial conduit for coronary surgery: early and midterm outcomes. *J Thorac Cardiovasc Surg* 2003; **126**(1):39–47.
177. Buxton BF, Raman JS, Ruengsakulrach P, *et al.* Radial artery patency and clinical outcomes: five-year interim results of a randomized trial. *J Thorac Cardiovasc Surg* 2003; **125**(6):1363–71.
178. Desai ND, Cohen EA, Naylor CD, *et al.* A randomized comparison of radial-artery and saphenous-vein coronary bypass grafts. *N Engl J Med* 2004; **351**(22):2302–9.
179. Fremes SE. Multicenter radial artery patency study (RAPS). Study design. *Control Clin Trials* 2000; **21**(4): 397-413.
180. Risk factors for deep sternal wound infection after sternotomy: a prospective, multicenter study. *J Thorac Cardiovasc Surg* 1996; **111**(6):1200–7.
181. Lu JC, Grayson AD, Jha P, *et al.* Risk factors for sternal wound infection and mid-term survival following coronary artery bypass surgery. *Eur J Cardiothorac Surg* 2003; **23**(6):943–9.
182. Suselbeck T, Latsch A, Siri H, *et al.* Role of vessel size as a predictor for the occurrence of in-stent restenosis in patients with diabetes mellitus. *Am J Cardiol* 2001; **88**(3):243–7.
183. Lau KW, Ding ZP, Sim LL, *et al.* Clinical and angiographic outcome after angiography-guided stent placement in small coronary vessels. *Am Heart J* 2000; **139**(5):830–9.
184. Randomised placebo-controlled and balloon-angioplasty-controlled trial to assess safety of coronary stenting with use of platelet glycoprotein-IIb/IIIa blockade. *Lancet* 1998; 352(9122):87–92.
185. Steinhubl SR, Berger PB, Mann JT III, *et al.* Early and sustained dual oral antiplatelet therapy following percutaneous coronary intervention: a randomized controlled trial. *JAMA* 2002; **288**(19):2411–20.
186. Inhibition of the platelet glycoprotein IIb/IIIa receptor with tirofiban in unstable angina and non-Q-wave myocardial infarction. Platelet Receptor Inhibition in Ischemic Syndrome Management in Patients Limited by Unstable Signs and Symptoms (PRISM-PLUS) Study Investigators. *N Engl J Med* 1998; **338**(21): 1488–97.
187. Kleiman NS, Lincoff AM, Kereiakes DJ, *et al.* Diabetes mellitus, glycoprotein IIb/IIIa blockade, and heparin: evidence for a complex interaction in a multicenter trial. EPILOG Investigators. *Circulation* 1998; **97**(19):1912–20.
188. Topol EJ, Moliterno DJ, Herrmann HC, *et al.* Comparison of two platelet glycoprotein IIb/IIIa inhibitors, tirofiban and abciximab, for the prevention

of ischemic events with percutaneous coronary revascularization. *N Engl J Med* 2001; **344**(25):1888–94.
189. Roffi M, Moliterno DJ, Meier B, *et al.* Impact of different platelet glycoprotein IIb/IIIa receptor inhibitors among diabetic patients undergoing percutaneous coronary intervention: Do Tirofiban and ReoPro Give Similar Efficacy Outcomes Trial (TARGET) 1-year follow-up. *Circulation* 2002; **105**(23):2730–6.
190. Labinaz M, Madan M, O'Shea JO, *et al.* Comparison of one-year outcomes following coronary artery stenting in diabetic versus nondiabetic patients (from the Enhanced Suppression of the Platelet IIb/IIIa Receptor With Integrilin Therapy [ESPRIT] Trial). *Am J Cardiol* 2002; **90**(6):585–90.
191. Kapur A, Hall RJ, Malik IS, *et al.* Randomized comparison of percutaneous coronary intervention with coronary artery bypass grafting in diabetic patients. 1-Year results of the CARDia (Coronary Artery Revascularization in Diabetes) trial. *J Am Coll Cardiol* 2010; **55**:432–40.
192. Yusuf S, Zhao F, Mehta SR, *et al*. Effects of clopidogrel in addition to aspirin in patients with acute coronary syndromes without ST-segment elevation. *N Engl J Med* 2001; **345**(7):494–502.
193. Mehta SR, Yusuf S, Peters RJ, *et al.* Effects of pretreatment with clopidogrel and aspirin followed by long-term therapy in patients undergoing percutaneous coronary intervention: the PCI-CURE study. *Lancet* 2001; **358**(9281):527–33.
194. A randomised, blinded, trial of clopidogrel versus aspirin in patients at risk of ischaemic events (CAPRIE). CAPRIE Steering Committee. *Lancet* 1996; **348**(9038):1329–39.
195. Bhatt DL, Marso SP, Hirsch AT, *et al.* Amplified benefit of clopidogrel versus aspirin in patients with diabetes mellitus. *Am J Cardiol* 2002; **90**(6):625–8.
196. Mehilli J, Kastrati A, Schuhlen H, *et al.* Randomized clinical trial of abciximab in diabetic patients undergoing elective percutaneous coronary interventions after treatment with a high loading dose of clopidogrel. Circulation 2004; **110**(24):3627–35.
197. Serebruany VL, Steinhubl SR, Berger PB, *et al.* Variability in platelet responsiveness to clopidogrel among 544 individuals. *J Am Coll Cardiol* 2005; **45**(2):246–51.
198. Angiolillo DJ, Shoemaker SB, Desai B, *et al.* Randomized comparison of a high clopidogrel maintenance dose in patients with diabetes mellitus and coronary artery disease: results of the Optimizing Antiplatelet Therapy in Diabetes Mellitus (OPTIMUS) study. *Circulation* 2007; **115**(6):708–16.
199. Fuster V, Farkouh ME. Acute coronary syndromes and diabetes mellitus: a winning ticket for prasugrel. *Circulation* 2008; **118**(16):1607–8.
200. Ferreira IA, Mocking AI, Feijge MA, *et al.* Platelet inhibition by insulin is absent in type 2 diabetes mellitus. *Arterioscler Thromb Vasc Biol* 2006; **26**(2):417–22.
201. Brandt JT, Payne CD, Wiviott SD, *et al.* A comparison of prasugrel and clopidogrel loading doses on platelet function: magnitude of platelet inhibition is related to active metabolite formation. *Am Heart J* 2007; **153**(1): 66–16.
202. Jernberg T, Payne CD, Winters KJ, *et al.* Prasugrel achieves greater inhibition of platelet aggregation and a lower rate of non-responders compared with clopidogrel in aspirin-treated patients with stable coronary artery disease. *Eur Heart J* 2006; **27**(10):1166–73.
203. Wallentin L, Varenhorst C, James S, *et al.* Prasugrel achieves greater and faster P2Y12receptor-mediated platelet inhibition than clopidogrel due to more efficient generation of its active metabolite in aspirin-treated patients with coronary artery disease. *Eur Heart J* 2008; **29**(1):21–30.
204. Wiviott SD, Trenk D, Frelinger AL, *et al.* Prasugrel compared with high loading- and maintenance-dose clopidogrel in patients with planned percutaneous coronary intervention: the Prasugrel in Comparison to Clopidogrel for Inhibition of Platelet Activation and Aggregation-Thrombolysis in Myocardial Infarction 44 trial. *Circulation* 2007; **116**(25):2923–32.
205. Wiviott SD, Braunwald E, McCabe CH, *et al.* Prasugrel versus clopidogrel in patients with acute coronary syndromes. *N Engl J Med* 2007; **357**(20):2001–15.
206. Wiviott SD, Braunwald E, Angiolillo DJ, *et al.* Greater Clinical Benefit of More Intensive Oral Antiplatelet Therapy With Prasugrel in Patients With Diabetes Mellitus in the Trial to Assess Improvement in Therapeutic Outcomes by Optimizing Platelet Inhibition With Prasugrel-Thrombolysis in Myocardial Infarction 38. *Circulation* 2008; **118**(16):1626–36.
207. Morice MC, Serruys PW, Sousa JE, *et al.* A randomized comparison of a sirolimus-eluting stent with a standard stent for coronary revascularization. *N Engl J Med* 2002; **346**(23):1773–80.
208. Moses JW, Leon MB, Popma JJ, *et al.* Sirolimus-eluting stents versus standard stents in patients with stenosis in a native coronary artery. *N Engl J Med* 2003; **349**(14):1315–23.
209. Stone GW, Ellis SG, Cox DA, *et al.* One-year clinical results with the slow-release, polymer-based, paclitaxel-eluting TAXUS stent: the TAXUS-IV trial. *Circulation* 2004; **109**(16):1942-7.
210. Sabate M, Jimenez-Quevedo P, Angiolillo DJ, *et al.* Randomized comparison of sirolimus-eluting stent versus standard stent for percutaneous coronary revascularization in diabetic patients: the diabetes and sirolimus-eluting stent (DIABETES) trial. *Circulation* 2005; **112**(14):2175–83.
211. Finn AV, Palacios IF, Kastrati A, *et al.* Drug-eluting stents for diabetes mellitus: a rush to judgment? *J Am Coll Cardiol* 2005; **45**(4):479–83.
212. Windecker S, Remondino A, Eberli FR, *et al.* Sirolimus-eluting and paclitaxel-eluting stents for coronary revascularization. *N Engl J Med* 2005; **353**(7):653–62.
213. Dibra A, Kastrati A, Mehilli J, *et al.* Paclitaxel-eluting or sirolimus-eluting stents to prevent restenosis in diabetic patients. *N Engl J Med* 2005; **353**(7):663–70.

214. Camenzind E, Steg PG, Wijns W. Stent thrombosis late after implantation of first-generation drug-eluting stents: a cause for concern. *Circulation* 2007; **115**(11):1440–55.
215. Shuchman M. Debating the risks of drug-eluting stents. *N Engl J Med* 2007; **356**(4):325–8.
216. Spaulding C, Daemen J, Boersma E, *et al.* A pooled analysis of data comparing sirolimus-eluting stents with bare-metal stents. *N Engl J Med* 2007; **356**(10):989–97.
217. Kirtane AJ, Ellis SG, Dawkins KD, *et al.* Paclitaxel-eluting coronary stents in patients with diabetes mellitus: pooled analysis from 5 randomized trials. *J Am Coll Cardiol* 2008; **51**(7):708–15.
218. Stettler C, Allemann S, Wandel S, *et al.* Drug eluting and bare metal stents in people with and without diabetes: collaborative network meta-analysis. *BMJ* 2008; **337**:a1331.
219. Serruys PW, Lemos PA, van Hout BA. Sirolimus eluting stent implantation for patients with multivessel disease: rationale for the Arterial Revascularisation Therapies Study part II (ARTS II). *Heart* 2004; **90**(9):995–8.
220. Cutlip DE, Windecker S, Mehran R, *et al.* Clinical end points in coronary stent trials: a case for standardized definitions. *Circulation* 2007; **115**(17):2344–51.
221. Serruys PW, Daemen J, Morice MC, *et al.* Three year follow up of the ARTS 2 – sirolimus eluting stents for the treatment of multivessel coronary artery disease. *EuroIntervention* 2007; **3**:450–9.
222. Daeman J, Kuck KH, Macaya C, *et al.* Multivessel coronary revascularization in patients with and without diabetes mellitus 3-year follow-up of the ARTS-II (Arterial Revascularization Therapies Study–Part II) trial *J Am Coll Cardiol,* 2008; **52**:1957–67.
223. Farkouh ME, Dangas G, Leon MB, *et al.* Design of the Future REvascularization Evaluation in patients with Diabetes mellitus: Optimal management of Multivessel disease (FREEDOM) Trial. *Am Heart J* 2008; **155**(2): 215–23.
224. Serruys PW. The Synergy between Percutaneous Coronary Intervention with TAXUS and Cardiac Surgery:The SYNTAX Study Primary Endpoint Results at One Year in the Randomized Cohort. European Society of Cardiology 2008; Hotline session 2 (http://www.escardio.org).
225. Norhammar A, Malmberg K, Ryden L, *et al.* Under utilisation of evidence-based treatment partially explains for the unfavourable prognosis in diabetic patients with acute myocardial infarction. *Eur Heart J* 2003; **24**(9): 838–44.
226. Mueller C, Buerkle G, Buettner HJ, *et al.* Prevention of contrast media associated nephropathy:randomised comparison of 2 hydration regimes in 1620 patients undergoing coronary angioplasty. *Arch Int Med* 2002; **162**:329–36.
227. Merten GJ, Burgess WP, Gray LV, *et al.* Prevention of contrast induced nephropathy with sodium bicarbonate: a randomised controlled trial. *JAMA* 2004; **291**: 2328–34.
228. Tepel M, van der Giet M, Schwarzfeld C, *et al.* Prevention of radiographic contrast agent induced reductions in renal function by acetylcysteine. *N Engl J Med* 2000; **343**: 180–4.
229. Rydén L, Standl E, Bartnik M, *et al.* Guidelines on diabetes, pre-diabetes, and cardiovascular diseases: executive summary. The Task Force on Diabetes and Cardiovascular Diseases of the European Society of Cardiology (ESC) and of the European Association for the Study of Diabetes (EASD). *Eur Heart J* 2007; **28**(1):88–136.

SECTION 5

Adjunctive therapies in percutaneous coronary intervention

CHAPTER 22

Current status of oral antiplatelet therapies

Alex Hobson and Nick Curzen

Introduction

As our understanding of the pathophysiology of adverse cardiovascular events evolves, the integral role of the platelet is increasingly recognized. Plaque rupture, platelet activation and aggregation, and thrombus formation occur as a result of complex interactions between platelets, vascular endothelium, inflammatory cells, and circulating proteins. These processes can result in vascular occlusion, ischaemia, and infarction. Similarly during percutaneous coronary intervention (PCI) and stent implantation, coronary vessel trauma and inflammation, as well as the poorly understood process of stent endothelialization, combine to make some patients susceptible to adverse thrombotic events, including stent thrombosis (ST).

Clinical studies have repeatedly shown that antiplatelet therapies improve outcomes in cardiovascular disease, including those patients undergoing PCI. As a result there has been increased awareness of the importance of antiplatelet therapies in primary and secondary prevention of cardiovascular disease, in the treatment of acute events such as myocardial infarction (MI), and acute coronary syndrome (ACS), and as an adjunctive therapy in PCI.

Dual antiplatelet therapy with aspirin and a thienopyridine, usually clopidogrel, has contributed to the dramatic improvements in outcomes that have led to the emergence of PCI and stenting as the treatment strategy of choice in many patients with ACS and as a viable alternative to coronary bypass surgery in many patients with stable angina.

However, even with current therapies, platelet activation, adhesion, and aggregation continue to contribute to adverse events after PCI, including MI and ST. As a result there has been a trend towards increased intensity of antiplatelet therapy. However, all antiplatelet therapies increase the bleeding risk and with modern invasive management strategies bleeding rates are increasing[1]. Importantly, it is now known that bleeding is associated with an increased risk of recurrent ischaemic events and death even when the bleeding episode itself is not life-threatening[2]. Data from the CRUSADE registry suggests that the commonest adverse event post non-ST segment elevation MI (NSTEMI) is now bleeding[3]. In addition, post hoc analysis of ACUITY has shown that bleeding after PCI conveys a greater mortality risk than peri-procedural MI[4]. In addition, in-hospital bleeding in ACUITY (Acute Catheterization and Urgent Intervention Triage Strategy trial) was shown to increase the risk of subsequent ST. A strong association is demonstrable between 30-day bleeding and 1-year mortality[5] and furthermore, major haemorrhage has been shown to be an independent predictor of 1-year mortality in both elective and urgent PCI[6]. In fact, even minor bleeding by the GUSTO criteria increases the risk of 30-day mortality by 60%[2].

In the light of these data it is perhaps no surprise that in some populations (e.g. CHARISMA[7] and ACUITY-PCI[8]) more intensive antiplatelet therapy has been associated with worse outcomes. It is therefore clear that the undoubted benefits of antiplatelet agents in terms of reducing ischaemic events need to be carefully balanced with the increased risk of bleeding.

An ideal antiplatelet agent would be safe, well tolerated, cheap, available in tablet form, and have predictable, rapid, long-lasting, measurable, and reversible effects. It must also be effective and improve patient outcomes. Whilst aspirin and clopidogrel have dramatically improved outcomes in PCI compared to previous therapies, this combination strategy is fallible in some patients with recurrent thrombotic and haemorrhagic events continuing to occur. It is counter-intuitive that current care pathways condone treating all patients with standard loading and maintenance doses of aspirin and clopidogrel, despite the well documented variation in individual responses to these agents. This raises the question: what can be done to improve on current therapy?

Many specific questions remain to be fully answered, including:

- When should loading doses of antiplatelet therapy be administered?
- What loading dose of clopidogrel should be administered?
- What maintenance dose should be prescribed?
- How long should dual antiplatelet therapy be continued after stent insertion?
- How should we manage patients with sensitivity or allergy to standard antiplatelet therapy?
- Will newer antiplatelet agents make any/many of these considerations obsolete?
- Should all or some patients have tests to determine if they have responded adequately to these therapies?

And if so:

- What tests should be utilized?
- Should we aim for the same level of platelet inhibition in all patients regardless of their presentation?
- How should therapy be altered when patients are found to respond poorly?

This chapter summarizes the current guidelines for antiplatelet drugs in the context of PCI; medications at our disposal, and we will attempt to answer these questions using the evidence that is currently available. We highlight some of these issues by discussing our management of a complex clinical case. In addition we will consider to what extent technologies, pharmaceuticals, and management strategies may alter in the near future.

Historical

Balloon angioplasty and coronary stenting cause trauma to the endothelium of the blood vessel wall exposing subendothelial contents such as collagen and von Willebrand factor to the blood. This invariably leads to platelet activation, aggregation, and activation and can result in subsequent thrombotic occlusion. Early stent trials used aspirin monotherapy or aspirin plus warfarin to reduce the risk of early thrombotic complications. However, rates of acute ST were 15–20% for aspirin monotherapy[9] and with aspirin and warfarin in combination these rates remained high (3.5% at the time of hospital discharge) and were also associated with very high bleeding rates. The introduction of dual antiplatelet therapy with aspirin and a thienopyridine (initially ticlopidine) reduced the risk of bare-metal ST to about 1% and also decreased bleeding rates[10]. Clopidogrel has now largely superseded ticlopidine in contemporary practice because of better tolerability and safety, no requirement for routine haematological monitoring, and robust evidence of at least equivalent efficacy[10,11].

Whilst the high levels of clinical restenosis seen with bare-metal stents (BMS) have been effectively attenuated by the advent of drug-eluting stents (DES), this development has challenged conventional antiplatelet strategies. As an inevitable side effect of the interference with the inflammatory healing response caused by drug elution, the rate at which the device is re-endothelialized is reduced, hence increasing the period of time that the stent surface is exposed to circulating platelets[12]. The requirement for a longer period of antiplatelet therapy to prevent the dreaded complication of ST, with its associated mortality of up to 45%[13], became apparent soon after their introduction, and more recently there have been concerns specifically related to late ST in patients with DES. It is unequivocal that premature discontinuation of antiplatelet therapy after PCI and DES insertion is particularly hazardous and associated with subsequent mortality[14].

Current guidelines

Aspirin

In patients undergoing PCI, American guidelines recommend 75–325mg of aspirin before the procedure (300–325mg if not on chronic maintenance therapy at least 2h and preferably 24h before the procedure) followed by 325mg daily for at least: 1) 1 month after BMS; 2) 3 months for sirolimus-eluting stents and 3) 6 months for paclitaxel-eluting stents. Chronic aspirin therapy should be continued indefinitely after this point at a dose of 75–162mg daily[15]. European guidelines recommend that an oral loading dose of 500mg aspirin is administered at least 3h prior to PCI, or at least 300mg given intravenously immediately prior to the procedure in patients not on chronic maintenance therapy[16]. They recommend that there is no need for doses greater than 100mg daily for maintenance therapy post PCI and stent insertion.

Clopidogrel

Current American and European guidelines, based on the results of the PCI-CURE study, suggest that a 300-mg loading dose of clopidogrel should be administered at least 6h before PCI followed by maintenance therapy[(17)]. However several studies suggest that 600-mg loading doses provide additional clinical benefit[(18)].

The optimal duration for clopidogrel therapy post PCI is still unknown but is the focus of active debate, particularly following concerns about ST occurring beyond the first 6 months after implantation of DES. For DES there is some evidence that 12 months of therapy is superior to 6 months[(19)] and data from the GHOST registry even suggests that more than 12 months' duration of dual antiplatelet therapy may be beneficial[(20)]. There is also increasing data to suggest a clustering of adverse events in the 90 days after clopidogrel cessation[(21)]. A cluster of thrombotic events in the 90 days after clopidogrel is stopped in PCI patients has led to the hypothesis that there is a 'rebound' vascular inflammatory response during this period. This is the subject of active research and will be specifically addressed by ongoing studies including DECADES.

Aspirin

Hippocrates left records of using an extract of willow bark to treat pain. The active compound (salicin) was isolated in the 1820s. Acetylsalicylic acid (aspirin) was first produced in the 1850s and patented and marketed by Bayer in 1889. Aspirin is known to cause platelet inhibition by irreversible acetylation of serine residue 529 of cyclooxygenase-1 (COX-1), preventing conversion of arachidonic acid (AA) to prostaglandin-H and subsequent formation of the potent vasoconstrictor and platelet activator thromboxane A2. Aspirin has a rapid onset of action. Its half-life in the circulation is only 20min but as its activity is irreversible the effects are relatively long-lasting allowing dosing every 24–48h. In normal adults the antithrombotic effect of aspirin is saturable at doses in the range of 75–100mg[(22)].

Long-term use of aspirin in patients with vascular disease decreases morbidity and mortality from cardiovascular events by 25% and it is a cornerstone of secondary prevention in coronary artery disease. In ACS aspirin reduces the risk of progression to death and MI by 50% and in ST segment elevation myocardial infarction (STEMI) aspirin reduces the risk of death by 23%[(22)]. The risk reduction observed with aspirin therapy appears consistent for a wide range of doses (75mg–1500mg daily) although doses lower than 75mg daily do appear to be associated with significantly increased risk and higher doses are associated with higher rates of bleeding[(23)]. Its role in PCI is sometimes underestimated. Its addition to heparin in early trials of PCI led to a 75% relative reduction in MACE rates[(24)].

Six months of maintenance therapy after PCI is supported by the M-Heart II study showing less re-infarction compared to placebo[(25)]. The data for supporting the benefit of aspirin in vascular disease in general, the benefit after acute MI, together with the elevated rates of observed ST in patients in whom aspirin is stopped all contribute to a strong 'circumstantial' case for continuing aspirin lifelong after stents.

Clopidogrel

Clopidogrel is a thienopyridine that, through irreversible inhibition of platelet P2Y12 receptors, inhibits adenosine diphosphate (ADP)-induced platelet aggregation and the conformational change of platelets so that fibrinogen can no longer bind to the glycoprotein (GP) IIb/IIIa receptor. It has largely superseded ticlopidine because of better tolerability and safety and several studies showing that it is at least as effective in preventing stent thrombosis, and has a faster onset of action[(10,11,26)]. It is a pro-drug that is metabolized by hepatic CYP3A4 to its active metabolite. As it takes a few days for clopidogrel to have its full effect a loading dose is usually administered in the context of PCI.

Data from CREDO and PCI-CURE support the use of a 300-mg loading dose prior to PCI[(17,27)]. In the CREDO trial outcomes were improved only when the 300mg loading dose was given at least 6h prior to intervention[(27)]. Further, a post hoc analysis of this trial suggests that 28-day outcomes were only significantly improved when the loading dose was administered at least 15h prior to angioplasty [(28)].

Several studies have now suggested that a 600-mg loading dose provides additional benefit. The ISAR-REACT and ISAR-SWEET trials strongly suggested a beneficial clinical effect from a 600-mg loading dose, but were not randomized trials comparing 600-mg to 300-mg doses. The ARMYDA-2 trial randomized 255 patients to either 300-mg or 600-mg loading doses of clopidogrel 4–8h prior to PCI. There was a significant decrease in cardiovascular events in the 600-mg group with no increase in the haemorrhagic risk[(29)]. A randomized trial of ACS patients receiving loading doses of clopidogrel at least 12h prior to PCI also found a significant decrease in cardiovascular events at 1 month in those receiving 600mg[(18)]. A non-randomized analysis of 4105 unselected patients undergoing PCI also showed a significant decrease in post-PCI MACE at 1 month without an increase in bleeding complications[30].

The licensed dose for maintenance therapy is 75mg daily. Data from CREDO and PCI-CURE support the use and long-term (9–12 months) maintenance therapy after stent insertion with diverging rates of death and MI with long-term therapy, although CREDO did suggest a slight increase in bleeding.

In summary there is evidence of considerable benefit from clopidogrel in large studies of PCI patients, although there remains important uncertainty about optimal dosing and duration of therapy. Furthermore, there is a large body of evidence that robustly demonstrates a wide variation in individual response to clopidogrel. No account of this is currently taken in routine clinical practice (See 'Assessment of response to antiplatelet therapy' section).

Other antiplatelet therapies

Several other antiplatelet therapies are currently available. These include ticlopidine, dipyridamole, and cilastozol.

Ticlopidine

Ticlopidine is a thienopyridine which irreversibly inhibits the platelet P2Y12 receptor. It is a pro-drug which is transformed into its active metabolite by metabolism by hepatic cytochrome P-450.

Ticlopidine is effective in the secondary prevention of MI and stroke[31] and has been shown to be effective in preventing stent occlusion when used in combination with aspirin. In the FANTASTIC study which compared aspirin and ticlopidine with aspirin and warfarin after implantation of BMS there was a dramatic reduction in cardiac events (mainly due to reductions in acute and subacute ST to less than 1%) in the ticlopidine arm. Haemorrhagic complications were also dramatically reduced in those on ticlopidine compared to warfarin[32].

The use of ticlopidine has now largely been superseded by clopidogrel due to side effects (principally neutropenia) and tolerability. Neutropenia occurs in 2.4% and can be fatal, although it usually resolves within 2–3 weeks of drug cessation. A full blood count is recommended every 2 weeks for the first 3 months of therapy and the compliance to this regimen is poor[33]. Thrombotic thrombocytopenic purpura, rashes, diarrhoea, nausea, vomiting, and abdominal pain also all limit its tolerability.

Dipyridamole

Dipyridamole exerts an antiplatelet effect through increasing platelet cyclic adenosine monophosphate (cAMP) levels. Adenosine modulates platelet function via its action on the platelet A2A receptor (which increases cAMP levels). By blocking adenosine uptake dipyridamole therefore increases the amount of adenosine having this inhibitory effect on platelet function. It is licensed as an adjunct to anticoagulants for patients with prosthetic heart valves and is also used together with aspirin in the secondary prevention of ischaemic stroke and transient ischaemic attacks.

There are limited and non-randomized data from the balloon angioplasty era that the addition of dipyridamole to aspirin reduced visible thrombus and acute vessel closure[34] but there is no evidence to support its use in the context of coronary stent implantation or as an alternative to aspirin or clopidogrel.

Cilostazol

Cilostazol inhibits c AMP phosphodiesterase III in platelets and also inhibits the production of platelet-derived growth factor from endothelial cells[35]. It inhibits platelet aggregation and also acts as an arterial vasodilator. Its main use (and licence in the UK) is in patients with intermittent claudication (as a vasodilator). There is some evidence however that it may be as effective as ticlopidine and clopidogrel as an antiplatelet agent after coronary stent implantation[36]. Concerns have been raised however by a study randomizing the use of BMS and paclitaxel-eluting stents in which cilostazol was used (not randomized) in some patients. In this study five out of 37 patients receiving cilostazol experienced ST compared to one of 138 receiving thienopyridines[37].

It has also been studied in combination with aspirin and clopidogrel as triple therapy. It leads to greater inhibition of ADP-induced platelet aggregation than aspirin and clopidogrel alone[38]. As well as the observed increased antiplatelet effect, the addition of cilostazol to standard dual antiplatelet therapy has been shown in one study to decrease the rate of ST after coronary artery stent insertion[39]. This study was however non-randomized, included only BMS, and had a relatively small sample size.

Emerging antiplatelet therapies

Whilst the widespread use of clopidogrel has led to dramatic improvements in outcome following PCI its relatively slow onset of action and the marked heterogeneity in observed responses (see 'Assessment of response to antiplatelet therapy' section) undoubtedly contribute to some of the residual risk post PCI. As a result several novel antiplatelet therapies are now in the late stages of development and show promise.

Prasugrel

Prasugrel is a thienopyridine but with important differences in its metabolism compared to Clopidogrel. Whilst both are pro-drugs, Prasugrel generates faster, more consistent and higher levels of active metabolite after its administration than clopidogrel. As a result there is a more rapid, potent and reliable inhibition of platelet activation and aggregation after prasugrel administration[40].

Post hoc analysis of JUMBO-TIMI 26 revealed that prasugrel may be associated with decreased thrombotic events when compared to clopidogrel[41]. More recently, the results of TRITON-TIMI 38[42], a larger phase III trial, have made an important case for the use of prasugrel in PCI in the context of acute coronary syndromes: a case that is currently being considered by both the FDA in USA and NICE in the UK. In the study, 13 608 patients with moderate- to high-risk ACS with scheduled PCI were randomized to receive prasugrel (60-mg loading dose followed by 10-mg maintenance) or clopidogrel (300-mg loading dose, then 75-mg maintenance) for 6–15 months. The primary endpoint was a combination of death from cardiovascular causes, non-fatal MI, or non fatal stroke, and occurred in 12.1% of the clopidogrel group and 9.9% of the prasugrel patients (hazard ratio for prasugrel versus clopidogrel 0.81; p <0.001). There were also significant reductions in the prasugrel group for individual prespecified endpoints, including MI (9.7% clopidogrel versus 7.4% prasugrel; p<0.001) and ST (2.4% versus 1.1%; p <0.001). However, the incidence of important bleeding complications was significantly higher in the prasugrel group. Thus, major bleeding was seen in 2.4% of prasugrel patients and 1.8% of the clopidogrel group (hazard ration 1.32; p = 0.03; life-threatening bleeding 1.4% versus 0.9% respectively (p = 0.01) and fatal bleeding was seen in 0.4% of the prasugrel group and 0.1% of the clopidogrel patients (p = 0.002). The benefit of prasugrel in terms of reduced ischaemic complications therefore are weighed against the increased risk of bleeding and an attempt is made to address this equation with the concept of 'net clinical benefit'. In this study therefore, a significant improvement in net clinical benefit is reported with prasugrel (all-cause death, MI, stroke, and major bleed) with a hazard ratio of 0.87[42], but this concept presents some intellectual challenges. The increase in bleeding complications was seen particularly in: 1) patients with previous stroke or transient ischaemic attacks in whom the bleeding risk outweighed the benefits; and 2) in the elderly; and 3) those with a low body weight in whom the benefits were balanced by the risks. It is estimated that overall treatment of 1000 patients with prasugrel would prevent 23 MIs at the expense of six non-CABG related TIMI major haemorrhage as compared with clopidogrel. There are some important reservations about the design of this study considering the potential enormous impact that it could have on clinical practice. Prasugrel was compared to a loading dose regimen of clopidogrel that is now known to be suboptimal in PCI. Firstly, the dose was 300mg. Secondly, this loading dose was administered 'anytime between randomization and 1h after leaving the catheterization laboratory'. Since randomization could not occur until the coronary anatomy was known (because there had to be certainty that the patient was suitable for PCI) and 'nearly all patients (99%) had PCI at the time of randomization' this means that in most cases the clopidogrel was given only very shortly before PCI was undertaken. Clearly, since it is well-established that prasugrel has a more rapid onset of action than clopidogrel, the use of a relatively low loading dose administered at the time of PCI rather than in advance of the procedure would undoubtedly have favoured prasugrel.

Coupled with the bleeding rates it appears that the case for prasugrel is not yet comprehensive.

Some of the potential weaknesses of this study have been answered with PRINCIPLE-TIMI 44. This study has evaluated the antiplatelet effects of prasugrel 60mg versus clopidogrel 600mg. This showed higher levels of platelet inhibition with prasugrel after 30min than clopidogrel at 6h[43]. Therefore prasugrel may have beneficial effects even when a 600mg loading dose of clopidogrel is administered in advance of the procedure.

A further trial, TRILOGY ACS is planned which will use a reduced dose of prasugrel in those sub-groups identified as at high risk of bleeding in TRITON-TIMI 38.

AZD 6140

AZD 6140 is an oral, directly acting and reversible antagonist of the P2Y12 receptor. It does not need to be metabolized although it is metabolized to an active metabolite which contributes to its effect. The DISPERSE and DISPERSE 2 trials were phase IIa, randomized and blinded studies of AZD 6140 against clopidogrel and showed faster and more consistent platelet inhibition with AZD 6140 (at doses of 100mg and 200mg twice daily) than clopidogrel 75mg daily[44].

The PLATO trial is an ongoing phase III trial comparing outcomes with the use of AZD 6140 and clopidogrel in ACS patients. Phase 2 trials have highlighted possible side effects of dyspnoea and pauses which may be due to effects of adenosine.

Other emerging therapies

There are other potential antiplatelet therapies which are in earlier stages of development including:

- *SCH 530348* is an oral PAR-1 inhibitor (thrombin receptor) which has completed phase 2 trials, the results of which have recently been published. Specifically, the drug blocks the protease-activated receptor 1 (PAR-1) on platelets on to which thrombin binds, thereby inhibiting thrombin-induced platelet activation. In this study[45], 1030 patients undergoing planned PCI were randomized to three different loading doses of SCH 530348 or placebo in a 3:1 ratio. Following PCI the study drug patients were further randomized to three different maintenance doses for 60 days. All patients had standard therapy that included aspirin and clopidogrel. TIMI major and minor bleeding represented the primary endpoint, and there was no significant difference between the groups. The study was not powered to assess clinical efficacy
- *PR-15; DZ-6976* are agents that inhibit the activity of platelet anti-collagen receptors
- *DG-041* is an EP3 receptor antagonist which potentiates the protective effects of prostaglandin E2
- *BX 667* is an orally active reversible P2Y12 inhibitor which has shown a wider therapeutic index than clopidogrel in preliminary animal studies[46].

Despite the undoubted ability of some of these agents to provide superior platelet inhibition, with the inherent increased risks of bleeding, large outcome trials are required to establish their optimal role in clinical practice.

Developments in PCI and stent technology

ST and other recurrent adverse thrombotic events are undoubtedly multifactorial. Procedural factors are important in many cases. Greater use of intravascular ultrasound and high-pressure balloon post-dilatation to reduce incomplete stent apposition and increase minimal stent area, both risk factors for ST[47], may reduce the incidence of ST. Developments in stent technology, such as endothelial progenitor cell capture could also reduce ST by encouraging rapid endothelialization[48]. Identification of cohorts of patients at increased risk of ST, such as those with malignancy[49], and increased risk of poor response to antiplatelet therapy, such as in diabetics[50] could influence the choice of antiplatelet therapy and procedure undertaken.

Assessment of response to antiplatelet therapy

Methods of assessing response

Conventional methods of measuring platelet activation and function are time consuming and cannot be performed at the bedside. The first test of platelet function developed in the early 1900s was the bleeding time. This utilizes a standardized *in vivo* wound and measures the time to cessation of bleeding. This is largely dependent on platelets but is not specific to platelet function, also depending, for example, on the concentration of von Willebrand factor. It is also insensitive, has high inter-operator variability, and can lead to scar formation and is therefore no longer recommended. Currently utilized assays are summarized in Table 22.1.

Optical aggregation

Optical aggregation is the historical gold standard test of platelet reactivity. The Global Platelet Function Working Group recommend that response to aspirin is assessed using light transmissance aggregation using stimulation with 1mmol AA with residual aggregation of >10% signifying lack of benefit. They also recommend its use to measure responses to clopidogrel using 10mmol ADP with an aggregation of >50% used to indicate lack of benefit. It can be performed on platelet rich plasma by turbidometry or on whole blood by electrical impedance. It measures platelet GP IIb/IIIa dependent aggregation. However, this is only one aspect of platelet function and it does not directly measure platelet adhesion, the platelets effect on thrombin generation, the release of granules, or the initiation of inflammation. From a clinical viewpoint this technique has disadvantages including: 1) high cost; 2) sample volume; 3) the need for sample preparation; 4) the length of the assay time; and 5) the level of skill required. As a result, and in common with most tests of isolated platelet function, it is not suitable as a rapid point-of-care test.

Table 22.1 Currently utilized assays of response to antiplatelet therapy

Assay	Pros	Cons	Ability to assess responses to aspirin (A) and/or clopidogrel (C)	Methodology
Platelet aggregometry	Highly specific for platelet aggregation in response to specific platelet agonists.	High cost, poor reproducibility, high required sample volume, need for sample preparation, length of assay time, skill required. Aggregation is only one aspect of platelet function	A + C	Measures *ex vivo* glycoprotein IIb/IIIa devpendent platelet aggregation. Can be performed on platelet rich plasma by turbidometry or on whole blood by electrical impedance. Response to aspirin is assessed using stimulation with arachidonic acid and response to clopidogrel using stimulation with ADP
VASP platelet reactivity index	Specific biomarker for platelet P2Y12 receptor activation	Costly, complex assay	C	VASP is a protein that is phosphorylated in the presence of P2Y12 stimulation. It is therefore a biomarker of P2Y12 stimulation and can be measured using flow-cytometric based techniques
Biomarkers of arachidonic acid metabolism	Largely dependent on platelet COX-1	Levels are not platelet specific. Little data to support use	A	Aspirin suppresses production of thromboxane B2, a stable metabolite of thromboxane A2 which can be measured in serum and 11-dehydro-thromboxane B2 levels a stable metabolite measurable in the urine
PFA-100	Ease of use. Whole blood assay	Non-specific as highly dependent on Von Willebrand factor	A	The PFA-100 is a whole blood assay that measures the time for occlusion of an aperture in a membrane under high stress shear conditions. A cartridge containing a membrane coated with collagen and epinephrine has been used to study the effects of aspirin
VerifyNow®	Ease of use, automated, rapid, whole blood assay	Further data required on optimal cut-off values	A + C	The Accumetrics VerifyNow® system is a rapid, automated whole blood assay that measures agglutination of fibrinogen-coated beads in response to specific agonists for aspirin, thienopyridines and Glycoprotein IIb/IIIa inhibitors
Plateletworks®	Whole blood assay. Ease of use	Requires cell counter. Little evidence for use	A + C	The Plateletworks® system calculates platelet aggregation by comparing platelet count in ethylenediamine tetra-acetic acid (EDTA) collection tubes with citrate tubes with collagen and ADP stimulation using a standard cell counter
Thromb-elastograph (TEG) PlateletMapping®	Whole blood assay. Information on plasmatic as well as cellular aspects of coagulation	Sample preparation	A + C	Blood is placed in an oscillating cup within which a torsion wire is suspended. As blood clots, fibrin strands link the cup and torsion wire. The resulting torque generates an electrical signal which is plotted as a function of time to produce a TEG trace. The use of specific platelet activators allows the effects of antiplatelet therapies to be detected.

Multiple electrode platelet aggregometry

Multiple electrode platelet aggregometry, which can be performed in whole blood in only 10min and has been shown to correlate with standard aggregometry[51], may be more suitable for widespread clinical use.

Biomarkers of aspirin metabolism

The response to aspirin can also be assessed by measuring products of AA metabolism such as thromboxane B2, a stable metabolite of thromboxane A2, which can be measured in serum, or 11-dehydro-thromboxane B2 in the urine.

Point-of-care assays

Recently several assays have been developed which show some potential as point of care tests of the effects of antiplatelet medication. These include the PFA-100® (Dade Behring), the Accumetrics VerifyNow® system, Plateletworks® (Helena Laboratories), the Cone and Plate(let)® analyser (DiaMed) and the modified Thrombelastography (TEG) PlateletMapping® system (Haemoscope). This area is summarized in detail in reference 11.

Short TEG

'ShortTEG' is a modification of the TEG PlateletMapping® system, providing: 1) rapid results based on both the speed and strength of clot formation, and 2) an assessment of response to therapy without the need for a baseline sample using the percentage clotting inhibition. Validation data suggest that it can provide aspirin and clopidogrel response data in a 15-min test [52–54].

VerifyNow®

The VerifyNow® system, formerly known as the Ultegra® rapid platelet function analyser, is a rapid, automated whole blood assay that measures agglutination of fibrinogen-coated beads in response to specific agonists for aspirin, the P2Y12 receptor (for thienopyridines) and GP IIb/IIIa inhibitors. It is easy to use, does not require sample preparation, only requires a small sample volume, and provides rapid results.

Vasodilator-stimulated phosphoprotein (VASP)

VASP is a protein that is phosphorylated and dephosphorylated in the presence of P2Y12 stimulation and can therefore be used as a biomarker of P2Y12 stimulation. It is increasingly utilized as it is highly specific for P2Y12 stimulation but is a costly and time-consuming laboratory based assay.

Correlation between assays of response to antiplatelet therapy and outcome

Regardless of the scientific basis for these assays the most important factor for the clinician is how the test can aid clinical practice. Therefore, the correlation of results with clinical outcomes and evidence that altering therapy on the basis of these results improves outcomes remain the clinically dominant factor.

Responses to aspirin

Just as there are large numbers of assays available to assess aspirin response there are huge discrepancies in quoted rates of aspirin 'resistance' with reported prevalences ranging from 1–59.5%[11]. This discrepancy depends on the assay utilized, the definition of resistance, the patient group studied, and the methods employed for analysing compliance. Studies using methods which specifically analyse platelet aggregation in response to AA, such as optical aggregation and TEG, suggest that the true incidence is low[51]. Non-specific assays of platelet reactivity whilst on aspirin (e.g. the PFA-100®) tend to give much higher levels of 'resistance', which raises a question mark about their direct clinical relevance.

Biochemical aspirin 'resistance' has been associated with a higher incidence of myonecrosis post PCI when assessed with the VerifyNow® aspirin assay, PFA-100®, and LTA[55–58]. Furthermore, relative resistance has been reported in patients with previous ST[59]. In patients on aspirin, urinary 11-dehydro thromboxane B2 levels have also been correlated with clinical outcome[60]. It is interesting in this context that the PFA-100®, whilst non-specific and more a marker of generalized platelet reactivity than response to aspirin, has been shown to have a higher sensitivity and specificity than AA-induced platelet aggregometry in predicting myocardial necrosis post stenting in the context of NSTEMI[57]. It is tempting to speculate that this may be because it focuses on platelet function in the context of whole blood rather than in isolation.

Responses to clopidogrel

Regardless of the method of assessment there is consistently demonstrable interindividual variability in platelet inhibition in response to clopidogrel[11], with a near normal distribution of response to clopidogrel in patients undergoing PCI and stent insertion[61].

600-mg loading doses have been shown to increase speed of onset and reduce variability in response compared to 300-mg doses[18,62,63]. By contrast, studies of 900-mg loading doses have not shown consistent benefits above 600-mg doses[64–66] but have confirmed the superiority over 300-mg of both 900-mg and 600-mg doses in terms of platelet inhibition without an increase in the bleeding risk. L'Allier *et al.* have shown that two 600-mg loading doses 12h apart achieves superior platelet inhibition[67].

The standard and licensed maintenance dose of clopidogrel is 75mg daily. However, maintenance therapy with 150mg clopidogrel leads to greater inhibition of platelet aggregation than a 75-mg daily dose[68,69].

Several studies have shown that the degree of ADP-induced platelet aggregation post PCI correlates with subsequent ischaemic events and even death. High platelet reactivity whilst on clopidogrel assessed with the VerifyNow® P2Y12 assay is associated with an increased risk of ischaemic events after PCI, including ST. Furthermore, studies have also specifically suggested that relative hypo-responsiveness to clopidogrel increases the risk of ST (all summarized in Table 22.2).

Treatment modification on the basis of results of assays of response to therapy

Studies have shown that therapeutic manipulation by repeating the loading dose[70], increasing the maintenance dose of clopidogrel[69,70], adding cilostazol[38], or changing to ticlopidine[69] or prasugrel[71] improves the observed antiplatelet response. These strategies have decreased the rate of poor responders by 60–78.9% [70].

Bonnello used a strategy of VASP-guided clopidogrel loading prior to PCI, with up to three further 600-mg clopidogrel loading doses administered, to obtain adequate response. In addition to improving biochemical response this strategy led to significantly improved MACE rates at 30 days without being associated with an increased risk of bleeding[72].

The ACC/AHA/SCAI 2005 guidelines recommended increasing the dose of clopidogrel maintenance therapy in patients at high risk from ST in whom clopidogrel response is suboptimal. However, there are few reported studies into therapeutic manipulation, particularly looking at outcome measures, and as a result the level of evidence for this recommendation is only IIb/C[15].

The concept that clopidogrel response can be inadequate and directly clinically relevant in some patients, and that the 'poor' response can be modified and tailored to the individual raises the question as to why current practice takes no account of this variability.

Dealing with drug sensitivity and allergy

Aspirin

The most frequent adverse reactions to aspirin are gastrointestinal irritation where coadministration of a proton pump inhibitor often allows treatment to be continued. Hypersensitivity to aspirin is reported in up to 10% of patients undergoing PCI. Symptoms include exacerbation of asthma, urticaria, and rashes to angio-oedema and anaphylaxis. Rapid desensitization protocols have been developed which are reported to allow subsequent long-term treatment with aspirin in 88–94% after a protocol taking only 3–6h[73,74]. This should therefore allow aspirin to be initiated before PCI in the vast majority of cases, with the exception of primary PCI. There is no evidence that alternative treatments such as clopidogrel monotherapy or the addition of dipyridamole or cilostazol improve outcomes in the minority who do not tolerate desensitization.

Clopidogrel

Potentially allergic reactions to clopidogrel have been reported in up to 4% of patients, usually requiring drug discontinuation[75]. Reported adverse reactions include generalized urticarial reactions, thrombotic thrombocytopenic purpura, aplastic anaemia, neutropenia (in 0.1% of patients), gastrointestinal disturbance, and serum sickness. Historically ticlopidine has been substituted for clopidogrel when adverse reactions have occurred. However, ticlopidine has potentially life-threatening side effects of its own and some cross-reactivity has been described. Clopidogrel desensitization protocols have also been reported which have allowed continuation of clopidogrel. Substitution for ticlopidine is the only currently available option supported by the evidence in patients who remain intolerant of clopidogrel.

The case of Mr DW

Mr DW, a current smoker with treated hypertension and dyslipidaemia, presented with typical angina aged 60 years. Following a positive exercise test he underwent diagnostic angiography which showed two-vessel coronary disease suitable for PCI. However, whilst waiting for this procedure he presented with an anterior STEMI. He received prompt thrombolysis but failed to reperfuse and therefore underwent rescue PCI with the insertion of a DES to the LAD. He received 300mg of aspirin on presentation and a 600-mg loading dose of clopidogrel immediately prior to PCI, and abciximab during and after the procedure. He also underwent stent implantation to a diseased right coronary artery. He made a good recovery and was discharged home on day 5 on aspirin 75mg and clopidogrel 75mg daily, with advice on smoking cessation.

Stent thrombosis 1

He represented with a further anterior STEMI 3 months later. He was still smoking and gave a history of vomiting for 24h. He admitted to vomiting after his medication the day before presentation but otherwise stated he was fully compliant with medication. He was treated

Table 22.2 Associations between results of assays of response to antiplatelet therapy and adverse outcome

Assay	Correlation of results with adverse clinical events?	Reference
Platelet aggregometry	The degree of ADP-induced aggregation post PCI is higher in those with subsequent ischaemic events	Gurbel *et al.* 2005[62]
	Those with poorest response to clopidogrel, assessed with ADP-induced aggregation after a 600-mg loading dose of clopidogrel and prior to PCI, have higher levels of adverse events within 30 days of PCI	Hochholzer 2006
	Low response to clopidogrel by ADP-induced aggregation significantly increased the occurrence of cardiovascular events and death within 3 months of PCI	Geisler 2006
	In a cohort of 60 consecutive patients undergoing primary PCI for STEMI, 7 of 8 recurrent ischaemic episodes in the 6-month follow up period occurred in patients in the lowest quartile of platelet inhibition	Matetzky 2004
	Poor response to aspirin and clopidogrel by light transmission aggregometry has been found in patients with previous ST	Wenawesar 2005
	Poor response to clopidogrel by light transmission aggregometry has been found in patients with previous ST	Gurbel *et al.* 2005[62]
	High ADP-induced aggregation whilst on clopidogrel is predictive of stent thrombosis	Buonamici 2007
VASP platelet reactivity index	Independent predictor of stent thrombosis in patients on clopidogrel	Blindt *et al.* 2007[57]
	Significant differences in VASP phosphorylation between patients with previous stent thrombosis and PCI controls	Frere 2007 Gurbel *et al.* 2005[62]
Biomarkers of arachidonic acid metabolism	In patients on aspirin high levels of urinary 11-dehydro thromboxane B2 are associated with a higher risk of cardiovascular death	Eikelboom *et al.* 2002[60]
PFA-100	Has been shown to have greater sensitivity and specificity than AA-induced platelet aggregometry in predicting myocardial necrosis post PCI in the context of NSTEMI.	Marcucci 2007
VerifyNow®	Poor response to aspirin has been correlated with an increased incidence of peri-procedural myocardial infarction post PCI.	Chen *et al.* Price M 2008
	High platelet reactivity whilst on clopidogrel associated with increased events, including stent thrombosis.	Hobson *et al.* 2008[49]
	Increased risk of death, ACS and stroke (adjusted hazard ratio 2.71) in aspirin non-responders with stable coronary artery disease.	Cheng 2005
Thrombelastography (TEG)	High platelet reactivity by TEG PlateletMapping® demonstrated in patients with previous stent thrombosis	Hobson *et al.* 2008[49]
	On combining two measures from standard TEG demonstrated an odds ratio of 38 for ischaemic events following PCI.	Gurbel 2005

with primary PCI, receiving balloon angioplasty to a thrombotic occlusion of his LAD stent, producing TIMI III flow. Again he made a swift recovery, and was discharged home on aspirin 150mg and clopidogrel 75mg daily.

Stent thrombosis 2

Six months later (9 months after the initial event) he represented with a further anterior STEMI. He underwent primary PCI with balloon angioplasty to a thrombotic occlusion of his LAD stent. Intravascular ultrasound revealed good stent expansion but some residual disease at the stent outlet which was treated with further stent implantation. He developed acute pulmonary oedema post procedure and had evidence of moderate left ventricular dysfunction prior to discharge. He was discharged home on aspirin 150mg and clopidogrel 150mg daily.

Stent thrombosis 3

He represented with a further anterior STEMI 3 months later (his third episode of stent thrombosis, now 12 months after the initial presentation). Again he underwent primary percutaneous intervention for a thrombotic occlusion of his LAD stents. He required intensive treatment for left ventricular failure prior to discharge as well as implantation of a defibrillator for poor left ventricular function and evidence of non-sustained ventricular tachycardia. After 2 weeks of witnessed drug administration we undertook tests of response to antiplatelet therapy using TEG PlateletMapping® (see 'Short TEG' section). This revealed poor response to clopidogrel even at the 150mg dose (Fig. 22.1). He was therefore prescribed aspirin 300mg, clopidogrel 150mg, and warfarin with a target INR of 2.5 long term.

Stent thrombosis 4

Fourteen months later (now 26 months from initial presentation) he represented with an acute inferior STEMI. During primary PCI he was found to have a thrombotic occlusion of his RCA stent which was successfully reopened (Fig. 22.2) and also visible thrombus in his LAD stent (Fig. 22.3). Tests of response to antiplatelet therapy were performed on admission using both short TEG and VerifyNow® and revealed poor response to both aspirin and clopidogrel. His INR on admission was 1.2.

Despite the current lack of evidence we believe that tests of response to antiplatelet therapy are useful, particularly in these very high-risk cases, and with the increasing array of thienopyridines becoming available, will soon become mandatory in cases of stent thrombosis.

The future

Whilst (1) several different assays have shown that levels of response to antiplatelet therapy correlate with clinical outcome (summarized in Table 22.2) and (2) studies have shown that therapeutic manipulation can improve the level of observed response there remain many unanswered questions.

First, conventional assays have low positive predictive values and it would therefore currently be necessary to modify therapy in large numbers of patients, most of whom would not have gone on to suffer an adverse event in order to try to improve outcomes. It is currently unclear whether assays that determine response to antiplatelet therapy by comparison with a baseline sample or assays assessing platelet reactivity as a snapshot whilst on treatment provide superior risk stratification or prognostic information. It also remains unclear whether highly specific assays (such as VASP phosphorylation for clopidogrel) or non-specific assays (e.g. PFA-100® for aspirin) are preferable. As there are significant differences in baseline platelet aggregation, with higher levels of aggregation correlating with total mortality at long-term follow-up post treatment platelet reactivity rather than a percentage change from baseline may prove to be a more appropriate measure. A whole blood assay may also be preferable as platelet count and fibrinogen levels have also been associated with outcome and it avoids the need for sample preparation.

Conclusion

Coronary stent insertion is now the commonest form of cardiac revascularization. Technological advances have been swift and have lead to an ever-expanding envelope for the type of coronary disease that can be treated in this manner. Particularly important in this evolution has been the development of DES because of their ability to limit clinical restenosis. However, the prevention of ST with its associated high mortality has become a clinical priority. Whilst we have robust evidence that the combination of aspirin and clopidogrel is effective at reducing the incidence of ST, this complication continues to occur with devastating consequences. The pathophysiology of ST is likely to be multifactorial but suboptimal antiplatelet therapy contributes in a substantial proportion of cases and this occurs in several ways: 1) early cessation of therapy

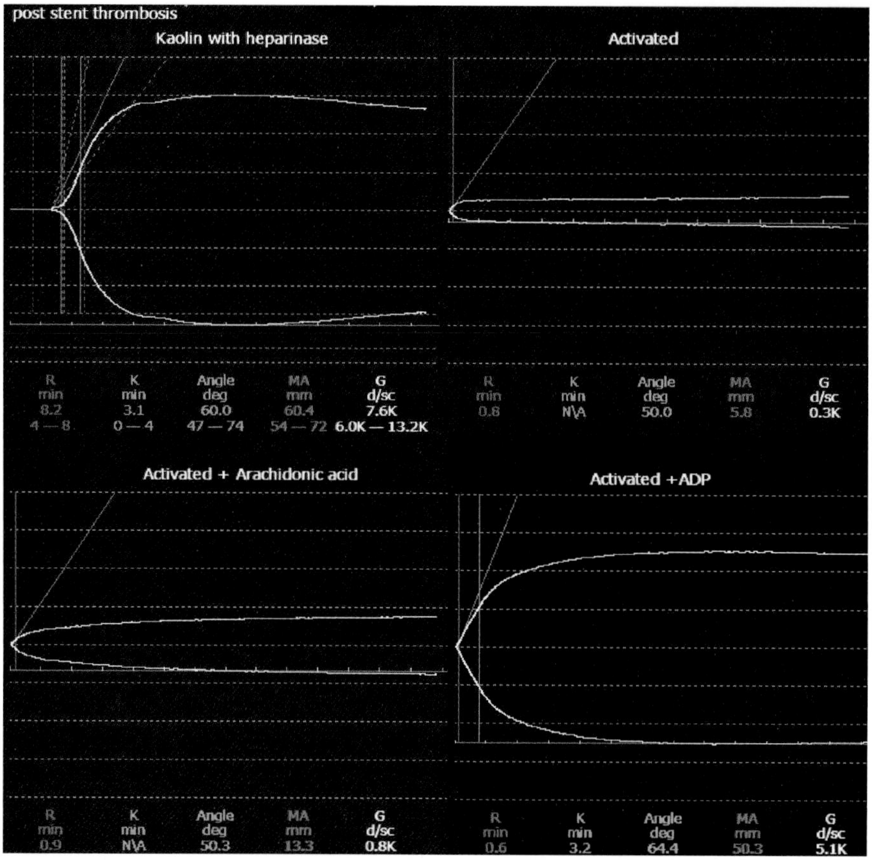

Fig. 22.1 TEG PlateletMapping® in Mr DW after ST3. The separation of the curve depends on the speed and strength of clot formation. The 4 channels are (i) a sample where platelets are maximally activated by reversing heparin and stimulating thrombin formation through the addition of kaolin; (ii) a heparinized sample with the addition of a fibrin activator—minimal platelet activation; (iii) a heparinized sample with fibrin activator and arachidonic acid (AA) to analyse response to aspirin and (iv) a heparinized sample with fibrin activator and ADP to analyse responses to clopidogrel. Whilst the addition of AA only leads to a small increase in clot formation compared to (ii), the addition of ADP leads to near maximal clot formation, signifying little effect of clopidogrel but a good response to aspirin.

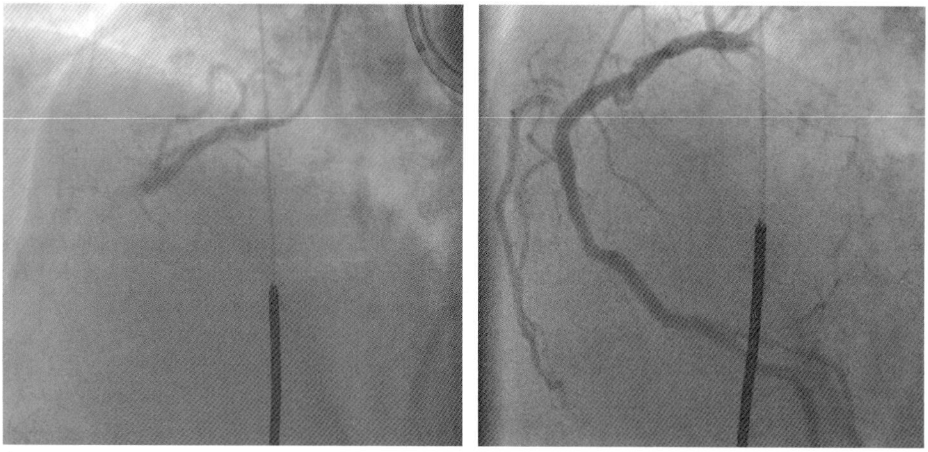

A B

Fig. 22.2 A coronary angiogram in LAO projection showing thrombotic occlusion at the ostium of the RCA stent (ST4) (A), and after treatment (B). The AICD lead and generator are also visible.

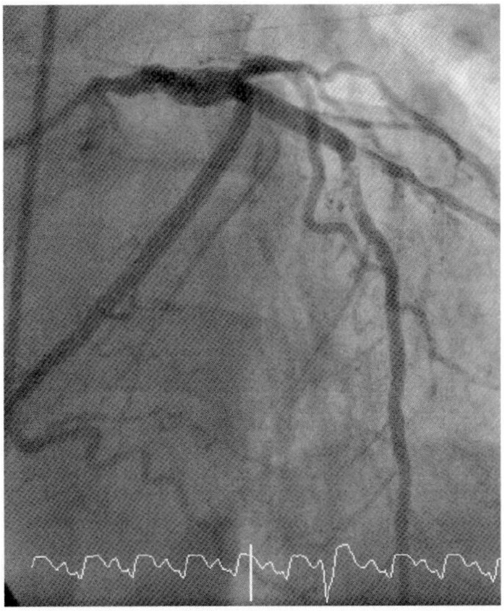

Fig. 22.3 Coronary angioram showing extensive thrombus within the LAD stents and ostium of diagonal at the time of RCA ST.

contravening accepted clinical practice guidelines; 2) cases with evidence of resistance to therapy, most commonly clopidogrel; and 3) there is the suspicion of a proinflammatory rebound effect upon cessation of clopidogrel therapy.

Ongoing trials such as GRAVITAS and OASIS-7 (investigating higher doses of clopidogrel), ISAR-SAFE (investigating the optimal duration of clopidogrel therapy post PCI), and DECADES (investigating clopidogrel cessation) will provide much needed evidence.

Our aim should, of course, be to minimize the contribution of suboptimal therapy on ST incidence. To prevent inappropriate early cessation of therapy requires excellent education of patients and other healthcare workers. However, to address 'resistance' it is likely that we need to individualize the antiplatelet therapy we administer to our stent patients, tailoring the drug and dose to the patient's response. That will only become possible in the intense and time-pressured world of clinical cardiology if rapid, easy-to-use, intuitive test(s) is/are available to facilitate such practice. Candidates for such a test all have potential disadvantages at present.

It may be that future antiplatelet therapy is delivered using agents to which the response is less heterogeneous, or even rendered obsolete by stent technology that does not require adjuvant antithrombotic treatment. For the foreseeable future, however, we continue to administer standard doses of drugs to stent patients despite the knowledge that variations in individual responses make it inevitable that we are not achieving therapeutic effect in some patients. The development of an ideal near-patient test with which to tailor antiplatelet therapy could represent an important therapeutic advance.

References

1. Moscucci M, Fox KAA, Cannon CP, *et al.* Predictors of major bleeding in acute coronary syndromes: the Global Registry of Acute Coronary Events (GRACE). *Eur Heart J* 2003; **24**:1815–23.
2. Rao SV, O'Grady K, Pieper KS, *et al.* Impact of bleeding severity on clinical outcome among patients with acute coronary syndromes. *Am J Cardiol* 2005; **96**:1200–6.
3. Yang X, Alexander KP, Chen AY, *et al.* The implications of blood transfusions for patients with non-ST-segment elevation acute coronary syndromes: Results from the CRUSADE National Quality Improvement Initiative. *J Am Coll Cardiol* 2005; **46**:1490–5.
4. Manoukian SV, Feit F, Mehran R, *et al.* Impact of major bleeding on 30-day mortality and clinical outcomes in patients with acute coronary syndromes: an analysis from the ACUITY trial. *J Am Coll Cardiol* 2007; **49**:1362–8.
5. Ndrepepa G, Berger PB, Mehilli J, *et al.* Periprocedural bleeding and 1-year outcome after percutaneous coronary interventions: appropriateness of including bleeding as a component of a quadruple end point. *J Am Coll Cardiol* 2008; **51**:690–7.
6. Feit F, Voeltz MD, Attubato MJ, *et al.* Predictors and impact of major haemorrhage on mortality following percutaneous coronary intervention from the REPLACE-2 trial. *Am J Cardiol* 2007; **100**:1364–9.
7. Bhatt DL, Fox KAA, Hacke W, *et al.* Clopidogrel and aspirin versus aspirin alone for the prevention of atherothrombotic events. *N Engl J Med* 2006; **354**:1706–17.
8. Stone GW, McLaurin BT, Cox DA, *et al.* for the ACUITY investigators. Bivalirudin for patients with acute coronary syndromes. *N Engl J Med* 2006; **355**:853–63.
9. Serruys PW, de Jaegere P, Kiemeneij F, *et al.* A comparison of balloon-expandable-stent implantation with balloon angioplasty in patients with coronary artery disease. Benestent Study Group. *N Engl J Med* 1994; **31**:489–95.
10. Bertrand ME, Rupprecht HJ, Urban, P, *et al.* Double-blind study of the safety of clopidogrel with and without a loading dose in combination with aspirin compared with ticlopidine in combination with aspirin after coronary stenting: the clopidogrel aspirin stent international cooperative study (CLASSICS). *Circulation* 2000; **102**:624–9.
11. Hobson AR, Curzen NP. Improving outcomes with antiplatelet therapies in percutaneous intervention. *Thromb Haemost* 2009; **101**:23–30.
12. Luscher T, Steffel J, Eberli F, *et al.* Drug-eluting stents and coronary thrombosis. Biological mechanisms and clinical implications. *Circulation* 2007; **115**:1051–8.
13. Iakovou I, Schmidt T, Bonizzoni E, *et al.* Incidence, predictors, and outcome of thrombosis after successful implantation of drug-eluting stents. *JAMA* 2005 **293**:2126–30.

14. Spertus JA, Kettelkamp R, Vance C, *et al.* (Prevalence, predictors, and outcomes of premature discontinuation of thienopyridine therapy after drug-eluting stent placement: results from the PREMIER registry. *Circulation* 2006; **113**:2803–9.
15. Smith SC Jr, Feldman TE, Hirshfeld JW Jr, *et al.* ACC/AHA/SCAI 2005 guideline update for percutaneous coronary intervention: a report of the American College of Cardiology / American Heart Association Task Force on Practice Guidelines (ACC/AHA/SCAI Writing Committee to Update 2001 Guidelines for Percutaneous Intervention). *Circulation* 2005; **113**:e166–e286.
16. Silber S, Albertsson P, Aviles FF, *et al.* Percutaneous coronary interventions: Guidelines for the European Society of Cardiology (ESC). *Eur Heart J* 2005; **26**:804–47.
17. Mehta SR, Yusuf S, Peters RJ, *et al.* Effects of pre-treatment with clopidogrel and aspirin followed by long-term therapy in patients undergoing percutaneous coronary intervention: the PCI-CURE study. *Lancet* 2001; **358**:527–33.
18. Cuisset T, Frere C, Quilici J, *et al.* Benefit of a 600-mg loading dose of clopidogrel on platelet reactivity and clinical outcomes in patients with non-ST segment elevation acute coronary syndrome undergoing coronary stenting. *J Am Coll Cardiol* 2006; **48**:1339–45.
19. Eisenstein EL, Anstrom KJ, Kong DF, *et al.* Clopidogrel use and long-term clinical outcomes after drug-eluting stent implantation. *JAMA* 2007; **297**:159–68.
20. Harjai K. GHOST: outcomes of drug-eluting compared to bare metal stents from the Guthrie Health System (2-3 year follow-up). Presented at Transcatheter Cardiovascular Therapeutics (TCT) meeting, 20-25 October 2007, Washington.
21. Ho MP, Peterson ED, Wang L, *et al.* Incidence of death and acute myocardial infarction associated with stopping clopidogrel after acute coronary syndrome. *JAMA* 2008; **299**:532–9.
22. Patrono C, Bachmann F, Baigent C, *et al.* Expert consensus document on the use of antiplatelet agents. *Eur Heart J* 2004; **25**:166–81.
23. Antithrombotic Trialists' Collaboration. Collaborative meta-analysis of randomised trials of antiplatelet therapy for prevention of death, myocardial infarction, and stroke in high risk patients. *BMJ* 2002; **324**:71–86.
24. Schwartz L, Bourassa MG, Lesperance J, *et al.* Aspirin and dipyridamole in the prevention of restenosis after percutaneous transluminal coronary angioplasty. *NEJM* 1998; **318**:1714–19.
25. Steinhubl SR, Berger P. What is the role for improved long-term antiplatelet therapy after percutaneous intervention? *Am Heart J* 2003; **145**:971–8.
26. Muller C, Buttner HJ, Peterson J, *et al.* A randomised comparison of clopidogrel and aspirin versus ticlopidine and aspirin after the placement of coronary-artery stents. *Circulation* 2000; **101**:590–3.
27. Steinhubl SR, Berger PB, Mann JT, *et al.* Early and sustained dual oral antiplatelet therapy following percutaneous coronary intervention: a randomized controlled trial. *JAMA*, 2002; **288**:2411–20.
28. Steinhubl SR, Berger PB, Brennan DM, *et al.* Optimal timing for the initiation of pre-treatment with 300mg clopidogrel before PCI. *J Am Coll Cardiol* 2006; **47**:939–43.
29. Patti G, Colonna G, Pasceri V, *et al.* Randomized trial of high loading dose of clopidogrel for reduction of periprocedural myocardial infarction in patients undergoing coronary intervention. *Circulation* 2005; **111**:2099–106.
30. Bonello L, Lemesle G, De Labriolle A, *et al.* Impact of a 600-mg loading dose of clopidogrel on 30-day outcome in unselected patients undergoing percutaneous coronary intervention. *Am J Cardiol* 2008; **102**:1318–22.
31. Balsano F, Rizzon P, Violi F *et al.* Antiplatelet therapy with ticlopidine in unstable angina: a controlled multicentre trial. *Circulation* 1990; **82**:17–26.
32. Bertrand ME, Legrand V, Boland J, *et al.* Randomized multicentre comparison of conventional anticoagulation versus antiplatelet therapy in unplanned and elective coronary stenting. The full anticoagulation vs aspirin and Ticlopidine (FANTASTIC) study. *Circulation* 1998; **98**:1597–603.
33. Richardson G, Curzen NP, Preston MA, *et al.* Failure to monitor ticlopidine: the case for clopidogrel. *Int J Cardiovasc Intervent* 2000; **3**:29–33.
34. Barnathan ES, Schwartz JS, Taylor L, *et al.* Aspirin and dipyridamole in the prevention of acute coronary thrombosis complicating coronary angioplasty. *Circulation* 1987; **76**:125–34.
35. Okuda K, Kimura Y, Yamashita K. Cilostazol. *Cardiovasc Drug Rev* 1993; **11**:451–65.
36. Lee SW, Park SW, Hong MK, *et al.* Comparison of cilostazol and clopidogrel after successful coronary stenting. *Am J Cardiol* 2005; **95**:859–62.
37. Park SJ, Shim WH, Ho DS *et al.* A paclitaxel-eluting stent for the prevention of coronary restenosis. *N Engl J Med* 2003; **348**:1537–45.
38. Lee BK, Lee SW, Park SW, *et al.* Effects of triple antiplatelet therapy (aspirin, clopidogrel, and cilostazol) on platelet aggregation and p-selectin expression in patients undergoing coronary artery stent implantation. *Am J Cardiol* 2007; **100**:610–14.
39. Lee SW, Park SW, Hong MK, *et al.* Triple versus dual antiplatelet therapy after coronary stenting: impact on stent thrombosis. *J Am Coll Cardiol* 2005; **46**:2833–7.
40. Brandt JT, Payne CD, Wiviott SD, *et al.* A comparison of prasugrel and clopidogrel loading doses on platelet function: magnitude of platelet inhibition is related to active metabolite formation. *Am Heart J* 2007; **153**:e9–16.
41. Wiviott SD, Antman EM, Winters KJ, *et al.*; JUMBO-TIMI 26 Investigators. Randomized trial of prasugrel (CS-747, LY640315), a novel thienopyridine P2Y12 antagonist, with clopidogrel in percutaneous intervention: results of the Joint Utilization of Medications to Block Platelets Optimally (JUMBO)-TIMI 26 trial. *Circulation* 2005; **111**:3366–73.
42. Wiviott SD, Brauwald E, McCabe CH, *et al.* for the TRITON-TIMI 38 Investigators (2007). Prasugrel vs clopidogrel in patients with acute coronary syndromes. *N Engl J Med*, **357**:2001–15.

43. Wiviott SD, Trenk D, Frelinger AL, *et al.* Prasugrel compared with high loading- and maintenance-dose clopidogrel in patients with planned percutaneous coronary intervention. The Prasugrel in Comparison to Clopidogrel for Inhibition of Platelet Activation and Aggregation – Thrombolysis in Myocardial Infarction 44 Trial. *Circulation* 2007; **116**:2923–2.
44. Husted S, Emanuelsson H, Hepinstall S, *et al.* Pharmacodynamics, pharmacokinetics, and safety of the oral reversible P2Y12 antagonist AZD6140 with aspirin in patients with atherosclerosis: a double-blind comparison to clopidogrel with aspirin. *Eur Heart J* 2006; **27**:1038–47.
45. Becker RC, Moliterno DJ, Jennings LK *et al.* Safety and tolerability of SCH 530348 in patients undergoing non-urgent PCI: a randomised, double-blind, placebo-controlled phase II study. *Lancet* 2009; **373**:919–28.
46. Wang YX, Vincelette J, da Cunha V, *et al.* A novel P2Y(12) adenosine diphosphate receptor antagonist that inhibits platelet aggregation and thrombus formation in rat and dog models. *Thromb Haemost* 2007; **97**:847–55.
47. Fujii K, Carlier S, Mintz G, *et al.* Stent underexpansion and residual reference vessel stenosis are associated with stent thrombosis after successful sirolimus-eluting stent implantation. *J Am Coll Cardiol* 2005; **45**:995–8.
48. Aoki J, Serruys PW, van Beusekom H, *et al.* Endothelial progenitor cell capture by stents coated with antibody against CD 34. *J Am Coll Cardiol* 2005; **45**:1574–9.
49. Hobson AR, McKenzie D, Kunadian V, *et al.* Malignancy: an unrecognised risk factor for coronary stent thrombosis? *J Inv Cardiol* 2008; **20**:E120–123.
50. Serebruany V, Pokor I, Kuliczkoski W, *et al.* Baseline platelet activity and response to clopidogrel in 257 diabetics among 822 patients with coronary artery disease. *Thromb Haemost* 2008; **100**:76–82.
51. Sibbing D, Braun S, Jawansky S, *et al.* Assessment of ADP-induced platelet aggregation with light transmission aggregometry and multiple electrode platelet aggregometry before and after clopidogrel treatment. *Thromb Haemost* 2008; **9**:121–6.
52. Hobson AR, Agarwala RA, Swallow RA, *et al.* Thrombelastography: Current clinical applications and its potential role in interventional cardiology. *Platelets* 2006; **17**:509–18.
53. Hobson A, Petley G, Dawkins K, *et* al. A novel fifteen minute test for assessment of individual time-dependent clotting responses to aspirin and clopidogrel using modified Thrombelastography. *Platelets* 2007; **18**:497–505.
54. Swallow R, Agarwala R, Dawkins K, *et* al. Thromboelastography: potential bedside tool to assess the effects of antiplatelet therapy? *Platelets* 2006; **17**:385–92.
55. Tantry US, Bliden KP, Gurbel PA. Overestimation of platelet aspirin resistance detection by thrombelastograph platelet mapping and validation by conventional aggregometry using arachadonic acid stimulation. *J Am Coll Cardiol* 2005; **46**:1705–9.
56. Crescente M, Di Castelnuovo A, Iacoviello L, *et al.* Response variability to aspirin as assessed by the platelet function analyzer (PFA)-100. A systematic review. *Thromb Haemost* 2008; **99**:14–26.
57. Chen WH, Lee PY, Ng W, *et al.* Aspirin resistance is associated with a high incidence of myonecrosis after non-urgent percutaneous intervention despite clopidogrel pre-treatment. *J Am Coll Cardiol* 2004; **43**:1122–6.
58. Marcucci R, Paniccia R, Antonucci E, *et al.* Residual platelet reactivity is an independent predictor of myocardial injury in acute myocardial infarction patients on antiaggregant therapy. *Thromb Haemost* 2007; **98**:844–51.
59. Wenaweser P, Dorffler MJ, Imboden K, *et al.* Stent thrombosis is associated with an impaired response to antiplatelet therapy. *J Am Coll Cardiol* 2005; **45**:1748–52.
60. Eikelboom JW, Hirsh J, Weitz JI, *et al.* Aspirin-resistant thromboxane biosynthesis and the risk of myocardial infarction, stroke or cardiovascular death in patients at high risk for cardiovascular events. *Circulation* 2002; **105**:1650–5.
61. Gurbel PA, Bliden KP, Hiatt BL, *et al.* Clopidogrel for coronary stenting: response variability, drug resistance and the effect of pre-treatment platelet reactivity. *Circulation* 2003; **107**:2908–13.
62. Gurbel PA, Bliden KP, Hayes KM, *et al.* The relation of dosing to clopidogrel responsiveness and the incidence of high post-treatment platelet aggregation in patients undergoing coronary stenting. *J Am Coll Cardiol* 2005; **45**:1392–6.
63. Angiolillo DJ, Fernandez OA, Bernardo E, *et al.* High clopidogrel loading dose during coronary stenting: effects on drug response and interindividual variability. *Eur Heart J* 2004; **25**:1903–10.
64. Montalescot G, Sideris G, Meulernan C, *et al.* A randomized comparison of high clopidogrel loading doses in patients with non-ST-segment elevation acute coronary syndromes: the ALBION (Assessment of the best loading dose of clopidogrel to blunt platelet activation, inflammation and ongoing necrosis) trial. *J Am Coll Cardiol* 2006; **48**:931–8.
65. Von Beckerath N, Taubert D, Pogatsa-Murray G, *et al.* Absorption, metabolization, and antiplatelet effects of 300-, 600-, and 900-mg loading doses of clopidogrel. Results from the ISAR-CHOICE trial. *Circulation* 2005; **112**:2946–50.
66. Price MJ, Coleman JL, Steinhubl SR, *et al.* Onset and offset of platelet inhibition after high-dose clopidogrel loading and standard daily therapy measured by a point-of-care assay in healthy volunteers. *Am J Cardiol* 2006; **98**:681–4.
67. L'Allier PL, Ducrocq G, Pranno N, *et al.* for the PREPAIR study investigators. Clopidogrel 600-Mg double loading dose achieves stronger platelet inhibition than conventional regimens. *J Am Coll Cardiol* 2008; **51**:1066–72.
68. Von Beckerath N, Kastrati A, Wieczorek A, *et al.* A double-blind, randomized study on platelet aggregation in patients treated with a daily dose of 150mg or 75mg od clopidogrel for 30 days. *Eur Heart J* 2007; **28**:1814–9.
69. Angiolillo DJ, Bernardo E, Palaguelos J, *et al.* Functional impact of high clopidogrel maintenance dosing in patients undergoing elective percutaneous intervention. *Thromb Haemost* 2008; **99**:161–8.

70. Neubauer H, Lask S, Engelhardt A, *et al.* How to optimise clopidogrel therapy? Reducing the low-response incidence by aggregometry-guided therapy modification. *Thromb Haemost* 2008; **99**:357–62.
71. Jakubowski JA, Payne CD, Li YG, *et al.* The use of the VerifyNow P2Y12 point-of-care device to monitor platelet function across a range of P2Y12 inhibition levels following prasugrel and clopidogrel administration. *Thromb Haemost* 2008; **99**:409–15.
72. Bonello L, Camoin JL, Armero S, *et al.* Tailored clopidogrel loading dose according to platelet reactivity monitoring to prevent acute and subacute stent thrombosis. *Am J Cardiol* 2009; **103**:5–10.
73. Silberman S, Neukirch-Stoop C, Steg PG. Rapid desensitisation procedure for patients with aspirin hypersensitivity undergoing coronary stenting. *Am J Cardiol* 2005; **95**:509–10.
74. Rossini R, Angiolillo DJ, Musumeci G, *et al.* Aspirin desensitisation in patients undergoing percutaneous interventions with stent implantation. *Am J Cardiol* 2008; **101**:786–9.
75. von Tiehl KF, Price MJ, Valencia R, *et al.* Clopidogrel desensitisation after drug-eluting stent placement. *J Am Coll Cardiol* 2007; **50**:2039–43.

CHAPTER 23

Current status of GP IIb/IIIa inhibitors

Tim Lockie and Simon Redwood

Introduction

The process of atheromatous plaque rupture is thought to underlie most acute coronary syndromes (ACS) and thus is a major cause of overall morbidity and mortality[1]. As a result, the costs in terms of healthcare expenditure of the consequences of acute plaque rupture are considerable[2]. The immediate and often catastrophic result of plaque rupture is intracoronary thrombosis resulting in vessel occlusion and myocardial infarction (MI)[3]. Over the last 20 years there has been a steady decline in the mortality rates from ACS[4] that has resulted from the successful implementation of therapies to attenuate the effects of plaque rupture that include fibrinolysis, percutaneous revascularization, antithrombotic therapy, and plaque stabilization. Glycoprotein (GP) IIb/IIIa receptor inhibitors are agents that have been developed to block the final common pathway that results in platelet aggregation, and following plaque rupture is a key process in coronary thrombosis. Despite the improvement in outcomes from ACS, however, the mortality rate still remains high and there is a need for critical appraisal of the use of currently available agents as well as the need for ongoing research and development of new agents and clinical techniques to improve outcomes further.

The pathophysiology of plaque rupture

Acute coronary syndromes

There is a wide variety of atheromatous lesion type found within the coronary arteries which are defined both by their histological and associated clinical features[5]. The first signs of atheromatous plaque formation can be seen within the first three decades of life; initially with infiltration of foam cells (type 1 lesions), followed by smooth muscle proliferation and lipid deposition (type II, 'fatty streaks'), and then the laying down of connective tissue (type III). These lesions tend not to be associated with any clinical features, such as angina pectoris, or form a substrate for ACS[5]. As they develop further these lesions become increasingly vulnerable to disruption with the formation of a soft, lipid-rich core and a progressively thinner fibrous cap that is prone to rupture (type IV–Va, 'atheroma')[6]. Progression in plaque development is accelerated by conditions such as hypertension, diabetes mellitus, hypercholesterolaemia, and smoking. Rupture of the fibrous cap exposes the highly thrombogenic material contained within the plaque to the circulating blood[7]. Platelets accumulate over a layer of fibrin forming the initial 'white clot' which lies directly above the disrupted plaque. In turn, this is enveloped by a fibrin and erythrocyte rich 'red clot' that propagates rapidly within the vessel lumen[8]. As the thrombus grows in size it reduces luminal blood flow leading to stasis and further expansion of the clot[9] with resultant unstable angina (UA) or MI[10]. Ruptured plaques with overlying thrombus are known as type VI, or 'complicated' lesions[i]. Vasospasm derived from underlying endothelial dysfunction in the atheromatous vessel wall together with local and systemic catecholamine release causes vasoconstriction and can impair flow further[12]. The microembolization of atherosclerotic and thrombotic debris into the coronary microcirculation also has an important effect and may cause continued attenuation of

---

[i] In the period after an ACS, thrombus over the disrupted lesion organizes and the lesion calcifies (type Vb) or fibroses (type Vc) into a chronic stenotic lesion[11].

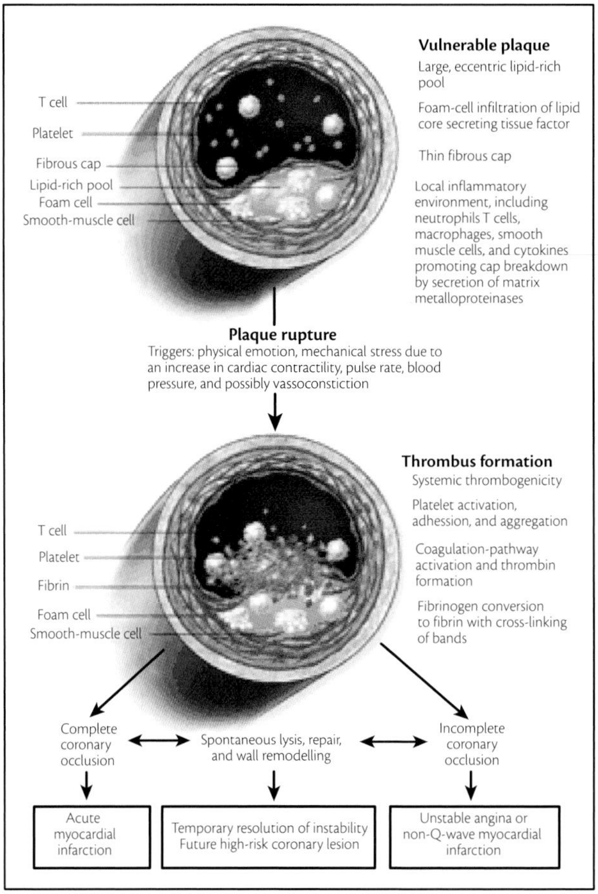

Fig. 23.1 Vulnerable plaque formation and rupture. Reproduced with permission from YeghiazariansY, Braunstein JB, Askari A, *et al.* Unstable angina pectoris. *NEJM* 2000; **342**(2):101–14.

myocardial blood flow even if the patency of the epicardial artery is restored(13). While fibrinolysis can dissipate the 'red' clot, additional antiplatelet therapy is required to attenuate formation of the platelet thrombus. Fibrinolysis can also have prothrombotic effects in the absence of antiplatelet agents and systemic anticoagulation by releasing thrombin that had been bound within the fibrin clot. Unopposed thrombin results in the conversion of fibrinogen to fibrin and stimulates further platelet aggregation (Fig. 23.1).

Percutaneous coronary intervention

While the spontaneous rupture of atherosclerotic plaque in a coronary artery can lead to ACS, plaque disruption also occurs during percutaneous coronary intervention (PCI) and is an inevitable part of the procedure in order to enlarge the lumen diameter. Such plaque disruption may cause thrombosis and vessel occlusion. Microembolization of atherosclerotic and thrombotic debris into the coronary microcirculation may also occur following PCI causing 'slow-flow' or 'no-reflow' and demonstrable myocardial necrosis as reflected by cardiac enzyme release, electrocardiographic abnormalities, and by contrast-enhanced cardiac magnetic resonance imaging(14). Given the increasing rates of PCI, especially in patients soon after ACS where the risk of these sequalae is increased, the use of adjunctive therapies that may minimize such complications is to be desired. Therapies that have been utilized include mechanical devices such as distal protection(15), and thrombus extraction(16). Concomitant pharmacotherapy includes optimum platelet blockade with clopidogrel(17) and glycoprotein IIb/IIIa inhibitors(18), and systemic anticoagulation with heparin-derived agents[19] and direct antithrombin agents such as bivalirudin[20]. While the benefit of mechanical devices is still to be established in large clinical trials there is an extensive body of evidence supporting the use of additional platelet inhibition and anticoagulation in selected patients scheduled for PCI.

The glycoprotein IIb/IIIa receptor (the $\alpha_{IIb}\beta_3$ integrin)

GP IIb/IIIa receptors are membrane glycoproteins with the $\alpha_{IIb}\beta_3$ integrin unique to the cell surface of platelets and megakaryocytes. Between 80 000–100 000 of these receptors are present on each platelet. Following plaque rupture, platelets are activated by coming into contact with the newly exposed subendothelium. Stimuli such as ADP, 5-HT, TXA_2, thrombin, and collagen activate the platelet through receptors present on its surface[21]. Once activated, the surface glycoproteins undergo conformational change that results in a high affinity for binding with fibrinogen, their principal ligand. This fibrinogen then links with GP IIb/IIIa receptors on other platelets and promotes platelet aggregation and the formation of a platelet plug that precipitates coronary thrombosis. Integrin binding affinity is dynamic and is dependent on the receptors' conformational status. In the resting state, the affinity for fibrinogen binding is low[22]. These changes to the GP IIb/IIIa receptor represent the final common pathway for platelet aggregation and thrombus formation (Fig. 23.2). Agents that block this receptor and prevent the binding of fibrinogen have been developed and extensively researched (Fig. 23.3). While there are logical reasons to suppose why such an approach would be expected to be beneficial, the results from the large clinical trials have been somewhat heterogeneous. The fundamental concept that appears to be essential to the effective reduction in ischaemic events by these agents is an adequate level of platelet GP IIb/IIIa receptor inhibition at the time of threatened thrombotic occlusion or atherothrombotic embolization. It was found from initial studies that greater than 80% receptor occupancy was considered optimal to maximize the benefits of these agents[23]. The apparent lack of consistency seen in the results from the large number of clinical trial examining the effects of these different agents possibly reflects the heterogeneity in the levels of inhibition that are obtained[24]. The following section will examine the different commercially available GP IIb/IIIa antagonists, their mode of action, and the major clinical trials examining their use.

The glycoprotein IIb/IIIa receptor inhibitors

There are three parenteral GP IIb/IIIa receptor inhibitors commercially available at present: abciximab (ReoPro®), eptifibatide (Integrelin®) and tirofiban (Aggrastat®).

Abciximab

Abciximab is a large chimeric monoclonal antibody that targets the GP IIb/IIIa receptor on the platelet surface in either the active or resting state. Although it has a high binding affinity for this receptor, abciximab is non-specific, also binding the vitronectin receptor on vascular smooth muscle cells and the MAC-1 receptor on monocytes[25]. The drug is administered intravenously at an initial bolus dose of 250mcg/kg body weight followed by a maintenance dose of 0.125mcg/kg/min (maximum 10mcg/min) for up to 36h, although it is commonly given as a 12-h infusion. Following the loading dose, a high proportion of the drug is rapidly taken up by platelet glycoprotein receptors with only a small amount remaining free in the plasma[26]. It is a large molecule and its strong binding results in a prolonged period of platelet inhibition that may last for up to 48h after the drug has been discontinued. This makes any reversal of the potent antiplatelet effect of abciximab difficult and can have important clinical implications. There is almost no renal excretion of the drug. It is dissipated slowly by being transferred to unoccupied receptor sites on other platelets, gradually reducing the antiplatelet effect and eventually undergoing protease degradation[27]. If rapid reversal of action is required then platelet transfusion is effective in speeding this process. Abciximab is a monoclonal antibody and has the potential for the formation of human antichimeric antibodies (HACA) that occurs in about 6–7% of patients[28]. Although the significance of this is unclear there is concern that this may predispose to immune-mediated hypersensitivity reactions and profound thrombocytopenia on subsequent re-administrations of the drug. The prevalence of severe and profound thrombocytopenia in patients who were re-administered abciximab (2.8% and 2% respectively) was 3–4 times greater than that observed after first-time administration[29]. Neither of the small-molecule GP IIb/IIIa inhibitors is immunogenic.

Eptifibatide and tirofiban

In contrast to abciximab, eptifibatide and tirofiban are synthetic small molecule GP IIb/IIIa receptor inhibitors

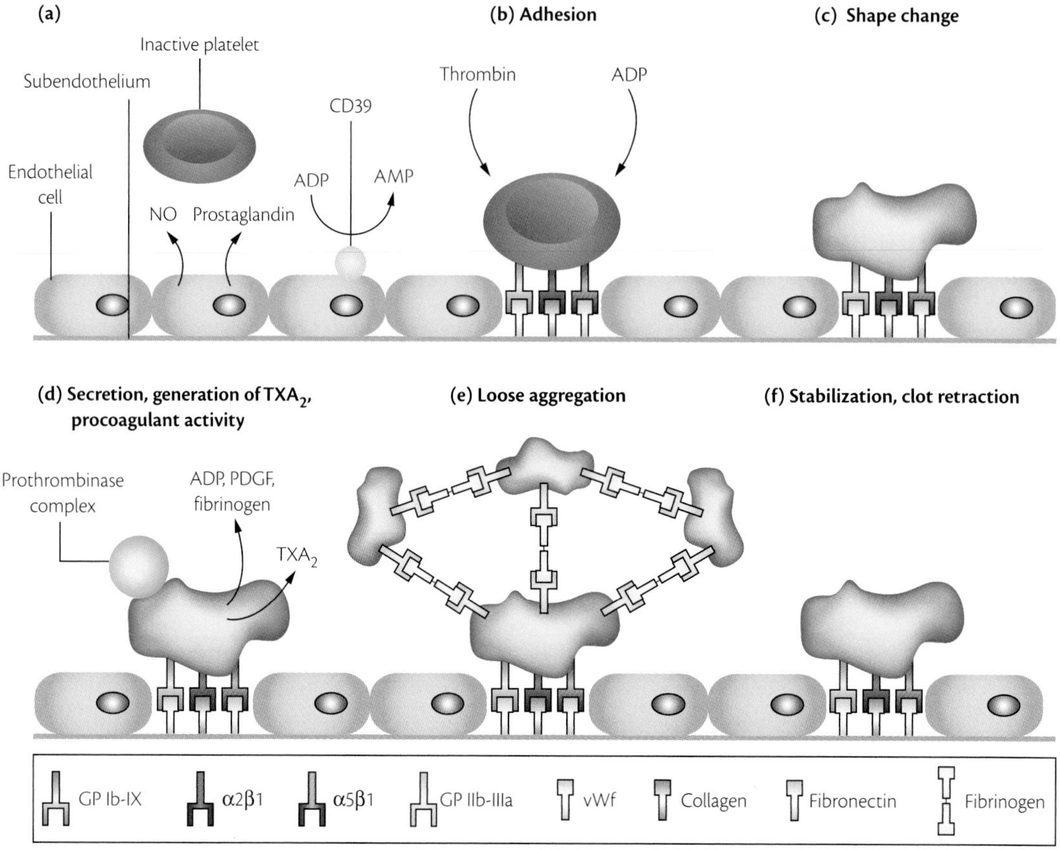

Fig. 23.2 A) Circulating platelets are usually kept in an inactive state by prostacyclin and nitric oxide (NO) released by the endothelial cells that line the walls of blood vessels. Endothelial cells also express CD39 on their surface, which inhibits platelet activation by converting adenosine diphosphate (ADP), a potent inducer of platelet activation, into adenosine monophosphate (AMP). B, C) At sites where the blood vessel wall has been injured, the platelets adhere to the exposed subendothelium through interactions between collagen, von Willebrand factor, and fibronectin and their receptors on the platelets, integrin alpha2beta1, glycoprotein Ib-IX (GP Ib-IX), and integrin alpha5beta1, respectively. Both thrombin and ADP cause platelets to change into an active conformation. D) Activated platelets secrete ADP, platelet-derived growth factor, and fibrinogen from storage granules in the platelet, and thromboxane A2 (TXA2), produced by immediate biosynthesis. ADP and TXA2 cause circulating platelets to change shape and become activated. E) Glycoprotein IIb/IIIa receptors on the surface of activated platelets bind fibrinogen, leading to the formation of fibrinogen bridges between the platelets, resulting in platelet aggregation. This, and the simultaneous formation of a fibrin mesh (not shown), lead to the formation of a platelet thrombus. F) Clot retraction then leads to formation of a stable thrombus. Reproduced with permission from MacMillan Publishers Ltd., from Bhatt DL, Topol EJ. Scientific and therapeutic advances in antiplatelet therapy *Nat Rev Drug Discov* 2003; **2**:15–28 © 2003

that bind with platelets only when they are in the active form. They exhibit differing pharmacokinetics to abciximab by binding the receptor with low affinity but in a much more specific and dose-dependent manner. This competitive and highly reversible mode of action results in a large proportion of the drug freely circulating in the plasma during steady-state. Eptifibatide is a cyclic heptapeptide small-molecule and is administered intravenously with an initial bolus dose of 180mcg/kg body weight followed by a maintenance dose of 2.0mcg/kg/min for up to 72h, although it has been used for longer periods of time up to 96h. Tirofiban is a non-peptide tyrosine derivative and is administered intravenously at an initial dose of 0.4mcg/kg/min for 30min followed by a maintenance dose of 0.1mcg/kg/min for at least 48h up to 108h maximum. Both eptifibatide and tirofiban exhibit first-order kinetics and are predominantly renally excreted. They have a short action of platelet

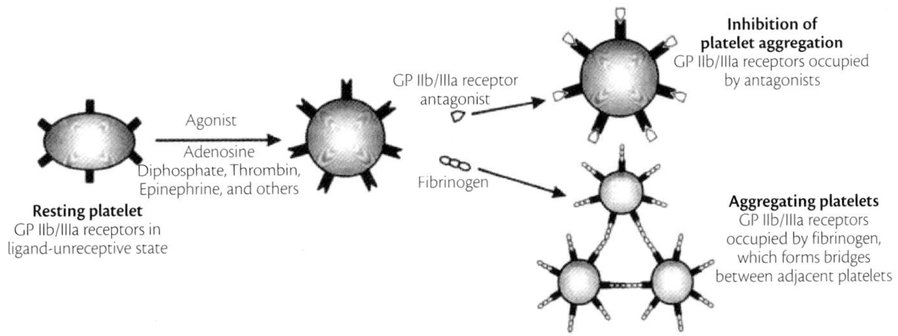

Fig. 23.3 Showing mechanism of action of GP IIb/IIIa inhibitors. Adapted with permission from Lefkovits J, Plow EF, Topol EJ. Platelet glycoprotein IIb/IIIa receptors in cardiovascular medicine. *N Engl J Med* 1995; **332**:1553–9. Copyright ©1995 Massachusetts Medical Society. All rights reserved.

inhibition compared to abciximab (eptifibatide, 2–4h; tirofiban 4–8h). In the case of the need for rapid reversal, platelet transfusion is of little benefit as a large proportion of the drug is non-receptor bound and the receptor sites on the new platelets are simply bound by the freely circulating drug. See Table 23.1.

Clinical use of glycoprotein IIb/IIIa inhibitors

PCI in stable coronary artery disease

The primary clinical endpoint of the clinical trials examining the role of GP IIb/IIIa inhibitors in conjunction with PCI has been the impact on the incidence of 30-day ischaemic composite endpoints. These endpoints generally comprise the clinical events of death, MI, and the need for urgent repeat revascularization procedures. Over 15 000 patients have been studied in several large randomized trials (see later sections). All three agents have been evaluated in this setting although abciximab has been studied the most thoroughly. There has been considerable variation in the duration of post-PCI infusions of agents between the different trials with generally shorter duration used for abciximab (12h) compared to eptifibatide (18–24h) or tirofiban (18–36h). These differences may explain in part some of the inconsistent

Table 23.1 Summary of GP IIb/IIIa inhibitor agents commonly used

	Abciximab	Eptifibatide	Tirofiban
Class	Monoclonal antibody fragment	Cyclic heptapeptide	Non-peptide
Mechanism of action	Binds receptor causing steric hindrance and conformational changes	Mimics native protein sequence in receptor	Mimics native protein sequence in receptor
Size	Large (48kDa)	Small (0.8kDa)	Small (0.5kDa)
Affinity and receptor binding	High affinity; non-specific	Low affinity; highly specific for GP IIb/IIIa receptor	Low affinity; highly specific for GP IIb/IIIa receptor
Duration of platelet inhibition	Long acting 24–48h	Short-acting 2–4h	Short acting 4–8h
Half-life	30min (plasma) 12–16h (platelet-bound)	0.85–2.8h Seconds	1.2–2h Seconds
Elimination	Protease degredation	Mostly renal	Renal
Dose	250mcg/kg bolus + infusion 0.125mcg/kg/min (max10mcg/min) for up to 36h	180mcg/kg bolus + infusion 2.0mcg/kg/min for up to 72h	0.4mcg/kg/min for 30min + maintenance dose of 0.1mcg/kg/min for at least 48h up to 108h

results from the trials due to potentially 'inadequate' platelet inhibition during and after PCI.

Abciximab

In the Evaluation in Percutaneous Transluminal Coronary Angioplasty to Improve Long-term Outcome with Abciximab GP IIb/IIIa Blockade (EPILOG) trial[30], a prospective, double-blind trial, patients at 69 centres were randomized to receive abciximab with standard-dose, weight-adjusted heparin (initial bolus of 100U per kg of body weight); abciximab with low-dose, weight-adjusted heparin (initial bolus of 70U per kg); or placebo with standard-dose, weight-adjusted heparin. The primary efficacy endpoint was death from any cause, MI, or urgent revascularization within 30 days of randomization. Interestingly, planned stenting was an exclusion criterion. The trial was terminated at the first interim analysis, with 2792 of the planned 4800 patients enrolled. At 30 days, the composite event rate was 11.7% in the group assigned to placebo with standard-dose heparin; 5.2% in the group assigned to abciximab with low-dose heparin (hazard ratio, 0.43; 95% confidence interval [CI], 0.30–0.60; p <0.001); and 5.4% in the group assigned to abciximab with standard-dose heparin (hazard ratio, 0.45; 95% CI, 0.32–0.63; p <0.001). There were no significant differences among the groups in the risk of major bleeding, although minor bleeding was more frequent among patients receiving abciximab with standard-dose heparin. The Evaluation of Platelet IIb/IIIa Inhibitor for Stenting (EPISTENT) trial[18], at 63 hospitals in the United States and Canada, randomly assigned 2399 patients undergoing percutaneous revascularization to stenting plus placebo (n = 809), stenting plus abciximab, a IIb/IIIa inhibitor (n = 794), or balloon angioplasty plus abciximab (n = 796). Again, the primary endpoint was a combination of death, MI, or need for urgent revascularization in the first 30 days. All patients received heparin, aspirin, and standard pharmacological therapy. Fifty-seven per cent of patients in the study had UA or recent MI. The primary endpoint occurred in 10.8% patients in the stent plus placebo group, 5.3% in the stent plus abciximab group (p<0.001), and 6.9% in the balloon plus abciximab group (p = 0.007).

Together these studies suggest that patients receiving abciximab showed a 4.5–6.5% absolute reduction in the risk for the 30-day composite endpoint of death, MI, or urgent revascularization. This translates to a 35–56% relative risk reduction for the composite endpoint. The majority of the effect was due to the reduction in non-fatal MI and the need for urgent repeat revascularization. Diabetic patients seem to derive particular benefit in the EPISTENT trial where they formed a pre-specified sub-group. Within this group the composite endpoint occurred in 25.2% of the stent-placebo group compared to 13% of the stent-abciximab group (p <0.005). A 51% reduction in target-vessel revascularization at 6 months (p = 0.02) was also noted in the diabetic group who received abciximab although these findings have yet to be replicated in other trials. Although there was a trend to a reduction in mortality in EPILOG, only the EPISTENT trial showed a statistically significant reduction in mortality at 1-year follow-up with a 60% relative risk reduction in the abciximab plus stent group compared to the other treatment groups[31]. Pooled-data of patients with diabetes mellitus was examined from the EPIC, EPILOG, and EPISTENT trials and abciximab was found to reduce the mortality of diabetic patients to the level of placebo-treated non-diabetic patients (4.5% vs. 2.5%). The effect was particularly noted in diabetic patients who were also obese and hypertensive and those patients with diabetes undergoing multi-vessel disease[32]. However, the ISAR-SWEET[33] prospective study examined diabetic patients undergoing elective PCI who received a 600-mg loading dose of clopidogrel and excluded patients with ACS and/or a visible thrombus. No improvement was found in the abciximab group, possibly because of the beneficial effect of the clopidogrel.

The effect of clopidogrel was investigated in the ISAR-REACT trial[34] which compared abciximab with placebo in a randomized trial in low-risk patients undergoing PCI who had been loaded with high-dose clopidogrel (600mg orally) 2h before the procedure and then continued the clopidogrel for 3 months (75mg od). At 30 days, there was no difference between the groups suggesting that the benefit of additional GP IIb/IIIa inhibitor therapy in low-risk PCI patients adequately loaded with clopidogrel may be limited. The study, however, may have been underpowered to demonstrate a benefit of abciximab in such a patient group. In select patients, however, with complex lesions and an unstable peri-procedural course abciximab may be useful[35].

Eptifibatide

The benefit of eptifibatide to reduce events in PCI was evaluated in the Integrelin to Manage Platelet Aggregation to prevent Coronary Thrombosis-II (IMPACT-II) trial[36]. This was a double-blind, placebo-controlled trial at 82 centres in the United States, enrolling 4010 patients undergoing elective, urgent, or emergency coronary intervention. Patients were assigned one of three treatments: placebo (n = 1328), a bolus of 135mcg/kg eptifibatide followed by an infusion of 0.5mcg/kg/min for 20–24h (n = 1349), or 135mcg/kg eptifibatide bolus with a 0.75mcg/kg/min infusion (n = 1333). The coronary procedure was started within 10–60min of the start of study treatment. The primary endpoint was the 30-day composite occurrence of death, MI, unplanned surgical or repeat percutaneous revascularization, or coronary stent implantation for abrupt closure (by intention to treat). By 30 days, the composite endpoint had occurred in 151 (11.4%) patients in the placebo group compared with 124 (9.2%) in the 135/0.5 eptifibatide group (p = 0.063) and 132 (9.9%) in the eptifibatide 135/0.75 group (p = 0.22). By treatment-received analysis, the 135/0.5 regimen produced a significant reduction in the composite endpoint (11.6 vs. 9.1%, p = 0.035), but the 135/0.75 regimen did not produce a significant reduction (11.6 vs.10.0%, p = 0.18). A potential reason for the reduced clinical effect seen in the IMPACT-II trial may have been problems with the assay used to measure platelet activity that resulted in lower than optimal doses of eptifibatide being used[37].

The Enhanced Suppression of the Platelet IIb/IIIa Receptor with Integrelin Therapy (ESPRIT) trial[38] re-examined the effect of eptifibatide on patients undergoing PCI but used a fourfold higher dose than in IMPACT-II. 2064 patients were recruited in a multicentre study. Immediately before PCI, patients were randomly allocated to receive eptifibatide, given as two 180mcg/kg boluses 10min apart and a continuous infusion of 2.0mcg/kg/min for 18–24h, or placebo, in addition to aspirin, heparin, and a thienopyridine. The primary endpoint was again the composite of death, MI, urgent target vessel revascularization, and thrombotic bailout glycoprotein IIb/IIIa inhibitor therapy within 48h after randomization. The trial was terminated early for efficacy. The primary composite endpoint was reduced from 10.5% to 6.6% with treatment (p = 0.0015). The key secondary endpoint (composite of death, MI, or urgent target vessel revascularization at 30 days) was also reduced, from 10.5% to 6.8% (p = 0.0034). The benefit of eptifibatide was sustained still being present at 6 months and 1 year[39,40]. The majority of the benefit, like many of these trials, was from reduction in MI and although there was a trend towards a reduction in mortality this was not statistically significant.

Tirofiban

There have been few trials examining the use of tirofiban in stable patients undergoing routine PCI. A small, single-centre study involving 93 patients served as a dose-ranging and safety study[41]. The Do Tirofiban And Reopro Give Similar Efficacy Outcomes Trial (TARGET)[42] used double-blind, double-dummy design at 149 hospitals in 18 countries and was designed and statistically powered to demonstrate the non-inferiority of tirofiban as compared with abciximab. Patients were randomly assigned to receive either tirofiban or abciximab before undergoing PCI with the intent to perform stenting. The primary endpoint was a composite of death, non-fatal MI, or urgent target-vessel revascularization at 30 days. The primary endpoint occurred more frequently among the 2398 patients in the tirofiban group than among the 2411 patients in the abciximab group (7.6% vs. 6.0%; hazard ratio, 1.26; one-sided 95% CI1.51, demonstrating lack of equivalence, and two-sided 95% CI 1.01–1.57, demonstrating the superiority of abciximab over tirofiban; p = 0.038). The majority of the difference in composite endpoint was due to a lower incidence of MI. The relative benefit of abciximab was consistent regardless of age, sex, the presence or absence of diabetes, or the presence or absence of pre-treatment with clopidogrel. There were no significant differences in the rates of major bleeding complications or transfusions, but tirofiban was associated with a lower rate of minor bleeding episodes and thrombocytopenia. It was suggested that an insufficient dosing regimeN and patients failing to reach adequate levels of platelet inhibition perhaps attenuated the clinical benefit of tirofiban in this study. This issue was due to be addressed in the TENACITY trial[43], a multicentre study comparing tirofiban at a higher dose to abciximab in patients undergoing PCI but was stopped early due to lack of funding.

Non ST-elevation acute coronary syndromes

A large number of patients have been studied in trials assessing the benefit of administration of GP IIb/IIIa inhibitors in ACS. These studies have utilized many different trial designs and definitions for clinical endpoints that must be considered in their evaluation. In some trials PCI was planned per protocol (CAPTURE[44], EPIC[32], RESTORE[45], ISAR-REACT 2[46], PRISM-PLUS[47]) and in others an invasive strategy was discouraged (GUSTO-IV[48], PRISM[49], and PARAGON[50]) or left to the discretion of the operator (PURSUIT[51]). Even in the older studies with planned PCI, stent rates were generally low, only 7.6% in CAPTURE and below 2% in EPIC and RESTORE where stenting was discouraged.

GP IIb/IIIa inhibitors without planned PCI in ACS

In the GUSTO-IV ACS trial, 7800 ACS patients treated with aspirin and either unfractionated heparin (UFH) or low-molecular weight heparin (LMWH) were randomized to an abciximab bolus and 24 h infusion, an abciximab bolus and 48-h infusion, or placebo. The trial found no reduction in the composite endpoints at 30 days and an increase in bleeding from abciximab treatment[(48)]. The PURSUIT trial was designed to allow investigators to treat patients according to institutional standard practice without mandated revascularization protocols. 10 948 ACS patients were randomly assigned, in a double-blind manner, to receive a bolus and infusion of either eptifibatide or placebo, in addition to standard therapy, for up to 72h (or up to 96h, if coronary intervention was performed near the end of the 72-h period). The primary endpoint was a composite of death and non-fatal MI occurring up to 30 days after the index event. As compared with the placebo group, the eptifibatide group had a 1.5% absolute reduction in the incidence of the primary endpoint (14.2% vs. 15.7% in the placebo group; p = 0.04). The benefit was apparent by 96h and was still apparent at 30 days. Benefits were most marked in those that underwent early PCI within the first 72h (n = 1228) with a 31% reduction in the incidence of the composite endpoint of death or non-fatal MI at 30 days in those treated with eptifibatide, as compared to placebo (11.6% vs. 16.6%, p = 0.01)[(51)]. Indeed, at 30 days eptifibatide had no significant effect over placebo in patients who did not receive early PCI[ii].

In the Platelet Receptor Inhibition in Ischemic Syndrome Management (PRISM) trial, a double-blind study, 3232 patients who were already receiving aspirin were randomly assigned to additional treatment with intravenous tirofiban for 48h. The primary endpoint was a composite of death, MI, or refractory ischemia at 48h. The incidence of the composite endpoint was 32% lower at 48h in the group that received tirofiban (3.8%, vs. 5.6% with heparin; risk ratio, 0.67; 95% CI, 0.48–0.92; p = 0.01). Percutaneous revascularization was only performed in 1.9% of the patients during the first 48h. At 30 days, the frequency of the composite endpoint (with the addition of readmission for UA) was similar in the two groups (15.9% in the tirofiban group vs. 17.1% in the heparin group, p = 0.34). There was a trend toward a reduction in the rate of death or MI with tirofiban and mortality was 2.3%, as compared with 3.6% in the heparin group (p = 0.02). Major bleeding occurred in 0.4% of the patients in both groups.

The Platelet IIb/IIIa Antagonism for the Reduction of Acute coronary syndrome events in a Global Organization Network (PARAGON A) study tested the benefit of different doses of lamifiban (an alternative small-molecule GP IIb/IIIa inhibitor) alone and in combination with heparin in ACS patients undergoing initial medical therapy without revascularization unless clinically necessitated[(50)]. The composite primary endpoint of death or non-fatal MI at 30 days was no different between the groups compared to standard therapy. By 6 months, this composite was lowest for those assigned to low-dose lamifiban (p = 0.027) and intermediate for those assigned to high-dose lamifiban (p = 0.450) compared with control (13.7%, 16.4%, and 17.9%, respectively).

A large meta-analysis of six trials that included 31 402 patients with ACS for whom an interventional strategy was not planned found a 9% relative reduction in the odds of death or MI at 30 days in patients treated with GP IIb/IIIa inhibitors compared to placebo (10.8 vs. 11.8%; OR, 0.91; 95% CI, 0.84–0.98; p = 0.015)[(52)]. The event reduction was greatest in patients at greatest risk of thrombotic complications as suggested by raised troponin levels. Major bleeding complications were increased by treatment with GP IIb/IIIa inhibitors (2.4% vs. 1.4%, p <0.0001). See Fig. 23.4.

GP IIb/IIIa inhibitors with planned PCI in ACS

The Chimeric c7E3 FAB Antiplatelet Therapy in Unstable Refractory Angina (CAPTURE) trial examined 1265 patients with refractory UA to investigate whether serum troponin T levels identify patients most likely to benefit from treatment with abciximab[(44)]. Serum troponin T levels at the time of study entry were elevated (above 0.1ng/mL) in 275 patients (30.9%). Among patients receiving placebo, the risk of death or non-fatal MI was related to troponin T levels. The 6-month cumulative event rate was 23.9% among patients with elevated troponin T levels, as compared with 7.5% among patients without elevated troponin T levels (p <0.001). Among patients treated with abciximab, the respective 6-month event rates were 9.5% for patients with elevated troponin T levels and 9.4% for

ii Some caution must be expressed in this subgroup analysis, as the patients were selected for early PCI in a non-randomized fashion.

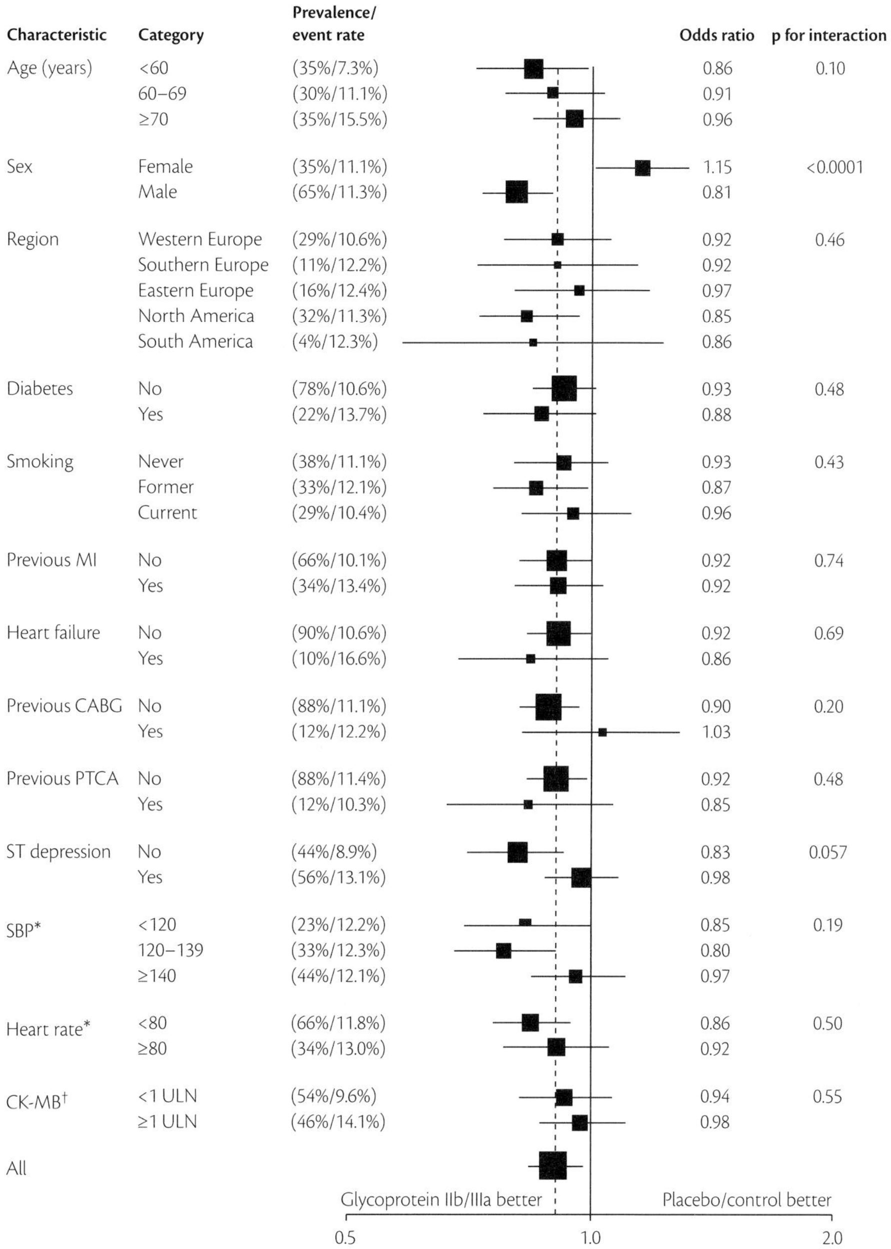
Characteristic
Category
Prevalence/ event rate
Odds ratio
p for interaction
Age (years) <60 (35%/7.3%) 0.86 0.10
60–69 (30%/11.1%) 0.91
≥70 (35%/15.5%) 0.96
Sex Female (35%/11.1%) 1.15 <0.0001
Male (65%/11.3%) 0.81
Region Western Europe (29%/10.6%) 0.92 0.46
Southern Europe (11%/12.2%) 0.92
Eastern Europe (16%/12.4%) 0.97
North America (32%/11.3%) 0.85
South America (4%/12.3%) 0.86
Diabetes No (78%/10.6%) 0.93 0.48
Yes (22%/13.7%) 0.88
Smoking Never (38%/11.1%) 0.93 0.43
Former (33%/12.1%) 0.87
Current (29%/10.4%) 0.96
Previous MI No (66%/10.1%) 0.92 0.74
Yes (34%/13.4%) 0.92
Heart failure No (90%/10.6%) 0.92 0.69
Yes (10%/16.6%) 0.86
Previous CABG No (88%/11.1%) 0.90 0.20
Yes (12%/12.2%) 1.03
Previous PTCA No (88%/11.4%) 0.92 0.48
Yes (12%/10.3%) 0.85
ST depression No (44%/8.9%) 0.83 0.057
Yes (56%/13.1%) 0.98
SBP* <120 (23%/12.2%) 0.85 0.19
120–139 (33%/12.3%) 0.80
≥140 (44%/12.1%) 0.97
Heart rate* <80 (66%/11.8%) 0.86 0.50
≥80 (34%/13.0%) 0.92
CK-MB† <1 ULN (54%/9.6%) 0.94 0.55
≥1 ULN (46%/14.1%) 0.98
All
Glycoprotein IIb/IIIa better
Placebo/control better
0.5
1.0
2.0

Fig. 23.4 Showing odds ratio of 30-day death or myocardial infarction in 31 402 presenting with ACS but not scheduled for early PCI. Odds ratio represents pooled trial-specific odds ratios by the method of Cochrane-Mantel-Haenszel. Data are presented on a logarithmic scale. p value corresponds with subgroup treatment interaction term in a logistic regression model, with adjustment for between-trial outcome differences. Blood pressure and heart rate not recorded in GUSTO-IV. †Data on creatine kinase MB missing in 7469 patients. CABG, coronary-artery bypass graft; CK, creatine kinase; MI, myocardial infarction; PTCA, percutaneous transluminal coronary angioplasty; SBP, systolic blood pressure. Reproduced from Boersma E, Harrington RA, Moliterno DJ, *et al.* Platelet glycoprotein IIb/IIIa inhibitors in acute coronary syndromes. *Lancet* 2003; **360**:342–3, with permission from Elsevier.

those without elevated levels. As compared with placebo, the relative risk of death or non-fatal MI associated with treatment with abciximab in patients with elevated troponin T levels was 0.32 (95% CI, 0.14–0.62; p = 0.002). The lower event rates in patients receiving abciximab were attributable to a reduction in the rate of MI (odds ratio [OR] 0.23; 95% CI 0.12–0.49; p <0.001). In patients without elevated troponin T levels, there was no benefit of treatment with respect to the relative risk of death or MI at 6 months (OR 1.26; 95% CI 0.74–2.31; p = 0.47). This study suggests that serum troponin T level can be used to identify a high-risk subgroup of patients with ACS who are scheduled for PCI who are likely to benefit particularly from treatment with abciximab[(44)].

The Evaluation of c73 for the Prevention of Ischaemic Complications (EPIC) trial was a prospective, randomized, double-blind trial involving 2099 patients treated at 56 centres scheduled to undergo coronary angioplasty or atherectomy in high-risk clinical situations involving severe UA, evolving acute MI, or high-risk coronary morphologic characteristics[(28,53)]. Abciximab was compared to placebo and patients received a bolus and an infusion of drug. At 30 days, a 35% relative reduction in the rate of the primary composite endpoint (12.8% vs. 8.3%, p = 0.008) was demonstrated. These effects were persistent and maintained at 3-year follow-up[(54)]. The majority of the impact on composite endpoint was due to a reduction in non-fatal MI and need for urgent revascularization.

The effect of tirofiban in 2139 patients undergoing PCI early after ACS (within 72h) was examined in the Randomized Efficacy Study of Tirofiban for Outcomes and Restenosis (RESTORE) trial[(45)]. The primary composite endpoint was used including death from any cause, MI, and urgent target vessel revascularization for recurrent ischemia at 30 days. Although patients receiving tirofiban experienced fewer events at 48h and at 7 days (38% and 27% relative reduction respectively), the reduction in primary composite endpoint was non-significant at 30 days. When repeat angioplasty or coronary artery bypass surgery procedures were included in the composite only if performed on an urgent or emergency basis, the composite 30-day event rates were 10.5% for the placebo group and 8.0% for the tirofiban group, a relative reduction of 24% (p = 0.052) suggesting more benefit in a higher-risk population. This was similar to findings from the EPIC and IMPACT-II studies where a more pronounced benefit was seen in high-risk patients.

The issue of the timing of administration of GP IIb/IIIa agents in ACS patients undergoing PCI was addressed in the Acute Catheterization and Urgent Intervention Triage Strategy (ACUITY) Timing trial[(55)]. Four hundred and fifty academic and community-based institutions in 17 countries recruited a total of 9207 patients with moderate- and high-risk ACS undergoing an invasive treatment strategy in a trial designed as a prospective, randomized, open-label trial with 30-day clinical follow-up. Patients were randomly assigned to receive either routine upstream (tirofiban or eptifibatide) or deferred selective (eptifibatide or abciximab) GP IIb/IIIa inhibitor administration just prior to PCI, respectively. The primary outcome was assessment of non-inferiority of deferred GP IIb/IIIa inhibitor use compared with upstream administration for the prevention of composite ischaemic events (death, MI, or unplanned revascularization for ischemia) at 30 days. Endpoints occurred in 7.9% of patients assigned to deferred use compared with 7.1% of patients assigned to upstream administration that, while not statistically significant, did not meet the criteria for non-inferiority. However, upstream use of GP IIb/IIIa inhibitors resulted in increased rates of major bleeding compared to the deferred group (6.1% vs. 4.9% respectively; p <0.001) as a result of more frequent usage and longer duration of therapy. Overall, the net clinical benefit was probably similar in both groups. The Early Glycoprotien IIb/IIIa Inhibition in Patients with Non-ST-Segment Elevation Acute Coronary Syndrome (EARLY-ACS) trial[56] examined the question of optimal timing of GP IIb/IIIa administration where early eptifibatide was compared with placebo (with provisional eptifibatide in the catheterization laboratory) in 9492 patients with high-risk ACS scheduled for early PCI (within 12–96 hours of randomization). The primary endpoint of all-cause mortality, MI, ischaemia-driven revascularization, or thrombotic bailout at 96h occurred in 9.3% in the early therapy group compared to 10% in the provisional eptifibatide arm (OR 0.92; 95% CI 0.8–0.16; P = 0.23). The secondary endpoint of all-cause, mortality or MI at 30 days slightly favoured the early GP IIb/IIIa inhibitor group (11.2% vs. 12.3% CI 0.79–1.01; P = 0.08), but at the cost of more TIMI major bleeding (2.6% vs. 1.8%; P = 0.02) and increased need for blood transfusion (8.6% vs. 6.7%; P = 0.001).

It has been suggested that GP IIb/IIIa inhibitors are most beneficial in high-risk ACS patients undergoing PCI and a meta-analysis by Roffi *et al.*[(57)] examined the diabetic populations enrolled in six large-scale platelet GP IIb/IIIa inhibitor ACS trials: PRISM, PRISM-PLUS, PARAGON A, PARAGON B, PURSUIT, and GUSTO IV. Among 6458 diabetic patients, platelet GP IIb/IIIa inhibition was associated with a significant mortality reduction at 30 days, from 6.2% to 4.6% (OR 0.74; 95% CI 0.59–0.92; p = 0.007). Conversely, 23 072 non-diabetic patients had no survival benefit (3.0% vs. 3.0%). The interaction between platelet GP IIb/IIIa inhibition and diabetic status was statistically significant (p = 0.036). The survival benefit was more apparent among the 1279 diabetic patients undergoing PCI during index hospitalization. The use of these agents was associated with a mortality reduction that was already apparent at 30 days from 4.0% to 1.2% (OR 0.30; 95% CI 0.14–0.69; p = 0.002).

ST-elevation myocardial infarction

The cornerstone of therapy for acute ST-elevation MI (STEMI) involves the rapid restoration of epicardial blood flow and myocardial tissue perfusion. Recent evidence suggests that primary PCI (PPCI) is the treatment of choice offering more definitive revascularization in a wider range of patients and with fewer bleeding complications[58]. In many regions, however, prompt PPCI is not available and fibrinolysis remains in widespread use around the world. In addition, even when PPCI is available problems of no/slow-reflow are widespread with impaired tissue perfusion in up to a third of patients following successful stent implantation. The use of adjunctive agents to improve outcomes for reperfusion therapy for STEMI includes GP IIb/IIIa inhibitors.

GP IIb/IIIa inhibitors as adjunctive therapy to fibrinolysis

Fibrinolytic agents fail to achieve optimum reperfusion in many patients with STEMI. The TIMI 14 trial[59] explored the hypothesis that the addition of abciximab would facilitate the rate and extent of thrombolysis when combined with a half dose of fibrinolytic. They examined 888 patients undergoing fibrinolysis with alteplase for STEMI that found that the addition of abciximab produced early, marked increases in TIMI 3 flow at 90min compared to alteplase alone. This improvement in reperfusion occurred without an increase in the risk of major bleeding. Modest improvements in TIMI 3 flow were seen when abciximab was combined with streptokinase, but there was a marked increased risk of bleeding. The Strategies for Patency Enhancement in the Emergency Department (SPEED) Group[60] found similar improvements in vessel patency using a combination of abciximab and low-dose reteplase. Again there were increased rates of minor bleeding rates in the combination group but major bleeding rates were similar.

The GUSTO V AMI trial[61] assessed the clinical benefits of GP IIb/IIIa inhibition as an adjunct to fibrinolysis. This was a randomized, open-label trial involving 16 588 patients in the first 6h of evolving STEMI to compare the effect of the standard-dose reteplase alone with half-dose reteplase plus abciximab. The primary endpoint was 30-day mortality, and secondary endpoints included various complications of MI. Analysis was by intention to treat. At 30 days, there was no difference in primary endpoint between the two groups (5.9% vs. 5.6%, p = 0.43). In the combination group there was a reduction in the composite endpoint of deaths or non-fatal reinfarction in the combination group compared to reteplase alone (8.8% vs. 7.4%, p = 0.0011). There also was less need for urgent revascularization (8.6% vs. 5.6%, p = 0.001) and fewer major non-fatal ischaemic complications of acute MI. On the other hand, these benefits were partly counterbalanced by increased non-intracranial bleeding complications in the combination group (4.3% vs. 1.9%, p <0.0001). The rates of intracranial haemorrhage and non-fatal disabling stroke were similar in both groups. ASSENT-3 randomized 6095 patients with STEMI of less than 6h to one of three regimens: full-dose tenecteplase and enoxaparin for a maximum of 7 days; half-dose tenecteplase with weight-adjusted low-dose unfractionated heparin and a 12-h infusion of abciximab; or full-dose tenecteplase with weight-adjusted unfractionated heparin for 48h. There was a reduction in the composite primary endpoints of 30-day mortality, in-hospital reinfarction, or in-hospital refractory ischaemia in the enoxaparin and abciximab groups compared to the unfractionated heparin group: 11.4% vs. 15.4%, p = 0.0002, for enoxaparin, and 11.1% vs. 15.4%, p <0.0001 for abciximab. Similar to GUSTO V, the combination of abciximab and half-dose tenecteplase did not have a mortality benefit compared to full-dose tenecteplase alone but did result in significantly reduced in-hospital infarction and refractory ischaemia. The need for urgent PCI was reduced in the GP IIb/IIIa and fibrinolytic combination group in both trials. In ASSENT-3, major bleeding (other than intracranial haemorrhage which was the same in both groups) was increased from 2.2% to 4.3% (p <0.005). In those over the age of 75 years the risk of major bleeds was the greatest with a threefold increase compared to younger patients.

Facilitated PCI refers to pharmacological reperfusion treatment delivered prior to a planned PCI in order to bridge the PCI-related time delay[62]. Full-dose fibrinolytic alone (ASSENT-4[63]), combinations of GP IIb/IIIa inhibitor and low-dose fibrinolytic (FINESSE[64]), or GP IIb/IIIa alone (On-TIME-2[65]) have been tested for this indication. In the Facilitated Intervention with Enhanced Reperfusion Speed to Stop Events (FINESSE) trial[64], primary PCI for patients with STEMI was preceded by early treatment with abciximab plus half-dose reteplase or with abciximab alone and compared with abciximab administered immediately before the procedure. 2452 patients were randomized into the study and although there were improved markers of reperfusion as suggested by early ST-segment resolution with the combination therapy, neither facilitation of PCI with reteplase plus abciximab nor facilitation with abciximab alone significantly improved the clinical outcomes, as compared with abciximab given at the time of PCI. Excess major bleeding was seen in the combination-facilitated group (14.5%) and abciximab-facilitated group (10.1%) compared to the primary PCI group (6.9%), (p <0.0001). The trial was troubled with slow recruitment that resulted in it being terminated early as well as a low event-rate that left it potentially underpowered to detect a clinical benefit of the intervention therapy. That said, the excess risk of bleeding (25 of 1000 patients treated) compared to the reduction in ischaemic composite endpoint (9 of 1000 patients treated) suggests that there is little role for facilitated PCI in this form, especially given recent data showing the strong relationship of in-hospital bleeding with long-term mortality[66].

GP IIb/IIIa inhibitors as adjunctive therapy to primary PCI

In the context of PPCI for the treatment of acute MI there are many reasons to suppose why additional antiplatelet therapy may be beneficial. The patient is in a pro-thrombotic state with activated platelets and inflammatory responses predisposing to potent platelet aggregation and further clot formation. Several randomized trials have assessed the value of abciximab given as adjunct therapy to PPCI. The RAPPORT study[67] examined the benefit of abciximab in a placebo-controlled trial in patients receiving primary angioplasty alone without stenting. They found a substantial reduction in the acute (30-day) combined endpoint of death, reinfarction, and urgent target vessel revascularization (TVR). However, the bleeding rates were excessive, and the 6-month primary endpoint, which included elective revascularization, was not favourably affected. In the stenting era, the Abciximab Before Direct Angioplasty and Stenting in Myocardial Infarction Regarding Acute and Long-Term Follow-Up (ADMIRAL) study[68] randomly assigned 300 patients with acute MI in a double-blind fashion either to abciximab plus stenting or placebo plus stenting. At 30 days, the primary endpoint, a composite of death, reinfarction, or urgent TVR, had occurred in 6.0% of the patients in the abciximab group, as compared with 14.6% of those in the placebo group (p = 0.01); at 6 months, the corresponding figures were 7.4% and 15.9% (p = 0.02). The better clinical outcomes in the abciximab group were related to the greater frequency of TIMI grade 3 coronary flow (according to the classification of the Thrombolysis in Myocardial Infarction trial[69]) in this group than in the placebo group before the procedure (16.8% vs. 5.4%, p = 0.01), immediately afterward (95.1% vs. 86.7%, p = 0.04), and 6 months afterward (94.3% vs. 82.8%, p = 0.04). One major bleeding event occurred in the abciximab group (0.7%); none occurred in the placebo group. The clinical benefits initially observed at 30 days were still apparent at 3-year follow up[70]. The CADILLAC trial[71] examined 2082 patients and also found a significant reduction in 6-month composite endpoints in the abciximab plus stenting group compared to stenting alone (10.2% vs. 11.5%, p <0.001). Like ADMIRAL the difference in the incidence of the primary endpoint was due almost entirely to differences in the rates of TVR. De Luca *et al.*[72] undertook a systematic review of 11 trials examining the use of abciximab in STEMI involving 27 115 patients. When compared with the control group, abciximab was associated with a significant reduction in short-term (30 days) mortality (2.4% vs. 3.4%, P = 0.047) and long-term (6–12 months) mortality (4.4% vs. 6.2%, p = 0.01) in patients undergoing PPCI. Abciximab was also associated with a significant reduction in 30-day reinfarction (1.0% vs. 1.9%, p = 0.03) in the PPCI group. Abciximab did not result in an increased risk of intracranial bleeding nor major bleeding complications[iii].

Outstanding questions regarding the use of GP IIb/IIIa inhibitors as adjunctive therapy in PPCI for STEMI remain. These include the use of tirofiban and eptifibatide where the data available regarding their use in this setting is much more limited than abciximab,

[iii] In the STEMI patients examined given abciximab and fibrinolysis there was a significant increase in major bleeding (5.2% vs. 3.1%, p <0.001).

the optimum timing of administration of these agents[iv], and the additional benefit of GP IIb/IIIa inhibition in patients who have received high-dose clopidogrel pre-loading as most trials have taken place in the era before such administration was routine in PPCI. Two recent meta-analyses of randomized trials have compared the use of the small-,molecule GPIIb/IIIa inhibitors with abciximab in STEMI patients undergoing PPCI[(73,74)]. Both found that there was no statistically significant difference in 30-day mortality, reinfarction, or major TIMI bleeding between the groups, nor death or reinfarction at 8 months, suggesting that based on the evidence to date the clinical effectiveness of the different GP IIb/IIIa inhibitor agents is similar. The MULTISTRATEGY trial[(75)] was an open label trial that randomized 745 patients with STEMI undergoing PPCI to high dose tirofiban versus abciximab. It also examined the effect of bare metal stents versus sirolimus-eluting stents in a 4x4 factorial design. All patients were pre-treated with aspirin and 300mg clopidogrel and then continued on dual antiplatelet therapy (including clopidogrel 75mg per day). Rates of ST-segment resolution at 90 minutes and all-cause mortality, reinfarction or target vessel revascularization at 8 months were similar between the different groups, as were major and minor bleeding rates. The On-TIME-2 trial[(65)] examined the benefit of pre-hospital, high-dose tirofiban in association with aspirin (500mg), and clopidogrel (600mg) and heparin (5000IU) in 984 patients with STEMI who were candidates for PPCI. They found improved ST-segment resolution in the high-bolus dose tirofiban group, although this was not associated with improved vessel patency rates on the initial angiogram when compared with placebo. There was no significant reduction in the composite endpoint of death, recurrent MI, or urgent TVR at 30 days, or an increase in major bleeding compared to placebo. In the Barvarian Reperfusion Alternatives Evaluation-3 (BRAVE-3) study[(76)] 800 patients who were being sent for PPCI for STEMI were pre-treated with 600mg clopidogrel and then randomly assigned in a double-blind manner to receive either abciximab or placebo, to be started before the patient arrived in the catheter lab. There was no difference in the primary endpoint of infarct size as determined by SPECT imaging before hospital discharge between the groups. There was also no difference in secondary endpoint, which consisted of a composite of death, MI or need for urgent revascularization at 30 days (abciximab 5% vs. placebo 3.8% CI 0.7–2.6; P = 0.4), or difference in major bleeding. There was also no benefit conferred by pre-hospital abciximab compared to abciximab administered at the time of PCI in the FINESSE trial (see previous section) although an excess of bleeding was observed in the pre-hospital arm. Overall, there does not appear to be a benefit in the use of upstream GP IIb/IIIa inhibitors as adjunctive therapy for patients undergoing PPCI for STEMI.

GP IIb/IIIa inhibitors and emergency coronary bypass grafting

In the early trials involving GP IIb/IIIa inhibitors there were relatively increased rates of emergency CABG after failed PCI. Single-centre, retrospective case series revealed concern over excess bleeding rates in patients receiving abciximab and undergoing emergency CABG[(77,78)]. The large trials showed excess rates of major bleeding in all patients undergoing surgery with data from EPIC[(28)], EPILOG[(30)], and EPISTENT[(18)] showing that 50–60% of the major bleeding episodes recorded were related to surgery. In the EPIC trial mortality rates in the abciximab-treated surgical arm where greater than control (29.4% vs. 8%, p <0.0001), but rates of major bleeding were similar. It should be noted that the median time from cessation of abciximab to surgery was >24h. Lincoff and colleagues examined the patients from the EPILOG and EPISTENT trials undergoing emergency CABG following PCI. In this case, 61% of the patients underwent surgery within 6h of the abciximab infusion being stopped. Although the group receiving abciximab required more platelet transfusions and surgical re-exploration for bleeding, there was no increase in major haemorrhagic risk in patients receiving abciximab compared to control[(79)]. In addition, the overall incidence of emergency surgery was significantly lower in the group that received abciximab (1.28% vs. 2.17% in the control group, p = 0.021). A similar reduction was found in pooled data from the EPIC, CAPTURE, and EPILOG trials[(80)]. An overall decline in rates of emergency CABG in the stenting era, together with careful regulation of perioperative heparin-dosing[(45)] and use of platelet transfusions[(79,81)] have all lead to a further reduction in bleeding rates in patients requiring emergency surgery. The use of antecedent GP IIb/IIIa inhibitors should not be seen as a major obstacle to surgery, and the evidence from the literature

[iv] *See previous section*

Table 23.2 Current guidelines for the use of GP IIb/IIIa inhibitors

Current guidelines for stable patients undergoing PCI*

ACC/AHA/SCAI Practice Guidelines (2005)[93]

Class IIa. In patients undergoing elective PCI with stent placement it is reasonable to administer a GP IIb/IIIa inhibitor (abciximab, eptifibatide, or tirofiban)—*level of evidence: B*

ESC Guidelines (2005)[94]

Class IIa. GP IIb/IIIa inhibitors are recommended in stable coronary artery disease (CAD) PCI with complex lesions, threatening/actual vessel closure, visible thrombus, slow/no reflow—*level of evidence: C*

Current guidelines for patients with acute coronary syndromes

ACC/AHA/SCAI Practice Guidelines (2005)[93]

Class I. In patients with UA/NSTEMI undergoing PCI without clopidogrel administration, a GP IIb/IIIa inhibitor (abciximab, eptifibatide, or tirofiban) should be administered*—*level of evidence: A*

Class IIa. In patients with UA/NSTEMI undergoing PCI with clopidogrel administration it is reasonable to administer a GP IIb/IIIa inhibitor (abciximab, eptifibatide, or tirofiban)*—*level of evidence: B*

* *In both of the above cases it is acceptable to administer the GP IIb/IIIa inhibitor before performance of the diagnostic angiogram ('upstream treatment') or just before PCI ('in-lab treatment').*

ESC Guidelines (2005)[94]

Class I. GP IIb/IIIa inhibitors are recommended in high-risk ACS patients with planned or performed PCI—*level of evidence: C*

Current guidelines for patients undergoing thrombolysis for STEMI

ACC/AHA/SCAI Practice Guidelines (2004, updated 2007)[58,95]

Class IIb:

- Combination pharmacological reperfusion with abciximab and half-dose reteplase or tenecteplase may be considered for prevention of re-infarction (*level of evidence: A*) and other complication of STEMI in selected patients: anterior location of MI, age <75 years old and no risk factors for bleeding. In two clinical trials of combination reperfusion, the prevention of re-infarction did not translate into survival benefit either at 30 days or 1 year[96]–*level of evidence: B*
- Combination pharmacological reperfusion with abciximab and half-dose reteplase or tenecteplase may be considered for prevention of re-infarction and other complication of STEMI in selected patients: anterior location of MI, age <75 years old and no risk factors for bleeding in whom an early referral for angiography and PCI (i.e. facilitated PCI) is planned—*level of evidence: C**

Class III. Combination pharmacological reperfusion with abciximab and half-dose reteplase or tenecteplase should not be given to patients >75 years of age because of an increased risk of intra-cranial haemorrhage—*level of evidence: B*

ESC Guidelines (2008)[97]

Does not recommend facilitated PCI with the combination of a fibrinolytic and GP IIb/IIIa inhibitor as a 'bridge' to PCI due to lack of clinical benefit and concerns over excess bleeding

Current guidelines for patients undergoing primary PCI for STEMI

ACC/AHA/SCAI Practice Guidelines (2004, updated 2007 and 2009)[58,95,98]

Class IIa. It is reasonable to start treatment with glycoprotein IIb/IIIa receptor antagonists (abciximab *[level of evidence: A]*, tirofiban *[level of evidence: B]* or eptifibatide [level of evidence: B] at the time of primary PCI (with or without stenting) in selected patients with STEMI

Class IIb. The usefulness of glyocaprotein IIb/IIIa receptor antagonists (as part of a preparatory pharmacological strategy for patients with STEMI before their arrival in the cardiac catheterization laboratory for angiography and PCI) is uncertain *[level of evidence: B]*

ESC Guidelines (2008)[97]

Class IIa. Abciximab should be used as antiplatelet co-therapy in primary PCI for reperfusion of STEMI–level of evidence: A

Class IIb. Tirofiban *[level of evidence: B]* or eptifibatide *[level of evidence: C]* could also be considered

* Class I: evidence and/or general agreement that a given diagnostic procedure/treatment is beneficial, useful, and effective; Class II: conflicting evidence and/or a divergence of opinion about the usefulness/efficacy of the treatment; Class IIa: weight of evidence/opinion is in favour of usefulness/efficacy; Class IIb: usefulness/efficacy is less well established by evidence/opinion.
Level of evidence A: data derived from multiple randomized clinical trials or meta-analyses; Level of evidence B: data derived from a single randomized clinical trial or large non-randomized studies; Level of evidence C: consensus of opinion of the experts and/or small studies, retrospective studies, registries.

* The 2005 guidelines do state that this remains to be tested prospectively in appropriately sized trials. The 2007 update was released prior to the results of the FINESSE trial being published; a trial that casts some doubt on the benefit of facilitated PCI.

suggests that surgery should not be delayed[v]. Once the decision to undergo surgery has been made, the GP IIb/IIIa inhibitor should be stopped immediately and activated clotting time carefully monitored. Platelet transfusion should be used for clinically significant bleeding. The effect of high-dose clopidogrel loading and concomitant use of GP IIb/IIIa inhibitors on bleeding risk in patients undergoing emergency CABG has yet to be fully evaluated[(82)].

Factors that may reduce efficacy in GP IIb/IIIa inhibition

The heterogenous results from the large clinical trials involving GP IIb/IIIa inhibitors could be explained by a variety of factors that result in suboptimal platelet inhibition within patients. It has been suggested, as mentioned previously, that at least 80% of the GP receptors on platelets need to be blocked in order for optimal clinical benefit to be apparent[(23)]. Up to 10–15% of patients undergoing PCI do not have adequate receptor blockade after a bolus dose of GP IIb/IIIa inhibitor, a figure that is increased in patients presenting with ACS[(27)]. Variation in the proportion of patients achieving optimum receptor-blockade has also been observed during the subsequent periods of GP IIb/IIIa infusion[(27)]. Because of the importance of achieving adequate receptor blockade on reducing platelet aggregation, individual variability in platelet number and function may have a significant impact on the clinical effect observed with the administration of GP IIb/IIIa inhibitors[(24)]. Platelet count and receptor number are affected by splenic size, age, gender, and diabetes and as a result all can significantly influence dose response. The expression of surface GP IIb/IIIa receptors also varies depending on platelet activation and the presence of factors such as thrombin and fibrinogen which can increase GP receptor frequency by 50%[(83)]. On the other hand, low-fibrin levels may enhance the antithrombotic effects of GP IIb/IIIa inhibitors, for example, after the administration of non-fibrin-specific fibrinolysis[(84)]. This may play a part in the excess bleeding rates seen in the clinical trials where GP IIb/IIIa inhibitors were given in combination with fibrinolytic agents[(63,64)]. Body mass, age, and renal function can also influence the pharmacokinetics of the GP IIb/IIIa inhibitors, especially the small-molecule agents which are predominantly renally excreted, and may affect levels of receptor blockade and clinical efficacy and safety[(36)].

Adverse effects of GP IIb/IIIa inhibitors

Bleeding

Bleeding is the most severe complication resulting from the administration of GP IIb/IIIa inhibitors. This can have a significant clinical impact in terms of morbidity and mortality[(66)]. Bleeding severity is most commonly based on the TIMI criteria[(69)][vi]. An increased rate of bleeding was noted in the EPIC trial[(28)] where major bleeding was observed in 14% of the abciximab-treated patients versus 7% in the placebo-control arm ($p = 0.001$). Most bleeding occurred at the vascular access site. Multivariate analysis suggested older age, low body weight, female sex, evolving MI, treatment with abciximab, and duration and complexity of the PCI as independent predictors of bleeding. There was a subsequent reduction in bleeding rates by using lower-dose, weight-adjusted heparin (70U/kg), avoiding routine post-procedural heparin, and early vascular sheath removal (4–6h post-procedure). Meta-analysis shows overall incidence of major bleeding in the GP IIb/IIIa trials examined of 2.5% compared to 1.3% in the placebo control ($p < 0.0001$)[(52)]. Intracranial haemorrhage was a rare complication occurring in only 0.08% of patients. GP IIb/IIIa inhibitors were not associated with a significantly higher rate of intracranial haemorrhage or total stroke. Safety results were similar in patients treated with and without heparin. There is some concern about increased bleeding risk in patients receiving GP IIb/IIIa inhibitors with chronic renal failure although studies

[v] Eli Liley (Indiana, IN), distributor of abciximab (ReoPro®), suggest that because of its anticoagulant activity consideration should be given to delaying CABG in the patient who has received abciximab if possible. This decision, however, lies within the realm of the physician's judgement based upon the clinical situation and appropriate consideration of the risks and benefits.

[vi] Major bleeding: intracranial bleeding, a decrease in haemoglobin by >5g/dL or a decrease in haematocrit of >15%. Minor bleeding: spontaneous gross haematuria, or haematemesis, a decrease in haemoglodin >3g/dL with observed bleeding, decrease in haemoglobin >4g/dL with no observed bleeding, and all other observed bleeding

Table 23.3 Showing contraindications and cautions relating to the use of GP IIb/IIIa inhibitors

Contraindications to use of GP IIb/IIIa inhibitors[94]	Caution to use
Active internal bleeding	Concomitant use of drugs that increase risk of bleeding
Major surgery	Discontinue if uncontrollable serious bleeding occurs or emergency cardiac surgery needed
Intracranial or intraspinal surgery or trauma within last 2 months	Elderly
Stroke within last 2 years	Hepatic impairment
Intracranial neoplasm	Renal impairment
Arteriovenous malformation or aneurysm	Pregnancy
Severe uncontrolled hypertension	Measure baseline prothrombin time, activated clotting time, activated partial thromboplastin time, platelet count, haemoglobin, and haematocrit
Haemorrhagic diathesis,	
Thrombocytopenia	Monitor haemoglobin and haematocrit 12h and 24h after start of treatment and platelet count 2–4h and 24h after start of treatment
Vasculitis	
Hypertensive retinopathy	
Breast-feeding	
Severe hepatic impairment	

have yielded conflicting results. Best and colleagues found no increase in bleeding complications in patients receiving abciximab with renal impairment[85], but other studies have suggested increased risk[86,87]. Caution is advised, especially when patients have received clopidogrel loading and enoxaparin which have been associated with a further increment in bleeding risk[88].

Thrombocytopenia

Thrombocytopenia (less than 100×10^9/L) is an uncommon, rarely fatal, but nevertheless concerning complication of GP IIb/IIIa inhibitor usage. The incidence across the clinical trials is approximately 5% of patients involving all agents although the incidence is greater in patients receiving abciximab than the small-molecule agents. The precise mechanism of thrombocytopenia is not well understood but it is possibly immune mediated given the increased prevalence of acute severe[vii] and profound[viii] thrombocytopenia on readministration of abciximab (2.8% and 2% respectively) compared to the incidence after first-time administration of 1% for severe, and 0.4% for profound is observed[29]. Patients who form human antichimeric antibodies following abciximab administration (approximately 6%) are more prone to develop severe thrombocytopenia on subsequent occasions[28].

Because heparin is often administered concomitantly with GP IIb/IIIa inhibitors, heparin-induced thrombocytopenia (HIT) must be excluded. HIT tends to occur 5–10 days after the heparin therapy has been initiated rather that a precipitous reduction in platelet count within 24h of initiation of the GP IIb/IIIa inhibitor. Following HIT immunoglobulin G antibodies against platelet factor 4 complexes may be detectable for 4–6 weeks after the episode. If HIT and other causes of platelet consumption (such as disseminated intravascular coagulopathy) have been excluded, GP IIb/IIIa inhibitor-induced thrombocytopenia should be treated by the immediate discontinuation of the agent. In the case of abciximab, platelet transfusion can be given if there is evidence of clinical bleeding, but not if small-molecule agents have been administered. In this case, because of their weak binding and short duration of action platelet counts will normally return to normal within 12–124h after the cessation of the drug.

[vii] Platelet count drop to less than 50×10^9/L within 24h of infusion

[viii] Platelet count drop to less than 20×10^9/L within 24h of infusion

Table 23.4 Summary of GP IIb/IIIa trials

Trial	Year	Study population	Drug	Groups**	Placebo		GP IIb/IIIa inhibitor		ARR, %	RR	95% CI	P value	Notes
					N	%	N	%					
PCI trials													
EPIC[28]	1994	High risk PCI; including ACS	Abciximab	Bolus; bolus + infusion	72/696	10.3	49/708	6.9*	3.4	0.68	0.47–0.95	0.022	↑Bleeding rates due to high dose UH
EPILOG[30]	1997	All PCI; ACS excluded	Abciximab	+ Standard or low dose UH	85/939	9.1	35/935	3.7*	5.4	0.41	0.28–0.61	<0.001	No ↑bleeding
CAPTURE[44]	1997	Refractory UA; within 24h angio	Abciximab	18–24-h infusion pre-PCI, 1h post	57/635	9.0	30/630	4.8	4.2	0.53	0.35–0.81	0.003	Study closed early; ↑bleeding in abciximab group
IMPACT II[36]	1997	Any PCI	Eptifibatide	Bolus + 24h 0.5 or 0.75mcg/kg/min	112/1328	8.4	93/1349	6.9*	1.5	0.83	0.63–1.06	0.134	No ↑bleeding
RESTORE[45]	1997	PCI within 72h of ACS	Tirofiban	36hr infusion	69/1070	6.4	54/1071	5.0	1.4	0.78	0.55–1.10	0.162	
EPISTENT[18]	1998	57% ACS; 43% stable AP	Abciximab	+ Stent or +PTCA; 12-h infusion post	83/809	10.2	38/794	4.8*	5.4	0.46	0.32–0.68	<0.001	Mortality benefit at 1year in stent + abciximab group
ESPRIT[38]	2000	51% ACS; 49% stable AP	Eptifibatide	Bolus + infusion for 18–24h	104/1024	10.2	66/1040	6.3	3.9	0.62	0.46–0.84	0.0016	Study stopped early due to sigt ↓death and MI at 48h
ISAR-REACT[100]	2004	Low risk PCI; ACS excluded	Abciximab	+ Pre-treatment with clopidogrel	42/1080	3.9	43/1079	4.0	-0.1	1.02	0.68–1.55	0.91	Diabetics and visible thrombus excluded
ACS trials													
PRISM-PLUS[47]	1998	NSTE-ACS; PCI encouraged after 48h	Tirofiban	± UH; >48h pre-PCI, then 12–24h post	95/797	11.9	67/733	9.1*	2.8	0.70	0.51–0.96	0.03	Tirofiban alone stopped as excess mortality
PRISM[49]	1998	NSTE-ACS; PCI discouraged	Tirofiban	+ASA; ASA + UH alone	115/1616	7.1	94/1616	5.8§	1.3	0.82	0.61–1.05	0.11	PCI in only 1.9% cases
PURSUIT[51]	1998	NSTE-ACS	Eptifibatide	<72h pre-PCI	744/4739	15.7	670/4722	14.2*	1.5	0.90	0.82–1.00	0.004	Variable UH dosing; 11.9% PCI rates

(Continued)

Table 23.4 (Continued) Summary of GP IIb/IIIa trials

Trial	Year	Study population	Drug	Groups**	Placebo		GP IIb/IIIa inhibitor		ARR, %	RR	95% CI	P value	Notes
					N	%	N	%					
PARAGON A(50)	1998	NSTE-ACS	Lamifiban	High/low dose ± UH	89/758	11.7	80/755	10.6§	1.1	0.9	0.68–1.20	0.48	PCI rates 10–15%
GUSTO IV ACS(101)	2001	NSTE-ACS; PCI discouraged	Abciximab	Bolus + infusion for 24 or 48h	209/2598	11.4	450/5202	8.7§§	-0.7	1.08	0.92–1.26	0.36	PCI rates 1.6% within 48h, 19% within 30 days
ISAR-REACT 2(46)	2006	NSE-ACS; PCI in all patients	Abciximab	+ Clopidogrel pre-treatment	116/1010	11.5	87/1012	8.6	2.9	0.75	0.57–0.97	0.03	
All ACS trials					1164/14115	11.7	1726/16668	10.4	1.3	0.86	0.81–0.93	<0.0001	
All PCI trials					624/7581	8.2	408/7606	5.4	2.8	0.65	0.58–0.74	<0.0001	
All trials combined					2288/21274	10.5	2134/24274	8.8	1.7	0.83	0.83–0.84	<0.0001	

ASA, aspirin; CI, confidence interval; NSE-ACS, non ST-segment elevation acute coronary syndrome; PTCA, percutaneous transluminal coronary angioplasty; UH, unfractionated heparin.

Modified from Anderson J, Adams C, Antman E, *et al.* ACC/AHA 2007 Guidelines for the Management of Patients With Unstable Angina/Non–ST-Elevation Myocardial Infarction – Executive Summary. *J Am Coll Cardiol* 2007; **50**:652–726, with permission of Elsevier.

**as compared to placebo unless specifically stated.

*Best treatment group selected for analysis.

*Best treatment group selected for analysis.

*Best treatment group selected for analysis.

*Best treatment group selected for analysis.

*Best treatment group selected for analysis.

§GP IIb/IIIa inhibitor without heparin

*Best treatment group selected for analysis.

§GP IIb/IIIa inhibitor without heparin

§§pooled results for 24-h and 48-h treatment arms

Other adverse reactions

Side effects of nausea, vomiting, hypotension, bradycardia, chest pain, back pain, headache, fever, puncture site pain, and, rarely cardiac tamponade, adult respiratory distress, hypersensitivity reactions have all been reported with GP IIb/IIIa inhibitors[28,30,38] (Table 23.3).

Other uses of GP IIb/IIIa inhibitors

Stroke

Two trials involving 474 patients were examined in a recent Cochrane review on the use of GP IIb/IIIa inhibitors in acute ischaemic stroke[89]. Only data for 414 patients treated within 6h were considered. Treatment with abciximab was associated with a non- significant reduction of death and dependency combined (OR 0.79; 95% CI 0.54–1.17) and of death alone (OR 0.67; 95% CI 0.36–1.25). Treatment with abciximab was associated with a non- significant increase of symptomatic intracranial haemorrhages (OR 4.13; 95% CI 0.86–19.67) and of major extracranial haemorrhages (OR 1.51; 95% CI 0.25–9.12). The authors therefore conclude that there is not enough data regarding efficacy or safety from randomized controlled trials to warrant the use of these agents in acute ischaemic stroke. The results from ongoing trials are awaited.

Peripheral vascular disease

There has been sparse data examining the benefit of adjunctive antiplatelet therapy with GP IIb/IIIa inhibitors in peripheral percutaneous interventions, in particular for critical limb ischaemia and peripheral vascular disease[90]. To date, trials have been small, single-centre studies but initial results have been encouraging showing a reduction in need for reintervention and improved angiographic patency at 6 months[91,92].

Conclusion

GP IIb/IIIa inhibitors have been extensively used in large clinical trials for a whole range of coronary syndromes and have found to confer considerable benefit when administered in concert with percutaneous revascularization (Table 23.4). As such, they have established themselves as part of the armamentarium of contemporary therapy for such syndromes. Although GP IIb/IIIa inhibitors are associated with proven benefits, an understanding of their mechanism of action as well as appropriate patient selection is essential to minimize the risk of adverse events, especially bleeding complications, associated with their use. With the use of adequate antiplatelet pre-treatment, the use of GP IIb/IIIa inhibitors in elective PCI has diminished. However, they remain useful adjuncts to high-risk PCI in the setting of acute coronary syndromes, especially in patients who have not received adequate thienopyridine loading. The use of these agents in the field of stroke and peripheral vascular disease remains undetermined.

References

1. Braunwald E, Jones RH, Mark DB, *et al.* Diagnosing and managing unstable angina. Agency for Health Care Policy and Research. *Circulation* 1994; **90**(1): 613–22.
2. Pedersen TR, Kjekshus J, Berg K, *et al.* Cholesterol lowering and the use of healthcare resources. Results of the Scandinavian Simvastatin Survival Study. *Circulation* 1996; **93**(10):1796–802.
3. Davies MJ. The composition of coronary-artery plaques. *N Engl J Med* 1997; **336**(18):1312–14.
4. Gillum RF. Trends in acute myocardial infarction and coronary heart disease death in the United States. *J Am Coll Cardiol* 1994; **23**(6):1273–7.
5. Stary HC, Chandler AB, Dinsmore RE, *et al.* A definition of advanced types of atherosclerotic lesions and a histological classification of atherosclerosis. A report from the Committee on Vascular Lesions of the Council on Arteriosclerosis, American Heart Association. *Circulation* 1995; **92**(5):1355–74.
6. Loree HM, Tobias BJ, Gibson LJ, *et al.* Mechanical properties of model atherosclerotic lesion lipid pools. *Arterioscler Thromb* 1994; **14**(2):230–4.
7. Mizuno K, Satomura K, Miyamoto A, *et al.* Angioscopic evaluation of coronary-artery thrombi in acute coronary syndromes. *N Engl J Med* 1992; **326**(5):287291.
8. Moreno PR, Bernardi VH, Lopez-Cuellar J, *et al.* Macrophages, smooth muscle cells, and tissue factor in unstable angina. Implications for cell-mediated thrombogenicity in acute coronary syndromes. *Circulation* 1996; **94**(12):3090–7.
9. Burke AP, Farb A, Malcom GT, *et al.* Coronary risk factors and plaque morphology in men with coronary disease who died suddenly. *N Engl J Med* 1997; **336**(18):1276–82.

10. Fuster V, Fallon JT, Nemerson Y. Coronary thrombosis. *Lancet* 1996; **348**(Suppl.1):s7–10.
11. Gutstein DE, Fuster V. Pathophysiology and clinical significance of atherosclerotic plaque rupture. *Cardiovasc Res* 1999; **41**(2):323–33.
12. Bogaty P, Hackett D, Davies G, *et al.* Vasoreactivity of the culprit lesion in unstable angina. *Circulation* 1994; **90**(1):5–11.
13. Topol EJ, Yadav JS. Recognition of the importance of embolization in atherosclerotic vascular disease. *Circulation* 2000; **101**(5):570–80.
14. Selvanayagam JB, Cheng AS, Jerosch-Herold M, *et al.* Effect of distal embolization on myocardial perfusion reserve after percutaneous coronary intervention: a quantitative magnetic resonance perfusion study. *Circulation* 2007; **116**(13):1458–64.
15. Dangas G, Stone GW, Weinberg MD, *et al.* Contemporary outcomes of rescue percutaneous coronary intervention for acute myocardial infarction: comparison with primary angioplasty and the role of distal protection devices (EMERALD trial). *Am Heart J* 2008; **155**(6):1090–6.
16. Vlaar PJ, Svilaas T, van der Horst IC, *et al.* Cardiac death and reinfarction after 1 year in the Thrombus Aspiration during Percutaneous coronary intervention in Acute myocardial infarction Study (TAPAS): a 1-year follow-up study. *Lancet* 2008; **371**(9628):1915–20.
17. Steinhubl SR, Berger PB, Mann JT, 3rd, *et al.* Early and sustained dual oral antiplatelet therapy following percutaneous coronary intervention: a randomized controlled trial. *JAMA* 2002; **288**(19):2411–20.
18. Randomised placebo-controlled and balloon-angioplasty-controlled trial to assess safety of coronary stenting with use of platelet glycoprotein-IIb/IIIa blockade. *Lancet* 1998; **352**(9122):87–92.
19. Brener SJ, Moliterno DJ, Lincoff AM, *et al.* Relationship between activated clotting time and ischemic or hemorrhagic complications: analysis of 4 recent randomized clinical trials of percutaneous coronary intervention. *Circulation* 2004; **110**(8):994–8.
20. Lincoff AM, Bittl JA, Harrington RA, *et al.* Bivalirudin and provisional glycoprotein IIb/IIIa blockade compared with heparin and planned glycoprotein IIb/IIIa blockade during percutaneous coronary intervention: REPLACE-2 randomized trial. *JAMA* 2003; **289**(7):853–63.
21. Ferguson JJ, Waly HM, Wilson JM. Fundamentals of coagulation and glycoprotein IIb/IIIa receptor inhibition. *Eur Heart J* 1998; **19**(Suppl D):D3–9.
22. Cierniewski CS, Byzova T, Papierak M, *et al.* Peptide ligands can bind to distinct sites in integrin alphaIIbbeta3 and elicit different functional responses. *J Biol Chem* 1999; **274**(24):16923–32.
23. Tcheng JE, Ellis SG, George BS, *et al.* Pharmacodynamics of chimeric glycoprotein IIb/IIIa integrin antiplatelet antibody Fab 7E3 in high-risk coronary angioplasty. *Circulation* 1994; **90**(4):1757–64.
24. Chew DP, Moliterno DJ. A critical appraisal of platelet glycoprotein IIb/IIIa inhibition. *J Am Coll Cardiol* 2000; **36**(7):2028–35.
25. Kleiman NS. Pharmacokinetics and pharmacodynamics of glycoprotein IIb-IIIa inhibitors. *Am Heart J* 1999; **138**(4 Pt 2):263–75.
26. Scarborough RM, Kleiman NS, Phillips DR. Platelet glycoprotein IIb/IIIa antagonists. What are the relevant issues concerning their pharmacology and clinical use? *Circulation* 1999; **100**(4):437–44.
27. Mascelli MA, Lance ET, Damaraju L, *et al.* Pharmacodynamic profile of short-term abciximab treatment demonstrates prolonged platelet inhibition with gradual recovery from GP IIb/IIIa receptor blockade. *Circulation* 1998; **97**(17):1680–8.
28. Use of a monoclonal antibody directed against the platelet glycoprotein IIb/IIIa receptor in high-risk coronary angioplasty. The EPIC Investigation. *N Engl J Med* 1994; **330**(14):956–61.
29. Dery JP, Braden GA, Lincoff AM, *et al.* Final results of the ReoPro readministration registry. *Am J Cardiol* 2004; **93**(8):979–84.
30. Platelet glycoprotein IIb/IIIa receptor blockade and low-dose heparin during percutaneous coronary revascularization. The EPILOG Investigators. *N Engl J Med* 1997; **336**(24):1689–96.
31. Topol EJ, Mark DB, Lincoff AM, *et al.* Outcomes at 1 year and economic implications of platelet glycoprotein IIb/IIIa blockade in patients undergoing coronary stenting: results from a multicentre randomised trial. EPISTENT Investigators. Evaluation of Platelet IIb/IIIa Inhibitor for Stenting. *Lancet* 1999; **354**(9195):2019–24.
32. Bhatt DL, Marso SP, Lincoff AM, *et al.* Abciximab reduces mortality in diabetics following percutaneous coronary intervention. *J Am Coll Cardiol* 2000; **35**(4):922–8.
33. Mehilli J, Kastrati A, Schuhlen H, *et al.* Randomized clinical trial of abciximab in diabetic patients undergoing elective percutaneous coronary interventions after treatment with a high loading dose of clopidogrel. *Circulation* 2004; **110**(24):3627–35.
34. Kastrati A, Mehilli J, Schuhlen H, *et al.* A clinical trial of abciximab in elective percutaneous coronary intervention after pretreatment with clopidogrel. *N Engl J Med* 2004; **350**(3):232–8.
35. Wijpkema JS, Jessurun GA, Van Boven AJ, *et al.* Clinical impact of abciximab on long-term outcome after complex coronary angioplasty. *Catheter Cardiovasc Interv* 2003; **60**(3):339–43.
36. Randomised placebo-controlled trial of effect of eptifibatide on complications of percutaneous coronary intervention: IMPACT-II. Integrilin to Minimise Platelet Aggregation and Coronary Thrombosis-II. *Lancet* 1997; **349**(9063):1422–8.

37. Phillips DR, Teng W, Arfsten A, *et al.* Effect of Ca2+ on GP IIb-IIIa interactions with integrilin: enhanced GP IIb-IIIa binding and inhibition of platelet aggregation by reductions in the concentration of ionized calcium in plasma anticoagulated with citrate. *Circulation* 1997; **96**(5):1488–94.
38. Novel dosing regimen of eptifibatide in planned coronary stent implantation (ESPRIT): a randomised, placebo-controlled trial. *Lancet* 2000; **356**(9247):2037–44.
39. O'Shea JC, Hafley GE, Greenberg S, *et al.* Platelet glycoprotein IIb/IIIa integrin blockade with eptifibatide in coronary stent intervention: the ESPRIT trial: a randomized controlled trial. *JAMA* 2001; **285**(19):2468–73.
40. Labinaz M, Madan M, O'Shea JO, *et al.* Comparison of one-year outcomes following coronary artery stenting in diabetic versus nondiabetic patients (from the Enhanced Suppression of the Platelet IIb/IIIa Receptor With Integrilin Therapy [ESPRIT] Trial). *Am J Cardiol* 2002; **90**(6):585–90.
41. Kereiakes DJ, Kleiman NS, Ambrose J, *et al.* Randomized, double-blind, placebo-controlled dose-ranging study of tirofiban (MK-383) platelet IIb/IIIa blockade in high risk patients undergoing coronary angioplasty. *J Am Coll Cardiol* 1996; **27**(3):536–42.
42. Topol EJ, Moliterno DJ, Herrmann HC, *et al.* Trial TIDTaRGSE. Comparison of two platelet glycoprotein IIb/IIIa inhibitors, tirofiban and abciximab, for the prevention of ischemic events with percutaneous coronary revascularization. *N Engl J Med* Vol 2001; **344**:1888–94.
43. Serebruany V, Malinin A, Pokov A, *et al.* Effects of escalating doses of tirofiban on platelet aggregation and major receptor expression in diabetic patients: hitting the TARGET in the TENACITY trial? *Thromb Res* 2007; **119**(2):175–81.
44. Hamm CW, Heeschen C, Goldmann B, *et al.* Benefit of abciximab in patients with refractory unstable angina in relation to serum troponin T levels. c7E3 Fab Antiplatelet Therapy in Unstable Refractory Angina (CAPTURE) Study Investigators. *N Engl J Med* 1999; **340**(21):1623–9.
45. Effects of platelet glycoprotein IIb/IIIa blockade with tirofiban on adverse cardiac events in patients with unstable angina or acute myocardial infarction undergoing coronary angioplasty. The RESTORE Investigators. Randomized Efficacy Study of Tirofiban for Outcomes and REstenosis. *Circulation* 1997; **96**(5):1445–53.
46. Kastrati A, Mehilli J, Neumann FJ, *et al.* Abciximab in patients with acute coronary syndromes undergoing percutaneous coronary intervention after clopidogrel pretreatment: the ISAR-REACT 2 randomized trial. *JAMA* 2006; **295**(13):1531–8.
47. Inhibition of the platelet glycoprotein IIb/IIIa receptor with tirofiban in unstable angina and non-Q-wave myocardial infarction. Platelet Receptor Inhibition in Ischemic Syndrome Management in Patients Limited by Unstable Signs and Symptoms (PRISM-PLUS) Study Investigators. *N Engl J Med* 1998; **338**(21):1488–97.
48. Simoons ML. Effect of glycoprotein IIb/IIIa receptor blocker abciximab on outcome in patients with acute coronary syndromes without early coronary revascularisation: the GUSTO IV-ACS randomised trial. *Lancet* 2001; **357**(9272):1915–24.
49. A comparison of aspirin plus tirofiban with aspirin plus heparin for unstable angina. Platelet Receptor Inhibition in Ischemic Syndrome Management (PRISM) Study Investigators. *N Engl J Med* 1998; **338**(21):1498–505.
50. International, randomized, controlled trial of lamifiban (a platelet glycoprotein IIb/IIIa inhibitor), heparin, or both in unstable angina. The PARAGON Investigators. Platelet IIb/IIIa Antagonism for the Reduction of Acute coronary syndrome events in a Global Organization Network. *Circulation* 1998; **97**(24):2386–95.
51. Inhibition of platelet glycoprotein IIb/IIIa with eptifibatide in patients with acute coronary syndromes. The PURSUIT Trial Investigators. Platelet Glycoprotein IIb/IIIa in Unstable Angina: Receptor Suppression Using Integrilin Therapy. *N Engl J Med* 1998; **339**(7):436–43.
52. Boersma E, Harrington RA, Moliterno DJ, *et al.* Platelet glycoprotein IIb/IIIa inhibitors in acute coronary syndromes. *Lancet* 2002; **360**:342–3.
53. Topol EJ, Califf RM, Weisman HF, *et al.* Randomised trial of coronary intervention with antibody against platelet IIb/IIIa integrin for reduction of clinical restenosis: results at six months. The EPIC Investigators. *Lancet* 1994; **343**(8902):881–6.
54. Topol EJ, Ferguson JJ, Weisman HF, *et al.* Long-term protection from myocardial ischemic events in a randomized trial of brief integrin beta3 blockade with percutaneous coronary intervention. EPIC Investigator Group. Evaluation of Platelet IIb/IIIa Inhibition for Prevention of Ischemic Complication. *JAMA* 1997; **278**(6):479–84.
55. Stone GW, Bertrand ME, Moses JW, *et al.* Routine upstream initiation vs deferred selective use of glycoprotein IIb/IIIa inhibitors in acute coronary syndromes: the ACUITY Timing trial. *JAMA* 2007; **297**:591–602.
56. Mehta SR, Granger CB, Boden WE, *et al.* Early versus delayed invasive intervention in acute coronary syndromes. *N Engl J Med.* 2009; **360**(21):2165–75.
57. Roffi M, Chew DP, Mukherjee D, *et al.* Platelet glycoprotein IIb/IIIa inhibitors reduce mortality in

diabetic patients with non-ST-segment-elevation acute coronary syndromes. *Circulation* 2001; **104**(23):2767–71.

58. Antman E, Hand M, Armstrong P, *et al.* 2007 Focused Update of the ACC/AHA 2004 Guidelines for the Management of Patients With ST-Elevation Myocardial Infarction: A Report of the American College of Cardiology/American Heart Association Task Force on Practice Guidelines: Developed in Collaboration With the Canadian Cardiovascular Society Endorsed by the American Academy of Family Physicians: 2007 Writing Group to Review New Evidence and Update the ACC/AHA 2004 Guidelines for the Management of Patients With ST-Elevation Myocardial Infarction, Writing on Behalf of the 2004 Writing Committee. *Circulation* 2008; **117**:296–329.
59. Antman EM, Giugliano RP, Gibson CM, *et al.* Abciximab facilitates the rate and extent of thrombolysis: results of the thrombolysis in myocardial infarction (TIMI) 14 trial. The TIMI 14 Investigators. *Circulation* 1999; **99**(21): 2720–32.
60. Trial of abciximab with and without low-dose reteplase for acute myocardial infarction. Strategies for Patency Enhancement in the Emergency Department (SPEED) Group. *Circulation* 2000; **101**(24):2788–94.
61. Topol EJ. Reperfusion therapy for acute myocardial infarction with fibrinolytic therapy or combination reduced fibrinolytic therapy and platelet glycoprotein IIb/IIIa inhibition: the GUSTO V randomised trial. *Lancet* 2001; **357**(9272):1905–14.
62. Keeley EC, Boura JA, Grines CL. Comparison of primary and facilitated percutaneous coronary interventions for ST-elevation myocardial infarction: quantitative review of randomised trials. *Lancet* 2006; **367**(9510): 579–88.
63. Primary versus tenecteplase-facilitated percutaneous coronary intervention in patients with ST-segment elevation acute myocardial infarction (ASSENT-4 PCI): randomised trial. *Lancet* 2006; **367**(9510):569–78.
64. Ellis SG, Tendera M, de Belder MA, *et al.* Facilitated PCI in patients with ST-elevation myocardial infarction. *N Engl J Med* 2008; **358**(21):2205–17.
65. Van't Hof AW, Ten Berg J, Heestermans T, *et al.* Prehospital initiation of tirofiban in patients with ST-elevation myocardial infarction undergoing primary angioplasty (On-TIME 2): a multicentre, double-blind, randomised controlled trial. *Lancet* 2008; **372**(9638):537–46.
66. Manoukian SV, Feit F, Mehran R, *et al.* Impact of major bleeding on 30-day mortality and clinical outcomes in patients with acute coronary syndromes: an analysis from the ACUITY Trial. *J Am Coll Cardiol* 2007; **49**(12): 1362–8.
67. Brener SJ, Barr LA, Burchenal JE, *et al.* Randomized, placebo-controlled trial of platelet glycoprotein IIb/IIIa blockade with primary angioplasty for acute myocardial infarction. ReoPro and Primary PTCA Organization and Randomized Trial (RAPPORT) Investigators. *Circulation* 1998; **98**(8):734–41.
68. Montalescot G, Barragan P, Wittenberg O, *et al.* Platelet glycoprotein IIb/IIIa inhibition with coronary stenting for acute myocardial infarction. *N Engl J Med* 2001; **344**(25):1895–903.
69. Chesebro JH, Knatterud G, Roberts R, *et al.* Thrombolysis in Myocardial Infarction (TIMI) Trial, Phase I: A comparison between intravenous tissue plasminogen activator and intravenous streptokinase. Clinical findings through hospital discharge. *Circulation* 1987; **76**(1): 142–54.
70. Three-year duration of benefit from abciximab in patients receiving stents for acute myocardial infarction in the randomized double-blind ADMIRAL study. *Eur Heart J* 2005; **26**(23):2520–23.
71. Stone GW, Grines CL, Cox DA, *et al.* Comparison of angioplasty with stenting, with or without abciximab, in acute myocardial infarction. *N Engl J Med* 2002; **346**(13):957–66.
72. De Luca G, Suryapranata H, Stone GW, *et al.* Abciximab as adjunctive therapy to reperfusion in acute ST-segment elevation myocardial infarction: a meta-analysis of randomized trials. *JAMA* 2005; **293**(14):1759–65.
73. Gurm H, Tamhane U, Meier P, *et al.* A comparison of abciximab and small molecule glycoprotein IIb/IIIa inhibitors in patients undergoing primary percutaneous intervention; a meta-analysis of contemporary randomized trials. *Circ Cardiovasc Intervent* 2009; **2**: 230–6.
74. De Luca G, Ucci G, Cassetti E, Marino P. Benefits from small molecule administration as compared with abciximab among patients with ST-segment elevation myocardial infarction treated with primary angioplasty: a meta-analysis. *J Am Coll Cardiol.* 2009; **53**(18): 1668–73.
75. Valgimigli M, Campo G, Percoco G, *et al.* Comparison of angioplasty with infusion of tirofiban or abciximab and with implantation of sirolimus-eluting or uncoated stents for acute myocardial infarction: the MULTISTRATEGY randomized trial. *JAMA.* 2008; **299**(15):1788–99.
76. Mehilli J, Kastrati A, Schulz S, *et al.* Abciximab in patients with acute ST-segment-elevation myocardial infarction undergoing primary percutaneous coronary intervention after clopidogrel loading: a randomized double-blind trial. *Circulation.* 2009; **119**(14): 1933–40.
77. Alvarez JM. Emergency coronary bypass grafting for failed percutaneous coronary artery stenting: increased costs and platelet transfusion requirements after the use of abciximab. *J Thorac Cardiovasc Surg.* 1998; **115**(2): 472–3.

78. Gammie JS, Zenati M, Kormos RL, *et al.* Abciximab and excessive bleeding in patients undergoing emergency cardiac operations. *Ann Thorac Surg.* 1998; **65**(2):465–9.
79. Lincoff AM, LeNarz LA, Despotis GJ, *et al.* Abciximab and bleeding during coronary surgery: results from the EPILOG and EPISTENT trials. Improve Long-term Outcome with abciximab GP IIb/IIIa blockade. Evaluation of Platelet IIb/IIIa Inhibition in STENTing. *Ann Thorac Surg.* 2000; **70**(2):516–26.
80. Pang JT, Fort S, Della Siega A, *et al.* Vmergency coronary artery bypass surgery in the era of glycoprotein IIb/IIIa receptor antagonist use. *J Card Surg* 2002; **17**(5): 425–431.
81. Juergens CP, Yeung AC, Oesterle SN. Routine platelet transfusion in patients undergoing emergency coronary bypass surgery after receiving abciximab. *Am J Cardiol* 1997; **80**(1):74–5.
82. De Carlo M, Maselli D, Cortese B, *et al.* Emergency coronary artery bypass grafting in patients with acute myocardial infarction treated with glycoprotein IIb/IIIa receptor inhibitors. *Int J Cardiol* 2008; **123**(3):229–33.
83. Wagner CL, Mascelli MA, Neblock DS, *et al.* Analysis of GPIIb/IIIa receptor number by quantification of 7E3 binding to human platelets. *Blood* 1996; **88**(3): 907–14.
84. Combining thrombolysis with the platelet glycoprotein IIb/IIIa inhibitor lamifiban: results of the Platelet Aggregation Receptor Antagonist Dose Investigation and Reperfusion Gain in Myocardial Infarction (PARADIGM) trial. *J Am Coll Cardiol* 1998; **32**(7):2003–10.
85. Best PJ, Lennon R, Gersh BJ, *et al.* Safety of abciximab in patients with chronic renal insufficiency who are undergoing percutaneous coronary interventions. *Am Heart J* 2003; **146**(2):345–50.
86. Freeman RV, Mehta RH, Al Badr W, *et al.* Influence of concurrent renal dysfunction on outcomes of patients with acute coronary syndromes and implications of the use of glycoprotein IIb/IIIa inhibitors. *J Am Coll Cardiol* 2003; **41**(5):718–24.
87. Frilling B, Zahn R, Fraiture B, *et al.* Comparison of efficacy and complication rates after percutaneous coronary interventions in patients with and without renal insufficiency treated with abciximab. *Am J Cardiol* 2002; **89**(4):450–2.
88. Macie C, Forbes L, Foster GA, *et al.* Dosing practices and risk factors for bleeding in patients receiving enoxaparin for the treatment of an acute coronary syndrome. *Chest* 2004; **125**(5):1616–21.
89. Ciccone A, Abraha I, Santilli I. Glycoprotein IIb-IIIa inhibitors for acute ischaemic stroke. *Cochrane Database Syst Rev* 2006; **4**:CD005208.
90. Shammas NW. An overview of antithrombins in peripheral vascular interventions. *J Invasive Cardiol* 2004; **16**(8):440–3.
91. Allie DE, Hebert CJ, Lirtzman MD, *et al.* A safety and feasibility report of combined direct thrombin and GP IIb/IIIa inhibition with bivalirudin and tirofiban in peripheral vascular disease intervention: treating critical limb ischemia like acute coronary syndrome. *J Invasive Cardiol* 2005; **17**(8):427–32.
92. Rocha-Singh KJ, Rutherford J. Glycoprotein IIb-IIIa receptor inhibition with eptifibatide in percutaneous intervention for symptomatic peripheral vascular disease: the circulate pilot trial. *Catheter Cardiovasc Interv* 2005; **66**(4):470–3.
93. Smith SC, Jr, Feldman TE, Hirshfeld JW, Jr, *et al.* ACC/AHA/SCAI 2005 Guideline Update for Percutaneous Coronary Intervention-Summary Article: A Report of the American College of Cardiology/American Heart Association Task Force on Practice Guidelines (ACC/AHA/SCAI Writing Committee to Update the 2001 Guidelines for Percutaneous Coronary Intervention). *J Am Coll Cardiol* 2006; **47**(1):216–35.
94. Silber S, Albertsson P, Aviles FF, *et al.* Guidelines for percutaneous coronary interventions. The Task Force for Percutaneous Coronary Interventions of the European Society of Cardiology. *Eur Heart J* 2005; **26**(8):804–47.
95. Antman EM, Anbe DT, Armstrong PW, *et al.* ACC/AHA guidelines for the management of patients with ST-elevation myocardial infarction: a report of the American College of Cardiology/American Heart Association Task Force on Practice Guidelines (Committee to Revise the 1999 Guidelines for the Management of Patients with Acute Myocardial Infarction). *Circulation* 2004; **110**(9):e82–292.
96. Morrow DA, Antman EM, Parsons L, *et al.* Application of the TIMI risk score for ST-elevation MI in the National Registry of Myocardial Infarction 3. *JAMA* 2001; **286**(11):1356–9.
97. Van de Werf F, Bax J, Betriu A, *et al.* Management of acute myocardial infarction in patients presenting with persistent ST-segment elevation: the Task Force on the Management of ST-Segment Elevation Acute Myocardial Infarction of the European Society of Cardiology. *Eur Heart J* 2008; **29**(23):2909–45.
98. Kushner FG, Hand M, Smith SC, *et al.* Focused Updates: ACC/AHA Guidelines for the Management of Patients With ST-Elevation Myocardial Infarction (Updating the 2004 Guideline and 2007 Focused Update) and ACC/AHA/SCAI Guidelines on Percutaneous Coronary Intervention (Updating the 2005 Guideline and 2007 Focused Update). A Report of the American College of Cardiology Foundation/American Heart Association Task Force on Practice Guidelines. *Circulation.* 2009.
99. Anderson J, Adams C, Antman E, *et al.* ACC/AHA 2007 Guidelines for the Management of Patients With Unstable Angina/Non–ST-Elevation Myocardial Infarction – Executive Summary. A Report of the American College of Cardiology/American Heart Association Task Force

on Practice Guidelines (Writing Committee to Revise the 2002 Guidelines for the Management of Patients With Unstable Angina/Non–ST-Elevation Myocardial Infarction) Developed in Collaboration with the American College of Emergency Physicians, the Society for Cardiovascular Angiography and Interventions, and the Society of Thoracic Surgeons Endorsed by the American Association of Cardiovascular and Pulmonary Rehabilitation and the Society for Academic Emergency Medicine. *J Am Coll Cardiol* 2007; **50**:652–726.

100. Gratsianskii NA. [Do low risk patients undergoing percutaneous coronary intervention after pretreatment with clopidogrel need abciximab infusion? Results of ISAR-REACT study]. *Kardiologiia* 2004; **44**(3):80–1.
101. Cohen M. Glycoprotein IIb/IIIa receptor blockers in acute coronary syndromes: Gusto IV-ACS. *Lancet* 2001; **357**(9272):1899–900.

CHAPTER 24

The contemporary use of antiplatelet therapy in interventional cardiology

Aung Myat and Tony Gershlick

Introduction

Accepting that the adhesion, activation, and aggregation of platelets plays a central role in the initial formation and subsequent propagation of intracoronary thrombi, antiplatelet therapy (APT) has become central to the management of a number of manifestations of cardiovascular (CV) disease; not least in preventing the deleterious effects of stent thrombosis (ST) that can follow percutaneous coronary intervention (PCI) with stent deployment. PCI causes significant local trauma to the vessel wall leading to exposure of the subendothelium and release of its thrombogenic constituents into the intravascular environment resulting in an increased risk of vaso-occlusive complications. Exposure of the stent struts can further stimulate platelet adherence to the non-endothelialized vessel wall and accelerate activation and aggregation. Furthermore, PCI can also potentiate the release of vasoactive agents from the platelet-rich thrombus. This may be of particular importance when PCI is undertaken in those presenting with acute coronary syndromes (ACS) where plaque disruption has already locally activated platelets by exposing the flowing blood constituents to thrombogenic plaque contents.

The two overriding phenomena that remain serious clinical challenges to the predictable success of intracoronary stenting are in-stent restenosis (ISR) secondary to intimal hyperplasia and ST. Much of the literature suggests that an intact and functionally viable endothelium is not only non-thrombogenic but also prevents the smooth muscle cell proliferation that leads to the late luminal loss caused by intimal hyperplasia. Hence the trial-driven clinical success of drug-eluting stents (DES) which reduce restenosis by inhibiting this smooth muscle hyperplasia. At the same time, however, DES can cause bystander endothelial cell inhibition thus potentially delaying the protective re-endothelialization which would otherwise normally occur within a month or so following bare metal stent (BMS) deployment. DES implantation is also thought to cause more inflammation, hypersensitivity, thrombus formation, and outward remodelling which may all augment the susceptibility to ST.

According to the Academic Research Consortium (ARC) ST can be defined as acute (within 24h), subacute (in the first 30 days), late (out to 1 year), and very late (over 12 months). Whenever it occurs ST can lead to significant major adverse cardiac events (MACE) including up to a 50% risk of acute myocardial infarction (AMI) or death. It is widely accepted that DES pose a greater risk of ST compared to BMS in the longer term. As a result those individuals receiving DES require a protracted course of dual antiplatelet therapy (DAPT); a fact borne out of a number of landmark clinical trials which have looked at the complementary inhibition of different segments of the platelet aggregatory pathway affected by various antiplatelet therapies. It is important to note that the length of re-endothelialization delay may well vary according to the stent platform, the polymer used to carry the drug and the drug itself. Adequate prevention of ST requires optimization of four key areas, all of which are intimately interrelated: the patient–physician dynamic; the antiplatelet drug(s) used and the ability of the patient to adequately respond to APT; platelet function and reactivity; and the characteristics of the stent following optimal deployment.

As our understanding of the pathophysiology and molecular interactions that underlie thrombosis formation in those presenting with, and treated for, atheromatous disease has increased, so has the number of potential targets for APT to inhibit. In this chapter we give an overview of the pivotal role of platelets in the coagulation and inflammatory processes that trigger the interaction of a multitude of cell-surface and intracellular platelet receptors, ligands, agonists, chemotactic agents, and inflammatory mediators, the coming together of which, during episodes of platelet stimulation, have the potential to result in life-threatening intracoronary thrombosis. We will examine trial data for APT used in the management of ACS and the prevention of ST post PCI with stent deployment and how this has evolved over time. There will also be particular emphasis on how patient response to APT is measured and a detailed exploration of the phenomenon of APT drug resistance. To conclude, future APT therapies, available now and those on the horizon, will be discussed and how these will supplement the drug armamentarium available to the interventional cardiologist.

Platelets: friend and foe?

Platelets are anucleate fragments of large bone marrow-derived cells called megakaryocytes. Once beyond the bone marrow, platelets circulate in the blood and under normal homeostatic conditions do not interact with other cells. They have a life-span of approximately 8–10 days and pass through the circulation only being activated by sites of endothelial damage[(1)]. Platelets adhere to the site of vascular injury and promote several key elements of the coagulation cascade which ultimately culminates in the formation of a growing haemostatic plug. As such, platelets are absolutely crucial to the body's vascular repair processes.

The role of platelets in atherothrombosis

The deleterious consequences of atherothrombosis are initiated when the fibrous cap that covers a mature plaque situated in the medium- to large-diameter vessels of the coronary, cerebral, and peripheral arterial trees either ruptures or the lesion surface erodes, thereby exposing the highly prothrombotic contents to the luminal microenvironment[(2)]. The process of atherothrombosis can be summarized in five phases (Fig. 24.1) although such a simplistic plan belies the highly complex nature of the interaction between atherogenesis, inflammation, oxidative stress, and plaque rupture. Indeed not all plaques rupture or erode and not all plaque rupture results in ischaemic sequelae. Intense research has elucidated a cycle of repeated rupture, thrombosis, and healing with continual renovation of the fibrous plaque surface akin to normal haemostasis[(3)]. The central catalyst that binds these processes together, however, is the adhesion, activation, and aggregation of platelets. Plaque rupture only leads to clinical events if it leads to the intiation and propagation of thrombus. This might depend on the degree of rupture and exposure of intraplaque contents (minor erosion versus complete de-capping); the size of the plaque, so that a small amount of thrombus from a large plaque will cause temporary or permanent occlusion if the remaining non-plaque lumen is narrow; or the thrombogenicity of the patient's blood—a minor plaque and its disruption may cause complete vessel occlusion if there is high platelet reactivity; for example in those with hypercholesterolaemia, obesity, or in smokers.

Platelet adhesion

Upon being exposed to a site of vascular injury, platelets attach to the exposed subendothelium via a glycoprotein (GP) Ib/V/IX receptor complex along with several other collagen receptors expressed on their cell surface[(4)]. The primary catalyst for this interaction is collagen, stabilized by von Willebrand factor (vWF); along with fibronectin, laminin, and thrombospondin found in the extracellular matrix of the subendothelium[(1)]. The adherent platelets undergo a conformational change from smooth disc to spiky sphere allowing them to roll across the subendothelial surface which, in turn, stimulates a further change in morphology to a hemisphere via an internal signalling network. This shape transition firmly anchors the platelet to the vessel wall by increasing the surface area for contact, allowing it to overcome the high shear forces of blood flowing through the lumen. Subsequent signalling cascades flatten the platelet further thus promoting irreversible adhesion to the injured vessel wall (Fig. 24.2).

Platelet activation and the coagulation cascade

Following platelet adhesion to the extracellular matrix, the vessel wall repair process is activated through a combination of circulating paracrine and autocrine mediators, primarily thromboxane A_2 (TXA_2), adenosine diphosphate (ADP), thrombin, and adrenaline which propagate the haemostatic response by binding to adherent platelets and synergistically inducing their activation and recruiting further circulating platelets to

Phase 1

Deposition, accumulation, and oxidation of low-density lipoprotein cholesterol within the arterial intima as a result of endothelial dysfunction.

Phase 2 and Phase 3 (Plate A)

Recruitment of inflammatory cells to the growing plaque with accumulation of lipid-laden foam cells and migrating smooth muscle cells linked together by a meshwork of extracellular matrix molecules such as collagen and elastin. The plaque surface begins to calcify to form a fibrous cap. Healthy endothelium secretes nitric oxide and prostacyclin which help keep platelets in an inactive state. CD39 on the endothelial surface also converts ADP, a potent platelet agonist, to adenosine monophosphate (AMP) which is then degraded to adenosine by CD73; therefore preventing the activation of platelets yet further.

Phase 4 (Plates A and B)

Plaque breakdown begins to occur as more smooth muscle is broken down than is formed. Under certain conditions the fibrous cap surface begins to erode or the plaque ruptures exposing the prothrombotic contents, such as the ligands von Willebrand factor and collagen which can then bind their respective platelet receptors, to the luminal microenvironment. This triggers the adhesion, conformational change, and activation of platelets from the passing circulation. As platelets begin to aggregate several positive secondary feedback loops are initiated which promote the formation of a platelet-rich clot.

Phase 5 (Plate C)

Formation of a platelet-rich thrombus at the site of vascular injury with mechanical disruption of the diseased artery. If blood flow is sufficiently impeded this can then manifest as a clinical syndrome leading to coronary, cerebral or peripheral arterial ischaemia.

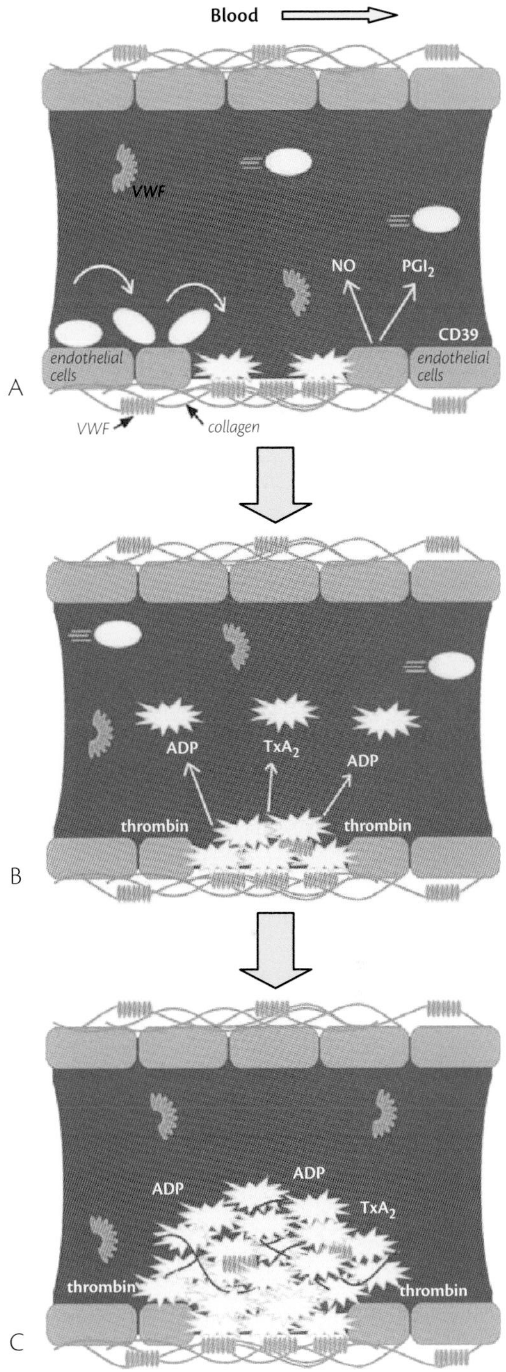

Fig. 24.1 Five phases of atherothrombosis[1]. ADP, adenosine diphosphate; NO, nitric oxide; PGI_2, prostacyclin; TXA_2, thromboxane A_2; VWF, von Willebrand factor. Adapted with permission from Michelson AD (ed). *Platelets*, 2nd edn. Elsevier Inc/Academic Press, © 2007.

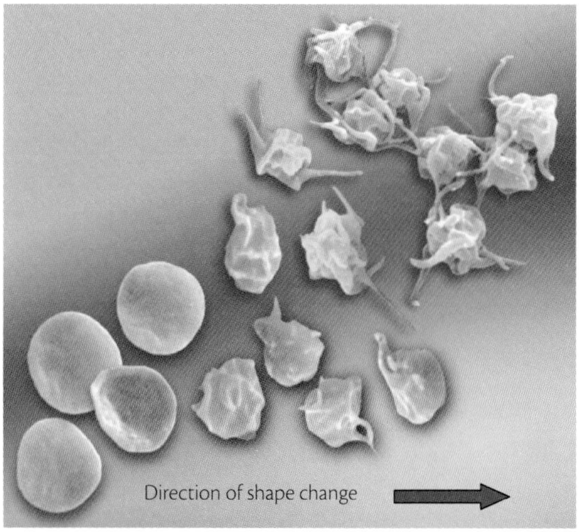

Fig. 24.2 Conformational platelet change from disc to spiky sphere to hemisphere, ultimately resulting in a flattened cell to allow maximum surface area for aggregation to other platelets. Adapted with permission from Michelson AD (ed). *Platelets*, 2nd edn. Elsevier Inc/Academic Press, © 2007.

the growing intraluminal plug. Within the platelet there is degranulation of storage vesicles which releases ADP and serotonin; further synthesis of TXA_2 and an increase in the cell-surface expression of the GP $\alpha_{IIb}\beta_3$ (IIb/IIIa) receptor—the purpose being to prevent major external haemorrhage through the development of a haemostatic plug. It is when this plug starts to form within a vessel, which is still intact (i.e. there is no leak to the outside) but injured through either spontaneous or iatrogenic plaque damage, that they then become problematic since they can potentially lead to life-threatening vessel occlusion.

It is not only platelet activation and the platelet plug that is important. The coagulation cascade is stimulated by exposure of negatively-charged elements within the phospholipid membrane on the platelet's surface. This ultimately results in the generation of insoluble fibrin which acts to form stabilizing cross linkages between adjacent platelets. The combination of activated platelets and coagulation cofactors along with their associated enzymes act to generate increasing amounts of thrombin which itself is a potent platelet activator[1]. Platelets also impede fibrinolysis by secretion of factors such as plasminogen activation inhibitor 1[5].

Platelet aggregation

The final stage in the formation of a persistent platelet-rich intraluminal thrombus is mediated primarily through upregulation of the GP IIb/IIIa receptor on the platelet surface and its interaction with various adhesion proteins such as fibrinogen, vWF, fibronectin, and vitronectin. Fibrinogen acts to stabilize the forming thrombus by bridging adjacent GP IIb/IIIa integrins between platelets through its thrombin-mediated conversion to fibrin (Fig. 24.3). This process is further augmented by platelet-derived bioactive tissue factor which is the primary initiator of the coagulation cascade and stimulates the conversion of prothrombin to thrombin and fibrinogen to fibrin. In effect, several positive secondary feedback loops work in unison and serve to recruit more platelets to the growing thrombus which is then strengthened by fibrin cross-linking, thus promoting further propagation of the clot[1,4].

The extent to which a thrombus grows largely depends on four factors:

- The degree of plaque rupture or erosion
- The degree of luminal stenosis
- The physicochemical properties of the surface exposed to the circulation, and
- Site of the lesion relative to blood flow[6].

Platelets cluster to the greatest extent at the lesion apex and continued narrowing of the artery and slower blood flow stimulates a larger, more platelet-rich clot to form which may eventually occlude the vessel to such a degree that a clinical syndrome is manifest in the absence of appropriate APT or mechanical intervention.

The role of inflammation in the formation of intraluminal thrombus has often been underestimated. It is now widely recognized that inflammation and atherothrombosis are intimately linked when once it was thought the two were situated at opposite ends of a continuum. A detailed exploration of this topic, however, is beyond the scope of this review. Suffice to say activated platelets secrete several inflammatory mediators such as: CD40 ligand, P-selectin, cyclooxygenase (COX), interleukin 1β, platelet factor 4, and platelet-derived growth factor amongst others which serve to alter the chemotactic and adhesive properties of endothelial cells[1,4]. There is now extensive research being conducted on the use of inflammatory markers as predictors of CV risk in addition to being potential targets for antiplatelet drugs[2]. It is likely that detection of the severity and degree of inflammation may become part of the clinical assessment in patients with ACS and may even have a role as a predictor for outcome. Management of those with high levels of inflammatory response such that the natural history is altered is more problematic.

Current targets for APT include the agonists TXA_2 and ADP via inhibition of COX and the $P2Y_{12}$ receptor respectively along with direct blockade of the GP IIb/IIIa receptor which, as previously mentioned, promotes

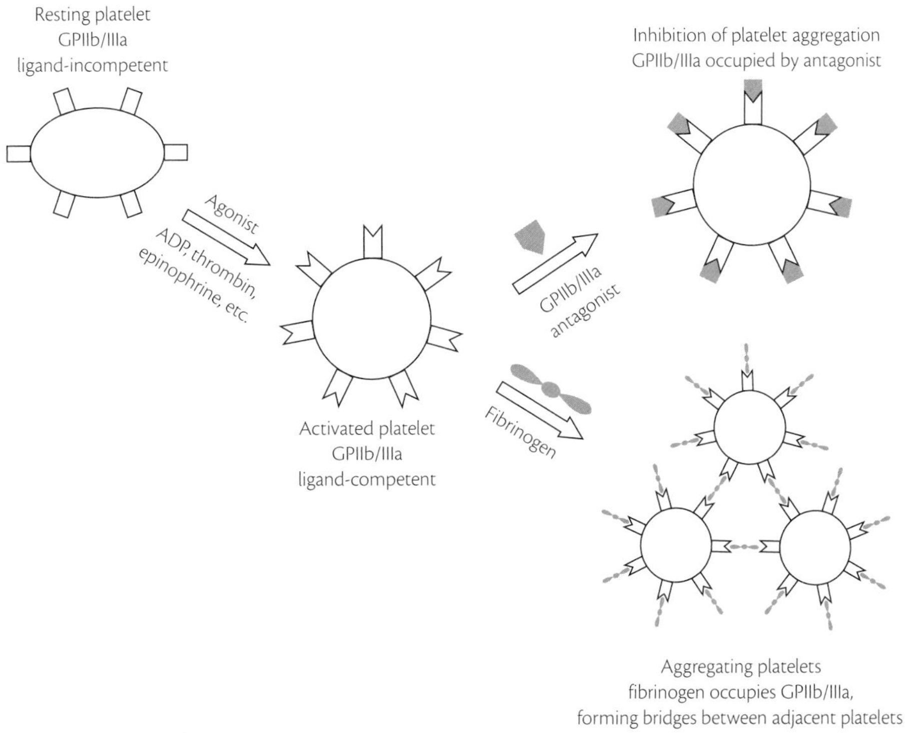

Fig. 24.3 Activation of platelet GPIIb/IIIa receptors followed by cross-linking to adjacent platelets mediated by fibrinogen in the final common pathway of platelet aggregation. Reproduced from Moliterno DJ, Topol EJ. Conjunctive use of platelet glycoprotein IIb/IIIa antagonists and thrombolytic therapy for acute myocardial infarction. *Thromb Haemost* 1997; **78**:214–19 with permission.

the final common platelet aggregatory pathway. Drugs that attenuate the pro-aggregatory action of thrombin through inhibition of G-protein-linked protease-activated receptors (PARs) present on the platelet surface are also under investigation (Fig. 24.4).

Aspirin

Acetyl-salicylic acid was patented under the trade name of Aspirin by Bayer & Co in 1899 and was first used as an analgesic and an antipyretic. Its effects on haemostasis, however, were demonstrated as early as 1945[5]. Its antithrombotic action is mediated through the irreversible acetylation of COX enzymes secreted by activated platelets. As such COX-mediated TXA_2 synthesis from arachidonic acid (AA) release, following phospholipase A_2 activation, is inhibited for the entire life span of the platelet (≈120 days). TXA_2 is a potent platelet agonist and vasoconstrictor and can induce platelet α-granule secretion and aggregation via G-protein coupled TPα and TPβ receptors found on the platelet surface[4]. It should be noted, however, that phospholipase A_2 activation and AA release have a relatively small role to play in the mechanism of action of many platelet agonists, other than collagen which is a notable exception. Indeed there are many who would not class aspirin as a true antiplatelet agent since its antiplatelet action is limited and comparatively weak. In situations of potent platelet stimulation aspirin, irrespective of dose, is not sufficient. Furthermore the balance between the beneficial antiaggregatory effects of aspirin against the negative impact of its dose-dependent inhibition of prostacyclin biosynthesis (the same pathway to PGI_2 production is inhibited) alongside the well established side effects on the gastrointestinal tract have limited standard aspirin dose to between 75–160mg once daily. Prostacyclin is a beneficial endothelial cell-derived vasodilator prostanoid that inhibits platelet activation in response to a variety of agonists and specifically modulates the platelet response to TXA_2[4].

Nevertheless aspirin has become the cornerstone of APT over the last two decades. It is antithrombotic at a wide range of daily doses, from 30–1500mg, although a low dose (75mg per day) is sufficient to reduce platelet production of TXA_2 by 97–99%[4]. In 1988 the Physicians' Health Study in the United States was the first primary prevention study to assess whether aspirin (325mg on alternate days) was able to avert AMI in over

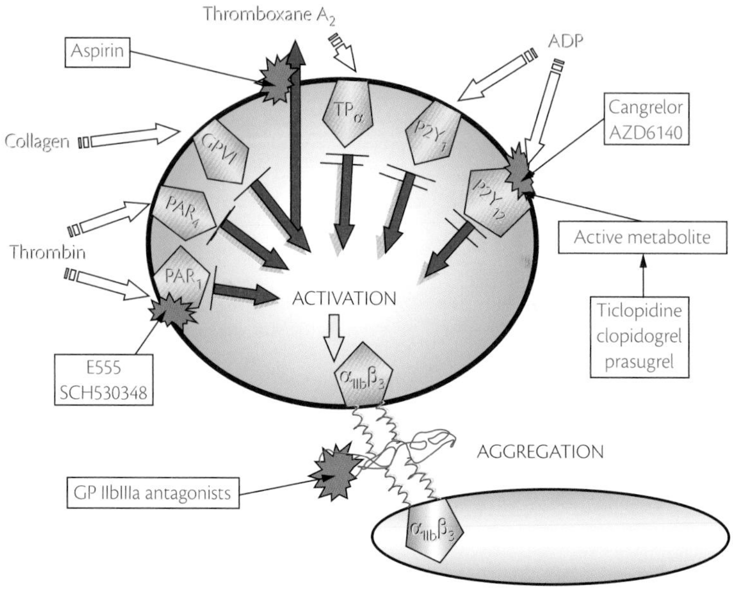

Fig. 24.4 Targets for platelet inhibition. Adapted with permission from 'Platelets, Second Edition' Alan D Michelson MD (eds), Elsevier Inc/Academic Press, © 2007.

20 000 male doctors. Aspirin reduced the risk of fatal MI by 75% and non-fatal MI by 44% although the absolute risk reduction was a modest 0.9% in previously healthy men with no significant reduction in CV mortality in those aged over 50 years[7]. Interestingly this trial also showed that aspirin was more effective in reducing future CV risk in those healthy men with high rather than low C-reactive protein (CRP) levels. Men with CRP levels in the highest quartile were found to have three times the risk of AMI and twice the risk of ischaemic stroke lending further support to the idea that atherothrombosis has an inflammatory substrate[2]. Overall a meta-analysis of aspirin primary prevention trials (including the Physicians' Health Study) demonstrated an absolute risk reduction of 0.7% for first MI in both men and women but not that of non-fatal stroke or vascular death alone[8]. This is countered by the fact that long-term aspirin therapy is associated with an increased incidence of gastrointestinal haemorrhage, as was the case in this study, through erosion or ulceration of the gut wall, and a propensity to increase the risk of haemorrhagic stroke.

Unlike primary prevention, the role of aspirin in the secondary prevention of ischaemic sequelae due to atherothrombosis is undoubted. The landmark Antithrombotic Trialists' Collaboration meta-analysis of 287 studies of APT, primarily with aspirin, involving some 140 000 high-risk individuals with vascular disease demonstrated an overall 25% reduction in the incidence of non-fatal MI, non-fatal stroke, and vascular death[9]. The Second International Study of Infarct Survival (ISIS-2) affirmed the benefit of aspirin therapy in the context of ST-elevation MI (STEMI) treated with streptokinase fibrinolytic therapy. It had previously been shown that the administration of streptokinase lead to increased production of TXA_2 resulting in rebound platelet activation. As such the concomitant use of aspirin would hypothetically nullify this adverse reaction. Over 17 000 patients with STEMI were randomized to four arms: placebo, aspirin, streptokinase, or streptokinase plus aspirin. Aspirin or streptokinase, as single agents, were equally good in reducing mortality compared with placebo (10.7% and 10.4% respectively compared to 13.2% in the placebo group). Combination aspirin and streptokinase, however, reduced mortality to 8.0% leading to an overall risk reduction of 42%[10].

The role of aspirin in ACS is undisputed. It is given routinely to those patients with STEMI, non-ST-elevation MI (NSTEMI), and unstable angina (UA) and is thought to benefit equally those undergoing or not undergoing PCI. A daily dose of 75–160mg of aspirin is adequate for the long-term prevention of serious vascular sequelae in high-risk patients. An additional bolus dose of 300mg, however, is recommended in acute clinical scenarios where an immediate antithrombotic effect is necessary, although this remains empiric.

The thienopyridines

The agonist ADP is crucial in platelet activation and therefore its G-protein coupled cell-surface receptors $P2Y_1$ and $P2Y_{12}$ are potential targets for antiplatelet drugs

(Fig. 24.4). The $P2Y_1$ receptor is a target receptor for many of the processes that occur in acute vessel injury; its activation triggers the mobilization of calcium from internal platelet stores which results in conformational change and transient aggregation in response to ADP. It is also involved in the aggregation response to collagen. Overall, however, the $P2Y_1$ receptor mediates relatively weak responses to ADP and other agonists although it remains an essential component of the platelet activation pathway when there is collagen-induced activation.

The $P2Y_{12}$ receptor is responsible for completion of the platelet activation response to ADP initiated by $P2Y_1$ and is the molecular target of the antiplatelet drug group the thienopyridines: ticlopidine, clopidogrel, and prasugrel (Fig. 24.5). It is central to amplification of the aggregatory pathways stimulated by all known platelet agonists including collagen, thrombin, immune complexes, TXA_2, adrenaline, and serotonin, and therefore is pivotal in stabilizing and propagating the growth of the platelet-rich intraluminal thrombus.

The thienopyridines selectively and irreversibly inhibit the $P2Y_{12}$ inhibitor with no direct effects on AA metabolism and as such work on a completely separate portion of the platelet aggregatory pathway with respect to aspirin. They require hepatic transformation to an active metabolite by the cytochrome P450 enzyme system to acquire their antiplatelet activity.

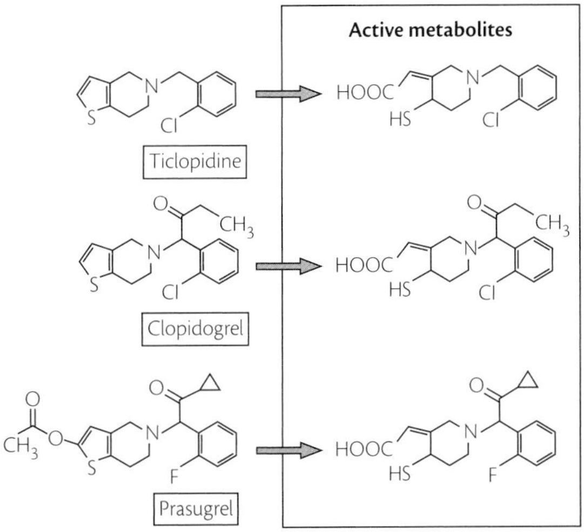

Fig. 24.5 Chemical structures of the first, second, and third generation of thienopyridines and their active metabolites. Reproduced from Peters RJH. *Circulation* 2003; **108**:1682–7.

Ticlopidine: a first-generation thienopyridine

Ticlopidine, the first thienopyridine to be developed, given as a twice-daily dose of 250mg has been shown to be just as effective as aspirin and significantly superior to placebo for the secondary prevention of ischaemic events in patients at high atherothrombotic risk(11). There is, however, a clear rationale for combining aspirin with a thienopyridine since they work via complementary mechanisms and have the potential to provide synergistic inhibition of the platelet aggregatory pathway; hence the evolution of DAPT.

The combination of aspirin plus oral anticoagulation (OAC), in the form of a coumadin derivative, was the first antithrombotic strategy used to prevent vaso-occlusive complications after percutaneous transluminal coronary angioplasty (PTCA) with stenting. This was until four landmark trials were published in the late 1990s: ISAR(12), STARS(13), FANTASTIC(14), and MATTIS(15). Together these studies clearly demonstrated the superiority of DAPT over OAC and aspirin in the prevention of ST and other MACE following PCI, and further significantly reduced the risk of bleeding complications. All four trials used a combination of ticlopidine and aspirin and compared them to OAC plus aspirin. Although patients were randomized to either treatment arm, each study had an open-label design. Different patient populations were studied, with variation in disease severity. Differences in peri-procedural anticoagulation and definitions of safety endpoints were also potential confounders. Despite this, all four studies came to the same conclusion: DAPT was superior to OAC plus aspirin in terms of reducing the incidence of adverse events and the rate of haemorrhagic/vascular complications following stent deployment. A subsequent meta-analysis of these trials confirmed the net clinical benefit of DAPT over OAC and aspirin(16). This advantage was essentially driven by significant reductions in non-fatal MI and the need for repeat target vessel revascularization (TVR). Interestingly there was no significant difference in mortality between the two treatment regimens.

The association of ticlopidine with hypercholesterolaemia and, more seriously, adverse haematological effects such as neutropenia, thrombocytopenia, aplastic anaemia, and thrombotic thrombocytopenic purpura (TTP) along with its relative expense means that it has been largely superseded by clopidogrel. Its use is now reserved primarily for those who are allergic to clopidogrel.

Clopidogrel: a second-generation thienopyridine

Clopidogrel is now well established as the current thienopyridine of choice, used in combination with low-dose aspirin, as DAPT to prevent the deleterious effects of ST in the coronary stenting era and for the secondary prevention of ischaemic vascular sequelae in high-risk individuals following an atherothrombotic event such as NSTEMI. It is a pro-drug which requires two cytochrome P450-dependent oxidative steps during its metabolism by the liver to produce its active moiety. Like ticlopidine it irreversibly binds to the $P2Y_{12}$ receptor and therefore inhibits ADP-induced platelet aggregation and the clustering of platelet-monocyte pairings therefore also interfering with the inflammatory response which, as previously indicated, is intimately linked with the atherothrombotic cascade that follows plaque rupture/erosion.

The superior tolerability of clopidogrel when compared to ticlopidine was first established by the CLASSICS trial[17]. A cohort of 1020 patients were randomized to a regimen of either: aspirin 325mg once a day plus ticlopidine 250mg twice daily; or aspirin plus clopidogrel 75mg once daily; or aspirin plus a 300-mg loading dose (LD) of clopidogrel followed by a maintenance dose (MD) of 75mg per day after coronary stenting. The study demonstrated an essentially equivalent efficacy of clopidogrel, with or without an LD, compared to ticlopidine in terms of MACE rates between the three groups (0.9% ticlopidine, 1.5% clopidogrel 75mg per day and 1.2% clopidogrel 300mg loading followed by 75mg daily) but importantly demonstrated a much improved safety profile for clopidogrel. Consequently, due to its adverse side-effect profile and slower onset of action, ticlopidine use fell dramatically and was replaced by the much safer, equally effective and, when a loading dose was given, significantly faster-acting clopidogrel.

Subsequent trials then proceeded to prove the benefits of clopidogrel use in the secondary prevention of atherothrombotic vascular disease (Table 24.1).

The CAPRIE trial compared clopidogrel to aspirin in 19 185 individuals who had recently suffered an MI, ischaemic stroke, or had established peripheral arterial disease. Clopidogrel use inferred a modest 0.51% absolute risk reduction in the composite endpoint of MI, ischaemic stroke, or vascular death but effectively the safety and tolerability of aspirin and clopidogrel were similar[18]. These results, therefore, did not effect a change in clinical practice but certainly revealed that clopidogrel was an appropriate alternative to aspirin, for instance, in those with aspirin allergy.

The landmark CURE study was the first to demonstrate the superiority of DAPT when compared to a single antiplatelet agent acting alone[19]. A total of 12 562 patients presenting within 24h of symptoms indicating UA/NSTEMI were randomized to receive clopidogrel (300mg LD followed by 75mg/day MD) or placebo in addition to aspirin (75–325mg/day MD) for 3–12 months. The primary endpoint; a composite of CV death, non-fatal MI, or stroke, occurred in 9.3% of individuals taking DAPT and 11.4% taking aspirin plus placebo, giving rise to a 2.1% absolute risk reduction overall. Of note the anti-ischaemic benefits of clopidogrel were apparent within the first 24h of drug administration, suggesting the LD was rapidly effective. They were also observed across a variety of subgroups and maintained throughout the 12-month treatment period. Conversely, however, DAPT was associated with a significant 1.0 and 2.7% increase in major and minor bleeding respectively, giving an early indication that with effective inhibition of the platelet aggregatory pathway comes the danger of excess bleeding, the need for transfusion, and vascular access complications. Surprisingly, however, a post hoc analysis of the CURE trial results revealed the observed increase in major bleeding events due to DAPT was primarily caused by increasing aspirin dose as opposed to the addition of clopidogrel (Fig. 24.6).

The role of clopidogrel in PCI for UA/NSTEMI patients was established following a subgroup analysis of some 2658 patients in the CURE study who subsequently proceeded to in-hospital coronary stenting as a consequence of refractory ischaemia or MACE: the PCI-CURE study[20]. Within the cohort 1313 patients were randomized to a 300-mg LD of clopidogrel followed by 75mg/day MD and 1345 randomized to placebo. PCI was conducted within a median 10-day pre-treatment period. Those patients receiving stents were then given open-label thienopyridine therapy (clopidogrel or ticlopidine) for 2–4 weeks after which time they were switched back to their pre-PCI treatment regimen. Again, the early beneficial effect of thienopyridine therapy was demonstrated in the clopidogrel arm in which significantly fewer individuals had an MI or refractory ischaemia pre-PCI when compared to placebo. At 30 days and a mean of 8 months post PCI the primary combined endpoint of CV death, MI, or urgent TVR was significantly lower in clopidogrel patients compared with the placebo arm. Since the vast majority of patients received open-label thienopyridine treatment for 4 weeks after stent deployment it follows that the period of clopidogrel treatment *pre-PCI* was pivotal in reducing MACE rates in the short- and long-term post procedure. The benefits were spread throughout all clinical and demographic subgroups and were

Table 24.1 Landmark clopidogrel trials in atherothrombotic vascular disease

Study (year)	Patients (n)	Clinical presentation	Treatment arms	Mean follow-up period	Primary endpoint	Event rate (%)		Relative risk reduction (%)	*p*-value
						Rx*	Ctrl†		
CAPRIE (1996)	19 185	Recent MI, CVA or PAD	Clopidogrel 75mg od vs. aspirin (ASA) 325mg od	1.9 years	Ischaemic stroke, MI, vascular death	5.32	5.83	8.7	0.043
CURE (2001)	12 562	UA/NSTEMI	Clopidogrel 300mg bolus then 75mg od + ASA 75 to 325mg od vs placebo + ASA 75 to 325mg od	9 months	Cardiovascular death, non-fatal MI, CVA	9.3	11.4	20.0	<0.001
PCI-CURE (2001)	2658	UA/NSTEMI proceeding to PCI	Clopidogrel 300mg bolus then 75mg od + ASA 75 to 325mg od vs placebo + ASA 75 to 325mg od	8 months	Cardiovascular death, MI, urgent target vessel revascularization	4.5	6.4	30.0	0.03
CREDO (2002)	2116	Elective PCI or at high likelihood to undergo PCI	Clopidogrel 300mg bolus then 75mg od + ASA 325mg od vs placebo + ASA 325mg od	1 year	Death, MI, CVA	8.4	11.5	26.9	0.02
COMMIT/CCS-2 (2005)	45 852	Suspected acute MI; 54% thrombolysed + heparin	Clopidogrel 75mg od + ASA 162mg od vs placebo + ASA 162mg od	28 days	Death, reinfarction, CVA	9.2	10.1	9.0	0.002
CLARITY-TIMI-28 (2005)	3491	Acute STEMI (<12h) Thrombolysis ± heparin	Clopidogrel 300mg bolus then 75mg od + ASA od vs placebo + ASA od	3.5 days	Occluded infarct-related artery, death, MI prior to angiography	14.9	21.7	30.9	<0.001
PCI-CLARITY (2005)	1863	Acute STEMI (<12h) Thrombolysis ± heparin proceeding to PCI	Clopidogrel 300mg bolus then 75 mg od + ASA od vs placebo + ASA od	30 days	Cardiovascular death, recurrent MI, stroke	3.6	6.2	41.9	0.008

*Clopidogrel arm.

†Aspirin ± placebo arm.

ASA, Acetyl-salicylic acid; CVA, cerebrovascular accident; MI, myocardial infarction; NSTEMI, non-ST elevated MI; PAD, peripheral arterial disease; STEMI, ST elevated MI; UA, unstable angina.

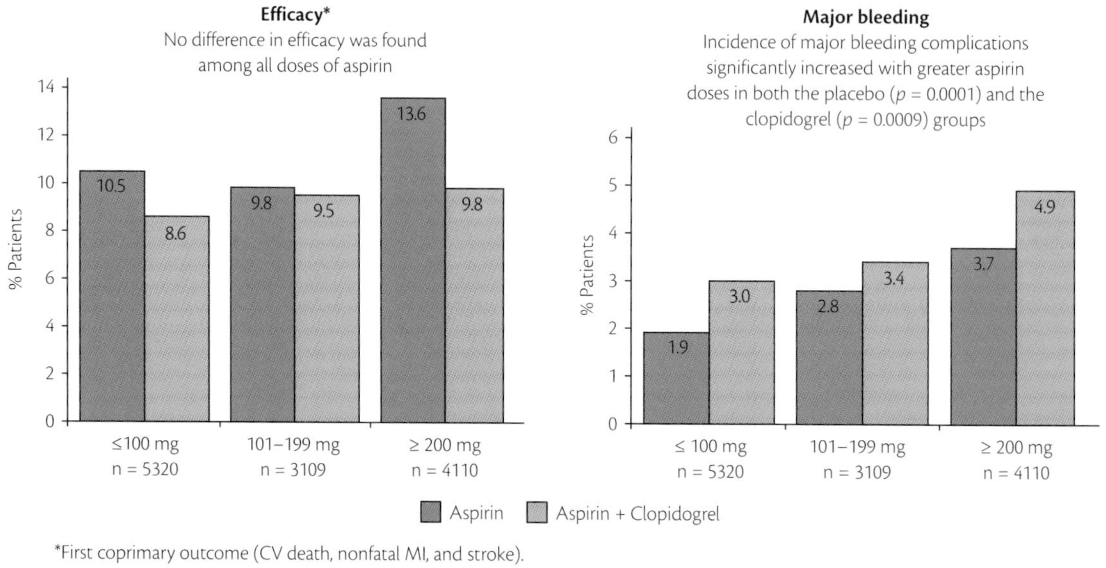

Fig. 24.6 Post hoc analysis of the CURE Trial demonstrating an association between increasing aspirin dose, rather than clopidogrel, with the increase in major bleeding complications. Adapted with permission from: Bhatt DL. Aspirin resistance: more than just a laboratory curiosity. *J Am Coll Cardiol* 2004; **43**:1127–9. Copyright © 2004 American College of Cardiology Foundation Published by Elsevier Inc.

maintained regardless of the timing of PCI. As with the CURE study there were more minor bleeding events in the clopidogrel arm but no significant increase in major bleeding.

The benefit of pre-PCI thienopyridine treatment was further substantiated by the CREDO study which randomized 2116 ACS patients to a 300-mg LD of clopidogrel or placebo 3–24h before planned PCI; all patients received aspirin[(21)]. Following PCI patients were administered a 28-day regimen of clopidogrel 75mg/day and were then switched back to the treatments arms to which they had been randomized pre-procedure. Similar to PCI-CURE there was a 26.9% relative risk reduction of death, MI, or stroke in those on clopidogrel after 1-year follow-up. However, there was no significant difference in the rate of death, MI, or TVR at 28 days. On closer post hoc inspection of the statistical data it appeared that the benefits in the short term were only gained in those pre-treated with clopidogrel ≥6h before PCI. Furthermore a significant (statistically just) improvement in short-term outcomes was only achieved if clopidogrel was administered at least 12h and ideally almost 24h before coronary stenting.

The role of clopidogrel in preventing adverse sequelae following STEMI was elucidated from the COMMIT/CCS-2 and CLARITY-TIMI 28 trials[(22,23)]. The COMMIT trial randomized 45 852 patients presenting within 24h of symptom onset with AMI (i.e. ST-segment elevation or new left bundle branch block) to clopidogrel 75mg/day during hospitalization (mean of 16 days) or placebo plus standard aspirin therapy with or without fibrinolysis. Those proceeding to primary PCI or at high risk of bleeding were excluded. There was a significant 9.0% relative risk reduction in the primary composite endpoint of death, reinfarction or stroke at hospital discharge; this was not accompanied by an increased risk of major bleeding or haemorrhagic stroke.

CLARITY-TIMI 28 studied the addition of clopidogrel (300-mg LD plus 75mg/day MD) to a standard regimen of aspirin at the time of fibrinolysis compared with placebo in 3491 individuals presenting within 12h of acute STEMI. Clopidogrel therapy resulted in a significant absolute reduction of 6.7% in the primary efficacy endpoint (a composite of occluded infarct-related artery at angiography – Thrombolysis In Myocardial Infarction [TIMI] grade 0/1, death or recurrent MI before angiography) and a 2.5% absolute reduction in the composite endpoint of CV death, recurrent MI or urgent TVR. This was, in some ways, an odd study since the primary endpoint was measured at 8 days and was based on angiographic data. Therefore the intervention undertaken as a result of the angiography would have influenced the clinical endpoints at 1 month, which were not impressive. Although benefits were achieved with no significant increase in major bleeding including intracranial haemorrhage, clopidogrel in the absence of

PCI for STEMI has not really taken off. Thus despite these two trials, if a patient receives thrombolysis there appears to be little conviction amongst clinicians that post lytic clopidogrel is mandated. However, if patients go for PCI whether it be for failed thrombolysis (i.e. rescue PCI) or post successful lysis as a means of risk stratification, as is becoming standard practice, then clopidogrel should be used.

Like the CURE study, a subgroup analysis of those 1863 patients who proceeded to PCI after fibrinolysis in the CLARITY-TIMI 28 cohort was also performed: the PCI-CLARITY trial(24). Patients were randomized to receive a 300-mg LD followed by a 75mg/day MD of clopidogrel or placebo. The median time from drug initiation to PCI was 3 days. At 30-day follow-up patients pre-treated with clopidogrel (since most patients who received coronary stenting were given open-label thienopyridine) had a 46% reduction in the rate of CV death, recurrent MI, or stroke. The benefit of clopidogrel pre-treatment remained consistent regardless of the fibrinolytic agent used, whether a GP IIb/IIIa inhibitor was added or whether PCI was emergent or planned.

It is important to note that large-scale randomized controlled trials of clopidogrel versus placebo in the setting of primary PCI have not been conducted. It is accepted, however, that primary PCI is the treatment of choice if STEMI patients present within 90 minutes of symptom onset to an interventional centre. The combined evidence from PCI-CURE, CREDO, and PCI-CLARITY has been implemented to justify the use of DAPT before, during, or after primary PCI to positively impact on ischaemic events.

Resistance to dual antiplatelet therapy

Theoretically, inhibition of the two main amplification pathways of platelet aggregation should be superior to inhibition of either pathway alone. Despite appropriate DAPT, however, a significant minority of patients continue to suffer MACE following ACS and coronary stenting. Late ST, especially in the era of DES, can occur in 1–2% of individuals following PCI and is reported to progress at 0.3–0.6% each year. In real terms this can account for 30 000 MACE per annum worldwide. Death, MI, or stroke occur in 8.5%, and 21.4% require revascularization a year after the index PCI procedure(21). This has lead to the postulation that those individuals suffering further events may represent a cohort of patients who have less than adequate response to aspirin and clopidogrel.

The term 'resistance' is controversial in this context since it has been used to encompass both the failure of an agent to prevent the clinical condition for which it is intended and also failure to achieve its full pharmacokinetic and/or pharmacodynamic effect. Since the pathophysiology of atherothrombosis is complex, comprising thrombosis, inflammation, innate vascular biology, and changing haemodynamics, no single type of agent can be expected to abolish ischaemic events completely. Furthermore, a patient may have the appropriate platelet response to a given therapy but have recurrent events mediated by non-platelet factors. For these reasons it would seem reasonable to categorize patients suffering recurrent events on therapy as having *treatment failure*, while limiting the term *resistance* to those for whom the antiplatelet drug does not achieve its pharmacological effect which is inhibition of platelet aggregation (IPA). Resistance in its broadest sense can be referred to as the continued occurrence of ischaemic events despite adequate duration of APT, dosing, and compliance alongside optimal stent deployment.

Aspirin resistance

The concept of aspirin resistance is made more problematic since there is a lack of definitive evidence to suggest that altering therapy in response to discovering this phenomenon actually improves clinical outcomes. Indeed, although aspirin strongly inhibits the production of TXA_2, it may still fail to inhibit platelet aggregation since there are a number of other potent agonists that will continue to activate platelets. Furthermore no standard has been set or widely accepted for determining biochemical aspirin resistance; as such an estimated incidence of between 5–45% has been postulated depending on the specificity of the assay and the definition of resistance used along with the population under study. At present, AA-stimulated platelet aggregation assessed by light transmittance aggregometry (LTA) or platelet mapping by thromboelastography are the most commonly used laboratory assays, but these putative tests may not be specific or sensitive enough to fully establish so called 'aspirin resistance'.

The cause of aspirin resistance, if it truly exists, remains contentious and is most likely multi-factorial (Fig. 24.7). Ultimately, however, given the issues listed here it is perhaps more appropriate to refer to the occurrence of adverse ischaemic events despite aspirin therapy as 'treatment failure' rather than hyporesponsiveness or resistance. There is also no evidence to suggest that increasing the dose of aspirin will overcome treatment failure. Indeed doses of 75–150mg per day may be more effective at preventing MACE compared to doses up to 10 times as high(25). Additionally increasing doses of aspirin have consistently been shown to increase bleeding complications.

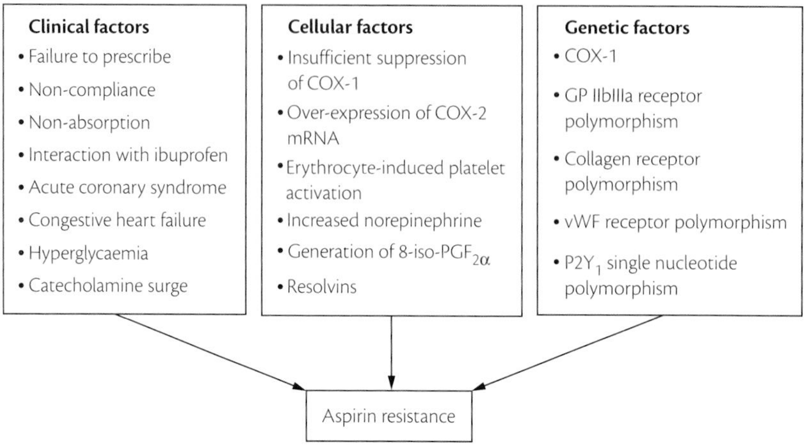
Clinical factors
• Failure to prescribe
• Non-compliance
• Non-absorption
• Interaction with ibuprofen
• Acute coronary syndrome
• Congestive heart failure
• Hyperglycaemia
• Catecholamine surge
Cellular factors
• Insufficient suppression of COX-1
• Over-expression of COX-2 mRNA
• Erythrocyte-induced platelet activation
• Increased norepinephrine
• Generation of 8-iso-PGF$_{2\alpha}$
• Resolvins
Genetic factors
• COX-1
• GP IIbIIIa receptor polymorphism
• Collagen receptor polymorphism
• vWF receptor polymorphism
• P2Y$_1$ single nucleotide polymorphism
Aspirin resistance

Fig. 24.7 Potential causes of aspirin resistance. Adapted with permission from Bhatt DL. Aspirin resistance: more than just a laboratory curiosity. *J Am Coll Cardiol* 2004; **43**:1127–9.

Clopidogrel resistance

In contrast to the phenomenon of aspirin resistance there is evidence to suggest that clopidogrel resistance is a definite pathopharmacotherapeutic entity that can lead to adverse clinical outcomes. There is wide interindividual variation in clopidogrel response. Currently, no laboratory definition of true clopidogrel resistance has been universally accepted. It is agreed that clopidogrel resistance occurs when the drug is unable to achieve adequate IPA. Since there are a number of different assays that can be used to assess this phenomenon it follows that there are a number of empiric cut-off values that have been adopted to suggest non-responsiveness. None of these tests have been fully standardized to measure clopidogrel responsiveness, leading to significant interlaboratory variation in results. Prevalence figures for non-responders to clopidogrel range from 4–30% 24h after drug administration depending on the technique used to measure platelet aggregation and the presence of factors contributing to greater baseline platelet reactivity.

Optical LTA is considered the historical gold standard for assessing platelet function. It uses spectrophotometric measurement of platelet aggregation in platelet-rich plasma in response to ADP as an agonist. The procedure carries with it a number of drawbacks: it is labour-intensive, requires expert personnel, has time-consuming centrifugation steps which may injure platelets, tests in an artificial milieu devoid of red and white blood cells, and can be subject to several interlaboratory differences.

Impedance aggregometry, on the other hand, uses electrical resistance between two electrodes immersed in whole blood to measure platelet aggregation. It offers improved sensitivity over LTA since it requires no centrifugation step and therefore no platelet 'injury' occurs; inclusion of giant platelets for functional assessment; and a shorter time to perform the test under more physiological conditions. The Multiplate® analyzer, for instance, allows measurement of platelet function in whole blood by using impedance aggregometry and can be used for a variety of applications such as monitoring of APT and assessment of perioperative platelet function disorders in a near-patient environment (Fig. 24.8).

Since clopidogrel is specific for P2Y$_{12}$, the P2Y$_1$ receptor can still be activated and contribute to platelet aggregation.

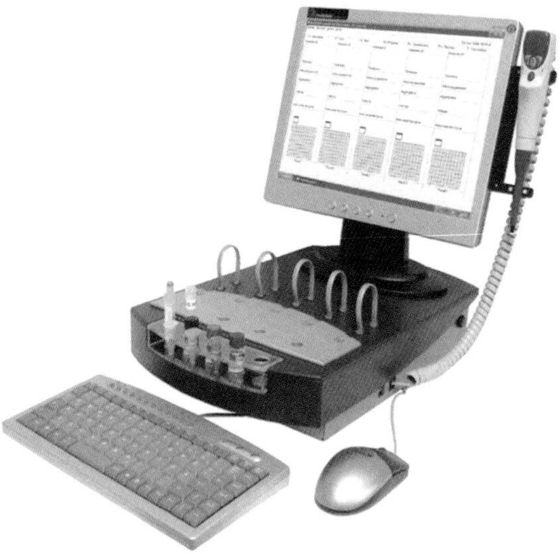

Fig. 24.8 The Multiplate® analyzer can be used to monitor response to antiplatelet therapy using whole blood impedance aggregometry.

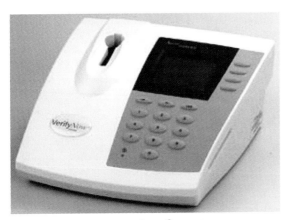

Fig. 24.9 The Point-of-Care VerifyNow® $P2Y_{12}$ Assay.

This can be a confounding factor when using LTA or impedance aggregometry. The vasodilator-stimulated phosphoprotein phosphorylation (VASP-P) assay is more specific to the $P2Y_{12}$ pathway. Levels of VASP-P and dephosphorylation reflect $P2Y_{12}$ inhibition and activation respectively and can be measured quite easily by quantitative flow cytometry. This is fast-becoming the only standardized $P2Y_{12}$-specific assay available. Furthermore, point-of-care assays for platelet aggregation have a promising role in guiding future APT. The VerifyNow® $P2Y_{12}$ system uses a similar principle to that employed by the VASP-P assay by using a combination of ADP and PGE_1 as agonists in order to specifically evaluate inhibition of the $P2Y_{12}$ pathway (Fig. 24.9). PGE_1 increases VASP-P by stimulation of adenylate cyclase. Binding of ADP to $P2Y_{12}$ leads to inhibition of adenylate cyclase thereby reducing PGE_1-induced VASP-P levels. If, however, $P2Y_{12}$ receptors are successfully blocked by clopidogrel, addition of ADP will have no theoretical effect on PGE_1-stimulated VASP-P levels. The VerifyNow® $P2Y_{12}$ system has recently been approved by the Food and Drug Administration in the United States but remains primarily a research tool and is yet to be used widely in the clinical forum.

Several studies have established clopidogrel resistance as an emerging clinical entity and proposed a link with adverse clinical outcomes. What are common to all of them, however, are relatively small sample sizes and short follow-up periods. They have not been sufficiently powered to detect a causal association between clopidogrel resistance and MACE. One of the largest studies found a normal distribution of clopidogrel responsiveness amongst 544 individuals consisting of healthy volunteers, patients post coronary stenting, those with heart failure, and after stroke[26]. The authors subsequently categorized hyporesponders, hyperresponders, and the remaining individuals as standard responders using the mean IPA achieved as a reference point. Another prospectively studied 60 patients who underwent primary PCI following presentation with STEMI to determine whether variability in response to clopidogrel affected clinical outcomes. Patients were stratified into four quartiles according to the percentage reduction of ADP-induced platelet aggregation. Forty per cent of patients in the first quartile, who were considered non-responders, sustained a MACE during 6-month follow-up compared to one patient in the second quartile and none in the third and fourth[27]. The largest study thus far looked at platelet reactivity following clopidogrel administration in 804 patients who had received DES during PCI. They found that patients with over 70% post-clopidogrel platelet aggregation *in vitro* had a nearly fourfold increase in definite or probable ST as compared with clopidogrel responders[28]. More recently Price and colleagues measured post-clopidogrel treatment platelet reactivity with the VerifyNow® $P2Y_{12}$ assay in 380 patients undergoing PCI with sirolimus-eluting stents to determine whether there was an optimal cut-off value for platelet reactivity in predicting 6-month MACE rates. They found that those patients with high post-treatment platelet reactivity had significantly higher rates of CV deaths, ST and overall MACE[29].

Several mechanisms of clopidogrel resistance have been postulated and encompass genetic, cellular, and clinical factors either acting alone or in conjunction (Table 24.2). Clinical factors can range from poor drug compliance to suboptimal stent deployment and increased baseline platelet reactivity due to increased body mass index, diabetes mellitus, and insulin resistance. Again a common thread of small sample sizes, empirical cut-off points for responsiveness, lack of robust clinical outcome data, differing methods of assessing platelet aggregation, and contradictory findings exists. No one mechanism has been accepted as the true cause of clopidogrel resistance. Particular interest has, however, focussed recently on several functional polymorphisms found in genes encoding cytochrome P450 isoenzymes involved in the hepatic biotransformation of clopidogrel to its active form. Abnormal function variants of the CYP2C9 and CYP2C19 genotypes have been associated with a decreased pharmacodynamic response to clopidogrel resulting in less exposure to the active metabolite[30]. The relationship between these genotypes and their corresponding pharmacodynamic

Table 24.2 Proposed mechanisms leading to variability in individual responsiveness to clopidogrel

Genetic factors	Polymorphisms of hepatic CYP3A4, CYP2C9, CYP2C19
	Polymorphisms of GPIa
	Polymorphisms of $P2Y_{12}$
	Polymorphisms of GPIIIa
Cellular factors	Accelerated platelet activity
	Reduced CYP3A4/CYP3A5 metabolic activity
	Increased ADP exposure
	Upregulation of the $P2Y_{12}$ pathway
	Upregulation of the $P2Y_1$ pathway
	Upregulation of P2Y-independent pathways(collagen, adrenaline, thromboxane A_2, thrombin)
Clinical factors	Failure to prescribe or underdosing
	Poor compliance
	Poor absorption
	Suboptimal stent deployment
	Drug–drug interactions involving CYP3A4(e.g. lipophilic statins such as atorvastatin and simvastatin)
	Increased baseline platelet reactivity (e.g. ACS, increased body mass index, diabetes mellitus and insulin resistance)
	Clopidogrel side effects such as thrombotic thrombocytopenic purpura (i.e. creation of a pro-thrombotic state)

effect must now be confirmed in larger cohorts and a link to clinical outcomes established.

Optimizing the dose of clopidogrel

The potential clinical validity of clopidogrel resistance has led to several studies designed to elucidate the optimal loading and maintenance doses for clopidogrel that could overcome hyporesponsiveness and yet remain safe in terms of bleeding rates. The ARMYDA-2 study indicated the benefit of pre-treatment with a 600-mg LD when compared with 300mg in reducing peri-procedural MI in patients with stable angina or NSTEMI undergoing planned PCI, without any increase in bleeding hazards[31].

The ALBION and ISAR-CHOICE studies looked at increasing the LD further to 900mg[32,33]. A higher LD did display a greater degree of platelet inhibition; more rapid onset of action (approximately 2h although maximal IPA may not be achieved until 3–4h); and a lower percentage of non-responders compared to the standard 300-mg strategy but the differences observed between the 600mg and 900mg regimens were less remarkable and *not significant*. These studies confirm the dose-dependent inhibitory effects of clopidogrel but also show there is a threshold for the platelet inhibitory function that can be achieved which may be linked to saturation of intestinal absorption as opposed to a limit on hepatic metabolism.

To establish further the mechanistic aspects of clopidogrel resistance Bonello and colleagues undertook a prospective, randomized, multicentre study of 162 patients due to undergo coronary stenting. Clopidogrel resistance was defined as a VASP-P index of >50% after a 600-mg LD. Patients who were non-responsive to clopidogrel were randomized to a control group or to a VASP-guided group; the latter received additional boluses of clopidogrel to reduce the VASP-P index to below 50% as measured by the VerifyNow® $P2Y_{12}$ assay. Although the study sample was small there was a significantly lower MACE rate in the VASP-guided group suggesting that adjusting the LD according to clopidogrel response was appropriate, safe (i.e. there was no difference in bleeding between the two groups) and could potentially improve clinical outcome[34].

The standard 75mg/day MD of clopidogrel requires 3–7 days to achieve maximal IPA. The ISAR-CHOICE-2 study revealed the advantage of a 150-mg clopidogrel MD over standard dosing in patients 1 month after low-risk PCI[35]. Additionally the OPTIMUS study showed that a 150-mg MD of clopidogrel resulted in pronounced platelet inhibition of numerous platelet function measures compared to the standard 75mg daily in patients with diabetes mellitus; although a significant number of patients continued to display high post-treatment platelet reactivity[36]. More definitive data on the optimal dosing of clopidogrel has come from the CURRENT-OASIS 7 trial, the results of which were first reported at the European Society of Cardiology (ESC) Annual Congress in September 2009. Over 25 000 patients presenting with ST and non-ST-elevation ACS intended for early (≤72h) revascularization were enrolled into a 2 × 2 factorial trial and randomized to either 600-mg LD followed by 150mg/day for 1 week then 75mg/day MD of clopidogrel or a 300-mg LD followed by 75mg/day MD[37]. Individuals were also randomized to receive either high-dose (300–325mg) or low-dose (75–100mg) aspirin in an open-label manner.

Of the 17 232 patients who did receive early intervention the primary composite endpoint of CV death, MI,

Table 24.3 Current European Society of Cardiology guidelines on the use of DAPT in patients requiring PCI

European Society of Cardiology guideline recommendations for antiplatelet therapy used in percutaneous coronary intervention (PCI) for STEMI patients[38,39]	
Aspirin	Patients already on daily aspirin should be given a 75–325mg stat dose before PCI Patients not on regular aspirin should be given 500mg at least 3h before PCI or 300mg intravenously at the time of the procedure Following PCI patients should continue on a maintenance dose of 75–160mg per day indefinitely
Clopidogrel	Patients should be given a 300-mg loading dose at least 6h before PCI; if this is not possible then a 600-mg loading dose at least 2h before the procedure Following BMS implantation patients should continue clopidogrel at a maintenance dose of 75 mg/day for 4–6 weeks Following DES implantation patients must continue clopidogrel for at least 12 months
European Society of Cardiology guideline recommendations for antiplatelet therapy in percutaneous coronary intervention (PCI) for NSTEMI/UA patients[38,39]	
Aspirin	A loading dose of 160–325 mg should be given to all patients presenting with NSTEMI/UA. A long-term maintenance dose of 75–100mg/day should be given indefinitely
Clopidogrel	All patients undergoing PCI should receive a loading dose of 600mg Following BMS implantation patients should continue clopidogrel at a maintenance dose of 75 mg/day for 4–6 weeks Following DES implantation patients must continue clopidogrel for at least 12 months
General advice	
Physicians and patients must be made aware that clopidogrel should not be discontinued too early, even for minor procedures like dental care, and that the opinion of a cardiologist should be sought if the patient is considering non-emergent non-cardiac surgery.	
In general, elective non-cardiac surgery should be deferred for 1 year after DES implantation. Conversely if it is known that a non-cardiac operation is required prior to PCI then all efforts should be made to implant a BMS so that clopidogrel need only be continued for 4–6 weeks as opposed to 1 year.	
Strict compliance to dual antiplatelet therapy must be maintained	
The issue of clopidogrel cards to patients that detail the PCI procedure and the recommended length of clopidogrel therapy should be strongly encouraged	
In patients treated with clopidogrel in whom it is decided that coronary artery bypass grafting is more favourable, the surgery should be delayed for 5 days if possible to reduce the risk of bleeding	

and stroke at 30 days occurred in 4.5% of those on the 'standard' clopidogrel regimen and 3.9% on the 'augmented' regimen (p = 0.036); the benefit primarily driven by a reduction in MI. Of the 7855 patients who did not proceed to PCI, through no significant CAD identified on angiography or those scheduled for CABG, there was no significant difference in the primary endpoint. Overall the rate of ST was significantly higher in the standard group compared to the augmented clopidogrel therapy cohort (1.2 vs. 0.7%; p = 0.001). There was no significant difference in the primary endpoint between a high- or low-dose aspirin strategy although, conversely, there was also no difference in bleeding indices between the two strategies either.

Data from CURRENT-OASIS 7 suggests that those patients scheduled to undergo PCI following an ACS should receive a 600-mg LD of clopidogrel which is already advocated in Europe and is current practice. A MD of 150mg for 1 week following PCI would be simple enough to institute thereafter and then patients could return to the 75-mg MD that we are all familiar with. Whether this practice will become commonplace in the 'real world' is yet to be seen. In the meantime current European guidelines on the use of DAPT in patients undergoing PCI are listed in Table 24.3 and indicate 600-mg preloading and 75mg/day maintenance doses.

Dual antiplatelet therapy for patients on long-term oral anticoagulation requiring PCI

By far the most common indication for OAC is atrial fibrillation (AF). It affects 5% of those aged over 65 years and almost 10% of people above the age of 80. This is thought to double over the next two generations. Since AF commonly coexists with vascular disease it follows that the incidence of patients in AF on warfarin therapy presenting with an ACS or requiring scheduled PCI is set to rise exponentially. To date, the decision to continue or withdraw OAC following PCI has largely been empiric and generally based on the 'guesstimated' risk by the physician of the thromboembolic complications balanced against the putative risk of bleeding. General consensus might suggest that there are very few instances in which OAC can be stopped safely and a complete switch to DAPT be made after coronary stenting: low thromboembolic-risk AF and low risk venous thromboembolism being the only likely scenarios.

There is marked heterogeneity in the use of antithrombotic regimens in warfarin-eligible patients post coronary stenting. A survey of 24 internationally-renowned interventional centres revealed that just over half used standardized protocols leaving the remainder to operator-directed decisions based on the balance between thromboembolic versus haemorrhagic risk[(40)]. The study did reveal triple therapy (DAPT plus OAC) to be the most prescribed regimen in the majority (83%) of centres.

Current joint European and US guidelines for the management of AF recommend triple therapy for a 'brief period' following PCI. This should then be followed by a maintenance regimen of OAC and clopidogrel for 3–12 months, depending on the stent platform used, after which clopidogrel is stopped and warfarin therapy continued indefinitely. Owing to a lack of robust randomized controlled trial (RCT) data these recommendations can only be assigned a level of evidence C and grade IIB (i.e. benefits ≥ risks)[(41)].

To date, the majority of published data on triple therapy post PCI has taken the form of small, observational, single-centre retrospective studies or registry analysis where safety endpoints have predominated over clinical efficacy measures. What is clearly needed, therefore, is a large multicentre RCT that is sufficiently powered for clinical outcomes to determine which antithrombotic strategy provides net clinical benefit for this expanding cohort of patients on chronic OAC undergoing PCI. The 'Finding Appropriate anti-Coagulation strategies to improve Outcomes after coRonary Stenting: The FACTORS Trial, is being planned in the UK.

Prasugrel: a third-generation thienopyridine

With the emergence of clopidogrel resistance as a probable clinical entity and the increasingly interventional treatment of ACS including STEMI, it has become apparent that there is a need for more potent antiplatelet agents which display less interindividual variability, have a faster onset of action and a good tolerability profile. Prasugrel, like clopidogrel, is a thienopyridine pro-drug which causes irreversible inhibition of the $P2Y_{12}$ receptor; has time- and dose-dependent antiplatelet effects, and requires hepatic biotransformation to form the active metabolite from the parent molecule *in vivo* (see Fig. 24.5). Unlike clopidogrel it requires *only one* oxidative step to form its active moiety which is, therefore, generated much faster, more efficiently, and in much higher concentration, giving rise to approximately 10 times more antiplatelet potency and a more consistent IPA despite both metabolites displaying similar antiplatelet activity *in vitro*. Indeed, in patients with stable atherosclerosis a 60-mg LD of prasugrel has been shown to achieve a more rapid and greater degree of IPA within 30min than that achieved by a 600-mg LD of clopidogrel over 24h[(42)]. In addition the metabolism of prasugrel is less likely to be affected by polymorphisms in CYP2C19 P450 iso-enzymes.

The JUMBO-TIMI 26 trial compared three different dose regimens of prasugrel against the standard dosing of clopidogrel in 904 patients due to undergo PCI. There was a comparable safety profile in terms of bleeding between all four groups and a trend, albeit not statistically significant, towards benefit in favour of prasugrel for the secondary composite endpoint of MACE at 30 days[(43)]. The PRINCIPLE-TIMI 44 two-phase crossover trial compared prasugrel to high-dose clopidogrel in 201 patients undergoing planned PCI[(44)]. Patients were initially randomized to a 60-mg LD of prasugrel or 600-mg LD of clopidogrel with a primary endpoint of ADP-induced platelet aggregation, as measured by optical LTA, the VASP-P index, and VerifyNow® $P2Y_{12}$ assays, at 6h. In the second phase of the trial, post-PCI patients entered a 28-day crossover comparison in which they were randomized to 14 days of prasugrel at 10mg/day followed by 14 days of clopidogrel at 150mg/day or vice versa. In both of the loading and maintenance phases, prasugrel was shown to cause significantly greater IPA compared to a high-dose clopidogrel strategy.

These Phase II clinical trials lead to the Phase III TRITON-TIMI 38, a large randomized multicentre head-to-head study of prasugrel (60-mg LD followed by 10mg/day MD) versus clopidogrel (300-mg LD followed by 75mg/day MD) in 13608 patients presenting with the entire spectrum of moderate- to high-risk ACS due to undergo primary or delayed PCI[(45)]. Initial results were promising: the primary efficacy endpoint of CV death, non-fatal MI, and stroke occurred in 12.1% of clopidogrel patients and 9.9% receiving prasugrel ($p < 0.001$). A significant difference between the two strategies had already emerged by day 3, presumably secondary to prasugrel's more potent and rapid onset of action and persisted throughout the entire 15-month follow-up period. There were also significant reductions in the secondary endpoints of ST (1.1% versus 2.4%; $p < 0.001$) and urgent TVR (2.5% versus 3.7%; $p < 0.001$) in favour of prasugrel. On more

Table 24.4 Factors that may underlie the association between bleeding and mortality

Forced discontinuation of antiplatelet therapy leading to ischaemia, haemodynamic compromise, stent thrombosis, arrhythmia, MI, urgent TVR, or death
Bleeding can lead to hypovolaemia, anaemia, and impaired oxygen carriage which may precipitate tachycardia, hypotension, and cardiac failure
Blood product transfusions have been associated with adverse outcomes
Bleeding complications lead to longer, more complex, hospital admissions
Patients may require invasive monitoring, intra-aortic balloon counterpulsation, intubation, endoscopy, anaesthesia, and surgical procedures, all of which can result in adverse outcomes

detailed analysis, however, benefits in the primary composite endpoint were driven predominantly by a reduced rate of non-fatal MI (7.3% versus 9.5%; p <0.001); there was indeed no significant difference in the rate of CV death, non-fatal stroke, or all-cause mortality. The other major issue with this trial was that it was US-based and patients were randomized once the angiogram had been done—in the UK and Europe as has been clearly outlined earlier, pre-loading with clopidogrel (600mg >24h) is thought, albeit on non-prospective comparative data, to be the standard of care. It is unclear whether prasugrel would have demonstrated the same advantages if it had been compared with patients pre-loaded with clopidogrel. However the reduction in opportunity for pre-loading in the time-dependant STEMI patient has prompted the National Institute of Health and Clinical Excellence (NICE) to support its use in this group of patients.

With greater platelet inhibition there is the inevitable hazard of more bleeding events (Table 24.4). Significantly more major bleeding (2.4% versus 1.8%; p = 0.03); life-threatening bleeding (1.4% versus 0.9%; p=0.01); and fatal bleeding (0.4% versus 0.1%; p = 0.002) was seen in the prasugrel arm of the trial. Post hoc analysis identified the following subgroups particularly at risk:

- Patients with known cerebrovascular disease
- Those aged ≥ 75 years, and
- Body weight <60kg.

In a pre-specified subgroup analysis the 3421 patients presenting with STEMI who received either primary or delayed PCI demonstrated a significant reduction in the primary efficacy endpoint (9.8% versus 12.3%; p = 0.02) without a significant increase in major bleeding at 15 months(46). Prasugrel also demonstrated greater efficacy in patients at higher risk of ST, for instance: those needing longer stents, bifurcation lesions, those with renal dysfunction, diabetes, and those presenting with STEMI; again with no significant increase in major bleeding(47). A further subanalysis looked at the diabetic cohort of patients who are known to have high platelet reactivity and a greater risk of being poorly responsive to clopidogrel therapy (see Table 24.2). Of the 2947 patients with diabetes the primary efficacy endpoint was reached in 12.2% of patients with prasugrel and 17.0% taking clopidogrel at 15 months (p <0.001). The occurrence of major bleeding, however, was not statistically significantly different between the groups(48). There was significantly less incidence of ST in the prasugrel group which has led NICE to provisionally recommend its use in those suffering ST. Individuals thought to be at high risk of suffering ST may be better served by giving them prasugrel as a primary agent as opposed to after the adverse event occurring first. The ultimate role of prasugrel remains undefined. NICE have produced its final Appraisal Consultation Document on prasugrel in August 2009 and will issue formal guidance in October 2009(49). Salient points that have arisen from the consultation so far are summarized in Table 24.5. In effect the NICE recommendations are for prasugrel to be used in those patients suffering STEMI, those who have evidence of previous ST and in diabetics.

Glycoprotein IIb/IIIa inhibitors

The role of GP IIb/IIIa inhibitors in modern-day PCI has become less well defined due to the emergence of DAPT in the clopidogrel era and, more recently, the increasing use of direct thrombin inhibitors such as bivalirudin for adjuvant anticoagulation during coronary stenting. Intravenous GP IIb/IIIa inhibitors act by blocking the binding of fibrinogen to the platelet GP IIb/IIIa receptor—an interaction which represents the final common pathway of platelet aggregation (see Fig. 24.3). Interestingly, following the initial success of intravenous agents in the setting of ACS and coronary stenting, their orally active counterparts were developed. Surprisingly these oral agents were found to increase the risk of major bleeding and were therefore associated with excess mortality, but did not reduce the incidence of ischaemic events. Three GP IIb/IIIa receptor antagonists are approved for intravenous use in ACS and those undergoing PCI: abciximab, which is a monoclonal antibody that has a relatively long duration of action; and eptifibatide and tirofiban which are low-molecular-weight,

Table 24.5 Summary of the NICE Appraisal Consultation Document on Prasugrel for the treatment of acute coronary syndromes with PCI (April 2009)

Appraisal Committee's preliminary recommendations:
1. Prasugrel in combination with aspirin is recommended as an option for preventing atherothrombotic events in individuals presenting with ACS having PCI, only when: ◆ Immediate primary PCI for STEMI is necessary, or ◆ Previous ST has occurred despite adequate clopidogrel treatment.
2. People currently receiving prasugrel for treatment of ACS whose circumstances do not meet the criteria above should have the option to continue therapy until they and their clinicians consider it appropriate to stop.
Recognition of Appraisal Committee's caveats:
1. Differences in the efficacy of prasugrel and clopidogrel in the trial were largely dependent on statistically significant differences in non-fatal MI, which included both clinical MI (which is symptom driven) and non-clinical MI (based on biomarkers and ECG readings). The Evidence Review Group (ERG) commented that if only clinical MIs were compared between treatment arms, the differences between prasugrel and clopidogrel may not remain.
2. The loading dose of clopidogrel (300mg) used in the trial does not reflect current practice in England and Wales of pre-loading patients with 600 mg ≥24h prior to PCI. As a result, the advantages of prasugrel over clopidogrel in preventing cardiovascular events may have been overstated, especially for NSTEMI patients for whom there would be adequate time to give a preloading dose of clopidogrel.
3. Practice in the trial did not reflect the growing trend in England and Wales for PCI to be conducted via radial artery access. The ERG referred to evidence that major bleeding rates can be reduced when PCI is peformed this way.
4. Concern was raised over the use of composite endpoints. The Committee noted that, although common in cardiovascular clinical research, they were difficult to interpret. It noted that non-clinical MIs were included in non-fatal MIs and that this would have increased composite endpoint event rates reported in the trial.
5. The Committee then considered the use of prasugrel compared with clopidogrel in patients with diabetes who were having PCI. It noted the subanalysis in diabetes patients which demonstrated a significant benefit with prasugrel in this patient cohort. However the Committee were mindful of the lack of an adequate preloading dose, combined with the dose of clopidogrel used in the trial, may have disadvantaged clopidogrel in the diabetes population. It agreed that the evidence presented on the efficacy of prasugrel in diabetes patients was highly uncertain and did not show a clear advantage over clopidogrel as used in current practice in England and Wales.
6. In summary, the ERG considered prasugrel and clopidogrel to be broadly equivalent in terms of clinical effectiveness at 15 months for patients with acute coronary syndromes having percutaneous coronary intervention.

rapidly-acting synthetically produced agents that have short half-lives of only approximately 2h.

There have been a multitude of trials examining the 'upstream' use of these agents in NSTEMI prior to PCI but none were conducted at a time when there was routine administration of clopidogrel given on admission in those with a high likelihood of ACS (chest pain + ECG changes and subsequent troponin positivity and definitely pre-PCI; undertaken now routinely in those with high likelihood of ACS within 72h). Patients who are likely to benefit most from these agents given at the time of PCI include: those with troponin-positive coronary events and/or those who have ST-segment depression on admission electrocardiogram (ECG) and diabetics. In the ISAR-REACT 2 study, 2022 high-risk NSTEMI patients were given a LD of 600mg clopidogrel plus standard aspirin and then randomized in the catheterization laboratory to receive heparin plus bolus abciximab followed by a 12-h infusion or placebo. The composite endpoint of death, MI, or TVR at 30 days was significantly reduced in the GP IIb/IIIa arm although on further analysis patients with elevated troponin levels were found to benefit the most from abciximab therapy[(50)]. It is important to note the administration of abciximab in this case was peri-procedural rather than being 'upstream'.

Current European guidelines advocate the use of eptifibatide or tirofiban during and after PCI in patients at intermediate to high risk (raised troponin, ST-segment depression, or diabetes) awaiting their procedure. Those not receiving an upstream agent should receive abciximab immediately following angiography[(39)]. There is much less use of up-front eptifibatide and tirofiban in the oral thienopyridine era.

Most data for GP IIb/IIIa inhibitors in primary PCI has been gathered for abciximab with current European guidelines supporting its administration upstream or peri-procedurally[38]. The BRAVE-3 trial, however, recently demonstrated no added benefit or reduction in infarct size with the administration of abciximab compared to placebo when 800 patients with acute STEMI were pre-loaded with 600mg clopidogrel prior to primary PCI[51].

Abciximab has also been compared to bivalirudin in the HORIZONS-AMI trial of 3602 STEMI patients presenting within 12h of symptom onset prior to primary PCI. Bivalirudin is a direct thrombin inhibitor and, since thrombin is one of the most potent platelet agonists, it therefore has a significant indirect effect on platelet reactivity. Patients were randomized to heparin plus abciximab or bivalirudin alone. There were two primary endpoints: major bleeding alone and combined adverse clinical events (bleeding plus death, MI, TVR, and stroke). Treatment with bivalirudin alone resulted in a reduced rate of both endpoints at 30 days owing predominantly to lower major bleeding rates. There was also a significant decrease in all-cause and CV mortality in the bivalirudin arm. Subsequent multivariate analyses of the data suggested that major bleeding as well as reinfarction were both significant predictors of 30-day all-cause mortality in the trial[52]. In this study much of the benefit was borne directly out of the adverse bleeding outcomes, which were significantly reduced with bivalirudin compared to abciximab. However, on closer inspection, there appeared to be an early hazard with excess ST which may in part be due to the adverse culmination of pro-thrombotic milieu; the inadequacy of clopidogrel-induced IPA and there being less time to pre-load (i.e. these were acute STEMI patients). In such circumstances use of a more potent antiplatelet agent such as prasugrel may have overcome the early ST. This is the basis of the BRAVE-4 trial. The continued use of GP IIb/IIIa inhibitors in the context of ACS and PCI seems less predictable now with the advent of more potent antiplatelet therapies like prasugrel.

Emerging antiplatelet therapies

Ticagrelor

Ticagrelor or AZD6140 is the first oral reversible ADP receptor antagonist which directly inhibits the $P2Y_{12}$ receptor but does not require hepatic metabolism for its activity. It is a non-thienopyridine which blocks platelet reactivity more consistently and completely than clopidogrel with a lower degree of inter-individual response variability. Additionally, a reversible antiplatelet effect may confer a clinical advantage for patients awaiting coronary artery bypass graft surgery since rapid recovery of platelet function can occur without having to wait for 5 days due to irreversible inhibition caused by thienopyridine administration.

The PLATO Phase III clinical trial which compared AZD6140 (180mg LD then 90-mg twice daily MD) with clopidogrel (300-mg LD plus a further bolus at time of PCI then 75mg/day MD) in 18 624 NSTEMI and STEMI ACS patients has now been completed[53]. Results reported first at the ESC Annual Congress in September 2009 were encouraging. Like the landmark CURE trial, PLATO enrolled the entire continuum of ACS with or without ST-segment elevation unlike TRITON-TIMI 38 which was predominantly a PCI trial. At 12 months there was a significant difference in the primary endpoint of death from vascular causes, MI, or stroke in patients taking ticagrelor compared with clopidogrel (9.8% vs 11.7%; $p < 0.001$) regardless of whether patients had received a higher dose of clopidogrel or whether they proceeded to PCI or not. There were also significant differences in individual secondary end-points such as death from vascular causes and MI but no difference in the rate of stroke between the two groups. Although known to have a more potent antiplatelet effect, ticagrelor did not cause a significant increase in overall major bleeding (11.6% vs 11.2%; $p = 0.43$) although there was a higher rate of non procedure-related major bleeding when compared to clopidogrel (4.5% vs 3.8%; $p = 0.03$). Interestingly, although much has been said about the reversibility of AZD6140, there was no difference in bleeding between the two drugs in those patients who proceeded to CABG surgery. Perhaps most striking, however, was the significant difference in the rate of all-cause mortality which was 4.5% with ticagrelor and 5.9% with clopidogrel ($p < 0.001$). The authors have equated this to saving 14 lives per 1000 treated patients although it must be remembered that the study was not adequately powered to detect such a difference. All in all, ticagrelor may well represent a paradigm shift in APT but care must be taken not to forget the ramifications of compliance issues with twice-daily dosing and quality of life concerns raised by an increased incidence of dyspnoea associated with the drug. This is the first published trial for this agent—others will be needed. We will need to await the PCI subgroup data to be presented at the Transcatheter Cardiovascular Therapeutics meeting in September 2009 to allow comparisons with the Prasugrel TRITON data.

Cangrelor

Cangrelor is a selective and competitive $P2Y_{12}$ antagonist suitable for intravenous administration. It is an adenosine triphosphate analogue with more potent antiplatelet activity than clopidogrel. CHAMPION PCI and CHAMPION PLATFORM are two currently ongoing prospective multi-centre phase III clinical trials evaluating the efficacy of cangrelor against clopidogrel. The CHAMPION study has (in June 2009) been stopped for lack of efficacy. Details will follow in due course.

Protease-activated receptor antagonists

Thrombin-induced platelet aggregation can occur in the absence of TXA_2 and ADP thus giving an idea of how potent a platelet agonist it is. Thrombin activates platelets via two protease-activated receptors (PARs): PAR1 and PAR4; the former mediates platelet activation at low concentrations of thrombin whereas the latter requires high concentrations of thrombin for its activity (see Fig. 24.4). Currently two experimental PAR1 antagonist compounds: E555 and SCH530348 are under phase II investigation. In addition the currently ongoing TRANSCENDENCE PCI multi-centre randomized trial has been designed to evaluate the effects of SCH530348 against those of a GP IIb/IIIa inhibitor in terms of major and minor bleeding. The results should tell us more on the safety and efficacy of thrombin receptor blockade.

Conclusions

The centrality of platelet activation in the deleterious processes leading to ACS and the events following PCI is now well established. Effective inhibition of platelet function has evolved from intravenous to potent effect oral agents, but there is still a way to go. Tailoring of the agent and dose to take account of pharmacological resistance and to minimize bleeding consequent on narrow therapeutic windows is now the clinical goal.

There are a multitude of biological processes and pathways involved in the formation of a growing haemostatic plug and so it seems slightly over optimistic to expect an agent to combat all of them single-handedly. Conversely, the more potent the antiplatelet effect the greater the tendency to bleed which is clearly an independent risk factor for morbidity and mortality. Interventional cardiologists, however, will soon have a greater arsenal of old and new antiplatelet agents available to them and so will be able to make specific choices dependent on individual patient requirements. Ticagrelor may be preferred in those whose coronary anatomy is unknown and may well require subsequent CABG surgery. Similarly those patients needing surgical intervention but already on clopidogrel or prasugrel could be switched to ticagrelor 5–7 days before. Those patients at high risk of bleeding or who have a history of cerebrovascular disease should avoid prasugrel or ticagrelor. There remains a place for clopidogrel especially if point-of-care antiplatelet response measuring becomes widely available and the dose can be optimized. We must also remember that PLATO and TRITON, although at first glance, may signal a paradigm shift in APT, are nonetheless single studies. Further trials are needed to compare all three ADP receptor antagonists at their optimal doses in patients manifesting the entire spectrum of ACS to adequately determine which patient cohorts receive greatest benefit from a particular agent. The future, however, appears bright!

References

1. Vorchheimer DA, Becker R. Platelets in atherothrombosis. *Mayo Clin Proc* 2006; **81**(1):59–68.
2. Yeh ETH, Khan BV. The potential role of antiplatelet agents in modulating inflammatory markers in atherothrombosis. *J Thromb Haemost* 2006; **4**:2308–16.
3. Pasterkamp G, Falk E. Atherosclerotic plaque rupture: an overview. *J Clin Basic Cardiol* 2000; **3**:81–6.
4. Davi G, Patrono C. Platelet activation and atherothrombosis. *N Engl J Med* 2007; **357**:2482–94.
5. Behan MWH, Storey RF. Antiplatelet therapy in cardiovascular disease. *Postgrad Med J* 2004; **80**:155–64.
6. Cimminiello C, Toschi V. Atherothrombosis: the role of platelets. *Eur Heart J Suppl* 1999; **1**(A):A8–A13.
7. Steering Committee of the Physicians' Health Study Research Group. Preliminary report: findings from the aspirin component of the ongoing Physicians' Health Study. *N Engl J Med* 1988; **318**:262–4.
8. Eidelman RS, Hebert PR, Weisman SM, *et al.* An update on aspirin in the primary prevention of cardiovascular disease. *Arch Intern Med* 2003; **163**:2006–10.
9. Antithrombotic Trialists' Collaboration. Collaborative meta-analysis of randomised trials of antiplatelet therapy for prevention of death, myocardial infarction, and stroke in high risk patients. *BMJ* 2002; **324**:71–86.
10. ISIS-2 (Second International Study of Infarct Survival) Collaborative Group. Randomised trial of intravenous streptokinase, oral aspirin, both, or neither among 17187 cases of suspected acute myocardial infarction: ISIS-2. *Lancet* 1988; **ii**:349–60.
11. Patrono C, Coller B, Fitzgerald GA, *et al.* Platelet-active drugs: The relationships among dose, effectiveness, and side effects: The Seventh ACCP Conference on Antithrombotic and Thrombolytic Therapy. *Chest* 2004; **126**:234–64.

12. Schömig A, Neumann FJ, Kastrati A, *et al.* A randomised comparison of antiplatelet and anticoagulant therapy after the placement of coronary-artery stents. *N Engl J Med* 1996; **334**:1084–19.
13. Leon MB, Baim DS, Popma JJ, *et al.* A clinical trial comparing three antithrombotic-drug regimens after coronary-artery stenting. *N Engl J Med* 1998; **339**:1665–71.
14. Bertrand ME, Legrand V, Boland J, *et al.* Randomised multicenter comparison of conventional anticoagulation versus antiplatelet therapy in unplanned and elective coronary stenting. The Full Anticoagulation Versus Aspirin and Ticlopidine (FANTASTIC) Study. *Circulation* 1996; **98**:1597–603.
15. Urban P, Macaya C, Rupprecht HJ, *et al.* Randomised evaluation of anticoagulation versus antiplatelet therapy after coronary stent implantation in high-risk patients. The Multicenter Aspirin and Ticlopidine Trial after Intracoronary Stenting (MATTIS). *Circulation* 1998; **98**:2126–32.
16. Rubboli A, Milandri M, Castelvetri C, *et al.* Meta-analysis of trials comparing oral anticoagulation and aspirin versus dual antiplatelet therapy after coronary stenting. Clues for the management of patients with an indication for long-term anticoagulation undergoing coronary stenting. *Cardiology* 2005; **104**:101–6.
17. Bertrand M, Rupprecht HJ, Urban P, *et al* for the CLASSICS Investigators. Double-blind study of the safety of clopidogrel with and without a loading dose in combination with aspirin compared with ticlopidine in combination with aspirin after coronary stenting: the clopidogrel aspirin stent international cooperative study (CLASSICS). *Circulation* 2000; **102**:624–9.
18. CAPRIE Steering Committee. A randomised, blinded, trial of clopidogrel versus aspirin in patients at risk of ischaemic events (CAPRIE). *Lancet* 1996; **348**:1329–39.
19. CURE Study Investigators. Effects of clopidogrel in addition to aspirin in patients with acute coronary syndromes without ST-segment elevation. *N Engl J Med* 2001; **345**:494–502.
20. Mehta SR, Yusuf S, Peters RJG, *et al.* Effects of pre-treatment with clopidogrel and aspirin followed by long-term therapy in patients undergoing percutaneous coronary intervention: the PCI-CURE study. *Lancet* 2001; **358**:527–33.
21. Steinhubl SR, Berger PB, Mann JT III, *et al.* Early and sustained dual oral antiplatelet therapy following percutaneous coronary intervention: a randomized controlled trial. *JAMA* 2002; **288**:2411–20.
22. Chen ZM, Jiang LX, Chen YP, *et al.* Addition of clopidogrel to aspirin in 45852 patients with acute myocardial infarction: randomised placebo-controlled trial. *Lancet* 2005; **366**:1607–21.
23. Sabatine MS, Cannon CP, Gibson CM, *et al.* for the CLARITY-TIMI 28 Investigators. Addition of clopidogrel to aspirin and fibrinolytic therapy for myocardial infarction with ST-segment elevation. *N Engl J Med* 2005; **352**:1179–89.
24. Sabatine MS, Cannon CP, Gibson CM, *et al.* for the Clopidogrel as Adjunctive Reperfusion Therapy (CLARITY) – Thrombolysis in Myocardial Infarction (TIMI) 28 Investigators. Effect of clopidogrel pre-treatment before percutaneous coronary intervention in patients with ST-elevation myocardial infarction treated with fibrinolytics: the PCI-CLARITY study. *JAMA* 2005; **294**:1224–32.
25. Patrono C. Aspirin resistance: definition, mechanisms and clinical read-outs. *J Thromb Haemost* 2003; **1**:1710–13.
26. Serebruany VL, Steinhubl SR, Berger PB, *et al.* Variability in platelet responsiveness to clopidogrel among 544 individuals. *J Am Coll Cardiol* 2005; **45**:246–51.
27. Matetzky S, Shenkman B, Guetta V, *et al.* Clopidogrel resistance is associated with increased risk of recurrent atherothrombotic events in patients with acute myocardial infarction. *Circulation* 2004; **109**:3171–5.
28. Buonamici P, Marcucci R, Migliorini A, *et al.* Impact of platelet reactivity after clopidogrel administration on drug-eluting stent thrombosis. *J Am Coll Cardiol* 2007; **49**:2312–7.
29. Price MJ, Endemann S, Raghava G, *et al.* Prognostic significance of post-clopidogrel platelet reactivity assessed by a point-of-care assay on thrombotic events after drug-eluting stent implantation. *Eur Heart J* 2008; **29**:992–1000.
30. Brandt JT, Close SL, Iturria SJ, *et al.* Common polymorphisms of CYP2C19 and CYP2C9 affect the pharmacokinetic and pharmacodynamic response to clopidogrel but not prasugrel. *J Thromb Haemost* 2007; **5**(12):2429–36.
31. Patti G, Colonna G, Pasceri V, *et al.* Randomised trial of high loading dose of clopidogrel for reduction of periprocedural myocardial infarction in patients undergoing coronary intervention: results from the ARMYDA-2 (Antiplatelet therapy for Reduction of MYocardial Damage during Angioplasty) study. *Circulation* 2005; **111**:2099–106.
32. Montalescot G, Sideris G, Meuleman C, *et al.* A randomised comparison of high clopidogrel loading doses in patients with non-ST-elevation acute coronary syndromes: the ALBION trial. *J Am Coll Cardiol* 2006; **48**:931–8.
33. von Beckerath N, Taubert D, Pogatsa-Murray G, *et al.* Absorption, metabolization, and antiplatelet effects of 300-, 600-, and 900-mg loading doses of clopidogrel: results of the ISAR-CHOICE (Intra-coronary Stenting and Antithrombotic Regimen: Choose between 3 High Oral doses for Immediate Clopidogrel Effect) trial. *Circulation* 2005; **112**:2946–50.
34. Bonello L, Camoin-Jau L, Arques S, *et al.* Adjusted clopidogrel loading doses according to vasodilator-stimulated phosphoprotein phosphorylation index decrease rate of major adverse cardiovascular events in patients with clopidogrel resistance. *J Am Coll Cardiol* 2008; **51**:1404–11.
35. von Beckerath N, Kastrati A, Wieczorek A, *et al.* A double-blind randomized study on platelet aggregation in patients treated with a daily dose of 150 or 75mg of clopidogrel for 30 days (ISAR-CHOICE-2 Trial). *Eur Heart J* 2007; **28**:1814–19.

36. Angiolillo DJ, Shoemaker SB, Desai B, *et al.* Randomised comparison of a high clopidogrel maintenance dose in patients with diabetes mellitus and coronary artery disease: Results of the optimising antiplatelet therapy in diabetes mellitus (OPTIMUS) study. *Circulation* 2007; **115**(6):708–16.
37. Mehta SR, Bassand JP, Chrolavicius S, *et al.* Design and rationale of CURRENT-OASIS 7: a randomized 2x2 factorial trial evaluating optimal dosing strategies for clopidogrel and aspirin in patients with ST and non-ST-elevation acute coronary syndromes managed with an early invasive strategy. *Am Heart J* 2008; **156**:1080–8.
38. Silber S, Albertsson P, Aviles FF, *et al.* Guidelines for percutaneous coronary interventions. *Eur Heart J* 2005; **26**:804–47.
39. Bassand JP, Hamm CW, Ardissino D, *et al.* Guidelines for the treatment of non-ST-segment elevation acute coronary syndromes. *Eur Heart J* 2007; **28**:2–63.
40. Rubboli A, Colletta M, Sangiorgio P, *et al.* Antithrombotic treatment after coronary artery stenting in patients on chronic oral anticoagulation: an international survey of current clinical practice. *Ital Heart J* 2004; **5**:851–6.
41. Fuster V, Ryden LE, Cannom DS, *et al.* ACC/AHA/ESC 2006 guidelines for the management of patients with atrial fibrillation – executive summary: a report of the American College of Cardiology/American Heart Association Task Force on Practice Guidelines and the European Society of Cardiology Committee for Practice Guidelines (Writing Committee to Revise the 2001 Guidelines for the management of patients with atrial fibrillation). *J Am Coll Cardiol* 2006; **48**:854–906.
42. Wallentin L, Varenhorst C, James S, *et al.* Prasugrel achieves greater and faster P2Y12 receptor-mediated platelet inhibition than clopidogrel due to more efficient generation of its active metabolite in aspirin-treated patients with coronary artery disease. *Eur Heart J* 2008; **29**:21–30.
43. Wiviott SD, Antman EM, Winters KJ, *et al.* Randomised comparison of prasugrel, a novel thienopyridine P2Y12 antagonist, with clopidogrel in percutaneous coronary intervention: results of the Joint Utilization of Medications to Block Platelets Optimally (JUMBO)-TIMI 26. *Circulation* 2005; **111**:3366–73.
44. Wiviott SD, Trenk D, Frelinger AL, *et al.* Prasugrel compared with high loading- and maintenance-dose clopidogrel in patients with planned percutaneous coronary intervention; the Prasugrel in Comparison to Clopidogrel for Inhibition of Platelet Activation and Aggregation-Thrombolysis in Myocardial Infarction 44 Trial. *Circulation* 2007; **116**:2923–32.
45. Wiviott SD, Braunwald E, McCabe CH, *et al.* Prasugrel versus clopidogrel in patients with acute coronary syndromes. *N Engl J Med* 2007; **357**:2001–15.
46. Montalescot G, Wiviott SD, Braunwald E, *et al.* for the TRITON-TIMI 38 Investigators. Prasugrel compared with clopidogrel in patients undergoing percutaneous coronary intervention for ST-elevation myocardial infarction (TRITON-TIMI 38): double-blind, randomised controlled trial. *Lancet* 2009; **373**(9665):723–31.
47. Wiviott SD, Braunwald E, McCabe CH, *et al.* Intensive oral antiplatelet therapy for reduction of ischaemic events including stent thrombosis in patients with acute coronary syndromes treated with percutaneous coronary intervention and stenting in the TRITON-TIMI 38 trial: a sub-analysis of a randomised trial. *Lancet* 2008; **371**(9621):1353–63.
48. Wiviott SD, Braunwald E, Angiolillo DJ, *et al.* TRITON-TIMI 38 Investigators. Greater clinical benefit of more intensive oral antiplatelet therapy with prasugrel in patients with diabetes mellitus in the trial to assess improvement in therapeutic outcomes by optimising platelet inhibition with prasugrel – Thrombolysis in Myocardial Infarction 38. *Circulation* 2008; **118**(16): 1626–36.
49. Greenhalgh J, Bagust A, Boland A, *et al.* *Prasugrel for the treatment of acute coronary syndromes with percutaneous coronary intervention: A Single Technology Appraisal.* Liverpool Reviews and Implementation Group, The University of Liverpool, 2009.
50. Kastrati A, Mehilli J, Neumann FJ, *et al.* For the Intracoronary Stenting Antithrombotic Regimen: Rapid Early Action for Coronary Treatment 2 (ISAR REACT 2) Trial Investigators. Abciximab in patients with acute coronary syndrome undergoing percutaneous coronary intervention after clopidogrel pre-treatment: the ISAR-REACT 2 randomised trial. *JAMA* 2006; **295**:1531–8.
51. Mehilli J, Kastrati A, Schulz S, *et al.* Abciximab in patients with acute ST-segment-elevation myocardial infarction undergoing primary percutaneous coronary intervention after clopidogrel loading: a randomized double-blind trial. *Circulation* 2009; **119**(14):1933–40.
52. Stone GW, Witzenbichler B, Guagliumi G, *et al.* for the HORIZONS-AMI Trial Investigators. Bivalirudin during primary PCI in acute myocardial infarction. *N Engl J Med* 2008; **358**:2218–30.
53. Wallentin L, Becker RC, Budaj A, *et al.* Ticagrelor versus clopidogrel in patients with acute coronary syndromes. *N Engl J Med* 2009; **361**(11):1045–57.

CHAPTER 25

The role of bivalirudin in percutaneous coronary intervention

Steffen Massberg, Julinda Mehilli, and Adnan Kastrati

Introduction

Rapid progress has been made in interventional cardiology over the past years, and many patients with coronary artery disease, even those with complex lesions, are nowadays being treated with percutaneous coronary interventions (PCI). As a result, a major focus of current cardiovascular research is on reducing negative peri-procedural clinical events associated with PCI, particularly in high-risk patients. Among the most dangerous peri-procedural events are thrombotic complications, leading to recurrent myocardial or cerebral ischaemia, often with fatal outcome. Anticoagulant and antithrombotic treatment, therefore, is an integral part of current PCI strategies. It is needless to say that prevention of procedural thrombotic events with the use of anticoagulants occurs at the expense of severe bleeding complications[1]. Hence, there has been a strong effort over recent years to develop and validate novel anticoagulant regimens that provide protection against thrombotic complications, but have only minor effects on normal haemostasis[2].

Until recently, the standard anticoagulation therapy during PCI consisted in either unfractionated (UFH) or low-molecular-weight heparin (LMWH) that prevent coagulation *indirectly* by activation of antithrombin (AT)[3]. Once activated, AT inactivates thrombin and other proteases involved in blood clotting[4]. However, only recently *direct* thrombin inhibitors (DTI) have been introduced as an alternative anticoagulant strategy in patients undergoing PCI. Bivalirudin is the most prominent member of the DTI class, *directly* inhibiting free- and clot-bound thrombin[5]. Use of bivalirudin has recently been shown to result in a significant reduction of bleeding without an increase in thrombotic or ischaemic endpoints compared to heparin and glycoprotein (GP) IIb/IIIa inhibitors in patients presenting with acute coronary syndromes (ACS)[5–14].

This chapter will give an overview of the pharmacology and mechanism of action of bivalirudin and summarize results from recent clinical trials evaluating the use of bivalirudin in patients undergoing PCI.

The role of thrombin in patients undergoing PCI

Thrombotic events, including myocardial infarction (MI) and stroke, are among the leading causes of peri-procedural deaths following PCI, particularly in patients with ACS. Peri-procedural strokes are uncommon, but potentially devastating and are usually caused by emboli released from atherosclerotic plaques on the aortic wall disrupted during catheterization or from thrombi that form directly on or within the material used for catheterization (diagnostic and guiding catheters, wires etc.). In contrast, peri-procedural MIs most frequently result from luminal thrombosis within the coronary artery secondary to plaque erosion or rupture[15,16]. Plaque rupture occurs either during balloon angioplasty or spontaneously in patients with ACS. In fact, the vast majority of ACS cases are considered to be due to spontaneous disruption of the endothelial lining that covers atherosclerotic plaques[17]. A necrotic core and a thin overlying fibrous cap containing a dense concentration of macrophages and only few smooth muscle cells, characterize 'vulnerable plaques' that predispose atherosclerotic lesions to rupture[18–20].

Plaque rupture allows direct contact between the extremely thrombogenic necrotic core and circulating platelets, monocytes, as well as clotting factors[18–20]. In a process generally referred to as 'thrombus initiation' circulating platelets adhere to the exposed subendothelial components, particularly to collagen and von Willebrand factor (vWF) through specific adhesion receptors including glycoprotein (GP) Ib , GPVI, and GP IIb/IIIa, respectively[4,21,22]. During adhesion platelets become activated and release an array of highly potent platelet agonists including adenosine diphosphate (ADP) and thromboxane A2, which promote recruitment of additional platelets from the circulation. Besides platelets, leucocytes, particularly neutrophils and monocytes, accumulate at the site of plaque rupture. Recruited myeloid leukocytes, but also platelets, as well as macrophages, and smooth muscle cells from the exposed necrotic core, release tissue factor (TF)[4,23,24]. TF triggers the activation of the coagulation cascade resulting in the generation of thrombin by activation of the zymogen prothrombin[25] (Fig. 25.1).

Thrombin plays a fundamental role in propagating thrombus growth after initial platelet accumulation[26]. Thrombin is the chief effector of the coagulation cascade and at the same time acts as highly potent endogenous platelet activator. Thrombin is a protease that binds to and cleaves fibrinogen into fibrin (Fig. 25.1). Fibrin in turn polymerizes and binds to the platelet fibrin(ogen) receptor GP IIb/IIIa, a step that is critical for stabilization and consolidation of the platelet-rich thrombus. Thrombin also activates factors V, VIII, and XIII, which further stimulate thrombin production in a positive feedback loop and stabilize the fibrin-bound thrombin[27]. Moreover, thrombin activates carboxypeptidase B, a potent inhibitor of fibrinolysis[28]. Together this leads to profound and rapid fibrin generation within the growing thrombus.

In addition to starting coagulation, thrombin directly triggers platelet activation through surface expressed receptors. Thrombin predominantly associates with platelet protease-activated receptors (PARs), G protein-coupled receptors with specific thrombin cleavage sites[29]. When thrombin cleaves the amino-terminal of PARs on platelets (in humans particularly PAR-1 and PAR-4), several signalling pathways are activated. As a result, platelets release additional potent platelet agonists, including ADP. In a concerted action, this leads to profound activation of additional circulating platelets that are incorporated into the growing thrombus[29]. Hence, thrombin-dependent activation of both platelets and the coagulation cascade is essential for thrombus growth and consolidates the platelet-rich thrombus and prevents dissolution. To accomplish these multiple tasks, thrombin contains three distinct receptor sites: one active catalytic and two exosites[30–32]. While the catalytic site mediates the conversion of fibrinogen to fibrin and triggers the activation of platelets and clotting factors[32], exosites 1 and 2 are positively charged and promote thrombin binding to negatively charged compounds, such as fibrinogen and heparin-antithrombin (AT)-III complex.

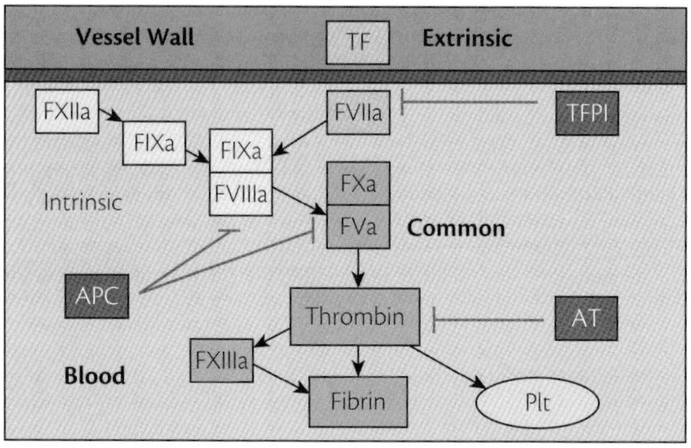

Fig. 25.1 Simplified version of the clotting cascade. The extrinsic pathway of the coagulation cascade consists of tissue factor (TF) and FVIIa. FXIIa, FXIa, FIXa, and FVIIIa are members of the intrinsic pathway. The common pathway is made up of FVa, FXa, and thrombin. Thrombin cleaves fibrinogen, activates FXIII, and activates platelets (Plt). The clotting cascade is regulated by three major pathways: TF pathway inhibitor (TFPI) that inhibits the TF:FVIIa complex; activated protein C (APC) that cleaves and inactivates FVa and FVIIIa; and antithrombin (AT) that inhibits thrombin and other proteases in the cascade. For simplicity only activated proteases and cofactors are shown. Reproduced with permission from Mackman N. The role of tissue factor and factor VIIa in hemostasis. *Anesth Analg* 2009;**108**(5):1447–52.

Anticoagulant treatment regimens in PCI patients

In patients with coronary artery disease undergoing PCI, particularly in those presenting with ACS, it is mandatory to reduce the risk of MI and death. This is achieved most efficiently by inhibiting platelet function. Currently, platelet aggregation and activation is prevented by a dual antiplatelet strategy, consisting of aspirin and ADP receptor (P2Y12) antagonists (e.g., clopidogrel or prasugrel)[33–36]. However, as outlined earlier, in addition to the recruitment of platelets, the activation of thrombin also substantially contributes to thrombotic processes in patients undergoing PCI. Hence, apart from antiplatelet drugs, anticoagulants are required to prevent thrombin-driven thrombus propagation and growth (see earlier section). Correspondingly, randomized trials have demonstrated that UFH in combination with aspirin (ASA) is superior to ASA alone, resulting in an approximate 33–50% reduction in short-term rates of MI or death in patients undergoing PCI[36–42]. Likewise, trials evaluating the combination of ASA with LMWH (e.g. nadroparin, dalteparin, enoxaparin) have demonstrated a significant reduction in ischaemic endpoints including MI, stroke, and need for re-revascularization procedures in patients with ACS[43,44].

Until recently, heparin, therefore, was the treatment of choice to achieve efficient anticoagulation in patients undergoing PCI. However, anticoagulant therapy using heparin unfortunately results in higher rates of major and minor bleeding in PCI patients[45]. Heparin acts by binding to AT-III and thereby multiplies AT-III's efficacy to inhibit thrombin and factor Xa[32, 46]. Notably, heparins mostly inhibit free thrombin, but have virtually no effect on thrombin bound to fibrin degradation products[31,47,48]. Moreover, heparin attaches to endothelial cells as well as a number of plasma proteins, which limits its anticoagulant efficacy[49]. Also, due to its non-specific binding to endothelium and plasma proteins, the half-life of heparin is dose-dependent and there is a high intra- and interpatient variability. In addition, both UFH and LMWH can be inactivated by platelet factor 4 (PF4)[50] and the resulting heparin-PF4 complex can trigger IgG-mediated heparin-induced thrombocytopenia (HIT type II)[8,51].

Given these limitations of heparin, another group of anticoagulants, the direct thrombin inhibitors (DTIs), was recently introduced and evaluated for the treatment of arterial thrombosis. In contrast to heparin, DTIs inhibit thrombin *directly* and independent of the cofactor AT-III. The class of DTIs includes hirudin, a naturally occurring peptide found in the salivary glands of leeches, synthetic hirudin derivatives ('hirulogs') such as bivalirudin, lepirudin, and desirudin, as well as synthetic non-hirulogs targeting the active-site of thrombin (e.g. argatroban, melagatran, and ximelagatran, and thrombin-binding DNA aptamers)[52]. While univalent DTIs, such as argatroban bind only to the catalytic domain of thrombin, bivalent DTIs, including hirudin and bivalirudin, interact with the active site as well as the exosite 1[52].

DTIs have three major advantages over heparin: 1) they inactivate both free as well as fibrin-bound thrombin; 2) they do not attach to endothelial cells or plasma proteins; and 3) as a result, they have better predictability of pharmacokinetics[53]. Among the DTIs, bivalirudin, the focus of this chapter, is characterized by a particularly wide therapeutic window and due to its safety profile can be administered at higher doses resulting in greater availability and hence greater inhibition of thrombin[54]. As a consequence, bivalirudin is now frequently used for anticoagulation in the mainstream setting of invasive cardiology, whereas other marketed DTIs are used for selected indications, such as HIT (e.g. lepirudin, argatroban) or for thromboprophylaxis following orthopaedic surgery (e.g. desirudin). In the remainder of this chapter we will focus on the role of bivalirudin in PCI patients.

Pharmacological considerations on bivalirudin

Molecular structure and mechanisms of action

Bivalirudin is a semisynthetic oligopeptide analogue of hirudin with a molecular mass of 2180 Da[52,55]. The size of bivalirudin is only approximately one-third the size of hirudin (20 vs. 65 amino acids). The bivalirudin molecule consists of two segments, linked together by four glycine residues[55]. A carboxy-terminal segment of 12 amino acids is derived from native hirudin (residues 53–64) and binds to the fibrino(gen)-binding exosite 1 of thrombin. The amino-terminal tetrapeptide sequence (D-Phe–Pro–Arg–Pro) of bivalirudin specifically binds to the active site of thrombin with high affinity. This indicates that the 'hirulog' bivalirudin, like hirudin itself, is a bivalent DTI that binds specifically to thrombin at two sites, the exosite 1 and the catalytic site (Fig. 25.2). Like the other DTIs, bivalirudin does not require a cofactor for thrombin binding. The affinity of bivalirudin for human thrombin is intermediate (Ki = 2 nM) between hirudin (Ki = 0.0001 nM) and the synthetic DTI, argatroban (40 nM)[56,57]. Unlike hirudin, which binds to thrombin irreversibly, the binding of bivalirudin to thrombin is reversible. Besides non-covalent bond formation, the major reason for the reversibility of the bivalirudin-thrombin interaction is that thrombin cleaves bivalirudin close to its amino-terminal end. As a result the amino-terminal segment of bivalirudin detaches from the active site of thrombin[58], thereby also weakening the binding of the carboxy-terminal segment to exosite 1. This facilitates displacement of bivalirudin from thrombin by a fibrinogen molecule[58].

Because bivalirudin is a bivalent DTI, it acts as a competitive inhibitor of both, the fibrinogen binding to

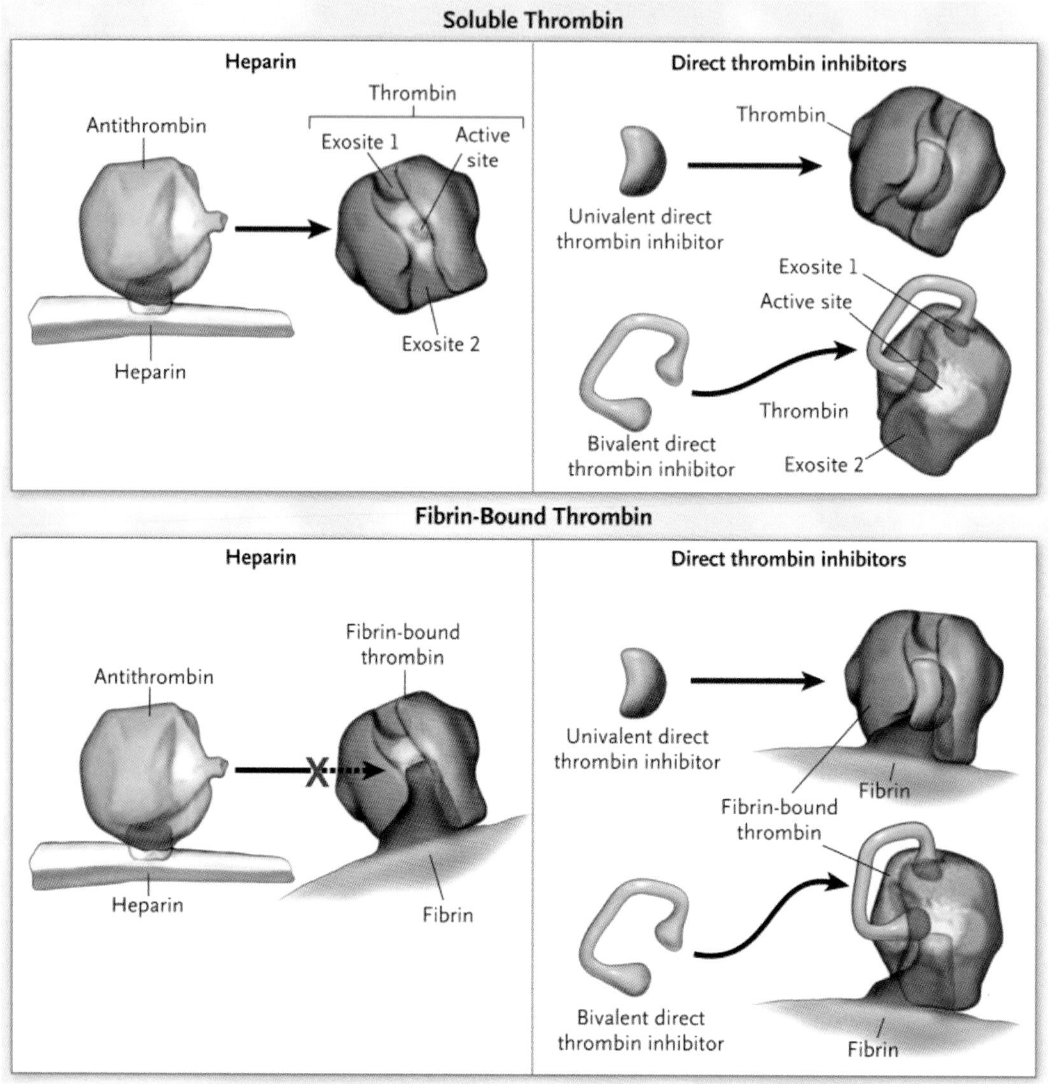

Fig. 25.2 Mechanism of action of direct thrombin inhibitors as compared with heparin. In the absence of heparin, the rate of thrombin inactivation by antithrombin is relatively low, but after conformational change induced by heparin, antithrombin irreversibly binds to and inhibits the active site of thrombin. Thus, the anticoagulant activity of heparin originates from its ability to generate a ternary heparin–thrombin–antithrombin complex. The activity of direct thrombin inhibitors (DTIs) is independent of the presence of antithrombin and is related to the direct interaction of these drugs with the thrombin molecule. Although bivalent DTIs simultaneously bind the exosite 1 and the active site, the univalent drugs in this class interact only with an active site of the enzyme. In the lower panel, the heparin–antithrombin complex cannot bind fibrin-bound thrombin, whereas given their mechanism of action, DTIs can bind to and inhibit the activity not only of soluble thrombin but also of thrombin bound to fibrin, as is the case in a blood clot. Reprinted with permission from Di Nisio M, Middeldorp S, Buller HR. Direct thrombin inhibitors. *N Engl J Med* 2005; **353**(10):1028–40.

thrombin and fibrinogen cleavage by thrombin. It competitively inhibits fibrinogen binding to exosite 1 as well as the catalytic domain of thrombin, resulting in complete inhibition of thrombin's catalytic function and hence of thrombin-dependent fibrin formation[55]. In contrast to bivalirudin, lepirudin binds to thrombin irreversibly and argatroban, an univalent DTI, binds only reversibly to thrombin's active site[59].

As already mentioned earlier, bivalirudin has several major advantages over heparin[52]: 1) it inhibits thrombin independent of whether thrombin is in solution or bound to fibrin; this is in contrast to heparin, which binds fibrin-bound thrombin poorly. 2) In contrast to heparin, inhibition of thrombin by bivalirudin does not require a cofactor and is not inactivated by PF4. 3) Whereas immune HIT is a rare but potentially dangerous complication of heparin therapy, bivalirudin has low if any immunogenic potential. 4) Binding of bivalirudin to plasma proteins or endothelial cells is negligible, resulting in better predictability of pharmacokinetics.

Monitoring of bivalirudin therapy

Bivalirudin is characterized by dose-dependent, linear pharmacokinetics and produces a rapid, almost immediate anticoagulant effect. Because of this, predetermined dosage regimens are recommended for the use of bivalirudin and there is no general need for monitoring of bivalirudin therapy. Monitoring may be valuable, however, in certain clinical conditions, including patients with renal dysfunction (see later section).

Several indices of coagulation, such as the activated clotting time (ACT), the activated partial thromboplastin time (aPTT), the prothrombin time (PT) or international normalized ratio (INR), as well as the thrombin time (TT) all rise in a linear fashion with infusion of bivalirudin[(5)]. In contrast, the aPTT has been used in patients treated for HIT. However, measurement of aPTT may not be valid for monitoring of bivalirudin therapy in patients that have additional factors contributing to aPTT prolongation (including HIT-associated disseminated intravascular coagulation [DIC], liver dysfunction, or warfarin administration).

Pharmokinetics and pharmacodynamics

Bivalirudin is administered intravenously and produces a rapid, almost immediate anticoagulant effect. It has linear pharmacokinetics with only a small volume of distribution (0.24L/kg), indicating that the majority of bivalirudin distributes extracellularly[(60)]. Correspondingly, the anticoagulant effects of bivalirudin, as assessed by aPTT, ACT, INR, or TT, rise in a linear manner with increasing doses of bivalirudin. Bivalirudin is rapidly cleared from plasma (3–4mL/min/kg). Bivalirudin clearance substantially exceeds the average glomerular filtration rate (~1.0–1.7mL/min/kg), reflecting its dual clearance by intravascular proteolysis and renal elimination. In healthy subjects, the *in vivo* half-life of bivalirudin is approximately 22min. Correspondingly, after discontinuation of bivalirudin infusion, its anticoagulant effects reverse rapidly and coagulation indices approach baseline within 1–2h in healthy patients with normal kidney function[(61–65)]. However, in patients with renal dysfunction, the half-life of bivalirudin may

Table 25.1 Recommended dosages for bivalirudin. *Renal function based on estimated glomerular filtration rate (GFR)

Patient subgroup	Initial bolus (mg/kg)	Infusion during PCI (mg/kg/h)
Normal renal function (>90mL/min*)	0.75	1.75
Mild or moderate kidney dysfunction (30–90mL/min*)	0.75	1.75
Severe kidney dysfunction (10–29mL/min*)	0.75	1.00
Patients on dialysis	0.75	0.25
HIT/HITTS undergoing PCI	0.75	1.75

HIT/HITTS, heparin-induced thrombocytopenia/heparin-induced thrombocytopenia with thrombotic syndrome; PCI, percutaneous coronary intervention.

be prolonged to up to 210min in end-stage renal failure, and it has been reported that compared to normal healthy subjects, bivalirudin clearance is approximately 40% in patients with a creatinine clearance of 10–60mL/min, and 10% in haemodialysis patients[(66,67)]. This implicates that patients with renal dysfunction require lower doses of bivalirudin and more frequent anticoagulant monitoring. It is recommended to maintain the standard bolus dosing and reduce the infusion rate to 1mg/kg/h if the creatinine clearance is less than 30mL/min or to 0.25mg/kg/h if the patient is on haemodialysis. Current dosage recommendations for bivalirudin are summarized in Table 25.1.

Drug interactions and safety considerations

Bivalirudin is not metabolized by the cytochrome P450 isoenzyme system and most likely does not bind to plasma proteins other than thrombin[(52)]. Therefore, the potential for drug–drug interactions is low. Nevertheless, bivalirudin could potentially exhibit a pharmacodynamic interaction, when it is given concomitantly with other antithrombotic, antiplatelet, or thrombolytic reagents during PCI. However, bivalirudin does not appear to have a pharmacodynamic interaction with the thienopyridine ticlopidine, LMWHs, UFH, or GP IIb/IIIa inhibitors[(11,52)]. Moreover, bivalirudin has been safely administered together with clopidogrel and aspirin in clinical trials and it has been reported that bivalirudin's anticoagulant actions are not affected by concurrent aspirin use[(62)]. Moreover, at therapeutic dosages bivalirudin unlike heparin does not directly activate platelets, but rather decreases platelet adhesion to the injured vessel wall in patients undergoing PCI[64,68–70].

Bleeding is the major adverse effect of bivalirudin, and occurs more commonly in patients with renal impairment. Bivalirudin is therefore contraindicated in patients with active major bleeding. Besides bleeding, the most frequent adverse effects of bivalirudin reported in initial studies were nausea, back pain, headache, and hypotension (Hirulog Angioplasty Study[71]). Less common effects include insomnia, nervousness, anxiety, hypertension, vomiting, dyspepsia, bradycardia, abdominal pain, fever, and pelvic pain[64]. So far, there has been no reported association of bivalirudin with thrombocytopenia. Also, no evidence of fetal harm has been reported for bivalirudin in animal teratogenicity studies. However, well-controlled studies in pregnant women are lacking and it is not known whether bivalirudin passes the placenta, or is excreted in breast milk. Therefore, caution is advised when giving bivalirudin to nursing women.

Bivalirudin is a small semisynthetic polypeptide and is therefore likely to have minimal antigenic potential. Correspondingly, there is currently no clear evidence for antibody formation against bivalirudin. In clinical trials of bivalirudin allergic reactions considered by the investigator to be related to bivalirudin were exceedingly rare[64,71]. This contrasts somewhat the experiences with lepirudin, for which several fatal post-bolus anaphylactic reactions have been reported, usually in the context of re-exposure following recent use[72]. Therefore, it remains possible that re-exposure or prolonged treatment with bivalirudin might be associated with risk of anaphylaxis. In addition, it is noteworthy that bivalirudin shares an 11-amino acid sequence with lepirudin. Hence, in theory it is possible that anti-lepirudin antibodies resulting from treatment with lepirudin could cross-react with bivalirudin. Hence, caution should be used if bivalirudin is used in patients previously treated with lepirudin.

Reversal of bivalirudin therapy

Currently, there is no specific antidote to counteract the anticoagulant effects of bivalirudin[60]. However, haemodialysis, haemofiltration, and plasmapheresis can remove significant amounts of bivalirudin and may be helpful in some situations of overdosing.

Clinical use of bivalirudin

Bivalirudin has been extensively tested and is currently recommended according to the American College of Cardiology (ACC)/The American Heart Association (AHA) guidelines for use in patients with non-ST-elevation MI (NSTEMI) or ST-elevation MI (STEMI) undergoing PCI (class IB and IC indication, respectively). In addition, bivalirudin is also recommended (class I) in patients with heparin-induced thrombocytopenia (HIT) without or with thrombotic syndrome (HITTS) requiring PCI or coronary artery bypass surgery (CABG)[3,73,74]. The current clinical indications according to the ACC/AHA guidelines are summarized in Table 25.2.

In addition to the discussed indications, bivalirudin has also been tested for non-interventional treatment of ACS including MI, and as an anticoagulant during cardiac surgery, particularly in clinical settings, in which heparin is contraindicated, but also for routine use. Another clinical application that has emerged recently is in the treatment and prevention of thrombotic events complicating HIT.

For the purpose of this chapter we will discuss predominantly the role during PCI. We will also report on the use of bivalirudin in patients with HIT undergoing PCI. We will, however, not discuss the use of bivalirudin in other clinical situations, including peripheral percutaneous interventions, the prevention and treatment of venous thromboembolism, or non-invasive treatment of ACS.

Unstable angina or NSTEMI patients: initial trials

In 1993, Topol and co-workers published the first report describing the use of bivalirudin (formerly named hirulog), instead of heparin in PCI patients[64]. It was a multicentre, open-label, dose-finding trial that enrolled 291 patients undergoing PCI. Patients were treated with an intravenous bolus followed by continuous infusion of bivalirudin for 4h after the PCI procedure. Different dosing strategies were tested. The authors reported that hirulog was associated with an almost immediate onset and dose-dependent anticoagulant effect. The primary endpoint of abrupt vessel closure occurred in 3.9% of patients at doses of 1.0–2.2mg/kg. No significant bleeding complications were observed in any patient.

After this initial demonstration that it was possible to safely perform PCI with a DTI instead of heparin in aspirin-pre-treated patients, the first randomized comparison of bivalirudin versus heparin in patients undergoing PCI was reported in the Hirulog Angioplasty Study (HAS Trial)[71]. In this trial, a total of 4,312 patients with unstable or post-infarction angina were randomly assigned to receive heparin or bivalirudin immediately prior to PCI. The reported primary endpoints were any combination of death in the hospital,

Table 25.2 ACC/AHA guideline for the use of bivalirudin in ACS patients[3,74]

Clinical setting	Description	ACC/AHA indication
HIT/HITTS	For patients with known HIT/HITTS and undergoing PCI or CABG	Class I
UA/NSTEMI	For patients in whom an invasive strategy is selected, bivalirudin is started upon hospital presentation	Class I, LoE B
	For patients in whom PCI has been selected as a post-angiography management strategy, bivalirudin is used with at least 300mg of clopidogrel administered at least 6h earlier	Class IIa, LoE B
	For patients in whom PCI has been selected as a post-angiography management strategy, bivalirudin is used with a GP IIb/IIIa inhibitor if at least 300mg of clopidogrel was NOT administered at least 6h earlier	Class IIa, LoE B
	For patients in whom a conservative strategy is selected, bivalirudin is started upon hospital presentation	No current recommendation.
STEMI	For patients undergoing primary PCI or rescue PCI, bivalirudin is started prior to intervention	No current recommendation.
	For patients undergoing primary PCI or rescue PCI who have received UFH up to the time of intervention, bivalirudin is used during the intervention	Class I, LoE C

ACC/AHA, American College of Cardiology/American Heart Association; ACS, acute coronary syndrome; CABG, coronary artery bypass surgery; HIT/HITTS, heparin-induced thrombocytopenia/heparin-induced thrombocytopenia with thrombotic syndrome; LoE, level of evidence; NSTEMI, non-ST-elevation myocardial infarction; PCI, percutaneous coronary intervention; STEMI, ST-elevation myocardial infarction; UA, unstable angina.

abrupt vessel closure, or rapid clinical deterioration of cardiac origin requiring emergency CABG, intra-aortic balloon counterpulsation (IABP), or repeated PCI. The HAS Investigators reported that there was no significant difference between the two groups in the combined primary endpoint (11.4% in the bivalirudin arm vs. 12.2% in the heparin arm, p = 0.44), but that bivalirudin was associated with a lower incidence of bleeding (3.8% vs. 9.8%; p <0.001). In a prospectively stratified subset of 704 patients with post-infarction angina enrolled in the HAS trial, bivalirudin resulted in a lower rate of the primary efficacy endpoint (9.1% vs. 14.2%; p = 0.04) and bleeding (3.0% vs. 11.1%; p<0.001)[54,71].

In 2001, Bittl and co-workers published a Food and Drug Administration (FDA)-endorsed re-analysis of the HAS patients, the Bivalirudin Angioplasty Trial (BAT)[75]. The BAT study included an additional 214 patients enrolled in the HAS trial, who had not undergone PCI, and who therefore had been excluded in the original per-protocol analysis, but who were now included per intention-to-treat principle in the subsequent report. The composite endpoint (at day 7) of death, MI, or revascularization occurred in 6.2% of bivalirudin-treated patients, and 7.9% of UFH-treated patients (p = 0.039). Further, major bleeding occurred in 3.5% of bivalirudin-treated patients, but 9.3% of heparin-treated patients (p <0.001). Thus, bivalirudin appeared to be non-inferior to heparin in preventing ischaemic complications in patients undergoing PCI for unstable angina, but was associated with a reduction in major bleeding[75].

In a subsequent randomized trial, the TIMI-8 study, the efficacy and safety of low-dose bivalirudin versus UFH in patients presenting with unstable angina or NSTEMI was evaluated in 133 patients (prior to early termination of the trial). The results showed a trend towards less combined non-fatal MI or death or major haemorrhage at 14 days in patients receiving bivalirudin (2.9% vs. 9.2% and 0% vs. 4.6%, respectively)[76].

Based on these trials, particularly the BAT trial, bivalirudin was FDA-approved. The recommended dose regimen included an intravenous bolus of 1.0mg/kg followed by 4h intravenous infusion at a rate of 2.5mg/kg/h. If needed, an additional infusion could be initiated at a rate of 0.2mg/kg/h for up to 20h after completion of the initial 4h infusion. Based upon subsequent studies, the FDA-approved dose was reduced in 2005 to a bolus of 0.75mg/kg and an infusion rate of 1.75mg/kg/h administered for the duration of the PCI, rather than for a 4h period (see Table 25.2).

Unstable angina or NSTEMI patients: the CACHET and REPLACE trials

After the introduction of stents, clopidogrel, and GP IIb/IIIa antagonist therapy into modern PCI procedures, bivalirudin underwent several clinical re-evaluations.

In the CACHET Trial (Comparison of Abciximab Complications with Hirulog for Ischemic Events Trial), a pilot trial that enrolled 268 patients undergoing PCI, the efficacy of different doses of bivalirudin (phase A: bolus, 1.0mg/kg; infusion, 2.5mg/kg/h for 4h, phase B: bolus, 0.50mg/kg; infusion 1.75mg/kg/h for duration of procedure, and phase C: bolus, 0.75mg/kg; infusion, 1.75mg/kg/h for the duration of the PCI) with and without abciximab was evaluated and compared to standard therapy consisting of UFH therapy plus abciximab[77]. In the initial course of CACHET the optimal dosing regimen (bolus, 0.75mg/kg; infusion, 1.75mg/kg/h for the duration of the PCI) was identified. When all three bivalirudin dosing regimens were pooled in a post hoc analysis, bivalirudin was found to be significantly more effective than heparin, using a combined endpoint of death, MI, surgical/interventional revascularization, or major bleeding (3.4% vs. 10.6%; p = 0.018). Later on, the results of CACHET also suggested that bivalirudin with provisional abciximab (i.e. use for indications such as coronary dissection, new or suspected thrombus formation, impaired or slow coronary flow, and distal embolization), is as safe and effective as standard UFH plus abciximab in patients undergoing PCI[77]. In none of the bivalirudin-treated patients that received abciximab on a provisional basis was the composite endpoint of death, MI, or surgical/interventional revascularization observed, but it occurred in 6.4% of the UFH-treated controls.

These promising pilot studies triggered the subsequent evaluation of bivalirudin for PCI in larger phase III trials. Initially, bivalirudin was evaluated in the Randomized Evaluation in PCI Linking Angiomax to Reduced Clinical Events Trials (REPLACE-1 and REPLACE-2). The REPLACE trials enrolled patients undergoing urgent or elective PCI. Almost 85% of the patients included into the REPLACE trials received clopidogrel before the procedure and stent implantation during the procedure. In REPLACE-1, a pilot study, heparin was compared to bivalirudin (0.75mg/kg bolus, 1.75mg/kg/h infusion) in 1056 patients undergoing elective or urgent PCI with any one of the GP IIb/IIIa inhibitors. In both groups, 72% of the patients received GP IIb/IIIa inhibitors at the discretion of the physician. Bivalirudin use was required only for the duration of the PCI procedure. The results showed a non-significant reduction of the combined endpoint of death, MI, or surgical/interventional revascularization, and major bleeding in bivalirudin-treated patients[78]. This was further addressed in REPLACE-2[79,80], a randomized trial that compared 6010 patients receiving UFH (65U/kg) plus planned administration of GP IIb/IIIa inhibitor (abciximab (Reopro®, Centocor Inc., PA, USA) or eptifibatide (Integrillin®, Millenium Pharmaceuticals, Inc, MA, USA)) for 12–18h or bivalirudin (dosing as in REPLACE-1: 0.75mg/kg bolus with 1.75mg/kg/h infusion during PCI) with only provisional use of GP IIb/IIIa inhibitors. As outlined earlier, indications for provisional use of GP IIb/IIIa inhibitors were abrupt vessel closure, obstructive dissection, new or suspected thrombus, slow coronary flow, distal embolization, persistent residual stenosis, unplanned stent placement, or prolonged ischaemia. All patients included in REPLACE-2 received aspirin and most also an ADP receptor antagonist, predominantly clopidogrel. Provisional GP IIb/IIIa was administered to 7.2% of bivalirudin-treated patients.

The primary composite endpoint of death, MI, severe ischaemia requiring repeat revascularization, or in-hospital major bleeding within 30 days of randomization showed no significant difference between the two groups of patients (9.2% bivalirudin versus 10.0% GP IIb/IIIa inhibitors, odds ratio [OR] 0.92; 95% confidence interval [CI] 0.77–1.09; p = 0.32)). Importantly though, there were less major bleedings (2.4% versus 4.1%, p = 0.001) in those patients initially treated with bivalirudin. In addition, significantly less bivalirudin-treated patients developed a drop in platelet count below 100×10^9/L (0.7 vs. 1.7%; p <0.001). Another important conclusion from REPLACE-2 is that clopidogrel therapy did not influence the relative efficacy of bivalirudin versus UFH plus GP IIb/IIIa blockade. Instead, clopidogrel therapy reduced the primary endpoint in patients receiving bivalirudin (8.7% pretreatment vs. 12.9% no pre-treatment; p = 0.0007)[81]. This implies that clopidogrel pretreatment improved clinical outcomes without compromising safety. However, clopidogrel is not required for bivalirudin to achieve efficacy similar to UFH plus GP IIb/IIIa blockade. Notably, the 6-month and 1-year follow-up results of REPLACE-2[79,80] also found similar incidences of death, MI, and repeat vascularization in the UFH- and the bivalirudin-treated groups. Hence, long-term clinical outcomes with bivalirudin and provisional GP IIb/IIIa blockade appeared to be similar to that of heparin plus planned GP IIb/IIIa inhibition in all patient subgroups analyzed.

Another study, evaluating the efficacy of bivalirudin in PCI patients was the PROTECT-TIMI-30 study. This randomized trial compared eptifibatide plus UFH or LMWH versus bivalirudin alone in 857 patients that underwent PCI for ACS. Specifically, three treatment arms were evaluated: 1) bivalirudin alone; 2) eptifibatide plus a reduced-dose of UFH; or 3) eptifibatide plus reduced-dose LMWH. The results indicated that bivalirudin was associated with higher coronary flow reserve following PCI. Secondary endpoint analysis suggested that patients undergoing PCI who were randomized to eptifibatide experienced an improve in Thrombolysis In Myocardial Infarction (TIMI) myocardial perfusion rate following PCI, shorter duration of ischaemia on continuous Holter monitoring after PCI, more minor bleeding events, a higher transfusion rate, and no difference in biomarkers for myonecrosis, inflammation, and thrombin generation[82].

Intermediate- and high-risk ACS patients: the ACUITY trial

The current medical treatment of patients with moderate- or high-risk ACS typically includes an early invasive strategy in conjunction with an aggressive antiplatelet and antithrombotic strategy, consisting in a combination of ADP receptor antagonism, predominantly clopidogrel, GP IIb/IIIa receptor antagonists, as well as UFH or LMWH. In the Acute Catheterization and Urgent Intervention Triage strategY (ACUITY) trial, it was therefore evaluated whether bivalirudin, in addition to acute catheterization and urgent intervention, might provide further improvement. In contrast to the REPLACE-2 trial, which included mainly low-risk ACS patients, the ACUITY trial enrolled moderate- as well as high-risk ACS patients. This prospective, randomized trial enrolled 13 819 patients with ACS in whom early invasive strategy was planned (i.e. angiography within 72h) and assigned them to three treatment regimens: 1) UFH plus GP IIb/IIIa inhibitors; 2) bivalirudin plus GP IIb/IIIa inhibitors; and 3) bivalirudin alone (with provisional GP IIb/IIIa inhibition). Bivalirudin was administered as a 0.1-mg/kg bolus, followed by 0.25-mg/kg/h infusion during angiography. An additional bolus of 0.5mg/kg was given, if after angiography PCI was performed, and the infusion increased to 1.75mg/kg/h until the end of the PCI. Optionally, bivalirudin infusion was continued at 0.25mg/kg/h for up to 12h at the discretion of the physician. The endpoint was a composite ischaemia endpoint including death, MI, unplanned revascularization at 30 days, the primary safety endpoint was major bleeding. A net clinical outcome endpoint was defined as the combination of these endpoints. The outcomes at day 30 after PCI revealed non-inferior rates of the composite ischaemic endpoint including death, MI, unplanned revascularization (7.3% vs. 7.8%, respectively, p = ns), but a significant reduction in major bleedings and the net clinical outcome endpoint (3.0% vs. 5.7%, $p < 0.001$, and 10.1% vs. 11.7%, $p = 0.02$) in patients who received bivalirudin alone when compared to UFH plus GP IIb/IIIa inhibitors. When bivalirudin plus a GP IIb/IIIa inhibitor was compared with heparin plus a GP IIb/IIIa inhibitor, ACUITY demonstrated a non-inferior rate of the composite ischaemic endpoint (7.7% and 7.3%, respectively), major bleeding (5.3% and 5.7%, respectively), as well as the net clinical outcome endpoint (11.8% and 11.7%, respectively). At 1 year, no statistically significant difference in rates of composite ischaemia or mortality among patients with moderate- and high-risk ACS undergoing invasive treatment with the three therapies was found[12].

In a substudy of ACUITY, the optimum strategy for use of GP IIb/IIIa inhibitors in patients enrolled in the ACUITY trial was evaluated by a second randomization procedure. Patients assigned to receive GP IIb/IIIa inhibitors were sub-randomized to two subgroups: 1) early initiation of the GP IIb/IIIa antagonist immediately after randomization, or 2) initiation of GP IIb/IIIa inhibitor in the catheterization laboratory starting immediately prior to PCI. A total of 7789 of the 13 918 patients in ACUITY underwent a PCI after angiography and were included into this substudy. Little effect was seen depending on whether the GP IIb/IIIa inhibitor was given initially or only prior to PCI. Similar to the main ACUITY trial, the rates of composite ischaemia, major bleeding, and the net clinical outcome among the patients who underwent PCI did not differ significantly between those who received bivalirudin plus GP IIb/IIIa inhibitors versus those who received heparin plus a GP IIb/IIIa inhibitor. In those patients who received bivalirudin alone versus those who received heparin plus GP IIb/IIIa inhibitors, there were significantly less major bleedings (3.5% vs. 6.8%; RR 0.52; 95% CI 0.40–0.66; $p<0.0001$), while the rates of the composite ischaemia endpoint did not differ significantly[13].

Another pre-specified analysis of the ACUITY trial showed that patients with an age ≥75 years treated with bivalirudin alone had similar ischaemic outcomes, but significantly lower rates of bleeding compared with those treated with heparin and GP IIb/IIIa inhibitors. The number needed to treat with bivalirudin alone to avoid one major bleeding event was lower in this age group than in younger patients[83].

Particularly the ACUITY data resulted in a Class I indication for the use of bivalirudin in patients presenting with unstable angina and NSTEMI[73].

An important caveat in the ACUITY study however is, that not all patients were treated with clopidogrel and that those patients who received bivalirudin monotherapy, but not clopidogrel, had a trend to increased ischaemic events, when compared with those patients that were treated with a GP IIb/IIIa antagonist. The results of this pre-specified subgroup analysis suggest that patients treated with bivalirudin alone might benefit from pre-treatment with clopidogrel prior to PCI[84]. Hence, further evaluation of the benefit of bivalirudin, particularly in clopidogrel pre-treated patients was mandatory.

Use of bivalirudin in patients with STEMI

In contrast to patients presenting with unstable angina and NSTEMI, the efficacy of bivalirudin in patients with STEMI is less well investigated.

The first study to address the use of bivalirudin in patients with STEMI receiving fibrinolytic therapy was the HERO-2 trial published in 2001. More than 17 000 STEMI patients were randomly assigned to receive either bivalirudin or UFH, each in conjunction with standard thrombolytic (streptokinase). There was no significant difference in overall mortality at 30 days between the two groups revealed, however patients randomized to bivalirudin therapy had a reduced incidence of re-infarction within 96h (RR 0.70; CI 0.56–0.87; p = 0.001)[85].

The efficacy and safety of bivalirudin in STEMI patients undergoing PCI was addressed in the BiAMI Trial. This prospective, single-arm study assigned patients presenting with STEMI to receive bivalirudin infusion for the duration of the PCI. The GP IIb/IIIa inhibitor abciximab was used as a provisional approach if TIMI 3 flow was not established after stent placement. When the data were compared to a historic control of patients receiving UFH plus GP IIb/IIIa inhibitors, bivalirudin appeared to provide a comparable ischaemic protection with fewer bleeding complications[86].

The first randomized trial investigating the efficacy of bivalirudin in STEMI patients undergoing PCI was the Harmonizing Outcomes with RevascularIZatiON and Stents in Acute Myocardial Infarction (HORIZONS AMI) trial, presented in 2007 and published in May 2008[87]. The HORIZONS AMI trial randomized 3602 patients with STEMI who presented within 12h after the onset of symptoms and who were undergoing primary PCI to receive either: 1) UFH plus GP IIb/IIIa inhibitors or 2) bivalirudin monotherapy with provisional use of GP IIb/IIIa inhibitors. Major bleeding and combined adverse clinical events (defined as the combination of major bleeding or major adverse cardiovascular events, including death, reinfarction, target vessel revascularization for ischaemia, and stroke) were the two primary endpoints of the study. At 30 days, treatment with bivalirudin alone resulted in a reduced rate of combined adverse clinical events, when compared with heparin plus GP IIb/IIIa inhibitors (9.2% vs. 12.1%; RR 0.76; 95% CI 0.63–0.92; p = 0.005). This was due to a lower rate of major bleeding (4.9% vs. 8.3%; RR 0.60; 95% CI, 0.46–0.77; p <0.001). However, there was an increased risk of acute stent thrombosis within 24h in the bivalirudin group, but no significant increase was present by 30 days. The 30-day rates of death from cardiac causes (1.8% vs. 2.9%; RR 0.62; 95% CI 0.40–0.95; p = 0.03) and death from all causes (2.1% vs. 3.1%; RR 0.66; 95% CI 0.44–1.00; p = 0.047) was significantly lower in patients treated with bivalirudin alone, as compared to patients assigned to treatment with heparin plus GP IIb/IIIa inhibitors[87].

The long-term efficacy of bivalirudin in STEMI patients in particular in combination with novel antiplatelet regimens (see later section) will have to be established in future.

Bivalirudin in HIT/HITTS patients undergoing PCI

Besides bleeding, a major complication of heparin therapy is the development of HIT without or with thrombotic syndrome (HITTS). Among patients treated with heparin, up to 5% develop HIT or HITTS. In the past years, off-label use of bivalirudin to treat HIT was evaluated, beginning with an initial case report by Chamberlin and co-workers[88], describing this treatment in three patients with acute HIT. Subsequently, additional patients with HIT were treated with bivalirudin[89]. The bivalirudin doses used depended on the clinical setting, which most often was PCI and venous thrombosis and/or pulmonary embolism. Four patients died due to complications of HIT. Further studies have evaluated the use of bivalirudin to treat HIT. However, although bivalirudin is a promising therapy for treatment of acute HIT, none of the studies have employed a control group of non-bivalirudin-treated patients. Further, its preferential use in the critically-ill (a setting where thrombocytopenia is usually explained by non-HIT factors) and the failure to document HIT (through use of high-quality laboratory assays for HIT antibodies) means that its efficacy and safety in HIT remains speculative and will have to be evaluated further[90].

Several studies have addressed the use of bivalirudin in patients with HIT or HITTS undergoing PCI.

The Anticoagulant Therapy with Bivalirudin to Assist in the Performance of PCI in patients with Heparin-induced Thrombocytopenia (ATBAT) trial, a prospective, single-arm, open-label study, determined the safety and efficacy of bivalirudin in patients with newly diagnosed or previous HIT/HITTS undergoing PCI. A total of 52 patients were enrolled in this trial and received bivalirudin during and up to 4h following the PCI procedure. The initial dosing regimen consisted in a bolus of 1.0mg/kg followed by an infusion of 2.5mg/kg/h for 4h and was later changed to reflect dosing in non-HIT patients (see above) to a bolus of 0.75mg/kg followed by an infusion of 1.75mg/kg/h for 4h. The primary efficacy endpoint was defined as procedural success (<50% stenosis) and clinical success without death, emergency bypass surgery, or Q-wave MI. Major bleeding within 48h after completion of bivalirudin was the primary safety endpoint. Only one out of 52 patients required a blood transfusion. Procedural and clinical success was achieved in 98% and 96% of the patients, respectively. No abrupt closures or thrombus formation were reported during or after PCI. One patient died of cardiac arrest about 46h after successful PCI. There was no significant thrombocytopenia observed in the 52 patients following PCI after administration of bivalirudin. These data triggered the Class I indication for use of bivalirudin in patients with or at high-risk of HIT/HITTS during treatment for ACS or undergoing PCI[3,91].

Role of bivalirudin in combination with modern antiplatelet regimens

In recent years, pretreatment with clopidogrel (300–600mg) prior to PCI instead of GP IIb/IIIa antagonists is increasingly being used in patients at low-to-intermediate risk, because it has been demonstrated to result in similar outcome[92]. One major problem of all of the studies outlined earlier, therefore, is that bivalirudin has been compared almost exclusively with heparin plus a GP IIb/IIIa antagonist. The only exception is the HAS trial (see 'Unstable angina or NSTEMI patients: initial trials' section). However, the conclusions that can be drawn from the HAS study for current peri-procedural antithrombotic therapy are also limited, mainly because of the exclusive use of balloon angioplasty, the lack of pre-treatment (or any treatment) with clopidogrel, the high dose of heparin administered, and the outdated regimen of bivalirudin.

In a recent randomized trial, the Intracoronary Stenting and Antithrombotic Regimen: Rapid Early Action for Coronary Treatment 3 trial (ISAR-REACT-3), we therefore compared bivalirudin with UFH in patients with stable or unstable angina pectoris that were undergoing PCI with subsequent stent placement after pre-treatment with 600mg of clopidogrel[93]. We enrolled 4570 patients with normal levels of troponin T and creatine kinase MB who were undergoing PCI. All patients were pre-treated with a 600-mg dose of clopidogrel at least 2h before the procedure and were randomly assigned in a double-blind manner to receive either bivalirudin or unfractionated heparin. The combined 30-day endpoint of death, MI, urgent target-vessel revascularization, or major bleeding occurred in 8.3% of the bivalirudin-treated patients and in 8.7% of the patients treated with UFH (RR 0.94; 95% CI 0.77–1.15; p = 0.57). The incidence of major bleeding was 3.1% in the bivalirudin group and 4.6% in the UFH group (RR 0.66; 95% CI 0.49– 0.90; p = 0.008).

This indicates that in patients presenting with stable or unstable angina with low or intermediate risk without elevated levels of biomarkers and that undergo PCI after pre-treatment with clopidogrel, bivalirudin does not appear to reduce the incidence ischaemic adverse events as compared with UFH, and there is a trend toward a higher incidence of post-procedural MI. However, also in this population of patients, bivalirudin does significantly reduce the incidence of major bleeding[93].

Impact of bleeding and transfusions on outcome after PCI

Even if bivalirudin did not reduce the risk of ischaemic adverse events in most of the studies discussed here, the reported reduction in the incidence of major bleeding events reported in patients receiving bivalirudin alone versus heparin plus GP IIb/IIIa inhibitor is of potential clinical relevance. Indeed, a recent subgroup analysis[94] of data from REPLACE-2 indicates that patients with major hemorrhage have a higher 30-day mortality rate, compared to patients without major bleeding (5.1% vs. 0.2%; p <0.001). In this study, major bleeding was an independent predictor of 1-year mortality (OR 2.66; 95% CI 1.44– 4.92; p = 0.002). Similarly, a subgroup analysis from the ACUITY trial[95] revealed that patients with major bleeding had a higher 30-day mortality rate compared with such patients that did not have major bleeding (7.3% vs. 1.2%; p <0.0001). Major bleeding was an independent predictor of 30-day mortality (OR 7.55; 95% CI 4.68– 12.18; p <0.0001). Notably though, in this largest study of bivalirudin use, no difference in 1-year mortality with bivalirudin was seen[12], suggesting that reduction of bleeding events by bivalirudin does not affect long-term survival.

In a substudy to the ISAR-REACT-3 trial we identified a subset of patients at high risk of bleeding or MI after PCI and investigated whether such high-risk subsets derive preferential benefit from heparin or bivalirudin. The study included 4570 ISAR-REACT-3 patients with coronary artery disease randomized to receive bivalirudin or heparin. Primary outcomes were in-hospital incidence of major bleeding and 30-day incidence of MI. Compared with heparin, bivalirudin was associated with a reduction in major bleeding (3.1 vs. 4.6%, $p = 0.008$), but mostly in low-risk patients. A reduction in the bleeding risk inversely correlated with an increase in the risk of MI with bivalirudin ($R = -0.61$). This suggests that bivalirudin and UFH have a differential effect on risk of bleeding and MI across various subsets of patients[96].

Open questions to be addressed in ongoing or future studies

The available evidence suggests, that bivalirudin is a safe and effective anticoagulant in patients with ACS considered for bail-out GP IIb/IIIa inhibitor use that have not been treated with a high dose of clopidogrel. In contrast, bivalirudin does not appear to be superior to UFH in patients with stable or unstable angina pectoris that undergo PCI after pretreatment with a high dose of clopidogrel[93].

Major open questions particularly involve the role of bivalirudin in NSTEMI and STEMI patients that are treated with modern antiplatelet regimens. These include pre-treatment with a high dose of clopidogrel or the use of novel antiplatelet drugs, such as prasugrel or cangrelor. Studies are underway that will address some of these issues. For example, in the ongoing ISAR-REACT-4 trial, we are currently investigating the role of bivalirudin compared to abciximab in combination with UFH in patients with NSTEMI after treatment with a high dose of clopidogrel. The role of bivalirudin in combination with the novel platelet antagonist prasugrel in STEMI patients undergoing PCI will be addressed in the Bavarian Reperfusion AlternatiVes Evaluation-4 (BRAVE-4) trial. Additional studies will have to focus particularly on the efficacy of bivalirudin when used in combination with antiplatelet drugs that are currently being clinically evaluated. One promising candidate in this context is cangrelor (formerly denoted as AR-C69931MX), a short-acting, potent, competitive P2Y12 platelet receptor antagonist[97].

Conclusions

In patients, that present with intermediate- or high-risk ACS and that are selected for an early, invasive PCI-therapy, aggressive antiplatelet and antithrombotic medications are required to prevent adverse ischaemic events. These potent anticoagulants pose risks of increased bleeding events. Bivalirudin, a member of the DTI class, has recently been shown to have: 1) predictable pharmacokinetics; 2) ability to inhibit free- and clot-bound thrombin; 3) avoidance of platelet activation; and 4) avoidance of HIT. Available evidence shows that bivalirudin is not superior to UFH in patients with stable or unstable angina undergoing PCI after pretreatment with a high dose of clopidogrel. In patients with NSTEMI or STEMI, bivalirudin in combination with bailout GP IIb/IIIa inhibitors present a valuable antithrombotic regimen during PCI. Ongoing studies including ACS patients will better clarify the role of bivalirudin in the era of novel antiplatelet regimens.

References

1. Doyle BJ, Rihal CS, Gastineau DA, *et al.* Bleeding, blood transfusion, and increased mortality after percutaneous coronary intervention: implications for contemporary practice. *J Am Coll Cardiol* 2009; **53**(22):2019–27.
2. Holmes DR, Jr., Kereiakes DJ, Kleiman NS, *et al.* Combining antiplatelet and anticoagulant therapies. *J Am Coll Cardiol* 2009; **54**(2):95–109.
3. Anderson JL, Adams CD, Antman EM, *et al.* ACC/AHA 2007 guidelines for the management of patients with unstable angina/non-ST-Elevation myocardial infarction: a report of the American College of Cardiology/American Heart Association Task Force on Practice Guidelines (Writing Committee to Revise the 2002 Guidelines for the Management of Patients With Unstable Angina/Non-ST-Elevation Myocardial Infarction) developed in collaboration with the American College of Emergency Physicians, the Society for Cardiovascular Angiography and Interventions, and the Society of Thoracic Surgeons endorsed by the American Association of Cardiovascular and Pulmonary Rehabilitation and the Society for Academic Emergency Medicine. *J Am Coll Cardiol* 2007; **50**(7):e1–e157.
4. Mackman N. Triggers, targets and treatments for thrombosis. *Nature* 2008; **451**(7181):914–18.
5. Warkentin TE, Greinacher A, Koster A. Bivalirudin. *Thromb Haemost* 2008; **99**(5):830–9.
6. Coons JC, Battistone S. 2007 Guideline update for unstable angina/non-ST-segment elevation myocardial infarction: focus on antiplatelet and anticoagulant therapies. *Ann Pharmacother* 2008; **42**(7):989–1001.
7. Hartmann F. Safety and efficacy of bivalirudin in acute coronary syndromes. *Curr Pharm Res* 2008; **14**(12):1191–6.
8. Lehman SJ, Chew DP. Bivalirudin in percutaneous coronary intervention. Vasc *Health Risk Manag* 2006; **2**(4):357–63.

9. Mukherjee D, Eagle KA. Pharmacotherapy of acute coronary syndrome: the ACUITY trial. *Expert Opin Pharmacother* 2009; **10**(3):369–80.
10. Stone GW, Bertrand M, Colombo A, *et al.* Acute Catheterization and Urgent Intervention Triage strategY (ACUITY) trial: study design and rationale. *Am Heart J* 2004; **148**(5):764–75.
11. Stone GW, McLaurin BT, Cox DA, *et al.* Bivalirudin for patients with acute coronary syndromes. *N Engl J Med* 2006; **355**(21):2203–16.
12. Stone GW, Ware JH, Bertrand ME, *et al.* Antithrombotic strategies in patients with acute coronary syndromes undergoing early invasive management: one-year results from the ACUITY trial. *JAMA* 2007; **298**(21):2497–506.
13. Stone GW, White HD, Ohman EM, *et al.* Bivalirudin in patients with acute coronary syndromes undergoing percutaneous coronary intervention: a subgroup analysis from the Acute Catheterization and Urgent Intervention Triage strategy (ACUITY) trial. *Lancet* 2007; **369**(9565):907–19.
14. White HD, Ohman EM, Lincoff AM, *et al.* Safety and efficacy of bivalirudin with and without glycoprotein IIb/IIIa inhibitors in patients with acute coronary syndromes undergoing percutaneous coronary intervention 1-year results from the ACUITY (Acute Catheterization and Urgent Intervention Triage strategY) trial. *J Am Coll Cardiol* 2008; **52**(10):807–14.
15. Burke AP, Farb A, Malcom GT, *et al.* Coronary risk factors and plaque morphology in men with coronary disease who died suddenly. *N Engl J Med* 1997; **336**(18): 1276–82.
16. Virmani R, Kolodgie FD, Burke AP, *et al.* Lessons from sudden coronary death: a comprehensive morphological classification scheme for atherosclerotic lesions. *Arterioscler Thromb Vasc Biol* 2000; **20**(5):1262–75.
17. Virmani R, Burke AP, Farb A, *et al.* Pathology of the vulnerable plaque. J *Am Coll Cardiol* 2006; **47**(8 Suppl):C13–8.
18. Lusis AJ. Atherosclerosis. *Nature*. 2000; **407**(6801): 233–41.
19. Rader DJ, Daugherty A. Translating molecular discoveries into new therapies for atherosclerosis. *Nature* 2008; **451**(7181):904–13.
20. Hansson GK. Inflammation, atherosclerosis, and coronary artery disease. *N Engl J Med* 2005; **352**(16):1685–95.
21. Ruggeri ZM. Platelets in atherothrombosis. *Nat Med* 2002; 8(11):1227–34.
22. Massberg S, Gawaz M, Gruner S, *et al. et al.* A crucial role of glycoprotein VI for platelet recruitment to the injured arterial wall in vivo. *J Exp Med* 2003; **197**(1):41–9.
23. Engelmann B, Luther T, Muller I. Intravascular tissue factor pathway – a model for rapid initiation of coagulation within the blood vessel. *Thromb Haemost* 2003; **89**(1):3–8.
24. Manukyan D, von Bruehl ML, Massberg S, *et al.* Protein disulfide isomerase as a trigger for tissue factor-dependent fibrin generation. *Thromb Res* 2008; **122**(Suppl.1):S19–22.
25. Mackman N. The role of tissue factor and factor VIIa in hemostasis. *Anesth Analg* 2009; **108**(5):1447–52.
26. Steffel J, Luscher TF. Novel anticoagulants in clinical development: focus on factor Xa and direct thrombin inhibitors. *J Cardiovasc Med* (Hagerstown) 2009; **10**(8):616–23.
27. Kumar R, Beguin S, Hemker HC. The influence of fibrinogen and fibrin on thrombin generation–evidence for feedback activation of the clotting system by clot bound thrombin. *Thromb Haemost* 1994; **72**(5):713–21.
28. Sakharov DV, Plow EF, Rijken DC. On the mechanism of the antifibrinolytic activity of plasma carboxypeptidase *Br J Biol Chem* 1997; **272**(22):14477–82.
29. Coughlin SR. Protease-activated receptors in hemostasis, thrombosis and vascular biology. *J Thromb Haemost* 2005; **3**(8):1800–14.
30. Becker DL, Fredenburgh JC, Stafford AR, *et al.* Exosites 1 and 2 are essential for protection of fibrin-bound thrombin from heparin-catalyzed inhibition by antithrombin and heparin cofactor II. *J Biol Chem* 1999; **274**(10):6226–33.
31. Hogg PJ, Bock PE. Modulation of thrombin and heparin activities by fibrin. *Thromb Haemost* 1997; **77**(3):424–33.
32. Sciulli TM, Mauro VF. Pharmacology and clinical use of bivalirudin. *Ann Pharmacother* 2002; **36**(6):1028–41.
33. Kereiakes DJ, Gurbel PA. Peri-procedural platelet function and platelet inhibition in percutaneous coronary intervention. *JACC Cardiovasc Interv* 2008; **1**(2):111–21.
34. CAPRIE. A randomised, blinded, trial of clopidogrel versus aspirin in patients at risk of ischaemic events (CAPRIE). CAPRIE Steering Committee. *Lancet* 1996; **348**(9038):1329–39.
35. Mehta SR, Yusuf S, Peters RJ, *et al.* Effects of pretreatment with clopidogrel and aspirin followed by long-term therapy in patients undergoing percutaneous coronary intervention: the PCI-CURE study. *Lancet* 2001; **358**(9281):527–33.
36. Yusuf S, Zhao F, Mehta SR, *et al.* Effects of clopidogrel in addition to aspirin in patients with acute coronary syndromes without ST-segment elevation. *N Engl J Med* 2001; **345**(7):494–502.
37. Telford AM, Wilson C. Trial of heparin versus atenolol in prevention of myocardial infarction in intermediate coronary syndrome. *Lancet* 1981; **1**(8232):1225–8.
38. Williams DO, Kirby MG, McPherson K, *et al.* Anticoagulant treatment of unstable angina. *Br J Clin Pract* 1986; **40**(3):114–16.

39. Cohen M, Adams PC, Parry G, *et al.* Combination antithrombotic therapy in unstable rest angina and non-Q-wave infarction in nonprior aspirin users. Primary end points analysis from the ATACS trial. Antithrombotic Therapy in Acute Coronary Syndromes Research Group. *Circulation* 1994; **89**(1):81–8.
40. Theroux P, Ouimet H, McCans J, *et al.* Aspirin, heparin, or both to treat acute unstable angina. *N Engl J Med* 1988; **319**(17):1105–11.
41. Theroux P, Waters D, Qiu S, *et al.* Aspirin versus heparin to prevent myocardial infarction during the acute phase of unstable angina. *Circulation* 1993; **88**(5 Pt 1):2045–8.
42. Oler A, Whooley MA, Oler J, *et al.* Adding heparin to aspirin reduces the incidence of myocardial infarction and death in patients with unstable angina. A meta-analysis. *JAMA* 1996; **276**(10):811–15.
43. FRISC. Low-molecular-weight heparin during instability in coronary artery disease, Fragmin during Instability in Coronary Artery Disease (FRISC) study group. *Lancet* 1996; **347**(9001):561–8.
44. Gurfinkel EP, Manos EJ, Mejail RI, *et al.* Low molecular weight heparin versus regular heparin or aspirin in the treatment of unstable angina and silent ischemia. *J Am Coll Cardiol* 1995; **26**(2):313–8.
45. Ferguson JJ, Califf RM, Antman EM, *et al.* Enoxaparin vs unfractionated heparin in high-risk patients with non-ST-segment elevation acute coronary syndromes managed with an intended early invasive strategy: primary results of the SYNERGY randomized trial. *JAMA* 2004; **292**(1):45–54.
46. Hirsh J. Heparin. *N Engl J Med* 1991; **324**(22):1565–74.
47. Furie B, Furie BC. Molecular and cellular biology of blood coagulation. *N Engl J Med* 1992; **326**(12):800–6.
48. Mirshahi M, Soria J, Soria C, *et al.* Evaluation of the inhibition by heparin and hirudin of coagulation activation during r-tPA-induced thrombolysis. *Blood* 1989; **74**(3):1025–30.
49. de Romeuf C, Mazurier C. Heparin binding assay of von Willebrand factor (vWF) in plasma milieu – evidence of the importance of the multimerization degree of vWF. *Thromb Haemost* 1993; **69**(5):436–40.
50. Eitzman DT, Chi L, Saggin L, *et al.* Heparin neutralization by platelet-rich thrombi. Role of platelet factor 4. *Circulation* 1994; **89**(4):1523–9.
51. Chong BH. Heparin-induced thrombocytopenia. *J Thromb Haemost* 2003; **1**(7):1471–8.
52. Di Nisio M, Middeldorp S, Buller HR. Direct thrombin inhibitors. *N Engl J Med* 2005; **353**(10):1028–40.
53. Arora UK, Dhir M. Direct thrombin inhibitors (part 1 of 2). *J Invasive Cardiol* 2005; **17**(1):34–8.
54. Bittl JA. Comparative safety profiles of hirulog and heparin in patients undergoing coronary angioplasty. The Hirulog Angioplasty Study Investigators. *Am Heart J* 1995; **130**(3 Pt 2):658–65.
55. Maraganore JM, Bourdon P, Jablonski J, Ramachandran KL, Fenton JW, 2nd. Design and characterization of hirulogs: a novel class of bivalent peptide inhibitors of thrombin. *Biochemistry* 1990; **29**(30):7095–101.
56. Warkentin TE, Greinacher A, Craven S,. Differences in the clinically effective molar concentrations of four direct thrombin inhibitors explain their variable prothrombin time prolongation. *Thromb Haemost* 2005; **94**(5):958–64.
57. Warkentin TE. Bivalent direct thrombin inhibitors: hirudin and bivalirudin. *Best Pract Res Clin Haematol* 2004; **17**(1):105–25.
58. Parry MA, Maraganore JM, Stone SR. Kinetic mechanism for the interaction of Hirulog with thrombin. *Biochemistry* 1994; **33**(49):14807–14.
59. Bates SM, Weitz JI. Direct thrombin inhibitors for treatment of arterial thrombosis: potential differences between bivalirudin and hirudin. *Am J Cardiol* 1998; **82**(8B):12P–8P.
60. Bates ER. Bivalirudin: an anticoagulant option for percutaneous coronary intervention. *Expert Rev Cardiovasc Ther* 2004; **2**(2):153–62.
61. Cannon CP, Maraganore JM, Loscalzo J, *et al.* Anticoagulant effects of hirulog, a novel thrombin inhibitor, in patients with coronary artery disease. *Am J Cardiol* 1993; **71**(10):778–82.
62. Fox I, Dawson A, Loynds P, *et al.* Anticoagulant activity of Hirulog, a direct thrombin inhibitor, in humans. *Thromb Haemost* 1993; **69**(2):157–63.
63. Lidon RM, Theroux P, Juneau M, Initial experience with a direct antithrombin, Hirulog, in unstable angina. Anticoagulant, antithrombotic, and clinical effects. *Circulation* 1993; **88**(4 Pt 1):1495–501.
64. Topol EJ, Bonan R, Jewitt D, *et al.* Use of a direct antithrombin, hirulog, in place of heparin during coronary angioplasty. *Circulation* 1993; **87**(5):1622–9.
65. Sharma GV, Lapsley D, Vita JA, *et al.* Usefulness and tolerability of hirulog, a direct thrombin-inhibitor, in unstable angina pectoris. *Am J Cardiol* 1993 Dec 15; **72**(18):1357–60.
66. Robson R. The use of bivalirudin in patients with renal impairment. *J Invasive Cardiol* 2000; **12**(Suppl.F):33F–6.
67. Robson R, White H, Aylward P, Bivalirudin pharmacokinetics and pharmacodynamics: effect of renal function, dose, and gender. *Clin Pharmacol Ther* 2002; **71**(6):433–9.
68. Anand SX, Kim MC, Kamran M, *et al.* Comparison of platelet function and morphology in patients undergoing percutaneous coronary intervention receiving bivalirudin versus unfractionated heparin versus clopidogrel pretreatment and bivalirudin. *Am J Cardiol* 2007; **100**(3):417–24.
69. Busch G, Steppich B, Sibbing D, *et al.* Bivalirudin reduces platelet and monocyte activation after elective percutaneous coronary intervention. *Thromb Haemost* 2009; **101**(2):340–4.

70. Sibbing D, Busch G, Braun S, *et al.* Impact of bivalirudin or unfractionated heparin on platelet aggregation in patients pretreated with 600mg clopidogrel undergoing elective percutaneous coronary intervention. *Eur Heart J* 2008; **29**(12):1504–9.
71. Bittl JA, Strony J, Brinker JA, *et al.* Treatment with bivalirudin (Hirulog) as compared with heparin during coronary angioplasty for unstable or postinfarction angina. Hirulog Angioplasty Study Investigators. *N Engl J Med* 1995; **333**(12):764–9.
72. Greinacher A, Lubenow N, Eichler P. Anaphylactic and anaphylactoid reactions associated with lepirudin in patients with heparin-induced thrombocytopenia. *Circulation* 2003; **108**(17):2062–5.
73. Anderson JL, Adams CD, Antman EM, *et al.* ACC/AHA 2007 guidelines for the management of patients with unstable angina/non ST-elevation myocardial infarction: a report of the American College of Cardiology/American Heart Association Task Force on Practice Guidelines (Writing Committee to Revise the 2002 Guidelines for the Management of Patients With Unstable Angina/ Non ST-Elevation Myocardial Infarction): developed in collaboration with the American College of Emergency Physicians, the Society for Cardiovascular Angiography and Interventions, and the Society of Thoracic Surgeons: endorsed by the American Association of Cardiovascular and Pulmonary Rehabilitation and the Society for Academic Emergency Medicine. *Circulation* 2007; **116**(7):e148–304.
74. King SB, 3rd, Smith SC, Jr, Hirshfeld JW, Jr, *et al.* 2007 Focused Update of the ACC/AHA/SCAI 2005 Guideline Update for Percutaneous Coronary Intervention: a report of the American College of Cardiology/American Heart Association Task Force on Practice Guidelines: 2007 Writing Group to Review New Evidence and Update the ACC/AHA/SCAI 2005 Guideline Update for Percutaneous Coronary Intervention, Writing on Behalf of the 2005 Writing Committee. *Circulation* 2008; **117**(2):261–95.
75. Bittl JA, Chaitman BR, Feit F, Bivalirudin versus heparin during coronary angioplasty for unstable or postinfarction angina: Final report reanalysis of the Bivalirudin Angioplasty Study. *Am Heart J* 2001; **142**(6):952–9.
76. Antman EM, McCabe CH, Braunwald E. Bivalirudin as a replacement for unfractionated heparin in unstable angina/non-ST-elevation myocardial infarction: observations from the TIMI 8 trial. The Thrombolysis in Myocardial Infarction. *Am Heart J* 2002; **143**(2):229–34.
77. Lincoff AM, Kleiman NS, Kottke-Marchant K, *et al.* Bivalirudin with planned or provisional abciximab versus low-dose heparin and abciximab during percutaneous coronary revascularization: results of the Comparison of Abciximab Complications with Hirulog for Ischemic Events Trial (CACHET). *Am Heart J* 2002; **143**(5):847–53.
78. Lincoff AM, Bittl JA, Kleiman NS, *et al.* Comparison of bivalirudin versus heparin during percutaneous coronary intervention (the Randomized Evaluation of PCI Linking Angiomax to Reduced Clinical Events [REPLACE]-1 trial). *Am J Cardiol* 2004; **93**(9):1092–6.
79. Lincoff AM, Kleiman NS, Kereiakes DJ, *et al.* Long-term efficacy of bivalirudin and provisional glycoprotein IIb/ IIIa blockade vs heparin and planned glycoprotein IIb/IIIa blockade during percutaneous coronary revascularization: REPLACE-2 randomized trial. *JAMA* 2004; **292**(6):696–703.
80. Lincoff AM, Bittl JA, Harrington RA, *et al.* Bivalirudin and provisional glycoprotein IIb/IIIa blockade compared with heparin and planned glycoprotein IIb/IIIa blockade during percutaneous coronary intervention: REPLACE-2 randomized trial. *JAMA* 2003; **289**(7):853–63.
81. Saw J, Lincoff AM, DeSmet W, *et al.* Lack of clopidogrel pretreatment effect on the relative efficacy of bivalirudin with provisional glycoprotein IIb/IIIa blockade compared to heparin with routine glycoprotein IIb/IIIa blockade: a REPLACE-2 substudy. *J Am Coll Cardiol* 2004; **44**(6):1194–9.
82. Gibson CM, Morrow DA, Murphy SA, *et al.* A randomized trial to evaluate the relative protection against post-percutaneous coronary intervention microvascular dysfunction, ischemia, and inflammation among antiplatelet and antithrombotic agents: the PROTECT-TIMI-30 trial. *J Am Coll Cardiol* 2006; **47**(12):2364–73.
83. Lopes RD, Alexander KP, Manoukian SV, *et al.* Advanced age, antithrombotic strategy, and bleeding in non-ST-segment elevation acute coronary syndromes: results from the ACUITY (Acute Catheterization and Urgent Intervention Triage Strategy) trial. *J Am Coll Cardiol* 2009; **53**(12):1021–30.
84. Bittl JA. Accounting for ACUITY. *N Engl J Med* 2006; **355**(21):2249–50.
85. White H. Thrombin-specific anticoagulation with bivalirudin versus heparin in patients receiving fibrinolytic therapy for acute myocardial infarction: the HERO-2 randomised trial. *Lancet* 2001; **358**(9296):1855–63.
86. Stella JF, Stella RE, Iaffaldano RA, *et al.* Anticoagulation with bivalirudin during percutaneous coronary intervention for ST-segment elevation myocardial infarction. *J Invasive Cardiol* 2004; **16**(9):451–4.
87. Stone GW, Witzenbichler B, Guagliumi G, *et al.* Bivalirudin during primary PCI in acute myocardial infarction. *N Engl J Med* 2008; **358**(21):2218–30.
88. Chamberlin JR, Lewis B, Leya F, al. Successful treatment of heparin-associated thrombocytopenia and thrombosis using Hirulog. *Can J Cardiol* 1995; 11(6):511–14.
89. Campbell KR, Mahaffey KW, Lewis BE, *et al.* Bivalirudin in patients with heparin-induced thrombocytopenia undergoing percutaneous coronary intervention. *J Invasive Cardiol* 2000; **12**(Suppl.F):14F–9.
90. Warkentin TE, Greinacher A, Koster A, *et al.* Treatment and prevention of heparin-induced thrombocytopenia: American College of Chest Physicians Evidence-Based Clinical Practice Guidelines (8th Edition). *Chest* 2008; **133**(6 Suppl):340S–80S.

91. Mahaffey KW, Lewis BE, Wildermann NM, *et al.* The anticoagulant therapy with bivalirudin to assist in the performance of percutaneous coronary intervention in patients with heparin-induced thrombocytopenia (ATBAT) study: main results. *J Invasive Cardiol* 2003; **15**(11):611–16.
92. Kastrati A, Mehilli J, Schuhlen H, *et al.* A clinical trial of abciximab in elective percutaneous coronary intervention after pretreatment with clopidogrel. *N Engl J Med* 2004; **350**(3):232–8.
93. Kastrati A, Neumann FJ, Mehilli J, *et al.* Bivalirudin versus unfractionated heparin during percutaneous coronary intervention. *N Engl J Med* 2008; **359**(7):688–96.
94. Feit F, Voeltz MD, Attubato MJ, *et al.* Predictors and impact of major hemorrhage on mortality following percutaneous coronary intervention from the REPLACE-2 Trial. *Am J Cardiol* 2007; **100**(9):1364–9.
95. Manoukian SV, Feit F, Mehran R, *et al.* Impact of major bleeding on 30-day mortality and clinical outcomes in patients with acute coronary syndromes: an analysis from the ACUITY Trial. *J Am Coll Cardiol* 2007; **49**(12):1362–8.
96. Iijima R, Ndrepepa G, Mehilli J, *et al.* Profile of bleeding and ischaemic complications with bivalirudin and unfractionated heparin after percutaneous coronary intervention. *Eur Heart J* 2009; **30**(3):290–6.
97. Norgard NB. Cangrelor: a novel P2Y12 receptor antagonist. *Expert Opin Investig Drugs* 2009; **18**(8):1219–30.

CHAPTER 26

Optimal medical therapy in percutaneous coronary intervention patients: statins and ACE inhibitors as disease-modifying agents

Simon J. Corbett, Nick Curzen, and Kim F. Fox

Introduction

The majority of this textbook is concerned with the indications for, and applications of, the numerous techniques that interventional cardiologists have at their disposal to assess and treat significant coronary stenoses. However, it is well recognized that atherosclerosis is far from being a discrete pathological process, such that by the time a person presents with clinically apparent coronary artery disease (CAD), they will often have widespread atheroma throughout their coronary tree[1]. Combined with the reproducible observation that the majority of acute coronary syndromes arise from lesions that were not previously flow-limiting[2], much research effort has been directed at identifying treatment strategies that will favourably modify all of the patient's atherosclerotic burden, not just that which can be targeted by percutaneous or surgical revascularization. In this chapter, we focus on the rationale and evidence base supporting the use of statins and renin–angiotensin–aldosterone system (RAAS) inhibition in patients with CAD.

The roles of cholesterol and inflammation in the pathophysiology of coronary artery disease

The self-evident accumulation of lipid seen within atherosclerotic plaques by histopathologists has been well recognized since the first part of the 20th century. Yet it took many decades before large epidemiological investigations such as the Framingham study showed a direct relationship between blood cholesterol levels and cardiovascular risk, and it was not until 1984 that a clinical trial showed for the first time that lowering cholesterol levels (with cholestyramine) reduced the risk of subsequent CAD events[3]. While it is clear that cholesterol is pivotal to the development and progression of atherosclerosis, histology has also long demonstrated that mature atherosclerotic plaques contain many active inflammatory cells, and there has been an increasing recognition that a fuller understanding of the pathophysiology of the condition will only come with a greater appreciation of how inflammation drives and interacts with cholesterol accumulation[4,5].

The initial stages of atherosclerosis remain obscure, particularly the differential distribution of plaques throughout the arterial tree, but there is increasing evidence to suggest that one of the earliest steps is the development of endothelial dysfunction, which can be promoted by a number of risk factors including hyperlipidaemia, hypertension, diabetes mellitus, and smoking[6]. Endothelial dysfunction is characterized by a diminution of nitric oxide activity, promoting not only unopposed vasoconstriction but also leucocyte adhesion, smooth muscle cell proliferation and platelet activation. In the midst of this inflammatory milieu, low density lipoprotein (LDL) cholesterol within the vessel wall is likely to be oxidized and/or glycated. It is this process that intimately links cholesterol and inflammation in the pathophysiology of atherosclerosis, because modified LDL is a potent stimulator of macrophages via their cell-surface scavenger receptors. This not only triggers phagocytosis of the modified LDL, ultimately converting the macrophage into the lipid-laden foam cell that is a hallmark of the mature atherosclerotic plaque, but perhaps more importantly it also activates the macrophage, thereby promoting chronic inflammation within the vessel wall that ultimately leads to development of mature atherosclerotic plaques with their central lipid core, walled off from the arterial lumen by a fibrous cap of smooth muscle cells and extracellular matrix[(5)].

There are two principal ways in which coronary atherosclerosis is pathogenic: obstructive encroachment of the plaque into the lumen such that distal perfusion of the myocardium is reduced at times of increased oxygen demand (ischaemia), and acute occlusive thrombus formation on exposed lipid core secondary to a breach in the fibrous cap (infarction). The former is generally considered to be a stable situation, while the latter is clearly acute. Although this pathophysiological paradigm has served cardiologists well as a basis for therapeutic decision making for some years, it has become increasingly clear that these two scenarios are opposite ends of a spectrum of disease progression and activity, with the conversion of a stable situation into an unstable one being driven by inflammation. Many markers of active inflammation including C-reactive protein (CRP), interleukins 6, 7, and 8, and soluble CD40-ligand have all been repeatedly shown to be elevated in patients with acute coronary syndromes, and also to a lesser extent to be markers of future risk in stable or even asymptomatic patients. It seems likely that chronic inflammatory activity within plaques, particularly the release of proteases which can degrade extracellular matrix, is a key process in plaque destabilization, promoting the rupture of thin-cap fibroadenomas that is thought to underlie most acute coronary syndromes (Fig. 26.1)[(5,7,8)].

It is not surprising therefore that much research endeavour has gone into the search for agents that can suppress this inflammatory activity with the aim of not only stabilizing 'vulnerable plaques', but even leading to their regression. It is serendipitous that by far and away the most potent anti-inflammatory agents currently available for atherosclerosis modification are the statins that were developed and promoted for their cholesterol-lowering properties.

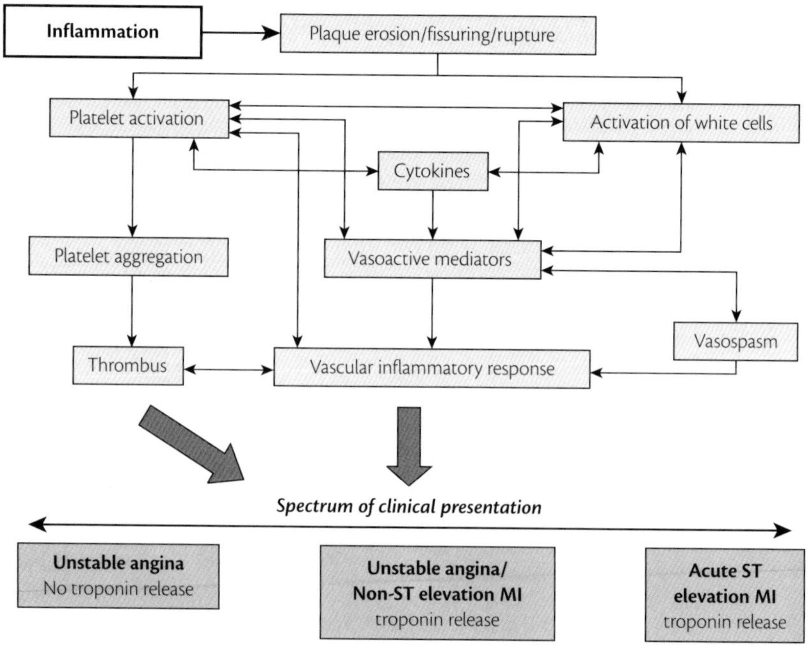

Fig. 26.1 Schematic diagram illustrating the cross-talk and inter-relation between inflammatory mediators and thrombotic pathways that occurs in acute coronary syndromes.

Statins as cholesterol-lowering and anti-inflammatory drugs

The discovery of the first statin in 1976 came from a laborious trial and error analysis by Akira Endo at Sankyo Pharmaceuticals of over 6000 fungal broths for a compound that inhibited cholesterol synthesis. Once identified, he established that his compound ML-236B (later called compactin, then mevastatin, and ironically never marketed by Sankyo), worked by inhibiting 3-hydroxy-3-methylglutaryl-coenzyme A (HMG-CoA) reductase, which was already known to be the rate-limiting enzymatic step in cholesterol biosynthesis within the liver. The resultant lower cholesterol levels within hepatocytes leads to increased cell-surface expression of LDL-receptors, which avidly clear LDL from the bloodstream thereby producing a sustained reduction in plasma LDL levels[9]. Despite Sankyo's failure to bring mevastatin to clinical practice, a number of pharmaceutical companies realised the utility of HMG-CoA reductase inhibition and developed their own statins, all of which competitively inhibit HMG-CoA reductase similarly, albeit with different potency, and have proved themselves to be one of the most effective (and safe) drug classes of all time (Fig. 26.2).

While it is undoubtedly true that the majority of clinical trials of statins in CAD and the prevention thereof have been predicated on their ability to lower LDL cholesterol levels, an increasing body of evidence has also accumulated to support the notion that they have a range of potentially beneficial, additional or 'pleiotropic' properties, including a marked anti-inflammatory action. A wide number of anti-inflammatory and lipid-independent activities of statins have now been demonstrated *in vitro*[10], including decreased expression of inflammatory cell adhesion molecules, matrix degrading enzymes, and cytokines. While statin therapy has been repeatedly shown to decrease markers of inflammation such as CRP levels *in vivo*[11,12], it is a source of ongoing controversy and debate as to what proportion of this activity is independent of lipid lowering, bearing in mind that oxidized LDL is a key driver of the whole inflammatory process within plaques.

Clinical studies of statins in coronary artery disease

There is perhaps a greater wealth of clinical evidence to support the use of statins in patients with, or at risk of, CAD than for any other currently available pharmacological intervention in modern medicine[13]. What is even more striking, are the repeatedly positive findings

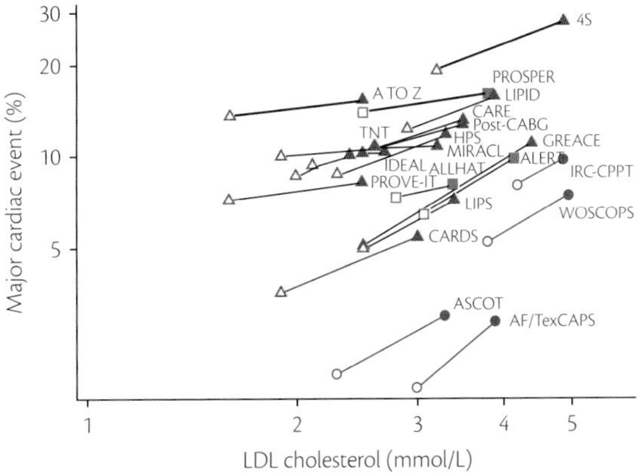

Fig. 26.2 Major adverse cardiac event rates plotted against LDL cholesterol levels (both on a logarithmic scale) in the control and statin arms of major clinical statin trials demonstrating the repeated observation that LDL lowering with statins reduces adverse events. Reproduced from Joint British Societies' guidelines on prevention of cardiovascular disease in clinical practice. *Heart* 2005; **91**;v1–v52 with permission from BMJ Publishing Group Ltd.

across a broad range of patients and clinical scenarios that have been reported with statins, such that international practice guidelines unsurprisingly uniformly award the use of statins in CAD patients with a Class IA recommendation[14,15]. Such consistency of clinical outcome across so many heterogenous populations of study patients indicates a potent biological effect. There are enough data showing the benefits of statins in atherosclerotic disease to fill a textbook in its own right, therefore for reasons of clarity and concision we have had to concentrate on the major, individual studies that we consider to be most relevant to the daily clinical practice of interventional cardiologists.

Statins in patients with established coronary artery disease

Initial statin studies were limited to angiographic analyses of lesion progression in patients with significantly elevated cholesterol levels[16], but the era of widespread clinical utility of statins can be considered to date from the publication of the landmark Scandinavian Simvastatin Survival Study (4S) in 1994[17]. This placebo-controlled, randomized, double-blind trial in 4444 patients with either angina or previous (but not recent) myocardial infarction (MI), who were on a lipid-lowering diet and had a total cholesterol between 5.5–8.0mmol/L, reported a highly significant reduction in overall mortality (relative risk 0.70; 95% confidence interval [CI] 0.58–0.85; p = 0.0003) over a median follow-up of 5.4 years, in patients randomized to receive

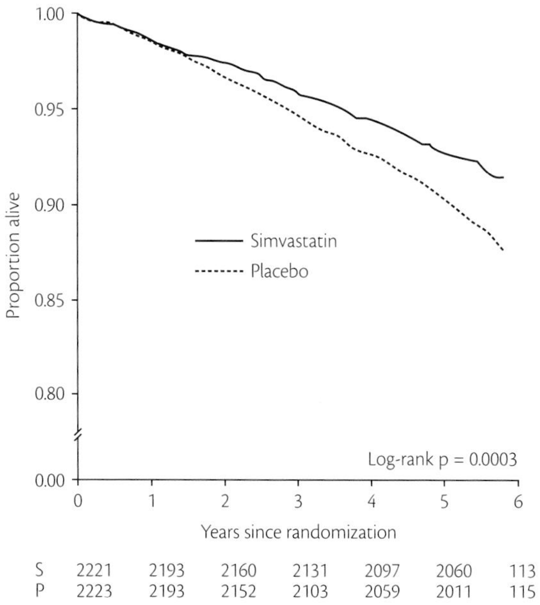

Fig. 26.3 Kaplan–Meier survival curves for all cause mortality up to 6 years follow-up in the statin and placebo arms of the 4S study. Reproduced from Scandinavian Simvastatin Survival Study Group. Randomized trial of cholesterol lowering in 4,444 patients with coronary heart disease. *Lancet* 1994; **344**:1383–8. © 1994 with permission from Elsevier.

simvastatin versus placebo (Fig. 26.3). The dose of simvastatin was started at 20mg once daily and titrated to achieve a total cholesterol level of 3.0–5.2mmol/L, with 37% of patients being uptitrated to 40mg simvastatin. Treatment with simvastatin was associated with 25% and 35% reductions in total and LDL cholesterol respectively, while the reduction in coronary deaths with simvastatin was even more pronounced with a relative risk of 0.58 (95% CI 0.46–0.73). Importantly, by demonstrating a reduction in total mortality, 4S put the first nail into the coffin of the prevalent notion that lowering cholesterol might be benefit-neutral, or even harmful, by raising the incidence of non-cardiac mortality. A single case of non-fatal rhabdomyolysis was reported in a woman taking 20mg simvastatin, while overall there were six patients who suffered a greater than 10× increase in creatine kinase level in the statin group as compared to one patient in the placebo group. There was no significant difference in the number of patients with a greater than 3× increase in aminotransferase levels in the statin and placebo groups. Such safety data have been typical of the large randomized studies yet the perception that statins are potentially dangerous because of life-threatening muscle and liver effects continues to be a feature of their everyday use.

The findings of 4S were quickly followed up and expanded to patients with lower baseline cholesterol levels in the placebo-controlled, randomized, double-blind Cholesterol And Recurrent Events (CARE)[18] and the Long-term Intervention in Patients with Ischaemic Disease (LIPID)[19] studies. In the CARE study, 4159 patients, all of whom had suffered a myocardial infarction in the previous 3–20 months, were randomized to receive 40mg pravastatin once daily or placebo provided their total cholesterol was less than 6.2mmol/L and their LDL cholesterol was between 3.0–4.5mmol/L. Over a median follow-up of 5.0 years, total and LDL cholesterol were lowered by 20% and 28% respectively in the pravastatin arm, which was associated with a relative risk of 0.76 (95% CI 0.64–0.91; p = 0.003) for the primary endpoint of coronary heart disease death or non-fatal MI. In contrast to 4S there was no reduction in overall mortality, but this was not due to an increase in cancer or non-cardiac mortality. By contrast, the substantially larger LIPID study, in which 9014 patients with a history of myocardial infarction or unstable angina (in an approximately 2:1 distribution) within the preceding 3–36 months, randomized to receive 40mg pravastatin once daily or placebo provided their total cholesterol was between 4.0–7.0mmol/L, did report a significant decrease in total mortality with statin therapy (relative risk 0.78; 95% CI 0.69–0.87; p <0.001). During a mean follow-up period of 6.1 years, the primary endpoint of death from coronary heart disease was reached in 6.4% of the pravastatin arm patients as compared to 8.3% in the placebo group, a relative reduction of 24% (95% CI 12–35%, p <0.001). The median total cholesterol level at baseline was 5.6mmol/L, and over the study period there were proportionately 18% and 25% greater reductions in total and LDL cholesterol respectively in the pravastatin than placebo arms (the study did not report the actual reductions in cholesterol levels).

Pre-specified subgroup analysis in the CARE study showed the benefits of pravastatin to be consistent in women, older patients, diabetics, patients with previous revascularization, and patients with total cholesterol level at baseline <5.4mmol/L (the mean total cholesterol level at baseline). However, in patients with a baseline LDL cholesterol of <3.2mmol/L, pravastatin therapy was not associated with any benefit. A similar finding was confirmed in the subgroup analysis of the LIPID study, in which patients with a baseline LDL cholesterol of <3.5mmol/L did not benefit. Women, patients aged over 70 and non-smokers also failed to show a benefit with pravastatin in this subgroup analysis. Such results appropriately spark debate about 1) whether statins exert their biological effect in all patients, especially women, and 2) whether the 'biological effect' is shared by the whole class of drug or is statin specific. In terms of safety, once again, in both CARE and LIPID there was no difference in the rates of liver or muscle enzyme rise in the statin and placebo groups. Importantly, in terms of drug tolerance, it is notable that more people discontinued placebo than pravastatin in CARE.

Interestingly, it took close to 2 years of follow-up for the event curves to separate in 4S, CARE and LIPID. This may help to explain why the similarly conceived, but shorter GISSI Prevenzione study[20] failed to show any reduction the endpoint of death, non-fatal MI, or non-fatal stroke. 4271 Italian patients with a recent myocardial infarction within the past 6 months, who had a total cholesterol level of > 5.2mmol/L, were randomized to low-dose pravastatin 20mg once daily or no treatment (not placebo) for a median follow-up of 24 months. This study was further limited by a number of factors including a change in the study protocol after the publication of 4S to treat patients with total cholesterol levels >6.5mmol/L with open label statin, lack of placebo and blinding, and the low dose of pravastatin used with its correspondingly lesser reduction in cholesterol levels.

Of direct relevance to this textbook, a principal inclusion criterion of the Lescol Intervention Prevention Study (LIPS)[21] was that the patients had to have undergone successful PCI prior to randomization. In this randomized, placebo-controlled, double-blind trial, 1677 PCI patients with total cholesterol levels between 3.5–7.0mmol/L were randomized to receive fluvastatin 40mg twice or day or placebo over a median follow-up of 3.9 years. The median time between PCI and treatment assignment was 2 days. The incidence of the primary endpoint, a combination of cardiovascular death, non-fatal MI, or repeat revascularization was reduced from 26.7% in the placebo arm to 21.4% in the fluvastatin arm (relative risk 0.78; 95% CI 0.64–0.95; p = 0.01), corresponding to a 27% reduction in LDL cholesterol levels with fluvastatin therapy. While it may seem superfluous, or stating the obvious, to pass comment on the need to treat PCI patients with concomitant medical therapy at the end of the first decade of the 21st century, LIPS was an important trial that highlighted the need to do more than simply revascularize patients with CAD. Another interesting incidental observation from this study which recruited patients after the publication of 4S, CARE and LIPID, was the prescription of open label lipid-lowering therapy to 24% of patients in the placebo group at the end of follow-up, thereby demonstrating the reluctance of physicians to run the risk of their patients with CAD not receiving such therapy by the late 1990s. Indeed since that time it has been considered unethical to run placebo-controlled trials of statins in patients with definite CAD.

Statins in patients at risk of coronary artery disease

Encouraged by the lipid hypothesis and the proven biological efficacy of statins in reducing LDL cholesterol levels, a number of investigators have looked for a benefit of statins in primary prevention, i.e. reducing the risk of subsequent coronary events in patients deemed to be at risk of future CAD. The landmark trial which first showed a convincing benefit of statins in this context, was the West Of Scotland COronary Prevention Study (WOSCOPS)[22]. 6595 Scottish men aged 45 to 64 with no prior history of myocardial infarction, and who had a sustained LDL cholesterol level of 4.0mmol/L despite a lipid lowering diet, were randomized to receive pravastatin 40mg once daily or placebo in a double-blind fashion and followed-up for a mean of 4.9 years for the development of death due to coronary heart disease or non-fatal myocardial infarction. It should be noted that a history of stable angina was allowed but only 5% of the patients enrolled reported this. The patients were what would be considered today to be significantly hypercholesterolaemic with a mean total cholesterol level at baseline of 7.0mmol/L, and in common with CARE and LIPID, pravastatin produced a 20% and 26% reduction in total and LDL cholesterol levels respectively. Unsurprisingly, this translated into a 31% reduction in the incidence of the primary endpoint in the statin arm (95% CI 17–43%; p <0.001). The justification to use statins to modify cardiovascular risk, regardless of whether the patient has already had an event or not was thus clearly established. However, up until the early years of the 21st century, there remained relatively less justification to use statins in certain subgroups of the population at risk of CAD, notably, diabetics, women, and the elderly, all of whom had been relatively under-represented in recruitment to the trials discussed earlier. Furthermore, it was unclear at which threshold of cholesterol level treatment should be targeted.

Epidemiological studies had suggested a linear relationship between cholesterol level and CAD risk, yet CARE and LIPID had suggested that pravastatin might not provide any significant benefit in those patients with lower LDL cholesterol levels at baseline.

The publication of the Heart Protection Study megatrial[23] has made a significant contribution to our understanding of these contentious issues. This study recruited 20 536 patients deemed to be at high risk of CAD over 5 years and who had a total cholesterol level of 3.5mmol/L or more. Patients were randomized to simvastatin 40mg once daily or placebo in a double-blind fashion. The inclusion criteria were: any history of CAD including revascularization, or a history of occlusive non-coronary vascular disease including ischaemic stroke and peripheral vascular disease, or diabetes mellitus, or male hypertensives aged 65 or older. The study recruited substantial proportions of previously under-represented groups including 25% women, 29% diabetics, and 28% aged 70 or older. Overall, 35% of the patients had no previous history of CAD. Over the mean follow-up period of 5 years, patients allocated to simvastatin had a reduction of 1.2mmol/L and 1.0mmol/L in total and LDL cholesterol respectively, and showed a highly significant reduction in the primary endpoint of overall mortality from 14.7% in the placebo group to 12.9% (relative risk 0.87; 95% CI 0.81–0.94; p = 0.0003). This outcome was driven primarily by a highly significant decrease in the coronary death rate from 6.9% to 5.7% (p = 0.0005). Similarly significant reductions in secondary coronary endpoints such as non-fatal myocardial infarction, hospitalization with unstable angina, and revascularization were also seen. In an array of pre-specified subgroup analyses, the benefits of simvastatin therapy (i.e. the 'biological effect') were preserved in women, diabetics, the elderly, patients with no prior CAD, patients with lower total and LDL cholesterols, non-smokers, and in patients taking other prognostically important therapies such as aspirin, angiotensin-converting enzyme (ACE) inhibitors, and beta-blockers (Fig. 26.4). Furthermore, for the first time, it emerged that there was unlikely to be a lower threshold of cholesterol level below which statin therapy was not beneficial, provided the patient's overall risk profile placed them at high risk.

A number of other large primary prevention trials have also helped reinforce the benefits of statins in at risk patients and extend our knowledge of which patients are likely to benefit. The Air Force/Texas Coronary Atherosclerosis Prevention Program study[24], in which 5608 and 997 generally healthy men and women respectively with a mean total cholesterol level of 5.7mmol/L were randomized in a double blind fashion to lovastatin 20–40mg once daily or placebo, demonstrated the benefits of statin therapy in primary prevention in patients with lower cholesterol levels than previously studied and also in women for the first time. There was a 37% reduction in first acute major coronary event rates over an average follow-up of 5.2 years ($p < 0.001$). The utility of statins in primary prevention in elderly patients was proved in the double blind, PROspective Study of Pravastatin in the Elderly at Risk (PROSPER) study[25] in which 2804 men and 3000 women aged 70–82 years with a history of, or risk factors for cardiovascular disease were randomized to receive pravastatin 40mg once daily or placebo. PROSPER demonstrated a 15% reduction in coronary death, non-fatal MI, or stroke over 3.2 years of average follow-up (p = 0.014). The synergistic benefit of statin therapy in patients with diabetes with no prior history of CAD was further confirmed in the Collaborative Atorvastatin Diabetes Study (CARDS)[26]. This study recruited 2838 patients with type 2 diabetes mellitus and at least one of retinopathy, albuminuria, smoking, or hypertension and they were randomized to 10mg atorvastatin once daily or placebo. Over a median follow-up of 3.9 years there was a 37% risk reduction in the primary event rate of acute coronary event, revascularization or stroke (p = 0.001), and the treatment benefits were seen in all patients regardless of their baseline LDL cholesterol level.

The synergistic benefit of adding statin therapy to high risk hypertensive patients was clearly shown in the lipid-lowering arm of the Anglo-Scandinavian Cardiac Outcomes Trial (ASCOT)[27], in which 19 342 patients with hypertension and at least three additional risk factors out of left ventricular hypertrophy, type 2 diabetes mellitus, smoking, family history of premature CAD, cerebrovascular disease, age >55, proteinuria or microalbuminuria, or a total cholesterol:HDL cholesterol ratio of 6 or more, were randomized to receive atorvastatin 10mg once daily or placebo in addition to their randomly allocated anti-hypertension therapy, provided their total cholesterol was less than 6.5mmol/L. After a median follow-up of 3.3 years there was a 36% reduction in the primary endpoint of coronary death or non-fatal MI (p = 0.0005). This was in contrast to the results of the Antihypertensive and Lipid-Lowering Treatment to Prevent Heart Attack Trial (ALLHAT)[28] in which the randomized addition of pravastatin 40mg once daily to 5170 hypertensive patients failed to show any reduction in the rates of all cause mortality or coronary

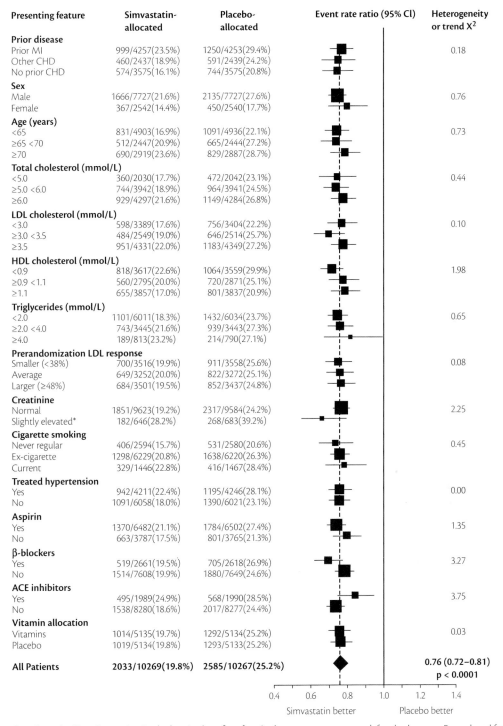

Presenting feature	Simvastatin-allocated	Placebo-allocated	Heterogeneity or trend X^2
Prior disease			
Prior MI	999/4257(23.5%)	1250/4253(29.4%)	0.18
Other CHD	460/2437(18.9%)	591/2439(24.2%)	
No prior CHD	574/3575(16.1%)	744/3575(20.8%)	
Sex			
Male	1666/7727(21.6%)	2135/7727(27.6%)	0.76
Female	367/2542(14.4%)	450/2540(17.7%)	
Age (years)			
<65	831/4903(16.9%)	1091/4936(22.1%)	0.73
≥65 <70	512/2447(20.9%)	665/2444(27.2%)	
≥70	690/2919(23.6%)	829/2887(28.7%)	
Total cholesterol (mmol/L)			
<5.0	360/2030(17.7%)	472/2042(23.1%)	0.44
≥5.0 <6.0	744/3942(18.9%)	964/3941(24.5%)	
≥6.0	929/4297(21.6%)	1149/4284(26.8%)	
LDL cholesterol (mmol/L)			
<3.0	598/3389(17.6%)	756/3404(22.2%)	0.10
≥3.0 <3.5	484/2549(19.0%)	646/2514(25.7%)	
≥3.5	951/4331(22.0%)	1183/4349(27.2%)	
HDL cholesterol (mmol/L)			
<0.9	818/3617(22.6%)	1064/3559(29.9%)	1.98
≥0.9 <1.1	560/2795(20.0%)	720/2871(25.1%)	
≥1.1	655/3857(17.0%)	801/3837(20.9%)	
Triglycerides (mmol/L)			
<2.0	1101/6011(18.3%)	1432/6034(23.7%)	0.65
≥2.0 <4.0	743/3445(21.6%)	939/3443(27.3%)	
≥4.0	189/813(23.2%)	214/790(27.1%)	
Prerandomization LDL response			
Smaller (<38%)	700/3516(19.9%)	911/3558(25.6%)	0.08
Average	649/3252(20.0%)	822/3272(25.1%)	
Larger (≥48%)	684/3501(19.5%)	852/3437(24.8%)	
Creatinine			
Normal	1851/9623(19.2%)	2317/9584(24.2%)	2.25
Slightly elevated*	182/646(28.2%)	268/683(39.2%)	
Cigarette smoking			
Never regular	406/2594(15.7%)	531/2580(20.6%)	0.45
Ex-cigarette	1298/6229(20.8%)	1638/6220(26.3%)	
Current	329/1446(22.8%)	416/1467(28.4%)	
Treated hypertension			
Yes	942/4211(22.4%)	1195/4246(28.1%)	0.00
No	1091/6058(18.0%)	1390/6021(23.1%)	
Aspirin			
Yes	1370/6482(21.1%)	1784/6502(27.4%)	1.35
No	663/3787(17.5%)	801/3765(21.3%)	
β-blockers			
Yes	519/2661(19.5%)	705/2618(26.9%)	3.27
No	1514/7608(19.9%)	1880/7649(24.6%)	
ACE inhibitors			
Yes	495/1989(24.9%)	568/1990(28.5%)	3.75
No	1538/8280(18.6%)	2017/8277(24.4%)	
Vitamin allocation			
Vitamins	1014/5135(19.7%)	1292/5134(25.2%)	0.03
Placebo	1019/5134(19.8%)	1293/5133(25.2%)	
All Patients	**2033/10269(19.8%)**	**2585/10267(25.2%)**	**0.76 (0.72–0.81) p < 0.0001**

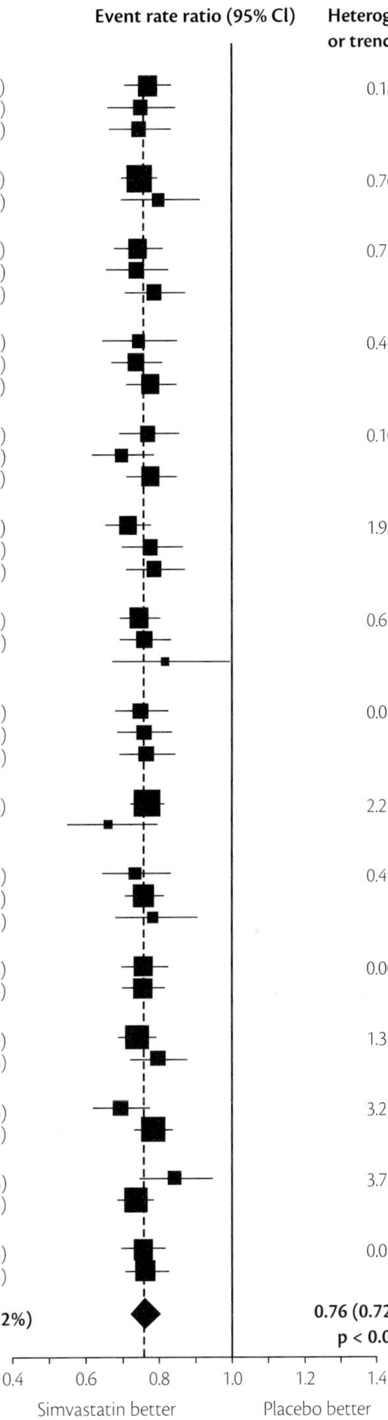

Fig. 26.4 Data from the Heart Protection Study showing benefits of statin therapy across many predefined subgroups. Reproduced from Heart Protection Study Collaborative Group. MRC/BHF Heart Protection Study of cholesterol lowering with simvastatin in 20,536 high-risk individuals: a randomized placebo-controlled trial. *Lancet* 2002; **360**:7–22. © 2002 with permission from Elsevier.

events as compared to the 5185 patients who received usual care over an average follow-up of 4.8 years. The principal reason underlying this negative result is likely to be the fact that during the trial 61% of the usual care group started taking open-label statins, such that there was only a very modest 9% additional reduction in cholesterol levels in the pravastatin group.

A common characteristic of the trialists responsible for these studies has been their willingness to share patient level data in a prospective patient-level meta-analysis, through the formation of the Cholesterol Treatment Trialists (CTT) collaboration in 1994. Pooled data from 90 056 patients in 14 randomized trials was duly published in a meta-analysis in 2005[13]. Unsurprisingly, given the predominantly positive findings of the individual studies, statin use was associated with highly significant reductions in many important clinical endpoints including all cause mortality, cardiac mortality, non-fatal MI, stroke, and revascularization, with relative risk reductions in the order of 12–25%. Subgroup analysis showed the benefits of statin therapy to be preserved in all subgroups studied including prior MI or CAD, age >65, women, hypertensives, diabetics, and all baseline cholesterol levels. With the pooled data, the authors were also able to show a linear relationship between the reduction in LDL cholesterol observed in the individual trials and the proportional reduction in major coronary and vascular events that occurred. This suggests that each 1mmol/L reduction in LDL cholesterol over 5 years should produce a 23% reduction in major vascular events, with the further implication that there may not be a lower cut-off LDL cholesterol level, below which further outcomes benefits do not accrue.

One important contemporary area of uncertainty about the mechanism of the biological effect of statins relates to whether it is achieved via the reduction of cholesterol levels or whether it is an anti-inflammatory property, measured by markers of vascular inflammation such as CRP, and that cholesterol reduction is a side effect. This is the subject of considerable debate, particularly in the context of a disease process, the pathophysiology of which features inflammation and lipid deposition. Clearly, these two mechanisms of action are not mutually exclusive. This issue has been recently been brought into focus with the publication of the Justification for the Use of statins in Prevention: an Intervention Trial Evaluating Rosuvastatin (JUPITER)[29]. This study sought to evaluate the role of CRP level as a marker of cardiovascular risk by randomizing 17 802 apparently healthy men and women with LDL cholesterol levels below 3.4mmol/L and high sensitivity CRP levels of 2.0mg/L or greater to receive rosuvastatin 20mg once daily or placebo in a double blind fashion. After a median follow-up of only 1.9 years, the trial was stopped early as the data and safety monitoring board found that rosuvastatin was associated with a 44% relative reduction in the primary endpoint of MI, stroke, arterial revascularization, unstable angina, or cardiovascular death (95% CI 31–54%, $p < 0.00001$). The potency of rosuvastatin as a lipid reducing agent is borne out by the 50% reduction in LDL cholesterol that was achieved, even in people with below average levels at baseline. In common with many prior studies showing that LDL cholesterol lowering with statins is associated with a reduction in CRP levels[11], the high sensitivity CRP level also fell by 37%. On the basis of the observed reduction in events with rosuvastatin being almost twice what would be expected on the basis of previous studies for the degree of LDL cholesterol lowering that was obtained, the authors conclude that rosuvastatin's anti-inflammatory activity, as demonstrated by the reduction in CRP levels, contributed to the clinical benefit seen. This is an attractive hypothesis, but it is by no means proven and teasing out the relative contributions of the lipid-lowering and pleiotropic properties of statins to their net clinical benefit *in vivo* remains to be elucidated.

Statins in patients with acute coronary syndromes

An important feature of all the studies discussed in previous sections was that patients were excluded if they had recently suffered an acute coronary syndrome (ACS). However, with increasing evidence to support the pleiotropic benefits of statin therapy, it was hypothesized that early statin administration in ACS patients may help stabilize the culprit ruptured plaque and prevent recurrent ischaemia in this high-risk patient group, even though many of the studies in stable patients had taken up to 2 years of statin therapy to demonstrate an effect.

The first study to address this question was the randomized, placebo-controlled, double blind Myocardial Ischaemia Reduction with Aggressive Cholesterol Lowering (MIRACL) study[30], in which 3086 patients with unstable angina or non-Q-wave myocardial infarction within the previous 24–96h were randomized to receive atorvastatin 80mg once daily or placebo. Patients were excluded if they had, or were planned to undergo revascularization as treatment of their ACS (this study was recruiting in the days before the wealth of evidence showing benefit from early revascularization in ACS was available), and if their total cholesterol was greater than 7.0mmol/L. The primary endpoint was defined as the incidence of death, non-fatal MI, cardiac arrest, or recurrent ischaemia during 16 weeks of follow-up and just reached statistical significance with a reduction from 17.4% in the placebo group to 14.8% in the statin group (relative risk 0.84; 95% CI 0.70–1.00; p = 0.048), at least supporting the concept in principle. Of the individual components of the primary endpoint, only recurrent ischaemia showed a statistically significant reduction with statin therapy in its own right. While there was no difference in the rate of discontinuation of study drug in the statin and placebo groups, it is noteworthy that the incidence of a >3× rise in liver transaminases was significantly more common in the statin group, which is perhaps unsurprising given the relative potency of atorvastatin 80mg as compared to pravastatin 40mg and simvastatin 40mg so extensively studied in stable patients.

The potential benefit of aggressive statin therapy during the index admission of patients with ACS was assessed in more detail in the Pravastatin or Atorvastatin Evaluation and Infection Therapy (PROVE-IT)[31]. 4162 patients who had been hospitalized with an ACS (including ST-elevation MI) within the previous 10 days and who had a total cholesterol level of <6.21mmol/L, were randomized in a double blind fashion to receive a pravastatin 40mg once daily versus a more intensive regimen of atorvastatin 80mg once daily. In contrast to MIRACL, patients were allowed to have been acutely revascularized, and just under 70% of the patients did indeed undergo PCI for treatment of their index ACS. The presenting ACS was essentially evenly divided three ways between unstable angina, non-ST-elevation MI, and ST-elevation MI. During a mean follow-up of 2 years, the median LDL cholesterol level in the pravastatin group was 2.46mmol/L which was substantially higher than the 1.60mmol/L level seen in the atorvastatin arm (p <0.001). The composite primary endpoint of all cause mortality, MI, unstable angina, revascularization after 30 days, and stroke occurred in 26.3% of the pravastatin group and 22.4% of the atorvastatin group (risk reduction 16%; 95% CI 5–26%, p = 0.005). Not only did this study fail to show non-inferiority of the less intensive regimen with pravastatin as per the initial study design, but it actually confirmed statistically significant superiority of the intensive atorvastatin regimen. In contrast to JUPITER, the additional benefit in clinical outcomes seen with atorvastatin in the PROVE-IT study closely correlates with the additional LDL cholesterol lowering it achieved, arguing against a significant dose-related pleiotropic statin effect. There was no difference in tolerability between the two regimens, although it is worth noting that more than 20% of patients in both arms discontinued their study drug.

In contrast, the subsequently published A to Z study failed to show a significant benefit of early, aggressive statin therapy in patients with ST-elevation and non-ST-elevation MI[32]. 4497 patients with a total cholesterol level of <6.48mmol/L were randomized to receive either an early intensive regimen of simvastatin 40mg once daily for 30 days before uptitration to simvastatin 80mg once daily thereafter, or a less aggressive strategy of placebo for 4 months followed by simvastatin 20mg once daily thereafter. Patients were followed up for up to 24 months. There was a non-significant reduction in the incidence of the primary endpoint of cardiovascular death, non-fatal MI, further ACS, and stroke in the early intensive group from 16.7% to 14.4% (p = 0.14). Interestingly when compared to the results of the PROVE-IT study, the LDL cholesterol level in the intensive arm of the A to Z study (1.63mmol/L) was very similar to that seen with atorvastatin in PROVE-IT (1.60mmol/L), whereas the less intensive regimen of placebo followed by simvastatin 20mg achieved a considerably lower LDL cholesterol level of 1.99mmol/L as compared to the 2.46mmol/L seen with 40mg pravastatin in PROVE-IT, which may help explain why the intensive regimen in A to Z failed to reach significance. Overall event rates were considerably lower in A to Z than PROVE-IT suggesting that the baseline risk of the population recruited to A to Z was lower than in PROVE-IT. Both of these trials have been combined in a meta-analysis along with the Treating to New Targets (TNT) and Incremental Decrease in End Points Through Aggressive Lipid-Lowering (IDEAL) studies to further address the issue of whether aggressive lipid-lowering with high dose statin is superior to less intensive therapy[33]. For the combined endpoint of coronary death or MI, high-dose statin therapy is associated with a highly significant 16% odds reduction (p <0.00001). However, despite combining data on 27 548 patients, this meta-analysis failed to show a significant reduction in individual endpoints such as MI or coronary death, suggesting that the benefit of such aggressive statin therapy, over and above that already produced by less intensive therapy, may be modest in many clinical scenarios.

Regression of atherosclerosis with statins

A number of early statin studies reported atheroma regression in statin-treated patients using quantitative coronary angiographic analysis[(16)]. However, such methodology is severely limited. Firstly, it cannot take account of the now well-described Glagovian phenomenon of compensatory enlargement of the coronary artery at the point of atheroma deposition, and secondly QCA cannot measure atheroma volume within the vessel wall. For these reasons this methodology has been superseded for such study purposes by quantitative intravascular ultrasound (IVUS).

The Reversal of Atherosclerosis with Aggressive Lipid Lowering (REVERSAL) trial was the first to address this issue in detail[(34)]. In this double-blind study, 654 patients who had LDL cholesterol levels between 3.24–5.44mmol/L with a coronary stenosis of between 20–50% angiographic severity (and that was therefore suitable for repeated IVUS evaluation), were randomized to the same moderate and intensive lipid-lowering regimens used in PROVE-IT i.e. pravastatin 40mg once daily and atorvastatin 80mg once daily. Motorized IVUS pullback at 0.5mm per second was performed from a distal side-branch marker and images were recorded at a rate of 30 frames per second. An IVUS pullback was recorded at baseline and repeated from the same marker point after 18 months of treatment. The primary endpoint in the study was the change in total atheroma volume per patient during treatment. For analysis, the atheroma volume at 1.0mm intervals along the target vessel was measured at baseline, summated for the patient to give a total atheroma volume at baseline and then used as the denominator against which to compare a paired set of measurements from the same vessel after 18 months and expressed as a percentage. Given the complexity of this IVUS methodology and analysis it is perhaps not surprising that a substantial number of the originally randomized patients did not have evaluable paired IVUS measurements and only 502 patients were included in the final analysis. Median total atheroma volumes at baseline in the pravastatin and atorvastatin groups were 168.6mm^3 and 161.0mm^3 respectively ($p = 0.20$). After 18 months, these measurements had changed to 180.0mm^3 and 160.9mm^3 in the pravastatin and atorvastatin groups respectively, representing a 2.7% increase versus a 0.4% decrease change in the primary endpoint which was statistically significant ($p = 0.02$). While it is perhaps over-interpreting the results to call this a regression of atherosclerosis with high dose atorvastatin, it certainly demonstrates lack of progression. This was associated with significantly greater reductions of both LDL cholesterol and CRP with atorvastatin than pravastatin (46.3% vs. 25.2% and 36.4% vs. 5.2% respectively; $p < 0.001$ for both), and at least shows a biological effect *in vivo* of more aggressive statin therapy and lipid lowering.

On the basis of these results, the same investigators used the same methodology to evaluate whether yet more potent LDL cholesterol lowering could produce an actual regression of atherosclerosis in the ASTEROID study (A Study to Evaluate the Effect of Rosuvastatin on Intravascular Ultrasound-Derived Coronary Atheroma Burden)[(35)]. As for REVERSAL, patients had to have an angiographic stenosis between 20–50% severity, but any baseline cholesterol level was allowed. There was no randomization in this study and all patients received rosuvastatin 40mg once daily for 24 months. The IVUS methodology and analysis were the same as in REVERSAL. 507 patients were recruited but only 349 had evaluable paired IVUS data. Although any cholesterol level was allowed at entry, baseline median LDL cholesterol levels were lower in ASTEROID than REVERSAL (3.3mmol/L versus 3.9mmol/L), and there was a greater 53.2% reduction during treatment with rosuvastatin in ASTEROID than the 46.3% achieved with atorvastatin in REVERSAL. In contrast to REVERSAL, this greater reduction in LDL cholesterol was associated with an unequivocal regression of atheroma with a median 6.8% reduction in total atheroma volume. While it is undoubtedly an achievement to have demonstrated a genuine reversal in plaque burden for the first time, the fact that it was necessary to reduce LDL cholesterol levels to such low levels, well below those achieved in any of the major outcome trials with statins discussed previously, indicates that a substantial portion of the biological effect of statins must be derived from other mechanisms such as plaque stabilization and reducing plaque progression.

The role of the renin–angiotensin–aldosterone system in coronary artery disease and atherosclerosis

Since the initial discovery of renin over a century ago, much has been learned about the RAAS and its crucial physiological role in the regulation of extracellular fluid volume and blood pressure (BP) homeostasis. In the classical circulatory description of the RAAS, the proteolytic hormone renin, is primarily released from the juxtaglomerular apparatus of the kidney in response to extracellular volume depletion. Renin's substrate is the circulating glycoprotein, *angiotensinogen*, from which it cleaves a decapeptide, *angiotensin I*. Angiotensin I's principal physiological role appears to be as the substrate for *angiotensin converting enzyme (ACE)*, which cleaves two carboxyterminal amino acids from angiotensin I to create the main physiological effector molecule of the RAAS, *angiotensin II*, a potent vasoconstrictor and stimulator of aldosterone release (and hence promoter of salt and water retention by the kidney) through its activation of specific, cell-surface, G-protein-linked AT_1 receptors. In this originally elucidated model, circulating angiotensin I was converted by ACE located on endothelial cells in capillary beds, particularly in the pulmonary circulation, with circulating angiotensin II then going onto have systemic effects. A further action of ACE is to breakdown bradykinin, a nonapeptide with vasodilatory activity via endothelial production of nitric oxide.

Overactivation of the RAAS has long been recognized to have an important pathophysiological role in both hypertension and heart failure, prompting the development of numerous pharmacological agents that block or reduce angiotensin II activity. The impressive and recurrent success of ACE inhibition at improving outcomes in randomized clinical trials of heart failure in particular[(36)], is well recognized and beyond the scope of this chapter. However, it was the repeated observation of a reduction of myocardial infarction rates during follow-up in the ACE inhibitor arms of both the SAVE and SOLVD trials of patients with heart failure that prompted investigators to hypothesize whether ACE inhibition also had specific effects on the coronary vasculature over and above the already recognized benefits of pre- and after-load reduction, and left ventricular remodelling.

Indeed, it has become increasingly apparent that angiotensin II formation can also take place outside of the circulation in many tissues, including the heart and blood vessel walls. Local effects include the promotion of inflammation, cell growth and extracellular matrix deposition[(37)]. With the finding of ACE in human coronary atherosclerotic plaques[(38)], and numerous experimental observations linking AT_1 receptor activation by angiotensin II to pro-atherosclerotic and plaque destabilization processes including endothelial dysfunction, interleukin-6 production, oxidation of low-density lipoprotein, matrix metalloproteinase production, and induction of oxidative stress via NADP(H) oxidase [(37)], there is an increasing case to justify the use of RAAS blockade as a rational therapeutic intervention in CAD. Furthermore, the potentiation of bradykinin and hence nitric oxide activity that comes with ACE inhibition is another way in which these agents may have a beneficial effect in CAD, by improving endothelial function.

Therapeutic blockade of the RAAS can now be achieved with ACE inhibitors which block ACE activity, Angiotensin II receptor blockers (ARB) which are specific inhibitors of the AT_1 receptor, and the newly introduced direct renin inhibitors which prevent renin from converting angiotensinogen into angiotensin I. We will now examine in some detail the key studies that have evaluated the strategy of RAAS blockade in patients with CAD without overt heart failure or left ventricular (LV) dysfunction.

Clinical studies of ACE inhibitors in coronary artery disease

The publication of both the Heart Outcomes Prevention Evaluation (HOPE) and the subsequent EURopean trial On reduction of cardiac events with Perindopril in stable coronary Artery disease (EUROPA) studies, demonstrated for the first time that ACE inhibition reduced the long-term risk of MI and cardiac death in patients with preserved LV systolic function, who had, or were at high risk for CAD[(39,40)]. These studies in conjunction thereby provided a substantial evidence base to support the notion that ACE inhibition can modify atherosclerotic disease progression in a clinically meaningful way.

In the HOPE study, 9297 patients aged 55 or older who had no symptoms or signs of heart failure (or were not known to have an ejection fraction less than 40%), and who had to have a history of CAD, stroke, peripheral vascular disease, or diabetes (with one or more additional risk factor of hypertension, raised total cholesterol, low high density lipoprotein cholesterol, smoking, or microalbuminuria), were randomized to receive 10mg once daily ramipril or placebo and followed-up for a mean of 5 years. The study was designed to identify a 13.5% reduction in the primary endpoint, defined as the composite of myocardial infarction, stroke, or cardiovascular death, at 90% power in the ramipril group in a total study population of 9000 patients followed up for 5 years. Patients were recruited in 267 centres in North and South America, and Europe between December 1993 and June 1995 with 4645 patients randomly allocated to ramipril, and the remaining 4652 allocated to placebo. 78.8% of patients allocated to

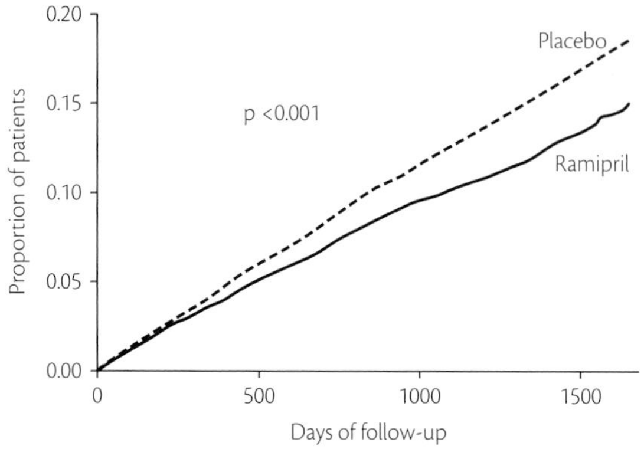

Fig. 26.5 Kaplan–Meier estimates of the incidence of the primary endpoint in the HOPE trial (the composite of cardiovascular death, myocardial infarction or stroke) out to 1500+ days follow-up. Reproduced with permission from The Heart Outcomes Prevention Evaluation Study Investigators. Effects of an angiotensin-converting–enzyme inhibitor, ramipril, on cardiovascular events in high-risk patients. *N Engl J Med* 2000; **342**:145–53.

ramipril were still taking the study medication or open label ACE inhibitor at the last follow-up visit. At baseline, the mean age and BP of the patients were 66 years and 139/79 respectively, while 25.7% were women, 43.6% had undergone prior coronary revascularization (18% having had PCI), 38.5% had diabetes, 76.1% were taking antiplatelet therapy, and 28.6% were on lipid lowering therapy. The primary endpoint was defined as the composite of myocardial infarction, stroke, or cardiovascular death, and occurred in 651 patients (14.0%) who were assigned to receive ramipril, as compared to 826 patients (17.8%) assigned to placebo (relative risk 0.78; 95% CI 0.70–0.86; p <0.001) (Fig. 26.5). In contrast to many clinical trials in which the composite endpoint is either driven by reduction in a particular component, or none of the individual components reaches significance on its own, all three of MI, stroke, and cardiovascular death were significantly reduced by at least 20% in the ramipril arm with p-values of <0.001. Furthermore, there were also significant reductions with ramipril in other clinically relevant secondary outcomes including death from any cause (10.4% vs. 12.2%; relative risk 0.84; p = 0.005), revascularization procedures (16.0% vs. 18.3%; relative risk 0.85; p = 0.002), cardiac arrest (0.8% vs. 1.3%; relative risk 0.63; p = 0.03), heart failure (9.0% vs. 11.5%; relative risk 0.77; p <0.001), new diagnosis of diabetes mellitus (3.6% vs. 5.4%; relative risk 0.66; p <0.001), and complications related to diabetes (6.4% vs. 7.6%; relative risk 0.84; p = 0.03).

In the even larger EUROPA study, 12 218 patients aged 18 or older who had no symptoms or signs of heart failure, and who had either documented CAD or were men with proven inducible ischaemia, were randomized to receive 8mg once daily perindopril or placebo and followed-up for a mean of 4.2 years. The study recruited patients between December 1993 and June 1995 in 24 European countries with 6110 patients randomly allocated to perindopril and the remaining 6108 allocated to placebo. At baseline, the mean age and BP of the patients were 60 years and 137/82 respectively, while 14.6% were women, 58.6% had undergone prior coronary revascularization, 12.3% had diabetes, 92.3% were taking antiplatelet therapy, and 57.6% were on lipid lowering therapy. 78.2% of patients allocated to perindopril were still taking the study medication at the end of follow-up. The primary endpoint was initially defined as the composite of total mortality, non-fatal myocardial infarction, unstable angina, and cardiac arrest with successful resuscitation. Somewhat controversially, the primary endpoint definition was changed during the trial, principally as a result of the widespread adoption of troponin levels into clinical practice, and also the interim finding that the cardiovascular proportion of total mortality was lower than expected. The new definition was the composite of cardiovascular mortality, non-fatal myocardial infarction, and cardiac arrest with successful resuscitation, with the removal of unstable angina, which was felt to be a subjective diagnosis with favourable prognosis. To the authors' credit, the original primary endpoint became the first secondary endpoint and it still showed a similar result to the changed primary endpoint. The study was designed to identify a 22.1% reduction in the (redefined) primary endpoint at 90% power in the perindopril group assuming an overall event rate of 775. 488 patients (8.0%) who were assigned to receive perindopril reached the primary endpoint, as compared to 603 patients (9.9%) assigned to placebo (relative risk 0.80; 95% CI 0.71–0.91; p = 0.0003). In contrast to the HOPE study in which all the components of the primary endpoint were significantly reduced in the ramipril arm, only non-fatal MI was significantly reduced by perindopril in EUROPA. While many secondary endpoints were reduced in the perindopril arm, only the incidence of heart failure requiring hospital admission reached significance. In contrast to the HOPE study, the reduction of stroke was not significant with perindopril. As evidenced by the lower event rates in the EUROPA study, it can be concluded that it recruited a population at lower overall risk to HOPE which is to be expected with its younger cohort with less diabetes and hypertension which was also more likely to be treated with aspirin, beta-blockers, and statins.

Interestingly, when the Kaplan–Meier estimates for the primary endpoints up to more than 4 years of follow-up in both HOPE and EUROPA are examined, it can be seen that the curves are still diverging at this time. Furthermore, it also took 2 years of treatment with ACE inhibitor in both studies before the reduction in event rates reached significance. The consistency of this finding in both trials suggests not only that long-term treatment with ACE inhibitor is necessary to achieve a biological effect, but also that benefits may continue to accrue over even longer treatment periods. A further consistent finding in the two studies was the benefit of ACE inhibitor therapy across many predefined subgroups including gender and age.

These landmark trials led to changes in international guidelines advising the use of ACE inhibitors for all patients with stable CAD regardless of whether they had LV impairment or not[14,15]. However, the publication of the similarly large Prevention of Events with Angiotensin Converting Enzyme (PEACE) trial, which found no outcomes benefit for ACE inhibition in a similar CAD patient population without heart failure, put this treatment strategy back in the spotlight in a debate which continues to this day[41]. PEACE randomized 8290 patients aged 50 or more with documentation of both CAD and an ejection fraction >40% to receive 4mg once daily trandolapril or placebo and followed-up for a median of 4.8 years. Similarly to EUROPA, the initial primary endpoint of cardiovascular death or non-fatal MI was changed during the trial when it became apparent that it would not be feasible to recruit the initially planned 14 100 patients that were originally estimated to be needed to prove the hypothesis. The primary endpoint was therefore expanded to include coronary revascularization and the sample size recalculated as 8100 patients, giving the study a 90% power to identify an 18% relative reduction in the primary endpoint assuming a 19% incidence in the placebo group. Patients were recruited in 187 centres in North America and Italy between November 1996 and June 2000 with 4158 patients randomly allocated to trandolapril and the remaining 4132 allocated to placebo. At baseline, the mean age and BP of the patients were 64 years and 134/78 respectively, while 18% were women, 72% had undergone prior coronary revascularization, 17% had diabetes, 90% were taking antiplatelet therapy, and 70% were on lipid lowering therapy. 74.5% of patients allocated to trandolapril were still taking the study medication or open label ACE inhibitor at 3 years (compliance data beyond this are not provided), although only 57.8% of patients were taking the target dose of 4mg trandolapril at this time. In marked contrast to HOPE and EUROPA, the primary endpoint occurred in 909 patients (21.9%) who were assigned to receive trandolapril, as compared to 929 patients (22.5%) assigned to placebo (relative risk, 0.96; 95% CI 0.88–1.06; p = 0.43). None of the other pre-specified secondary composite endpoints which included the addition of unstable angina, stroke, heart failure, and peripheral vascular disease to the primary endpoint in various combinations, nor post hoc analyses of the same primary endpoints used in HOPE or EUROPA reached significance or even approached a trend for benefit with trandolapril. The only positive benefits with trandolapril were found in post-hoc analyses of the data looking at the development of diabetes and heart failure requiring hospitalization (no doubt prompted by the findings of the HOPE study), both of which were significantly reduced in the trandolapril arm.

How then can the results of PEACE be reconciled with those of HOPE and EUROPA, when the inclusion and exclusion criteria of all three trials were remarkably similar? The most simplistic explanation is of course that the benefits of ACE inhibition found in HOPE and EUROPA are not generalizable to all ACE inhibitors and this is not a class effect. While trandolapril has previously been shown to be beneficial in heart failure[42], it should be borne in mind that much of the presumed benefit of ACE inhibitors in CAD with preserved LV function relates to direct effects on atherosclerotic plaques (see earlier discussion) and it is currently unknown whether ramipril, perindopril, and trandolapril have similar plaque-penetrating properties[43]. On this point, it is worth considering whether the dose of trandolapril used in PEACE was adequate? The dose of 4mg once daily was chosen as it had been shown to be efficacious in the TRACE study of post-MI patients with impaired LV function[42]. However, the doses of ramipril and perindopril used in HOPE and EUROPA were higher than those often used at the time to treat heart failure and hypertension, and have comparatively higher plasma ACE activity inhibition than 4mg trandolapril[44]. As patients without heart failure usually do not have excessive activation of the circulatory RAAS, it is not unreasonable to suggest that higher doses of ACE inhibitor are required to penetrate the atherosclerotic plaques and modify disease progression in this setting, as compared to patients with heart failure. It has therefore been suggested that the 4-mg dose of trandolapril used in the PEACE study was inadequate to produce a therapeutic effect in enough patients with CAD without heart failure, particularly when it is borne in mind that only 57.8% of patients were taking the target dose of 4mg trandolapril at 3 years[43,44].

The primary issue to address when questioning the result of any clinical study is to examine whether it was appropriately powered to investigate the study hypothesis? Technically, the PEACE study had a high level of statistical power to identify an 18% relative risk reduction in the primary endpoint, and the event rate in the placebo arm was higher than estimated. However, it should be remembered that the study size was dramatically reduced with the expansion of the original primary endpoint to include coronary revascularization, a much 'softer'endpoint which could be influenced by external confounders unrelated to ACE inhibition (such as physician preferences) than the 'harder'clinical endpoints of death, MI, stroke, and cardiac arrest used in HOPE and EUROPA. The PEACE study authors concentrate much of their discussion highlighting the lower risk population taking more optimal medical therapy recruited in their trial. It is undoubtedly true that when the study populations recruited to PEACE and HOPE are specifically examined, it can be seen that there was a 14% and 42% greater adherence to antiplatelet and lipid-lowering therapy respectively, combined with 5/1mmHg lower BP, 21% less diabetes, and 28% more prior revascularization in PEACE, but is this enough to account for the greater than 50% reduction in cardiovascular mortality that was observed in the placebo arms (3.7% vs. 8.1%), and negate any additional benefit of ACE inhibition? Or was PEACE simply underpowered to detect a benefit of ACE inhibition in its lower risk population? The observation that the populations recruited to EUROPA and PEACE were much more similar than in HOPE and PEACE, not only in terms of the patients' demographics at baseline, but also the cardiovascular mortality in the placebo arms during follow-up (4.1% and 3.7% respectively), adds further weight to the notion that PEACE was underpowered since the 4000 patient larger EUROPA study found a significant benefit with ACE inhibition[45].

While it is tempting to hypothesize that the negative findings of PEACE may be largely explained by the superior prescription of lipid-lowering therapy, there are substantial theoretical reasons and experimental evidence to support a synergistic interaction between ACE inhibition and statin therapy in atherosclerosis[43,46]. Furthermore, a subgroup analysis of the HOPE and EUROPA study populations showed significant reductions in cardiovascular death, non-fatal MI or stroke in the 9489 and 12 026 patients concurrently treated with lipid-lowering therapy or not respectively[47].

Where then does the balance of evidence lie? Unsurprisingly, a number of groups have turned to meta-analysis in an attempt to answer this question[44,47,48]. Dagenais and colleagues limited their analysis to the 29 805 patients in HOPE, EUROPA, and PEACE, whereas the other two groups included a number of smaller studies which individually were not powered to detect differences in individual hard clinical endpoints, and indeed none of which reached significance for their primary endpoints. These additional, placebo-controlled, randomized trials of ACE inhibitor therapy in patients with CAD but no heart failure added over 4000 additional patients to the meta-analysis. They were the: Quinapril Ischaemic Event Trial (QUIET), in which 1750 patients were randomized to 20mg quinapril or placebo and followed for a mean of 2 years for the occurrence of cardiac death, resuscitated cardiac arrest, non-fatal MI, revascularization or hospitalization for angina[49]; the PART-2 study[50] in which 617 patients were randomized to 5–10mg ramipril or placebo and followed for a mean of 4 years to evaluate changes in carotid artery thickness; the CAMELOT study[51] in which 1997 patients were randomized to enalapril 10mg twice daily, amlodipine 5mg once daily, or placebo and followed for a mean of 2 years for the occurrence of cardiovascular death, non-fatal MI, resuscitated cardiac arrest, revascularization, stroke or TIA, hospitalization for angina or heart failure, or new peripheral vascular disease; and the SCAT study[52] in which 460 patients were randomized to enalapril 10mg twice daily or placebo (in a factorial design with simvastatin 40mg) and followed for a mean of 4 years for a change in coronary angiographic dimensions.

A consistent finding in all three meta-analyses is a statistically significant reduction in all cause mortality, and non-fatal MI with ACE inhibitor therapy, while similarly significant reductions in cardiovascular death and stroke are also reported in two of the meta-analyses. Unfortunately, none of these meta-analyses use patient-level data and all the results are based on the data published in the original papers of each study. As a result, subgroup analyses which may shed light on particular patient characteristics that benefit (or not) from ACE inhibition cannot be performed. However, Dagenais *et al.* did have access to patient-level data from

HOPE and EUROPA and present a subgroup analysis showing that in these two studies the benefits of ACE inhibition are preserved across a number of subgroups including: patients taking antiplatelet, lipid-lowering, and beta-blocker therapy (alone or in combination), and patients with prior revascularization[47].

While these analyses undoubtedly show a benefit with ACE inhibition in patients with CAD without heart failure, a consistent finding is that this benefit is modest at best with <20% reductions in death and MI. This translates into a need to treat 100 patients for an average of 4.4 years to prevent one death, MI or revascularization procedure[48]. As with many therapeutic interventions, it is highly likely that the higher the patient's baseline risk, the greater the benefit of ACE inhibition will be. Extrapolating from the HOPE data, diabetes, older age, higher systolic BP, female gender, and less optimal medical therapy, with less lipid-lowering treatment in particular, all appear to increase a patient's risk. Certainly, CAD patients with an additional indication for ACE inhibition such as LV impairment or diabetic nephropathy should receive an ACE inhibitor indefinitely. Nevertheless, the findings of the meta-analyses on top of HOPE and EUROPA support the *long-term* utilization of ACE inhibitors in all patients with CAD. We feel that this should be regardless of their risk profile or LV function and we concur with international guidelines[14,15] that it is reasonable to do so, provided there are no major issues with tolerability. As the event curves were still diverging at the end of long-term follow-up in both HOPE and EUROPA, it is important to stress that indefinite therapy should be the treatment goal, with a minimum of 2 years' therapy before any benefit is likely to accrue on an individual basis.

Finally with regard to ACE inhibitors in CAD, a frequent criticism of many of the studies is that some authorities have argued that the benefits of ACE inhibition are due to BP lowering alone, as was unsurprisingly seen in all the studies. This seems unlikely for a number of reasons. The HOPE study authors have shown that the benefits of ramipril were not only greater than would have been expected for the modest BP reduction observed, but also regardless of whether the patients were normotensive or not[53]. Furthermore, BP reduction does not necessarily translate into a reduction in death and MI in stable CAD patients, as shown in both PEACE and also the CAMELOT study, in which patients in the amlodipine arm had an equivalent BP reduction to those in the enalapril arm and did show a significant reduction in cardiovascular events whereas those in the enalapril arm did not.

Clinical studies of angiotensin receptor blockers in coronary artery disease

A further consistent finding of the HOPE, EUROPA, and PEACE studies, was the relatively high rate of discontinuation of ACE inhibitor during follow-up, ranging from 22.8% in EUROPA, to 28.9% in HOPE, although in both of these studies these rates were within 2 percentage points of those for placebo discontinuation. An undoubted compliance advantage of ARBs over ACE inhibitors is their low incidence of cough as a side-effect. However, this may be a double-edged sword, as the potentiation of bradykinin, which causes the so-called 'ACE inhibitor cough', may be particularly advantageous in the CAD setting with its contribution to vasodilatation and endothelial function. Nevertheless, given the success of ACE inhibition in reducing clinical events in patients with CAD, it is unsurprising that investigators have also turned their attention to ARBs in this regard. There have been two major randomized studies of ARB in patients with, or at high risk for CAD: the Ongoing Telmisartan Alone and in Combination with Ramipril Global Endpoint Trial (ONTARGET)[54], and the Telmisartan Randomized AssessmeNt Study in ACE iNtolerant subjects with cardiovascular Disease (TRANSCEND)[55].

In the ONTARGET study, 25 620 patients aged 55 or older who did not have congestive cardiac failure, and who had to have a history of CAD, stroke, peripheral vascular disease or diabetes with end-organ damage, were randomized to receive 10mg once daily ramipril, 80mg once daily telmisartan, or both and followed-up for a median of 56 months. The study was designed to demonstrate non-inferiority of telmisartan versus ramipril and superiority of combination- over mono-therapy at power of 89% and 93% respectively. Patients were recruited in 733 centres in 40 countries worldwide with 8576 patients randomly allocated to ramipril, 8542 to telmisartan, and the remaining 8502 to dual therapy. At baseline, the mean age and BP of the patients were 66 years and 142/82mmHg respectively, while 26% were women, 51% had undergone prior coronary revascularization, 37.5% had diabetes, 81% were taking antiplatelet therapy, and 62% were on lipid lowering therapy. The primary endpoint was defined as the composite of myocardial infarction, stroke, cardiovascular death, or hospitalization for heart failure and occurred in 1412 patients (16.5%) in the ramipril group, as compared to 1423 patients in the telmisartan group (16.7%; relative risk 1.01; 95% CI 0.94–1.09), which comfortably met the predefined non-inferiority criteria for telmisartan. In terms of compliance issues, the permanent discontinuation of study medication rates were 24.5% for ramipril, 23.0% for telmisartan, and 29.3% for dual therapy ($p = 0.02$ for telmisartan versus ramipril comparison) with the telmisartan group having both lower rates of cough (1.1% vs. 4.2%, $p < 0.001$) and angio-oedema (0.1% vs. 0.3%, $p = 0.01$). However, there was no additional benefit and even harm in the dual therapy group compared to ramipril, with the primary outcome occurring in 1386 patients (16.3%; relative risk 0.99; 95% CI 0.92–1.07), with increased hypotensive symptoms (4.8% vs. 1.7%, $p < 0.001$), syncope (0.3% vs. 0.2%, $p = 0.03$), and renal dysfunction (13.5% vs. 10.2%, $p < 0.001$). Therefore the authors' principal conclusion from this study was that telmisartan was a viable alternative to ramipril in patients with CAD or at high risk for it, with some potential benefits in terms of increased compliance and decreased angio-oedema.

However, the potential danger of basing treatment decisions on non-inferiority studies which apparently demonstrate equivalence of two therapies, rather than placebo controlled trials is borne out by the TRANSCEND study. In this sister study to ONTARGET with the same inclusion and exclusion criteria with the caveat that all patients were intolerant to ACE inhibitor, 5,926 patients were randomized to receive 80mg once daily telmisartan or placebo and followed-up for a median of 56 months. The study was designed to have 94% power to detect a 19% relative risk reduction in the primary endpoint of the composite of myocardial infarction, stroke, cardiovascular death, or hospitalization for heart failure, in a sample size of 6000 patients with an event rate of 5% per year in the placebo arm. Patients were recruited in 630 centres in 40 countries worldwide with 2954 randomly allocated to telmisartan and the remaining 2972 to placebo. At baseline, the mean age and BP of the patients were 67 years and 141/82mmHg respectively, while 43% were women, 45% had undergone prior coronary revascularization, 36% had diabetes, 79% were taking antiplatelet therapy, and 55% were on lipid lowering therapy. The primary endpoint occurred in 465 patients (15.7%) in the telmisartan group, as compared to 504 patients in the placebo group (17.0%; relative risk, 0.92; 95% CI 0.81–1.05; $p = 0.216$). The primary endpoint used in the HOPE study (the composite of myocardial infarction, stroke, or cardiovascular death), which was predefined as the main secondary endpoint, just reached statistical significance in the telmisartan arm with a relative risk of 0.87 (95% CI 0.76–1.00; $p = 0.048$), but when adjusted for overlap with the primary endpoint and multiplicity of comparisons was no longer significant with a p-value of 0.068.

Given that TRANSCEND recruited a very similar population to ONTARGET, apart from more women, and did not demonstrate any significant benefit of telmisartan in reducing subsequent events as compared to placebo, its role as an alternative agent to ACE inhibitor is currently far from proven. As with PEACE, it can be argued that the population recruited was too low risk to allow a beneficial effect of telmisartan to be demonstrated, and the event rate in the placebo arm was indeed lower than estimated during study design. However, at the present time one has to conclude that telmisartan does not have a role as standard therapy in the way that can be argued for ACE inhibitors, but that it may have a role in higher risk patients, although this would require a larger, appropriately powered randomized trial to prove this.

Conclusions

Almost by definition, any patient who has undergone PCI is extremely likely to have significant CAD (with the possible exception of the minority of patients with spontaneous coronary dissections or embolization). On the basis of the sum of the published data discussed in this chapter, there is a strong evidence base mandating the prescription of statins, and to a lesser extent ACE inhibitors, in patients with both stable and unstable CAD, with important reductions in hard clinical endpoints which are likely to be meaningful to individual patients. The overwhelming positivity of studies with many different statins argues strongly that there is a class effect which is linked to the LDL cholesterol reduction produced by HMG-CoA reductase inhibition. It is therefore unlikely to make a significant difference which statin is used in individual patients, provided that a substantial reduction in LDL cholesterol is achieved. Nevertheless, the results of more recent studies such as MIRACL, PROVE-IT, and JUPITER, do suggest that at the very least, greater LDL cholesterol reductions produce greater clinical benefits, possibly through additional anti-inflammatory activity. However, for the majority of our patients this has yet to be defined, and more specific recommendations to use particular agents for their purported anti-inflammatory properties or advantages over competing drugs cannot be supported at present and requires further research.

The situation is less clear cut for the ACE inhibitors and ARBs given the heterogeneity of trial results, and on this basis if faced with a patient with CAD but no other overt reason to use RAAS inhibition, the balance of evidence favours use of ramipril or perindopril at the present time, with much less evidence of an overall class effect than is seen for RAAS inhibition in patients with LV dysfunction.

Finally, it should be noted that despite the notable success of statins and ACE inhibitors, that the event rates in the treatment arms of all of the major studies discussed here remain substantial and there is considerable room for therapeutic improvement. However, the disappointingly negative results of both the ENHANCE study in which ezetimibe was added to simvastatin in patients with familial hypercholesterolaemia, and the ILLUMINATE and ILLUSTRATE studies with torcetrapib suggest that this may not come from additional non-statin modifications of LDL and HDL cholesterol levels in favourable directions. It remains to be seen whether other anti-inflammatory agents may have synergistic effects with statins, but for the time being there can be little doubt that statins and ACE inhibitors represent the best available agents at our disposal for favourably modifying atherosclerosis. It is tempting to consider that these disease-modifying agents have solved the problem, but the event rates in the treatment arms of any of the clinical outcome studies discussed here testify to the need for continued research into the identification of individuals truly at risk of events and methods to further modify that risk. The complexities of trial design in pursuit of this goal, as well as the enormous cost of prosecution of the studies, represent important challenges. Criticism of the role of pharmaceutical companies in financing such trials has to be balanced by the simplest of enquiries: if not them, then who?

References

1. Schoenhagen P, Ziada KM, Kapadia SR, *et al.* Extent and direction of arterial remodelling in stable versus unstable coronary syndromes: an intravascular ultrasound study. *Circulation* 2000; **101**:598–603.
2. Falk E, Shah PK, Fuster. V. Coronary plaque disruption. *Circulation* 1995; **92**:657-71.
3. Lipid Research Clinics Program, The Lipid Research Clinics Coronary Primary Prevention Trial results. *JAMA* 1984; **251**:351–74.
4. Ross R. Atherosclerosis – an inflammatory disease. *N Engl J Med* 1999; **340**:115–26.
5. Hansson GK. Inflammation, atherosclerosis and coronary artery disease. *N Engl J Med* 2005; **352**:1685–95.
6. Mahmoudi M, Curzen N, Gallagher PJ. Atherogenesis: the role of inflammation and infection. *Histopathology* 2007; **50**:535–46.
7. Davies MJ, Thomas A. Thrombosis and acute coronary-artery lesions in sudden cardiac ischemic death. *N Engl J Med* 1984; **310**:1137–40
8. Libby P, Theroux P. Pathophysiology of coronary artery disease. *Circulation* 2005; **111**:3481–8.
9. Steinberg D. The statins in preventive cardiology. *N Engl J Med* 2008; **359**:1426–7.
10. Schonbeck U, Libby P. Inflammation, immunity, and HMG-CoA reductase inhibitors: statins as antiinflammatory agents? *Circulation* 2004; **109**:II-18–II-26.
11. Albert MA, Danielson E, Rifai N, *et al.*, for the PRINCE Investigators. Effect of statin therapy on C-reactive protein levels: the pravastatin inflammation/CRP evaluation (PRINCE): a randomized trial and cohort study. *JAMA* 2001; **286**:64–70.
12. Nissen SE, Tuzcu EM, Schoenhagen P, *et al.*, for the Reversal of Atherosclerosis with Aggressive Lipid Lowering (REVERSAL) Investigators. Statin therapy, LDL cholesterol, C-reactive protein, and coronary artery disease. *N Engl J Med* 2005; **352**:29–38.
13. Baigent C, Keech A, Kearney, *et al.*, for the Cholesterol Treatment Trialists' collaboration. Efficacy and safety of cholesterol-lowering treatment: prospective meta-analysis of data from 90,056 participants in 14 randomized trials of statins. *Lancet* 2005; **366**:1267–78.
14. Fox K, Garcia MAA, Ardissino D, *et al.* Guidelines on the management of stable angina pectoris: executive summary. *Eur Heart J* 2006; **27**:1341–81.
15. Fraker TD, Fihn SD, for the 2002 chronic stable angina writing committee. 2007 chronic angina focused update of the AHA/ACC 2002 guidelines for the management of patients with chronic stable angina. *Circulation* 2007; **116**:2762–72.
16. Steinberg D, Gotto AM. Preventing coronary artery disease by lowering cholesterol levels: fifty years from bench to bedside. *JAMA* 1999; **282**:2043–50.
17. Scandinavian Simvastatin Survival Study Group. Randomized trial of cholesterol lowering in 4,444 patients with coronary heart disease. *Lancet* 1994; **344**:1383–8.
18. Sacks FM, Pfeffer MA, Moye LA, *et al.* The effect of pravastatin on coronary events after myocardial infarction in patients with average cholesterol levels. *N Engl J Med* 1996; **335**:1001–9.
19. Long-Term Intervention with Pravastatin in Ischaemic Disease (LIPID) Study Group. Prevention of cardiovascular events and death with pravastatin in patients with coronary heart disease and a broad range of initial cholesterol levels. *N Engl J Med* 1998; **339**:1349–57.
20. GISSI Prevenzione Investigators. Results of the low-dose (20mg) pravastatin GISSI Prevenzione trial in 4271 patients with recent myocardial infarction: do stopped trials contribute to overall knowledge? *Ital Heart J* 2000; **1**:810–20.

21. Serruys PW, de Feyter P, Macaya C, *et al*, for the Lescol Intervention Prevention Study (LIPS) Investigators. Fluvastatin for prevention of cardiac events following successful first percutaneous coronary intervention: a randomized controlled trial. *JAMA* 2002; **287**:3215–22.
22. Shepherd J, Cobbe SM, Ford I, *et al*. Prevention of coronary heart disease with pravastatin in men with hypercholesterolemia. *N Engl J Med* 1995; **333**:1301–7.
23. Heart Protection Study Collaborative Group. MRC/BHF Heart Protection Study of cholesterol lowering with simvastatin in 20,536 high-risk individuals: a randomized placebo-controlled trial. *Lancet* 2002; **360**:7–22.
24. Downs JR, Clearfield M, Weis S, *et al*. Primary prevention of acute coronary events with lovastatin in men and women with average cholesterol levels: results of AFCAPS/TexCAPS. Air Force/Texas Coronary Atherosclerosis Prevention Study. *JAMA* 1998; **279**:1615–22.
25. Shepherd J, Blauw GJ, Murphy MB, *et al*, the PROSPER study group. Pravastatin in elderly individuals at risk of vascular disease (PROSPER): a randomised controlled trial. *Lancet* 2002; **360**:1623–30.
26. Colhoun HM, Betteridge DJ, Durrington PN, *et al*, for the CARDS investigators. Primary prevention of cardiovascular disease with atorvastatin in type 2 diabetes in the Collaborative Atorvastatin Diabetes Study (CARDS): multicentre randomized placebo-controlled trial. *Lancet* 2004; **364**:685–96.
27. Sever PS, Dahlöf B, Poulter NR, *et al*, for the ASCOT investigators. Prevention of coronary and stroke events with atorvastatin in hypertensive patients who have average or lower-than-average cholesterol concentrations, in the Anglo-Scandinavian Cardiac Outcomes Trial – Lipid Lowering Arm (ASCOT-LLA): a multicentre randomized controlled trial. *Lancet* 2003; **361**:1149–58.
28. ALLHAT Officers and Coordinators for the ALLHAT Collaborative Research Group. Major outcomes in moderately hypercholesterolemic, hypertensive patients randomized to pravastatin vs usual care: The Antihypertensive and Lipid-Lowering Treatment to Prevent Heart Attack Trial (ALLHAT-LLT). *JAMA* 2002; **288**:2998–3007.
29. Ridker PM, Danielson E, Fonseca FA, *et al*, for the JUPITER Study Group. Rosuvastatin to prevent vascular events in men and women with elevated C-reactive protein. *N Engl J Med* 2008; **359**:2195–207.
30. Schwartz GG, Olsson AG, Ezekowitz MD, *et al*, for the Myocardial Ischemia Reduction with Aggressive Cholesterol Lowering (MIRACL) Study Investigators. *JAMA* 2001; **285**:1711–18.
31. Cannon CP, Braunwald E, McCabe CH, *et al*, for the Pravastatin or Atorvastatin Evaluation and Infection Therapy-Thrombolysis in Myocardial Infarction 22 Investigators. Intensive versus moderate lipid lowering with statins after acute coronary syndromes. *N Engl J Med* 2004; **350**:1495–504.
32. de Lemos JA, Blazing MA, Wiviott SD, *et al*, for the A to Z Investigators. Early intensive vs a delayed conservative simvastatin strategy in patients with acute coronary syndromes: phase Z of the A to Z trial. *JAMA* 2004; **292**(11):1307–16.
33. Cannon CP, Steinberg BA, Murphy SA, *et al*. Meta-analysis of cardiovascular outcomes trials comparing intensive versus moderate statin therapy. *J Am Coll Cardiol* 2006; **48**:438–45.
34. Nissen SE, Tuzcu EM, Schoenhagen P, *et al*, for the REVERSAL Investigators. Effect of intensive compared with moderate lipid-lowering therapy on progression of coronary atherosclerosis: a randomized controlled trial. *JAMA* 2004; **291**:1071–80.
35. Nissen SE, Nicholls SJ, Sipahi I, *et al*, for the ASTEROID Investigators. Effect of very high-intensity statin therapy on regression of coronary atherosclerosis: the ASTEROID trial. *JAMA* 2006; **295**:1556–65.
36. Flather MD, Yusuf S, Kober L, *et al*, for the ACE-inhibitor myocardial infarction collaborative group. Long-term ACE-inhibitor therapy in patients with heart failure or left-ventricular dysfunction: a systematic overview of data from individual patients. *Lancet* 2000; **355**:1575–81.
37. Schmieder RE, Hilgers KF, Schlaich MP, *et al*. Renin-angiotensin system and cardiovascular risk. *Lancet* 2007; **369**:1208–19.
38. Ribichini F, Pugno F, Ferrero V, *et al*. Cellular immunostaining of angiotensin-converting enzyme in human coronary atherosclerotic plaques. *J Am Coll Cardiol* 2006; **47**:1143–9.
39. The Heart Outcomes Prevention Evaluation Study Investigators. Effects of an angiotensin-converting enzyme inhibitor, ramipril, on cardiovascular events in high-risk patients. *N Engl J Med* 2000; **342**:145–53.
40. Fox K, for the EUROPA trial investigators. Efficacy of perindopril in reduction of cardiovascular events among patients with stable coronary artery disease: randomized, double-blind, placebo-controlled, multicentre trial (the EUROPA study). *Lancet* 2003; **362**:782–8.
41. The PEACE Trial Investigators. Angiotensin-converting–enzyme inhibition in stable coronary artery disease. *N Engl J Med* 2004; **351**:2058–68.
42. Køber L, Torp-Pedersen C, Carlsen JE, *et al*. A clinical trial of the angiotensin-converting-enzyme inhibitor trandolapril in patients with left ventricular dysfunction after myocardial infarction. Trandolapril Cardiac Evaluation (TRACE) Study Group. *N Engl J Med* (1995); **333**:1670–6.
43. Fox K, Ferrari R, Yusuf S, Borer JS. Should angiotensin-converting enzyme-inhibitors be used to improve outcome in patients with coronary artery disease and 'preserved' left ventricular function? *Eur Heart J* 2006; **27**:2154–7.
44. Danchin N, Cucherat M, Thuillez C, *et al*. Angiotensin-converting enzyme inhibitors in patients with coronary artery disease and absence of heart failure or left ventricular systolic dysfunction: an overview of long-term randomized controlled trials. *Arch Int Med* 2006; **166**:787–96.

45. Yusuf S, Pogue J. ACE inhibition in stable coronary artery disease. *N Engl J Med* 2005; **352**:937–9.
46. Chiong JR, Miller AB. Renin-angiotensin system antagonism and lipid-lowering therapy in cardiovascular risk management. *J Renin Angiotensin Aldosterone Syst* 2002; **3**:96–102.
47. Dagenais GR, Pogue J, Fox K, *et al*. Angiotensin-converting-enzyme inhibitors in stable vascular disease without left ventricular systolic dysfunction or heart failure: a combined analysis of three trials. *Lancet* 2006; **368**:581–8.
48. Al-Mallah MH, Tleyjeh IM, Abdel-Latif AA, *et al*. Angiotensin-converting enzyme inhibitors in coronary artery disease and preserved left ventricular systolic function: a systematic review and meta-analysis of randomized controlled trials. *J Am Coll Cardiol* 2006; **47**:1576–83.
49. Pitt B, O'Neill B, Feldman R, *et al*, for the QUIET study group. The QUinapril Ischemic Event Trial (QUIET): evaluation of chronic ACE inhibitor therapy in patients with ischemic heart disease and preserved left ventricular function. *Am J Cardiol* 2001; **87**:1058–63.
50. MacMahon S, Sharpe N, Gamble G, *et al*, for the PART-2 Collaborative Research Group. Randomized, placebo-controlled trial of the angiotensin-converting enzyme inhibitor, ramipril, in patients with coronary or other occlusive arterial disease. *J Am Coll Cardiol* 2000; **36**:438–43.
51. Nissen SE, Tuzcu EM, Libby P, *et al*, for the CAMELOT Investigators. Effect of antihypertensive agents on cardiovascular events in patients with coronary disease and normal blood pressure. The CAMELOT study: a randomized controlled trial. *JAMA* 2004; **292**:2217–26.
52. Teo KK, Burton JR, Buller CE, *et al*. Long-term effects of cholesterol lowering and angiotensin-converting enzyme inhibition on coronary atherosclerosis: The Simvastatin/Enalapril Coronary Atherosclerosis Trial (SCAT). *Circulation* 2000; **102**:1748–54.
53. Sleight P, Yusuf S, Pogue J, *et al*, for the HOPE study investigators. Blood-pressure reduction and cardiovascular risk in HOPE study. *Lancet* 2001; **358**:2130–1.
54. Yusuf S, Teo KK, Pogue J, *et al*, for the ONTARGET Investigators. Telmisartan, ramipril, or both in patients at high risk for vascular events. *N Engl J Med* 2008; **358**:1547–59.
55. Yusuf S, Teo K, Anderson C, *et al*, for the Telmisartan Randomized AssessmeNt Study in ACE iNtolerant subjects with cardiovascular Disease (TRANSCEND) Investigators. Effects of the angiotensin-receptor blocker telmisartan on cardiovascular events in high-risk patients intolerant to angiotensin-converting enzyme inhibitors: a randomized controlled trial. *Lancet* 2008; **372**:1174–83.

SECTION 6

Complications of percutaneous coronary intervention

CHAPTER 27

Contrast-induced acute kidney injury

Peter A. McCullough

New terms and definitions

Contrast-induced acute kidney injury (AKI), previously known as contrast-induced nephropathy (CIN) is an important complication in the catheterization laboratory[1–3]. The most commonly used definition in clinical trials was a rise in serum creatinine (Cr) of 44.2mmol/L (0.5mg/dL) or a 25% increase from the baseline value, assessed at 48h after the procedure. In 2007, the Acute Kidney Injury Network proposed the definition to a rise in serum Cr ≥26.5mmol/L (0.3mg/dL) or a 50% rise in Cr with oliguria which is compatible with previous definitions and is a new standard to follow. If there is a sustained reduction in estimated glomerular function (eGFR) from a baseline above 60 to a new baseline below 60mL/min/1.73m^2 at 90 days after the procedure, then a definition of chronic kidney disease (CKD) (Stage 3) would be met as a late outcome of this complication.

Consensus on contrast-induced acute kidney injury

Table 27.1 gives the 10 consensus statements on contrast-induced AKI agreed upon by multidisciplinary panels[4]. Fortunately, the frequency of contrast-induced AKI has decreased over the past decade from a general incidence of approximately 15% to approximately 7% of patients[5]. This decrease in frequency may be due to the advent of lower toxicity agents, greater awareness of the problem, and improved prevention measures in patients at high risk undergoing percutaneous coronary intervention (PCI).

Pathophysiology

CKD is both necessary and sufficient for the development of contrast-induced AKI. In patients with CKD, identified by an eGFR <60mL/min/1.73m^2 (which approximates in the elderly [≥75 years] to a serum Cr >88.4mmol/L [1.0mg/dL] in a woman and >111.4mmol/L [1.3mg/dL] in a man), there is a considerable loss of nephron units and the residual renal function is vulnerable to decline with renal insults (iodinated contrast, cardiopulmonary bypass, renal-toxic medications, atheroembolism, etc.). Diabetes mellitus (DM) is an accepted risk amplifier, so that at any level of decreased eGFR, patients with DM have a higher risk of contrast-induced AKI. Thus, the pathophysiology of contrast-induced AKI assumes baseline reduced nephron number, with superimposed acute vasoconstriction caused by the release of adenosine, endothelin, and other renal vasoconstrictors triggered by iodinated contrast. After a very brief increase in renal blood flow, via these mechanisms, there is an overall approximately 50% sustained reduction in renal blood flow lasting for several hours. There is concentration of iodinated contrast in the renal tubules and collecting ducts, resulting in a persistent nephrogram on fluoroscopy. This stasis of contrast in the kidney allows for direct cellular injury and death to renal tubular cells. The degree of cytotoxicity to renal tubular cells is directly related to the length of exposure those cells have to iodinated contrast, hence, the importance of high urinary flow rates before, during, and after contrast procedures. The sustained reduction in renal blood flow to the outer medulla leads to medullary hypoxia, ischaemic injury, and death of renal tubular cells. By these two mechanisms, it is believed that other organ injury processes including oxidative stress and inflammation may play a further role. Importantly, many reactions involved in oxidative stress are dependent on sources of intracellular labile iron, including the cytochrome p450 chain and mitochondria. Any superimposed insult such as sustained hypotension in the catheterization laboratory, microshowers of atheroembolic material from catheter

Table 27.1 Consensus statements concerning contrast-induced AKI[4]

Consensus Statement 1
Contrast-induced AKI is a common (5–15%) and potentially serious complication following the administration of contrast media in patients at risk for acute renal injury
Consensus Statement 2
The risk of contrast-induced AKI is elevated and of clinical importance in patients with CKD (particularly when diabetes is also present), recognized by an eGFR <60mL/min/1.73m^2
Consensus Statement 3
When serum creatinine or eGFR is unavailable, then a history of kidney disease risk factors can identify patients at higher risk for contrast-induced AKI than the general population
Consensus Statement 4
In the setting of emergency procedures, where the benefit of very early imaging outweighs the risk of waiting, the procedure can be performed without knowledge of serum creatinine or eGFR
Consensus Statement 5
The presence of multiple contrast-induced AKI risk factors in the same patient or high-risk clinical scenarios can create a very high risk (~50%) for contrast-induced AKI and (~15%) acute renal failure requiring dialysis after contrast exposure
Consensus Statement 6
In patients at increased risk for contrast-induced AKI undergoing intra-arterial administration of contrast, ionic high-osmolality agents pose a greater risk for contrast-induced AKI than low-osmolality agents. Current evidence suggests that for intra-arterial administration in very high-risk patients with CKD, particularly those with diabetes mellitus, non-ionic, iso-osmolar contrast may be associated with the lowest risk of contrast-induced AKI
Consensus Statement 7
Higher contrast volumes (>100mL) are associated with higher rates of contrast-induced AKI in patients at risk. However, even small (~30mL) volumes of iodinated contrast in very high risk patients can cause contrast-induced AKI and acute renal failure requiring dialysis, suggesting the absence of a threshold effect
Consensus Statement 8
Intra-arterial administration of iodinated contrast appears to pose a greater risk of contrast-induced AKI above that with intravenous administration
Consensus Statement 9
Adequate intravenous volume expansion with isotonic crystalloid (1.0–1.5mL/kg/h) for 3–12h before the procedure and continued for 6–24h afterwards can lessen the probability of contrast-induced AKI in patients at risk. The data on oral as opposed to intravenous volume expansion as a contrast-induced AKI prevention measure are insufficient
Consensus Statement 10
No adjunctive medical or mechanical treatment has been proven to be efficacious reducing the risk of AKI after exposure to iodinated contrast. Prophylactic haemodialysis or haemofiltration has not been validated as an effective strategy

Adapted from McCullough PA, Stacul F, Davidson C, *et al.* Overview. *Am J Cardiol* 2006; **98:**2K–4K.

exchanges or the use of intra-aortic balloon counterpulsation (IABP), or a bleeding complication can amplify the injury processes occurring in the kidney.

Classification of iodinated contrast agents

The osmolality, or particle concentration in solution, is the major physiochemical property by which contrast agents are classified. Therefore, contrast media can be categorized according to osmolality (high-osmolal [HOCM] ~2000 mOsm/kg, low-osmolal [LOCM] 600-800 mOsm/kg, and isosmolal [IOCM] 290 mOsm/kg) with decreasing levels of renal toxicity according to these classifications. The American College of Cardiology/American Heart Association guidelines for the management of ACS patients with CKD listed the use of IOCM as a class I, level of evidence A recommendation[6].

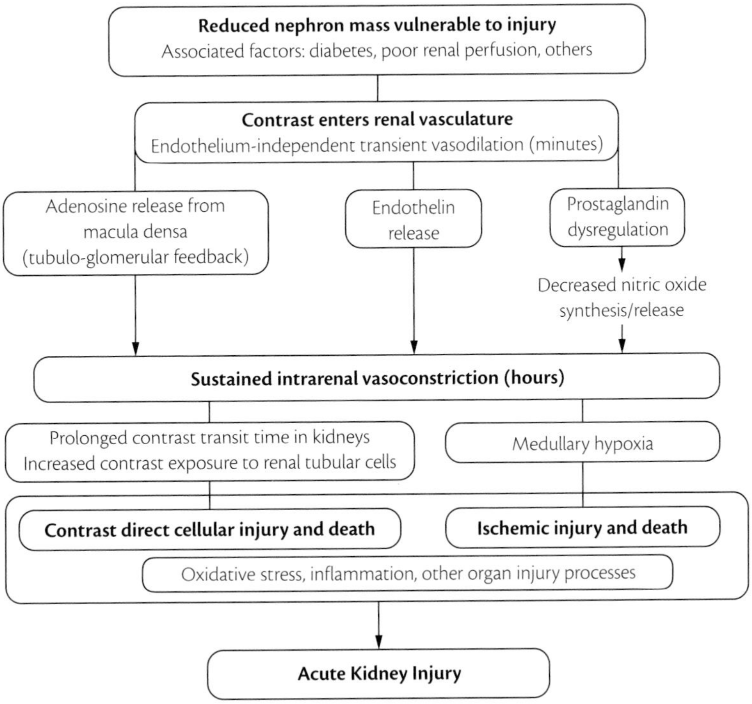

Fig. 27.1 Pathophysiology of contrast-induced AKI demonstrating in the presence of a reduced nephron mass, the remaining nephrons are vulnerable to injury. Iodinated contrast, after causing a brief (minutes) period of vasodilation, cause sustained (hours to days) intrarenal vasoconstriction and ischaemic injury. The ischaemic injury sets off a cascade of events largely driven by oxidative injury causing death of renal tubular cells. If a sufficient mass of nephron units are affected, then a recognizable rise in serum creatinine will occur. Adapted from McCullough PA. Contrast-induced acute kidney injury. *J Am Coll Cardiol* 2008; **51**:1419–28.

The use of IOCM is also recommended in renal dialysis patients to minimize the chances of volume overload and complications prior to the next dialysis session. Most other societies concur with these recommendations for intra-arterial administration and allow the use of LOCM in lower risk patients and intravenous administration.

The volume of contrast is an important predictor of contrast-induced AKI. Even small volumes (~30cc) of contrast medium can have adverse effects on renal function in patients at particularly high risk[7]. As a general rule, the volume of contrast (mL) received should not exceed twice the baseline level of eGFR[8]. This means for patients with significant CKD reasonable goals would be <30cc for diagnostic cardiac catheterization and <100cc for PCI, computed omography (CT), and other intravascular studies.

The risk of contrast-induced AKI is generally higher following intra-arterial than after intravenous injection[9,10]. However, in CT studies, where a comparatively large volume of contrast medium is given as a compact intravenous (80–120cc) bolus rather than an infusion, the risk of AKI may be increased.

Finally, it is believed that serial exposures of contrast and subsequent administration in the setting of AKI further worsens renal function and may be more likely to cause persistent renal dysfunction. Therefore, when faced with the option, a limited diagnostic catheterization and PCI in the same setting is favoured over a diagnostic catheterization and then a scheduled PCI within 10 days. It should be noted, there are no published sources of comparative data on this topic. In addition, the optimal waiting period after a first contrast exposure before a second, is also unstudied and unknown.

Intravascular volume expansion to improve renal blood flow

Volume expansion and treatment of dehydration has a well established role in prevention of contrast-induced AKI, although few studies address this strategy directly. The benefits of volume expansion include an increase

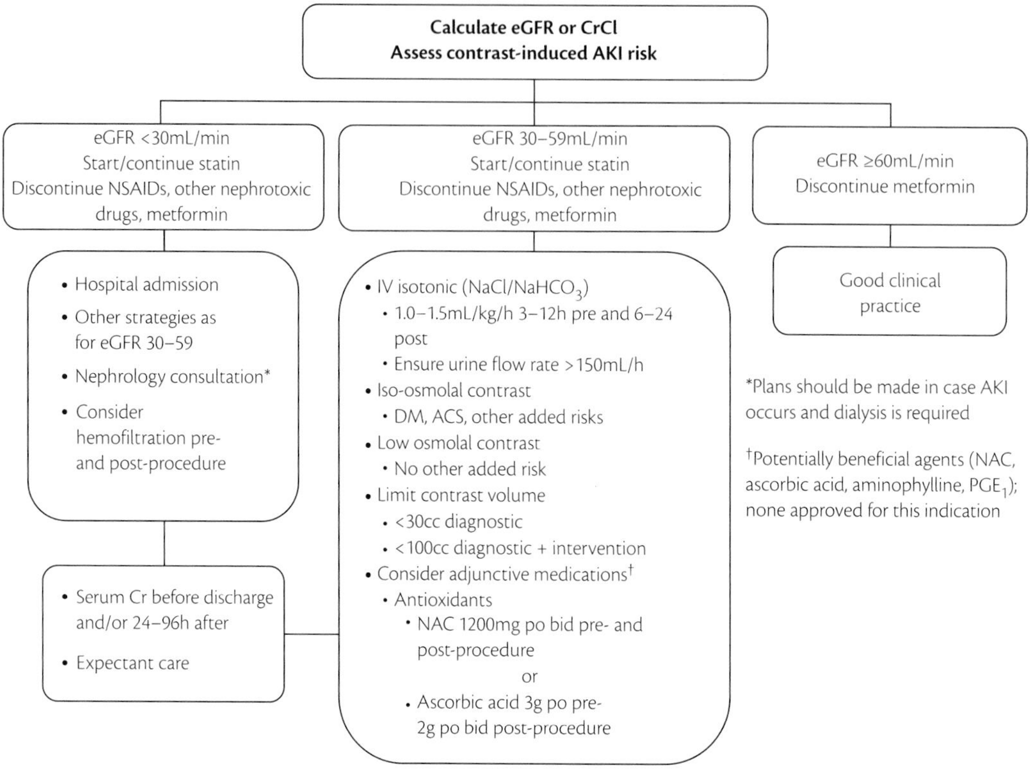

Fig. 27.2 Algorithm for management of patients receiving iodinated contrast media, suggesting a multidimensional approach with assessment of risk based on eGFR and then volume expansion and use of cytoprotective drugs in patients at risk. Discontinuation of metformin is advised to reduce the risk of lactic acidosis if AKI develops. AKI, acute kidney injury; Cr, creatinine; CrCl, creatinine clearance; eGFR, estimated glomerular filtration rate; NSAIDs, non-steroidal anti-inflammatory drugs; NAC, N-acetylcysteine; PGE1, prostaglandin E1). Adapted from McCullough PA. Contrast-induced acute kidney injury. *J Am Coll Cardiol*, 2008; **51**:1419–28.

in renal blood flow and a reduction in tubular and peritubular stasis of contrast in the outer medulla. In theory, this works to limit the exposure of iodinated contrast to tubular and peritubular cells, and thus, reduces the degree of direct cytotoxicity of all forms of iodinated contrast to the kidney (Fig. 27.3). There are limited data on the most appropriate choice of intravenous fluid, but the evidence indicates that isotonic crystalloid (saline or bicarbonate solution) is probably more effective than half-normal saline since a greater degree remains in the intravascular space for a longer period of time[11]. Additional confirmatory trials with sodium bicarbonate[12] are needed since the largest trial to date showed no benefit of sodium bicarbonate over normal saline[13]. There is also no clear evidence to guide the choice of the optimal rate and duration of infusion. However, good urine output (>150mL/h) in the 6h after the procedure has been associated with reduced rates of AKI in one study[14]. Conversely, oliguria in the face of intravenous hydration can be a sign of AKI. Since not all of intravenously administered isotonic crystalloid remains in the vascular space, in order to achieve a urine flow rate of at least 150mL/h, ≥1.0–1.5mL/kg/h of intravenous fluid has to be administered for 3–12h pre- and 6–12h after contrast exposure.

Dialysis and haemofiltration

Iodinated contrast is water soluble and removed by dialysis. Patients who are already receiving renal replacement therapy with haemodialysis should have a dialysis session shortly after intravascular contrast administration to remove contrast media from the body and avoid the risk of volume overload and late contrast reactions. In patients with advanced CKD but not on dialysis, there is no clinical evidence that prophylactic dialysis reduces the risk of AKI, even when carried out within 1h or simultaneously with contrast administration. Haemofiltration,

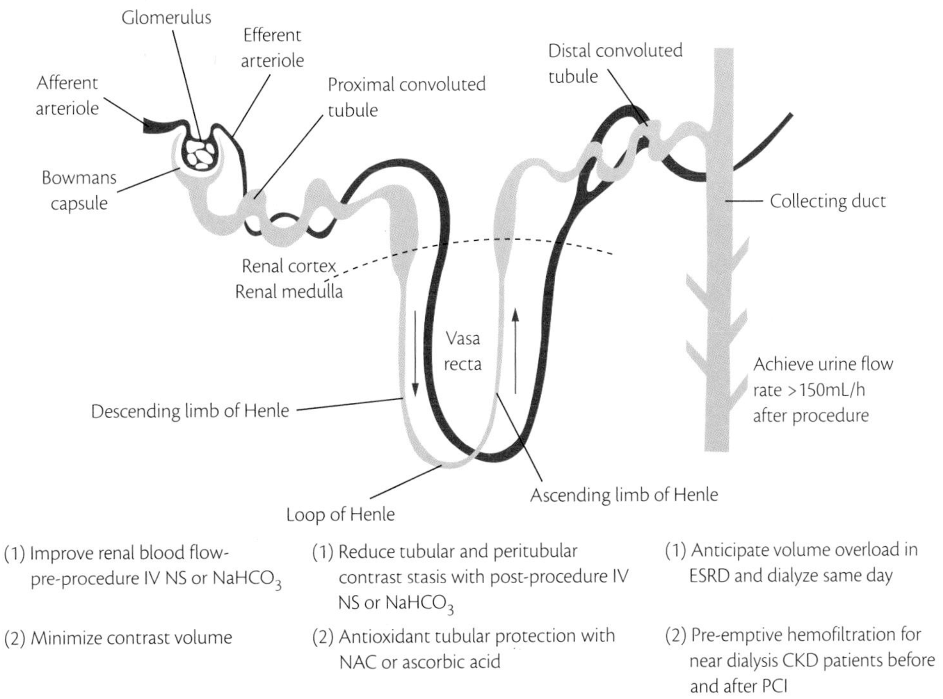

Fig. 27.3 Rationale for steps taken as protective measures against nephron injury in patients undergoing coronary angiography and PCI. NAC, N-acetylcysteine, ESRD, end-stage renal disease on dialysis, IV, intravenous, NS, normal saline, $NaHCO_3$, sodium bicarbonate, CKD, chronic kidney disease.

however, performed 6h before and 12–18h after contrast deserves consideration given reports of reduced mortality and need for haemodialysis in the post-procedure period in very high-risk patients (serum Cr 3.0–4.0mg/dL, eGFR 15–20mL/min/1.73m^2) (Fig. 27.3)[15,16], The interventionalist should be aware that haemofiltration calls for a 5000IU heparin bolus before initiation followed by a continuous heparin infusion of 500–1000IU/h through the inflow side of the catheter. At the time of the cardiac procedure, the haemofiltration treatment should be stopped, and the circuit temporarily filled with a saline solution and short-circuited to exclude the patient without interruption of the flow.

Prophylactic agents

In the absence of a non-toxic radio-opaque contrast agent, there is considerable interest in pharmacologic prophylaxis for iodinated contrast procedures. There are no currently approved pharmacological agents for the prevention of contrast-induced AKI. The pharmacological agents tested in small trials that deserve further evaluation include the antioxidants ascorbic acid and N-acetylcysteine (NAC), statins, aminophylline/theophylline, and prostaglandin E_1. Although popular, NAC has not been consistently shown to be effective in protecting renal tubular cells to the toxic effects of iodinated contrast. To date, 11 meta-analyses have been published on this subject[17–27], and seven of these reports found a net benefit for NAC in the prevention of AKI. However, a recent review by Bagshaw and colleagues found marked heterogeneity in study results in 10 of the 11 meta-analyses[28]. Importantly, only in those trials where NAC reduced serum Cr below baseline values did renal injury rates appear to be reduced. Thus, because NAC reduces the skeletal muscle production of Cr into the bloodstream, it may falsely lower post-contrast Cr and not fundamentally protect against AKI. However, NAC as an antioxidant has been shown to lower rates of AKI and mortality after primary PCI in one trial[29]. Dosing of NAC has varied in the trials; however, the most successful approach has been with high-dose 1200mg PO bid on the day before and after the procedure and this strategy is suggested for clinical practice in those at risk for contrast-induced AKI, particularly in the setting of urgent angiography and PCI[30].

The use of 3-hydroxy-3-methyl-glutaryl-CoA reductase inhibitors, or statins, is an evidence-based approach for the reduction of myocardial infarction and cardiovascular death when administered over the course of several years. The reduction of low-density lipoprotein cholesterol with statins probably confers the majority of this benefit. However, statins have been shown to improved endothelial function and may have protective effects on the kidney. The vast majority of cardiovascular patients undergoing contrast procedures should be on statin therapy before they present to the catheterization laboratory. It has been demonstrated that patients continued on statins during cardiovascular procedures including PCI and coronary artery bypass surgery have lower rates of AKI(31). Small randomized trials published to date support this concept, demonstrating reduced rates of contrast-induced AKI in those treated with statins in the peri-procedural period; however, conclusive trials have not been reported to date(32). Preservation of endothelial function at the level of the glomerulus and reductions in systemic inflammatory factors are postulated mechanisms by which statins may have renoprotective effects(32).

Nephrotoxic drugs including non-steroidal anti-inflammatory agents, gentamicin, amphotericin, and cyclosporin should be discontinued 72h prior to contrast exposure if possible and resumed after renal function has been re-evaluated after the procedure. In addition, metformin should be withheld to minimize the theoretical risk of lactic acidosis should AKI develop and the metformin be continued.

After care

All patients at risk for contrast-induced AKI should have follow-up Cr and electrolyte monitoring daily while in hospital, and then at 48–96h after discharge. Rehospitalization is reasonable for uremic symptoms, hyperkalaemia, and volume overload in the setting of AKI.

Novel biomarkers for contrast-induced AKI

Neutrophil gelatinase-associated lipocalin (NGAL), a member of the lipocalin family, is readily excreted and detected in both blood and urine, due to its small molecular size (25kDa) and resistance to degradation. NGAL production is upregulated in the human kidney cortical tubules, and released into blood and urine after nephrotoxic and ischemic injuries such as exposure to iodinated contrast. Thus, whole blood NGAL might represent an early, sensitive, biomarker for AKI being developed for point-of-care use in the catheterization laboratory, analogous to the use of troponin for myocardial injury(33,34). Alternatively, the urine NGAL to creatinine ratio in the urine may become a clinical measure for the early detection of contrast-induced AKI. All studies to date indicate the rise in NGAL is detected in a matter of hours and much earlier than markers indicating a decline in renal filtration function such as Cr and cystatin C(35).

Future approaches

Future approaches include large planned studies of oral and intravenous antioxidants (including a potent oral antioxidant, deferiprone), intrarenal infusions of renal vasodilators using flow-directed catheters in the procedural suite or intensive care unit, forced hydration using a balancing pump with marked elevations of urine output to reduce the transit time of iodinated contrast in the renal tubules, systemic cooling, and novel, hopefully less toxic forms of radio-opaque contrast agents. One such approach is Veropaque® (Verrow Pharmaceuticals, Inc., Lenexa, KS) which is a reformulation of an existing low-osmolar contrast agent designed for greater direct exit in the urine and less extravasation in the peritubular space, and hence, reduced opportunity for persistent exposure of contrast to the tubules in the outer medulla.

Conclusion

Contrast-induced AKI is a predictable and partially preventable complication after PCI. Reasonable steps should be taken to anticipate and minimize risk. Novel diagnostic and therapeutic approaches are needed to manage the ever-increasing numbers of patients at-risk undergoing interventions using iodinated contrast media(36).

References

1. McCullough PA, Soman SS. Contrast-induced nephropathy. *Crit Care Clin* 2005; **21**(2):261–80.
2. Gleeson TG, Bulugahapitiya S. Contrast-induced nephropathy. *AJR Am J Roentgenol* 2004; **183**(6):1673–89.
3. Nash K, Hafeez A, Hou S. Hospital-acquired renal insufficiency. *Am J Kidney Dis* 2002; **39**(5):930–6.
4. McCullough PA, Stacul F, Davidson C, *et al.* Overview. *Am J Cardiol* 2006; **98**:2K–4K.
5. Bartholomew BA, Harjai KJ, Dukkipati S, *et al.* Impact of nephropathy after percutaneous coronary intervention and a method for risk stratification. *Am J Cardiol* 2004; **93**(12):1515–19.

6. Anderson JL, Adams CD, Antman EM, *et al.* ACC/AHA 2007 Guidelines for the Management of Patients With Unstable Angina/Non-ST-Elevation Myocardial Infarction-Executive Summary A Report of the American College of Cardiology/American Heart Association Task Force on Practice Guidelines (Writing Committee to Revise the 2002 Guidelines for the Management of Patients With Unstable Angina/Non-ST-Elevation Myocardial Infarction) Developed in Collaboration with the American College of Emergency Physicians, the Society for Cardiovascular Angiography and Interventions, and the Society of Thoracic Surgeons Endorsed by the American Association of Cardiovascular and Pulmonary Rehabilitation and the Society for Academic Emergency Medicine. *J Am Coll Cardiol* 2007; **50**(7):652–726.
7. Manske CL, Sprafka JM, Strony JT, *et al.* Contrast nephropathy in azotemic diabetic patients undergoing coronary angiography. *Am J Med* 1990; **89**(5):615–20.
8. Laskey WK, Jenkins C, Selzer F, *et al.* Volume-to-creatinine clearance ratio: a pharmacokinetically based risk factor for prediction of early creatinine increase after percutaneous coronary intervention. *J Am Coll Cardiol* 2007; **50**(7):584–90.
9. Campbell DR, Flemming BK, Mason WF, *et al.* A comparative study of the nephrotoxicity of iohexol, iopamidol and ioxaglate in peripheral angiography. *Can Assoc Radiol J* 1990; **41**(3):133–7.
10. Moore RD, Steinberg EP, Powe NR, *et al.* Nephrotoxicity of high-osmolality versus low-osmolality contrast media: randomized clinical trial. *Radiology* 1992; **182**(3):649–55.
11. Mueller C, Buerkle G, Buettner HJ, *et al.* Prevention of contrast media-associated nephropathy: randomized comparison of 2 hydration regimens in 1620 patients undergoing coronary angioplasty. *Arch Intern Med* 2002; **162**(3):329–36.
12. Merten GJ, Burgess WP, Gray LV, *et al.* Prevention of contrast-induced nephropathy with sodium bicarbonate: a randomized controlled trial. *JAMA* 2004; **291**(19):2328–34.
13. Brar S. A randomized controlled trial for the prevention of contrast induced nephropathy with sodium bicarbonate vs. sodium chloride in persons undergoing coronary angiography (the MEENA trial). Abstract 209-9. Presentation at the 56th Annual Scientific Session of the American College of Cardiology, New Orleans, LA, USA, 24–27 March 2007.
14. Stevens MA, McCullough PA, Tobin KJ, *et al.* A prospective randomized trial of prevention measures in patients at high risk for contrast nephropathy: Results of the P.R.I.N.C.E. study. *J Am Coll Cardiol* 1999; **33**(2):403–11.
15. Marenzi G, Marana I, Lauri G, *et al.* The prevention of radiocontrast-agent-induced nephropathy by hemofiltration. *N Engl J Med* 2003; **349**(14):1333–40.
16. Marenzi G, Lauri G, Campodonico J, *et al.* Comparison of two hemofiltration protocols for prevention of contrast-induced nephropathy in high-risk patients. *Am J Med* 2006; **119**(2):155–62.
17. Birck R, Krzossok S, Makowetz F, *et al.* Acetylcysteine for prevention of contrast nephropathy: Meta-analysis. *Lancet* 2003; **362**:598–603.
18. Isenbarger D, Kent S, O'Malley P. Meta-analysis of randomized clinical trials on the usefulness of acetylcysteine for prevention of contrast nephropathy. *Am J Cardiol* 2003; **92**:1454–8.
19. Alonso A, Lau J, Jaber B, *et al.* Prevention of radiocontrast nephropathy with N-acetylcysteine in patients with chronic kidney disease: A meta-analysis of randomized, controlled trials. *Am J Kidney Dis* 2004; **43**:1–9.
20. Kshirsagar A, Poole C, Mottl A, *et al.* N-acetylcysteine for the prevention of radiocontrast induced nephropathy: A meta-analysis of prospective controlled trials. *J Am Soc Nephrol* 2004; **15**:761–9.
21. Pannu N, Manns B, Lee H, *et al.* Systematic review of the impact of N-acetylcysteine on contrast nephropathy. *Kidney Int* 2004; **65**:1366–74.
22. Guru V, Fremes S. The role of N-acetylcysteine in preventing radiographic contrast-induced nephropathy. *Clin Nephrol* 2004; **62**:77–83.
23. Bagshaw S, Ghali WA. Acetylcysteine for prevention of contrast-induced nephropathy: A systematic review and meta-analysis. *BMC Med* 2004; **2**:38.
24. Misra D, Leibowitz K, Gowda R, *et al.* Role of N-acetylcysteine in prevention of contrast-induced nephropathy after cardiovascular procedures: a meta-analysis. *Clin Cardiol* 2004; **27**:607–10.
25. Nallamothu BK, Shojania KG, Saint S, *et al.* Is acetylcysteine effective in preventing contrast-related nephropathy? A meta-analysis. *Am J Med* 2004; **117**:938–47.
26. Liu R, Nair D, Ix J, *et al.* N-acetylcysteine for prevention of contrast-induced nephropathy: A systematic review and meta-analysis. *J Gen Intern Med* 2005; **20**:193–200.
27. Duong M, MacKenzie T, Malenka D. N-Acetylcysteine prophylaxis significantly reduces the risk of radiocontrastinduced nephropathy. *Catheter Cardiovasc Interv* 2005; **64**:471–9.
28. Bagshaw SM, McAlister FA, Manns BJ, *et al.* Acetylcysteine in the prevention of contrast-induced nephropathy: A case study of the pitfalls in the evolution of evidence. *Arch Intern Med* 2006; **166**:161–6.
29. Marenzi G, Assanelli E, Marana I, *et al.* N-acetylcysteine and contrast-induced nephropathy in primary angioplasty. N Engl J Med 2006; 354(26):2773–82.
30. Briguori C, Airoldi F, D'Andrea D, *et al.* Renal insufficiency following contrast media administration Trial (REMEDIAL): a randomized comparison of 3 preventive strategies. *Circulation* 2007; **115**(10):1211–17.
31. Khanal S, Attallah N, Smith DE, *et al.* Statin therapy reduces contrast-induced nephropathy: an analysis of contemporary percutaneous interventions. *Am J Med* 2005; **118**(8):843–9.

32. McCullough PA, Rocher LR. Statin therapy in renal disease: Harmful or protective. *Curr Atheroscler Rep* 2007; **9**(1):18–24.
33. Bachorzewska-Gajewska H, Malyszko J, Sitniewska E, *et al.* Neutrophil-gelatinase-associated lipocalin and renal function after percutaneous coronary interventions. *Am J Nephrol* 2006; **26**(3):287–92.
34. Mishra J, Dent C, Tarabishi R, *et al.* Neutrophil gelatinase-associated lipocalin (NGAL) as a biomarker for acute renal injury after cardiac surgery. *Lancet* 2005; **365**(9466):1231–8.
35. Endre ZH. Acute kidney injury: definitions and new paradigms. *Adv Chronic Kidney Dis* 2008; **15**(3):213–21.
36. McCullough PA. Contrast-induced acute kidney injury. *J Am Coll Cardiol* 2008; **51**(15):1419–28.

CHAPTER 28

In-stent restenosis in the drug-eluting stent era

Adriano Caixeta, Philippe Généreux, George Dangas, and Roxana Mehran

Introduction

For the last two decades, restenosis has been considered the most significant problem in interventional cardiology. Drug-eluting stents (DES) have reduced rates of restenosis and target lesion revascularization (TLR) by 50–90% compared with bare-metal stents (BMS) across all lesion and patient subsets[1–5]. However, a small number of patients have in-stent restenosis (ISR) after DES treatment. DES efficacy has been limited by suboptimal polymer biocompatibility, suitability of pharmacological agents, suboptimal *in vivo* pharmacokinetic properties, and local drug resistance and toxicity. The first two DES (sirolimus-eluting stents [SES] and paclitaxel-eluting stents [PES]) have the longest clinical follow-up, whereas the zotarolimus-eluting stents [ZES], everolimus-eluting stents [EES], and biolimus-eluting stents [BES] have only recently been introduced in daily practice. Although the low frequency of ISR events with DES makes it difficult to fully investigate this syndrome, many studies have been conducted or are ongoing to find the mechanism, incidence, predictors, and optimal treatment of DES restenosis. This review discusses the data relevant to DES restenosis and the perspective on the current treatment of this condition.

Incidence of DES restenosis

As shown in the pivotal randomized trials comparing DES and BMS, ISR is only observed in a small number of patients (Table 28.1). However, randomized head-to-head DES comparisons have shown higher restenosis rates when compared with the pivotal randomized trials on restenosis in complex lesions[6–11]. It is well known that complex lesions have a higher risk of restenosis even with DES[12], and it should be realized that the real-world performance of DES is not quite the same as that seen in randomized trials, which were largely restricted to de novo coronary lesions with visually moderate lesion length and moderate reference vessel diameter. Clinical registries or observational studies also have been conducted by single or multiple centres to ascertain the efficacy of DES in routine clinical settings[13–19]. The potential for under-reporting clinical events and the low rate of follow-up angiography are the main limitations when using these studies to determine the frequency of restenosis occurring after implantation with DES. One study, the Rapamycin-Eluting Stent Evaluated At Rotterdam Cardiology Hospital (RESEARCH) registry, included a subgroup with mandatory angiographic follow-up in a real-world (unselected) setting[20]. In this registry, both the ISR and clinically-driven TLR rates following SES implantation were reported. Patients with acute myocardial infarction (MI), ISR, 2.25mm diameter SES, left main coronary stenting, chronic total occlusion, stented segment >36mm, or bifurcation stenting were selected to comprise the mandatory angiographic follow-up group. The in-segment restenosis rate at 6 months (238 patients, 441 lesions) was 7.9%. Currently, follow-up angiography after DES implantation usually is recommended at 8–9 months. Therefore, the true ISR rate may be underestimated. Furthermore, the TLR rate was 9.5% at 6 months (486 patients, 1027 lesions) in a large, single-centre experience with SES from Milan[14]. In addition, the target vessel revascularization (TVR) rate was 8.7% at an average of 6.6 months in the multicentre

Table 28.1 Incidence of restenosis after DES implantation in the randomized trials

	Number of DES-treated patients	Follow-up angiography rate	Follow-up period	In-stent restenosis	In-segment restenosis
SES					
RAVEL (5)	120	89%	6 months	0%	0%
SIRIUS (1)	533	66%	8 months	3.2%	8.9%
E-SIRIUS (58)	175	92%	8 months	3.9%	5.9%
C-SIRIUS (57)	50	88%	8 months	0%	2.3%
SES SMART (108)	129	95%	8 months	4.9%	9.8%
DIABETES (109)	80	93%	9 months	3.9%	7.8%
PES					
TAXUS II SR (110)	131	98%	6 months	2.3%	5.5%
TAXUS II MR (110)	135	96%	6 months	4.7%	8.6%
TAXUS IV (75)	662	44%	6 months	5.5%	7.9%
TAXUS V (12)	577	86%	9 months	13.7%	18.9%
TAXUS V ISR (101)	195	88%	9 months	7.0%	14.5%
TAXUS VI (111)	219	96%	9 months	9.1%	12.4%
SES vs. PES					
REALITY(7) SES	648	93%	8 months	7.0%	9.6%
PES	669	91%	8 months	8.3%	11.1%
SIRTAX(8) SES	503	53%	8 months	3.2%	6.6%
PES	569	54%	8 months	7.5%	11.7%
ISAR-DIABETIC(9) SES	180	86%	6–8 months	8.0%	11.4%
PES	180	88%	6–8 months	14.9%	19.0%
ISAR-SMART 3(10) SES	100	91%	6–8 months	11.0%	14.3%
PES	100	92%	6–8 months	18.5%	21.7%
ISAR-DESIRE(11) SES	125	82%	6–8 months	4.9%	6.9%
PES	125	82%	6–8 months	13.6%	16.5%
ZES					
ENDEAVOR II (112)	598	88.5%	8 months	9.4%	13.2%
ZES vs. SES					
ENDEAVOR III ZES	323	87.3%	8 months	9.2%	11.7%
SES	113	83.2%	8 months	2.1	4.3%
ZES vs. PES					
ENDEAVOR IV(113) ZES	770	18.7%	8 months	13.3%	15.3%
PES	772	17.5%	8 months	6.7%	10.4%
EES vs. PES					
SPIRIT II(114) EES	223	92%	6 months	1.3%	3.4%
PES	77	92%	6 months	3.5%	5.8%
EES vs. PES					
SPIRIT III(115) EES	669	51%	8 months	2.3%	4.7%
PES	332	50%	8 months	5.7%	8.9%
BES vs. SES					
LEADERS(116) BES	857	20%	9 months	17.5%	16.4%
SES	850	20%	9 months	19.6%	18.5%

BES, biolimus-eluting stents; EES, everolimus-eluting stents; PES, paclitaxel-eluting stents; SES, sirolimus-eluting stents; ZES, zotarolimus-eluting stents.

prospective German Cypher stent registry, in which 7445 patients were enrolled at 122 hospitals[21], and 6.0% at 1 year in the DEScover registry, which collected data on 6509 patients who underwent DES implantation at 140 medical centres[22]. Long-term clinical outcomes after DES and BMS in the Massachusetts registry[19], including a total of 11 556 patients treated with DES and 6237 treated with BMS, demonstrated TLR rates of 11.0% vs. 16.8% ($P < 0.0001$). Considering that there was no mandatory follow-up coronary angiography in these registries, the true angiographic restenosis rates would be even higher than the figures discussed here. In clinical practice, restenosis rates have been higher after DES implantation in more complex lesions that were excluded from the pivotal randomized trials, probably exceeding 10%.

Clinical presentation of in-stent restenosis

Given its gradual and progressive onset, ISR has been perceived as a benign phenomenon. However, while some cases of ISR are clinically silent, the majority lead to recurrent symptoms, including unstable angina in up to 35% and MI in up to 20% of patients, resulting in repeat revascularization procedures, increased costs, and a substantial increase in patient morbidity[23,24]. Futhermore, in patients presenting with acute coronary syndromes (ACS), the treatment of ISR seems to increase the risk of adverse clinical events during follow-up. The Prevention of REStenosis with Tranilast and its Outcomes (PRESTO) trial compared outcomes in patients presenting with ACS versus stable angina who had previously developed ISR after successful PCI (824 patients had ACS and 617 patients had stable angina). The study showed that an ACS presentation in patients with ISR is associated with a higher incidence of recurrent MACE (35% vs. 22%, $P < 0.001$) and angiographic restenosis (56% vs. 42%, $P = 0.043$) at 9-month follow-up[25].

Of note, some authors have shown that with BMS-related recurrent clinical ischaemia, ISR has occurred at an average of 5.5 months after the previous intervention, with a shorter interval for MI patients than non-MI patients. Futhermore, diffuse ISR also was more frequent in MI patients[26]. On the other hand, there is a paucity of published data on the clinical presentation of ISR related to DES. In one study of 39 ISR cases associated with DES, Lee and colleagues[27] showed that the mean time from PCI to ISR detection was approximately 12 months. Indeed, the time frame to develop clinical signs of restenosis after DES may be longer than after BMS because antiproliferative drugs might delay the biological response to injury. Furthermore, 5% of patients with DES-related ISR presented with unstable angina and 10% with non-ST-segment elevation MI.

The mechanism of late MI associated with ISR is unclear. The most likely explanations are late stent thrombosis due to incomplete neointimal coverage of the stent, early discontinuation of antiplatelet therapy, or increased thrombogenic tissue factor in the neointimal tissue raising the likelihood of thrombosis. Another potential explanation for MI could be the restenosis itself; a profuse and critical ISR may be associated with diminished flow in the vessel that leads to MI.

These studies suggest that ISR observed with DES, similar to BMS-related ISR, is not a benign clinical entity and requires adequate treatment[27].

The pathophysiologic mechanism of restenosis after DES implantation

The clinical effect of each DES model is highly dependent on its components: the platform, the active pharmacologic compound, and the drug carrier. DES technology enables anti-inflammatory, immunomodulatory, and/or anti proliferative agents to be released in appropriate amounts and distributed at the site of arterial injury during the initial 30-day healing period[28]. The rate-controlling system ensures drug retention during stent deployment and modulates drug-elution kinetics[29]. Unless an appropriate dose of the drug is eluted to the target at the proper times, DES lose their ability to reduce neointimal growth. Initial reports suggested that SES restenosis was associated not with intrinsic drug resistance but instead with a discontinuity in stent coverage and local barotrauma outside the stent[30]. However, the precise reasons why DES fail in some patients and in some lesions are still controversial. Multiple factors—biological, mechanical, and technical—may all contribute to restenosis after DES implantation (Table 28.2).

Biological factors

Drug resistance

Sirolimus inhibits the function of the mammalian target of rapamycin (mTOR) and may suppress smooth-muscle-cell migration and proliferation by arresting cells in G1 phase or by inducing apoptosis[31]. However, recent data indicate that genetic mutations or compensatory changes influence sensitivity to the drug, conferring rapamycin resistance[32]. Mutations of

Table 28.2 Possible mechanisms of restenosis after DES

Biological related factors
Drug resistance
Hypersensitivity
Mechanical related factors
Stent underexpansion
Non-uniform stent strut distribution
Stent fracture
Over dilatation of undersized stent
Non-uniform drug deposition
Polymer peeling
Technical related factors
Barotrauma outside the stented segment
Stent gap
Residual uncovered atherosclerotic plaques

mTOR or FKBP12 prevent rapamycin from binding to mTOR. Mutations or defects of mTOR-regulated proteins, including S6K1, 4E-BP1, PP2A-related phosphatases, and p27 (Kip1), also contribute to rapamycin insensitivity. In addition, ATM, p53, PTEN/Akt, and 14-3-3 are associated with rapamycin sensitivity.

Laboratory investigations have revealed a wide variety of mechanisms contributing to paclitaxel resistance[33]. Paclitaxel binds specifically to the β-tubulin subunit of microtubules, and its principal action is to interfere with microtubule dynamics, preventing their depolymerization[31]. Resistance to paclitaxel is associated with increased expression of the mdr-1 gene and its product P-glycoprotein, mutation of β-tubulin, and changes in apoptotic regulatory proteins and mitosis checkpoint proteins as well as possibly with overexpression of interleukin 6 (IL-6)[34,35]. How these drug resistance issues affect restenosis after DES implantation remains unknown.

Hypersensitivity

For BMS and first-generation DES, the predominant platform material is 316L stainless steel. In the BMS era, allergic reactions to nickel and molybdenum released from 316L stainless steel stents was one of the triggering mechanisms for ISR[36]. In DES, the triggers are more complex. DES consist of 3 components: the anti-restenotic drug, the drug carrier vehicle (polymer), and the stent platform. A hypersensitivity reaction to any 1 of these components may lead to restenosis after implantation. In the Research on Adverse Drug/Device events And Reports (RADAR) project, hypersensitivity symptoms were identified in 262 patients among 5,783 adverse event reports from the Food and Drug Administration (FDA) DES database[37]. In those 262 patients, the authors identified 17 cases in which the DES themselves appeared to be a probable cause of hypersensitivity. In other studies, pathology findings from 4 autopsies presented the strongest evidence yet that DES can cause a hypersensitivity reaction. Because the exact incidence is unclear, any patient suspected of having a hypersensitivity reaction after DES implantation should be carefully monitored[38,39]. Nonetheless, the platform material used in many novel balloon-expandable DES is cobalt chromium, which can provide superior radial force and better radiopacity with significantly thinner struts. Cobalt chromium does not appear to trigger the adverse proliferative response and hypersensitivity that accompanies the incorporation of other alloys.

Mechanical factors

Stent underexpansion and non-uniform stent strut distribution

Serial intravascular ultrasound (IVUS) has shown that ISR is primarily caused by neointimal proliferation (Fig. 28.1). However, stent underexpansion is commonly found in restenotic stents, resulting from poor expansion at implantation rather than from chronic stent recoil. The lack of full stent expansion, IVUS-measured stent length > 40 mm, and non-uniform strut distribution (e.g. non-uniform/circular lumen expansion) contribute to increased ISR risk after DES implantation[40–44]. An IVUS study indicates that non-uniform strut distribution—possibly increasing inter-strut space and drug underdosing—contributes to intimal hyperplasia after SES implantation[45]. Still, an IVUS substudy of the SIRIUS trial showed that a post-procedure minimum stent area (MSA) < 5.0 mm^2 was responsible for the majority of cases of restenosis[42].

Stent fracture

A stent fracture can occur in conjunction with restenosis, resulting from a decrease in local drug delivery at the fracture point; it also may be a marker of severe non-uniform stent expansion. Initial case reports and small registries of SES fractures suggested that implantation of long stents concomitantly with post-dilatation using larger balloons at higher pressures is related to coronary stent fractures and that fractured stents are more commonly located in the right coronary artery[46–48]. One observational study reported an incidence of SES fracture of 2.6%[49]. In an additional paper[50], significant predictors of stent fracture were saphenous vein graft location, length of implanted stent, and right

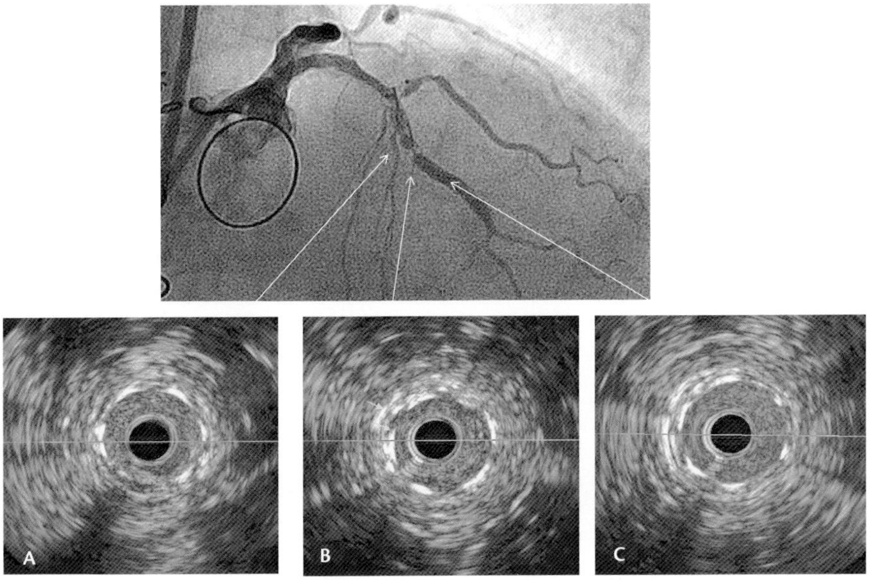

Fig. 28.1 This patient underwent a previous Cypher® implantation at mid left anterior descending artery for the treatment of Cypher® in-stent restenosis (same DES approach to treat DES in-stent restenosis). The angiogram and IVUS show diffuse in-stent re-restenosis with 2 layers of Cypher® stents. Neointimal tissue is packed around the IVUS catheter at panels (A) and (B) where the maximum amount of intimal hyperplasia occurs. Note the two layers of stent on IVUS (arrows). In (C), there is a mild intimal hyperplasia.

coronary artery location. ISR was observed in 37.5% of stent fracture lesions. Stent fracture itself was likely influenced by mechanical stress provoked by rigid structures and locations that served as hinges during vessel movement in the cardiac contraction cycle; both SES and PES fractures have been reported. In another observational study, by Shaikh and colleagues[51], stent fracture was identified by angiography in 19% of all ISR cases; stenting on a bend > 75°, SES implantation, and overlapping stented segments were independent predictors of stent fracture, while larger stent diameter was protective. However, compared with angiography, IVUS more reliably detects stent fracture during follow-up evaluation (Figs. 28.2 and 28.3)[52].

Over-dilatation of an undersized stent

Stent underexpansion is related to DES restenosis. Paradoxically, overdilatation has also been related to a possible increase in restenosis. Extreme post-dilatation of the stent can impair the effectiveness of DES in different ways, such as: by enhancing tissue proliferation in response to greater vessel injury, by altering the mechanical properties of the stent, by disrupting the polymer coating, and by increasing the distance between the stent struts. However, 2 observational, prospective studies concluded that overdilatation of undersized SES with oversized balloons is both safe and effective[53,54]. Despite the rationale behind this hypothesis, it remains unclear what role overdilatation plays in DES ISR.

Non-uniform drug delivery and deposition

The effectiveness of local drug delivery requires transmural and circumferential distribution across and within the vessel walls. After DES implantation, the drug is deposited not only beneath the regions of arterial contact with the stent struts but also beneath the standing pools of drug created where the struts disrupt blood flow. Physiological and computational models have shown that local blood flow alterations and the location of drug elution from the struts are more important in determining arterial wall drug deposition and distribution than drug load or arterial wall contact with the drug-coated strut surface[55]. It appears that alterations in blood flow pattern caused by stent strut conditions such as strut thickness, the depth of strut penetration into the arterial wall, and strut overlap may play an important role in the efficacy of DES. In addition, even small amounts of local mural thrombus attached to the stent struts can affect arterial wall drug uptake and retention. Hwang and colleagues[56] have shown that clots between artery and stent reduce arterial drug uptake, whereas clots overlying the stent can shield drug from washout, thus increasing drug uptake. Furthermore, polymer damage may hamper the

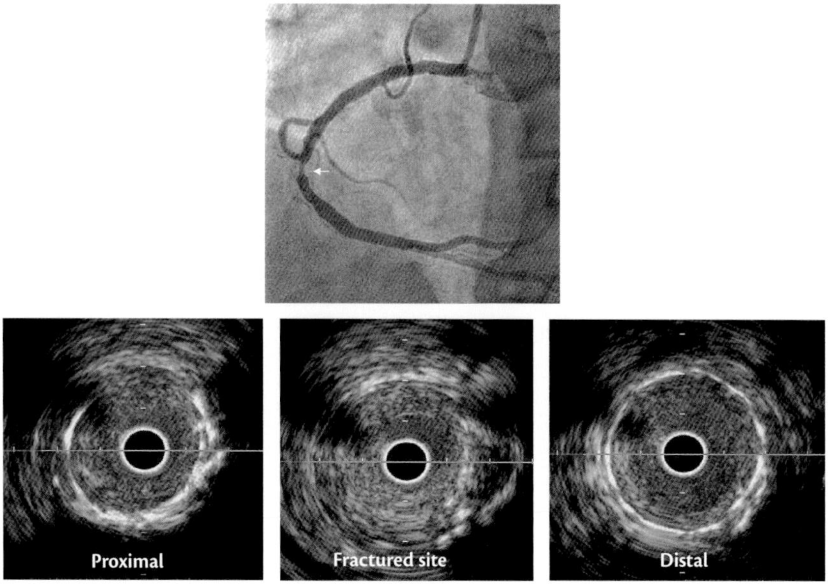

Fig. 28.2 A patient presented with focal in-stent restenosis at follow-up after Taxus® stent implantation in the right coronary artery (arrow on angiogram). On IVUS, all stent struts were seen at proximal and distal references, whereas no stent struts were seen at the fracture site. Note the neointimal tissue at the fracture site.

uniformity of drug elution when DES cross severely calcified lesions.

Technical factors

Barotrauma outside the stented segment

Subgroup analyses in the SIRIUS trial first indicated that the exposed margins of the stents that did not cover the entire balloon-injury region were the primary sites of restenosis. Restenosis occurred predominantly at the proximal stent margin after SES placement[1]. Currently, the recommended technique includes pre-dilatation with shorter balloons, use of a longer single stent in order to cover the entire area of balloon injury, and dilatation within the stented regions using short, high-pressure balloons. Following these recommendations, proximal margin restenosis rates decreased in subsequent studies that followed a revised implantation protocol: the decreased incidence was 5.9% in E-SIRIUS and 2.3% in C-SIRIUS, compared with 5.8% in SIRIUS[57,58]. The use of direct stenting in E-SIRIUS

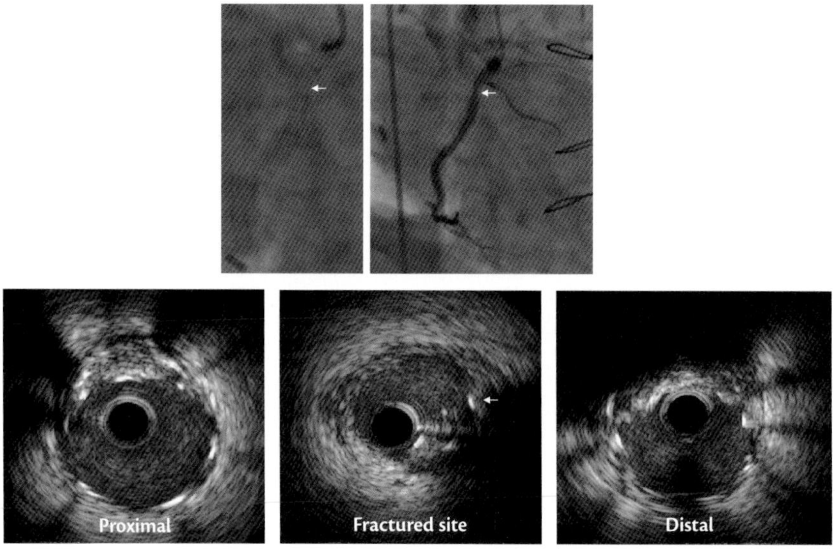

Fig. 28.3 An example of in-stent restenosis at follow-up after Cypher® stent implantation in the right coronary artery (arrows on angiogram). Note the stent fracture with acquired transaction of fluoroscopy. On IVUS, all stent struts were seen at proximal and distal references, whereas only one stent strut was seen at the fracture site (arrow).

and C-SIRIUS also may have limited proximal edge trauma and subsequent restenosis in some patients.

Stent gap

Similar to stent fracture, stent gap can cause discontinuous DES coverage. Theoretically, the amount of local drug deposition in the vessel wall decreases at the gap site. In general, considering the reported safety and efficacy of overlapping DES, stent gap should be avoided[30,59].

Residual uncovered atherosclerotic plaques

When treating ostial and bifurcation lesions, it is sometimes difficult to avoid incomplete lesion coverage. In bifurcation lesions, the recent introduction of DES has resulted in a lower incidence of main branch restenosis compared with historical BMS controls. However, side-branch ostial restenosis remains a problem due to the difficulty of full lesion coverage[60,61]. Various techniques using 1 or 2 stents have been developed to optimize the treatment of bifurcation lesions, such as T-stenting, Y-stenting, V-stenting, crush-stenting, and skirt-stenting[62]. Kissing balloon post-dilatation after crush-stenting increases stent strut apposition as much as possible in the carina and reduces side-branch restenosis, but the optimal technique for treating bifurcation lesions with DES remains controversial[49,63].

The prospective evaluation of the impact of Stent deployment Techniques on cLinicaL outcomes of patients treated with the cypheR stent (STLLR trial)[64] evaluated the frequency of suboptimal PCI and its impact on the long-term outcomes of 1,557 patients treated with SES. The presence of 'geographic miss' during the procedure (i.e. injured or diseased segment not covered by DES or balloon-artery size ratio < 0.9 or >1.3) was associated with an increased risk of TVR and MI at 1 year.

Predictors of DES restenosis

In the DES era, specific characteristics still confer an increased risk for ISR (Table 28.3). The TAXUS V trial has shown that small vessels receiving small-diameter and multiple stents were associated with a higher ISR rate[12]. Several studies focusing on daily clinical practice have also investigated predictors of restenosis after DES implantation[20,65–69]. Initial reports from a multivariate logistic regression analysis of 441 lesions indicated that ISR ostial lesions, diabetes mellitus, total stent length, vessel size, and left anterior descending coronary artery are significant predictors of restenosis after SES implantation[20]. Berenguer and colleagues showed in 263 lesions that female sex and lesion length >30mm were multivariate independent predictors of restenosis after SES implantation[65]. One study evaluated the significant predictors of SES ISR, including clinical, angiographic, procedural, and IVUS predictors[40]. Notably, the only independent predictors of restenosis were IVUS parameters: post-procedural final minimum stent area and stent length.

Recent studies investigating predictors of restenosis after SES and PES implantation have been published by 2 independent centers. In one of the studies, multivariate logistic regression analysis based on angiographic follow-up of 1,703 available lesions revealed that vessel size, type of DES, and final stenosis diameter were significant predictors of binary angiographic restenosis[66]. The other study found that DES type, post-minimal lesion diameter, and lesion length were significant predictors of angiographic restenosis in 2,405 lesions[67]. Predictive factors for DES restenosis, identified from real-world data, including small vessels, longer stents, and stent underexpansion, seem to be similar to those for BMS restenosis[70–72]. Considering that post-minimal lumen diameter is a major factor in restenosis, it is still important to obtain optimal acute angiographic results after DES implantation.

Morphological pattern of DES restenosis

Both the incidence and angiographic patterns of restenosis differ between DES and BMS. After SES implantation, the most common angiographic restenosis pattern is focal. In the SIRIUS trial, 26 of 31 (83.9%) restenotic lesions were focal[73], and this tendency persisted in 2 series from Rotterdam and Milan, showing that in 'real-world' practice settings, 15 of 20 (75%) and 14 of 14 (100%) restenotic lesions were focal[30,74]. In the TAXUS IV study, the pattern of restenosis after PES implantation was predominantly focal (62.5%), yet a considerable percentage (37.5%) of ISR lesions were non-focal (Table 28.4)[75]. In a series of 977 consecutive patients after PES implantation, 98 lesions were identified as ISR, and half of these were focal[76]. In data from 2 independent centres that reported restenosis patterns after SES and PES implantation in an unselected real-world population, there was a significantly higher incidence of diffuse and occlusive restenosis in the PES cohort compared with the SES cohort (Fig. 28.4)[77,78]. Therefore, angiographic restenosis patterns following SES and PES implantation may not be identical, and

Table 28.3 Independent predictors of TLR or ISR after DES implantation

Randomized trials	Independent predictors of TLR	Observational studies	Independent predictors of restenosis
SES arm in the SIRIUS trial[117]	Post procedure in-stent MLD Total implanted stent length	Lemos *et al.*[20]	In-stent restenosis lesion Ostial lesion
PES arm in the TAXUS IV trial[2]	No study stents implanted No prior MI Female gender Lesion length		Diabetes mellitus Vessel size LAD
		Kastrati *et al.*[66]	Vessel size Final diameter stenosis DES type
		Lee *et al.*[67]	DES type Post-intervention MLD Lesion length
		Roy *et al.*[68]	Age Hypertension Procedural length Lack of IVUS guidance Total stented length
		Corbett *et al.*[69]	Diabetes mellitus Unstable angina Reference vessel diameter Number of stents per lesion

DES, drug-eluting stents; IVUS, intravascular ultrasound system; LAD, left anterior descending coronary artery; MI, myocardial infarction; MLD, minimal lumen diameter; PES, paclitaxel-eluting stents; SES, sirolimus-eluting stents; TLR, target lesion revascularization.

Table 28.4 Morphological pattern of DES versus BMS restenosis

	SES (n = 31)	Control (n = 128)	P-value
SIRIUS[73]			
I: focal	83.9%	43.0%	<0.001
II/III: diffuse or proliferative	9.7%	49.2%	<0.001
IV: total occlusion	6.5%	7.8%	0.90
	PES (n = 16)	**Control (n = 65)**	**P-value**
TAXUS IV[75]			
I: focal	62.5%	30.8%	<0.001
II/III: diffuse or proliferative	25.0%	66.2%	<0.001
IV: total occlusion	12.5%	3.1%	0.25

The pattern of restenosis was defined according to the classification of Mehran *et al.*[79]

further investigation in large, head-to-head randomized studies is required before definitively judging any differences.

Prognostic implications for morphologic patterns of ISR

After BMS implantation, the classification of angiographic patterns of ISR has important prognostic significance. Mehran and colleagues reported that TLR at 1 year after repeat intervention for ISR increased progressively with ISR classification (focal 19%, intrastent 35%, proliferative 50%, total occlusion 83%, $P < 0.001$)[79]. After DES implantation, it is unknown whether the morphologic pattern of DES ISR has any impact on the outcome of percutaneous re-treatment. Some studies have shown that the morphologic pattern of DES ISR being treated is an important predictor of outcomes[80,81]. In one study, the rate of restenosis recurrence following previous successful DES ISR PCI was 17.8% in the focal group and 51.1% in the non-focal group ($P = 0.001$); the incidence of TLR at a

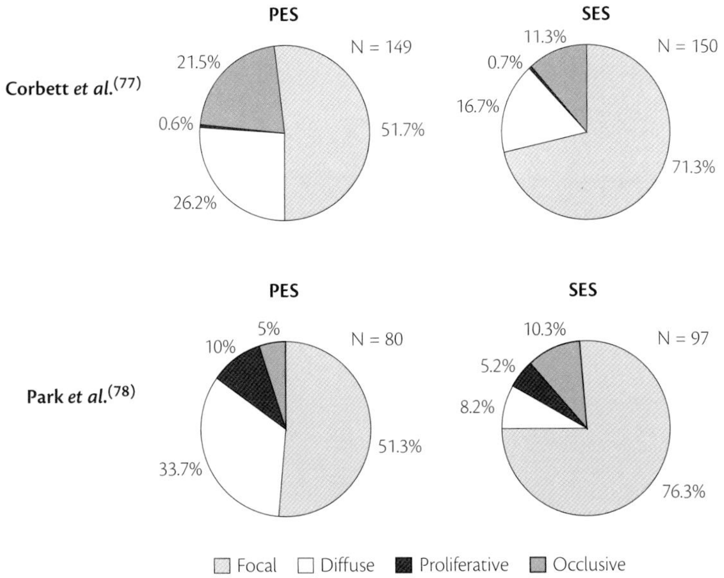

Fig. 28.4 Morphological pattern of DES restenosis (SES vs. PES). Adapted from Corbett SJ, Cosgrave J, Melzi G, *et al.* Patterns of restenosis after drug-eluting stent implantation: Insights from a contemporary and comparative analysis of sirolimus- and paclitaxel-eluting stents. *Eur Heart J* 2006; **27**(19):2330–7 and Park CB, Hong MK, Kim YH, *et al.* Comparison of angiographic patterns of in-stent restenosis between sirolimus- and paclitaxel- eluting stent. *Circulation* 2006; **114**(18,Suppl.):II-642.

median of 13.7 months was 9.8% and 23.0%, respectively (P = 0.007). Similar to BMS, the morphologic pattern of DES restenosis may have an impact on clinical outcomes (Fig. 28.5).

The issue of delayed restenosis

DES dramatically reduce neointimal growth at 6 and 9 months compared with BMS. Although long-term follow-up after DES implantation shows a sustained clinical benefit in several trials, little is known about neointimal growth beyond the first 6–9 months[82–84]. The phenomenon of 'late catch-up' has not been fully investigated with DES. Preclinical porcine studies have consistently demonstrated that the inhibition of neointimal growth after DES implantation does not persist beyond 90 days[85,86]. Previous serial angiographic analyses showed that intimal hyperplasia peaks at 12–16 weeks after intervention and that restenosis rarely occurs beyond 6 months after BMS implantation in humans[87,88]. Furthermore, neointimal hyperplasia regression beyond 6 months after BMS implantation has been described in several reports[88–90]. Histological analyses of post-mortem coronary arteries demonstrate that neointima regression occurs due to the replacement of water-trapping proteoglycans by decorin and type I collagen[91,92]. After DES implantation, however, late restenosis and persistent neointimal growth have been reported. Wessely and colleagues reported on 2 patients with recurrent angina symptoms who were treated with SES at 13 and 19 months, respectively[93]. Of note, both patients had undergone follow-up angiography at 7 months, which revealed excellent angiographic results. Another report, by the Rotterdam team, noted persistent neointimal growth 12 months after intervention and occurrences of delayed restenosis[94]. In 15 patients with left main coronary artery disease treated with DES, average late loss increased from 0.29 mm at 6 months to 0.63 mm at 12 months (P < 0.001). One patient with mild hyperplasia at 6 months received TLR at 12 months due to severe focal restenosis. The finding that neointima may persistently grow beyond 6 months after the index procedure casts doubt on current judgement about the validity of using late loss at 6–9 months as an indicator of post-DES efficacy. Both serial angiographic and IVUS analyses can depict persistent neointimal growth after several kinds of DES implantation (see Table 28.3)[95]. In the TAXUS II study, serial IVUS analyses were performed in 161 patients up to 2 years after deployment of BMS and PES[96]. Whereas the BMS group showed neointimal growth over time, only modest increases occurred in the PES group between 6 months and 2 years. The precise reason for this observation is still unclear

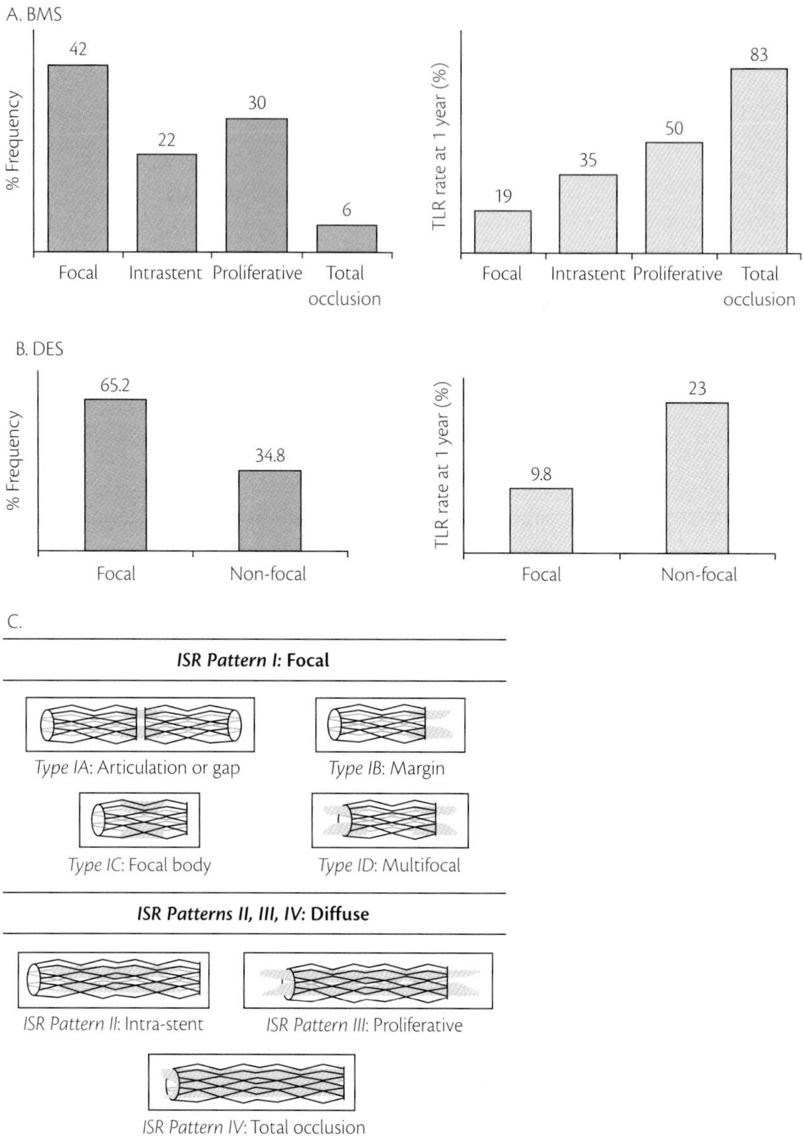

Fig. 28.5 Morphological pattern of ISR predicts clinical outcomes after BMS and DES implantation. Adapted from Mehran R, Dangas G, Abizaid AS, *et al.* Angiographic patterns of in-stent restenosis: classification and implications for long-term outcome. *Circulation* 1999; **100**(18).

but may be related to a delayed healing response, persistent biological reaction caused by the drug soon after implantation, and/or a hypersensitivity reaction to the polymer carried on the stent. Another study showed coronary artery response 4 years after SES implantation using serial IVUS and computer-assisted greyscale value analysis. Neointima kept growing over the entire 4 years, but no statistically significant changes occurred between years 2 and 4. In addition, peri-stent tissue began to shrink with a concomitant increase in echogenicity between 2–4 years. These observations may suggest that the biological phenomenon of delayed healing response begins to subside by 2 years[97]. Further study is warranted to investigate the clinical relevance of this persistent neointimal growth and establish the appropriate length of follow-up after DES implantation.

Approaches to DES restenosis

The optimal treatment for DES restenosis is unknown. Although many observational studies have evaluated clinical and angiographic outcomes after percutaneous treatment for DES restenosis, the numbers of enrolled patients in these studies have been too small and the results too inconsistent to draw any conclusions (Table 28.5). A first report from the team at Rotterdam showed that

Table 28.5 Clinical and angiographic outcomes after percutaneous treatment of DES failure

Author	Restenosis	Treatment	Number of patients (lesions)	Follow-up period	TLR	Angiographic follow-up rate	ISR
Lemos *et al.*[98]	SES	DES	– (23)	490 days	20.8%*	78% (281 days)	42.0%*
		POBA	– (3)				
		BMS	– (1)				
Moussa *et al.*[118]	SES	BMS	18 (18)	12 months	16.7%	–	–
		CBA	2 (2)		0%	–	–
		VBT	1 (1)		100%	–	–
		POBA	1 (1)		100%	–	–
Lee *et al.*[119]	SES	PES	125 (140)	7.2 months	14%	–	–
Nakamura *et al.*[120]	SES	SES	156 (198)	12 months	6.4%	– (12 months)	7.7%
		PES	152 (161)		15.7%		15.7%
Stone *et al.*[121]	PES	DES	7 (7)	2 years	0%	–	–
		BMS	12 (12)		17%	–	–
		POBA	13 (13)		23%	–	–
		VBT	9 (9)		11%	–	–
Kim *et al.*[102]	DES	SES	31 (33)	21.4 months	3.2%	82.8% (6 months)	4%
		CB or VBT	24 (25)		8.3%		35%
Torguson *et al.*[103]	DES	DES	50 (50)	8 months	8%	–	–
		VBT	61 (62)		10%	–	–
Kwak *et al.*[122]	DES	DES	– (31)	–	–	67% (6 months)	10.5%
		CBA	– (21)	–	–		53.8%
Mishkel *et al.*[104]	DES	DES (same)	59 (64)	12 months	28.5%	–	–
		DES (different)	18 (22)		19.0%	–	–
		POBA, BMS, or VBT	15 (22)		36.5%	–	–
Cosgrave *et al.*[81]	DES	DES (same)	96 (107)	25.7 months	16.7%	69.7% (9 months)	26.4%
		DES (different)	78 (94)		16.7%		25.8%
Solinas *et al.*[105]	DES	DES (same)	– (61)	13 months	0%	–	–
		DES (different)	– (36)		8.3%	–	–
de Lezo *et al.*[123]	DES	DES (same)	– (32)	15 months	5.6%*	–	–
		DES (different)	– (47)			–	–
		POBA	– (32)			–	–
Garg *et al.*[106]	DES	DES (same)	62 (–)	12 months	22.5%	–	–
		DES (different)	54 (–)		21.4%	–	–
Solinas *et al.*[124]	DES	DES (same)	37 (–)	12 months	6.7%	–	–
		DES (different)	62 (–)		3.9%		
		POBA	19 (–)		25%		

* Overall incidence.

BMS, bare-metal stents; CBA, cutting balloon angioplasty; DES, drug-eluting stents; ISR, in-stent restenosis; PES, paclitaxel-eluting stents; POBA, plain old balloon angioplasty; SES, sirolimus-eluting stents; TLR, target lesion revascularization; VBT, vascular brachytherapy.

percutaneous treatment for DES restenosis had a high recurrence rate (42%)[98]. In the randomized SIRIUS trial and the meta-analysis of the TAXUS trials, the TLR rate after percutaneous re-treatment was 22.7% at 1 year and 11.5% at 2 years. The variety of treatment options (balloon, cutting balloon, BMS, same DES, different DES, vascular brachytherapy [VBT], or bypass surgery) and varied aetiologies of DES restenosis (as mentioned previously) make it difficult for interventional cardiologists to find an optimal therapy for the condition.

DES for DES restenosis

Since clinical and angiographic results with DES for BMS restenosis were superior to those with conventional therapy (balloon or VBT) in several randomized trials[99–101], DES are used as a re-treatment modality for DES restenosis. Several studies compared the clinical or angiographic effect of repeat DES placement with conventional therapies[102–104] In the Radiation for Eluting Stents in Coronary FailUrE (RESCUE) trial, TLR rates at 8 months in 112 DES restenotic lesions were not significantly different between repeat-DES and conventional VBT groups (8% vs. 10%, P = 1.00)[103]. On the other hand, Kim and colleagues reported a restenosis rate of 4% at 6 months in 58 consecutive lesions with SES treatment compared with 35% with conventional treatment (cutting balloon angioplasty [CBA] and/or VBT) (P = 0.006)[102]. Mishkel and colleagues reported similar results in 108 DES-failure lesions[104]. The 1-year TLR rate was 28.5% in patients given the same DES, 19.0% in patients given a different DES, and 36.5% in patients receiving conventional (CBA, BMS, or VBT) treatments. The efficacy of DES re-treatment seems to render it a feasible option compared with conventional percutaneous treatments. However, no studies have compared DES re-treatment and coronary artery bypass surgery for this indication.

Same or different DES

One of the aetiologies of DES restenosis is drug resistance. Therefore, the placement of a different DES model might more effectively treat DES restenosis than the use of the same DES. Few studies have investigated same or different DES implantation for DES restenosis; in general, these studies have compared SES and PES. To date, there have been no reports on the use of ZES, EES, or BES for this indication. As mentioned previously, the data show that treatment with a different DES tends to result in more favorable outcomes at 12 months than treatment with the same DES[104]. A group from New York has also presented data showing that implantation of a different DES results in more favorable outcomes compared with re-treatment with the same DES[105]. However, data from Milan[81] and Washington[106] showed no difference between implantation of the same DES vs. a different DES in 201 DES restenotic lesions. The randomized GISE-CROSS trial is currently evaluating same vs. different DES as alternate therapies for DES restenosis[107].

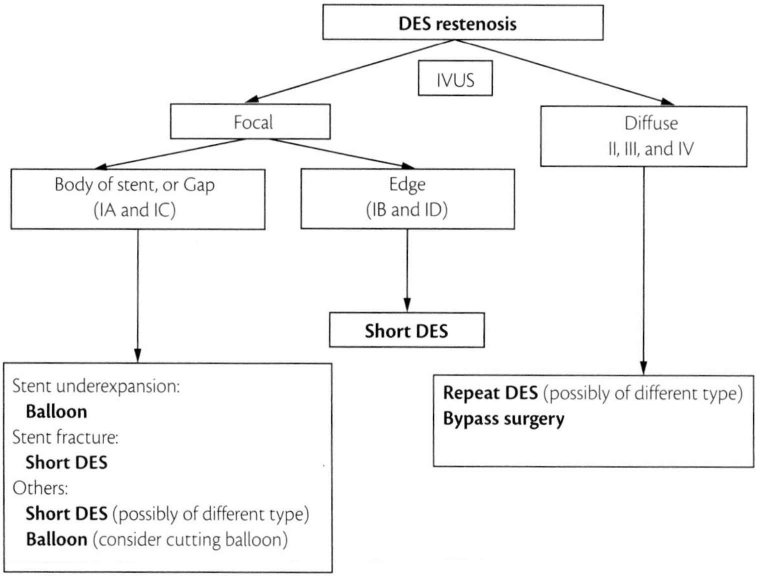

Fig. 28.6 Algorithm for the treatment of DES restenosis.

Proposed treatments of DES restenosis

It is important to consider that therapeutic options for DES restenosis are somewhat controversial as there are few data comparing interventional modalities (balloon, cutting balloon, BMS, same DES, different DES, or VBT) to surgery. The aetiologies of DES restenosis are diverse. Therefore, we recommend that treatment of DES restenosis be 'individualized' using IVUS analysis. Fig. 28.6 depicts a proposed algorithm for the current approach to DES restenosis. There are several known origins of focal DES restenosis. Percutaneous treatments for focal ISR caused by stent underexpansion or fracture and for focal edge restenosis have gained general consensus. However, treatments for focal ISR caused by unclear etiology and for diffuse DES ISR have not met with widespread agreement.

Conclusions

DES result in reduced restenosis rates compared with BMS across all lesion and patient subsets. Angiographic coronary restenosis rates after DES implantation have fallen below 10% in several randomized trials. However, this rate increases when treating complex lesions. Whereas predictors of restenosis after BMS deployment—such as diabetes mellitus, small vessels, and stenting long lesions—are still significant in the era of DES, the morphologic pattern of restenosis is different following BMS vs. DES implantation. The predominant pattern of angiographic restenosis is focal, which is related to better prognosis. However, a diffuse pattern type still exists and is associated with a high incidence of recurrent restenosis. In addition, delayed restenosis and the mechanisms of restenosis with DES have not been fully investigated. Further detailed studies are warranted to understand the development of restenosis in DES and its precise treatment. We anticipate that these studies will become more complex with the emergence of new DES types.

References

1. Moses JW, Leon MB, Popma JJ, *et al.* Sirolimus-eluting stents versus standard stents in patients with stenosis in a native coronary artery. *N Engl J Med* 2003; **349**(14):1315–23.
2. Stone GW, Ellis SG, Cox DA, *et al.* One-year clinical results with the slow-release, polymer-based, paclitaxel-eluting TAXUS stent: the TAXUS-IV trial. *Circulation* 2004; **109**(16):1942–7.
3. Kastrati A, Mehilli J, Pache J, *et al.* Analysis of 14 trials comparing sirolimus-eluting stents with bare-metal stents. *N Engl J Med* 2007; **356**(10):1030–9.
4. Sousa JE, Costa MA, Abizaid AC, *et al.* Sustained suppression of neointimal proliferation by sirolimus-eluting stents: one-year angiographic and intravascular ultrasound follow-up. *Circulation* 2001; **104**(17):2007–11.
5. Morice MC, Serruys PW, Sousa JE, *et al.* A randomized comparison of a sirolimus-eluting stent with a standard stent for coronary revascularization. *N Engl J Med* 2002 Jun 6; **346**(23):1773–80.
6. Rogers C, Edelman ER. Pushing drug-eluting stents into uncharted territory: simpler than you think–more complex than you imagine. *Circulation* 2006; **113**(19):2262–5.
7. Morice MC, Colombo A, Meier B, *et al.* Sirolimus- vs paclitaxel-eluting stents in de novo coronary artery lesions: the REALITY trial: a randomized controlled trial. *JAMA* 2006; **295**(8):895–904.
8. Windecker S, Remondino A, Eberli FR, *et al.* Sirolimus-eluting and paclitaxel-eluting stents for coronary revascularization. *N Engl J Med* 2005; **353**(7):653–62.
9. Dibra A, Kastrati A, Mehilli J, *et al.* Paclitaxel-eluting or sirolimus-eluting stents to prevent restenosis in diabetic patients. *N Engl J Med* 2005; **353**(7):663–70.
10. Mehilli J, Dibra A, Kastrati A, *et al.* Randomized trial of paclitaxel- and sirolimus-eluting stents in small coronary vessels. *Eur Heart J* 2006; **27**(3):260–6.
11. Kastrati A, Mehilli J, von Beckerath N, *et al.* Sirolimus-eluting stent or paclitaxel-eluting stent vs balloon angioplasty for prevention of recurrences in patients with coronary in-stent restenosis: a randomized controlled trial. *JAMA* 2005; **293**(2):165–71.
12. Stone GW, Ellis SG, Cannon L, *et al.* Comparison of a polymer-based paclitaxel-eluting stent with a bare metal stent in patients with complex coronary artery disease: a randomized controlled trial. *JAMA* 2005; **294**(10):1215–23.
13. Lemos PA, Serruys PW, van Domburg RT, *et al.* Unrestricted utilization of sirolimus-eluting stents compared with conventional bare stent implantation in the "real world": the Rapamycin-Eluting Stent Evaluated At Rotterdam Cardiology Hospital (RESEARCH) registry. *Circulation* 2004; **109**(2):190–5.
14. Mikhail GW, Airoldi F, Tavano D, *et al.* The use of drug eluting stents in single and multivessel disease: results from a single centre experience. *Heart* 2004; **90**(9):990–4.
15. Zahn R, Hamm CW, Schneider S, *et al.* Incidence and predictors of target vessel revascularization and clinical event rates of the sirolimus-eluting coronary stent (results from the prospective multicenter German Cypher Stent Registry). *Am J Cardiol* 2005; **95**(11):1302–8.
16. Urban P, Gershlick AH, Guagliumi G, *et al.* Safety of coronary sirolimus-eluting stents in daily clinical practice: one-year follow-up of the e-Cypher registry. *Circulation* 2006; 113(11):1434–41.
17. Abizaid A, Chan C, Lim YT, *et al.* Twelve-month outcomes with a paclitaxel-eluting stent transitioning from controlled trials to clinical practice (the WISDOM Registry). *Am J Cardiol* 2006; **98**(8):1028–32.

18. Russell ME, Friedman MI, Mascioli SR, *et al.* Off-label use: An industry perspective on expanding use beyond approved indications. *J Interv Cardiol* 2006; **19**(5):432–8.
19. Mauri L, Silbaugh TS, Wolf RE, *et al.* Long-term clinical outcomes after drug-eluting and bare-metal stenting in Massachusetts. *Circulation* 2008; **118**(18):1817–27.
20. Lemos PA, Hoye A, Goedhart D, *et al.* Clinical, angiographic, and procedural predictors of angiographic restenosis after sirolimus-eluting stent implantation in complex patients: an evaluation from the Rapamycin-Eluting Stent Evaluated At Rotterdam Cardiology Hospital (RESEARCH) study. *Circulation* 2004; **109**(11):1366–70.
21. Zahn R, Hamm CW, Schneider S, *et al.* Predictors of death or myocardial infarction during follow-up after coronary stenting with the sirolimus-eluting stent. Results from the prospective multicenter German Cypher Stent Registry. *Am Heart J* 2006; **152**(6):1146–52.
22. Williams DO, Abbott JD, Kip KE. Outcomes of 6906 patients undergoing percutaneous coronary intervention in the era of drug-eluting stents: report of the DEScover Registry. *Circulation* 2006; **114**(20):2154–62.
23. Chen MS, John JM, Chew DP, *et al.* Bare metal stent restenosis is not a benign clinical entity. *Am Heart J* 2006; **151**(6):1260–4.
24. Walters DL, Harding SA, Walsh CR, *et al.* Acute coronary syndrome is a common clinical presentation of in-stent restenosis. *Am J Cardiol* 2002; **89**(5):491–4.
25. Assali AR, Moustapha A, Sdringola S, *et al.* Acute coronary syndrome may occur with in-stent restenosis and is associated with adverse outcomes (the PRESTO trial). *Am J Cardiol* 2006; **98**(6):729–33.
26. Nayak AK, Kawamura A, Nesto RW, *et al.* Myocardial infarction as a presentation of clinical in-stent restenosis. *Circ J* 2006; **70**(8):1026–9.
27. Lee MS, Pessegueiro A, Zimmer R, *et al.* Clinical presentation of patients with in-stent restenosis in the drug-eluting stent era. *J Invasive Cardiol* 2008; **20**(8):401–3.
28. Kamath KR, Barry JJ, Miller KM. The Taxus drug-eluting stent: a new paradigm in controlled drug delivery. *Adv Drug Deliv Rev* 2006; **58**(3):412–36.
29. Acharya G, Park K. Mechanisms of controlled drug release from drug-eluting stents. *Adv Drug Deliv Rev* 2006; **58**(3):387–401.
30. Lemos PA, Saia F, Ligthart JM, *et al.* Coronary restenosis after sirolimus-eluting stent implantation: morphological description and mechanistic analysis from a consecutive series of cases. *Circulation* 2003; **108**(3):257–60.
31. Costa MA, Simon DI. Molecular basis of restenosis and drug-eluting stents. *Circulation* 2005; **111**(17):2257–73.
32. Huang S, Houghton PJ. Mechanisms of resistance to rapamycins. *Drug Resist Updat* 2001; **4**(6):378–91.
33. Yusuf RZ, Duan Z, Lamendola DE, *et al.* Paclitaxel resistance: molecular mechanisms and pharmacologic manipulation. *Curr Cancer Drug Targets* 2003; **3**(1):1–19.
34. Orr GA, Verdier-Pinard P, McDaid H, *et al.* Mechanisms of Taxol resistance related to microtubules. *Oncogene* 2003; **22**(47):7280–95.
35. Cabral FR. Isolation of Chinese hamster ovary cell mutants requiring the continuous presence of taxol for cell division. *J Cell Biol* 1983; **97**(1):22–9.
36. Koster R, Vieluf D, Kiehn M, *et al.* Nickel and molybdenum contact allergies in patients with coronary in-stent restenosis. *Lancet* 2000; **356**(9245):1895–7.
37. Nebeker JR, Virmani R, Bennett CL, *et al.* Hypersensitivity cases associated with drug-eluting coronary stents: a review of available cases from the Research on Adverse Drug Events and Reports (RADAR) project. *J Am Coll Cardiol* 2006; **47**(1):175–81.
38. Virmani R, Guagliumi G, Farb A, *et al.* Localized hypersensitivity and late coronary thrombosis secondary to a sirolimus-eluting stent: should we be cautious? *Circulation* 2004; **109**(6):701–5.
39. Azarbal B, Currier JW. Allergic reactions after the implantation of drug-eluting stents: is it the pill or the polymer? *J Am Coll Cardiol* 2006; **47**(1):182–3.
40. Hong MK, Mintz GS, Lee CW, *et al.* Intravascular ultrasound predictors of angiographic restenosis after sirolimus-eluting stent implantation. *Eur Heart J* 2006; **27**(11):1305–10.
41. Mintz GS, Weissman NJ. Intravascular ultrasound in the drug-eluting stent era. *J Am Coll Cardiol* 2006; **48**(3):421–9.
42. Sonoda S, Morino Y, Ako J, *et al.* Impact of final stent dimensions on long-term results following sirolimus-eluting stent implantation: serial intravascular ultrasound analysis from the sirius trial. *J Am Coll Cardiol* 2004; **43**(11):1959–63.
43. Fujii K, Mintz GS, Kobayashi Y, *et al.* Contribution of stent underexpansion to recurrence after sirolimus-eluting stent implantation for in-stent restenosis. *Circulation* 2004; **109**(9):1085–8.
44. Takebayashi H, Mintz GS, Carlier SG, *et al.* Nonuniform strut distribution correlates with more neointimal hyperplasia after sirolimus-eluting stent implantation. *Circulation* 2004; **110**(22):3430–4.
45. Sano K, Mintz GS, Carlier SG, *et al.* Volumetric intravascular ultrasound assessment of neointimal hyperplasia and nonuniform stent strut distribution in sirolimus-eluting stent restenosis. *Am J Cardiol* 2006; **98**(12):1559–62.
46. Umeda H, Gochi T, Iwase M, *et al.* Frequency, predictors and outcome of stent fracture after sirolimus-eluting stent implantation. *Int J Cardiol* 2009; **133**(3):321–6.
47. Sianos G, Hofma S, Ligthart JM, *et al.* Stent fracture and restenosis in the drug-eluting stent era. *Catheter Cardiovasc Interv* 2004; **61**(1):111–6.
48. Halkin A, Carlier S, Leon MB. Late incomplete lesion coverage following Cypher stent deployment for diffuse right coronary artery stenosis. *Heart* 2004; **90**(8):e45.

49. Hoye A, Iakovou I, Ge L, *et al.* Long-term outcomes after stenting of bifurcation lesions with the "crush" technique: predictors of an adverse outcome. *J Am Coll Cardiol* 2006; **47**(10):1949–58.
50. Hamilos MI, Papafaklis MI, Ligthart JM, *et al.* Stent fracture and restenosis of a paclitaxel-eluting stent. *Hellenic J Cardiol.* 2005; **46**(6):439–42.
51. Shaikh F, Maddikunta R, Djelmami-Hani M, *et al.* Stent fracture, an incidental finding or a significant marker of clinical in-stent restenosis? *Catheter Cardiovasc Interv* 2008; **71**(5):614–8.
52. Yamada KP, Koizumi T, Yamaguchi H, *et al.* Serial angiographic and intravascular ultrasound analysis of late stent strut fracture of sirolimus-eluting stents in native coronary arteries. *Int J Cardiol* 2008; **130**(2):255–9.
53. Saia F, Lemos PA, Arampatzis CA, *et al.* Clinical and angiographic outcomes after overdilatation of undersized sirolimus-eluting stents with largely oversized balloons: an observational study. *Catheter Cardiovasc Interv* 2004; **61**(4):455–60.
54. Iakovou I, Stankovic G, Montorfano M, *et al.* Is overdilatation of 3.0 mm sirolimus-eluting stent associated with a higher restenosis rate? *Catheter Cardiovasc Interv* 2005; **64**(2):129–33.
55. Balakrishnan B, Tzafriri AR, Seifert P, *et al.* Strut position, blood flow, and drug deposition: implications for single and overlapping drug-eluting stents. *Circulation* 2005; **111**(22):2958–65.
56. Hwang CW, Levin AD, Jonas M, *et al.* Thrombosis modulates arterial drug distribution for drug-eluting stents. *Circulation* 2005; **111**(13):1619–26.
57. Schampaert E, Cohen EA, Schluter M, *et al.* The Canadian study of the sirolimus-eluting stent in the treatment of patients with long de novo lesions in small native coronary arteries (C-SIRIUS). *J Am Coll Cardiol* 2004; **43**(6):1110–5.
58. Schofer J, Schluter M, Gershlick AH, *et al.* Sirolimus-eluting stents for treatment of patients with long atherosclerotic lesions in small coronary arteries: double-blind, randomised controlled trial (E-SIRIUS). *Lancet* 2003; **362**(9390):1093–9.
59. Kereiakes DJ, Wang H, Popma JJ, *et al.* Periprocedural and late consequences of overlapping Cypher sirolimus-eluting stents: pooled analysis of five clinical trials. *J Am Coll Cardiol* 2006; **48**(1):21–31.
60. Tanabe K, Hoye A, Lemos PA, *et al.* Restenosis rates following bifurcation stenting with sirolimus-eluting stents for de novo narrowings. *Am J Cardiol* 2004; **94**(1):115–8.
61. Colombo A, Moses JW, Morice MC, *et al.* Randomized study to evaluate sirolimus-eluting stents implanted at coronary bifurcation lesions. *Circulation* 2004; **109**(10):1244–9.
62. Iakovou I, Ge L, Colombo A. Contemporary stent treatment of coronary bifurcations. *J Am Coll Cardiol* 2005; **46**(8):1446–55.
63. Ge L, Airoldi F, Iakovou I, *et al.* Clinical and angiographic outcome after implantation of drug-eluting stents in bifurcation lesions with the crush stent technique: importance of final kissing balloon post-dilation. *J Am Coll Cardiol* 2005; **46**(4):613–20.
64. Costa MA, Angiolillo DJ, Tannenbaum M, *et al.* Impact of stent deployment procedural factors on long-term effectiveness and safety of sirolimus-eluting stents (final results of the multicenter prospective STLLR trial). *Am J Cardiol* 2008; **101**(12):1704–11.
65. Berenguer A, Mainar V, Bordes P, *et al.* Incidence and predictors of restenosis after sirolimus-eluting stent implantation in high-risk patients. *Am Heart J* 2005; **150**(3):536–42.
66. Kastrati A, Dibra A, Mehilli J, *et al.* Predictive factors of restenosis after coronary implantation of sirolimus- or paclitaxel-eluting stents. *Circulation* 2006; **113**(19):2293–300.
67. Lee CW, Park DW, Lee BK, *et al.* Predictors of restenosis after placement of drug-eluting stents in one or more coronary arteries. *Am J Cardiol* 2006; **97**(4):506–11.
68. Roy P, Raya V, Okabe T, *et al.* Clinical correlates of restenosis following coronary implantation of drug-eluting stents. *J Am Coll Cardiol* 2007; **49**(9,Suppl.B):4B.
69. Corbett SJ, Cosgrave J, Melzi G, *et al.* Clinical, angiographic and procedural predictors of angiographic restenosis after drug-eluting stent implantation. *Circulation* 2006; **114**(18,Supplement):II-688.
70. Kastrati A, Schomig A, Elezi S, *et al.* Predictive factors of restenosis after coronary stent placement. *J Am Coll Cardiol* 1997; **30**(6):1428–36.
71. Cutlip DE, Chauhan MS, Baim DS, *et al.* Clinical restenosis after coronary stenting: perspectives from multicenter clinical trials. *J Am Coll Cardiol* 2002; **40**(12):2082–9.
72. Cutlip DE, Chhabra AG, Baim DS, *et al.* Beyond restenosis: five-year clinical outcomes from second-generation coronary stent trials. *Circulation* 2004; **110**(10):1226–30.
73. Popma JJ, Leon MB, Moses JW, *et al.* Quantitative assessment of angiographic restenosis after sirolimus-eluting stent implantation in native coronary arteries. *Circulation* 2004; **110**(25):3773–80.
74. Colombo A, Orlic D, Stankovic G, *et al.* Preliminary observations regarding angiographic pattern of restenosis after rapamycin-eluting stent implantation. *Circulation* 2003; **107**(17):2178–80.
75. Stone GW, Ellis SG, Cox DA, *et al.* A polymer-based, paclitaxel-eluting stent in patients with coronary artery disease. *N Engl J Med* 2004; **350**(3):221–31.
76. Iakovou I, Schmidt T, Ge L, *et al.* Angiographic patterns of restenosis after paclitaxel-eluting stent implantation. *J Am Coll Cardiol* 2005; **45**(5):805–6.

77. Corbett SJ, Cosgrave J, Melzi G, *et al.* Patterns of restenosis after drug-eluting stent implantation: Insights from a contemporary and comparative analysis of sirolimus- and paclitaxel-eluting stents. *Eur Heart J* 2006; **27**(19):2330–7.
78. Park CB, Hong MK, Kim YH, *et al.* Comparison of angiographic patterns of in-stent restenosis between sirolimus- and paclitaxel- eluting stent. *Circulation* 2006; **114**(18,Suppl.):II-642.
79. Mehran R, Dangas G, Abizaid AS, *et al.* Angiographic patterns of in-stent restenosis: classification and implications for long-term outcome. *Circulation* 1999; **100**(18):1872–8.
80. Cosgrave J, Melzi G, Biondi-Zoccai GG, *et al.* Drug-eluting stent restenosis the pattern predicts the outcome. *J Am Coll Cardiol* 2006; **47**(12):2399–404.
81. Cosgrave J, Melzi G, Corbett S, *et al.* Repeated drug-eluting stent implantation for drug-eluting stent restenosis: the same or a different stent. *Am Heart J* 2007; **153**(3):354–9.
82. Sousa JE, Costa MA, Abizaid A, *et al.* Four-year angiographic and intravascular ultrasound follow-up of patients treated with sirolimus-eluting stents. *Circulation* 2005; **111**(18):2326–9.
83. Fajadet J, Morice MC, Bode C, *et al.* Maintenance of long-term clinical benefit with sirolimus-eluting coronary stents: three-year results of the RAVEL trial. *Circulation* 2005; **111**(8):1040–4.
84. Weisz G, Leon MB, Holmes DR, Jr, *et al.* Two-year outcomes after sirolimus-eluting stent implantation: results from the Sirolimus-Eluting Stent in de Novo Native Coronary Lesions (SIRIUS) trial. *J Am Coll Cardiol* 2006; **47**(7):1350–5.
85. Carter AJ, Aggarwal M, Kopia GA, *et al.* Long-term effects of polymer-based, slow-release, sirolimus-eluting stents in a porcine coronary model. *Cardiovasc Res* 2004; **63**(4):617–24.
86. Farb A, Heller PF, Shroff S, *et al.* Pathological analysis of local delivery of paclitaxel via a polymer-coated stent. *Circulation* 2001; **104**(4):473–9.
87. Kimura T, Yokoi H, Nakagawa Y, *et al.* Three-year follow-up after implantation of metallic coronary-artery stents. *N Engl J Med* 1996; **334**(9):561–6.
88. Kimura T, Abe K, Shizuta S, *et al.* Long-term clinical and angiographic follow-up after coronary stent placement in native coronary arteries. *Circulation* 2002; **105**(25):2986–91.
89. Asakura M, Ueda Y, Nanto S, *et al.* Remodeling of in-stent neointima, which became thinner and transparent over 3 years: serial angiographic and angioscopic follow-up. *Circulation* 1998; **97**(20):2003–6.
90. Kuroda N, Kobayashi Y, Nameki M, *et al.* Intimal hyperplasia regression from 6 to 12 months after stenting. *Am J Cardiol* 2002; **89**(7):869–72.
91. Farb A, Sangiorgi G, Carter AJ, *et al.* Pathology of acute and chronic coronary stenting in humans. *Circulation* 1999; **99**(1):44–52.
92. Farb A, Kolodgie FD, Hwang JY, *et al.* Extracellular matrix changes in stented human coronary arteries. *Circulation* 2004; **110**(8):940–7.
93. Wessely R, Kastrati A, Schomig A. Late restenosis in patients receiving a polymer-coated sirolimus-eluting stent. *Ann Intern Med.* 2005; **143**(5):392–4.
94. Valgimigli M, Malagutti P, van Mieghem CA, *et al.* Persistence of neointimal growth 12 months after intervention and occurrence of delayed restenosis in patients with left main coronary artery disease treated with drug-eluting stents. *J Am Coll Cardiol* 2006; **47**(7):1491–4.
95. Aoki J, Abizaid A, Ong AT, Serial assessment of tissue growth inside and outside the stent after implantation of drug-eluting stent in clinical trials. Does delayed neointimal growth exist? *EuroIntervention* 2005; **1**(3):253–5.
96. Aoki J, Colombo A, Dudek D, *et al.* Peristent remodeling and neointimal suppression 2 years after polymer-based, paclitaxel-eluting stent implantation: insights from serial intravascular ultrasound analysis in the TAXUS II study. *Circulation* 2005; **112**(25):3876–83.
97. Aoki J, Abizaid AC, Serruys PW, *et al.* Evaluation of four-year coronary artery response after sirolimus-eluting stent implantation using serial quantitative intravascular ultrasound and computer-assisted grayscale value analysis for plaque composition in event-free patients. *J Am Coll Cardiol* 2005; **46**(9):1670–6.
98. Lemos PA, van Mieghem CA, Arampatzis CA, *et al.* Post-sirolimus-eluting stent restenosis treated with repeat percutaneous intervention: late angiographic and clinical outcomes. *Circulation* 2004; **109**(21):2500–2.
99. Alfonso F, Perez-Vizcayno MJ, Hernandez R, *et al.* A randomized comparison of sirolimus-eluting stent with balloon angioplasty in patients with in-stent restenosis: results of the Restenosis Intrastent: Balloon Angioplasty Versus Elective Sirolimus-Eluting Stenting (RIBS-II) trial. *J Am Coll Cardiol* 2006; **47**(11):2152–60.
100. Holmes DR, Jr, Teirstein P, Satler L, *et al.* Sirolimus-eluting stents vs vascular brachytherapy for in-stent restenosis within bare-metal stents: the SISR randomized trial. *JAMA* 2006; **295**(11):1264–73.
101. Stone GW, Ellis SG, O'Shaughnessy CD, *et al.* Paclitaxel-eluting stents vs vascular brachytherapy for in-stent restenosis within bare-metal stents: the TAXUS V ISR randomized trial. *JAMA* 2006; **295**(11):1253–63.
102. Kim YH, Lee BK, Park DW, *et al.* Comparison with conventional therapies of repeated sirolimus-eluting stent implantation for the treatment of drug-eluting coronary stent restenosis. *Am J Cardiol* 2006; **98**(11):1451–4.
103. Torguson R, Sabate M, Deible R, *et al.* Intravascular brachytherapy versus drug-eluting stents for the treatment of patients with drug-eluting stent restenosis. *Am J Cardiol* 2006; **98**(10):1340–4.

104. Mishkel GJ, Moore AL, Markwell S, *et al.* Long-term outcomes after management of restenosis or thrombosis of drug-eluting stents. *J Am Coll Cardiol* 2007; **49**(2):181–4.
105. Solinas E, Kirtane A, Dangas G, *et al.* Long term (one year) follow-up after treatment of drug-eluting stent restenosis (DES-ISR) with repeat DES: to switch or not to switch? *J Am Coll Cardiol* 2007; **49**(9, Suppl.B):26B.
106. Garg S, Smith K, Torguson R, *et al.* Treatment of drug-eluting stent restenosis with the same versus different drug-eluting stent. *Catheter Cardiovasc Interv* 2007; **70**(1):9–14.
107. Costa MA. Treatment of drug-eluting stent restenosis. *Am Heart J* 2007; **153**(4):447–9.
108. Ardissino D, Cavallini C, Bramucci E, *et al.* Sirolimus-eluting vs uncoated stents for prevention of restenosis in small coronary arteries: a randomized trial. *JAMA* 2004; **292**(22):2727–34.
109. Sabate M, Jimenez-Quevedo P, Angiolillo DJ, *et al.* Randomized comparison of sirolimus-eluting stent versus standard stent for percutaneous coronary revascularization in diabetic patients: the diabetes and sirolimus-eluting stent (DIABETES) trial. *Circulation* 2005; **112**(14):2175–83.
110. Colombo A, Drzewiecki J, Banning A, *et al.* Randomized study to assess the effectiveness of slow- and moderate-release polymer-based paclitaxel-eluting stents for coronary artery lesions. *Circulation* 2003; **108**(7):788–94.
111. Dawkins KD, Grube E, Guagliumi G, *et al.* Clinical efficacy of polymer-based paclitaxel-eluting stents in the treatment of complex, long coronary artery lesions from a multicenter, randomized trial: support for the use of drug-eluting stents in contemporary clinical practice. *Circulation* 2005; **112**(21):3306–13.
112. Fajadet J, Wijns W, Laarman GJ, *et al.* Randomized, double-blind, multicenter study of the Endeavor zotarolimus-eluting phosphorylcholine-encapsulated stent for treatment of native coronary artery lesions: clinical and angiographic results of the ENDEAVOR II trial. *Circulation* 2006; **114**(8):798–806.
113. Leon M. ENDEAVOR IV. A randomized comparison of a zotarolimus-eluting stent and paclitaxel-eluting stent in patients with coronary artery disease: 8-month angiographic and 9- and 12-month clinical results. Presented at Transcatheter Cardiovascular Terapeutics, Washington, DC. October 2007.
114. Serruys PW, Ruygrok P, Neuzner J, *et al.* A randomized comparison of an everolimus-eluting coronary stent with a paclitaxel-eluting coronary stent: the SPIRIT II trial. *EuroIntervention* 2006; **2**:286–94.
115. Stone GW, Midei M, Newman W, *et al.* Comparison of an everolimus-eluting stent and a paclitaxel-eluting stent in patients with coronary artery disease: a randomized trial. *JAMA* 2008; **299**(16):1903–13.
116. Windecker S, Serruys PW, Wandel S, *et al.* Biolimus-eluting stent with biodegradable polymer versus sirolimus-eluting stent with durable polymer for coronary revascularisation (LEADERS): a randomised non-inferiority trial. *Lancet* 2008; **372**(9644):1163–73.
117. Holmes DR, Jr, Leon MB, Moses JW, *et al.* Analysis of 1-year clinical outcomes in the SIRIUS trial: a randomized trial of a sirolimus-eluting stent versus a standard stent in patients at high risk for coronary restenosis. *Circulation* 2004; **109**(5):634–40.
118. Moussa ID, Moses JW, Kuntz RE, *et al.* The fate of patients with clinical recurrence after sirolimus-eluting stent implantation (a two-year follow-up analysis from the SIRIUS trial). *Am J Cardiol* 2006; **97**(11):1582–4.
119. Lee SS, Price MJ, Wong GB, *et al.* Early- and medium-term outcomes after paclitaxel-eluting stent implantation for sirolimus-eluting stent failure. *Am J Cardiol* 2006; **98**(10):1345–8.
120. Nakamura S, Bae JH, Cahyadi YH, *et al.* Impact of sirolimus-eluting stent and paclitaxel-eluting stent on the outcome of patients with sirolimus-eluting stent failure: multicenter registry in asia. *J Am Coll Cardiol* 2007; **49**(9,Suppl.B):39B.
121. Stone GW, Colmbo A, Grube E, *et al.* Long-term outcomes following treatment of in-stent restenosis with drug-eluting stents: insight from the TAXUS meta-analysis. *Circulation* 2006; **114**(18,Suppl.):II-689.
122. KwaK JJ, Kim YS, Suh JW, *et al.* Drug-eluting stent implantation versus cutting balloon angioplasty for in-stent restenosis of drug-eluting stent. *Am J Cardiol* 2006; **98**(Suppl.8A):177M.
123. de Lezo JS, Segura J, Pan M, *et al.* Clinical outcome of patients with coronary restenosis after drug eluting stents. *Circulation* 2006; **114**(18,Suppl.):II-689.
124. Solinas E, Dangas G, Kirtane AJ, *et al.* Angiographic patterns of drug-eluting stent restenosis and one-year outcomes after treatment with repeated percutaneous coronary intervention. *Am J Cardiol* 2008; **102**(3):311–5.

CHAPTER 29

Stent thrombosis

Mariuca Vasa-Nicotera and
Tony Gershlick

Summary

Over the past three decades, new strategies have rapidly evolved to achieve coronary reperfusion of ischaemic myocardium in patients with coronary artery disease (CAD). Studies comparing percutaneous coronary intervention (PCI) with coronary artery bypass grafting (CABG) have shown that the long-term rates of death and/or myocardial infarction (MI) are substantially the same[1,2], justifying the increasing and widespread use of PCI. PCI is the dominant reperfusion therapy for such patients with the ratio of numbers of PCIs undertaken to CABG performed being 4:1 in the United Kingdom and up to 8:1 in other parts of Europe. A recurrent issue during the evolution of PCI has been the difference between PCI and CABG in the percentage of patients requiring a repeat procedure (reintervention). To date, the need of reintervention has been less with CABG and this is due to the development of in-stent restenosis that occurs after PCI. Restenosis is the re-narrowing of the vessel, which requires a repeat procedure. The rate of restenosis with early balloon angioplasty has been high. The implantation of bare metal stents (BMS) and then drug-eluting stents (DES) has reduced significantly the incidence of restenosis. While such improved overall clinical outcomes with DES has supported the use of these in preference to BMS, another long-term complication has somewhat tempered the enthusiasm for their use: the possibility that implantation of DES would result in an excess of occlusive stent thrombosis (ST).

This chapter will analyse the data on the incidence, causes, and clinical consequences of ST, and will outline the ongoing and future preventive and therapeutic initiatives. Finally, the risk/benefit of DES will be addressed.

Introduction

Progressive atheromatous narrowing of the coronary arteries can lead to pharmacotherpy-resistant angina pectoris. Patients who have significant symptoms despite medication and in whom objective evidence of ischaemia has been demonstrated should be referred for coronary angiography. For many years, and certainly until the mid 1990s, CABG was considered the gold standard revascularization treatment to relieve symptoms and improve prognosis. The introduction of percutaneous balloon angioplasty (in 1977) followed some 10 years later by the implantation of intracoronary stents has, despite initial drawbacks, revolutionized treatment of patients with coronary heart disease. Simple balloon angioplasty was associated with a high rate of restenosis (leading to a need for reintervention in up to 35% of patients). Furthermore, balloon inflation caused vessel wall/intimal dissection, potentially resulting in abrupt vessel closure and thus a need for emergency CABG. Coronary stents prevent abrupt vessel closure, reduce vessel recoil (one of the causes of restenosis), and thus reduce the rate of restenosis, to a rate with BMS of approximately 15%. BMS development therefore produced a major change in patient care with a shift from CABG towards PCI—for example, by 2007 there were 77 373 PCI, versus 23 000 CABG, performed per year in the UK.

BMS were, however, prone to restenosis due to in-stent scar tissue response with 15% of BMS cases still requiring reintervention. To attenuate restenosis after bare-metal stenting, DES (stent ± polymer coated with an eluting antiproliferative agent) were introduced, in 2000, following *in vitro*, animal and pilot, first-in-man, studies. Randomized trials and registries since 2002 have shown that DES reduce the need for subsequent

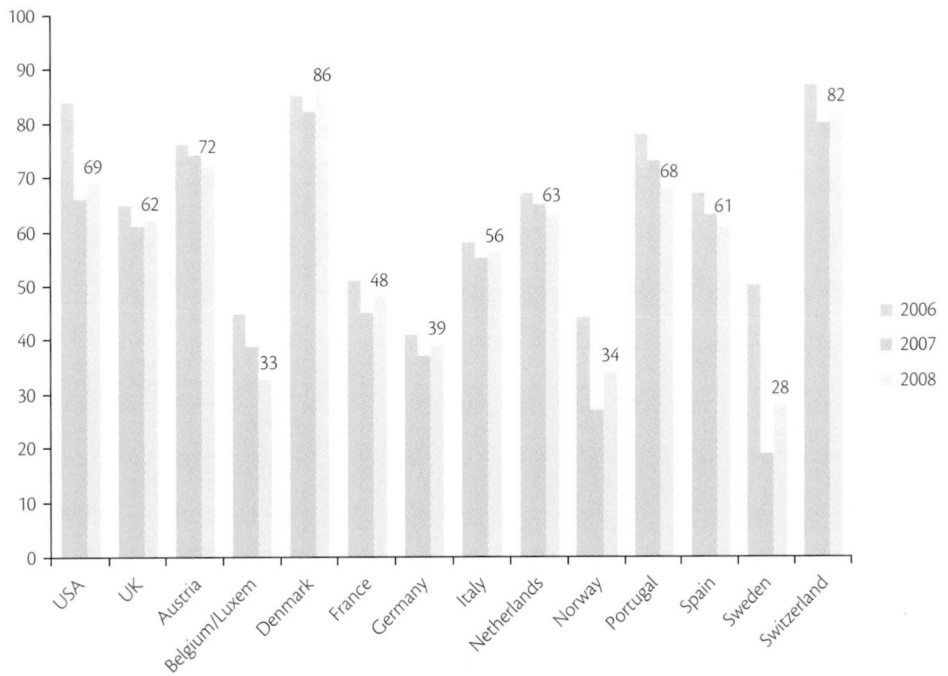

Fig. 29.1 Drug-eluting stent penetration (%) worldwide.

revascularization procedures by about 65%, when compared with BMS[3–8]. In 2006, coronary stents were deployed in 94.7% of the PCI performed in the United Kingdom, of which 63.5% were DES[9]. Similar patterns have been reported worldwide (Fig. 29.1). In the United Kingdom, the National Institute of Health and Clinical Excellence (NICE) recommends the use of DES based on the anatomy of the target vessel for stenting (less than 3mm in calibre–internal diameter, or lesion longer than 15mm).

As early as 2004, however, there appeared reports of cases of 'late' ST (Fig. 29.2). McFadden and colleagues[10] reported on four cases of late ST all of whom had stopped all antiplatelet therapy. In 2006 in a presentation to the European Society of Cardiology, Camenzind and colleagues suggested there may be a significant association between the use of DES and excess mortality, as a result of this late incidence of ST[11]. While this presentation has never been published as a full paper, it did however raise serious concerns and prompted a dramatic decrease in the use of DES to 55% in the United Kingdom in 2007 and even lower usage in other countries (e.g. to 17% in Sweden). ST occurring as an acute event and possible outside of the hospital was associated with serious cardiovascular events, including acute (thrombotic) myocardial infarction (AMI) and even death. The concerns regarding the potential for late ST initiated a major review of the available research data including re-analysis of all the previous randomized controlled clinical trials at individual patient data level and reconsideration of all previous registries. New prospective studies, such as the PROTECT trial which will investigate ST in two different DES over 3 years in more than 8000 patient were initiated, and such studies are designed to evaluate the long-term safety and efficacy outcome in patients treated with DES. What is clear is that irrespective of the incidence (and estimates have varied over the last 4–5 years due to changes in definition and determination of time of occurrence), the consequences of developing ST (with its sudden occlusion of the stent and interruption of blood flow) may be very serious indeed. If it occurs it can be associated with a 20% mortality and with non-fatal MI in 70% of cases[12]. The consequences of even a slight increase in the rates of death and MI are dramatic, considering the current high numbers

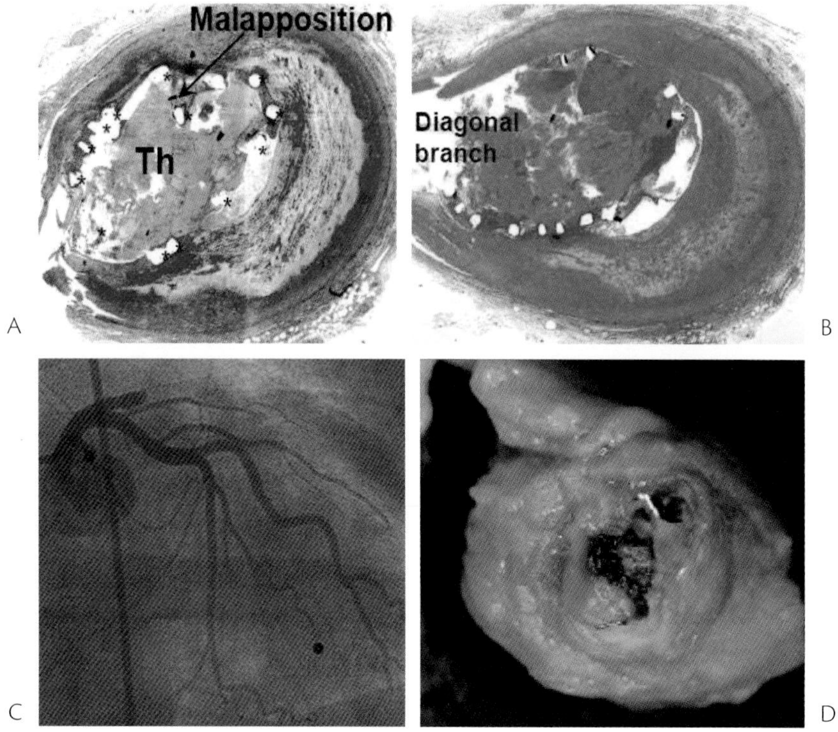

Fig. 29.2 Stent thrombosis.

of DES used—if two million DES are implanted worldwide each year and the incidence of ST is only 1%, then clearly many patients could be suffering important adverse clinical consequences.

What is stent thrombosis? How do we define it?

The Academic Research Consortium (ARC) have recently reviewed and published on the definition of ST and categorized this according to[13]:

- The timing after initial PCI
- The evidence for ST.

Timing of stent thrombosis

ST is considered as being 'acute' when it has occurred between 0–24h after stent implantation, 'subacute' between 24h and 30 days, 'late' between 30 days and 1 year, and 'very late' after 1 year. Acute and subacute ST are sometimes replaced with the term 'early' ST.

Definite ST is defined as when there is angiographic confirmation of ST (the presence of a thrombotic occlusion that originates in the stent or in the segment 5mm proximal or distal to the stent) together with the presence of at least one of the following criteria within a 48-h window: acute onset of ischaemic symptoms at rest; new ischaemic electrocardiographic changes that suggest acute ischaemia or a typical rise and fall in cardiac biomarkers; or in the presence of a pathological confirmation of ST (evidence or recent thrombus within the stent determined at autopsy or via examination of tissue retrieved following thrombectomy). The incidental angiographic documentation of stent occlusion in the absence of clinical signs or symptoms is not considered a confirmed ST (silent occlusion).

Probable ST is defined as the presence of any unexplained death within the first 30 days after stent implantation, or in the presence of any MI related to documented acute ischaemia in the territory of the implanted stent, without necessarily angiographic confirmation of ST and in the absence of any other obvious cause, irrespective of the time after the index procedure.

Possible ST is defined as any unexplained death from 30 days after PCI until the end of follow-up.

What is happening in the stent?

The pathophysiology of stent thrombosis

Several pathogenic factors may be important in the development of ST. In general these factors come into play at the different stages of interaction between the stent, the blood, and the vessel wall. There are those linked to the clinical procedure, those related to the patient's underlying comorbidities (such as the presence of diabetes), and factors associated with lesion characteristics, while others, such as platelet reactivity, vascular healing, stent-induced inflammation, and haemodynamic factors, e.g. vasoconstriction and shear stress, play an important mechanistic role in determining the onset of ST. In addition, the type of stent (BMS or DES), the polymer coating on the DES, and the drug that is being eluted can all have a major role in adversely affecting the healing process and thus potentially trigger ST.

Vascular reaction to injury

The vessel wall and platelet reactivity

The intact endothelium has an essential role in regulating thrombosis and haemostasis. Under physiological conditions, endothelial cells produce both pro- and antithrombotic factors. The former include von Willebrand and tissue factors, whereas nitric oxide and prostacyclins have both vasodilating and antithrombotic functions. Injury to the endothelial layer can result in the local loss of regulation of the balance between pro- and antithrombotic factors. Balloon angioplasty or stent implantation cause disruption of the endothelial layer. Exposure of subendothelial extracellular matrix and lipids to the blood flow and loss of the endothelial modulatory haemostasis function can promote thrombosis. The response to endothelial injury is well understood[14] and involves platelet adhesion, activation, and aggregation. This will lead to platelet deposition in the region of, and particularly to, the stent, which can initiate the process of ST. A causal relationship between the extent of platelet reactivity and the occurrence of ST has been proposed[15,16]. The mechanisms responsible for enhanced platelet reactivity in response to endothelial damage involve the interaction with, and the activation of, the coagulation cascade. Exposure of tissue factor after vascular injury triggers the formation of an active complex with the coagulation factor VIIa, which has proteolytic activity on factor X. The resulting product, factor Xa, activates prothrombin to thrombin on the surface of activated platelets. Platelet activation follows their adhesion to injured vessel wall triggered by exposure of collagen and von Willebrand factor. At this stage, platelets will release secondary mediators including ADP and thromboxane A2 that will recruit further platelets to the process. These will aggregate via glycoprotein (GP) IIb/IIIa mediated fibrinogen cross-linking.

While platelet reactivity has been implicated in both early and late ST, a confounding issue is the potentially wide inter-individual variability in the individual response to antiplatelet therapy. Following stenting, dual antiplatelet therapy (DAPT) with aspirin and clopidogrel is mandatory and its premature discontinuation when the stent struts are still exposed, is the most important predictor of ST[17]. However, even when antiplatelet therapy is prolonged, a residual heightened platelet activity may be linked to late occurrence of ST and thrombosis can occur when either of the components of the dual antiplatelet is discontinued. Variation in individual response to clopidogrel may be an important factor in ST, most of which occurs early (within the first few days) after the procedure when the prothrombotic influences are greatest. Changes in dose or agent especially during this early period may have significant beneficial influence on early and thus the overall burden of ST.

Re-endothelialization

Stent deployment causes disruption of the inner vessel wall with denudation of the endothelium exposing thrombogenic factors to the blood flow (Fig. 29.3). Thus, rapid re-endothelialization of the stented segment is a prerequisite to decreasing the risk of platelet aggregation and favouring vascular healing. Animal studies have shown that re-endothelialization is completed between 2-4 weeks after implantation of BMS[18]. These observations are supported by angioscopic and autopsy studies in humans[19,20]. In contrast, while DES reduce restenosis typical of BMS by inhibiting smooth muscle cell proliferation, they can adversely delay re-endothelialization through their bystander effect on the endothelial cell replication and regeneration and may also inhibit vessel healing through an inflammatory and/or hypersensitivity process caused either, or both, by the drug itself or, as is now believed, more likely the polymer. Both cellular and extracellular processes favouring thrombosis can therefore persist over a longer period of time if delayed re-endothelialization or inflammatory reactivity processes are ongoing. First-generation DES release the antiproliferative agents sirolimus or paclitaxel, which are potent drugs that may well have bystander inhibitory effects on re-endothelialization by blocking the cell cycle via different mechanisms—they

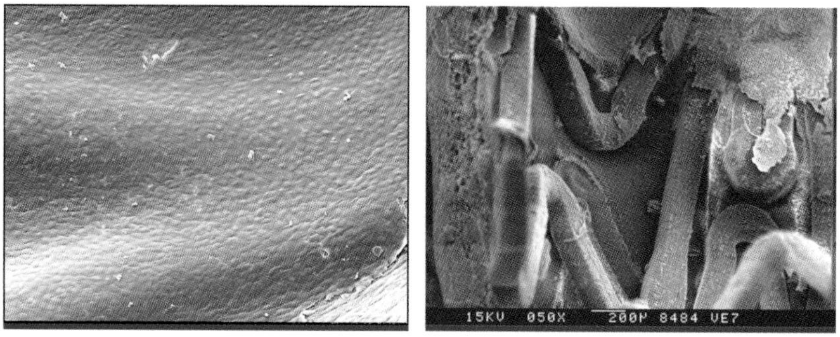

Fig. 29.3
Re-endothelialization following stent placement. A) Complete strut coverage. B) Stent strut exposure and endothelial denudation.

deliver the drug by being loaded onto the stent with polymers that may well have longer-term inflammatory responses (Fig. 29.4).

Sirolimus inhibits the mammalian target of rapamycin, mTOR, and prevents the degradation of p27kip1a cyclin-dependent kinase inhibitor that plays an important role in regulating vascular smooth muscle cell migration and proliferation[21,22]. In addition, sirolimus blocks endothelial cell proliferation by inhibiting the p70S6 kinase pathway, which mediates cell cycle progression in response to growth factors. Paclitaxel stabilizes microtubules inhibiting cell division in the G_0–G_1 and G_2–M phase. Hence, the effect of these drugs is not cell-type specific and endothelial cell division and migration is inhibited along with smooth muscle cell proliferation[23]. Decreased proliferation and migration of endothelial cells would impair endothelial coverage after stent deployment, leaving stent struts exposed to the circulating blood and thereby favouring thrombosis. Both drugs or congeners such as rapamycin can have a more direct prothrombogenic effect. Inhibition of the mTOR pathway by sirolimus or rapamycin and stimulation of the c-Jun terminal NH_2 kinase by paclitaxel enhance the expression of tissue factor (TF) one of the major triggers of coagulation. In addition, both rapamycin and paclitaxel can increase the expression of PAI-1 in coronary artery endothelial cells[24], a fast acting inhibitor of plasminogen activators, but also a key regulator of smooth muscle cell proliferation, migration, and apoptosis implicated in vascular remodelling.

Stent-induced inflammation

Stent implantation can trigger inflammatory reactions within the vessel wall. These are predominantly mediated by CD45-positive leucocytes and eosinophils and lead to the formation of eosinophilic infiltrates that reflect the hypersensitivity reaction to the stent, most likely the polymer[25]. Evidence from animal studies suggests that the inflammatory reactions are more pronounced after DES implantation as compared to BMS[26], with more fibrin deposition and an incomplete re-endothelialization. The non-erodible polymers used with first-generation DES are not biologically inert and can trigger a local hypersensitivity reaction and over a longer period, thereby favouring the occurrence of thrombotic events by altering vascular healing. In an

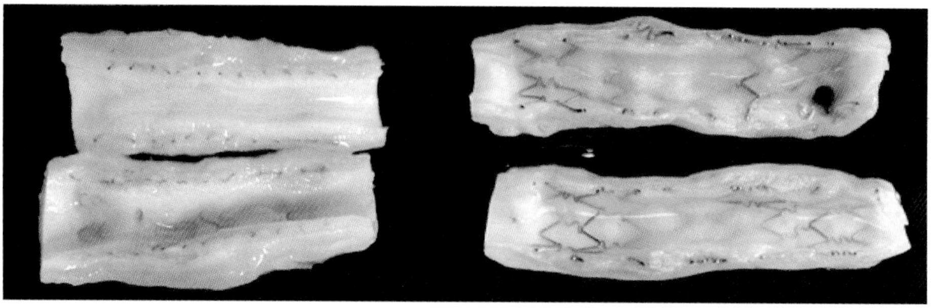

BMS 24 months after deployment   Cypher® 16 months after deployment

Fig. 29.4 Re-endothelialization following bare-metal stenting and drug-eluting stenting (Cypher®).

attempt to reduce the inflammatory reaction, which may in a major part be caused by the polymer, several companies have developed more biocompatible/bioneutral coatings. Medtronic, for example recently released the BioLinx® polymer system that contains a mixture of polymers which are lipophilic/hydrophobic, and hydrophilic to promote a controlled drug release while being more biocompatible because of their hydrophilicity. New concepts in stent development are the bioabsorbable stents made of poly-L-lactic acid and the initial results in clinical trials proved that their use is feasible, safe, and effective in humans. Biocompatible polymers are the focus of intense current research (Fig. 29.5).

Endothelial progenitor cells

Endothelial progenitor cells (EPCs) are the circulating precursors of mature endothelial cells that play an important role in vascular repair. EPCs are attracted to the site of endothelial injury both following acute coronary syndromes and during the early post-PCI period, and contribute to the process of re-endothelialization. However, the active compounds released from DES may affect the function and survival of EPCs. At concentrations significantly lower that those achieved *in vivo* both abluminally and endoluminally, sirolimus can cause EPCs senescence and apoptosis[27]. To accelerate the process of endothelialization and thereby reduce the risk of thrombosis an EPC-capture stent (Genous®, OrbusNeich) was developed. This stent is coated with CD34-positive antibody that targets EPC surface antigens. Again, initial results in humans show promising results with regard to restenosis and ST.

Shear stress and vasoconstriction

Shear stress is the frictional force acting on the endothelium due to the blood flow. Endothelial cells respond to shear stress by adapting their function (i.e. gene expression, production of antiatherogenic substances such as nitric oxide). Low or reduced turbulent flow may favour the development of atherosclerotic plaques. Stent implantation may modify shear stress by scaffolding of the arterial segments or because stent struts may modify stress at the local level. Shear stress can modulate both neointima proliferation and platelet activation enhancing their adhesion to the vessel wall. Platelet adhesion to regions of injury may be promoted in conditions of low-flow or low shear environment[28] favouring aggregation and thrombus formation. Shear stress can also be modified by vasoconstriction, which in turn can be triggered by the active drug and polymer components of DES. Indeed, DES can impair the endothelial response to acetylcholine- and exercise-mediated vasodilation, promoting endothelial dysfunction[29].

Incidence and outcome of stent thrombosis

The incidence and timing of ST with DES and how these compare to BMS is still unclear, not least since there are few comparative data from robust randomized trials nor real-life all-comers properly conducted sequential recruiting registry studies. From the data we do have however, it can probably be suggested that most ST with either stent type occurs *early*. Furthermore, the incidence of early ST is probably higher with BMS, while these stents appear to have a lower incidence of late and very late actual ST compared with DES. Whether this late excess with DES translates into real clinical disadvantage (i.e. produces overall more deaths and MIs) is less certain, since the restenosis associated with BMS can itself lead to late occlusive closure which can present as an acute event.

Incidence of stent thrombosis with BMS

Early definite ST was a common complication following BMS implantation in the early 1990s with an incidence ranging from 10–15%[30,31]. The combination of aspirin and ticlopidine reduced the risk of subacute ST and was found to be associated with a lower risk of bleeding than anticoagulant regimens (aspirin with heparin or warfarin) that were initially utilized after stent placement[32–36]. Treatment with DAPT (aspirin and thienopyridine) for 4 weeks after placement of BMS has thus reduced this risk of ST to *less than 2%* as has been reported in a review of 6058 patients[37]. In this review, the timing of BMS ST was acute in 11%, subacute in 64%, and late in 25% of the patients (for timing definitions see earlier section). Few data are available on the rate of very late ST after BMS implantation although there is a report of 0.2% in a large meta-analysis of 38 trials[38].

Incidence of stent thrombosis in BMS versus DES

To try and determine the comparative incidence of ST in patients treated with BMS versus DES several meta-analyses of the various randomized trials have been performed in the past few years. It should be noted that while meta-analyses are useful, they contain significant generic drawbacks including the comparative similarity or otherwise of the studies making up the meta-analysis and the acquisition of the cumulative statistical answer

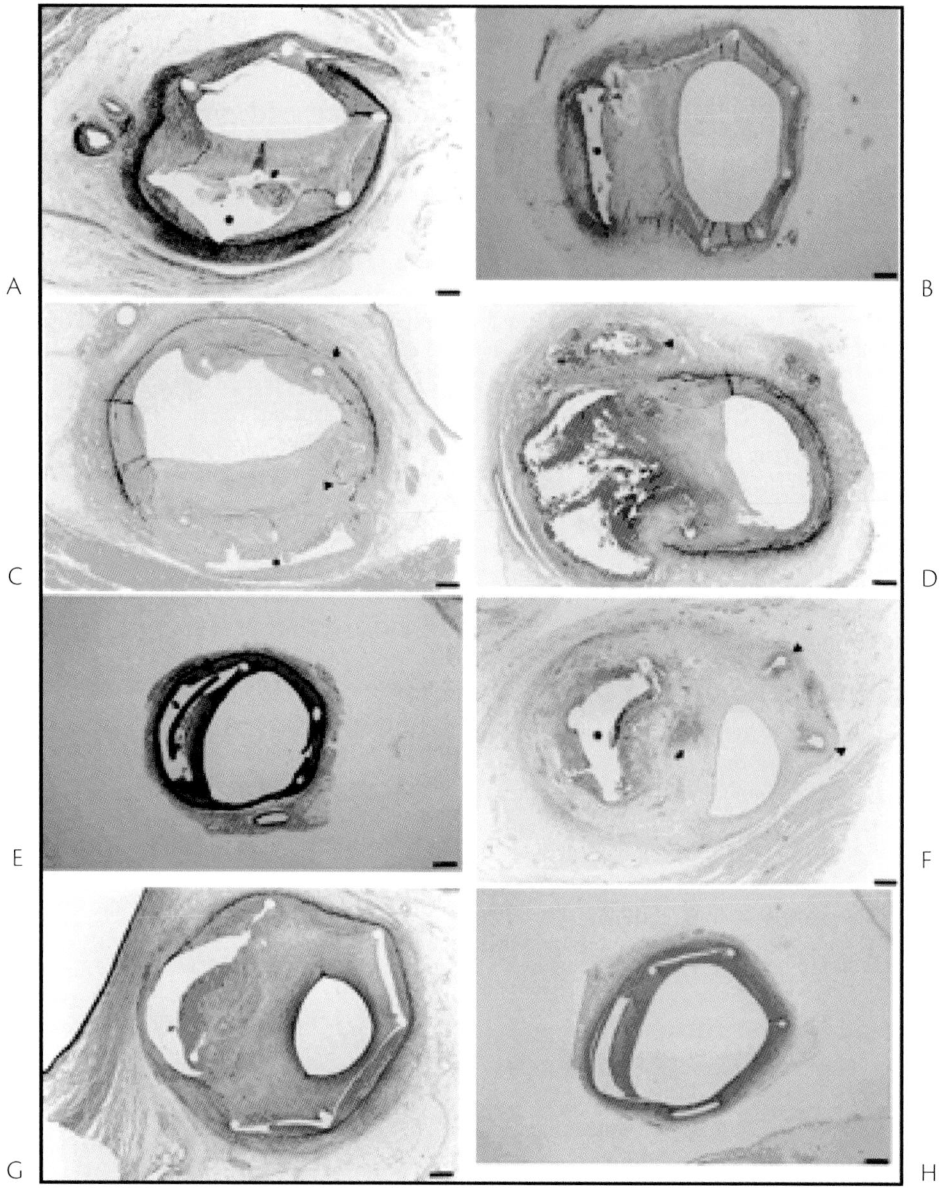

Fig. 29.5 Stent-induced inflammation.

from a potentially small number of non statistically-important studies.

- To date, the largest meta-analysis study has been published by Stetteler and colleagues[38]. This included 38 trials (18 023 patients) and compared sirolimus-eluting stents (SES) (6771 patients) versus paclitaxel eluting stents (PES) (6331 patients) versus BMS (4921 patients) with a 4-year follow-up. The study concluded that there was no significant difference in the risk of ST in the overall follow-up period. However, the risk of late definite ST increased with PES (HR 2.11; $p = 0.017$ vs. BMS and HR1.85; $p = 0.041$ vs. SES). Nevertheless, this outcome did not impact on mortality. There is again this important distinction to be made between the incidence of late ST and an overall adverse clinical consequence of any such overall background excess. SESs were, however, associated with the lowest risk of MI. To better understand the risk predicted by this study one should assume that in order to prevent one MI over 4 years, about 100 patients should receive SES, rather than BMS or PES. The authors concluded that SES seem to produce a better clinical outcome than BMS and PES. This study was, however, flawed somewhat by its comparison of the DES directly without serious account being taken of the difference in BMS control groups in the two stent types and the various trials inclusion data

- A further meta-analysis of 14 trials including data from 4958 patients compared SES versus BMS[39]. This meta-analysis also included acute MI in 24% of the cases, some chronic total occlusions, bypass grafts, and other complex lesions. The clinical outcome was all-cause mortality and the follow-up for 1–4.9 years. In this study there was no significant difference in the overall risk of ST between BMS and the SES–DES. However, there was a slight increase in the risk of ST associated with SES *after the first year*. ST was defined as per study protocols and *not* as per the ARC definitions and was observed overall in 65 patients (34 with SES and 31 with BMS). After the first year, ST occurred in nine patients, eight of whom had received SES. Over the 4-year follow-up period and following the first year after the procedure, the overall risk for ST was 0.6% in the SES group and 0.05% in the BMS group. This confirms the higher later incidence of ST with DES
- Stone and colleagues[40] analysed safety and efficacy as the major clinical endpoints in a pooled *patient-level analysis* from four double-blind trials in which 1748 patients were treated with either SES or BMS and five double-blind trials in which 3513 patients were treated with either PES or BMS. The follow-up was up to 4 years and the selected patients were clinically stable and had simple native lesions. The 4-year rates of ST were 1.2% in the SES vs. 0.6% in the BMS-group ($p = 0.20$) and 1.3% in the PES vs. 0.9% in the BMS group ($p = 0.30$). However, after 1 year, there were five episodes of ST in patients with SES vs. none in patients with BMS ($p = 0.025$) and nine episodes in patients with PES vs. two in patients with BMS ($p = 0.028$). The number of episodes of ST within the first year was identical among patients treated with SES, PES, or BMS. Again, while the incidence of ST was higher late with DES, the rates of death or MI did not differ significantly between the groups
- Using a hierarchical classification of ST as set by the ARC group, Mauri and colleagues[41] analyzed 878 patients treated with SES, 1400 treated with PES, and 2267 treated with BMS. Four-year follow-up data in clinically stable patients with simple native lesions were pooled and analysed for ST as primary outcome. The incidence of early, late, or very late ST did not differ significantly between patients with DES and those with BMS in these randomized clinical trials, although the power to detect small differences was limited. Clinical outcome in the 68 patients with definite or probable ST was poor, however, indicating the importance of prevention of any ST—21 patients died (30.9%) and 57 had MI (83.8%). Outcome rates after ST were similar among stent groups. At 4 years, the proportion of deaths from ST was 7.0% in the SES vs. 11.1% in the corresponding BMS group, and 8.2% in the PES group vs. 6.1% in the corresponding BMS group. The authors concluded that both longer and larger studies were needed to understand how these infrequent, but potentially deadly events could be predicted and/or prevented
- In a further pooled analysis of four randomized trials, Spaulding and colleagues[42] compared SES and BMS in 1748 patients with 4-year follow-up. Again, there were no significant differences in the rates of death, MI, or ST in the two groups. According to the ARC definition, 30 ST were found in the SES and 28 in the BMS group. ST was more frequent in the BMS group in the first year (11 vs. 3 in the SES group; $p = 0.03$), whereas very late ST was more frequent in the SES group (23 vs. 14 in the BMS group; $p = 0.14$). Significant heterogeneity was found in patients with diabetes. The 4-year cumulative survival rates was significantly lower in the SES group (87.8% vs. 95.6% in the BMS groups; $p = 0.008$) in patients with diabetes. Although no clear pattern of mortality was identified, among the patients with diabetes there was a small excess of very late ST in the SES group (11 patients vs. 3 in the BMS group).

In conclusion, the clinical outcomes of large-scale meta-analyses did not reveal any significant differences in death rates during long-term follow-up to 5 years (Table 29.1). It was hypothesized that compared to BMS the small increase *in very late* ST seen with DES was balanced by a somewhat smaller *early* ST rate, but additionally with DES there was less frequent need for repeated revascularization procedures, and fewer associated complications, compared with BMS. However, groups of DES and BMS differed widely with respect to cardiovascular risk factors such as diabetes, number of stents, stent diameter, stent length, and target lesion

Table 29.1 Clinical outcomes of large-scale meta-analyses

	N of patients	BMS	PES	SES	PES vs. BMS	SES vs. BMS	SES/PES	Mortality
Stettler *et al. Lancet* 2007[38] (4-year follow-up; safety and effectiveness, definite ARC ST)								
Total	12973	4003	4327	4643				**ns**
Overall ST	188	50	72	66	ns	ns	ns	
Early ST	94	28	30	36	ns	ns	ns	
Late ST	46	14	16	16	ns	ns	ns	
Very late ST	48	8	26	14	ns	ns	ns	
Late and very late ST	94	22	42	30	**p = 0.017**	ns	**p = 0.041**	
Kastrati *et al. NEJM* 2007[39] (1–4-year follow-up, primary endpoint—death from any cause, ST as per study protocol)								
Total	4958	2472	–	2486	–		–	**ns**
Overall ST	65	31	–	34	–	ns	–	
Early ST	na	na	–	na	–	na	–	
Late ST	na	na	–	na	–	na	–	
Very late ST	9	1	–	8	–	**p = 0.02**	–	
Stone *et al. NEJM* 2007[40] (4-year follow-up; trial endpoints—ST as per study protocol, death, cardiac and non-cardiac)								
Total	5261	870/1758	1755	878				**ns**
Overall ST	50	14/5	20*	10	ns	ns	na	
Early ST	23	10/1	8	4	ns	ns	na	
Late ST	11	2/4	4	1	ns	ns	na	
Very late ST	16	2/0	9	5	**p = 0.028**	**p = 0.025**	na	
Mauri *et al. NEJM* 2007[41] (4-year follow-up; ST as per any ARC criterion)								
Total	4545	1397/870	1400	878				
Overall ST	138	41/28	39	30	p = 0.84	p = 0.80	na	na
Early ST	21	7/3	7	4	na	na	na	
Late ST	38	13/11	12	2	na	na	na	
Very late ST	79	21/14	20	24	na	na	na	
Spaulding *et al. NEJM* 2007[42] (primary endpoint—survival at 4-year follow-up; ST as per ARC definition)								
Total	1748	870	–	878	–	–	–	**ns**
Overall ST	58	28	–	30	–	–	–	
Early ST	7	3	–	4	–	p = 0.70	–	
Late ST	14	11	–	3		p = 0.03	–	
Very late ST	3p	14	–	23	–	p = 0.14	–	

location, limiting the value of adjustments made by propensity score analysis. This and the fact that no matter what the incidence of ST is, it must be considered a serious clinical event that does not dissipate concern that the use of DES in more complex patients and lesion subsets, not represented in the randomized clinical trials included in the meta-analyses described earlier, may indeed be associated with higher adverse event rates.

The outcomes between DES and BMS seem more at variance in *real-world registries* where the off-label use of DES (i.e. in patients who fall outside the lesion types that the licence was originally considered for—the original licence is generally based on the early trials which tend to include simpler more straightforward patients) accounts for up to 60% of the population treated in the real world compared to the randomized trials, although again the limitation of registries is that many are not composed of sequential patients and therefore open to potentially worse selection bias than RCT.

- In the Western Denmark Heart Registry[43], 12 395 consecutive patients treated with stent implantation were followed for 15 months. DES were implanted in 3548 patients (5422 lesions) and BMS were implanted in 8847 patients (11 730 lesions). Definite, probable, or possible ST was found in 190 (2.1%) patients in the BMS group and in 64 (1.8%) patients in the DES. Very late definite ST occurred more frequently in patients receiving DES. The risk of MI between 12–15 months after implantation was higher in the DES group but mortality was similar in the two groups. The authors conclude that the minor risk of ST and MI within 15 months after implantation of DES seems unlikely to outweigh the benefits of these stents
- Long-term follow-up data of 8146 patients treated with DES (there were no BMS patients in this registry) in two academic institutions (Bern and Rotterdam)[44] showed that angiographically documented ST, observed in 152 patients, occurred at a median of 9 days and accrued at a steady rate of 0.6% per year between 30 days and 3 years of follow-up. Late ST was encountered steadily with no decrease up to 4 years follow-up. Most of the ST occurred very early after the procedure with a then slow increasing and unlevelling-off plateauing. Early and late ST was observed with SES and with PES. Acute coronary syndrome at presentation and diabetes were independent predictors of ST. During extension of the follow-up period, Wenaweser and colleagues[45] identified that late ST occurred steadily at an annual rate of 0.4–0.6% for up to 4 years with an incidence density of 1.0/100 patient-years and a cumulative total incidence of 3.3%. Rates of death, MI, and the composite of death or MI were 10.6%, 4.6%, and 14.6%, respectively, in the overall population. During the entire observation period of 4 years, 27 patients suffering from definite ST subsequently died
- The DEScover Registry[46] collected data from 6906 patients who underwent PCI in the United States with follow-up to 1 year. The majority of the patients were treated with DES (SES or PES). Substantial baseline differences were observed between patients receiving BMS compared with those treated with DES. In the BMS group the patients were older and more often had a previous history of CABG. Acute MI was more frequently the indication for stenting compared to the DES group. Finally, left ventricular function was lower among BMS patients. Rates for ST were low (<1%) for both groups and did not differ significantly. Adjusted 1-year HRs comparing BMS with DES did not differ significantly for either death or MI. This does suggest that even if the patients are chosen to receive DES because they are a higher-risk group or have more complex lesions subsets, outcome with DES is good
- In the Swedish Coronary Angiography and Angioplasty Registry (SCAAR)[47], 6033 patients were treated with DES and 13 738 patients with BMS with outcome analysis data up to 3 years. *In contrast* to the studies above, DES implantation was associated with an increased risk of death, as compared with BMS. This trend was evident after 6 months, when the risk of death was 0.5 % higher and a composite of death or MI was 0.5–1.0 % higher per year. However, this group reversed their findings beyond 1 year data review for reasons that remain uncertain
- Results from the Multicenter Spanish Registry ESTROFA have been published by de la Torre-Hernandez and colleagues[48]: 23 500 patients undergoing DES implantation were studied. Definite ST occurred in 301 patients with a cumulative incidence of 2% at 3 years. The mortality at 1 year follow-up was 16% and ST recurrence 4.6%. ST-segment elevation MI (STEMI) appeared to be the most potent predictor of ST, both in the acute/subacute phase and in the late phase.

While it is expected that higher rates of very late ST after DES implantation will place patients at higher risk for death and MI in the long term, the controversial findings of large real-world registries cannot be relied upon for conclusive evidence. Not least the highest risk patients (for restenosis) with the most complex disease will have been chosen for the DES use. This stresses the importance of properly randomized controlled trials of all comers which, apart from the PROTECT trial, are unfortunately currently lacking.

While the indication for stenting in most patients in the discussed studies was 'on-label' where DES have been shown to be safe up to 4 years, the off-label long-term safety has not yet been determined as the implication of DES stenting high-risk patients is unknown.

With the increasing availability of DES, several important CAD subsets, including stenoses of the unprotected left main coronary artery (ULMCA), previously considered unattractive or too high-risk for PCI, are being increasingly considered. In a 2004 survey of interventions for LMS stenosis, PCI was used in 29% of European and 18% of US patients[49]. Nevertheless, the approach to revascularizing patients with ULMCA percutaneously remains cautious and controversial. It could certainly be expected that patients with ST of the LMCA, whether early, late, or very late, would have a particularly high risk of dying. Although seven different groups have published results involving 599 patients, interpretations remains limited by small patient numbers, short duration of follow-up, and lack of a control group in four studies.

A recent meta-analysis published by Chieffo and colleagues[(50)] reports frequency and timing of ST in treatment of patients with DES for ULMCA. Data were collected from five centres' prospective registries with 4-year follow-up and included 731 patients undergoing elective DES-PCI for de novo ULMCA. This analysis did not include patients with acute MI as procedural indication but 46% of the patients had unstable angina. PCI was considered instead of surgery due to patients preference, a high (>6%) EuroSCORE, or failure of all previously placed bypass grafts conduits. Dual antiplatelet therapy was given for a median of 9 months. The incidence of definite or probable ST was 0.95% at 2.5 years which is remarkably low, while possible ST occurred in 2.7% of the cases. No case of ST was reported after 12 months, and, as such, all events occurred while taking dual antiplatelet therapy. More importantly, all four patients with definite ST survived. Cardiac-related mortality occurred in 4.2% of the cohort, and this should not be different from mortality expected had these patients undergone CABG (median EuroSCORE 3 and more than one-third of patients had a score of >6).

Use of DES in the setting of *acute MI* remains controversial according to some interventionists but in general has become the acceptable device to use in this condition. Data from GRACE[(51)] (The Global Registry of Acute Coronary Events) provides an opportunity to compare follow-up with DES and BMS in acute MI in a population from routine clinical practice as opposed to the highly selected population participating in randomized clinical trials. After comprehensive adjustment, early mortality was no different between patients receiving DES or BMS (from admission to 1 year), whereas late mortality was higher in patients receiving DES (from 6 months to 2 years). Although these observations should be interpreted with caution given the observational, non-randomized, registry data nature of the GRACE data set, increased mortality with DES following STEMI is biologically plausible. It may be attributed to the increased risk of late ST observed with DES use but also the potential for late acquired stent malapposition of the stent strut to the vessel wall may play a role. Once the vessel has been recanalized and the thrombosis subsided, the reference diameter may be larger then had appeared when the stent was deployed. Late-stent malapposition is a potential factor favouring late ST because of the thrombosis forming in the gap between the stent and the vessel wall where flow will be low, and the frequency of late malapposition appears greater after primary PCI with DES[(52)] then with BMS. On the other hand, data from a large meta-analysis published by Kastrati and colleagues[(53)] suggests that the use of DES in patients with STEMI is safe and improves clinical outcomes by reducing the risk of reintervention compared with BMS. Similarly, Pasceri and colleagues[(54)] indicates in a further meta-analysis that use of DES in STEMI shows a beneficial effect in terms of MACE as compared with BMS without increase in ST at 1 year follow-up.

After stent implantation, patients with *diabetes mellitus* (DM) are more likely to develop restenosis and require repeat revascularization procedures compared with those without DM, and are also at greater risk for ST, MI, and death. However, use of DES in diabetic patients has been associated with reduced rates or target lesion revascularization compared to BMS but the rates of death, MI, or ST remain the same when compared to BMS use[(55)]. In these trials comparisons were made between DES and BMS use and not between stent implantation and coronary artery bypass surgery or optimal medical therapy in stable patients. Ongoing large-scale randomized trials are underway to determine the relative safety and efficacy of DES compared with that of CABG in patients with DM (FREEDOM, BARI-2).

DES use for off-label indications

A substantial amount of data has proved the efficacy of DES for off-label indications like chronic total occlusion, in-stent restenosis, small vessels, and bypass grafts. However, the primary endpoints of these trials were most often angiographic, and the follow-up is still unreported beyond 1 year. The limited number of patients in these trials makes them underpowered for assessing hard clinical endpoints. Thus, the long-term safety for DES for off-label indications needs to be determined on the basis of both pooled meta-analyses of these trials and real-world registries. However, many of these indications for PCI (i.e. chronic total occlusion) are associated with high restenosis rates and use of DES would seem intuitive.

Predictors of stent thrombosis

We do not have a clear understanding as to why some patients suffer ST yet others do not, although some general predictors are available. There are not absolute markers of risk or risk score for ST. However, clinical trial data may provide some insights and 'profile' those at higher risk. Recent work has analysed different potential predictors for early and late ST.

In general, predictors of ST can be classified into three groups:

1) Those related to the patient: DM, renal failure, low left ventricular ejection fraction (LVEF), clinical setting (acute coronary syndrome at presentation), antiplatelet therapy discontinuation, antiplatelet therapy resistance.
2) Those linked to the treated lesion: lesion length and diameter, pre-procedural minimal lumen diameter (MLD) and stenosis percentage, type C (complex) lesion, bifurcation disease.
3) Those associated with the PCI procedure itself: stent length, maximal balloon diameter, post-procedural MLD and residual stenosis percentage, number of stent per lesion, DES use, stent underexpansion or malapposition, residual thrombus, residual dissection. This may be the most important group since obsessive acute post-procedure results may be an important factor in producing longer-term results.

Iakovou and colleagues[56] have analysed predictors for ST in a prospective observational cohort, where 2229 consecutive patients underwent successful implantation of SES or PES. Patients were given an antiplatelet regimen, with aspirin continued indefinitely and ticlopidine or clopidogrel for at least 3 months after SES and for at least 6 months after PES implantation. The study was designed using ST as the main outcome (early ST from procedure's end up to 30 days, late ST over 30 days, and cumulative ST). After 9-month follow-up, 29 patients had ST (9 with SES and 20 with PES, $p = 0.09$). Of these, 14 patients had early and 15 late ST. The study revealed that independent predictors of ST were: *premature discontinuation of antiplatelet therapy (HR 89.78)*, renal failure (HR 6.49), bifurcation lesion (HR 6.42), diabetes (HR 3.71), and a lower ejection fraction (HR 1.09) at entry. It is perhaps not surprising that complex lesions and patients are now treated with DES since their widespread availability has broadened the scope of PCI. In the Iakovu study, 27% of the population had diabetes and 79% of the lesions were complex. The clinical implications of ST were severe, with a case-fatality rate of 45% (amongst all the 29 patients with ST, 13 died). Overall the most important predictor of ST after implantation was premature discontinuation of the antiplatelet therapy. Thrombosis occurred in 29% of patients who prematurely discontinued DAPT, making adherence to treatment of paramount importance. The incidence of ST at 9 months after DES implantation in consecutive real-world patients was 1.3%.

A further major study assessing predictors for ST comes from Airoldi and colleagues[57]. Until this study was published the incidence and predictors of ST had been evaluated over relatively short follow-up periods, generally limited to a maximum of 12 months and few data were available on the incidence of DES ST 1 year after implantation. DAPT to prevent ST had been recommended at the time of trial publication for the first 3–6 months after DES implantation, and no data were available on whether prolonged DAPT was necessary, valuable or associated with risks over a longer time period. Airoldi and colleagues selected as study outcome 'delayed ST' in an 18-month follow-up study. This was a prospective observational study on 3021 patients consecutively collected and successfully treated with DES (this does not mean they were not a selected group of patients though). The incidence of ST throughout follow-up period and its relationship with thienopyridine therapy was analyzed. ST occurred in 58 patients (1.9%) at 18 months and out of these, 42 patients (1.4%) experienced the event within 6 months after stent implantation. Acute MI (fatal and non-fatal) occurred in 46 patients out of the total of 58 and death occurred in 23 patients of those 58 patients who developed ST. The median interval from discontinuation of thienopyridine therapy to ST was 13.5 days for the first 6 months and 90 days between 6 and 18 moths. On multivariate analysis, *the strongest predictor for ST within 6 months of stenting was discontinuation of thienopyridine therapy (HR 13.74)* but after 6 months this did not predict the occurrence of ST. A very important finding (stressing the relevance of other factors such as procedural variables) was that *50% of the thrombotic events occurred in the first 30 days after DES implantation*. This supports the view that improved implantation technique and screening for antiplatelet resistance may have a role in reducing early ST and thus its overall (longer-term) burden.

A recent very large registry reconfirms many of the concepts that have now evolved. In a study published in the *Journal of the American College of Cardiology* in April 2009[58], the authors demonstrate as has been previously suggested that discontinuation of clopidogrel and stent under-sizing were the most significant predictors of ST of an extensive list of clinical, procedural, and angiographic variables assessed. Of 19 840 patients followed to nearly 3 years (31 months) 437 (2.2%) presented with ST. Of these, 73% were within 30 days (32% within 24h), 13% were between 30 days and 1 year, and 13% presented >1 year. BMS ST was 2.2% and DES ST 2.0%. Compared to those who did not have ST independent predictors in hierarchical order were:

1) *Cessation of clopidogrel* (at various time points but highest risk within 30 days)
2) *Sent undersizing*
3) Current malignancy
4) Intermediate CAD (>50% stenosis) proximal to the culprit lesion
5) *Suboptimal procedural result (TIMI grade flow <3 after PCI)*
6) *Uncovered dissection*
7) *Bifurcation stenting*
8) LVEF <30%
9) Periphery artery disease
10) Intermediate CAD distal to the culprit lesion
11) *No aspirin therapy*
12) Any DES use
13) *DM*
14) Younger age (protective role).

In our clinical experience numbers 1, 2, 5, 6, 7, 11, and 13 are important predictors of ST in everyday clinical practice in the United Kingdom and are the factors that need attention being paid to when a patient is undergoing coronary intervention.

The interesting aspect of this registry study is that it confirms that, in general, ST is essentially an early issue, that technical aspects (care with stent deployment) are important but this is impacted on by thrombogenicity of the lesion. For patients who underwent elective PCI for stable angina, the cumulative rate of ST was 1%, while for those who were stented for unstable angina/non-STEMI (NSTEMI) the rate was 1.8%, and rose to 4.3% for those with STEMI. The timing of ST was significantly different for the different categories of patients: 79% of ST in STEMI patients occurred early (within 30 days) vs. 65% in NSTEMI and stable angina patients. On the other hand, the proportion of late and very late (beyond 30 days) ST was higher in the stable angina and NSTEMI groups. However, what the study doesn't tell us is which patients with DES suffer late ST since it would only be these who we would want to give longer term DAPT to (>1 year and beyond) (Table 29.2).

Unfortunately, many predictors of late ST are similar to those of restenosis. This similarity makes choosing a DES based on these criteria alone difficult, since many patients will be at increased risk for both restenosis and thrombosis. People with diabetes are a particular example, in whom risk for both restenosis and thrombosis is high. Efforts to reduce ST in diabetics are therefore important.

Dual antiplatelet therapy continuation as a major factor influencing the rate of ST

DAPT is currently recommended by the American College of Cardiology (ACC)/American Heart Association

Table 29.2 Predictors of early and late stent thrombosis

Predictors of early ST	Predictors of late ST
Acute coronary syndrome	Acute coronary syndrome
Diabetes mellitus	Diabetes mellitus
Chronic renal failure	Chronic renal failure
Left ventricular ejection fraction	Left ventricular ejection fraction
Discontinuation of anti-platelet therapy	Discontinuation of antiplatelet therapy
Bifurcation	Bifurcation
Total stent length	Total stent length
Number of stents	Number of stents
Post-procedural minimal lumen diameter	Post-procedural minimal lumen diameter
Stent underexpansion or malapposition	Stent underexpansion or malapposition
Residual dissection	–
Residual thrombus	–
–	Drug-eluting stent use (?)
–	Brachytherapy

(AHA)/Society for Cardiovascular Angiography and Interventions (SCAI) guidelines for 1 month after BMS, for 3 months after SES, and for 6 months after PES[59]. However, the FDA and British Cardiovascular Intervention Society, following the 2006 ST scare, recommended DAPT for a minimum of 1 year following DES. The rationale for this is a precautionary measure based on the assumption that DAPT should probably be continued for more then 3 months. For how long DAPT should be continued remains unclear. In the BASKET-LATE study, Pfisterer and colleagues[60] analysed consecutive series of 746 non-selected patients surviving 6 months without major events and followed them for 1 year after discontinuation of clopidogrel. Rates of 18-month cardiac death/MI were no different between DES and BMS patients. However, after discontinuation of clopidogrel, these events occurred in 4.9% after DES versus 1.3% after BMS implantation. Documented late ST and related death/target vessel MI were twice as frequent after DES compared to BMS (2.6% vs. 1.3%). Thrombosis-related events occurred between 15–362 days after discontinuation of clopidogrel, and presenting as MI or death in 88%. This prospective randomized comparison of DES versus BMS in a 'real-world' setting shows that the incidence of late cardiac death or non-fatal MI after discontinuation of clopidogrel after 6 months appears greater in DES- as compared with BMS-treated patients although the relationship between discontinuation of DAPT and incidence of ST, its timing, and predictability is really not so clear and these results are at variance with other studies. The findings of this study emphasized the implication of discontinuation of DAPT. However, it did not show that late thrombosis-related events could be prevented by prolonging such a therapy. Nevertheless, a prolonged antiplatelet strategy may be chosen empirically, at least for patients at increased risk for such events, until better strategies to prevent late thrombosis-related events have been found and shown to be effective.

More recently, in the 3-year follow-up of BASKET[62], all 826 consecutive BASKET patients were further studied after 3 years to assess the long-term benefit:risk ratio of DES versus BMS relative to stent size and risk of ST. Data were analysed separately for patients with small stents (<3mm vessel) versus only large stents (>3mm vessel) and clinical events related to ST. Cardiac death/MI rates were similar, however, death/MI beyond 6 months was higher with DES (9.1% vs. 3.8% BMS; $p = 0.009$), mainly due to increased late death/MI in patients with large stents. The results paralleled findings for ST. The findings of this long-term study suggest that baseline stent size seems to determine the long-term benefit:risk balance with patients with small stents having a larger benefit of DES in all clinical endpoints including ST. It remains uncertain how this will translate into even longer-term outcome balance which, however, will also be affected by the natural progression of underlying coronary disease. This uncertainty and the possible impact of newer DES on this benefit:risk balance, particularly regarding the large group of patients in need of large stents in daily practice, is addressed prospectively in the ongoing European multicentre BASKET-PROVE, in which 2323 consecutive patients with large-vessel stenting were randomized to a first- versus a second-generation DES versus a BMS (results expected in 2010).

Duration of dual antiplatelet treatment

The BASKET studies raise questions as to how long patients should be treated with DAPT for. In terms of the early ST, the role of antiplatelet therapy discontinuation is well recognized and not questioned. It is the strongest predictor for early ST and Iakovou and colleagues[56] reported a relative risk of 161.17 in this situation (i.e. patients who discontinue DAPT prematurely are 161.17-fold more likely to develop ST than those who do not). The current European and North American guidelines, which highlight the need for DAPT during the first 4 weeks after PCI, are derived directly from those results[63]. In contrast, the time at which antiplatelet therapy can be discontinued in relation to trying to prevent late and very late ST remains to be determined, although as stated above the Food and Drug Administration (FDA) advisory committee has advocated 12 months of uninterrupted treatment[64]. This proposal is supported by the AHA, ACC, and European Society for Cardiology (ESC)[65].

Treatment with aspirin and clopidogrel for 12 months provided a 27% reduction in the relative risk of death, MI, or stroke in patients undergoing PCI, compared with a 1-month regimen ($p = 0.02$) (CREDO trial: clopidogrel for the reduction of events during observation)[66]. In the DUKE study[67], which analysed 2-year mortality in patients treated with DES, the outcome was lowest for those who remained on clopidogrel for at least 1 year and was highest in individuals not on this drug at 1 year. Findings of other registry studies[47,60] have also confirmed an increase in mortality and MI with termination of clopidogrel 6–12 months after implantation of DES.

The optimum duration of DAPT must of course balance the benefit of reduced ischaemic events against the harm from increased bleeding episodes. Despite this there are those who believe that 12 months for all irrespective of ST risk is unnecessarily long for some patients receiving DES (putting them at risk of bleeding and adding to the overall cost of the procedure), although there are no data to support earlier discontinuation, while others would in certain higher-risk circumstances (e.g. LMS stenting) wish the patient to receive DAPT for >1 year (?indefinitely). A number of studies now suggest that, especially in higher-risk groups, treatment should be prolonged for at least 2 years. Whether this is cost-effective and outweighs the risk of spontaneous and non-cardiac surgery-induced bleeding is much less clear. How long DAPT should be continued for thus remains unresolved. Furthermore, there is the issue around the patients who do indeed need a non-cardiac surgical procedure at any time after stenting and while still on DAPT—should the DAPT be stopped to reduce the risk of surgical bleeding, and if that is done, what is then the excess risk of ST? Clearly if the patient has a known surgical procedure on the horizon then a BMS should be the most appropriate option.

Aside from the need to stop DAPT because of surgical bleeding risk there is also concern regarding spontaneous bleeding in patients on longer-term DAPT. Most of the bleeding risk associated with dual antiplatelet regimens seems to come fairly early after initiation of treatment. Data from the CHARISMA trial (clopidogrel for high atherothrombotic risk and ischaemic stabilization, management, and avoidance)[(68)] showed similar rates of moderate-to-severe bleeding after DAPT compared with aspirin alone after 270 days. Thus, a patient who has tolerated a dual regimen for 9–12 months, without occurrence of any bleeding episodes that led to a doctor stopping treatment or the patient discontinuing the regimen themselves, has essentially passed a so-called bleeding stress test. Therefore, available data lend to support to uninterrupted DAPT for *at least 1 year. Whether a longer regimen would provide additional benefit with acceptable bleeding risk is unknown.* Only a prospective randomized clinical trial can properly address this question. Such studies of short- versus longer-term DAPT duration are planned.

Clopidogrel resistance and novel thienopyridine

Despite DAPT with aspirin and clopidogrel in stented patients, ST can still occur and at any time but especially in the context of resistance to antiplatelet therapy, early. Platelet response to clopidogrel treatment may be highly variable and clinical, cellular, and genetic factors have been shown to be causative. Persisting high platelet reactivity, despite adequate pre-treatment with clopidogrel, is associated with an increased risk of adverse cardiovascular events after PCI, and this of course includes ST. Clopidogrel, an inactive pro-drug, requires oxidation by the hepatic cytochrome P450 system to generate its active compound, which targets and irreversibly inhibits the platelet P2Y12 receptor. Several hepatic enzymes are involved in this metabolization process of clopidogrel. Recent studies link mutation in the CYP2C19 enzyme in the form of a loss-of-function polymorphism with an increased risk of ST following PCI[(69)]. It is possible that further genetic alterations will prove significant in determining one's individual risk of developing ST and genetic determination of these mutations will help identify patients at risk and provide a rationale for administration of an intensified antiplatelet treatment. The risk of clopidogrel resistance is about 5–10% and such patients are at risk of ischaemic events.

The novel thienopyridine *prasugrel* provides greater level of, and less variance in, inhibition of platelet aggregation. In the laboratory prasugrel nearly abolishes clopidogrel variable responses. Its efficacy, safety, and net clinical benefit were evaluated in the TRITON-TIMI 38 analysis[(70)], a study of acute coronary syndromes. A reduction in hazard ratio for ST was observed with prasugrel (51% reduction by 3 days and 55% reduction from 3 days to the end of trial—maximum 15-month follow-up). During the maintenance phase, the absolute risk difference with prasugrel for ST was 0.94%. Inspection of the event curves showed a progressive widening of the differences between the two treatment groups for ST during the first 3 days and from 3 days to the end of trial. There was no effect of stent type (BMS vs. DES) on prevention of ST with prasugrel. Nevertheless, a higher rate of major bleeding, especially in the maintenance period, is still the principal limit of a systematic prasugrel prescription; this treatment is not currently recommended for routine practice. How we will use this more potent agent that reduces ST is still unclear but becoming clearer. Currently, we do not routinely measure clopidogrel unresponsiveness but if we did (and there are planned studies to assess the value of systems like VerifyNow®) then those with less than optimal response to clopidogrel could receive prasugrel. Alternatively, we could use the data on predictors of ST, outlined earlier, to create a 'profile' of those most likely to suffer ST on the basis of clinical criteria and attenuate the risk by the use of agents such as prasugrel. There are other agents in the pipeline such as ticagrelor and cangrelor—direct P2Y12 inhibitors that may be beneficial. Downsides to the more potent antiplatelet agents is always the risk of excess bleeding compared to clopidogrel, most prominent in TRITON in the >75-year-olds, those with previous cerebrovascular events, and those with low body weight. Benefits of prasugrel over clopidogrel appear also to be shown in diabetics and in the context of this article in reducing ST (2.4% vs. 1.1% at 450 days) but TRITON did not compare prasugrel with clopidogrel pre-treatment which is a major study flaw, since we pre-load all our patients with clopidogrel. Therefore much of the potential beneficial prasugrel data on diabetics may not be applicable since it may not have been shown to be beneficial if the right comparator (preloaded clopidogrel) had been used. One exception may be the STEMIs where there is less time for pre-loading.

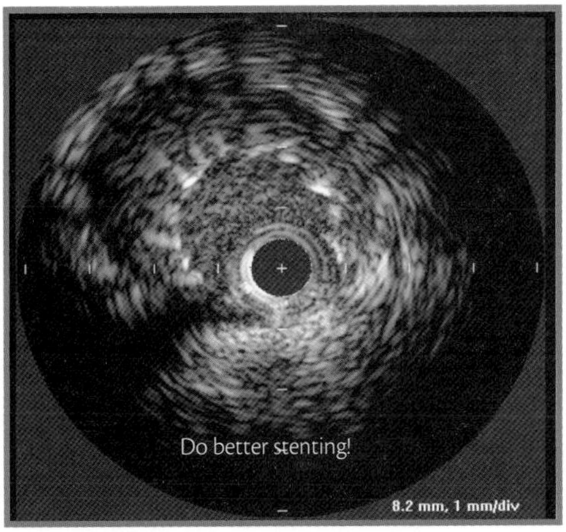

Fig. 29.6 Intravascular ultrasound showing stent underexpansion and malapposition.

Treatment of ST

Treatment is unsatisfactory since the event, coronary occlusion, has happened and thereafter any treatment is an attempt to retrieve the situation. Therefore all 'treatment' should be aimed at prevention in the first place.

- Above all, the first basis of preventive treatment for ST is good PCI technique, (Fig. 29.6) including good expansion and apposition of the stent with a low threshold for post-stenting dilatation at high pressure within the stent. In this context the role of intravascular ultrasound (IVUS), a technique that is significantly more sensitive than angiography in defining suboptimal stent deployment leading to ST, must be highlighted. IVUS studies have suggested that suboptimal stent deployment is a major aetiology underlying both DES restenosis and thrombosis[(71)]. The POST registry[(72)] suggests that stent malapposition, in-stent thrombus, and edge tears/dissection as determined by IVUS are important determinants of ST. However, *IVUS is not a cost-effective strategy to be performed in every stent deployment* and in cases where the clinical consequences of stent occlusion are great (such as with LMS disease) or where problems with antiplatelet therapy are anticipated, IVUS may be a useful adjunct to angiography in fully defining the optimal deployment of intracoronary stents
- Emerging technologies such as the intravascular optical coherence tomography (OCT) may provide new opportunities to perform a more refined analysis of vessel response to endovascular devices. The promise of OCT relies in its ability to generate ultra-high resolution cross-sectional images (down to 10 micron) of tissue layers using infrared back-reflected light, however with the drawback of a limited penetration. It is the optimal method for assessing stent strut apposition and subsequently during any follow-up stent strut coverage (Fig. 29.7). This does again not mean it is a routine clinical tool
- Regarding antiplatelet therapy, it may be important however to underscore the need of *compliance* with dual antiplatelet treatment. Predictors of premature discontinuation of thienopyridine therapy are older age, lower socioeconomic status, pre-existing cardiovascular disease, and lack of discharge instructions or cardiac rehabilitation. DES should be avoided in possible situations of potential non-compliance. In our institution, each patient undergoing PCI and stenting will receive at discharge a 'clopidogrel information card' indicating the date of the procedure, the type and name of the stent (BMS and/or DES) and the duration of clopidogrel treatment recommended
- As described previously, ST presents in most cases as an acute MI which can lead to death. Thus the principal objective in those presenting with ST must be to *obtain early effective reperfusion*. The thrombus quality in patients with ST differs from that in patients presenting with a usual acute MI. It is almost totally composed of platelets and contains very little fibrin and this fact may explain the poor efficacy of thrombolysis in obtaining reperfusion in this setting. Thus many interventionists rightly prefer emergency PCI for treatment of ST. The impact of thrombus aspiration for ST treatment is debated in the literature. According to the results of the TAPAS study[(73)], use of thrombus aspiration before stenting of the infarcted artery improves the 1-year clinical outcome after usual STEMI

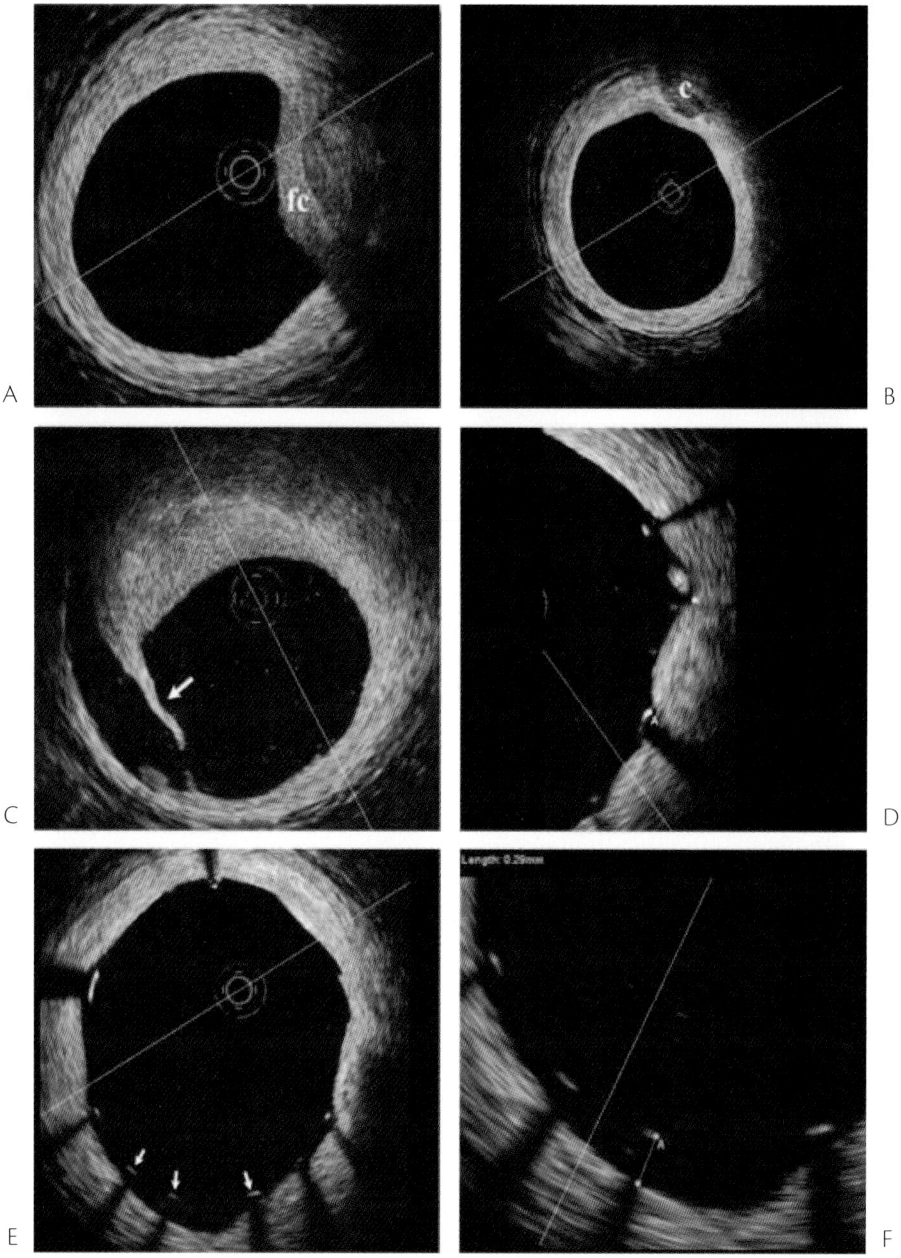

Fig. 29.7 Optical coherence tomography.

compared to conventional PCI. Thrombus quality in ST seems to be a good rationale for use of GP IIb/IIIa inhibitors. Indeed, some authors have shown efficacy with this treatment, with a reperfusion success rate of around 90% when associated with PCI. The most important point is to obtain an effective reperfusion, with TIMI flow grade 3, as quickly as possible

- Thus in a case of clear ST (recent stent and STEMI—see ARC definitions section) GP IIb/IIIa receptor inhibitors (such as abciximab/ReoPro®, Eli Lilly) should be considered as the patient arrives on the ward rather than wait till the patient comes to the cath lab. Aspiration should be considered and tried but wiring and achieving TIMI grade 3 flow is the prime objective

- Those with ST who survive should currently be treated with higher-dose clopidogrel (150mg daily) but in the future are likely to be treated with one of the newer thienopyridines, most likely prasugrel.

Future developments

ST may remain a problem even with newer second- or later-generation DES. Current trials with limited follow-up duration in low-risk patients preclude firm conclusion at this time[74]. Because durable polymers used in the first-generation DES are suspected to be responsible for some of the observed pathological changes, efforts concentrate on drug release via biodegradable polymers with reduced surface area through the use of reservoirs or coating of the abluminal surface only[75,76] and on polymer-free drug release[77]. However, the fact that early ST appears slightly lower in DES compared with BMS in randomized trials using identical patient management for both may be a hint that polymers protect from thrombosis during the phase when all stent struts are exposed to blood. Another approach concentrates on drugs with improved healing properties such as antibodies capturing CD34-positive endothelial progenitor cells[78]. Fully biodegradable stents based on polylactic acid or magnesium compounds are in clinical evaluation and may be the answer to longer-term ST. Finally, stent coating with improved biocompatibility such as titanium-nitride oxide have been shown to be more effective than conventional BMS in reducing restenosis and repeat revascularizaton[79].

The PROTECT trial (Patient-Related OuTcome with Endeavor versus Cypher stenting Trial) has just finished enrolling 8000 patients to compare safety and efficacy of the Endeavor® zotarolimus-eluting stent (Medtronic) to the Cypher® stent (Cordis Corporation, Johnson & Johnson), with ST as one of its primary endpoints at 3 years. Also currently ongoing are two prospective, randomized, multicentre trials that compare the Biolimus A9®-eluting (Nobori) stent Biomatrix® with a Cypher® SES (Limus Eluted From a Durable versus Erodable Stent Coating—LEADERS trial) and to a Taxus® Liberate PES (Boston Scientific) (Nobori-I study). Finally, the large-scale SPIRIT III, which was designed for further evaluation of the efficacy of the XIENCE V® everolimus-eluting stent (Abbott) compared to PES, published the 2-year clinical follow-up of the 1002 patients included[80]. With regard to ST this showed a differential pattern according to thienopyridine therapy. The rate of ST was comparable between the PES and EES within the first year after implantation; after 1 year, however, trends were present for fewer ST episodes within the EES than with the PES (0.3% versus 1.0%, respectively). Thienopyridine discontinuation within the first 6 months was associated with a nearly fivefold increase in the rate of thrombosis with both EES and PES, discontinuation for the first time after 6 months, however, was associated with a greater rate of subsequent ST with the PES than with the EES (2.6% vs. 0.4%), although given the relatively low rate of ST, this difference did not reach statistical significance ($p = 0.10$). Larger trials are required to confirm these observations. The event-free survival was improved in patients treated with EES rather than PES, with statistically significant 32% and 45% reductions, respectively.

Conclusions

PCI has become the treatment of choice in patients with ischaemic heart disease. The main risk attributable to bare-metal stenting was restenosis requiring repeat revascularization—a risk that largely ended within 1 year after stenting. The introduction of DES has reduced the occurrence of clinical restenosis by 50–70%. For both types of stents, ST is a serious clinical adverse event after PCI, potentially resulting in abrupt vessel closure with risk of MI and death. Although early ST and late ST occur with similar frequency after BMS or DES and outnumber very late ST by far, very late ST has emerged as a distinct clinical entity more germane to (at least the first-generation) DES than BMS. Decisions regarding percutaneous treatment of obstructive coronary disease have become increasingly challenging for patients and physicians since the observation of delayed ST in DES. Although there is no absolute marker of risk for ST or risk score, several predictors may help identify patients at risk and among those premature discontinuation of DAPT and poor stenting technique (i.e. stent undersizing and malapposition) require the most attention. Duration of DAPT remains largely unclarified, current guidelines recommend DAPT for 1 months after BMS and for 1 year after DES implantation. Randomized controlled trials are required to help establish the optimal duration and the benefit:risk ratio, as DAPT may be associated with increase risk of bleeding. Outcome to patients developing ST is poor with high mortality figures; therefore treatment of ST should be directed to achieving reperfusion fast, preferably by primary PCI. Finally, new antiplatelet agents and new-generation DES are available and initial results appear promising, but these have to be further studied in randomized controlled trials with adequate power and sufficient length of follow-up, until final conclusions can be drawn.

References

1. Comparison of coronary bypass surgery with angioplasty in patients with multivessel disease. The Bypass Angioplasty Revascularization Investigation (BARI) Investigators. *N Engl J Med* 1996; **335**:217–25.
2. Serruys PW, Ong AT, van Herwerden LA, *et al.* Five-year outcomes after coronary stenting versus bypass surgery for the treatment of multivessel disease: the final analysis of the Arterial Revascularization Therapies Study (ARTS) randomized trial. *J Am Coll Cardiol* 2005; **46**:575–81.
3. Morice MC, Serruys PW, Sousa JE, *et al.* A randomized comparison of a sirolimus-eluting stent with a standard stent for coronary revascularization. *N Engl J Med* 2002; **346**:1773–80.
4. Moses JW, Leon MB, Popma JJ, *et al.* Sirolimus-eluting stents versus standard stents in patients with stenosis in a native coronary artery. *N Engl J Med* 2003; **349**:1315–23.
5. Schampaert E, Cohen EA, Schluter M, *et al.* The Canadian study of the sirolimus-eluting stent in the treatment of patients with long de novo lesions in small native coronary arteries (C-SIRIUS). *J Am Coll Cardiol* 2004; **43**:1110–15.
6. Schofer J, Schluter M, Gershlick AH, *et al.* Sirolimus-eluting stents for treatment of patients with long atherosclerotic lesions in small coronary arteries: double-blind, randomised controlled trial (E-SIRIUS). *Lancet* 2003; **362**:1093–9.
7. Daemen J, Ong AT, Stefanini GG, *et al.* Three-year clinical follow-up of the unrestricted use of sirolimus-eluting stents as part of the Rapamycin-Eluting Stent Evaluated at Rotterdam Cardiology Hospital (RESEARCH) registry. *Am J Cardiol* 2006; **98**:895–901.
8. Urban P, Gershlick AH, Guagliumi G, *et al.* Safety of coronary sirolimus-eluting stents in daily clinical practice: one-year follow-up of the e-Cypher registry. *Circulation* 2006; **113**:1434–41.
9. Serruys PW, Kutryk MJ, Ong AT. Coronary-artery stents. *N Engl J Med* 2006; **354**:483–95.
10. McFadden EP, Stabile E, Regar E, *et al.* Late thrombosis in drug-eluting coronary stents after discontinuation of antiplatelet therapy. *Lancet* 2004; **364**:1519–21.
11. Camenzind E. Do drug-eluting stent increase death? ESC Congress News, Barcelona, Spain 2006.
12. Windecker S, Meier B. Late coronary stent thrombosis. *Circulation* 2007; **116**:1952–65.
13. Cutlip DE, Windecker S, Mehran R, *et al.* Clinical end points in coronary stent trials: a case for standardized definitions. *Circulation* 2007; **115**:2344–51.
14. Michelson AD. How platelets work: platelet function and dysfunction. *J Thromb Thrombol* 2003; **16**:7–12.
15. Farb A, Burke AP, Kolodgie FD, *et al.* Pathological mechanisms of fatal late coronary stent thrombosis in humans. *Circulation* 2003; **108**:1701–6.
16. Buonamici P, Marcucci R, Migliorini A, *et al.* Impact of platelet reactivity after clopidogrel administration on drug-eluting stent thrombosis. *J Am Coll Cardiol* 2007; **49**:2312–17.
17. Bhatt DL. Role of antiplatelet therapy across the spectrum of patients with coronary artery disease. *Am J Cardiol* 2009; **103**:11A–9A.
18. Finn AV, Nakazawa G, Joner M, *et al.* Vascular responses to drug eluting stents: importance of delayed healing. *Arterioscler Thromb Vasc Biol* 2007; **27**:1500–10.
19. Kotani J, Awata M, Nanto S, *et al.* Incomplete neointimal coverage of sirolimus-eluting stents: angioscopic findings. *J Am Coll Cardiol* 2006; **47**:2108–11.
20. Finn AV, Joner M, Nakazawa G, *et al.* Pathological correlates of late drug-eluting stent thrombosis: strut coverage as a marker of endothelialization. *Circulation* 2007; **115**:2435–41.
21. Tanner FC, Boehm M, Akyurek LM, *et al.* Differential effects of the cyclin-dependent kinase inhibitors p27(Kip1), p21(Cip1), and p16(Ink4) on vascular smooth muscle cell proliferation. *Circulation* 2000; **101**:2022–5.
22. Sun J, Marx SO, Chen HJ, *et al.* Role for p27(Kip1) in vascular smooth muscle cell migration. *Circulation* 2001; **103**:2967-72.
23. Garcia-Touchard A, Burke SE, Toner JL, *et al.* Zotarolimus-eluting stents reduce experimental coronary artery neointimal hyperplasia after 4 weeks. *Eur Heart J* 2006; **27**:988–93.
24. Muldowney JA, 3rd, Stringham JR, Levy SE, *et al.* Antiproliferative agents alter vascular plasminogen activator inhibitor-1 expression: a potential prothrombotic mechanism of drug-eluting stents. *Arterioscler Thromb Vasc Biol* 2007; **27**:400–6.
25. Nebeker JR, Virmani R, Bennett CL, *et al.* Hypersensitivity cases associated with drug-eluting coronary stents: a review of available cases from the Research on Adverse Drug Events and Reports (RADAR) project. *J Am Coll Cardiol* 2006; **47**:175–81.
26. Joner M, Finn AV, Farb A, *et al.* Pathology of drug-eluting stents in humans: delayed healing and late thrombotic risk. *J Am Coll Cardiol* 2006; **48**:193–202.
27. Imanishi T, Kobayashi K, Kuki S, *et al.* Sirolimus accelerates senescence of endothelial progenitor cells through telomerase inactivation. *Atherosclerosis* 2006; **189**:288–96.
28. Wenzel J, Gijsen, FJH, Schuubiers, JCH, *et al.* The influence of shear stress on in-stent restenosis and thrombosis. *EuroIntervention* 2008; **4**(Suppl.C):C27–32.
29. Togni M, Raber L, Cocchia R, *et al.* Local vascular dysfunction after coronary paclitaxel-eluting stent implantation. *Int J Cardiol* 2007; **120**:212–20.
30. Schatz RA, Baim DS, Leon M, *et al.* Clinical experience with the Palmaz-Schatz coronary stent. Initial results of a multicenter study. *Circulation* 1991; **83**:148–61.
31. Serruys PW, Strauss BH, Beatt KJ, *et al.* Angiographic follow-up after placement of a self-expanding coronary-artery stent. *N Engl J Med* 1991; **324**:13–17.
32. Schomig A, Neumann FJ, Kastrati A, *et al.* A randomized comparison of antiplatelet and anticoagulant therapy after the placement of coronary-artery stents. *N Engl J Med* 1996; **334**:1084–9.

33. Bertrand ME, Legrand V, Boland J, *et al.* Randomized multicenter comparison of conventional anticoagulation versus antiplatelet therapy in unplanned and elective coronary stenting. The full anticoagulation versus aspirin and ticlopidine (fantastic) study. *Circulation* 1998; **98**:1597–603.
34. Leon MB, Baim DS, Popma JJ, *et al.* A clinical trial comparing three antithrombotic-drug regimens after coronary-artery stenting. Stent Anticoagulation Restenosis Study Investigators. *N Engl J Med* 1998; **339**:1665–71.
35. Urban P, Macaya C, Rupprecht HJ, *et al.* Randomized evaluation of anticoagulation versus antiplatelet therapy after coronary stent implantation in high-risk patients: the multicenter aspirin and ticlopidine trial after intracoronary stenting (MATTIS). *Circulation* 1998; **98**:2126–32.
36. Bertrand ME, Rupprecht HJ, Urban P, *et al.* Double-blind study of the safety of clopidogrel with and without a loading dose in combination with aspirin compared with ticlopidine in combination with aspirin after coronary stenting: the clopidogrel aspirin stent international cooperative study (CLASSICS). *Circulation* 2000; **102**:624–9.
37. Wenaweser P, Rey C, Eberli FR, *et al.* Stent thrombosis following bare-metal stent implantation: success of emergency percutaneous coronary intervention and predictors of adverse outcome. *Eur Heart J* 2005; **26**:1180–7.
38. Stettler C, Wandel S, Allemann S, *et al.* Outcomes associated with drug-eluting and bare-metal stents: a collaborative network meta-analysis. *Lancet* 2007; **370**:937–48.
39. Kastrati A, Mehilli J, Pache J, *et al.* Analysis of 14 trials comparing sirolimus-eluting stents with bare-metal stents. *N Engl J Med* 2007; **356**:1030–9.
40. Stone GW, Moses JW, Ellis SG, *et al.* Safety and efficacy of sirolimus- and paclitaxel-eluting coronary stents. *N Engl J Med* 2007; **356**:998–1008.
41. Mauri L, Hsieh WH, Massaro JM, *et al.* Stent thrombosis in randomized clinical trials of drug-eluting stents. *N Engl J Med* 2007; **356**:1020–9.
42. Spaulding C, Daemen J, Boersma E, *et al.* A pooled analysis of data comparing sirolimus-eluting stents with bare-metal stents. *N Engl J Med* 2007; **356**:989–97.
43. Jensen LO, Maeng M, Kaltoft A, *et al.* Stent thrombosis, myocardial infarction, and death after drug-eluting and bare-metal stent coronary interventions. *J Am Coll Cardiol* 2007; **50**:463–70.
44. Daemen J, Wenaweser P, Tsuchida K, *et al.* Early and late coronary stent thrombosis of sirolimus-eluting and paclitaxel-eluting stents in routine clinical practice: data from a large two-institutional cohort study. *Lancet* 2007; **369**:667–78.
45. Wenaweser P, Daemen J, Zwahlen M, *et al.* Incidence and correlates of drug-eluting stent thrombosis in routine clinical practice. 4-year results from a large 2-institutional cohort study. *J Am Coll Cardiol* 2008; **52**:1134–40.
46. Williams DO, Abbott JD, Kip KE. Outcomes of 6906 patients undergoing percutaneous coronary intervention in the era of drug-eluting stents: report of the DEScover Registry. *Circulation* 2006; **114**:2154–62.
47. Lagerqvist B, James SK, Stenestrand U, *et al.* Long-term outcomes with drug-eluting stents versus bare-metal stents in Sweden. *N Engl J Med* 2007; **356**:1009–19.
48. de la Torre-Hernandez JM, Alfonso F, Hernandez F, *et al.* Drug-eluting stent thrombosis: results from the multicenter Spanish registry ESTROFA (Estudio ESpanol sobre TROmbosis de stents FArmacoactivos). *J Am Coll Cardiol* 2008; **51**:986–90.
49. Kappetein AP, Dawkins KD, Mohr FW, *et al.* Current percutaneous coronary intervention and coronary artery bypass grafting practices for three-vessel and left main coronary artery disease. Insights from the SYNTAX run-in phase. *Eur J Cardiothorac Surg* 2006; **29**:486–91.
50. Chieffo A, Park SJ, Meliga E, *et al.* Late and very late stent thrombosis following drug-eluting stent implantation in unprotected left main coronary artery: a multicentre registry. *Eur Heart J* 2008; **29**:2108–15.
51. Steg PG, Fox KA, Eagle KA, *et al.* Mortality following placement of drug-eluting and bare-metal stents for ST-segment elevation acute myocardial infarction in the Global Registry of Acute Coronary Events. *Eur Heart J* 2009; **30**:321–9.
52. Percoco G, Manari A, Guastaroba P, *et al.* Safety and long-term efficacy of sirolimus eluting stent in ST-elevation acute myocardial infarction: the REAL (Registro REgionale AngiopLastiche Emilia-Romagna) registry. *Cardiovasc Drugs Ther* 2006; **20**:63–8.
53. Kastrati A, Dibra A, Spaulding C, *et al.* Meta-analysis of randomized trials on drug-eluting stents vs. bare-metal stents in patients with acute myocardial infarction. *Eur Heart J* 2007; **28**:2706–13.
54. Pasceri V, Patti G, Speciale G, *et al.* Meta-analysis of clinical trials on use of drug-eluting stents for treatment of acute myocardial infarction. *Am Heart J* 2007; **153**:749–54.
55. Kirtane AJ, Ellis SG, Dawkins KD, *et al.* Paclitaxel-eluting coronary stents in patients with diabetes mellitus: pooled analysis from 5 randomized trials. *J Am Coll Cardiol* 2008; **51**:708–15.
56. Iakovou I, Schmidt T, Bonizzoni E, *et al.* Incidence, predictors, and outcome of thrombosis after successful implantation of drug-eluting stents. *JAMA* 2005; **293**:2126–30.
57. Airoldi F, Colombo A, Morici N, *et al.* Incidence and predictors of drug-eluting stent thrombosis during and after discontinuation of thienopyridine treatment. *Circulation* 2007; **116**:745–54.
58. van Werkum JW, Heestermans AA, Zomer AC, *et al.* Predictors of coronary stent thrombosis: the Dutch Stent Thrombosis Registry. *J Am Coll Cardiol* 2009; **53**:1399–409.

59. Smith SC, Jr, Feldman TE, Hirshfeld JW, Jr, *et al.* ACC/AHA/SCAI 2005 Guideline Update for Percutaneous Coronary Intervention–summary article: a report of the American College of Cardiology/American Heart Association Task Force on Practice Guidelines (ACC/AHA/SCAI Writing Committee to Update the 2001 Guidelines for Percutaneous Coronary Intervention). *Circulation* 2006; **113**:156–75.
60. Pfisterer M, Brunner-La Rocca HP, Buser PT, *et al.* Late clinical events after clopidogrel discontinuation may limit the benefit of drug-eluting stents: an observational study of drug-eluting versus bare-metal stents. *J Am Coll Cardiol* 2006; **48**:2584–91.
61. Kaiser C, Brunner-La Rocca HP, Buser PT, *et al.* Incremental cost-effectiveness of drug-eluting stents compared with a third-generation bare-metal stent in a real-world setting: randomised Basel Stent Kosten Effektivitats Trial (BASKET). *Lancet* 2005; **366**:921–9.
62. Pfisterer M, Brunner-La Rocca HP, Rickenbacher P, *et al.* Long-term benefit-risk balance of drug-eluting vs. bare-metal stents in daily practice: does stent diameter matter? Three-year follow-up of BASKET. *Eur Heart J* 2009; **30**:16–24.
63. Silber S, Albertsson P, Aviles FF, *et al.* Guidelines for percutaneous coronary interventions. The Task Force for Percutaneous Coronary Interventions of the European Society of Cardiology. *Eur Heart J* 2005; **26**:804–47.
64. Update to FDA statement on coronary drug-eluting stents. http://wwwfdagov/cdrh/news/010407html 2008.
65. Grines CL, Bonow RO, Casey DE, Jr, *et al.* Prevention of premature discontinuation of dual antiplatelet therapy in patients with coronary artery stents: a science advisory from the American Heart Association, American College of Cardiology, Society for Cardiovascular Angiography and Interventions, American College of Surgeons, and American Dental Association, with representation from the American College of Physicians. *J Am Coll Cardiol* 2007; **49**:734–9.
66. Steinhubl SR, Berger PB, Mann JT, 3rd, *et al.* Early and sustained dual oral antiplatelet therapy following percutaneous coronary intervention: a randomized controlled trial. *JAMA* 2002; **288**:2411–20.
67. Eisenstein EL, Anstrom KJ, Kong DF, *et al.* Clopidogrel use and long-term clinical outcomes after drug-eluting stent implantation. *JAMA* 2007; **297**:159–68.
68. Bhatt DL, Flather MD, Hacke W, *et al.* Patients with prior myocardial infarction, stroke, or symptomatic peripheral arterial disease in the CHARISMA trial. *J Am Coll Cardiol* 2007; **49**:1982–8.
69. Sibbing D, Stegherr J, Latz W, *et al.* Cytochrome P450 2C19 loss-of-function polymorphism and stent thrombosis following percutaneous coronary intervention. *Eur Heart J* 2009; **30**:916–22.
70. Antman EM, Wiviott SD, Murphy SA, *et al.* Early and late benefits of prasugrel in patients with acute coronary syndromes undergoing percutaneous coronary intervention: a TRITON-TIMI 38 (TRial to Assess Improvement in Therapeutic Outcomes by Optimizing Platelet InhibitioN with Prasugrel-Thrombolysis In Myocardial Infarction) analysis. *J Am Coll Cardiol* 2008; **51**:2028–33.
71. Roy P, Steinberg DH, Sushinsky SJ, *et al.* The potential clinical utility of intravascular ultrasound guidance in patients undergoing percutaneous coronary intervention with drug-eluting stents. *Eur Heart J* 2008; **29**:1851–7.
72. Uren NG, Schwarzacher SP, Metz JA, *et al.* Predictors and outcomes of stent thrombosis: an intravascular ultrasound registry. *Eur Heart J* 2002; **23**:124–32.
73. Vlaar PJ, Svilaas T, van der Horst IC, *et al.* Cardiac death and reinfarction after 1 year in the Thrombus Aspiration during Percutaneous coronary intervention in Acute myocardial infarction Study (TAPAS): a 1-year follow-up study. *Lancet* 2008; **371**:1915–20.
74. Fajadet J, Wijns W, Laarman GJ, *et al.* Randomized, double-blind, multicenter study of the Endeavor zotarolimus-eluting phosphorylcholine-encapsulated stent for treatment of native coronary artery lesions: clinical and angiographic results of the ENDEAVOR II trial. *Circulation* 2006; **114**:798–806.
75. Serruys PW, Sianos G, Abizaid A, *et al.* The effect of variable dose and release kinetics on neointimal hyperplasia using a novel paclitaxel-eluting stent platform: the Paclitaxel In-Stent Controlled Elution Study (PISCES). *J Am Coll Cardiol* 2005; **46**:253–60.
76. Grube E, Buellesfeld L. BioMatrix Biolimus A9-eluting coronary stent: a next-generation drug-eluting stent for coronary artery disease. *Expert Rev Med Devices* 2006; **3**:731–41.
77. Scheller B, Hehrlein C, Bocksch W, *et al.* Treatment of coronary in-stent restenosis with a paclitaxel-coated balloon catheter. *N Engl J Med* 2006; **355**:2113–24.
78. Aoki J, Serruys PW, van Beusekom H, *et al.* Endothelial progenitor cell capture by stents coated with antibody against CD34: the HEALING-FIM (Healthy Endothelial Accelerated Lining Inhibits Neointimal Growth-First In Man) Registry. *J Am Coll Cardiol* 2005; **45**:1574–9.
79. Windecker S, Simon R, Lins M, *et al.* Randomized comparison of a titanium-nitride-oxide-coated stent with a stainless steel stent for coronary revascularization: the TiNOX trial. *Circulation* 2005; **111**:2617–22.
80. Stone GW, Midei M, Newman W, *et al.* Randomized comparison of everolimus-eluting and paclitaxel-eluting stents: two-year clinical follow-up from the Clinical Evaluation of the Xience V Everolimus Eluting Coronary Stent System in the Treatment of Patients with de novo Native Coronary Artery Lesions (SPIRIT) III trial. *Circulation* 2009; **119**:680–6.

CHAPTER 30

Stent loss and retrieval

Adam de Belder and Mrinal Saha

It is a painful thing to look at your own trouble
and know that you yourself and no-one else
had made it.

Ajax. Sophocles, 447 BC.

In the right hands, percutaneous coronary intervention (PCI) is a relatively straightforward technique that is rewarding for both the operator and the patient. Success rates are high, and complications of PCI are unusual. Meticulous technique generally avoids problems. When complications occur, the consequences can be significant and understanding how to deal with them in order to secure satisfactory outcomes is key. One such complication is stent loss, whereby a stent becomes dislodged from the delivery balloon platform. Fortunately the phenomenon is rare. The methods used to manage stent loss can potentially be associated with significant morbidity. This chapter addresses the incidence, classification, and management of stent loss.

Incidence

The incidence of stent loss was greater when the operator was required to manually compress (crimp) a stent onto the delivery balloon (1.43–8.3%; see Table 30.1). In the era of factory-mounted stents, loss is less frequent. In the largest review to date[1], stent loss occurred in 38 (0.32%) of 11 773 procedures, with successful retrieval in 30 of these (86%). Five patients had failed attempts at externalization, although retrieval from the coronary tree was successful.

Of those in whom stent loss occurred, 24% required transfusion following access site complications, 5% emergency coronary artery bypass grafting (CABG), and 2.6% died.

There is thus a persistent but low reported incidence of stent loss that probably predominantly reflects the increasing complexity of cases which are undertaken rather more than a specific defect in the stent technology itself.

Stent loss is relatively rare, and fortunately significant clinical events occur only in exceptional cases. A broad message from the angioplasty literature is that the procedure should be kept simple. Increasing complexity of cases rarely leads to better results, but definitely leads to increasing complications.

Factors that may contribute to the risk of stent loss may be categorized as follows:

- Anatomical: 1) coronary anatomy that is tortuous and calcified, thus increasing the rigidity of the vessel making it more likely for a stent to be peeled off the balloon as increasing force is applied to advance the device[1]. Similarly a stent may be partially advanced within a lesion, but withdrawal is restricted by the anatomy leading to balloon removal with an undeployed stent left within the vessel. 2) Patients with previous coronary artery bypass grafting; or 3) in whom there is a coronary dissection also tend to have a greater risk of stent loss[1].
- Equipment: 1) stent delivery balloons may fail to expand properly leaving a partially deployed stent within the vessel as the balloon is withdrawn, with consequent partial failure of stent wall apposition. This may often occur because of calcified and eccentric plaque that resists stent expansion. 2) Poor guide support may contribute to stent loss in two ways. First, the lack of support may lead to stents being passed to the lesion but drawn back because of failure

Table 30.1 Reported episodes and retrieval success of stent loss[1]

Author (reference)	Publication year	Incidence of stent loss	Retrieval success rate
Foster-Smith KW[2]	1993	3/193 (1.6%)	3/3(100%)
Alfonso[3]	1996	17/11 495 (3.4%)	9/17 (53%)
Elsner[4]	1996	6/419 (1.43%)	4/6 (66%)
Cantor[5]	1998	108/1303 (8.3%)	60/134 (45%)
Eggebrecht[6]	2000	20/2211 (0.9%)	10/14 (71%)
Brilakis[1]	2005	38/11 773 (0.32%)	30/35 (86%)

to cross, with inadvertent slippage of the stent off the balloon during this process. Second, a common mechanism of stent loss occurs when a stent cannot be deployed and upon withdrawal the stent is caught by the edge of the guide, dislodging it from the balloon platform. A failure of the guide to be coaxial to the coronary makes this complication substantially more likely

- Operator decision-making:
  - Direct stenting of lesions in heavily calcified and/or tortuous vessels may lead to poor lesion access and inadequate stent expansion, with the same consequences as described earlier[1]. This emphasizes the basic PCI principle of ensuring optimal lesion preparation usually by modification either using balloon angioplasty or atherectomy
  - Bifurcation strategies: numerous techniques have been described to provide stent coverage of both limbs of a bifurcation. This often requires the passage of one stent through the struts of another or the manipulation of balloons through recently deployed stents. The requirement of such techniques for two wires and two balloons or stents in the vessel increases the chances of stent loss. Current randomized trial data do not support two-stent strategies in bifurcation disease[7]
  - Treatment of multivessel disease with stenting instead of bypass surgery: increasingly often patients are considered too high risk for bypass surgery, but have coronary disease requiring the use of multiple stents, thereby increasing the risk of procedure-related complications[1]

Brilakis and colleagues[1] confirm the theoretically intuitive prediction that the clinical factors that appear to be associated with stent loss include proximal tortuosity of the target vessel, lesions located on a bend, and the degree of lesion calcification.

Strategies to manage stent loss

A later section describes case reports of episodes in which operators have employed innovative and sometimes imaginative techniques to address stent loss. However, the best approach is to avoid stent loss. Once it has occurred there are four principal strategies (Fig. 30.1):

1) Assuming the guide wire remains in place, a small balloon or pair of balloons can be passed through the stent, expanded, and retracted (see Case 4, Fig. 30.19).
2) A snare or retrieval device can be used to drag the stent back into a sheath (see Case 1, Figs. 30.9 and 30.10)
3) A free stent in the intracoronary circulation may be associated with an increased risk of thrombosis or endothelial disruption leading to myocardial infarction[4], emergency CABG[4,6], or death. The stent may be either deployed (in the vessel segment where it has become dislodged), or crushed with a second stent without retrieval. Reports suggest few, if any, adverse consequences of this strategy[6,8] although this may not be the most suitable solution for stents dislodged in the left main stem or proximal LAD where restenosis is most critical. Ideally however, this strategy should be accompanied by intravascular ultrasound to ensure adequate strut apposition of the second stent following crushing[9]. As well as reducing both contrast load and fluoroscopy dose, the procedure may be far less complicated than stent retrieval, as previous authors report from their experience in complex stent strategies such as bifurcations[10,11].
4) The stent may be crushed in the peripheral circulation using a larger peripheral stent[12], or left as a distal embolic phenomenon, which appears to have had a benign clinical course in all patients receiving this strategy in previous series[1,3,6]. In the peripheral circulation, unless the patient is symptomatic from

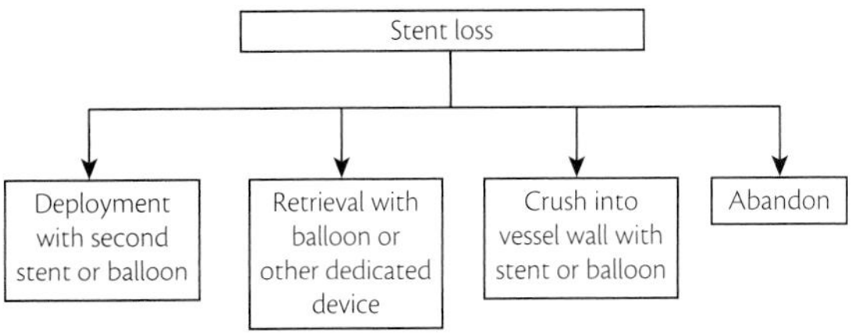

Fig. 30.1 Summary of strategies for managing stent loss.

the embolized material[13], or if there is a risk of cerebral embolization, a surgical intervention may not be required.

History: stent retrieval

The first .percutaneous retrieval of an intravascular foreign body was described in 1964[1]. Thomas *et al.* describe how a stainless steel guide wire was embolized into the inferior vena cava during right heart catheterization in a woman with mitral insufficiency. Surgery was avoided by introducing a bronchoscope forceps to the level of the wire through the saphenous vein, with successful retrieval. The majority of experience in non-surgical removal of embolized devices was gained in the venous system prior to the advent of routine cardiac catheterization, with the commonest methods being the snare, wire basket, and endoscopy forceps[15,16]. Correspondingly, some of those device designs were adapted for retrieval purposes in the arterial tree[2], with the first report of an intra-aortic retrieval of a fractured guide wire being described in 1985[17]. The first description of a successful retrieval of an embolized stent appeared in 1993, incorporating the use of both a balloon and biopsy forceps[18].

Principles and methods of stent retrieval

General considerations

Choice of guide catheter: maximizing guide support allows for more effective retrieval. One of the contributing factors to stent loss may be an inadequately supportive guide catheter. If no wire remains inside the lost stent, changing the guide over an exchange wire at this stage may be the most appropriate manoeuvre, the new catheter having a larger internal diameter allowing for a retrieval strategy to be used.

If the intention is to maintain the coronary guide wire position, but a larger gauge or different-shaped guide catheter or sheath is required, the procedure to exchange the guide catheter may be complicated by both loss of wire position and bleeding from the access point. One possible exchange method is as follows:

- Place an exchange dock wire on the distal end of an intracoronary guide wire. The dock wire has a hollow proximal end for receiving the distal end of the in situ coronary wire. This is attached by careful firm pressure of these two ends, minimizing the force applied in any direction other than parallel to the wires' long axis, thus reducing the risk of wire fracture
- Remove current guide catheter under screening, attempting to maintain wire position in the coronary artery
- Remove current sheath (if required) and exchange for larger sheath maintaining pressure over access point
- Introduce new guide catheter/retrieval sheath over the guide wire–dock wire combination
- Remove dock wire and proceed with retrieval.

This method may be compromised by the lack of support from the intracoronary guide wire, so the placement of a second intracoronary wire/dock system may be required to improve support during the exchange.

Given the prolonged nature of retrieval procedures, meticulous attention should be paid both to ensure adequate *anticoagulation* throughout the case with systemic heparinization, and also to prevent embolization of air through the large-bore devices required.

Imaging: biplane angiography provides more comprehensive three-dimensional imaging than monoplane as well as potentially reducing radiation dose.

Some *retrieval devices* may be packaged with their own carrier catheter, but the majority of cases require the use of a separate catheter to deliver the retrieval device. In general, a sheath 2–3F sizes larger than the original sheath may be required to retrieve the stent. The long sheath may have to be shaped by the operator prior to insertion to minimize trauma to the vascular system during advancement to the target location. In order to position these sheaths, a long 0.035-inch Super Stiff® wire (Boston Scientific Corp., USA) may be required. Accurate placement of the delivery sheath for the retrieval device may require the use of a separate guiding catheter, within which the retrieval catheter system may need to be placed. This double support may allow for extra force to be applied when pulling the retrieved stent into the sheath, preventing the tip of the retrieval catheter for collapsing as the retrieved stent is retracted (see Case 6). Once the stent has been captured, it should be withdrawn in its entirety into the retrieval

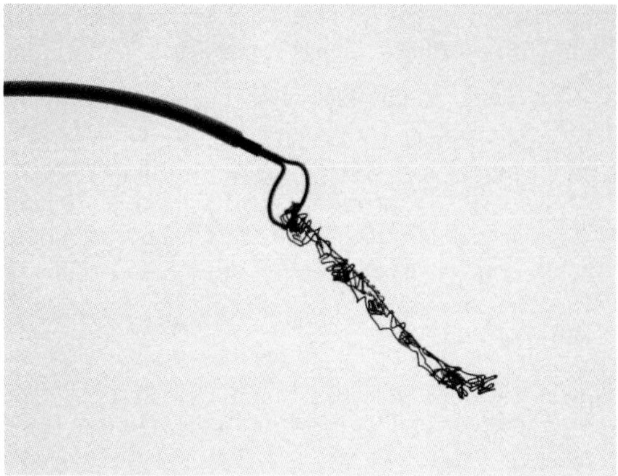

Fig. 30.2 A stent retrieved by a snare device, with obvious distortion of stent architecture.

sheath to prevent irregular edges from traumatizing the vessel (Fig. 30.2)

A short stiff recovery sheath may also be useful for withdrawing the retrieval sheath and device. These short sheaths are often used during implantation of ASD closure devices, and are effective for withdrawing objects which have not been fully crushed inside the retrieval sheath, thus minimizing skin trauma as the embolized stent/retrieval sheath/retrieval device combination is externalized.

If an attempt is made to *capture a stent that has embolized into the left ventricle*, the retrieval device should have the stent completely enclosed within the carrier sheath before the system is drawn back through the aortic valve to avoid damage or entanglement.

Retrieval methods using non-specialized equipment

Single-balloon technique

This technique is perhaps the most commonly used for stent retrieval and is practicable only if the stent remains on the angioplasty guide wire. After withdrawal of the stent balloon from which the stent has become dislodged, a second, smaller balloon (such as a 2 × 12mm) is passed through the same guide catheter as the first, and advanced through the stent. This balloon is then inflated, and drawn back with the stent buttressed between it and the guide catheter. The disadvantages are: 1) finding a balloon small enough to pass through the stent; 2) increasing the risk of the stent being pushed further down the vessel as the balloon is advanced; 3) externalizing the stent without upgrading to larger diameter sheath. Indeed, a feature common to most methods of stent salvage using non-dedicated retrieval devices is that the stent cannot be withdrawn back into the original sheath, which may result in the decision to deploy the stent or crush it in the peripheral circulation. There are few reported negative outcomes associated with this strategy.

Double-balloon technique

This utilizes the same principles as the single balloon technique, applied if the stent is retained on the guide wire but not deployed in the vessel, but requires two balloons if the stent diameter is too large for a single balloon to retract (see Case 4).

'Home-made' snares

A snare may also be fashioned by the operator in the catheter lab using a coronary catheter and a long intracoronary guide wire, if commercially made devices are unavailable. The loop of the snare is made by folding over the mid section of the guide wire. The doubled over portion is then the first part of the wire to the guide catheter, leaving the two ends trailing. The guide wire needs to be long enough to allow the two free ends of the wire to remain externalized even as the loop has exited the end hole of the catheter and entered the circulation. The guide catheter must therefore be large enough to accommodate the diameter of effectively two coronary guide wires and any retrieved stent. The device is then used in a similar fashion to commercial snares. The free ends of the wire are passed through a bleed back valve such as the Ketch® (Minvasys, France) or Tuohy-Borst to allow both control of the loop and also prevent internalization of these free ends. An angulation of the two ends of the wire at the base of the loop can be made to facilitate ensnaring of the stent in a manner similar to commercial snares, as otherwise the long axis of the loop remains parallel to both the guide catheter and blood vessel, which is less likely to result in successful retrieval. The main disadvantage of operator-fashioned snares is that they tend not to retain any preformed shape. Once deformed, they do not open out to produce as large an area for grasping as commercial snares, but instead take on a more slit-like configuration. A Terumo wire however will retain a more open loop after passage through the guide catheter, but will not be amenable to being angulated. Hence the preformed loop remains parallel but not perpendicular to the axis of the catheter, which may reduce the likelihood of ensnarement.

Wire braiding technique

This method is useful if the stent has come off the balloon but remains on the wire. A second, soft-tipped wire is passed alongside the stent, taking care not to push the stent off the wire, which is then passed into a branch distal to the stent and separate form the first wire. Torque is then applied to both wires, and the twisting action results in the wires wrapping around both sides of the stent, trapping the stent between the wrapped portions. Both wires are then retracted, pulling the stent out of -the coronary tree. This method requires the up-front use of a large enough sheath to allow retrieval and externalization of the guide catheter, wrapped wires and stent. There is a risk that the stent will still not come out of the vessel in which case the wires may also be trapped. Backward pressure on the wires may also pull the guide further into the coronary artery, hence running the risk of creating dissection. Finally the wires may break off if the stent will not come out.

Use of distal embolic protection devices (DEPD) for retrieval

Embolic protection devices, used to capture unwanted debris embolized from stent deployment in vein grafts, have also been used as stent capture devices (see Case 3). Typically their use has been serendipitous, with planned insertion during vein graft angioplasty[19,20]. Their open configuration is effective for trapping a free-floating stent, but as their primary purpose is to capture clots, their design does not allow for effective crushing. Hence the DEPD, stent, guide wire, and guide catheter are withdrawn as a single unit if possible. However, if the long axis of the stent is not co-axial with the vessel, the DEPD cannot be withdrawn unless it is re-sheathed, and an alternative strategy is sought.

Commercial retrieval devices

Snares

These are probably the most widely used tools for stent retrieval[2,6]. One widely used design consists of a halo-shaped ring of flexible wire attached at a single point to a second wire which can be manipulated by the operator (Fig. 30.3).

Other designs incorporate several loops attached to a wire, such as the EN Snare® system, thus potentially maximizing the chance of capturing the stent (Fig. 30.4).

The angle of the loop with respect to the connecting wire, and the material used to make the loop portion varies between manufacturers. The snare is opened and closed by advancing or retracting movements respectively while fixing the end hole catheter that ensheaths the snare, acting as the 'carrier' catheter. Typically, the method of retrieval involves either direct grasping proximal to the embolized stent, or passing the tip of carrier catheter distal to the stent with the retrieval device still fully sheathed within the catheter. The loop

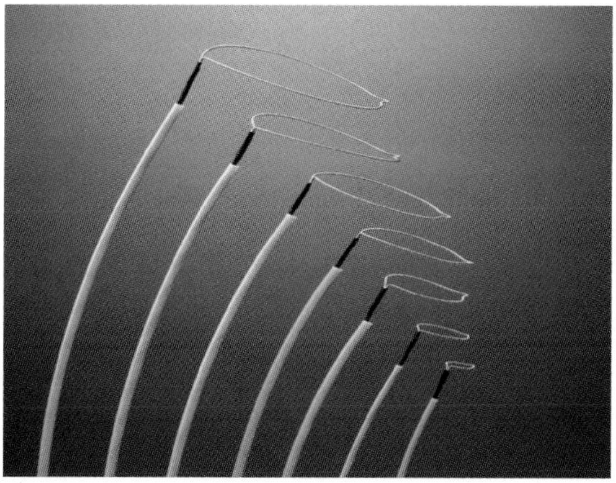

Fig. 30.3 Examples of snares with varying sizes (image courtesy of ev3).

is then advanced, keeping the catheter fixed. The snare and catheter are gradually withdrawn until the snare has encircled the stent. Then snare is then fixed while the carrier catheter is advanced, thus closing the loop and capturing the stent within the catheter (see Case 1).

Several snare sizes are available (Fig. 30.3), and typically the most efficient retrieval is determined by matching snare and vessel diameter. The main limitation of the snare design is that only stents with a free end can be encircled and captured. Thus these snares are often used in combination with a separate wire introduced from a separate vascular access point, which is used to pass through the embolized object. The distal end of the second wire is then grasped by the snare and may then be used to pull the stent free.

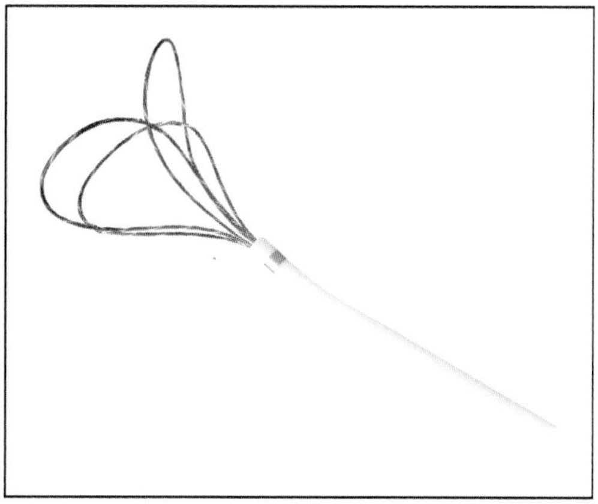

Fig. 30.4 The EN Snare® device (Image courtesy of Hatch Medical®, LLC).

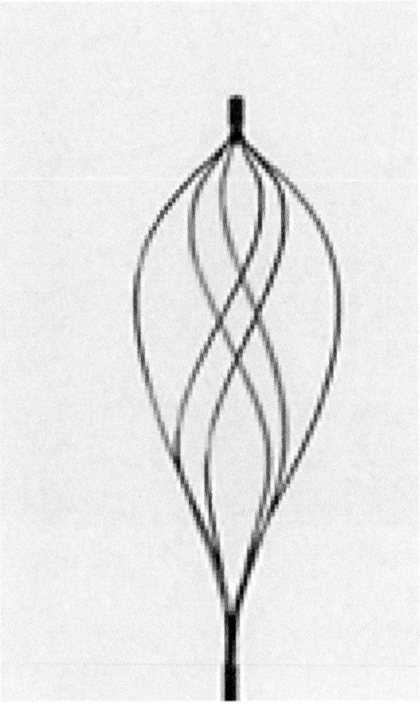

Fig. 30.5 Example of retrieval basket (courtesy of Global Laser Solutions).

Basket devices

These are comprised of between three and five separate wires, each of which has been curved at the distal end, and welded together at their tips (Fig. 30.5).

Similar to the snare systems, they are combined at the proximal point of convergence to form a single wire which can be withdrawn into a carrier catheter. As a consequence of the more numerous wires required in their construction, basket devices necessitate larger diameter delivery sheaths than their single-snare counterparts. They are useful for removal of larger diameter stents or objects that require compression before withdrawal, and cannot be used in the coronary tree. Manipulation of the basket device requires the distal tip to be advanced beyond the embolized stent, allowing the centre of the opened helix to lie adjacent. The device is then gently rotated and moved back and forth until the stent is caught. However, the initial manoeuvre of passing the basket beyond the stent may result in displacing the stent further distally which is perhaps the main drawback of this system. Yet the more robust construction of basket devices allows for more reliable compression of a retrieved stent than conventional snares following withdrawal into the carrier sheath.

As with the basket devices, these are too large to be used in the coronary tree. Their design consists of long, digit-like wire projections which can be extended and retracted to grasp a loose stent, without the necessity of encircling the stent entirely[19]. The device is delivered through a long sheath which should be 3–4F sizes greater to accommodate the retrieved object. If the device is unable to exert sufficient grip upon the grasped object, it may also be used in conjunction with a snare device. The snare is first passed into the same sheath as the forceps, and advanced until the loop of the snare encircles the forceps before the jaws are fully opened. The forceps then grip the stent, after which the open loop is passed distally to now ensnare the stent and pulled back into the sheath, grabbed by both snare and forceps devices.

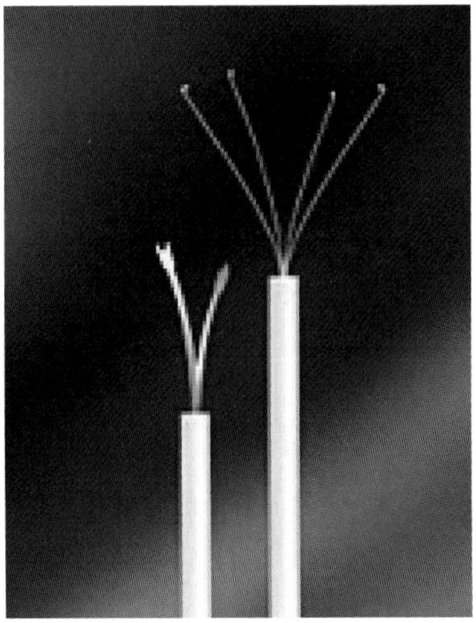

Fig. 30.6 Biliary Forceps (image courtesy of Sumayamed).

Complications of retrieval

- Prolonged manipulation of retrieval devices or catheters wires may increase risk of clot or air embolization
- Inability to remove a lost stent may lead to coronary ischaemia from vessel obstruction, or thrombosis
- Tearing of intravascular structures during stent removal may lead to vessel rupture and tamponade. Such complications may lead to emergency surgery with a high associated mortality
- Some retrieval devices may become self-entangled during the retrieval process, or caught upon heart valves
- Failure to withdraw the stent into access sheath may require the stent to be deployed in the peripheral circulation

- Guide catheter dissection due to pulling back on devices within the coronary when trying to move the stent backwards
- Vascular access site bleeding, haematoma, and tearing due to excessive trauma and larger sheath sizes.

Few data exist comparing the outcomes of patients in whom stent loss has occurred. As the incidence is so small, it is unlikely that any direct comparison can be made to patients without stent loss. This is suggested in the study by Brilakis[1], in which the stent loss group was reported to have significantly higher emergency CABG, retroperitoneal bleeding, and transfusion requirement. However the number in the stent loss and no stent loss groups were 38 and 11 735 respectively.

Case reports

Case 1

Tortuous calcified left main artery into circumflex increases the risk of stent loss (Fig. 30.7).

The undeployed stent is retained within the left main coronary artery (arrows) (Fig. 30.8).

The snare is looped over the distal end of the stent and withdrawn into the guiding catheter (Fig. 30.9).

The disrupted stent is removed with the help of a snare (Fig. 30.10).

Case 2

A stent has become stuck in the mid-course of this tortuous right coronary artery (Fig. 30.11).

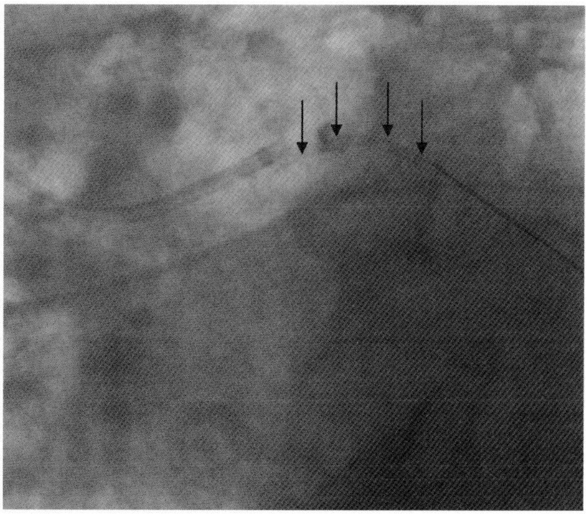

Fig. 30.8 Undeployed stent in left main/circumflex angle having come off the balloon.

A balloon is passed distal to the stent to encourage its passage back into the catheter—in this case, the manoeuvre failed (Fig. 30.12).

A mother-and-child catheter (arrows) within a left Amplatz guiding catheter (5F in 6F) used to gain support to increase traction. In this case the stent would still not budge from its position (Fig. 30.13).

Finally, a snare (arrows) has caught the proximal end of the stent which allows for its removal (Fig. 30.14).

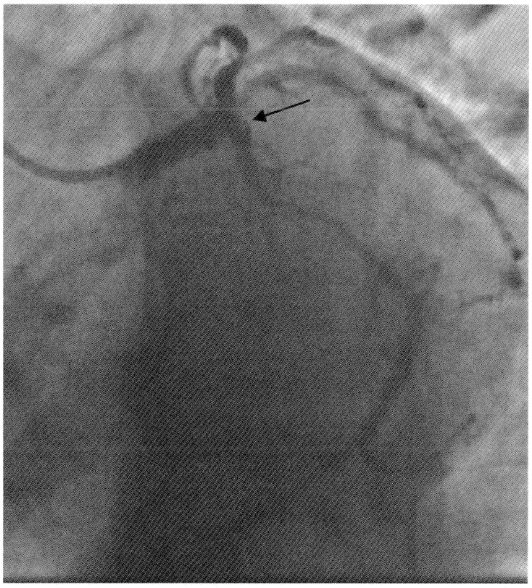

Fig. 30.7 Tortuous calcified left main/circumflex angle.

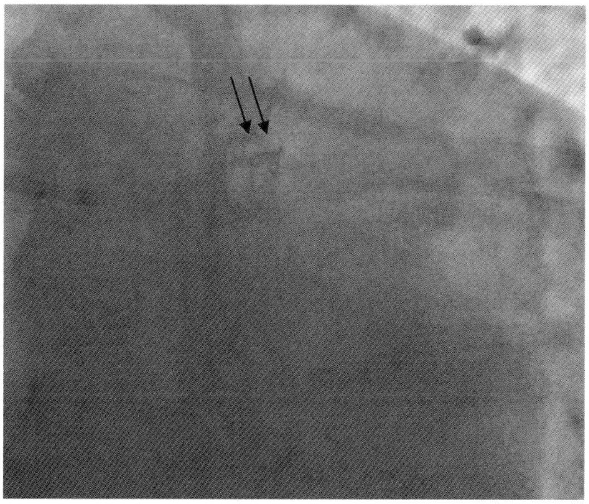

Fig. 30.9 Use of a snare looped over the distal end of the stent allows withdrawal into the guiding catheter.

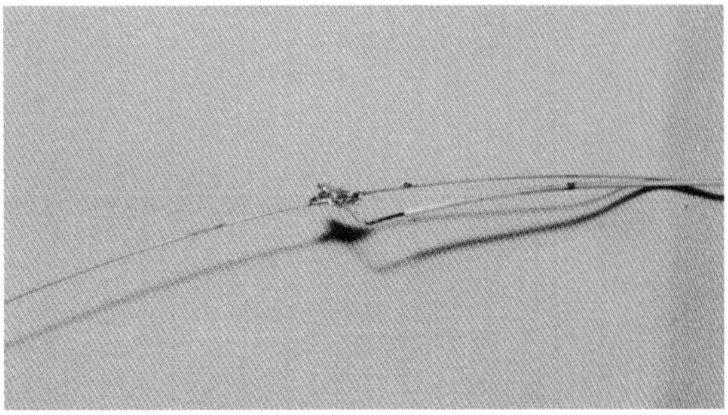

Fig. 30.10 Appearance of disrupted stent after removal.

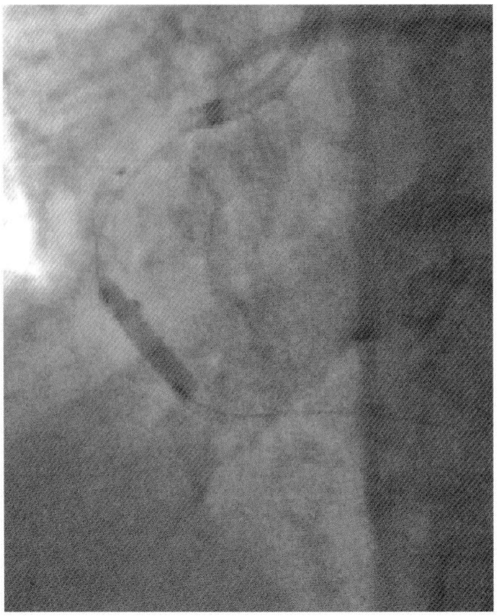

Fig. 30.12 A small balloon has been passed distally and inflated to low atmospheres to encourage removal of the stent—in this case it failed to work.

Case 3

A previously stented vein graft had developed in-stent restenosis (Fig. 30.15, before dye injection; Fig. 30.16, after dye injection). Previous stents are shown with black arrows. A distal embolic protection wire was placed distally to capture embolized fragments (white arrow). However, because of the tortuous, rigid nature of the stented region, the new stent could not be advanced. Removal of the stent balloon revealed the stent had been lost in the vein graft.

Withdrawal of the distal protection device resulted in crushing of the lost stent against the guide catheter and eventual externalization (Fig. 30.17).

Case 4

An attempt was made to deploy a covered stent within a vein graft. However, on withdrawal of the delivery balloon the stent was found not to be in the vessel but on the shaft of the guide catheter (Fig. 30.18).

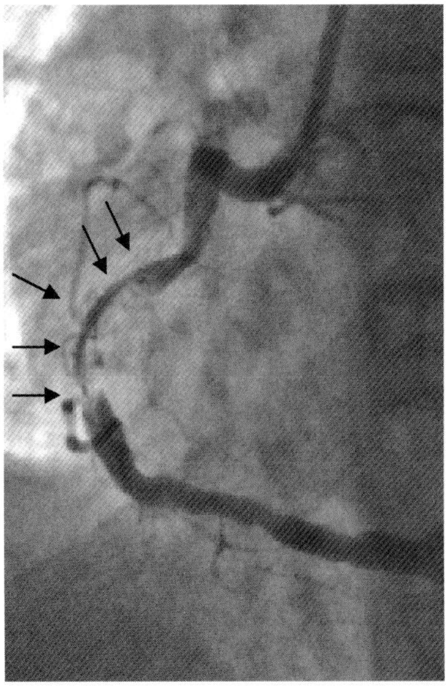

Fig. 30.11 Undeployed stent within tortuous right coronary artery (arrows).

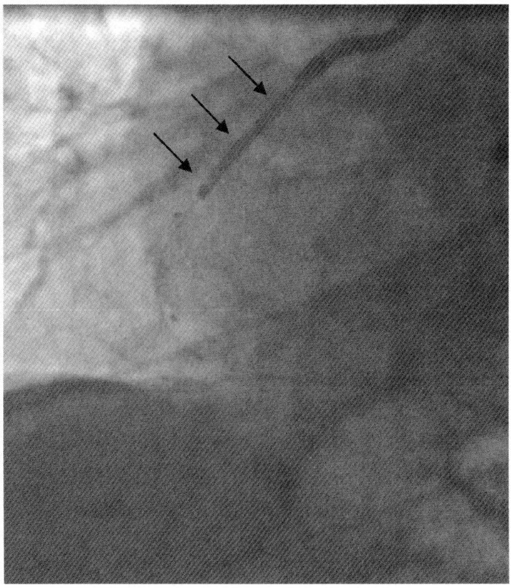

Fig. 30.13 More support is gained from a mother and child catheter to increase traction but stent still would not budge.

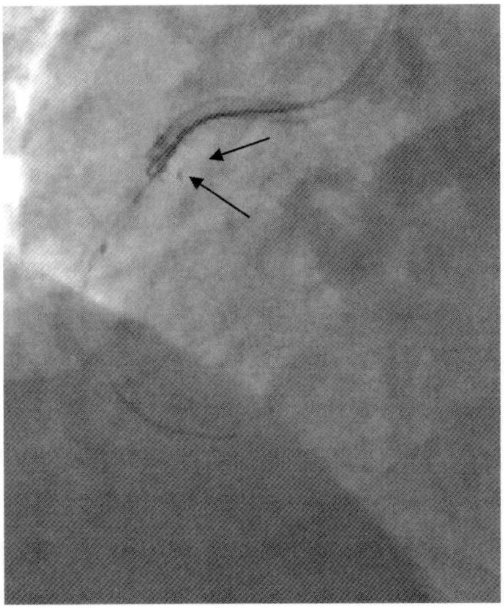

Fig. 30.14 Eventually a snare (arrows) catches the proximal end of the stent to allow safe removal.

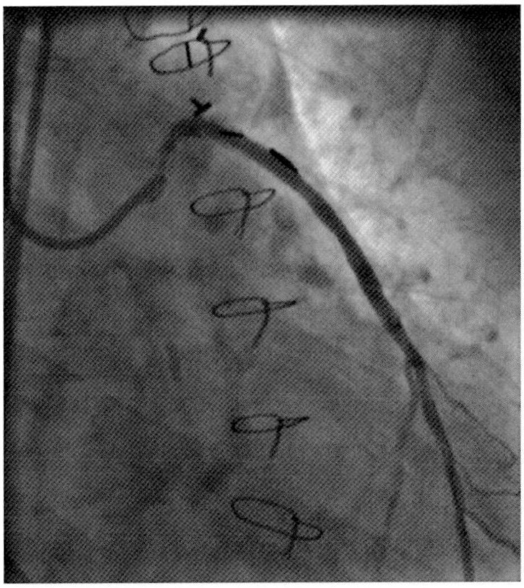

Fig. 30.16 Proximal in stent restenosis seen on dye injection. An underdeployed stent has been dislodged from its balloon.

A double balloon strategy was used to allow retrieval of the stent following which it was crushed in an iliac vessel (Fig. 30.19).

Case 5

Typical appearances of a challenging RCA with a combination of tortuosity and calcification (arrows) in the proximal bend prior to a distal stenosis (arrow), increasing the risk of stent displacement (Fig. 30.20).

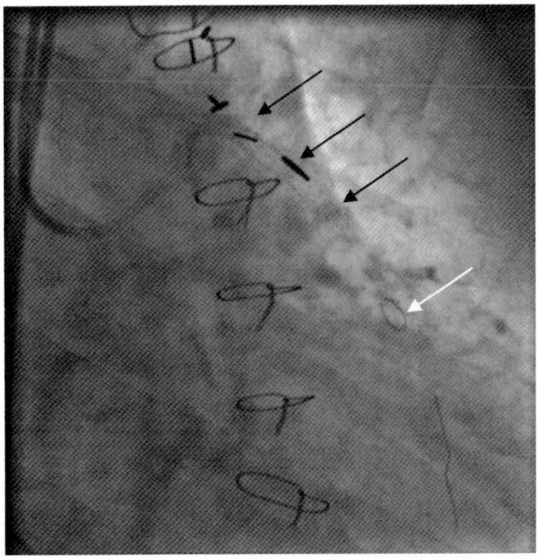

Fig. 30.15 In stent restenosis within a vein graft (black arrows). A distal protection device is in place (white arrow)

A stent has passed through the proximal bend with a supportive catheter and wire, but would not pass to the distal lesion (Fig. 30.21). On attempting to bring the stent back into the guide catheter, the stent was stripped off the balloon platform (arrows), with loss of the wire position. In this case, the stent was crushed by deployment of a further stent.

Case 6

An elderly patient with previous coronary artery bypass operation and severe aortic stenosis undergoing transcutaneous aortic valve replacement. The CoreValve® (CoreValve, California, USA) was being pulled gently

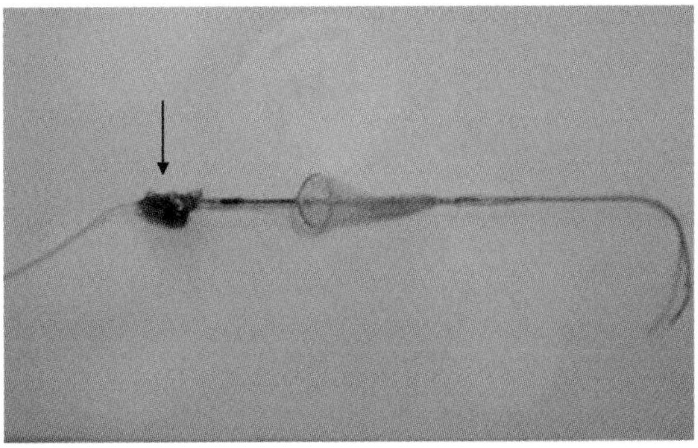

Fig. 30.17 The dislodged stent was dragged back into the guiding catheter by the distal protection mechanism, crushed and removed (black arrow)

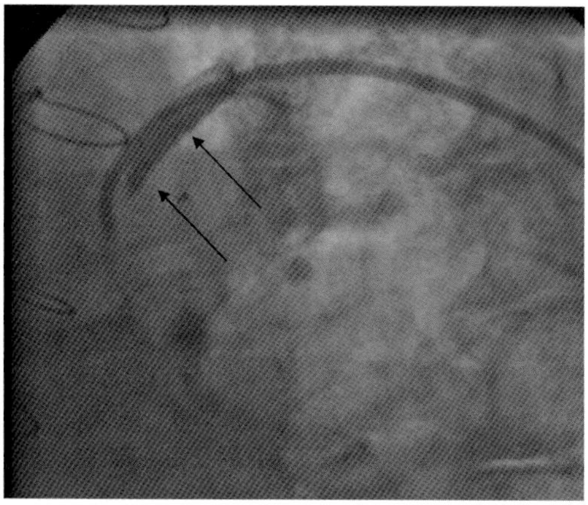

Fig. 30.18 Failed delivery of a self-expanding covered stent into a vein graft has led to the stent slipping over the guiding cather (black arrows).

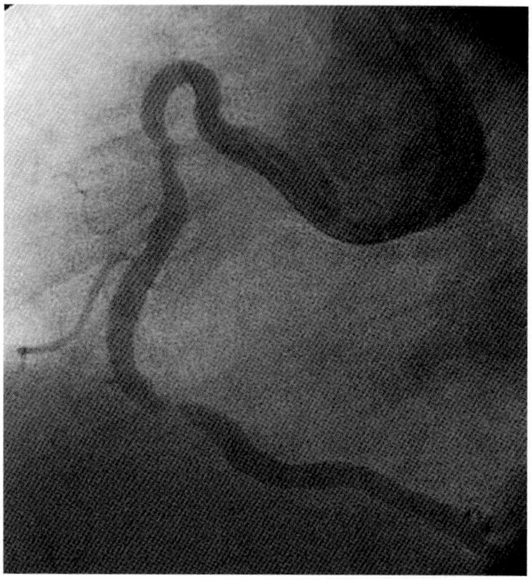

Fig. 30.20 A tortuous and calcified right coronary artery—a combination that increases the risk of stent dislodgement.

back into an appropriate position when it jumped back into the aorta, resting in the ascending aortic root (Fig. 30.22, see arrows). In order to allow the passage of a second valve into position the original valve had to be pulled back.

One limb of the CoreValve® was snared from the descending aorta, and the other limb was captured by passing a wire through the mesh of the valve skirt from the radial artery, into the descending aorta (Fig. 30.23).

The distal end of this wire was snared in the descending aorta to allow sufficient traction to pull the CoreValve® back (Fig. 30.24).

The second CoreValve® has now been placed, but there is still severe aortic regurgitation, and it needs to be manipulated further back into the ascending aorta. Two snares are placed on either side of the CoreValve® to allow an optimal position to be achieved (Fig. 30.25).

Manipulation of a CoreValve® using two snares (arrows) to optimize position of the valve in the aortic root to reduce aortic regurgitation (Fig. 30.26).

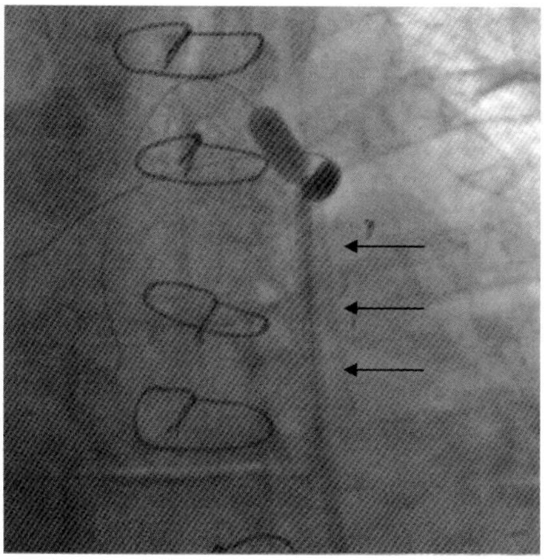

Fig. 30.19 Two balloons were inflated beyond the guiding catheter endhole to allow the stent to be dragged back into the iliac circulation where it was externalized by a further stent.

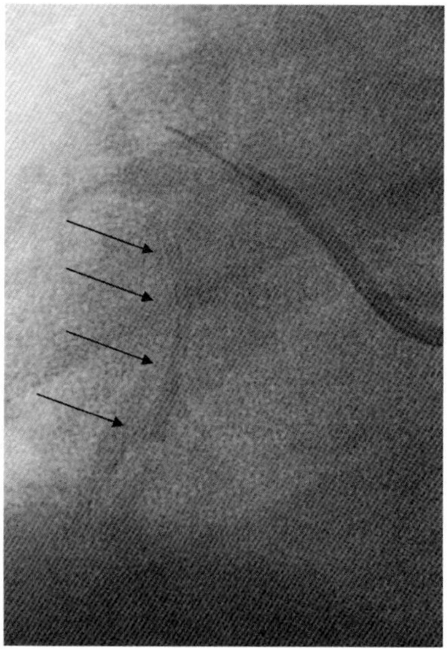

Fig. 30.21 A dislodged undeployed stent free within the right coronary artery. In this case it was externalized by deployment of a further stent.

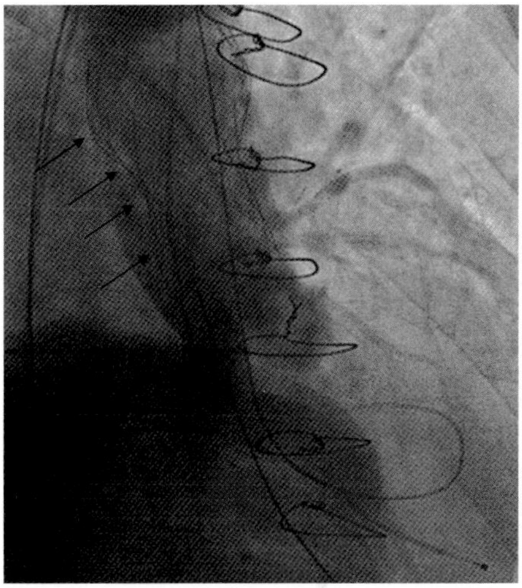

Fig. 30.22 Inadvertent slippage of CoreValve from aortic valve position into ascending aorta (black arrows).

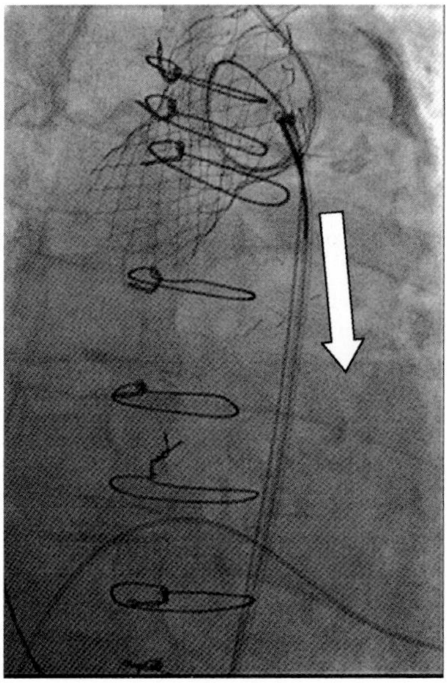

Fig. 30.24 The radial artery wire has passed through the skirt of the CoreValve and into the descending aorta, to allow sufficient traction to place within a 'safe' part of the aorta.

Summary

Successful stent deployment is customary using modern equipment, and stent embolization is a rare but potentially serious complication. Studies of stent loss are necessarily observational and retrospective, and the number of patients who experience this complication is small. Patient factors, operator decision-making, choice of equipment, and familiarity with retrieval equipment influences the strategy for dealing with stent loss. The majority of cases of intracoronary stent loss may be effectively managed by deployment or crushing. This may be a safer alternative than retrieval which can be

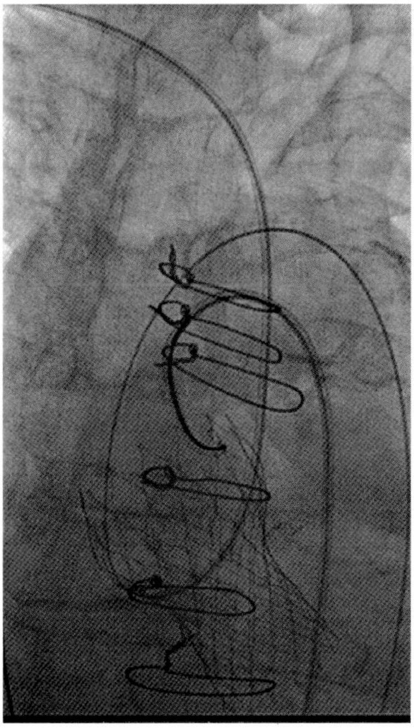

Fig. 30.23 The CoreValve has been snared from the descending aorta and radial artery.

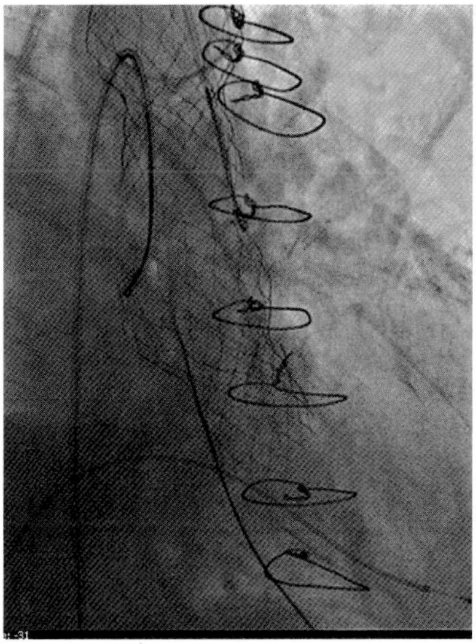

Fig. 30.25 A second CoreValve has been placed and manipulated into position using 2 snares.

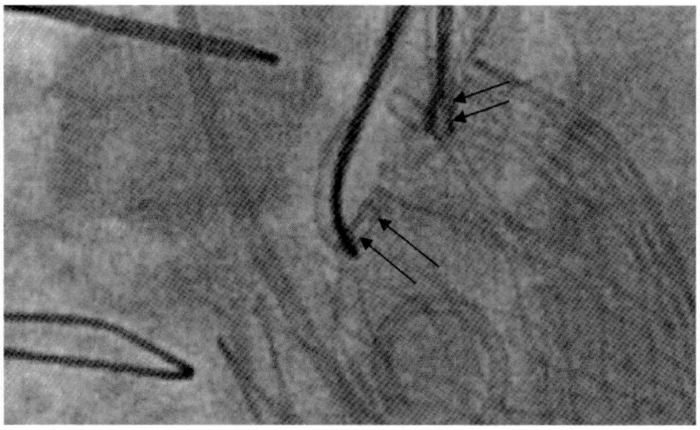

Fig. 30.26 A magnified view of the snares around the loops of the CoreValve skirt which allow for optimal manipulation.

associated with the need for emergency CABG and bleeding. Peripheral circulation embolization also appears to have a benign course when managed conservatively. Surgical retrieval may be required when the patient is symptomatic or if there is a risk of stent migration to the cerebral circulation. The best strategy is to avoid it.

Care and diligence bring luck.
Gnomologia. Thomas Fuller, 1732.

References

1. Brilakis ES, Best PJ, Elesber AA, *et al.* Incidence, retrieval methods, and outcomes of stent loss during percutaneous coronary intervention: a large single-center experience. *Catheter Cardiovasc Interv* 2005; **66**(3):333–40.
2. Foster-Smith KW, Garratt KN, Higano ST, *et al.* Retrieval techniques for managing flexible intracoronary stent misplacement. *Cathet Cardiovasc Diagn* 1993; **30**(1):63–8.
3. Alfonso F, Martinez D, Hernandez R, *et al.* Stent embolization during intracoronary stenting. *Am J Cardiol* 1996; **78**(7):833–5.
4. Elsner M, Peifer A, Kasper W. Intracoronary loss of balloon-mounted stents: successful retrieval with a 2 mm-"Microsnare"-device. *Cathet Cardiovasc Diagn* 1996; **39**(3):271–6.
5. Cantor WJ, Lazzam C, Cohen EA, *et al.* Failed coronary stent deployment. *Am Heart J* 1998; **136**(6):1088–95.
6. Eggebrecht H, Haude M, von BC, *et al.* Nonsurgical retrieval of embolized coronary stents. *Catheter Cardiovasc Interv* 2000; **51**(4):432–40.
7. Steigen TK, Maeng M, Wiseth R, *et al.* Randomized study on simple versus complex stenting of coronary artery bifurcation lesions: the Nordic bifurcation study. *Circulation* 2006; **114**(18):1955–61.
8. Bartorelli AL, Montorsi P, Ravagnani P, *et al.* Failure of fluoroscopy and success of intravascular ultrasound to locate an intracoronary embolized Palmaz-Schatz stent. *J Invasive Cardiol* 1997; **9**(1):25–9.
9. Wongpraparut N, Yalamachili V, Leesar MA. Novel implication of combined stent crushing and intravascular ultrasound for dislodged stents. *J Invasive Cardiol* 2004; **16**(8):445–6.
10. Daemen J, Lemos PA, Serruys PW. Multi-lesion culotte and crush bifurcation stenting with sirolimus-eluting stents: long-term angiographic outcome. *J Invasive Cardiol* 2003; **15**(11):653–6.
11. Colombo A, Stankovic G, Orlic D, *et al.* Modified T-stenting technique with crushing for bifurcation lesions: immediate results and 30-day outcome. *Catheter Cardiovasc Interv* 2003; **60**(2):145–51.
12. Meisel SR, DiLeo J, Rajakaruna M, *et al.* A technique to retrieve stents dislodged in the coronary artery followed by fixation in the iliac artery by means of balloon angioplasty and peripheral stent deployment. *Catheter Cardiovasc Interv* 2000; **49**(1):77–81.
13. Gahlen J, Koeppel T, Prosst RL. Vascular occlusion by ruptured balloon after percutaneous transluminal angioplasty. *J Endovasc Ther* 2003; **10**(6):1117–19.
14. Thomas J, Sinclair-Smith B, Bloomfield D, *et al.* Non-surgical retrieval of a broken segment of steel spring guide from the right atrium and inferior vena cava. *Circulation* 1964; **30**:106–8.
15. Bloomfield DA. The nonsurgical retrieval of intracardiac foreign bodies--an international survey. *Cathet Cardiovasc Diagn* 1978; **4**(1):1–14.
16. Fisher RG, Ferreyro R. Evaluation of current techniques for nonsurgical removal of intravascular iatrogenic foreign bodies. *AJR Am J Roentgenol* 1978; **130**(3):541–8.
17. Steele PM, Holmes DR, Jr, Mankin HT, *et al.* Intravascular retrieval of broken guide wire from the ascending aorta after percutaneous transluminal coronary angioplasty. *Cathet Cardiovasc Diagn* 1985; **11**(6):623–8.
18. Berder V, Bedossa M, Gras D, *et al.* Retrieval of a lost coronary stent from the descending aorta using a PTCA balloon and biopsy forceps. *Cathet Cardiovasc Diagn* 1993; **28**(4):351–3.
19. Guigauri P, Dauerman HL. A novel use for a distal embolic protection device: stent retrieval. *J Invasive Cardiol* 2005; **17**(3):183–4.
20. Hussain F, Rusnak B, Tam J. Retrieval of a detached partially expanded stent using the SpideRX and EnSnare devices – a first report. *J Invasive Cardiol* 2008; **20**(2):E44–E47.

CHAPTER 31

No-reflow

Julian Strange and Andreas Baumbach

Introduction

The no-reflow phenomenon is associated with significant cardiac consequences: poor functional recovery, ongoing or recurrent ischaemia, and increased short-term mortality[1,2]. It occurs rarely in elective percutaneous interventions, but far more frequently in patients who present with acute myocardial infarction (AMI). It is in these patients, where primary percutaneous coronary intervention (PPCI) has become the gold standard that has most recently highlighted the phenomenon as it is commonly visualized in real time by the interventional cardiologist.

Definition

The term 'no-reflow' was first used in the 1960s following animal experiments looking at restoration of cerebral perfusion after prolonged periods of ischaemia. Changes were seen in the microvasculature which impeded normal arterial blood flow to brain cells after the initial obstruction to flow was relieved. This phenomenon was also noted to occur in other organs, and finally described in the ischaemiac canine cardiac model by Kloner and colleagues in 1975[3]. It was noted that after occlusion of the canine coronary artery for 90min only partial recovery of flow was achieved to the myocardium, following complete restoration of vessel patency. 'Coronary' no-reflow is defined as the inability to adequately perfuse myocardium after temporary occlusion of an epicardial coronary artery without evidence of a persistent mechanical obstruction[1]. Other terms used to describe this phenomenon include slow-flow and slow-reflow and refer to absent or impaired flow into previously ischaemic tissue.

Pathophysiology

The pathophysiology of no-reflow is not entirely understood, but appears to be multifactorial[1,4]. Potential mechanisms responsible depend on the clinical or experimental setting. Many of the processes involved are interrelated with ischaemia due to coronary obstruction leading to sufficient damage of the microvasculature to prevent perfusion of cardiac myocytes. Subendocardial perfusion defects are seen and under electron microscopy there is severe capillary, interstitial, and myocardial cellular damage. Marked capillary damage can also be seen, with intraluminal obstruction due to endothelial swelling, capillary plugging, and microthrombi. Production of oxygen free radicals, altered calcium metabolism, complement and platelet activation, accumulation of leucocytes, and apoptosis all potentiate the microvascular dysfunction.

No-reflow is most pronounced in the subendocardium with expansion into the myocardium over the time of coronary occlusion. During a period of ischaemia, endothelial damage and myocyte oedema create initial no-reflow areas. With reperfusion these areas expand due to additional oedema, myocyte contraction, fibrin, and leucocyte plugging. Further embolization of atherosclerotic debris, thrombus, and platelet plugs can be released into the microcirculation at the time of restoration of coronary flow. Hence, the process of no-reflow starts during the ischaemic period, increases with reperfusion, and can be exacerbated by atheroembolization. This worsening or expansion of the no-reflow area at the point of restoration of coronary flow is termed 'reperfusion injury'. It describes not only the increased ischaemic damage, but also changes in the myocardial arrhythmogenic potential and contractile performance. Of note, expansion of the no-reflow zone can increase for several hours after complete restoration of coronary flow[5], associated with an increase in the area of myocardial infarction.

Increased myocardial damage after reperfusion is accompanied with a marked increase in neutrophil accumulation within the no-reflow areas. Experiments have demonstrated extensive capillary leucocyte plugging in the microvasculature. Depletion of leucocytes has in various studies lead to a reduction in anatomical no-reflow.

The main triggers of no-reflow during coronary intervention appear to be distal embolization of plaque and/or thrombus with subsequent release of vasoconstrictor substances. This concept is underlined by the fact that no-reflow is a major problem in the treatment of AMI, saphenous vein grafts, thrombus-containing lesions, and rotational atherectomy.

Incidence

The overall reported incidence for angiographic no-reflow in percutaneous coronary intervention (PCI) ranges between 0.2–2%. Higher rates have been reported for primary PCI (11.5%)[6], saphenous vein grafts (9%)[7], and rotational atherectomy (12%)[8].

Outcomes associated with no-reflow

The no-reflow phenomenon following PCI is associated with poor functional recovery, impaired ventricular remodelling, and increased recurrence of ischaemia. In particular, persistent no-reflow has been associated with increased mortality[1].

Diagnosis

Angiographic appearance: TIMI flow and myocardial blush grade

The definitive model of no-reflow is the AMI patient. Following presentation with ST-elevation myocardial infarction, attempts at restoration of coronary patency may result in slow- or no-reflow. This is likely to be associated with poor or no resolution of ST segments. Coronary angiography allows a grading of the degree of no-reflow and was defined by the Thrombolysis in Myocardial Infarction trial (TIMI) blood flow grades in the 1980s. The TIMI grade is a semiquantitative assessment of filling and clearing of contrast across the coronary artery which equates to the degree of myocardial perfusion. There are four grades: TIMI 0–3 (see Table 31.1). In a meta-analysis, mortality at 6 weeks was found to be lower in patients who achieved TIMI 3 flow (3.7%), compared with TIMI 2 or TIMI 1/0 (6.6% and 9.2%, respectively)[9]. Echocardiography contrast studies have demonstrated that TIMI 2 flow is associated with large areas of no-reflow[10]. No-reflow should therefore be suspected if TIMI flow is reduced.

Despite achieving TIMI 3 epicardial flow, myocardial perfusion can still be impaired. In patients with TIMI 3 flow the myocardial blush grade (MBG) allows further risk assessment. MBG is a densitometric, semiquantitative parameter which depends on the tissue phase of myocardial perfusion that appears as a 'blush' or a 'ground-glass' after a sufficiently long, 25 frames/s, X-ray acquisition. MBG is measured on patients with TIMI 3 flow and is based on the principle that a functionally preserved microvascular bed allows the injected contrast to pass easily from the arterial to the venous side of coronary circulation, showing an appreciable 'blush' at the myocardial level. The definitions of MBGs 0–3 are shown in Table 31.1.

12-lead electrocardiogram

The standard 12-lead ECG is a simple and inexpensive method to evaluate myocardial reperfusion in the setting of AMI. Rapid ST-segment resolution following restoration of TIMI 3 flow has been shown to be highly specific and reasonably sensitive for the absence of no-reflow as demonstrated by myocardial contrast echo[11]. In the setting of coronary angioplasty, no-reflow is often associated with persistent or new ST elevation in the monitor leads.

Myocardial contrast echocardiography

Myocardial contrast echocardiography (MCE) has increased our understanding of the functional significance of no-reflow. It is a powerful imaging tool for the bedside assessment of the myocardial microcirculation. It utilizes gas-filled micro bubbles that are inert and remain entirely within the vascular space to identify the course of red blood cells. This has allowed the clear identification of the area at risk, and also confirms the success of reperfusion in the acute myocardial setting. Several studies have shown that despite TIMI 3 epicardial flow there is clear evidence of tissue no-reflow in up to 16% of patients[10].

Functional recovery can be determined by MCE with the identification of microvascular integrity closely associated with myocyte viability. Factors associated with increased size of perfusion defects in STEMI on MCE are prolonged time from symptoms to reperfusion, older age, large anterior infarction, low admission blood pressure, and absence of angina pre-infarction.

Coronary Doppler imaging

The no-reflow phenomenon has a characteristic coronary blood flow pattern: systolic flow reversal, reduced

Table 31.1 Definitions of TIMI flow and myocardial blush grades

TIMI flow		Myocardial blush grade	
TIMI 0	There is no antegrade flow beyond the point of occlusion	MBG 0	No myocardial blush or staining of blush (due to leakage of dye into the extravascular space)
TIMI 1	The contrast material passes beyond the area of obstruction, but 'hangs up' and fails to opacify the entire coronary bed distal to the obstruction for duration of the cine run	MBG 1	Minimal myocardial blush
TIMI 2	The contrast material passes across the obstruction and opacifies the coronary bed distal to the obstruction. However, the rate of entry of contrast material into the vessel distal to the obstruction or its rate of clearance from the distal bed (or both) are perceptibly slower than its entry into or clearance from comparable areas not perfused by the previously occluded vessel, e.g. the opposite coronary artery or the coronary bed proximal to the obstruction	MBG 2	Moderate myocardial blush, less than that obtained during angiography of a contralateral or ipsilateral non-infarct-related artery
TIMI 3	Antegrade flow into the bed distal to the obstruction occurs as promptly as antegrade flow into the bed proximal to the obstruction, and clearance of contrast material from the involved bed is as rapid as clearance from an uninvolved bed in the same vessel or the opposite artery	MBG 3	Normal myocardial blush, comparable with that obtained during angiography of a contralateral or ipsilateral non-infarct-related artery

Reproduced from the ESC Guidelines. Van de Werf F, Bax J, Betriu A, *et al.* Management of acute myocardial infarction in patients presenting with persistent ST-segment elevation. *Eur Heart J* 2008;**29**:2909–45.

antegrade systolic flow, and forward diastolic flow with a rapid deceleration slope. The reduced antegrade flow leads to reduced TIMI flow on imaging.

Cardiovascular magnetic resonance

Cardiovascular magnetic resonance (CMR) allows a complete and accurate assessment of left ventricular status in patients after AMI. The use of gadolinium contrast enables visualization of total infarct size and areas of microvascular obstruction (MVO). The high spatial resolution of CMR has allowed accurate validation against histological microvascular injury. The extent of MVO as detected by CMR predicts extent of left ventricular remodelling and outcome.

Strategic approach to suspected no-reflow during PCI

No-reflow must be considered if there is reduced epicardial flow, absence of myocardial blush, and new, persistent, or worsening ST elevation on the electrocardiogram. Failure to establish TIMI 3 flow following balloon inflation or stent implantation can be caused by no-reflow. However, there can also be mechanical obstructions that prevent flow past the site of the lesion. Dissection and residual occlusive thrombus formation must be ruled out first. Another cause of decreased flow of contrast can be the injection of air bubbles into the coronary circulation. Dissection flaps can sometimes be identified by simply placing the uninflated balloon catheter into the lesion area. Repeat injection may reveal good flow past the obstruction.

A diagnosis can be reliably and quickly established by passing a double lumen catheter or over-the-wire balloon into the distal segment of the target vessel. Injection of contrast through the second lumen or through the wire lumen of the balloon catheter will provide information about flow in this part of the vessel. If the vessel fills with contrast past the suspected occlusion into the proximal segment and the contrast does not clear, the diagnosis of no-reflow is made. In case of mechanical obstructions, the distal flow will be normal and the vessel will fill back to the point of obstruction.

A major benefit of this approach is the potential to treat no-reflow immediately with the catheter positioned subselectively in the coronary artery.

Treatment of established no-reflow

Treatment aims at reducing MVO and platelet inhibition. Apart from antiplatelet agents, all pharmacological

Table 31.2 Approach to angiographic no-reflow following PCI

Establish diagnosis:
TIMI flow <3
12-lead ECG: persistent ST elevation
IC nitroglycerine to exclude epicardial spasm
OTW balloon/double lumen balloon and distal contrast injection
IVUS to document patent epicardial artery
Pharmacological treatment options:
Verapamil IC (0.25–2.5mg)
Nicorandil IC (2mcg)
Nitroprusside IC (50–200mcg)
Adenosine boluses IC (up to 50mcg)
Epinephrine IC (50–200mcg)
Abciximab IV (0.25mg/kg bolus followed by 10mcg/min infusion)
Consider intra-aortic balloon pump

IC, intracoronary application subselectively through double lumen or OTW balloon; IV, intravenous; IVUS, intravenous ultrasound; OTW, over-the-wire.

agents should be injected subselectively into the target vessel in order to reach the affected areas of myocardium. Systemic or proximal intracoronary injections are unlikely to yield benefits, as by definition there is no flow into the target zone.

The strategic approach to no-reflow during PCI and pharmacological options are summarized in Table 31.2.

Verapamil has been shown to reverse no-reflow in clinical studies[12,13]. Adenosine, especially given with high-velocity boluses and saline has been associated with improved outcomes[14]. Nitroprusside is a potent vasodilator but may be contraindicated in situations with low blood pressure[15]. Intracoronary injection of diluted adrenaline is an alternative approach, but must be handled with care because of the potential haemodynamic and arrhythmogenic effects[16].

The insertion of an intra-aortic balloon pump in situations with haemodynamic instability is an intuitive approach, but has never been proven to have a direct impact on the resolution of no-reflow.

Prevention of no-reflow

Measures to reduce the incidence of no-reflow include: devices to reduce embolization, antiplatelet agents, prophylactic pharmacology, and the adaptation of the technique of rotational atherectomy (Table 31.3).

Table 31.3 Prevention of no-reflow in different settings of PCI

Primary PCI
Thrombus extraction catheter*
Consider distal protection device in lesions with large thrombus burden
Saphenous vein grafts
Distal protection*
Proximal occlusion device
Rotational atherectomy
Low burr to artery ratio (0.6–0.8)**
Low rotational speed 140 000 rpm**
Abciximab*
Intracoronary adenosine (boluses 24–48mcg)**
Drug cocktail (verapamil (10mcg/mL) + nitroglycerin (4mcg/mL) + heparin (20IU/mL) through sheath**
Lesions with visible thrombus
Thrombus extraction
AngioJet/TEC
Excimer laser

*Evidence from randomized clinical trial.
**Suggested benefit from clinical evaluation.

Primary angioplasty

The routine use of a thrombus extraction catheter prior to dilatation of the target lesion in primary angioplasty for acute STEMI reduces the incidence of low MBGs and is associated with improved clinical outcomes[6].

Routine use of distal protection devices has not shown to be beneficial in randomized comparisons.

Saphenous vein grafts

The SAFER (Saphenous vein graft Angioplasty Free of Emboli Randomized) trial established that the routine use of a distal protection device is associated with a reduced incidence of no-reflow in the treatment of degenerated saphenous vein grafts[7]. In a later study, equivalence of proximal occlusion with the distal protection approach was reported[17].

Rotational atherectomy

Rotational atherectomy is associated with embolization of plaque debris, platelet activation, and an increased incidence of no-reflow. Measures to prevent angiographic no-reflow deserve special attention:

- Koch and colleagues showed that pre-treatment with abciximab leads to a reduced incidence, extent, and severity of myocardial hypoperfusion on subsequent myocardial perfusion scanning(18).
- Intracoronary adenosine(19) as well as a drug cocktail including nitrates, verapamil, and heparin delivered through the rotablator shaft have been suggested(20).
- A low burr to artery ratio and slower rotational speed have been suggested as methods to reduce the amount of debris produced which should limit the incidence of no-reflow in this setting.

References

1. Eeckhout E, Kern MJ. The coronary no-reflow phenomenon: a review of mechanisms and therapies. *Eur Heart J* 2001; **22**(9):729–39.
2. Ito H, Okamura A, Iwakura K, *et al.* Myocardial perfusion patterns related to thrombolysis in myocardial infarction perfusion grades after coronary angioplasty in patients with acute anterior wall myocardial infarction. *Circulation* 1996; **93**(11):1993–9.
3. Kloner RA, Ganote CE, Jennings RB, *et al.* Demonstration of the "no-reflow" phenomenon in the dog heart after temporary ischemia. *Recent Adv Stud Cardiac Struct Metab* 1975; **10**:463–74.
4. Reffelmann T, Kloner RA. The "no-reflow" phenomenon: basic science and clinical correlates. *Heart* 2002; **87**(2):162–8.
5. Ambrosio G, Weisman HF, Mannisi JA, *et al.* Progressive impairment of regional myocardial perfusion after initial restoration of postischemic blood flow. *Circulation* 1989; **80**(6):1846–61.
6. Vlaar PJ, Svilaas T, van der Horst, *et al.* Cardiac death and reinfarction after 1 year in the Thrombus Aspiration during Percutaneous coronary intervention in Acute myocardial infarction Study (TAPAS): a 1-year follow-up study. *Lancet* 2008; **371**(9628):1915–20.
7. Baim DS, Wahr D, George B, *et al.* Randomized trial of a distal embolic protection device during percutaneous intervention of saphenous vein aorto-coronary bypass grafts. *Circulation* 2002; **105**(11):1285–90.
8. Matsuo H, Watanabe S, Watanabe T, *et al.* Prevention of no-reflow/slow-flow phenomenon during rotational atherectomy – a prospective randomized study comparing intracoronary continuous infusion of verapamil and nicorandil. *Am Heart J* 2007; **154**(5):994–6.
9. Fath-Ordoubadi F, Huehns TY, Al-Mohammad A, *et al.* Significance of the Thrombolysis in Myocardial Infarction scoring system in assessing infarct-related artery reperfusion and mortality rates after acute myocardial infarction. *Am Heart J* 1997; **134**(1):62–8.
10. Ito H, Maruyama A, Iwakura K, *et al.* Clinical implications of the 'no reflow' phenomenon. A predictor of complications and left ventricular remodeling in reperfused anterior wall myocardial infarction. *Circulation* 1996; **93**(2):223–8.
11. Santoro GM, Valenti R, Buonamici P, *et al.* Relation between ST-segment changes and myocardial perfusion evaluated by myocardial contrast echocardiography in patients with acute myocardial infarction treated with direct angioplasty. *Am J Cardiol* 1998; **82**(8):932–7.
12. Kaplan BM, Benzuly KH, Kinn JW, *et al.* Treatment of no-reflow in degenerated saphenous vein graft interventions: comparison of intracoronary verapamil and nitroglycerin. *Cathet Cardiovasc Diagn* 1996; **39**(2):113–18.
13. Hang CL, Wang CP, Yip HK, *et al.* Early administration of intracoronary verapamil improves myocardial perfusion during percutaneous coronary interventions for acute myocardial infarction. *Chest* 2005; **128**(4):2593–8.
14. Fischell TA, Carter AJ, Foster MT, *et al.* Reversal of "no reflow" during vein graft stenting using high velocity boluses of intracoronary adenosine. *Cathet Cardiovasc Diagn* 1998; **45**(4):360–5.
15. Fischell TA. Pharmaceutical interventions for the management of no-reflow. *J Invasive Cardiol* 2008; **20**(7):374–9.
16. Baim DS. Epinephrine: a new pharmacologic treatment for no-reflow? *Catheter Cardiovasc Interv* 2002; **57**(3):310–11.
17. Mauri L, Cox D, Hermiller J, *et al.* The PROXIMAL trial: proximal protection during saphenous vein graft intervention using the Proxis Embolic Protection System: a randomized, prospective, multicenter clinical trial. *J Am Coll Cardiol* 2007; **50**(15):1442–9.
18. Koch KC, vom Dahl J, Kleinhans E, *et al.* Influence of a platelet GPIIb/IIIa receptor antagonist on myocardial hypoperfusion during rotational atherectomy as assessed by myocardial Tc-99m sestamibi scintigraphy. *J Am Coll Cardiol* 1999; **33**(4):998–1004.
19. Hanna GP, Yhip P, Fujise K, *et al.* Intracoronary adenosine administered during rotational atherectomy of complex lesions in native coronary arteries reduces the incidence of no-reflow phenomenon. *Catheter Cardiovasc Interv* 1999; **48**(3):275–8.
20. Cohen BM, Weber VJ, Blum RR, *et al.* Cocktail attenuation of rotational ablation flow effects (CARAFE) study: pilot. *Cathet Cardiovasc Diagn* 1996; Suppl 3:69–72.

CHAPTER 32

Coronary artery perforation

Mark Gunning and Martyn Thomas

There are few scenarios in the cardiac catheterization laboratory quite as dramatic as a coronary artery perforation. While some instances of this mishap are subtle, others are quite dramatic. Fortunately this occurrence is rare, but carries with it a significant risk of serious adverse events. The potential for harm may be reduced by the brisk identification of the problem within the catheter laboratory, together with early implementation of treatment.

Definition and classification

Coronary artery perforation is defined as evidence of extravasation of contrast medium or blood from the coronary artery, during or following percutaneous intervention. The usual means of identification include fluoroscopy or echocardiography.

Anatomically the perforation might be categorized as

- Proximal or mid-vessel—usually more profound with greater likelihood of significant sequelae.
- Distal vessel—where the aetiology is often the guide wire and the clinical course is frequently benign.

Thus the clinical spectrum ranges from mere puncture of the vessel by the guide wire (assigned the somewhat understated term 'wire exit'), leading to dye staining but no adverse haemodynamic consequences, through to vessel rupture, resulting in brisk extravasation of contrast and blood, and abrupt haemodynamic collapse. The management of the problem is dictated by the severity of the leak.

The most frequently adopted classification is that proposed by Ellis and colleagues in 1994[1]:

- Type I: extra-luminal crater without extravasation.
- Type II: pericardial or myocardial blush without contrast jet extravasation.
- Type III: extravasation through frank perforation ($\geq$1mm).
- Type III (cavity): extravasation into a cardiac chamber, or coronary sinus, but not into the pericardial space.

Although this classification is helpful in the clinical setting, there are cases where the angiographic appearance does not adequately predict the consequences. As described in later sections of this chapter, a seemingly trivial distal perforation of a minor coronary side-branch, perhaps with a hydrophilic wire, might result in cardiac tamponade 8–12h following the procedure, particularly where adjunctive glycoprotein IIb/IIIa inhibitors have been used. Using the above classification this event would be classed as type II, inaccurately inferring a more favourable outlook. Thus, caution should be exercised with any coronary perforation, and vigilant monitoring of the patient during the post-procedural stay is warranted.

Historical perspective

The first documented description of human coronary artery rupture, albeit spontaneous rather than iatrogenic, dates back to 1737 in Kesmark, Hungary[2]. The article pertaining to this case of sudden death is written in Hungarian, and alas it is somewhat beyond the scope of these authors to furnish further details on this report. Mention of coronary artery perforation related to diagnostic catheterization is seen in the literature as early as 1970[3]. Case reports on perforation in the context of percutaneous intervention emerge as early as 1982[4]. One is mindful that the methods and materials of the interventional cardiologist in the 1980s and in the early 1990s, are very different to those currently used in a contemporary catheter laboratory. However, a review of the frequency, pattern, and causes of this complication evolving through the decades provides us with valuable insight into how some of the previous problems have been surmounted.

This earliest report by Kimbiris describes coronary artery rupture and tamponade secondary to the use of an angioplasty balloon and catheter[4]. On that particular occasion pericardiocentesis and emergency bypass surgery were required in order to rescue the situation. A later report in 1985[5] refers to coronary perforation occurring on two separate occasions, where conservative management was sufficient. The literature during 1980s is peppered with numerous anecdotal reports, but there is no definitive article describing the scale of the problem at that time. There is no comprehensive description of issues particular to that early era of percutaneous intervention, where plain old balloon angioplasty (POBA) was the rule rather than exception. Thus the incidence of coronary perforation during this early period is poorly quantified.

The evolution of interventional cardiology over three decades has brought with it innovative devices. These have usually been embraced by a few enthusiasts. It is interesting that at least four publications are titled 'coronary perforation in the new device era', suggesting that the novel technology primarily influenced the frequency of this complication. However, it is important to also recognize that the nature of the coronary disease being treated via percutaneous means has become progressively more complex and challenging over time. Therefore the substrate has a significant bearing on any complication arising from its treatment.

Ellis and colleagues reported the first large-scale series derived from data obtained from 11 interventional centres, reflecting practice in 1990 and 1991[1]. Of 12 900 procedures carried out, 62 were complicated by coronary perforation (0.5%). The authors observed that use of 'new devices' accentuated the risk of perforation appreciably. None of the cases of perforation were associated with stent deployment. The term 'new devices' on this occasion referred to atherectomy and ablation technology (including excimer laser) as opposed to POBA. Thus only 14 out of 62 perforations (23%) occurred following POBA, while the remainder resulted from debulking techniques (see Table 32.1). Furthermore the proportion of all POBA cases complicated by perforation was only 0.1%, whereas the complication rate for excimer laser was 1.9%, and 1.3% for rotational atherectomy. Predisposing patient characteristics included female gender and increasing age. The early problems with novel technology such as excimer laser and rotational atherectomy were partly related to operator unfamiliarity with the potential pitfalls of the techniques. As cardiologists adjusted and improved their techniques, the results for the use of these devices also improved.

Other important information emerged from the Ellis report. Over-sizing of the angioplasty balloon was one of the key causes of perforation. The development of cardiac tamponade was associated with appreciable mortality (20%), particularly if this occurred within the catheter laboratory as a result of brisk extravasation (type III perforation). In two of the 15 patients who developed tamponade, it only became manifest more than 6h following the procedure. This is a cautionary point. Such patients have left the more intensive monitoring environment of catheter lab recovery at this point and have returned to the ward, where the problem of bleeding into pericardium may not be immediately obvious. The importance of this first publication should be emphasized as, for the first time, the scale of the problem was brought to the attention of the interventional community. The findings are largely reiterated in subsequent work.

Incidence and outcome

Somewhat surprisingly the incidence of coronary artery perforation has not changed significantly over two decades. It is reported between 0.2% and 0.93%. Tables 32.1 and 32.2 illustrate the results of the large published series on this topic over the past 15 years and most of these reflect contemporary interventional practice[1,6–19]. Thirteen of the 15 studies cited were conducted during the 'stent era' where the majority of interventions included the deployment of an intracoronary stent. The later studies include observational reports of practice using modern guide-wire technology and antiplatelet drug regimens.

The first report in 1994 indicates an overall incidence of perforation of 0.5 % and the most recent from 2007 is 0.4%[1,19]. The complexity of interventional cases has increased markedly over those 13 years, and yet perforation rates have not. Naturally there is a degree of variation in the incidence reported by the authors. This variation may, in part, be explained by a differing definition of coronary perforation for each article. Together with colleagues, the authors of this chapter reported an incidence of just under 0.8% in 6245 patients in 2002[12]. We incorporated the whole clinical spectrum in our definition of perforation, from mere vessel puncture ('wire exit') through to frank rupture and tamponade. On the other hand, Gruberg and colleagues reported an incidence of only 0.29% but the spectrum of pathology described is less clear[8]. Although free perforation was reported in 69% of these cases in this study, this was a retrospective observational study over a 10-year period so it is unlikely that benign

Table 32.1 Cause of coronary perforation

Study authors (reference)	Year	Guidewire	Balloon	Stent	DCA	Excimer laser	Rotational atherectomy	Temporary wire	Other
Ellis *et al.*[1]	1994	0	14/62 (23%)	0	12/62 (19%)	17/62 (27%)	10/62 (16%)	0	9/62 (15%)
Von Sohsten *et al.*[7]*	2000	3/15 (20%)	0	1/15 (7%)	0	0	3/15 (20%)	7/15 (46%)	1/15 (7%)
Dippel *et al.*[9]	2001	13/36 (36%)	8/36 (22%)	2/36 (6%)	3/36 (8%)	1/36 (3%)	8/36 (22%)	0	1/36 (3%)
Fukutomi *et al.*[11]	2002	27/69 (39%)	20/69 (29%)	4/69 (0.6%)	7 (10%)	0	0	0	11 (16%)
Fasseas *et al.*[13]	2003	29/95 (31%)	26/95 (27%)	20/95 (21%)	3/95 (4%)	8/95 (8%)	8/95 (8%)	0	0
Witzke *et al.*[15]	2004	20/39 (51%)	3/39 (8%)	7/39 (18%)	2/39 (5%)	0	7/39 (18%)	0	0
Stankovic *et al.*[16]	2004	22 (26%)	42 (50%)	4 (5%)	8 (9%)	0	3 (4%)	0	5 (6%)
Ramana *et al.*[17]	2005	17/25 (68%)	0	6/25 (24%)	0	0	2/25 (8%)	0	0
Javaid *et al.*[18]	2006	15/72 (21%)	18/72 (25%)	18/72 (25%)	0	7/72 (10%)	14/72 (19%)	0	0

Only studies where the aetiology is clearly identified are cited.
*Study focused solely on cases of tamponade.

Table 32.2 Incidence and in-hospital complications of coronary artery perforation

Study authors (reference)	Year	Size of cohort	No. of perforations (incidence)	No. of tamponade (proportion of perforations)	Emergency surgery	Mortality
Ellis *et al.*[1]	1994	12900	62 (0.5%)	15/62 (24%)	15/62 (24%)	3/62 (5%)
Ajluni *et al.*[6]	1994	8932	35 (0.4%)	3/35 (9%)	13/35 (37%)	2/35 (6%)
Von Sohsten *et al.*[7]	2000	6999	Not recorded	15	9	0
Gruberg *et al.*[8]	2000	30746	88 (0.3%)	26/88 (30%)	33/88 (38%)	8/88 (9%)
Dippel *et al.*[9]	2001	6214	36 (0.6%)	8/36 (22%)	8/36 (22%)	4/36 (11%)
Fejka *et al.*[10]	2002	25697	Not recorded	31	12	14
Fukutomi *et al.*[11]	2002	7443	69 (0.9%)	26/69 (38%)	2/69 (3%)	0
Gunning *et al.*[12]	2002	6245	52 (0.8%)	24/52 (46%)	8/52 (15%)	6/52 (12%)
Fasseas *et al.*[13]	2003	16298	95 (0.6%)	11/95 (12%)	10/95 (11%)	7/95 (7%)
Eggebrecht *et al.*[14]	2004	6433	19 (0.3%)	3/19 (16%)	2/19 (11%)	2/19 (11%)
Witzke *et al.*[15]	2004	12658	39 (0.3%)	7/39 (18%)	2/39 (5%)	1/39 (3%)
Stankovic *et al.*[16]	2004	5728	84 (1.5%)	10/84 (12%)	11/84 (13%)	7/84 (8%)
Ramana *et al.*[17]	2005	4886	25 (0.5%)	4/25 (16%)	3/25 (12%)	2/25 (8%)
Javaid *et al.*[18]	2006	38559	72 (0.2%)	14/72 (19%)	25/72 (35%)	12/72 (17%)
Shikarabe *et al.*[19]	2007	3415	12 (0.4%)	3/12 (25%)	1/12 (8%)	1/12 (8%)

events were incorporated into the analysis. Von Sohsten and colleagues, on the other hand, focused solely on cases of tamponade rather than perforation per se[7]. They identified 15 cases of tamponade occurring in 6999 coronary interventions (0.21%), but made no reference to minor perforation. The report of Fejka and colleagues is similar[10]. Nevertheless it is clear that coronary perforation is a rare complication, seldom amounting to more than 1% of all cases performed.

The development of pericardial tamponade should be taken seriously. A consistent finding in all of these publications is that the development of tamponade in the context of coronary perforation imparts a very poor prognosis. As shown in Table 32.2, the proportion of perforations which progress on to tamponade ranges between 10–50%. In Fejka's series from 2002, almost 50% of those developing tamponade died, despite emergency surgery to six of the cases who succumbed[10]. Several other important points emerge from this paper. Of 31 cases of tamponade, 14 presented more than 4h after the interventional procedure. The mortality in these late presenters was lower than those who had a more precipitous course within the catheter laboratory (21% vs. 59%), but it was still appreciable. Furthermore, even on retrospective analysis of the cases, it was not possible to identify the bleeding point leading to tamponade in 10 of the 14 late presenters. This would suggest that the likely mechanism was distal branch perforation from the guide wire. However, even with hindsight the angiogram did not show this. This is a salient point.

In a later report by Javaid and colleagues in 2006, 11 of the 14 cases of tamponade died (79%)[18]. We reported similar findings[12]. In our study the mortality of the 24 patients who developed tamponade following perforation was 25% even though half of these cases underwent emergency surgery prior to demise. Five of the 24 instances of tamponade presented more than 2h after the procedure, but fortunately all of these survived. All were related to distal wire perforation and four of the five procedures had involved co-administration of abciximab. Late onset and late identification of a pericardial collection is reported in a number of the other studies[1,7]. A high level of awareness should be maintained for the possible development of this late complication, even if perforation is not immediately obvious on angiography. The clinical manifestation may be rather non-specific, and the patient may simply develop progressive hypotension. There are a number of other plausible explanations for a fall in blood pressure following intervention, so a high index of suspicion should be maintained in order to secure the correct diagnosis in a timely fashion.

Although tamponade imposes a poor outlook, low-grade perforations usually fare well with conservative management. This is borne out by most of the studies. Fukutomi and colleagues reported excellent outcomes in 51 cases with type I perforation[11]. Similarly Javaid and colleagues found that all 14 cases of type I perforation in their series enjoyed an uneventful recovery, although one patient with very severe multi-vessel disease went forward for early bypass surgery[18]. However, in the 33 cases with type II perforation in their study, the clinical course was less favourable. Four patients developed tamponade, nine needed emergency surgery, and one died. Those with type III classification fared worse still—15 of the 25 cases required emergency surgery and 11 died. It is intuitive therefore that the angiographic appearance of the coronary perforation has some bearing on the ultimate outcome. Furthermore, the outlook is worse if tamponade develops abruptly within the catheter laboratory, rather than in a delayed fashion on the ward[10]. From these results it is clear that those cases who have the most precipitous haemodynamic deterioration, do worst. The bigger the vessel rupture, the more rapid the bleed into the pericardial space.

Associated comorbidity also influences outcome. Javaid and colleagues found that the presence of chronic renal dysfunction had a deleterious influence on mortality[18]. It is also likely that pre-procedural impairment of left ventricular function confers a worse outlook but this is less clear from the available data. There has been some change in the clinical pattern over successive decades. Stankovic and colleagues observed the changing pattern of coronary perforation over a 9-year period within their institution in Milan, Italy[16]. The in-hospital major adverse clinical event (MACE) rate was considerably higher in an early phase from 1993–1997, compared with later years from 1998–2001 (51.4% vs. 22.4%, $p = 0.006$). This included a very significant fall in the requirement for emergency coronary bypass and/or subsequent death (31.4% vs. 4.1%, $p = 0.001$). Furthermore, grade of perforation changed over time. The early phase was characterized by a higher incidence of type III perforations, whereas type II perforations were more common in the later phase.

Cavity spilling type III perforations have a good outlook on the whole. Favourable outcomes are reported by most authors without the need for recourse to surgery[1,13]. The reasons are fairly self explanatory. Blood flowing from the coronary circulation through the

Table 32.3 Coronary vessel and lesion characteristics predisposing to perforation

Calcification
Tortuosity
Eccentric plaque
AHA/ACC class B or C lesions
Small calibre vessel
Older patient

ACC, American College of Cardiology; AHA, American Heart Association.

perforation site is retained within the patient's intravascular space, and does not produce any extrinsic compression on the cardiac chambers such as tamponade. Furthermore this type of perforation constitutes a very small minority of those reported.

Lesion characteristics

The most complex coronary artery disease is the most vulnerable to complication during intervention. It would be reasonable to assume that treatment of a discreet, short lesion in the mid-segment of a 3-mm vessel, without undue tortuosity nor calcification, should present a low risk of perforation. Logically, therefore, the antithesis of this description represents the vessel at most risk of rupture or perforation. One should be most cautious when undertaking percutaneous coronary intervention (PCI) on a small calibre, tortuous, calcified coronary artery in an elderly patient. Table 32.3 lists those vessel and lesion characteristics which enhance the likelihood of perforation.

Coronary calcification is the lesion characteristic most worthy of respect. It is associated with concomitant renal disease, hypertension, and diabetes. Although calcification may develop early on in the process of atherosclerosis, it is usually a feature of longstanding coronary disease. Calcification of the intima presents a technical challenge for the interventionalist. If the treatment strategy for this type of disease is simple, i.e. balloon pre-dilatation followed by stent deployment, it often requires very high pressure balloon inflation in order to achieve success. Unlike a more forgiving elastic vessel, the calcified artery may initially be very resistant to balloon preparation, but will abruptly capitulate, often by dissecting or tearing. Intimal calcification is best dealt with by lesion preparation (debulking) prior to stenting. Rotational atherectomy is the most widely used technique for this purpose, and in some institutions excimer laser is employed. Both are enjoying a resurgence in the United Kingdom[20]. The relative merits and risks of both of these techniques are discussed in further detail in later sections of this chapter.

In their analysis of the characteristics of target lesions in vessels which were complicated by perforation, Javaid and colleagues found that 93% were complex, ACC/AHA class B or C. Of 72 lesions which were studied, 42 (58%) exhibited heavy calcification[18]. These findings are in keeping with the results of other published series[10,12,13]. In spite of this calcification only 21 of 72 cases (29%) in Javaid's report underwent debulking with atheroablative technology. Therefore a simple balloon/stent strategy was employed in the remainder. In a separate report, a similarly high proportion of the cases (61%) ending in tamponade following PCI occurred after the treatment of heavily calcified vessels[13]. Once again less than half of the lesions were debulked. This reinforces the point that the substrate (calcification) augments the risk of perforation and it is not all down to the 'new device' technology used in order to treat it. Dealing with these vessels by balloon and stent alone, is just as likely to result in this complication, if not more so.

Tortuosity is another well-recognized risk factor and is identified as characterizing between 39–46% of perforated coronary arteries[8,10,13,18]. A number of authors have also concluded that eccentric lesions are more likely to rupture[10,16,21]. In our report from 2002, a small but important proportion of cases ending in coronary perforation (17%) were undertaken on chronic total occlusions (CTO)[12]. This ties in with most of the other series[8,13,18] with the exception of Eggebrecht and colleagues who noted that 12 of 19 cases of perforation occurred when attempting to open a chronically occluded vessel[14]. The key point is that recanalization of a chronic occlusion is not without risk. While in some instances the perforations are simply classified as simple 'wire exit', higher grade perforations with more serious consequences have been reported in this type of intervention[12].

There is some debate as to whether coronary lumen size clearly predicts likelihood of problems. Nevertheless in the series reported by Javaid and colleagues just over 40% of perforation was seen in vessels of less than 2.5mm diameter[18]. These authors describe that device/lumen mismatch is more important than the vessel reference diameter. Ajluni and colleagues observed that balloon-induced perforation was more likely where the balloon to artery ration was 1.3 ± 0.3, compared with a ratio of 1.0 ± 0.3 where no problem ensued[6]. Ellis and colleagues recorded similar findings where lesions complicated by perforation had a ratio of 1.19 ± 0.7, compared with 0.92 ± 0.16 in those without complication[1]. Almost all studies report the mean age of the perforation cohort to be in the mid 60s. The only authors to demonstrate that this age was significantly higher than the group who did not perforate were Ellis and colleagues[1].

Platelet inhibitors

In the era of POBA, aspirin and unfractionated heparin were standard of care during the procedure. The heparin doses administered at that time were considerably higher than those currently used to meet the requirements of intracoronary stents. There is now a greater emphasis on platelet inhibition rather than anticoagulation. In current practice, the primary role of heparin is to avert thrombus formation on equipment (guide wires, balloons, and catheters) during the procedure. Reversal of the effects of unfractionated heparin by the administration of protamine is well documented as a first-line strategy when coronary perforation occurs. This has been shown to be of value, particularly in lower grade perforations[11,13,19].

The vast majority of coronary intervention now involves the dual antiplatelet therapy of aspirin combined with clopidogrel. The late 1990s witnessed the introduction of more powerful agents, glycoprotein IIb/IIIa inhibitors. Audit figures from the British Cardiovascular Intervention Society demonstrate a steady increase in the use of these agents from 1999 onwards, peaking in 2003 when just over 48% of all coronary intervention involved IIb/IIIa antagonists[22]. Abciximab binds irreversibly to platelet receptors, rendering platelet activity almost negligible for 24–36h. If coronary perforation occurs when these drugs have been administered, establishing control of the bleeding may prove difficult. A number of authors have explored whether the use of IIb/IIIa antagonists has any deleterious effect on the frequency and outcome of this complication. Rather surprisingly many authors find no adverse association. Dippel and colleagues examined the records of 6214 interventions between 1995–1999, complicated by 36 perforations[9]. In this group, 24 (67%) involved the use of abciximab. While proportionate use of this agent increased steadily over the 5 years analysed, there was no increase in the incidence of perforation or tamponade. These authors concluded that it was the angiographic appearance of the perforation which predicted an adverse clinical outcome, rather than the use of these drugs. However in their article they did not determine whether those receiving abciximab fared better or worse than those who had not. They simply examined the temporal relationship of complications to the increased use of abciximab.

Other authors who did explore comparative outcomes reported a modest adverse influence where IIb/IIIa inhibitors were used. Fasseas and colleagues compared 33 perforations where these agents had been administered, with 62 cases without administration[13]. Mortality and myocardial infarction did not differ between groups, but there was a trend towards a higher incidence of tamponade with IIb/IIIa antagonists (15.2 % vs. 9.7%, p = ns). There was also a significantly greater requirement for emergency surgery (24.2% vs. 3.2%, p = 0.003). Others report a negligible influence associated with the use of these agents[11,15]. However, in our study with colleagues in 2002, we reported some changes in the pattern seen[12]. Confining attention solely to those cases of perforation which culminated in tamponade, we observed an increased overall incidence of tamponade for the years analysed (1995–2001) which corresponded with the increased abciximab usage in our unit. Furthermore, the proportion of such cases of tamponade where abciximab administration was associated increased from 17% in 1999 to 86% in 2001. Overall abciximab usage in PCI cases in our unit was approximately 60% in that final year. It is important to note that in 40% of instances of tamponade where abciximab had been administered, it only became manifest more than 2h after the procedure. Retrospective analysis of the angiograms in these cases revealed little or no evidence of extravasation. Where it was identified, the mechanism was clearly wire-tip trauma to a distal sub-branch. Such events would be classified as Ellis type I or II. Our conclusion, therefore, was that great caution should be exercised if any perforation is identified, even if seemingly trivial, where IIb/IIIa inhibitors have been used.

Abciximab demonstrates a prolonged high affinity for the IIb/IIIa receptor binding site. Therefore, unlike the smaller molecules tirofiban and integrilin, simply discontinuing the infusion of abciximab will not reverse these effects. Platelet transfusion is of value in correcting the bleeding time and this has been clearly demonstrated[23]. However, administering platelets goes somewhat against the objective of maintaining stent patency by inhibiting this arm of the clotting process. Therefore a number of authors recommend either avoiding a transfusion where feasible[24] or even continuing abciximab in the most complex cases[24]. In reality the strategy chosen should be determined by the importance of either stopping a potentially life-threatening haemorrhage, or maintaining a crucial revascularization result in a complex case. This is, perhaps, a situation where interventional cardiology demands the art of medicine rather than the science.

Atheroablative devices

Even enthusiastic proponents of debulking techniques would not deny that the use of either atherectomy or laser technology is associated with a higher incidence of perforation than in conventional balloon and stent PCI. However, the point has been made earlier that the increased complication rate using these devices is strongly influenced by the complexity of the coronary disease being treated. More specialized equipment is necessary in order to treat more challenging cases. This should be kept in perspective when appraising the literature on this topic.

Ellis and colleagues were the first to highlight the potential problems with 'new devices' in their report of 1994[(1)]. The incidence of perforation with balloon angioplasty was a mere 14 out of 9080 cases (0.1%) whereas that of debulking techniques collectively was 48 out of 3820 cases (1.3%). Excimer laser fared the worst in this article with an incidence of 1.9%. The Ellis report covered interventional activity through 1990 and 1991. Therefore experience with all of the debulking techniques was still developing at this time. The excimer laser registry results published in 1993 identified perforation in 23 out of 764 patients (3%)[(25)]. While no patients died, nine of the 23 suffered a significant haemodynamic insult from this. The authors concluded that down-sizing the laser catheter, rendering the device at least 1mm smaller than the reference artery diameter, reduced the risk of perforation. This advice must have been heeded as the subsequent registry report on excimer laser the following year by Holmes and colleagues indicated an improvement, with 36 of 2759 (1.3%) cases complicated by perforation[(26)]. The authors specifically commented on the reduction in complication rates as operators became more experienced, with laser perforations declining from 1.6% in the first 1888 patients treated to only 0.4% in the latter 1000 patients of this registry.

Rotational atherectomy (rotablation) was first developed in the late 1980s. This involves the use of a rapidly rotating drill tipped with industrial diamond over a fine monofilament steel wire. Very little has changed in the equipment employed for this procedure in the 20 years that have elapsed since its inception. However, operator expertise and appropriate caution have evolved. Ellis reported that 10 of 771 rotablator cases were complicated by coronary perforation (1.3%)[(1)]. More favourable results were reported in subsequent publications. Reisman and colleagues described the outcome in two chronological registries, one between 1988–1993 and the other from 1994–1997[(27)]. In the first, the perforation rate was 0.8%, and this fell to 0.5% in the second. The results reported by Von Sohsten and colleagues highlighted an important issue[(7)]; while they identified tamponade in eight out of 743 rotablator procedures, seven of these eight instances were actually as a consequence of a temporary pacing wire puncturing the right ventricle, rather than coronary perforation per se. Softer, smaller calibre pacing wires are now available which are much less likely to produce this problem.

More favourable results for rotablation were reported by Gruberg and colleagues in their institution's interventional practice in the late 1990s[(8)]. The perforation rate was only 0.4% in this study, very similar to that reported by Fejka and colleagues in 2002 (0.3%)[(10)]. Thus despite an increase in the complexity of cases being treated, there has been no major increase in perforation rates secondary to rotational atherectomy. So far that is. The use of this device is enjoying a resurgence. In the United Kingdom it is the most commonly employed atheroablative technique. Across the nation in 2007, 844 procedures were performed in 42 units, which is part of a continuing pattern of increased uptake. In 2005, 479 cases were carried out in 37 units, compared to only 170 in 27 units in 2002([20]). Based on history alone, this technology should be accorded respect, and appropriate precautions observed in order to avert a rise in perforation rates as this expansion in activity continues.

The guide wire

The case for caution with respect to the angioplasty guide wire has become more pressing over the last decade. The major cause of perforation in early studies was either balloon barotrauma or the use of a debulking device. The range and specifications of guide wires which are currently available is impressive. More supportive equipment with a hydrophilic coating on the distal segment may pass easily through tortuous resistant anatomy, where older wires might have proven cumbersome. However, it is just this type of guide wire that appears more likely to induce trauma to the distal coronary vasculature, perhaps as a direct result of this more efficient tracking. The recommendation therefore must be to pay careful attention to these guide wires during the procedure.

Several authors have clearly pin-pointed the hydrophilic wire as a more risky iteration of this equipment. Javaid and colleagues found that 13 of 15 wire-associated perforations had a hydrophilic coating[18]. In the study by Ramana and colleagues on a cohort of 4886 cases treated between 2001–2004, the majority of the 25 perforations were caused by guide wires and these were usually hydrophilic and stiff[17]. Witzke's group found that 51% of perforations were wire mediated[15]. This shows the changing pattern of perforation over time. This has been observed by a number of authors. The Milan group reported on two different time periods at their institution[16]. When comparing perforations in the early phase from 1993–1997 with those in the late phase after 1998, they found that complications in the later years were much more likely to be attributable to the guide wire (19 cases vs. one case). This difference in cause of the complication also translated into a different angiographic appearance. The majority of the events in the later group were classified as Ellis type II, as opposed to type III in the early phase.

This trend is seen in other reports. Fasseas classified 86% of guide-wire mediated ruptures as Ellis type I or II on angiography[13]. Wires are much less likely to cause a breach in the proximal or mid vessel, but more likely to do so distally, perhaps in the terminal sub-branches. They are also less likely to cause frank rupture of the vessel than a high-pressure balloon barotrauma. So the appearance on angiography is usually more subtle when a wire is the culprit. However these events should not be regarded as innocuous. A proportion may go on to develop pericardial tamponade and in some instances this only becomes manifest late (between 2–26h post procedure). One way to minimize distal trauma is to create a loop at the end of the wire, rendering it less likely to inadvertently puncture the vessel wall. We have already highlighted the point that adjunctive use of IIb/IIIa antagonists may potentiate prolonged bleeding from a seemingly minor blemish in the vessel.

Where chronic total occlusions are treated percutaneously, there is always a risk that the guiding wire will pass out of the vessel. This is particularly true if heavy-weight, stiff-tipped equipment is used. Provided there is no balloon inflation when the wire is incorrectly positioned, the extravasation of dye or blood is usually minimal. It may be corrected by heparin reversal and conservative measures. Eggebrecht and colleagues described 19 cases of perforation in 6433 percutaneous interventions[14]. In 12 of these (63%) the operators were attempting to open a chronic occlusion. This represents a higher proportion than other studies. Not all of these had a benign course. In our study with colleagues in 2002, nine out of 52 identified perforations (17%) were related to the treatment of occlusions[12]. Six of these resulted in pericardial tamponade, and there was an association with the use of abciximab in these more complicated cases. There is a cautionary note here. Where possible, the administration of IIb/IIIa antagonists should be withheld until the occlusion is safely crossed and the operator is confident that the distal tip of the wire is seated intraluminally.

Treatment

The strategy for dealing with coronary artery perforation is determined by both the site of the perforation and the severity of the insult. In dealing with a mid-vessel rupture which threatens imminent tamponade, the objective is to rapidly seal that segment of artery, preserving distal perfusion as far as possible. The opposite may apply to a distal branch puncture where the aim may be to 'safely' occlude the smaller vessel, disregarding the tiny area of myocardial necrosis which will result. Either way, the management chosen will be influenced by features of the case such as haemodynamic instability or persistent bleeding into the pericardial space. Fig. 32.1 displays an algorithm for the management of coronary perforation.

Basic principles

The most important first step is to recognize and identify the presence of a perforation. While it may seem an obvious statement, these events are all too often missed where the index of suspicion is not high enough. Any unusual migration of a wire-tip, dye staining, or unexplained hypotension should alert the operator to the possibility of this problem. By scrutinizing the angiogram while in the catheter laboratory, and dealing with any complication on the spot, one can avert a return to the lab out of hours, perhaps when the patient is more unstable due to haemodynamic embarrassment. Intravenous fluids, oxygen, analgesia, and even inotropic support should be considered. Atropine should be administered where bradycardia occurs as a vagal mediated response.

At this stage the Ellis classification is a helpful tool guiding the approach but it should not be regarded as fool proof. Type I perforations will usually respond to conservative measures. This is supported by a number of studies[11,18]. In some instances no action is required and the case may simply be completed as per the original interventional strategy, with careful observation of the perforation. Deployment of an intracoronary stent over the visible blemish often successfully deals with the problem area. Nevertheless fastidious post-procedural

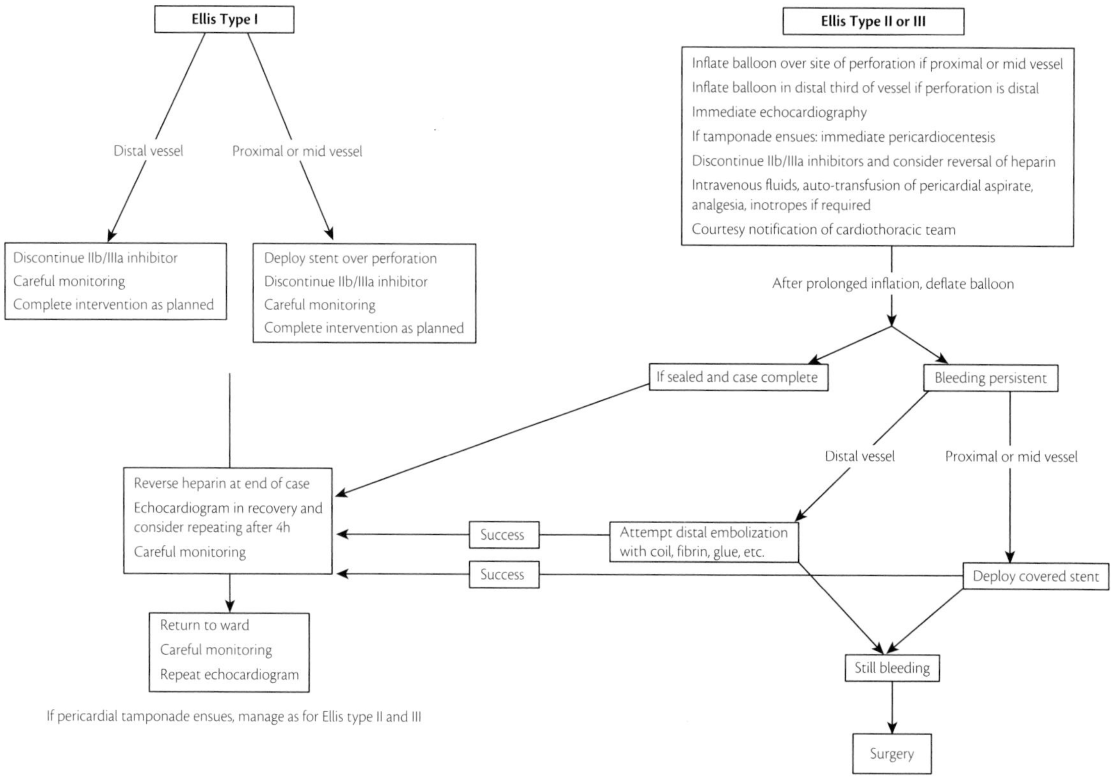

Fig. 32.1 Management algorithm for coronary perforation.

care is prudent, with cautious monitoring of haemodynamic parameters, and at least one echocardiographic assessment to rule out accumulation of fluid in the pericardial space. If the patient is entirely stable, there is some wisdom in delaying this echo study by around 30min post procedure in the stable patient, to capture those cases where the accumulation of pericardial fluid is insidious.

The initial management of a type II or a type III perforation should be similar. The first objective is to stop the bleeding. This may be a temporary measure, gaining valuable time before a definitive strategy can be implemented. It is best achieved by inflating an angioplasty balloon over the site of the rupture if it is in the mid or proximal vessel, and more distally for a remotely situated wire perforation. This manoeuvre may prevent the development of tamponade, which favourably alters the outlook of the situation. Furthermore, prolonged balloon inflation alone may be sufficient to treat the problem without need for any further action, The required duration of balloon inflation may approach 30min. If the patient cannot tolerate the associated ischaemia, a perfusion balloon may prove helpful. Fukotomi and colleagues reported excellent results using a perfusion balloon for Ellis type III rupture[11]. Other authors report that balloon tamponade is only a successful strategy in a minor proportion of cases[1,18]. A number of authors advocate the deployment of standard intracoronary stents in order to secure the perforation site[28]. This may involve the deployment of a number of layers of stent over the point of rupture before success is achieved.

While implementing these mechanical solutions, attention should also be paid to anticoagulant therapy and/or platelet inhibitors. A key question is whether dealing with the perforation signals the end of the case, or whether the operator aims to continue the revascularization procedure once control of the bleeding has been established. If the case is to be discontinued, reversal of heparin using protamine sulphate has been shown to be effective alongside other measures in numerous reports[11,19]. This should, however, be deferred while equipment such as balloons and wires remain in the coronary artery.

Conversely, intravenous IIb/IIIa antagonists should be discontinued in the majority of cases where perforation is identified. As described earlier, even seemingly trivial blushes of extravasation may progress later on to haemodynamic problems where these agents are in use. The use of a platelet infusion to counter the effects of abciximab should be carefully weighed against the possible deleterious effects of fresh platelets. If their activity is not inhibited, at least in part, they could provoke abrupt stent thrombosis. This introduces an unwelcome new complexion to an already complex case. For this reason, aspirin and clopidogrel are invariably continued whatever the predicament.

Tamponade

Tamponade should receive attention as soon as it is identified. Percutaneous drainage not only alleviates the haemodynamic problem, but also allows for an active evaluation of the rate of ongoing bleeding from the perforation site. Emergent echocardiography is required. In some instances the accumulation of a very small volume of pericardial blood may result in profound haemodynamic suppression or even cardiac arrest. Deploying a drain under these conditions demands considerable skill and experience. There is little to be gained from deliberation, but a clear rim of fluid should be present before the needle is passed as there is a risk of puncturing the free wall of the right ventricle, thereby compounding the problem. In cases which manifest after a few hours, there is usually a more sizeable collection of fluid, which proves easier to drain.

The route chosen for drainage is not crucial, and should be guided by the echo findings. The usual approach is from a point inferior and to the left of the xiphisternum, directed supero-posteriorly towards the left shoulder. Once the pig-tail catheter is positioned, active drainage to dryness should be undertaken using a large-volume syringe. Ample analgesia is important as this phase is often uncomfortable for the patient. It is not uncommon for several hundred millilitres of blood to be removed in this fashion. Rather than calling upon blood product resources, there is merit in transferring the pericardial blood directly back into the intravascular space. This is best achieved by creating a connection between the drainage catheter and a femoral vein sheath. Thus blood is taken off the heart and returned to the leg.

Once the pericardial space has been drained to dryness, the volume which continues to accumulate should be recorded every minute. In this manner the cardiologist can assess whether the treatment already undertaken has successfully dealt with the bleeding point, and whether the bleeding is subsiding. If there no resolution after approximately 30min, further action is required, and this may include surgery. We have already emphasized that pericardial tamponade in this context carries a mortality of between 20–50%. This is still true in the more recent reports[12,17–19]. Arresting the source of the bleeding is crucial.

Covered stents

Frank rupture of the proximal or mid coronary artery produces the most dramatic angiographic demonstration of the perforation. In the final analysis, such events often constitute a tear in the vessel, up to 5mm in length. Haemodynamic collapse is abrupt and expedient action is required. One solution is to deploy a covered stent, thereby isolating the point of haemorrhage from the circulation. The most widely used device is the polytetrafluoroethylene (PTFE) covered stent which is in effect a stent sandwich with a PTFE membrane housed between the two layers of metal. As such it is rather inflexible, and this is particularly relevant to those trying to deploy it without delay.

Favourable case reports on the use of covered stents abound in the literature[29,30]. Occasionally more than one stent is required to seal the leak. In an analysis of 3 years of clinical practice at their institution, Briguori and colleagues reported a series of 11 cases treated in this fashion, and compared the results with 17 cases which had been treated by bare-metal stent alone in the preceding 4 years[31]. In both groups ordinary balloon tamponade and reversal of anticoagulation had failed. The MACE rate was 18% in the covered stent group, compared to 88% in the bare-metal group ($p < 0.001$), suggesting that this is a very effective treatment for cases where conservative measures have proved unsuccessful. Stankovic reported a reduction in MACE for type III perforations using PTFE covered stents (33% vs. 91%, $p = 0.002$), but no benefit was gained in the treatment of type II perforations[16].

Not all authors support this view. Ly and colleagues achieved successful seal of the perforation using PTFE in 71% of cases[32]. However, there was no statistically significant reduction in the development of tamponade, nor the requirement for emergency surgery, when this treatment modality was compared to prolonged balloon inflation. One of the problems is the difficulty in delivering this inflexible device, and this is cited by other authors as well[12,18]. This is most troublesome in the calcified, tortuous vessel, which is the archetypal substrate for perforation in the first instance. An additional

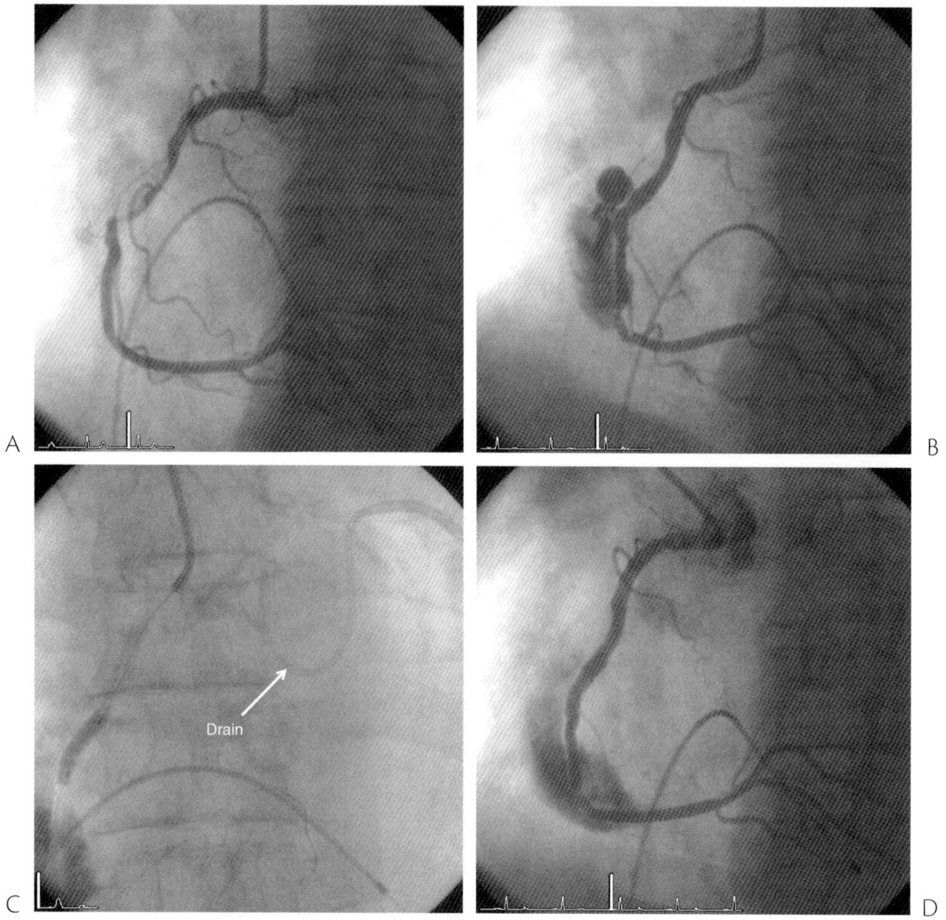

Fig. 32.2 Mid-vessel rupture of right coronary artery: A) vessel prior to treatment; B) brisk dye extravasation and distal spasm following rotablation, stenting, and post-dilatation; C) balloon inflation to arrest bleeding, pericardial drain indicated by arrow; D) appearance following the deployment of two PTFE-covered stents.

late concern is that of in-stent restenosis. This is poorly quantified, but in the small number who underwent angiographic follow-up in the Briguori study, 29% demonstrated restenosis[31].

On balance however, if the covered stent can be passed and deployed, it provides a valuable rescue option in selected cases. It should be considered early in the treatment strategy. Fig. 32.2 illustrates this point. A dramatic rupture of a right coronary artery is shown. It occurred after the calcified vessel was debulked using rotational atherectomy, and further treated by the deployment of two drug-eluting stents. Modest residual constraint in the middle of the stented segment was treated with a non-compliant balloon to optimize deployment, resulting in the impressive extravasation shown in Fig. 32.2B. This was rapidly sealed by the deployment of two PTFE-coated stents. The case was only briefly interrupted by this event, anticoagulation was not reversed, and the operator went on to successfully treat the left main stem, circumflex, and left anterior descending artery in this candidate who was deemed unsuitable for bypass surgery.

Distal perforation

Clearly, covered stents are of no benefit in dealing with haemorrhage from a distal sub-branch of a coronary artery. The vast majority of these events are caused by the angioplasty guide wire, but very occasionally they are due to distal work with a balloon. The objective is to seal off the leaking branch, and little concern need be given to the small region of myocardium supplied by it.

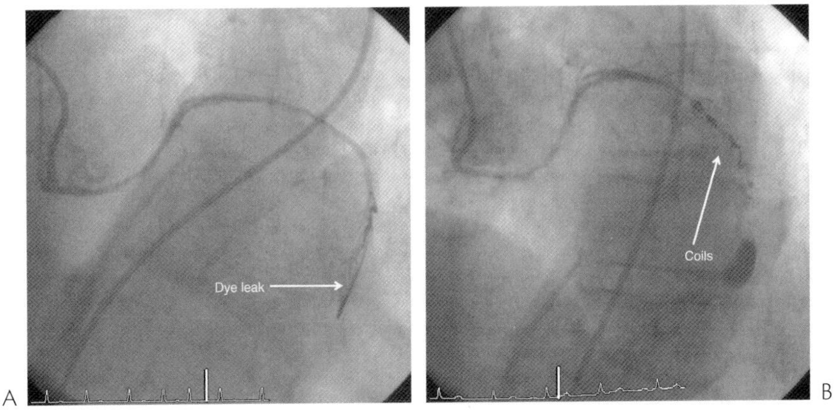

Fig. 32.3 Distal perforation of aberrant left circumflex vessel: A) extravasation of dye indicated by Arrow; B) perforation sealed by deployment of three platinum coils.

The risk from the bleed far exceeds the risk of the limited regional necrosis which occurs following occlusion. The conventional basic measures described earlier are often successful in stemming flow from the perforation. However, if these fail the vessel may be occluded by a variety of means. Platinum microcoils are designed to be thrombogenic. They are delivered through dedicated, trackable microcatheters and are ideally suited to this purpose[33,34]. Fig. 32.3A demonstrates a perforation in an aberrant left circumflex artery. This is successfully sealed using Trufill® (Terumo) platinum coils (see Fig. 32.3B). Other rather innovative methods of sealing the distal vessel have been reported in the literature. These include injection of thrombin[35], autologous clotted blood[36], tris-acryl gelatin microspheres[37], fibrin glue[38], subcutaneous adipose tissue[39], and polyvinyl alcohol foam[40]. The principle is simple: any material which will induce clotting and plug the leak will suffice.

The role of surgery

Surgery is the final recourse in the management algorithm. Cases not responding to the measures described earlier are referred for surgical repair of the ruptured vessel, possibly with concurrent bypass grafting. Not surprisingly the perforations referred on for this treatment are usually frank ruptures rather than modest distal perforations. In the report of Ellis and colleagues from 1994, 63% of type III perforations had to be treated surgically, but very few type I or II perforations required this treatment[1]. Fasseas and colleagues required surgical intervention for 8.6% of type II perforations, and a higher number, 27.7%, of type III[13]. No type I lesion needed an operation. Over time the requirement for surgery had declined but not disappeared, and this is illustrated in Table 32.2.

Not all authors have described the outcome of patients who are referred on to the operating theatre, but for those who have, the results are disappointing. The mortality of emergency surgery in the reports of both Fejka[10] and Witzke[15] was 50%. Our results were similar where three of eight patients (38%) referred for surgical repair succumbed[12]. So why is an operation such a poor option for these cases? In evaluating these findings one has to bear in mind that it is only cases where other treatment options have failed who are managed via this route. They are usually obtunded, with ongoing bleeding and haemodynamic compromise, requiring inotropic support. This precarious state may be further compounded by coagulopathy, myocardial infarction, and deterioration of renal function. Such cases are presented to surgical colleagues in the hopes of rescuing a bad situation. It is inevitable that this proves impossible in a proportion of them. For the cardiac surgeon the problem is the substrate, rather than the treatment.

If this is the case, should patients be considered earlier for surgery? While some groups refer remarkably few patients on for an operation, their overall mortality figures are impressively low. Fukutomi and colleagues reported on 69 instances of coronary perforation, with 29 progressing on to tamponade (42%)[11]. The mortality was zero. Only two of the 69 (3%) underwent surgery. Therefore either conservative or percutaneous treatment options were successful in the vast majority of cases. These are impressive results, but are not a reflection of usual findings.

It is always sensible to offer advance notice to surgical colleagues the moment one is dealing with a high-grade perforation via percutaneous means in the catheter lab. This will allow for expedient transfer should this prove necessary. There is no clear answer as to the optimal timing for calling in cardiothoracic involvement. However, if bleeding from a pericardial drain is persisting at a rate above 10mL per minute, despite all other action being taken, mechanical and pharmacological, it is prudent to call a surgeon.

Conclusions

It is fortuitous that coronary perforation remains a rare complication. However, in light of this, few interventional fellows will have the occasion to deal with this complication, first hand, during their training. In the most severe cases, remedial measures must be taken instantly in order to avert demise of the patient. Prevention remains the best of course of action. An awareness of those features which augment the potential risk of this complication allows for an adjustment in interventional practice in order to minimize the likelihood of it occurring.

References

1. Ellis SG, Ajluni S, Arnold AZ, *et al.* Increased coronary artery perforation in the new device era. Incidence, classification, management and outcome. *Circulation* 1994; **90**:2725–30.
2. Kiss L. [Sudden death caused by rupture of the coronary artery in 1737, verified by autopsy – a case report by Daniel Fischer from Kesmark (Hungary).] *Orv Hetil* 2008; **149**:89–91.
3. Morettin LB, Wallace JM. Uneventful perforation of a coronary artery during selective angiography. A case report. *Am J Roentgenol Ther Nucl Med* 1970; **110**:184–8.
4. Kimbiris D, Iskandrian AS, Goel I, *et al.* Transluminal coronary angioplasty complicated by coronary artery perforation. *Cathet Cardiovasc Diagn* 1982; **8**:481–7.
5. Meier B. Benign coronary perforation during percutaneous transluminal coronary angioplasty. *Br Heart J* 1985; **54**: 33–5.
6. Ajluni SC, Glazier S, Blankenship L, *et al.* Perforation after percutaneous coronary interventions: Clinical, angiographic, and therapeutic observations. *Cathet Cardiovasc Diagn* 1994; **32**:206–12.
7. Von Sohsten R, Kopitansky C, Cohen M, *et al.* Cardiac tamponade in the 'new device era: evaluation of 6999 consecutive percutaneous coronary interventions. *Am Heart J* 2000; **140**:279–83.
8. Gruberg L, Pinnow E, Flood R, *et al.* Incidence, management, and outcome of coronary artery perforation during percutaneous coronary intervention. *Am J Cardiol* 2000; **86**:680–2.
9. Dippel EJ, Kereiakes DJ, Tramuta DA, *et al.* Coronary perforation during percutaneous coronary intervention in the era of abciximab platelet glycoprotein IIb/IIIa blockade: An algorithm for percutaneous management. *Catheter Cardiovasc Interv* 2001; **52**:279–86.
10. Fejka M, Dixon SR, Safian RD, *et al.* Diagnosis, management, and clinical outcome of cardiac tamponade complicating percutaneous coronary intervention. *Am J Cardiol* 2002; **90**:1183–6.
11. Fukutomi T, Suzuki T, Popma JJ, *et al.* Early and late clinical outcomes following coronary perforation in patients undergoing percutaneous coronary intervention. *Circ J* 2002; **66**:349–56.
12. Gunning MG, Williams IL, Jewitt DE, *et al.* Coronary artery perforation during percutaneous intervention: incidence and outcome. *Heart* 2002; **88**:495–8.
13. Fasseas P, Orford JL, Panetta CJ, *et al.* Incidence, correlates, management, and clinical outcome of coronary perforation: analysis of 16298 procedures. *Am Heart J* 2004; **147**:140–5.
14. Eggebrecht H, Ritzel A, von Birgelen C, *et al.* Acute and long-term outcome after coronary artery perforation during percutaneous coronary intervention. *Z Kardiol* 2004; **93**:791–8.
15. Witzke CF, Martin-Herrero F, Clarke SC, *et al.* The changing pattern of coronary perforation during percutaneous coronary intervention in the new device era. *J Invasive Cardiol* 2004; **16**:297–301.
16. Stankovic G, Orlic D, Corvaja N, *et al.* Incidence, predictors, in-hospital, and late outcomes of coronary artery perforations. *Am J Cardiol* 2004; **93**:213–16.
17. Ramana R, Arab D, Joyal D, *et al.* Coronary artery perforation during percutaneous coronary intervention: Incidence and outcomes in the new interventional era. *J Invasive Cardiol* 2005; **17**:603–5.
18. Javaid A, Buch AN, Satler LF, *et al.* Management and outcomes of coronary artery perforation during percutaneous coronary intervention. *Am J Cardiol* 2006; **98**:911–14.
19. Shikarabe A, Takano H, Nakamura S, *et al.* Coronary perforation during percutaneous coronary intervention. *Int Heart J* 2007; **48**:1–9.
20. Ludman P. British Cardiovascular Intervention Society: Audit returns 2007 http://www.bcis.org.uk
21. Cohen BM, Weber VJ, Relsman M, *et al.* Coronary perforation complicating rotational ablation: The U. S. multicenter experience. *Cathet Cardiovasc Diagn* 1996; (Suppl)**3**:55–9.
22. Ludman P. British Cardiovascular Intervention Society: Audit returns 2003 http://www.bcis.org.uk
23. Juergens CP, Yeung AC, Oesterle SN. Routine platelet transfusion in patients undergoing emergency coronary bypass surgery after receiving abciximab. *Am J Cardiol* 1997; **80**:74–5.
24. Klein LW. Coronary artery perforation during interventional procedures. *Cathet Cardiovasc Interv* 2006; **68**:713–17.

25. Bittl JA, Ryan TJ Jr, Keaney JF Jr, *et al.* Coronary artery perforation during excimer laser coronary angioplasty. The percutaneous Excimer Laser Coronary Angioplasty Registry. *J Am Coll Cardiol* 1993; **21**:1158–65.
26. Holmes DR Jr, Reeder GS, Ghazzal ZM, *et al.* Coronary perforation after excimer laser coronary angioplasty: the Excimer Laser Coronary Angioplasty Registry experience. *J Am Coll Cardiol* 1994; **23**:330–5.
27. Reisman M, Harms V, Whitlow P, *et al.* Comparison of early and recent results with rotational atherectomy. *J Am Coll Cardiol* 1997; **29**:353–7.
28. Thomas MR, Wainwright RJ. Use of an intracoronary stent to control intrapericardial bleeding during coronary artery rupture complicating coronary angioplasty. *Cathet Cardiovasc Diagn* 1993; **30**:169–72.
29. Nageh T, Thomas MR. Coronary-artery rupture treated with a polytetrafluoroethylene-coated stent. *N Engl J Med* 2000; **342**:1922–24.
30. Ramsdale DR, Mushahwar SS, Morris JL. Repair of coronary artery perforation after rotastenting by implantation of the JoStent covered stent. *Cathet Cardiovasc Diagn* 1998; **45**:310–313.
31. Briguori C, De Gregorio J, Nishida T, *et al.* Emergency polytetrafluoroethylene-covered stent implantation to treat coronary ruptures. *Circulation* 2000; **102**:3028–31.
32. Ly H, Awaida JP, Lesperance J, *et al.* Angiographic and clinical outcomes of polytetrafluoroethylene covered stent use in significant coronary perforations. *Am J Cardiol* 2005; **95**:244–6.
33. Gaxiola E, Browne KF. Coronary artery perforation repair using microcoil embolisation. *Cathet Cardiovasc Diagn* 1998; **43**:474–6.
34. Mahmud E, Douglas JS Jr. Coil embolisation for successful treatment of perforation of chronically occluded proximal coronary artery. *Cathet Cardiovasc Interven* 2001; **53**:549–52.
35. Jamali AH, Lee MS, Makkar RR. Coronary perforation after percutaneous coronary intervention successfully treated with local thrombin injection. *J Invasive Cardiol* 2006; **18**:E143–5.
36. Hadjimiltiades S, Paraskeviades S, Kazinakis G, *et al.* Coronary vessel perforation during balloon angioplasty: a case report. *Cathet Cardiovasc Diagn* 1998; **45**:417–20.
37. To AC, El-Jack SS, Webster MW, *et al.* Coronary artery perforation successfully treated with tris-acryl gelatin microsphere embolisation. *Heart Lung Circ* 2008; **17**:423–6.
38. Storger H, Ruef J. Closure of guide-wire induced coronary artery perforation with a two component fibrin glue. *Cathet Cardiovasc Interv* 2007; **70**:237–40.
39. Oda H, Oda M, Makiyama Y, *et al.* Guide-wire induced coronary artery perforation treated with transcatheter delivery of subcutaneous tissue. *Cathet Cardiovasc Interv* 2005; **66**:369–74.
40. Iakovou I, Colombo A. Management of right coronary artery perforation during percutaneous coronary intervention with polyvinyl alcohol foam embolization particles. *J Invasive Cardiol* 2004; **16**:727–8.

SECTION 7

Special devices in percutaneous coronary intervention

CHAPTER 33

Rotational atherectomy

Adam de Belder and Martyn Thomas

Introduction

Since 1979, plain old balloon angioplasty (POBA) has provided relief of angina for many patients. Recurrent symptoms due to restenosis diminished with bare-metal stent and, more recently, drug-eluting technology. A limitation to achieving good results with POBA and stenting is calcification within the artery which not only can prevent passage of balloons and stents into a lesion but also may prevent adequate lumen expansion. Rotational atherectomy or rotablation (RA) can treat highly resistant calcified plaque within coronary arteries to allow adequate vessel expansion and ensure optimal stent deployment.

The concept of using a high-speed diamond-tipped drill spinning at 150 000rpm driven by compressed air to clear an artery that is 3mm in diameter is challenging, yet this technique has been available for use in coronary arteries since 1989 when M.E. Bertrand (Lille, France) and R. Erbel (Essen, Germany) first used it in humans.

Pathophysiology

RA ablates plaque—when properly utilized, it minimizes wall stretch in all plaque morphologies, not only calcified disease, and the end result is a smooth lumen, which allows further vessel modification with balloon and stent placement (see Figs. 33.1 and 33.2)

RA leads to pulverization of tissue rather than fragmentation—the debris is similar in size to red blood cells (5µm), which is taken up by the reticulo-endothelial system (see Fig. 33.3). In clinical use it is important to use appropriate sizing and good technique to ensure pulverization is the end-result – for example use of too big a burr size can lead to fragmentation and distal embolization leading to myocardial infarction.

Equipment

RA equipment (Fig. 33.4) consists of:

- Hardware: a console which controls and monitors the rotational speed, monitors the procedural and ablation time periods, and has an advancer stall warning light
- Disposables: these include an advancer, which provides housing for the air turbine, brake assemblies and the burr control knob, a guide wire, and a torquer.

Guide wire

The stainless steel guide wires are 0.009 inches in diameter and have an overall length of 325cm. The spring tip is atraumatic, radiopaque, and can be shaped to form a steerable system.

The RotaWire® is smaller in diameter than standard 0.014-inch coronary wires and is prone to damage if not carefully handled (Fig. 33.5). The Rotablator® system should not be used if there is a bend, kink, or loop in the guide wire or if the spring tip is prolapsed.

Manipulating the RotaWire® is highly operator-sensitive—it has different handling and its lubricity is inferior to modern coronary guide wires. Some operators choose to use a routine coronary guide wire to cross the lesion, and then use an over-the-wire balloon or exchange catheter to place the RotaWire® in the distal vessel.

Burr size

Burr sizes vary and are available in 1.25, 1.5, 1.75 (6F typically compatible, but related to internal diameter of the guiding catheter), 2.0, and 2.15mm (7F or above). The drive shaft is enclosed by a 4.3F sheath (Fig. 33.6).

The drive shaft has a simple advance mechanism, with three ports:

- One for high flow solution (see below) which bathes the artery during the procedure, as the heat generation during RA is quite significant

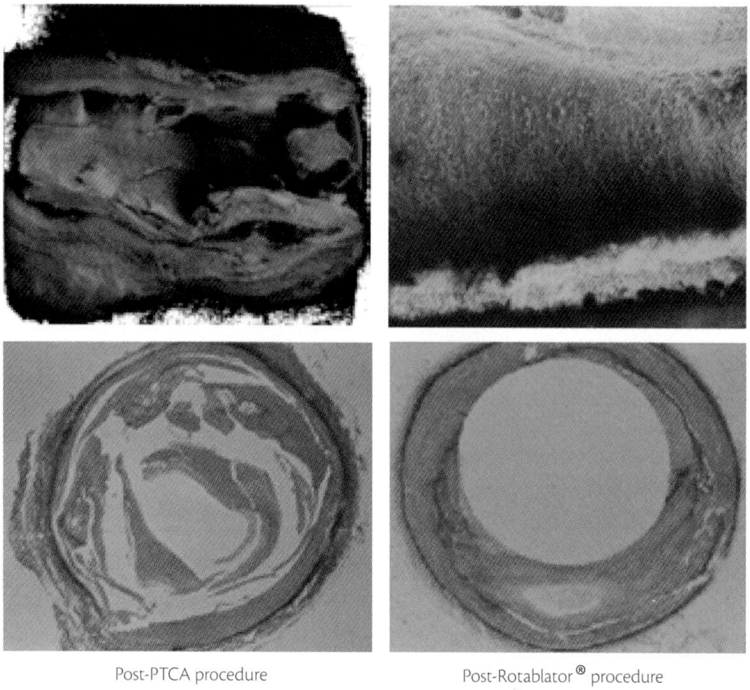

Fig. 33.1 Porcine model of angioplasty and rotablation emphasizing the difference in outcome to the vessel wall between the two techniques.

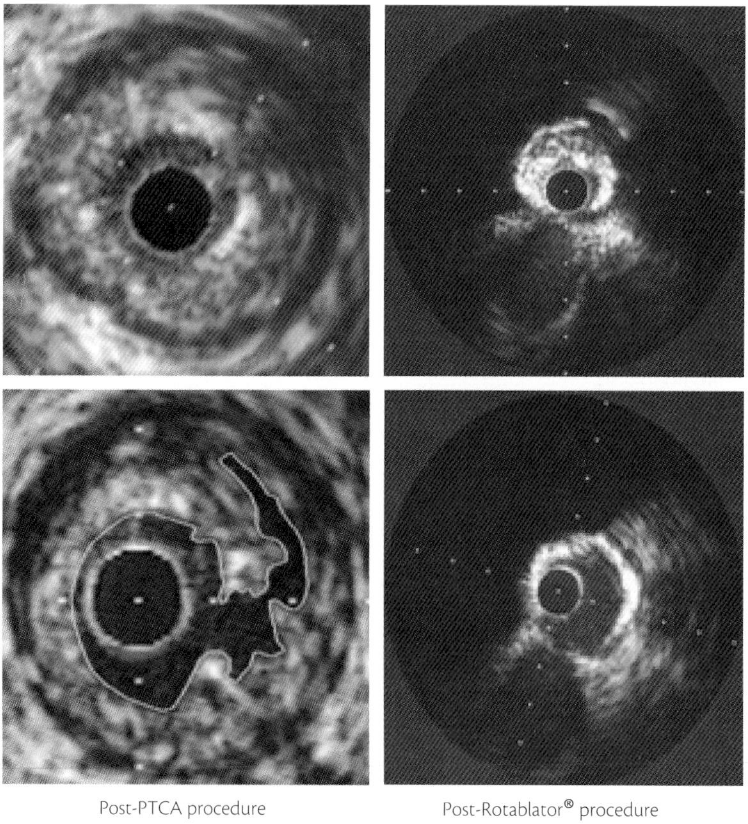

Fig. 33.2 Intravascular ultrasound images confirming the smooth intraluminal appearance after successful rotablation, in comparison to balloon angioplasty.

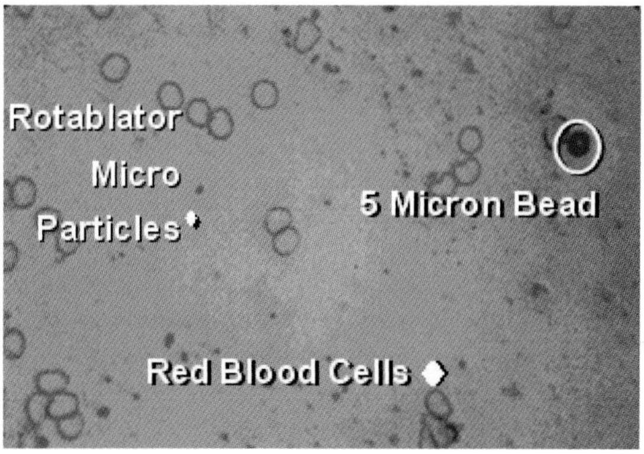

Fig. 33.3 Microparticles caused by RA, showing similar size to red blood cells.

- One fibreoptic cable to allow rotational speed measurement
- One for transmission of compressed air.

The newer systems (Rotalink®) allow for 1 advancer per case and multiple burr use using a simple exchange mechanism.

Air supply set up

The compressed air cylinder can be a source of technical failure. Failure of compressed air equipment at a critical time can lead to unwanted complications. An adequate supply in tank and regulation to working pressures are fundamental.

Technique for debulking

Compressed air generates rotational speeds of 140 000–150 000rpm—the ideal speed for ablation is debated with some operators suggesting lower speed may lead to less complications but the data for this is limited[1].

The debulking procedure is preferred as a 'pecking' motion rather than a continuous 'push' into the plaque. Generally, short engagements of RA, totalling no longer than 20s per run is recommended. Pausing adequately before the next run allows particle washout and vessel perfusion.

Tips on technique

Marked reductions in rotational speed (>5000rpm) generates heat in vessel wall. This can be avoided by the appropriate 'pecking' technique with very transient engagement of the plaque. Many operators use a single burr strategy (rather than a stepwise increase in size) but if this approach is used it is recommended that the lesion is subsequently 'tested' with a balloon (before stenting) because in some cases the ring of calcium has not been fully ablated to allow safe stenting and a larger burr has to be used.

There are a few things which can commonly happen to the inexperienced operator, which should be avoided:

- Do not stop the burr distal to the lesion
- Avoid dottering (forcing the burr through the lesion rather than ablating) the lesion
- Do not alter the rpm during RA
- Do not start RA with the burr in the lesion
- Avoid advancing the rotating burr to make contact with the guide wire spring tip
- Avoid RA in a forward motion within the guide catheter (although this can be difficult for ostial lesions.

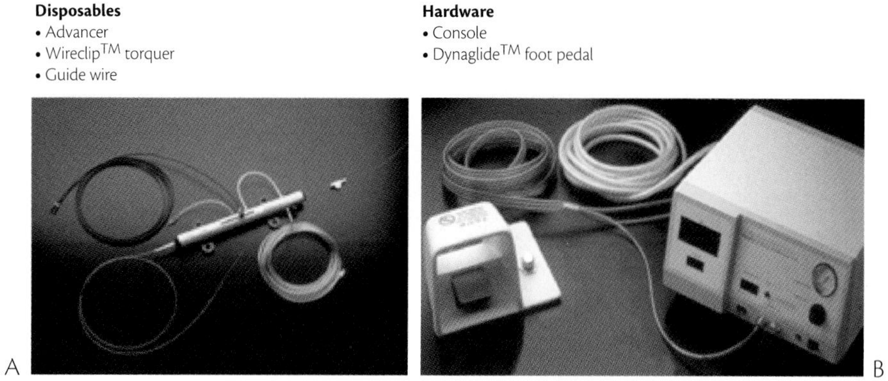

Fig. 33.4 A) Disposable and B) hardware equipment for rotablation.

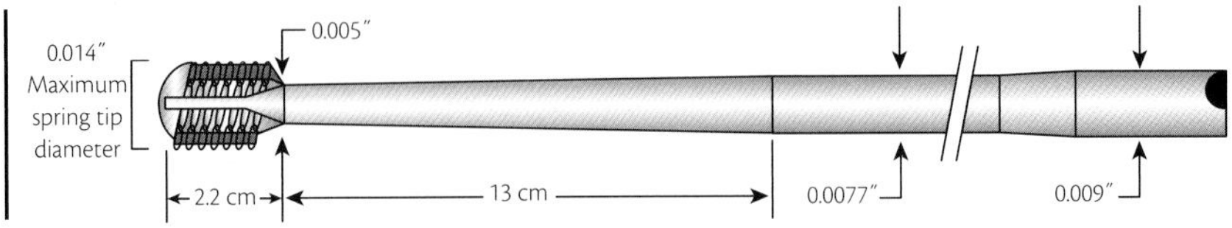

Fig. 33.5 Detailed view of the RotaWire® tip.

Good technique involves the gentle advancement and retraction of an appropriately sized burr at high speed.

Complications and their management

Even in the most competent of hands, RA is associated with more complications than routine angioplasty and stenting. This is principally because of the complexities of the lesions that are generally dealt with by the device rather than the technique itself. The management of these circumstances is central to good outcomes[2].

Vasospasm

RA procedures are performed with a constant heparinized saline flush (5000 IU heparin in 500mL normal saline) continually bathing the coronary vessel. 5mg verapamil and 5mg isosorbide dinitrate, can be added to the 500-mL bag to potentially deal with vasospasm[3].

Despite this, vasospasm does occur, but as long as good technique is used this complication is minimized and nearly always resolves with the passage of time and the delivery of intracoronary nitrate. Good technique ('big pecks and short runs') is the key to its prevention.

Dissection

This is uncommon but can occur at the lesion site. Fortunately the occurrence of vessel obstruction is very unusual. The most important thing is to recognize it, and don't do any further RA. Regular visualization of burr progress is advised. One of the limitations of using 6F catheters is that injecting dye past the burr to check progress is limited—it is the main reason why many RA operators choose 7F or 8F catheters from the outset of a procedure. Ultimately, stenting the vessel will deal with any dissection (Fig. 33.7), but if concentric calcium remains a limiting factor, prolonged balloon inflation at low atmospheres usually deals with the issue.

Slow flow/no flow phenomenon

RA leads to impairment of flow by the very nature of what it is trying to achieve. Showers of pulverized tissue take time to pass through the microvasculature, and as long as the appropriate decisions have been made about

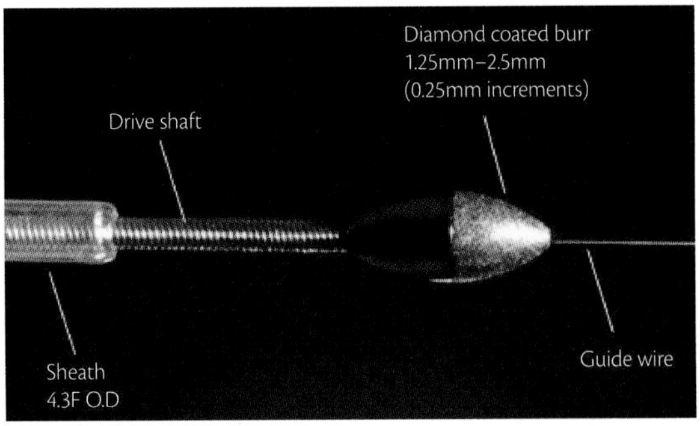

Fig. 33.6 Detailed view of the diamond tipped burr—the technique for ablating plaque is key to successful ablation.

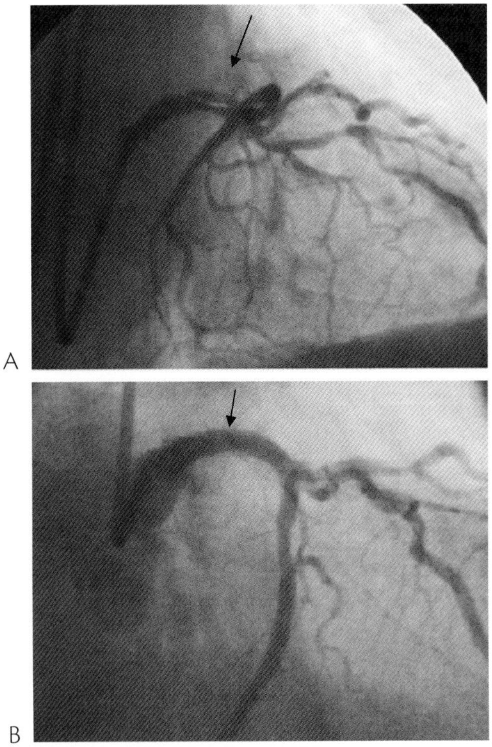

Fig. 33.7 A) Dissection seen in left main artery after 1.75mm burr into circumflex. B) Stent inserted to left main into circumflex.

size of burr and good technique applied, it nearly always resolves with the passage of time and intracoronary nitrates. If it occurs, adequate perfusion pressure is essential, and adequate hydration of the patient is recommended in all cases.

Other vasodilators may be used to prevent and treat this phenomenon, such as verapamil, nitroprusside or adenosine, sometimes delivered directly to the microvasculature via an over-the-wire balloon or microcatheter. Occasionally, a balloon pump will encourage the perfusion pressure required to restore flow. In general once 'slow flow' develops it is recommended to discontinue rotational atherectomy.

Abrupt closure

This is managed in the usual way to any other form of abrupt closure. The most important thing is to understand what the cause is—the management of vasospasm and no-flow phenomenon is quite different.

Perforation

This is uncommon, and is usually due to poor technique (oversizing of burr, 'pushing' of burr rather than pecking) or poor choice of vessel (extreme angulation).

Its management depends on the degree of perforation and cardiac compromise. It can range from a catastrophic emergency to a localized coronary injury. The use of covered stents can be lifesaving, as can sacrificing the disrupted vessel. Sometimes the perforated segment cannot be treated percutaneously, in which case, a balloon is inflated proximal to the perforated segment to staunch flow whilst arrangements are made to undergo urgent coronary bypass surgery (Fig. 33.8).

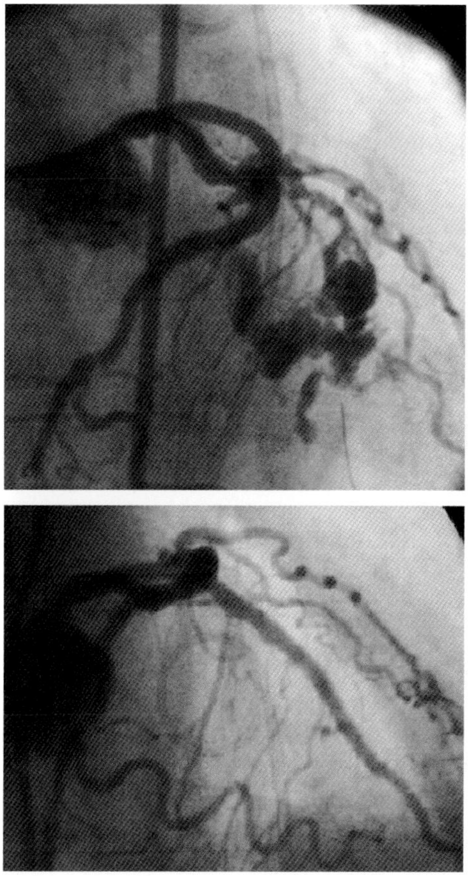

A

B

Fig. 33.8 A) Catastrophic perforation within LAD after rotablation of calcified lesion. B) As a covered stent would not pass into the LAD, the distal LAD was 'sacrificed' by stenting across it into the diagonal with three stents.

Burr stalling in lesion

This is a very unusual occurrence, and is often a reflection of poor technique, e.g. burr size too large, the increase in burr size too great, and using a 'pushing' rather than a 'pecking' technique. Once it is stuck, do not attempt to continue spinning as a torsion dissection maybe be induced. Pull the burr back while asking the patient to cough or take a very large breath in. Failing that a small balloon inflated to 1 atmosphere placed alongside may help dislodge the burr. A last resort is to seek the help of a cardiothoracic surgeon.

Clinical use

Initially RA was used quite widely in the belief that it would complement the use of balloon strategies. The COBRA trial[4] compared the use of RA with POBA for treating complex lesions, and showed little clinical benefit for using RA routinely (in terms of MACE and relief of angina), but the use of RA did allow more complex cases to be successfully treated when compared to the POBA arm. The STRATAS trial[1] found no advantage to a more aggressive RA technique, and the CARAT trial[5] showed that aggressive debulking with a higher burr:artery ratio led to higher complication rates and worse clinical outcomes. Its use in the bare-metal stent era declined to a niche technique only for patients with severe calcification that prevented a good balloon/stent result.

A meta-analysis of randomized trials of POBA versus different forms of atherectomy (directional atherectomy, cutting balloon atherotomy, RA, or laser angioplasty) concluded that '… the combined experience from randomized trials suggests that ablative devices failed to achieve predefined clinical and angiographic outcomes. This meta-analysis does not support the hypothesis that routine ablation or sectioning of atheromatous tissue is beneficial during percutaneous coronary interventions'[6,7].

It appeared logical that RA would have a role in the management of the diffuse intimal hyperplasia that characterizes in-stent restenosis. The ARTIST trial[8] showed a significantly worse outcome for RA when compared to POBA, but the ROSTER trial[9] suggested that MACE at 1 year was significantly better for the patients undergoing RA. Overall, the current situation would not advocate the routine use of RA for in-stent restenosis.

Routine stenting post RA gave superior results to POBA alone but the results at 6 months were still disappointing[10,11]. The advent of drug-eluting stents (DES) to inhibit the restenotic process has led to the re-emergence of this technology—interventional cardiologists feel more confident in dealing with the challenges of coronary calcification, knowing that the potential for restenosis has been blunted with the availability of DES. This is now reflected as a recommendation in the ESC Guidelines—'Recommendation for rotablation of fibrotic or heavily calcified lesions that cannot be crossed by a balloon or adequately dilated before planned stenting: I C'[12].

Who should perform RA and where?

On-site surgical cover

Complications of RA are uncommon in experienced hands. The nature of the device does mean that occasional high-risk complications can occur, and under these circumstances the availability of immediate bypass facilities can be lifesaving. However, the vast majority of cases performed do not require surgery, and it would seem restrictive to compel every case to be done in a surgical facility.

Many of these cases would have been discussed at a multidisciplinary forum, to decide whether RA is the appropriate strategy. As with all PCI cases, thorough documentation of procedures should be kept, and a forum for audit be available for the scrutiny of individual and unit results.

Certification

In some countries, physicians intending to perform RA must:

- Attend a rotablation certification course
- Complete some RA cases with a recognized RA proctor, and
- Be signed off by the RA training directorate.

In those countries where these safeguards are in place, equipment for RA is not supplied to a centre that does not have a certified operator.

Whatever system of governance is in place, RA is a procedure that requires regular use to ensure optimal outcomes.

Conclusions

RA is an extremely useful tool in interventional cardiology. It should be seen as a device which facilitates the rest of a complex case (improving immediate outcomes) rather than an anti-restenotic tool. Training and regular use are essential. The results of RA are undoubtedly experience and technique related. When used appropriately, RA expands the envelope of interventional cardiology.

Appendix I

Trials and registries

The Rotablator MultiCenter registry[13]

This registry evaluated the safety and efficacy of the Rotablator® system when used as a stand-alone device or with adjunctive PTCA. The following data is based on findings from 22 clinical sites through April 1993 (2953 procedures and 3717 lesions registered) (Fig. 33.9).

Inclusion criteria for the procedure included native vessel disease <25mm in length, and had to be candidates for CABG.

Exclusion criteria:

- Poor left ventricular function (<30%)
- Patients not suitable for CABG

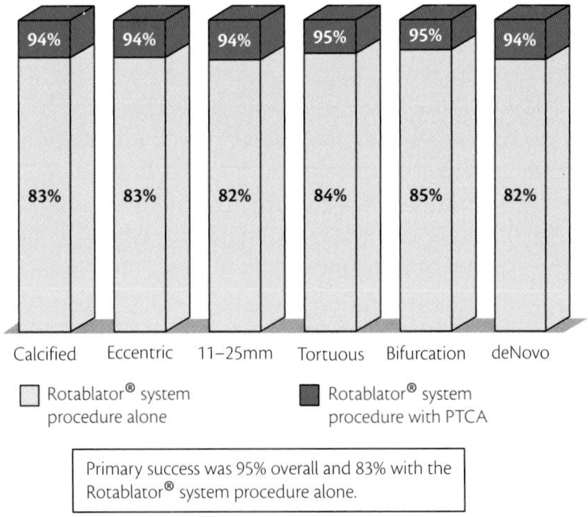

Fig. 33.9 Percentage procedural success—RA alone or RA and PTCA.

- Vein graft disease
- >25mm in length
- Visible thrombus
- Left main stem disease
- Extensive dissection in relation to recent POBA procedure within 1 month
- Severe diffuse three-vessel disease.

The complications were:

- Death: 1%
- Q-wave MI: 1.2%
- CABG:. 2.5%

Other complications included:

- Intimal dissection with dye stain: 3.1%
- Intimal dissection without dye stain: 10.6%
- Acute vessel closure: 5.1%
- Vessel perforation/tear: 0.8%
- Arrhythmia: 3.1%.

Further complications included slow flow, no-flow, cardiac tamponade distal embolization, and ventricular perforation.

Not surprisingly, the complexity of the case and the inexperience of the operator increased the likelihood of a complication arising.

This registry highlights the potential risks to the patient and the operator—the results from the registry were performed by experienced operators in high-volume centres. New operators should learn this technique after appropriate training and supervision.

New Approaches to Coronary Intervention (NACI) registry(2)

This was an American-based registry from November 1990 to March 1994 and included 525 patients with 670 lesions (Tables 33.1 and 33.2). The majority of the lesions were complex (57%B2/14% C lesions). This registry was pre-stents or modern antiplatelet drugs.

Table 33.1 Procedural results

Reference vessel	2.77 ± 0.51
% stenosis—pre	70.0 ± 12.2
% stenosis—post	25.8 ± 11.9
Slow flow/no flow	<1%
Death/MI/CABG at 30 days	8.4%

Table 33.2 Follow-up at 1 year

Death	5%
Any MI	10%
CABG	12%
TLR	26%
Death/MI/CABG at 1 year	30%

It must be remembered that the techniques used for this registry involved:

- Burr speed of 160–180 000rpm
- 9–10F guiding catheters
- Stepped burr approach to 75% enlargement in relation to the reference vessel
- Temporary pacemakers mandatory for all cases
- No stents available
- No glycoprotein inhibitors available.

Excimer Laser, Rotational Atherectomy and Balloon Angioplasty Comparison (ERBAC) Study(6)

The study examined 2 debulking strategies (excimer laser [EL] and RA) with POBA with respect to procedural and clinical outcome in 685 patients (Tables 33.3 and 33.4).

- This trial was pre-stenting and no glycoprotein inhibitors available
- The trial suggested that RA meant that procedural success was more likely but that restenosis rates were higher than in the POBA group
- It should be noted that no POBA balloon inflation was used after the RA/EL procedure.

Table 33.3 ERBAC results—acute

	EL	RA	POBA
Procedural success	77.2%	89.2%	79.2%
In-hospital MACE	4.3%	3.2%	3.1%
Dissections	56.7%	39.8%	46.7%

Table 33.4 ERBAC results at 1 year

	EL	RA	POBA
Death/MI/CABG	11.4%	12.1%	12.6%
TVR	46%	42.4%	31.9%
Restenosis at angio.	59%	57%	31.9%

Table 33.5 Procedural results

	Aggressive	Routine
Reference vessel	2.65 ± 0.46	2.64 ± 0.45
% stenosis—pre	69 ± 13	67±14
% stenosis—post	27 ± 14	26 ± 14
% slow flow/no flow	15.7	7.7
% death/MI/CABG at 30 days	6.1	6.5

Table 33.6 Follow-up results

	Aggressive	Routine
% TVR at 9 months	23.5	21.1
% TVR/MI/CABG at 9 months	24.9	23.5
% restenosis >50%	58	52

Study to determine Rotablator And Transluminal Angioplasty Strategy (STRATAS)[1]

This was a randomized trial to compare an aggressive rotablation technique (burr:artery ratio >0.7 ± balloon inflation<1 bar (n = 249) with routine rotablation (burr:artery ratio <0.7, balloon inflation >4 bar) (Table 33.5 and 33.6). The techniques were relatively comparable, but the procedure was still dogged by high restenosis and TVR rates.

Comparison of Balloon versus Rotational Angioplasty (COBRA) study[4]

This was a multicentre, prospective randomized comparison of RA versus POBA for the management of complex coronary lesions, and included 502 patients recruited between May 1992 and May 1996 (pre-stent) (Tables 33.7 and 33.8).

RA allowed more complete procedural success, but that did not translate into beneficial results at 6 months.

Table 33.7 Procedural results

	Rota	POBA
Reference vessel	2.6 ± 0.4	2.8 ± 0.5
% stenosis—pre	75 ± 8.7	76 ± 9.2
% stenosis—post	34 ± 14	33 ± 16
% slow flow/no flow	12	4.8
% need for stenting	6.4	14.9
% death/MI/CABG at 30 days	8.7	8.8
% procedural success	84	73

Table 33.8 Follow-up results at 6 months

	Rota	POBA
% TVR	21	23
% TVR/MI/CABG	28.2	26.2
% angina free	59.4	63.8
Restenosis >50%	48.9	51.1

Stent Implantation Post Rotational Atherectomy (SPORT) trial[14]

A multicentre prospective randomized comparison of RA as debulking versus POBA prior to stenting; 725 patients. See Tables 33.9 and 33.10.

This was a contemporary trial with liberal use of glycoprotein inhibitors in both arms. Little difference shown in the 6-month outcomes. The use of RA routinely prior to stenting offers little advantage.

The use of RA in the management of in-stent restenosis

Two randomized studies compared RA with balloon angioplasty—ARTIST[8] and ROSTER[9]—have shown that routine use of RA offers no advantage over other strategies to the management of this condition.

Table 33.9 Procedural results

	Rota	POBA
Reference vessel	2.85	2.85
Acute gain mm	1.94	1.86
% procedural success	94	88
Stents/lesion	1.3	1.3
No. burrs	1.9	–
Stent deployment atm	14	15
% SACT	0	0

Table 33.10 Sport trial—6 months

Follow-up at 6 months	Rota	POBA
% TLR	14.5	11.5
% restenosis rate (RR)	30.4	27.6
RR if vessel >3mm	5.3	14.3
RR if vessel <2.5mm	47.7	37.5
RR if diabetes	41.4	35.5
RR if calcium visible	23.3	30.4

Table 33.11 RA and stenting (bare metal)

	RA/stent	RA/POBA
% procedural success	94	96
Lesions length	26.4 ± 9.2	27.4 ± 14.5
% 3-year death/MI/TLR	21 ± 4	25 ± 3 (NS)

Early and late clinical outcomes after rotational atherectomy with stenting versus rotational atherectomy with balloon angioplasty for complex coronary lesions(11)

Not a randomized trial, but a retrospective analysis, with no routine angiographic follow up and a relatively small sample size (1997–1999; 323 patients with 357 lesions). N = 158 (RA + stent); N=165 (RA +POBA). Concluded that routine stenting post RA for complex anatomy offered little advantage (see Table 33.11).

Conclusions from the randomized trials and registry data

- RA is a useful technique which leads to improved procedural success in some complex cases
- A bigger burr:artery ratio does not translate into improved outcomes
- A smaller burr:artery ratio causes less dissection than POBA

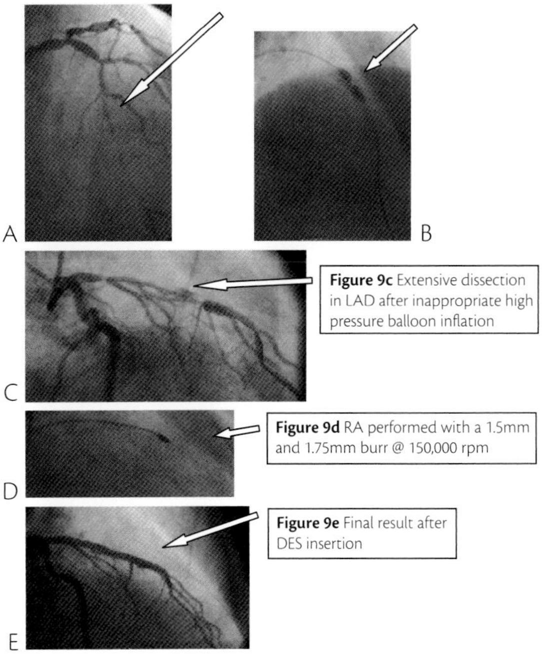

A
B
C
Figure 9c Extensive dissection in LAD after inappropriate high pressure balloon inflation
D
Figure 9d RA performed with a 1.5mm and 1.75mm burr @ 150,000 rpm
E
Figure 9e Final result after DES insertion

Fig. 33.10 Subtotal occlusion of LAD in heavily calcified artery

- Debulking before ballooning and stenting does not provide better long-term results, although it is advantageous in some subgroups (heavy calcification)
- All the trials have chosen a high rotational speed (usually >160 000rpm), and perhaps lower speeds may cause less disruption to the vessel
- The role of IIb/IIIa inhibitors to accompany RA procedures is far from clear
- The role of RA as an adjunct to the use of DES has not been characterized in a randomized trial.

Case studies

Case 1 (Fig. 33.10)

Case 2 (Fig. 33.11)

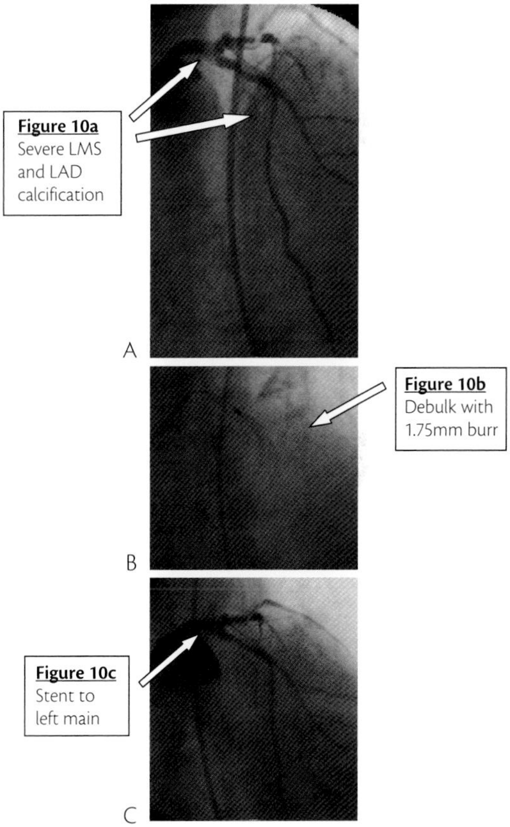

Fig. 33.11 It is increasingly common for elderly patients to present with intractable angina, with severe coronary disease where the option of bypass surgery is not appropriate due to age and comorbidity. Rotablation is invariably necessary under these circumstances to deal with the elderly heavily-calcified arteries. This patient was 89 years old with intractable angina despite extensive medication, with severe calcification of the left main stem and LAD coronary arteries.

References

1. Whitlow PL, Bass TA, Kipperman RM, *et* al. Results of the study to determine rotablator and transluminal angioplasty strategy (STRATAS). *Am J Cardiol* 2001; **87**:699–705
2. Brown DL, George CJ, Steenkiste AR, *et al.* High speed rotational atherectomy of human coronary stenoses: acute and one-year outcomes from the New Approaches to Coronary Intervention (NACI) registry. *Am J Cardiol* 1997; **80**(10A):60K–67K
3. Cohen BM, Weber VJ, Blum RR, *et al.* Cocktail attenuation of rotational ablation flow effects (CARAFE) study: pilot.*Cathet Cardiovasc Diagn* 1996; (Suppl 3):69–72.
4. Dill T, Dietz U, Hamm C, *et* al. A randomized compariaon of balloon angioplasty versus rotational atherectomy in complex coronary lesions (COBRA study). *Eur Heart J* 2000; **21**:1759–66.
5. Safian RD, Feldman T, Muller DW, *et* al. Coronary angioplasty and Rotablator atherectomy trial (CARAT): immediate and late results of a prospective multicentre randomized trial. *Catheter Cardiov Interv* 2001; **53**:213–20.
6. Reifart N, Vandormael M, Krajcar M, *et* al. Randomized comparison of angioplasty of complex coronary lesions at a single center – Excimer Laser, Rotational Atherectomy and Balloon Angioplasty Comparison (ERBAC) Study. *Circulation* 1997; **96**:91–8.
7. Bittl JA, Chew DP, Topol EJ, *et* al. Meta-analysis of randomized trials of percutaneous transluminal coronary angioplasty versus atherectomy, cutting balloon atherectomy or laser angioplasty. *J Am Coll Cardiol* 2004; **43**:936–42.
8. Vom Dahl J, Dietz U, Haager PK, *et* al. Rotational atherectomy does not reduce recurrent in-stent restenosis: results of the angioplasty versus rotational atherectomy for treatment of diffuse in-stent restenosis trial (ARTIST). *Circulation* 2002; **105**:583–8.
9. Sharma SK, Kini A, Mehran R, *et* al. Randomized trial of Rotational Atherectomy Versus Balloon Angioplasty for Diffuse In-stent Restonsis (ROSTER). *Am Heart J* 2004; **147**:16–22.
10. Moussa I, Di Mario C, Moses J. Coronary stenting after rotational atherectomy in calcified and complex lesions. Angiographic and clinical follow-up results. *Circulation* 1997; **96**:128–36.
11. Lee SW, Hong MK, Lee CW, *et* al. Early and late clinical outcomes after rotational atherectomy with stenting versus rotational atherectomy with balloon angioplasty for complex coronary lesions. *J Inv Cardiol* 2004; **16**:406–9.
12. Silber S, Albertsson P, Aviles FF, *et al.* Guidelines for percutaneous coronary interventions: the Task Force for Percutaneous Coronary Interventions of the European Society of Cardiology. *Eur Heart J* 2005; 26(8)**:**804–47.
13. Warth D, Leon M, O'Neill W, *et al.* Rotational atherectomy multicenter registry: acute results, complications and 6-month angiographic follow-up in 709 patients. *J Am Coll Cardiol* 1994; **24**:641–8.
14. Buchbinder M, Fortuna R, Sharma SK. Debulking prior to stenting improves acute outcomes: early results from the SPORT trial. *J Am Coll Cardiol* 2000; **35**(SupplA):8A.

CHAPTER 34

Laser

Peter O'Kane and Simon Redwood

Introduction

The first medical application of laser was reported by Dr Leon Goldman who, in 1962, reported the use of ruby and carbon dioxide (CO_2) lasers in dermatology[1]. In cardiovascular disease, early laser use was confined to cadaver vessels[2], animal models[3], and arteries located in freshly amputated limbs[4], until eventually work progressed to the use of laser energy to salvage an ischaemic limb[5] in 1984. The concept of using laser to remove atherosclerotic material in coronary arteries developed as an alternative strategy to simply modifying the shape of an obstructed lumen as occurs with simple balloon angioplasty. Expectations grew that this new biomedical technology may overcome the low success rate and high complication rate of lesions considered non-ideal for balloon angioplasty[6]. However, initial successful reports could not be replicated. Furthermore, underdeveloped catheter technology and limited appreciation of laser/tissue interactions meant that a cure for restenosis was not in fact discovered and laser coronary angioplasty became isolated to only a few centres in the world. However, more recently with advancement in both catheter technology and technique, excimer coronary laser angioplasty (ELCA) has been rediscovered for use in specific subsets of percutaneous coronary interventions (PCIs).

This chapter outlines the basic principles of ELCA and important practical aspects for using the device in contemporary PCI. A discussion of the current indications for clinical use follows and these are highlighted by clinical case examples.

Basic laser physics

LASER is an acronym for light amplification by stimulated emission of radiation. The concept exists when an excited state atom encounters a photon of the same energy resulting in the stimulated emission of another photon. Common features within all laser devices include an active lasing gain medium, an excitation mechanism, and a feedback mechanism.

The optical cavity within a laser's generator contains either a liquid, solid, or gaseous active gain medium which emits light of a particular wavelength to categorize the laser device (Table 34.1). Energy is supplied to electrons to move them from a low energy level to a higher, unstable energy level and photons are released as the excited electrons return to baseline. A photon can either strike an excited electron causing a stimulated release of two photons or strike an unexcited electron which elevates that electron into an excited state. Stimulated emission rather than absorption occurs because more atoms are kept in the excited state than in the ground state, a phenomenon termed population inversion. Mirrors placed either end of the optical cavity reflect the formed light and create the necessary feedback mechanism for amplification of stimulated emission. One mirror is a total reflector, while the other permits a predetermined number of photons to be emitted outside the optical cavity as coherent electromagnetic energy, which ultimately becomes the usable laser beam.

Understanding laser–plaque interactions

Endovascular use of lasers requires them to be able to produce a high energy, monochromatic light beam that is easily and precisely delivered through fibreoptic catheters to a small area of tissue. In addition, it is essential that light energy applied directly to obstructive atherosclerotic plaque only alters and/or dissolves this material without damaging the surrounding milieu.

The overall effects that a particular laser will have on local tissue will depend on a number of characteristics of the light energy laser emitted.

Table 34.1 Medical lasers have a number of properties which determine their use and safety profile. Only the excimer laser has FDA approval for therapeutic use in the cardiovascular system owing to its excellent safety profile. YAG lasers operate in a similar manner whether combined with the active lasing ion neodymium (Nd^{3+}) or holmium and are used in a variety of surgical procedures. Dye, ruby, and CO2 lasers are used in dermatology whilst argon laser is used in ophthalmology

Laser	Constituents/properties	Wave mode	Wavelength (nm)	Penetration depth (μm)
Ruby	Al_2O_3 with 0.05% trivalent chromium	Continuous	694	2000
Nd-YAG	$Y_2Al_5O_{12}$ with 1% neodymium in place of yttrium–poorly absorbed by water but deep penetration	Continuous & pulsed	1064	1000
CO_2	CO_2 lasers are strongly absorbed by haemoglobin and water and tend to vaporize tissue	Continuous & pulsed	10,600	100–2000
Holmium-YAG	$Y_2Al_5O_{12}$ with a variable % of holmium in place of yttrium	Pulsed	2090	500
Excimer	Xeon and HCl with strong absorption by protein with superior precision and less thermal spread to adjacent tissue	Pulsed	308	30–50
Argon	Poorly absorbed by water and energy is freely transmitted through the eye	Continuous	520	400
Dye	Strongly absorbed by their opposite colour so green light is absorbed by red colours	Pulsed	480	330

Wavelength

Individual lasers emit light with a characteristic wavelength determined by the laser medium (Fig. 34.1). For example, the Nd-YAG lasing medium is the colourless, isotropic crystal $Y_2Al_5O_{12}$ (yttrium–aluminum–garnet, YAG) where about 1% of the yttrium is replaced by neodymium. The energy levels of the Nd^{3+} ion are responsible for the fluorescent properties and light emitted has a wavelength of 1060nm. In contrast, the xeon chloride excimer lasing action is produced by high voltage electrical discharge placed across a mixture of inert gas (xeon) and a dilute halogen compound (hydrogen chloride). Light emitted has a wavelength of 308nm.

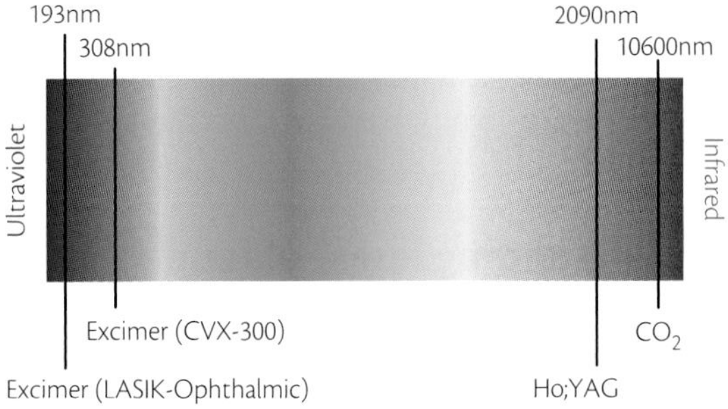

Fig. 34.1 The wavelength of light emitted from a laser is determined by the lasing medium and it is an important factor in determining the properties of the system. Laser light emitted from the Spectranectics CVX-300 excimer (XeCl) laser system is 'Cool' (308nm) which is similar to laser light employed for LASIK (193.3nm) used in Ophthalmic surgery. In contrast to infrared lasers, the excimer laser has a shallow penetration of depth and ablates tissue precisely without 'cooking'. Excimer energy interacts with intracellular molecules exploding cells from inside out and has minimal side effects.

An important parameter in determining the biological effect of laser on tissue is penetration depth. Expressed as absorption depth it is defined as the distance over which the tissue absorption diminishes the light to 37% of its original intensity and it is determined by wavelength of light and tissue density. In the near-infrared regions (2000–3000nm), water is the dominant absorber and light penetration depth varies from 1–0.1mm. This deep penetration is a major disadvantage since it makes ablation difficult to control and the dehydration effectively 'cooks' tissue leading to an inflammatory response. In contrast, light in the ultraviolet B (UVB) region (300nm), has shallow absorption depth owing to absorption by non-aqueous cellular macromolecules such as proteins and nucleic acids. Light emitted here is 'cool' and at 308nm where the excimer laser emits, the typical absorption depth is only 50 microns.

Continuous versus pulsed wave lasers

Early medical lasers (Nd-YAG and Argon) utilized continuous wavelengths in the infrared region with constant power output during laser–lesion contact to achieve tissue vaporization. However, successful ablation was offset by activation of the coagulation system and tissue carbonization resulting in charring. Histological examination found large craters with inside diameters greater than that of the surface opening[7] and radial extension of damage beyond the ablated plaque secondary to tissue temperatures reaching 300°C[8]. This thermal injury translated to thrombosis, vasospasm, and subsequent inflammation leading to high restenosis rates.

In contrast, the current excimer laser fires high-energy pulses that last only a fraction of a second confining the thermal effect to the irradiated tissue. The number of pulses generated during a 1-s interval (i.e. frequency) is known as the pulse repetition rate and the duration of each pulse termed the pulse width. The 'laser-on' time during each pulse is much shorter than the resting time allowing energy to dissipate and provide recovery time after initial exposure which prevents thermal injury to adjacent arterial structures. Pulse width can be varied according to tissue type being ablated with longer pulse duration selected for hard material such as calcium.

Effective power

The minimum pulse energy for a pulsed laser system is determined by the penetration depth of the light and by the need to form a steam bubble. This creates a unique threshold energy density for each laser type so for XeCl lasers, the fluence necessary for therapy ranges from 30–80mJ/mm^2. Delivering more energy may be advantageous in calcified lesions but it results in greater heat deposition. The earliest pulsed excimer lasers operated at lower energy parameters compared to contemporary catheters and as a result, they were pushed through the lesions with inadequate tissue ablation which may explain the suboptimal outcomes with the early experience.

Mechanisms of excimer laser ablation

Excimer laser ablates tissue through photochemical, photothermal and photokinetic mechanisms. UV light is highly absorbed during the 125 billionths of a second pulse and each photon carries sufficient energy to break a single carbon–carbon bond. However, only 2% of photons absorbed by intracellular proteins and lipids actually break chemical bonds to weaken or lyse cellular structures[9]. More importantly, as the molecular bonds are vibrated to breaking point by UV light, intracellular water is heated to vapour which causes the cells to rupture from the inside out[10]. A steam bubble is created that further dissolves plaque by expanding to approximately twice the diameter of the catheter tip. This photothermal effect lasts only a 100 millionths of a second so heat does not diffuse into the tissue itself[10]. Rapid expansion and implosion of the vapour bubble produces secondary cavitation bubbles with pressure effects that further break down tissue and assists in sweeping ablated debris from the tip of the catheter to maintain constant contact with the lesion. A shallow crater forms under the catheter with each laser pulse and a further layer of tissue only 10 microns at the bottom of the crater is removed. The debris byproducts consist of water, hydrocarbons (gases), and small particles. Notably absent are oxidative byproducts implying that the tissue does not burn. More than 90% of the particles are less than 10-micron diameter and are easily absorbed by the reticuloendothelial system minimizing the risk of distal embolization to the microcirculation[11].

Excimer laser catheter development

The design of fibreoptic catheters for delivery of laser has progressed significantly from the early metal-tipped probes and intraoperative single-fibre devices first evaluated in the 1980s[12]. Grundfest pioneered the delivery of excimer laser energy to vaporize plaque using less thermal injury and lower rates of perforation compared to alternative continuous-wave lasers[13]. Further safety improvements were demonstrated with the development of pulsed-wave excimer laser[14] which led to second-generation excimer catheters in the late 1980s. These featured flexible, multifibre construction which permitted percutaneous use. Third-generation catheters were enhanced by using larger number of small-diameter fibres densely packed into a flexible catheter shaft and were further developed to become rapid exchange catheters with lubricious coatings in a variety of sizes with both eccentric and concentric designs by the mid 1990s (Fig. 34.2A). Indeed, these design improvements led to increased success (87% to 94%) and lower complication rates (8% to 5%) when data from ELCA clinical registry was compared during the switch from second- to third- generation catheters[12].

Currently, each disposable ELCA catheter contains a bundle of very pure fused silica (synthetic quartz) fibres. Ordinary glass or polymer fibres such as that used for telecommunications will not conduct UV light at useful power levels. Up to 250 individual fibres are used in each catheter with a fibre diameter of 50–140 microns.

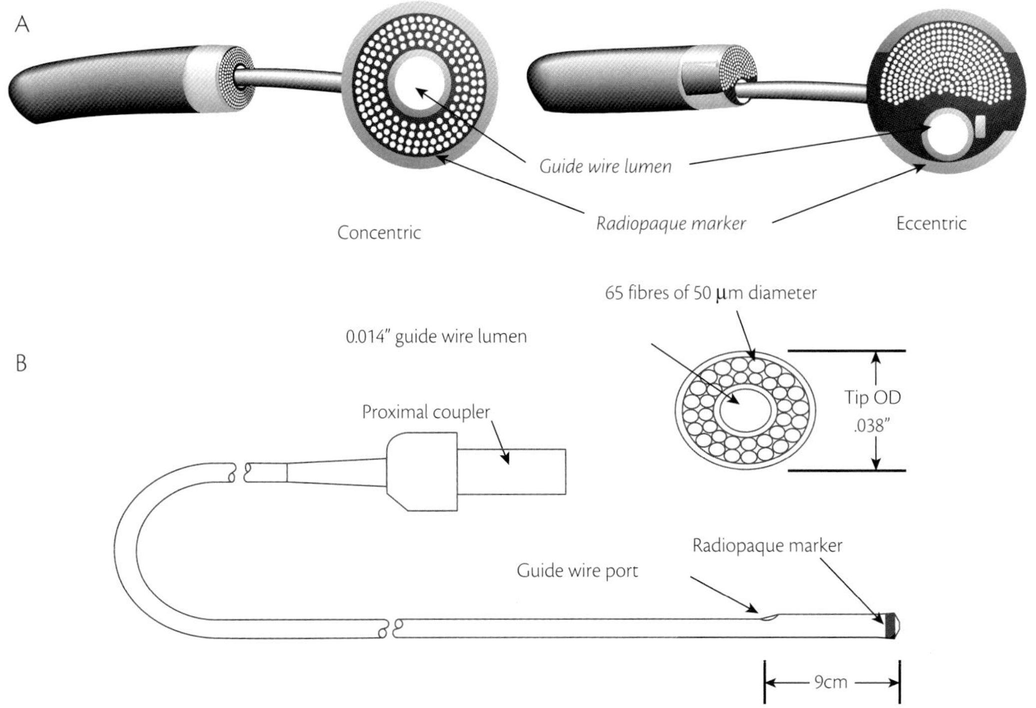

Fig. 34.2 (A) Excimer laser catheters may have either a concentric or eccentric array of upto 250 laser fibres depending on the diameter (B) The 0.9mm rapid exchange X80 catheter has a concentric array of 65 fibres with the radiopaque marker set back from the tip so the fibres can occupy this space.

The use of these multiple fibres is preferable since it permits catheter flexibility and improves deliverability. At the distal end of the concentric catheter the fibres are potted in epoxy around a guide wire lumen and polished to an optical finish. At the proximal end of the catheter, a laser coupler holds the fibres in a bundle to receive the laser beam.

The proximal coupler inserts into the CVX-300® system (Spectranectics Inc, Colorado Springs, CO, USA), which is a portable unit 89cm high, 124cm long, and 61cm wide, weighing approximately 295kg. The system can emit laser energy from 30–80mJ/mm^2 with repetition rate from 25–80Hz and a pulse width range of 125–200ns (nominal 135ns). Prior to introduction of the laser catheter, it should be calibrated by pointing the tip of the catheter towards the energy detector on the CVX 300 unit itself and activating the laser by pressing the foot pedal for 5s. The laser calibrates automatically and enters standby mode.

The eccentric catheter features an off-centre fibre bundle that can be directed by the operator to the target tissue. This catheter was originally designed for treating eccentric or bifurcation lesions but it may also be superior at debulking type B or C coronary lesions. A clinical study in 39 patients has demonstrated the ability to achieve greater residual lumen diameters in treatment of in-stent restenosis where the 1.7mm eccentric catheter created a 2.2mm lumen and 2.0mm eccentric catheter a 3.0mm lumen(15). The operators utilized a technique of pulling the tip back through the lesion after first pass and rotating the tip 40–60° before making a further pass.

The effectiveness of the concentric catheter was further improved by development of 'optimally spaced' (OS) fibres at the catheter tip as compared to the 'closest-packed' (CP) design(16). The diameter of craters ablated by the OS design was shown to be greater than that produced by the CP design with craters at least as large as the tip of the device produced when used in a bench model of porcine aorta(17). Furthermore, the ablation debris produced by the OS device contained fewer particles potentially making ablation less likely to disturb the microcirculation when used in clinical practice.

To specifically treat calcified lesions where there has been balloon failure from either an inability to dilate or cross the lesion, the 0.9mm catheter was developed (Fig. 34.2B). This device has a closest-packed array of fibres with two circular rows containing 65 fibres around a 0.014-inch guide wire lumen and remains low profile with good tracking qualities. The radiopaque marker band is moved further back from the tip to permit the fibres to occupy the tip space out to the edge distinguishing it from the other catheters in the range. The catheter is capable of being used at fluence 80mJ/mm^2 and repetition rate 80Hz to improve the penetrative potential and this has been shown to improve laser lesion recanalization in one study when compared with standard laser parameters (60mJ/mm^2 and 40Hz)[18]. In 36 patients with high-grade calcific lesions in which 22 had failed balloon angioplasty, standard laser parameters were successful in 26 patients with increased laser parameters required in 10 lesions with success in eight of these without any increase in procedural complications or in-hospital MACE.

The complete range of currently available ELCA coronary rapid exchange catheters are listed in Table 34.2. From a practical perspective, the CVX-300 system permits lasing for a maximum of 5s at a time with a 10-s standby period marked by an audible signal for all catheters except the 0.9mm X80 catheter. With this device, lasing time is 10s with a 5-s standby period.

Excimer lasing technique

An attention to lasing technique represents a crucial component for the success of coronary laser angioplasty. Important aspects for lasing include the use of saline infusion at the laser catheter/plaque interface, slow catheter advancement with multiple passes, and the selection of suitably sized catheter (Fig. 34.3).

Saline infusion technique

Both blood and iodinated dye, in comparison to water or saline, almost completely absorb the excimer laser energy. This results in the formation of cavity microbubbles at site of delivery which subsequently potentates the effects of pressure waves increasing the likelihood of vessel wall dissection[19]. Therefore, removal of contrast and blood at the laser catheter tip/plaque interface has become mandatory and this is achieved with saline flushing[20]. This allows the target atherosclerotic material to absorb the energy and has resulted in lower dissection rates in clinical practice[21].

In practical terms a 1-L bag of 0.9% saline is attached to the manifold via a three-way tap and saline can be injected with a 20mL Leur-lock syringe when required. It is important to visualize under fluoroscopy that all contrast is flushed from the guide catheter with the laser catheter in the selected starting position and that the saline syringe does not become mixed with contrast. Initially 5mL of saline is infused prior to laser activation and then a slow injection continued at a rate of 2–3mL/s throughout the pulsed activation (5s or 10s). It is important to ensure that the guide catheter is well intubated into the coronary artery to ensure saline is delivered to the laser catheter tip and extra care must be taken when lasing through chronic total occlusions.

Table 34.2 Excimer laser catheters available for cardiovascular applications

Device	0.9mm Rx	0.9mm Rx	1.4mm Rx	1.7mm Rx	2.0mm Rx	1.7mm E Rx	2.0mm E Rx
Tip design	C Concentric	X-80 catheter	Cos Concentric	Cos Concentric	Cos Concentric	Eccentric	Eccentric
Number of fibres	65	65	108	136	250	185	290
Maximum guide wire compatible	0.014″	0.014″	0.014″	0.014″	0.014″	0.014″	0.018″
Maximum tip outer diameter	0.038″	0.038″	0.057″	0.069″	0.080″	0.069″	0.079″
Working length (cm)	135	135	135	135	135	135	135
Maximum shaft diameter	0.049″	0.049″	0.062″	0.072″	0.084″	0.072″	0.084″
Guide compatibility	5F >0.056″	5F >0.056″	7F >0.073″	7F >0.073″	8F >0.086″	7F >0.073″	8F >0.086″
Maximum settings (mJ/mm^2/Hz)	60/40	80/80	60/40	60/40	60/40	60/40	60/40
Maximum timings	5s On 10s Off	10s On 5s Off	5s On 10s Off	5s On 10s Off	5s On 10s Off	5s On 10s Off	5s On 10s Off

Cos, optimally spaced; Rx, rapid exchange.

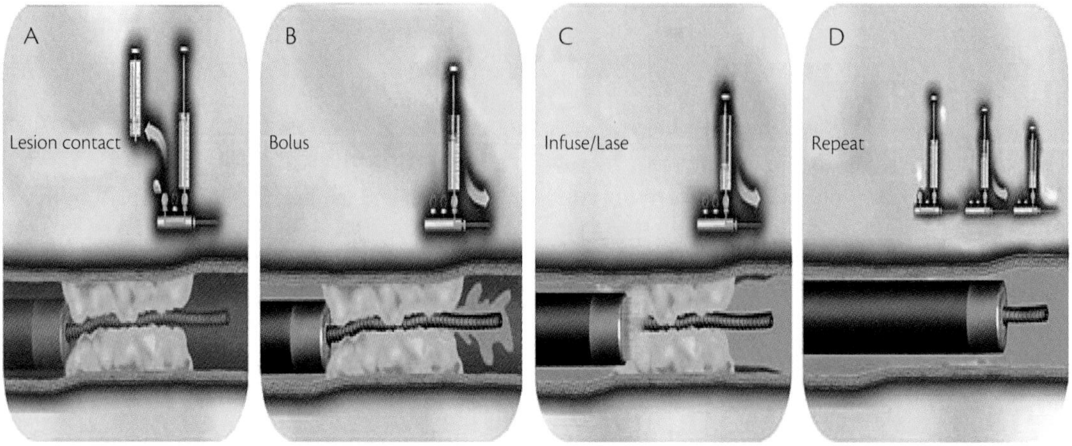

Fig. 34.3 (A) The laser catheter is advanced to the lesion over the guide wire. (B) Prior to activation of laser, saline is injected to completely remove contrast which can be confirmed on fluoroscopy. (C) Slow advancement at 0.5mm/s along the lesion with laser activation whilst injecting saline. (D) Repeat steps A–C but if lesion is longer than 10mm or if there is ischaemia, withdraw catheter to guide, inject nitrate and wait 30s before next lasing.

Slow catheter advancement

The ability of the excimer laser to successfully ablate atherosclerotic plaque and thrombus without damaging the vessel wall is largely the result of the shallow depth of penetration (30–50 microns) associated with this energy. It has been demonstrated that the slow advancement rate of 0.2mm/s results in maximal ablation compared with advancement rates of 0.5 or 1.0mm/s[17]. Furthermore, a small histopatholgical analysis of specimens obtained from intracoronary directional atherectomy after the lesions had been lased with a slow catheter advancement technique revealed that 76% had no laser-induced injury with the remaining showing only small foci of charring but no evidence of extensive tissue damage[22]. Any attempt to rapidly advance the catheter should be avoided since this defies the principles governing laser-induced plaque removal and simply leads to dilatation rather than lesion debulking[16].

Selection of an appropriately sized laser catheter

The size of the laser catheter (see Table 34.2) is best selected in relation to the severity of the lesion as opposed to the diameter of the normal reference vessel[23]. Thus, a more severe stenosis requires a smaller initial catheter size. Therefore, a 0.9mm or 1.4mm ELCA catheter is recommended for lesions with 95–100% stenosis whilst a 1.7mm catheter would be preferred for a lesion of 85%. However, this approach may require the use of more than one catheter for one procedure if more debulking is desired. In practice, 1.7mm and 2.0mm catheters may be used initially if the lesion has 'smooth shoulders' and is located in a straight segment of the artery. However, the 0.9mm catheter is safe and effective for the majority of lesions and these larger catheters are often reserved for thrombotic lesions or for use in saphenous venous grafts. Generally, the maximum catheter to artery ratio should not exceed 0.7. Catheter selection will also be determined by the indication for ELCA—for example, eccentric catheters have been preferred when debulking in-stent restenosis[15] although our clinical experience indicates that eccentric lesions can successfully be debulked using concentric catheters.

Multiple passes with the appropriately sized excimer laser catheter at a slow advancement rate are required to achieve maximum tissue removal. It is essential that the laser catheter is not advanced forcefully if it meets resistance from the lesion despite several passes. Instead, the fluence may be increased up to either 60mJ/mm^2 for 1.4, 1.7, and 2.0mm catheters or up to 80mJ/mm^2 for the 0.9mm X80 catheter to permit successful ablation. If still unsuccessful then the lasing option should be reconsidered.

Laser safety

The Spectranectics CVX-300® excimer laser system delivers an invisible therapeutic beam of coherent light radiation which diverges from the end of the delivery device. Permanently aligned with this therapeutic beam is a visible aiming beam of red coherent light from a helium–neon laser. The therapeutic beam is the source of hazard although the aiming beam could also be hazardous if stared at for prolonged periods.

The radiation of the therapeutic beam is absorbed by the cornea of the eye and this can potentially cause harm. In addition, skin erythema can result if the beam is intercepted by any part of the body. To protect against eye damage, it is mandatory that all catheter lab personnel, both staff required at the time of the procedure and patient, wear protective glasses when the laser is switched on. In addition, the room should be sealed to prevent unauthorized access during laser activation and appropriate warning signs should be displayed outside all entrances to the room. All operators of laser equipment should have attended a laser safety 'core of knowledge' training course and have suitable clinical training in excimer laser catheter use.

ELCA complications

The most severe complications of laser coronary angioplasty are perforation, major dissection, and abrupt vessel closure. There are no particular angiographic features that distinguish lesions complicated by perforation compared to those without this complication but there is a relationship with operator experience. Of 2759 consecutive patients in the ELCA registry, the frequency of coronary artery perforation declined over time from 1.6% among the first 1888 patients to only 0.4% among the subsequent 1000 patients treated[24]. Before the knowledge of safer lasing techniques, the major dissection rate was as high as 22% with excimer laser[25] but is more likely less than 1% when the aforementioned techniques are adopted. Similarly, acute vessel closure, thrombosis, and distal embolization or 'no-reflow' are rarely encountered in clinical use of laser coronary angioplasty.

ELCA clinical indications

There are a number of current clinical applications and contraindications for excimer laser (Table 34.3) which is the only US Food and Drug Administration (FDA)-approved system for delivering laser energy within the cardiovascular system. ELCA can be performed from either the femoral or radial artery and can be utilized in the presence of significantly impaired left ventricular impairment. Unlike rotational atherectomy, it will have no interaction with a second guide wire used, for example, to protect a side branch and in the treatment of dominant coronary arteries temporary pacing wires are not required. ELCA may be performed in the presence of glycoprotein IIb/IIIa inhibitors but is usually still very effective even when these agents are contraindicated since laser energy exhibits unique antiaggregatory effects on platelets and can successfully vaporize thrombus.

Early clinical studies

There were a number of prospective non-randomized studies of ELCA that generally demonstrated a substantial improvement in primary success rates and procedural complications compared to standard treatment of complex coronary lesions. In the Spectranectics excimer laser registry[26], 89% of 2432 patients treated with ELCA had clinical success defined as a <50% residual stenosis with no adverse complication (death, Q-wave or non-Q-wave MI, or need for further revascularization). The overall rate of complications decreased during the course of the study and clinical success was associated with operator experience with a superior success rate in those who had performed more than 25 procedures.

In a 3000-patient study[27], ELCA proved successful in 84% patients which increased to 90% with adjunctive balloon angioplasty. Major complications included death (0.5%), coronary artery bypass graft (CABG, 3.8%), Q-wave myocardial infarction (MI, 2.1%) and non-Q-wave MI (2.3%). Once again, the incidence of perforations decreased in time from 1.4% for the first 2592 patients to 0.3% for the last 1000 patients. Approximately two-thirds of perforations were safely managed medically. Six-month follow up angiography in 50% of the patients revealed a 58% angiographic restenosis rate.

These promising studies encouraged the development of randomized trials to evaluate the initial and long-term clinical and angiographic outcome of ELCA compared to conventional angioplasty modalities. The AMRO study (Amsterdam-Rotterdam Trial) enrolled 308 patients with stable angina and coronary lesions

Table 34.3 Current clinical indications and contraindications for the use of excimer laser

Indications	Contraindications
Saphenous venous grafts	Unprotected left main stem
Lesions that can not be crossed or dilated with balloon	Lesions in vessels with diameter smaller than catheter size
Thrombotic lesions	Coronary dissection or perforation before laser
Primary PCI	Extreme tortuosity of proximal target vessel
Moderately calcified lesions	Heavily calcified lesions
In-stent restenosis	Severe lesion angulation (>45)

longer that 10mm. Patients were randomized to either balloon angioplasty or ELCA (followed by balloon angioplasty in 98%) and 6-month angiographic follow-up was undertaken[28]. The procedural success was achieved in 80% of ELCA-treated patients compared to 79% treated with balloon angioplasty alone. At 6 months, with 98% follow up achieved, a primary end-point (death, MI, CABG, or repeat PCI) was reached in 33% patients treated with ELCA compared to 30% treated with balloon angioplasty alone. There was no significant difference in restenosis rate between the different treatment methods although there was a trend for a lower rate in the balloon angioplasty group. Although this study concluded that in patients with diffuse disease, ELCA did not provide any additional acute nor long-term clinical or angiographic benefits compared to balloon angioplasty, the lasing technique was very different to that currently recommended. For instance, the laser catheter was advanced at a speed of about 1mm/s and was performed without the saline infusion method.

Laser guide wire

In an attempt to improve on mechanical wire technology for treating chronic occlusions, a steerable laser guidewire (Prima® wire, Spectranectics Corp, Colorado Springs, CO, US) was developed. The laser wire consisted of a concentric array of 12 optical fibres (45 micron diameter) enclosed in a 0.018-inch hypotube. The wire could be steered using a torque device and the 3cm shapable tip was capable of delivering high-density excimer laser energy at a maximum fluence of 60mJ/mm^2 and a repetition rate of 25–40Hz when the proximal end of the guidewire was connected to the CVX-300 excimer laser console. Although this technology was used successfully by some operators, there was no difference in angioplasty success demonstrated in the Total Occlusion Trial with Angioplasty by using Laser guidewire (TOTAL) study over conventional wires in 303 patients from 18 European centres[29]. As manufacture of laser guide wires was both time consuming and expensive, and with a limited market, this technology has recently become unavailable and is unlikely to return in the near future.

Specific clinical scenarios and target lesions for ELCA

Saphenous vein grafts

Lesions within saphenous vein grafts (SVGs) tend to be multifocal, diffuse, friable, and degenerative containing significant atherosclerotic thrombotic material which makes them prone to distal embolization when being treated with PCI[30]. This may lead to the 'no-reflow' phenomenon and subsequent distal bed myonecrosis. ELCA has been successfully used to treat lesions within SVGs including aorto-ostial and focal thrombotic occlusions. Data for the 495 patients who had PCI to SVGs treated with ELCA and enrolled in the original ELCA registry reveals that distal embolization occurred in only 18 (3.3%) of the 545 SVG stenoses treated despite the lack of stenting and the use of old laser technology[31]. The authors observed that success and complication rates were superior when ELCA was used for ostial lesions of all vein grafts and for discrete stenoses in vein grafts <3.0mm in diameter. In addition, the presence of a target lesion within a SVG was actually a predictor of ELCA success from this non-randomized data in contrast to experiences with other devices[26]. Success rates reported are as high as 92%[31].

The Washington Hospital Centre group compared ELCA versus transluminal extraction catheter (TEC) with adjunct stenting in both groups[32]. Angiographic success was 100% in each group but the complication rate was higher in the TEC + stent group with a non-Q wave MI rate of 15.6% versus 8.7%. Although the TLR rate in the ELCA + stent group at 6 months was only 6.9%, the event free survival was low (67%) driven by a high mortality rate (9%). From a substudy of the Cohort of Acute Revascularization in Myocardial Infarction with Excimer Laser registry (CARMEL study) [33], 31 patients with ELCA-treated SVGs presenting with AMI had laser success in 87%, angiographic success in 97%, and overall procedural success in 84%[34]. Complications included significant dissections (10%) and no-reflow phenomenon (10%), although post-procedure CK-MB rise was only observed in 6%. These authors also describe data from 119 consecutive patients who underwent ELCA to SVGs with a mean age of 10.8 years, the success rate was 98.2% with a non-Q wave MI (defined as CPK-MB >3× upper limit of normal) rate of 0.8% and Q wave MI 1.7%[34]. This rate of MI is lower than that observed in the SAFER trial using distal protection devices which documented an MI rate of 8.4%[35].

In a retrospective analysis of 50 consecutive ELCA-treated SVGs at St.Thomas' Hospital, London (unpublished data) angiographic success was achieved in 98% with 6% having a peri-procedure rise in CK >3× and 10% between 2–3× upper limit of normal. Clinical follow up at mean 2.8 ± 1.6 years demonstrated 10% mortality, 10% further revascularization, and 22% rehospitalization with angina.

The importance of slow advancement of the laser catheter is none more so than in the treatment of lesions in SVGs. It is essential to allow the laser energy to gentle ablate the friable, atherosclerotic material without manual dilatation to avoid distal embolization. When the disease in the SVG is severely stenotic or particularly friable, passage of a distal protection device may be difficult and may occur at risk of distal embolization, ELCA provides a safe alternative. In the treatment of such lesions a 1.7mm or 2.0mm laser catheter can be advanced on a standard 0.014-inch guide wire to gently ablate sufficient material to then permit easy transition of a distal protection device. The intervention can then usually be completed with stenting without the need to predilate, before withdrawing the distal protection device.

Case examples of ELCA in treating saphenous venous graft lesions

Case 1 (Fig. 34.4A–C)

An 83-year-old gentleman underwent elective PCI to a 12-year-old SVG. An 8F JR4 guide was used with 5000U heparin. The lesion in the mid-graft was severe and crossing with a distal protection device may have been difficult. Instead, a Luge® guidewire (Boston Scientific, Natick, MA, USA) was advanced to the distal native RCA and ELCA performed on the mid-segment of SVG using the CVX-300® system with a 2.0mm Vitesse® C catheter (15 trains) to debulk the atherothrombitic material. There was a dramatic reduction in lesion severity following laser and after exchanging the Luge® wire for a Filterwire EZ® (Boston Scientific, Natick, MA, USA), a Cypher® 3.5 × 28mm stent (Cordis Corp., Miami, FL, USA) was delivered and deployed at 16atm. An excellent angiographic result was achieved with TIMI 3 flow and CK at 24h was normal.

Case 2 (Fig. 34.4D–F)

A 57-year-old male with diabetes, hypertension, and dyslipidaemia presented with troponin-positive unstable angina with inferior ECG ischemia. He had previous coronary revascularization with CABG ×2 (SVG-OM and SVG-RCA) 11 years previously and bare-metal stent PCI to SVG-RCA followed by drug-eluting stent PCI to SVG-RCA 1 year later. Cardiac magnetic resonance had revealed lateral wall full thickness infarction but a viable inferior wall a few months prior to the ACS.

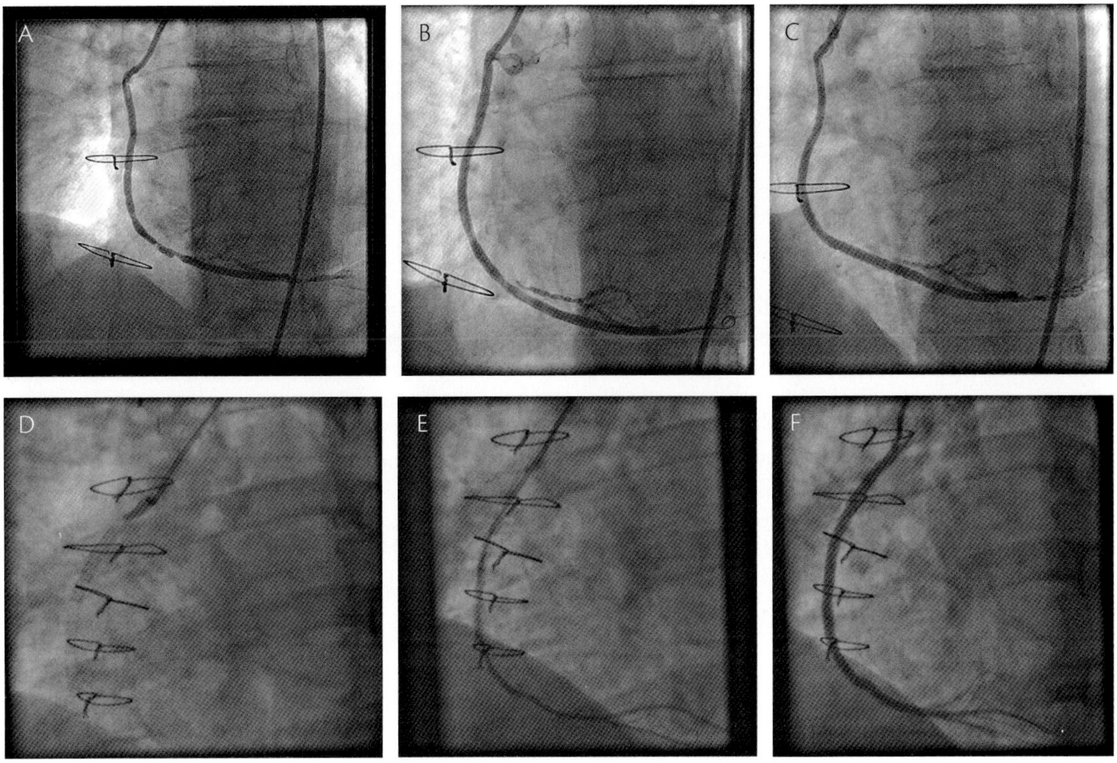

Fig. 34.4 Use of ELCA for SVG-PCI (A-C refer to case 1; D-F refer to case 2). (A) Severe mid-course lesion SVG-RCA (B) After 2.0mm excimer laser (C) Final image after single stent (D) Occluded SVG-RCA (E) After 1.4mm excimer laser (F) Final image.

At coronary angiography SVG-RCA was occluded and the native RCA appeared an unattractive option for PCI. The occluded SVG was wired with a Pilot 50® guidewire and ELCA performed on the entire length of SVG using the CVX-300® system with a 1.4mm Vitesse® C catheter (31 trains) to debulk the atherothrombitic material. This restored TIMI 3 flow and on IVUS there was extensive neo-intimal hyperplasia with a clear channel created by ELCA. 5 × Taxus® drug-eluting stents (2.5 × 20; 3.5 × 32; 3.5 × 32; 3.5 × 38 and 4.0 × 16mm [Boston Scientific, Natick, MA, USA]) were used and post dilated to high pressure with IVUS guidance which confirmed satisfactory stent expansion throughout, even in the section of the graft with three layers of stent. Six-month follow up angiography revealed a patent graft and he was without symptoms.

Acute coronary syndromes

Primary PCI for the treatment of ST elevated MI (STEMI) has clear advantages over pharmacological thrombolytic therapy(36) and a national programme is under development to offer such a service to the majority of the population in the future. Performing PCI in the milieu of thrombus is often associated with an increased complication rate. To combat this, adjunctive devices to stenting including those for thrombectomy and distal protection have been utilized although the only device with robust evidence that it improves outcome from a randomized trial is the simple thrombus aspiration catheter(40).

Application of excimer laser for adjunctive therapy in the setting of intracoronary thrombus has several potential advantages. ELCA facilitates rapid removal of target thrombus, vaporizes procoagulant mediators, augments tissue plasminogen factor(23), and suppresses platelet aggregation kinetics leading to the 'stunned platelet' phenomenon(37). This effect on platelets was demonstrated by *in vitro* exposure of whole blood from healthy volunteers to increasing levels of laser energy (30, 45, and 60mJ/mm^2) delivered from a 1.7mm concentric laser catheter. A dose-dependent suppression of both ADP and collagen-induced whole blood aggregation was observed in addition to a suppression of platelet contractile force with 60mJ/mm^2 energy. There was no difference in platelet concentration or any discernable morphological changes on scanning electron micrographs of platelet-rich plasma between platelets exposed to different levels of laser energy. The precise mechanism by which UV laser exerts its effect on platelets remains unknown.

Topaz and colleagues have published their experience of treating patients with acute coronary syndromes using excimer laser(38). Of a cohort of 256 patients treated between September 1997 and September 2000 they have reported on the results of 50 patients presenting with STEMI (56%) or non-STEMI (NSTEMI, 44%) who either failed to respond to lytic therapy (n = 29) or had contraindications to lyis or glycoprotein IIb/IIIa inhibitors (n = 16). Six patients presented with cardiogenic shock. Ninety per cent of the patients were male with mean age 60 ± 13 years and baseline left ventricular ejection fraction 44 ± 13%. Nearly half (48%) had single-vessel coronary disease and 54 lesions were treated. Eighty-four per cent of coronary lesions had visible thrombus at the time of coronary angiography and ELCA was successfully delivered to 98% or infarct related arteries using 1.4mm (n = 26), 1.7mm (n = 26), or 2.0mm (n = 7) catheters adopting the saline bolus lasing technique. The energy parameters for lasing were set at a fluence of 45mJ/mm^2 and repetition rate 25Hz with only one lesion requiring 60mJ/mm^2 because of resistance. Post-laser stenting was performed in 83% of target lesions with adjunctive glycoprotein IIb/IIIa receptor antagonists used in only 6% of patients. Procedural success was achieved in all patients.

By quantitative coronary angiography (QCA), the minimal luminal diameter increased from baseline of 0.7 ± 0.5 to 1.3 ± 0.5mm post lasing and then to 2.0 ± 0.6 with balloon dilation to a final 3.0 ± 0.5mm post stenting. Thrombolysis in myocardial infarction (TIMI) flow increased from baseline of 1.7 ± 1.1 to 2.8 ± 0.4 by laser to a final 2.9 ± 0.4 and importantly there was a reduction in thrombus burden area observed in 83%. There was one major dissection caused by laser and treated with stenting but no other significant complications. All 50 patients survived and were eventually discharged and it was concluded that the application of ELCA is safe, feasible and efficacious for treating selected patients with STEMI or NSTEMI, especially those with thrombotic target lesions who fail to respond to thrombolytics or have contraindications to these agents or glycoprotein IIb/IIIa receptor antagonists.

In the CARMEL registry(33), 151 patients with AMI (54% Q-wave and 46% non-Q-wave) underwent excimer laser atherectomy at eight intervention centres (six in the United States, one in Canada, and one in Germany.). Eleven per cent of patients had failed thrombolytic therapy, 17% had contraindications for lytics, 37% had TIMI 0 flow in the infarct related vessel, and 13% of patients were in cardiogenic shock. Baseline left ventricular ejection fraction was 44% ± 13%. A SVG was the target vessel in 21%. QCA and statistical analysis were performed by independent core laboratories. ELCA was successfully delivered in 95% of cases with the 1.7mm catheter used most commonly (43% of procedures).

Ninety-seven per cent angiographic success and 91% overall procedural success rate were attained with glycoprotein IIb/IIIa receptor antagonists used in 52% of patients. Sixty-five per cent of cases contained a large thrombus burden and maximal laser gain was achieved in lesions with extensive thrombus burden ($p < 0.03$ vs. small burden). TIMI flow grade was increased significantly by the laser: 1.2 ± 1.1 to 2.8 ± 0.5 ($p < 0.001$), reaching a final 3.0 ± 0.2 ($p < 0.001$ vs. baseline). Mean minimal luminal diameter increased by laser from 0.5 ± 0.5 to 1.6 ± 0.5mm ($p < 0.001$), followed by 2.7 ± 0.6mm after stenting ($p < 0.001$ vs. baseline and vs. after laser). The laser decreased target stenosis from 83% ± 17% to 52% ± 15% ($p < 0.001$ vs. baseline), followed by 20% ± 16% after stenting ($p < 0.001$ vs. baseline and vs. after laser). Six patients died with each presenting initially with cardiogenic shock. Complications included perforation (0.6%), dissection (5% major, 3% minor), acute vessel closure (0.6%), distal embolization (2%), and bleeding (3%). In a multivariate regression model, only absence of cardiogenic shock remained as a significant factor affecting procedural success. In was concluded from this registry that successful debulking by excimer laser in the setting of AMI gained maximal thrombus dissolution in lesions with extensive thrombus burden which was combined with a considerable increase in MLD and restoration of antegrade TIMI flow.

More contemporary studies of the utilization of excimer laser during PCI for patients presenting with AMI have been reported. Ambronsini *et al.* published their single-centre experience of ELCA in 66 patients during primary or rescue PCI cases [39]. They used optimal lasing technique (saline flushing with slow advancement 0.2–0.5mm/s) using the CVX-300® excimer laser system and treated the majority of lesions with a laser-stent strategy (only two patients required balloon angioplasty prior to stenting). Primary angiographic endpoints were myocardial blush grade, TIMI flow, and length-adjusted TIMI frame count. The group also analysed echocardiographic LV remodelling, electrocardiographic ST-segment resolution at 90min post PCI, and event-free survival at 6 months.

TIMI-score increased from baseline 0.2 ± 0.4 to 2.65 ± 0.5 post laser to 2.9 ± 0.3 post stent (both $p < 0.01$ vs. baseline). Similarly, myocardial blush grade increased from 0.12 ± 0.4 to 2.5 ± 0.6 post laser to 2.8 ± 0.4 post stent. Corrected TIMI frame count fell from 100 at baseline (occluded epicardial artery) to 29 ± 6 post laser and 22 ± 3 post stent (both $p < 0.01$ vs. baseline). No reflow was observed in 11% of cases after laser and a major dissection occurred in one case. There were no intra-procedural deaths and at 6 months there was 95% event-free survival with LV remodelling occurring in 8% patients.

The prognostic implications of myocardial blush grade in primary PCI were elegantly highlighted in the Thrombus Aspiration during Percutaneous Coronary Intervention in Acute Myocardial Infarction study (TAPAS)[40]. This trial of 1071 patients receiving primary PCI for treatment of STEMI were randomized to either thrombus-aspiration prior to stenting or conventional PCI without thrombus extraction. Although there were a small number of patients who crossed over, the results demonstrated significantly less patients had myocardial blush grade 0 or 1 (17.1%) following thrombus aspiration compared to conventional PCI (26.3%). This corresponded with a 30-day improvement in death and major adverse cardiac events in the thrombus-aspiration group and a clear correlation of myocardial blush score with rate of death or MACE identified for the whole cohort of patients. Since myocardial blush score achieved in the setting of primary PCI predicts clinical outcome the finding that excimer laser PCI significantly improves myocardial blush score suggests that this would also translate into improved outcome.

The only published randomized trial of excimer laser-PCI versus conventional PCI in consecutive patients presenting with STEMI is the LaserAMI study[41]. This small study of 27 patients was not powered to demonstrate superiority of ELCA over conventional PCI but did show that ELCA was both feasible and safe in all cases. There was no significant difference observed between the two groups in the decrease in diameter stenosis or the increase in either TIMI flow or myocardial blush score from baseline. Corrected TIMI frame count was also similar in both groups although the gain from baseline was higher in the ELCA group (53 ± 14% vs. 35 ± 20%; $p < 0.05$) perhaps suggesting that there was a greater benefit. It is clear that for the excimer laser to develop a role in routine primary PCI for STEMI, larger randomized control trials are required with specific comparison with the now accepted gold standard of simple thrombus aspiration utilized prior to stenting.

Case examples of ELCA during PCI at the time of an acute coronary syndrome

Case 3 (Fig. 34.5A–C)

A 67-year-old gentleman who had previous CABG 11 years before with LIMA-LAD; SVG-diagonal and SVG-RCA presented with 12h of unstable symptoms with >2mm ST segment depression in the anterior leads on ECG. Coronary angiography demonstrated an occluded LAD proximally with a patent LIMA graft to mid-vessel

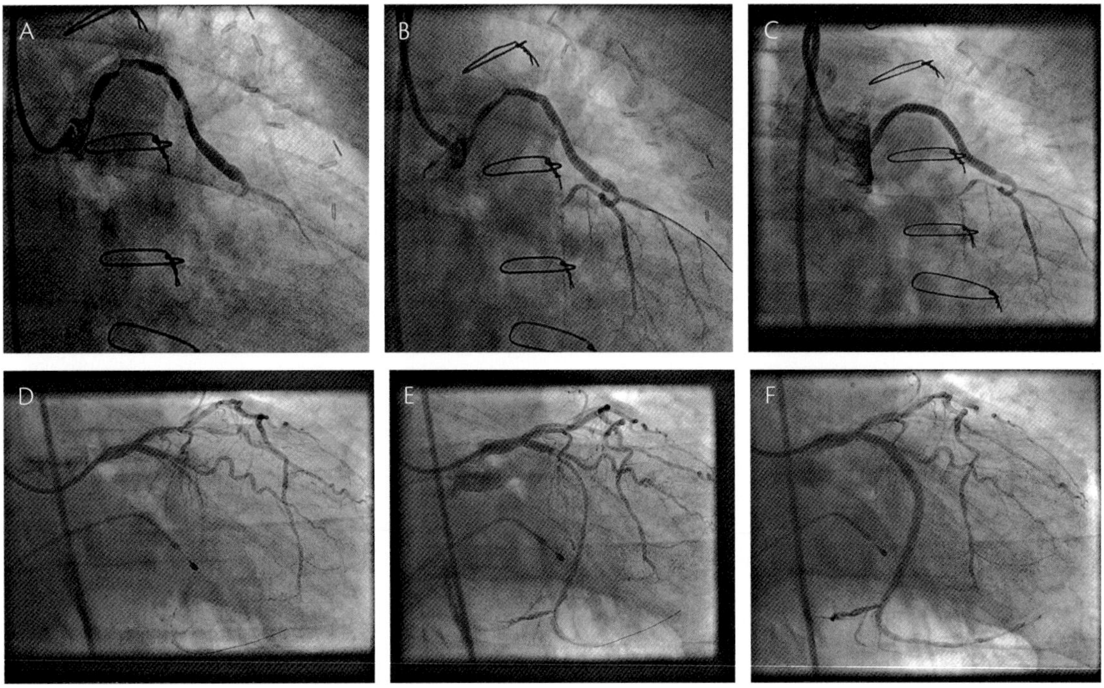

Fig. 34.5 Use of ELCA for PCI in ACS (A-C refer to case 3; D-F refer to case 4) (A) Severe lesion & thrombus in diagonal SVG (B) After 1.7mm ELCA with TIMI 3 flow to diagonal restored (C) Final stent result (D) Persistent occlusion of dominant circumflex after guide wire and balloon pre-dilation in a patient presenting with STEMI (E) TIMI 3 flow restored only after 1.4mm ELCA (F) Final stent result.

and diffuse mild disease in the distal LAD beyond the graft insertion. The major diagonal was grafted but the SVG contained extensive atheromatous material and thrombus with TIMI 0 flow beyond the insertion. The circumflex was aberrant arising from the proximal RCA and there was a moderate proximal lesion. Both the native RCA and SVG were occluded with faint anterograde flow through bridging collaterals. PCI was performed to the diagonal vein graft using an 8F JR4 guide with both heparin and abciximab pharmacotherapy. A BMW wire was advanced into the distal vessel and ELCA performed on the entire length of SVG using the CVX-300® system with a 1.7mm Vitesse® C catheter (16 trains) to debulk the atherothrombitic material. The post ELCA result was excellent with TIMI 3 flow into the distal diagonal which could now be seen as an important large epicardial vessel. The BMW wire was exchanged for a Filterwire EZ® and the graft was stented with bare metal overlapping Tsunami® (Terumo, Japan) stents (3.0 × 15; 3.0 × 15 and 3.0 × 23) with a bare metal Titan II® (Hexacath, Rueil-Malmaison, France) 3.5 × 10 stent overlapped to the ostium. The distal protection device was removed and there was no macroscopic evidence of thrombus. The final result was excellent.

Case 4 (Fig. 34.5D–F)

An 80-year-old gentleman presented with posterior STEMI, complete heart block, and cardiogenic shock. Coronary angiography demonstrated an occluded dominant circumflex. A temporary pacing wire had provided an improvement in cardiac output and blood pressure and PCI was undertaken to the infarct related artery. JL4 guide, heparin 5000U, Luge® guidewire advanced to distal vessel. 2.5 × 12mm balloon was advanced along the vessel and dilated throughout without any improvement in TIMI flow which remained 0. 1.4mm ELCA catheter then advanced throughout vessel and following this, TIMI 2 flow was restored before stent deployment.

Calcification and non-crossable or non-dilatable coronary lesions

Within an aging population the probability of encountering complex coronary disease when performing PCI is increasingly more likely. Calcified stenosis, chronic total occlusions and non-compliant plaques remain technically challenging and often require utilization of techniques other than balloon angioplasty in order to prepare the vessel for stenting. For severe calcification, rotational atherectomy is the most effective adjunctive treatment to debulk the lesion sufficiently to allow adequate stent delivery and expansion. In mildly calcified lesions an alternative device is the excimer laser. The 0.9mm X80 catheter is capable of operating at a fluence of 80mJ/mm^2 and repetition rate of 80Hz and this device has been compared in a multicentre, self-controlled comparative study against standard laser therapy defined by laser energy of 60mJ/mm^2 at 40Hz[18].

A total of 95 patients with 100 treated lesions were enrolled in this study. Patients participated according to one of three inclusion criteria: angiographic calcification (58%), failure to cross lesion with a 1.5mm balloon (37%), or chronic total occlusion crossable with a guidewire (5%). In five, lesions were abandoned because of failing to cross with the guidewire (n = 3) or laser software faults (n = 2). Standard laser therapy parameters were successful in 66 lesions. At least three laser trains at this energy were delivered to the remaining lesions before using increased energy. Of the 29 resistant lesions, 21 were successfully crossed after increased energy (12 lesions with 60mJ/mm^2 at 80Hz and further nine lesions at 80mJ/mm^2 at 80Hz). Of the eight lesions unsuccessfully crossed with the tip of the X80 0.9mm laser catheter, PCI was completed in four by adjunctive balloon angioplasty, one had successful rotational atherectomy, two were treated medically (including one failed rotational atherectomy), and one required CABG. There were five laser-related dissections which were treated by stenting except for one, and one patient had a VF arrest during laser and subsequently suffered a non-Q-wave MI. Increased laser energy was not associated with complications. Form this study and our own experience, if the catheter tip itself fails to cross the lesion completely, the lesion has often been modified sufficiently to allow a balloon to cross and dilate the lesion and complete the PCI.

In situations where passage of a RotaWire® is impossible, and the lesion is not crossable with a support catheter or over-the-wire (OTW) balloon, a potential advantage of the laser over the Rotablator® is the ability to use a conventional 0.014-inch wire. The use of the X80 excimer laser catheter to modify the lesion characteristics may permit subsequent successful passage of a RotaWire®, support catheter or OTW balloon to complete the PCI. We have termed this combined use of excimer laser and rotational atherectomy as 'The Raser'. Excimer laser catheter can also be deployed to successfully treat a non-dilated stent within a calcified coronary lesion.

Case examples of ELCA during PCI for non-crossable or non-dilatable lesion

Case 5 (Fig. 34.6A–C)

An 85-year-old gentleman underwent staged PCI to LAD having had successful PCI to the mid-RCA a few months before following an acute inferior STEMI which had initially been treated with thrombolyis. He had preserved LV systolic function and had exercise limiting angina. The LAD was a moderately calcified vessel with an angiographic severe lesion just distal to the first septal branch. A 6F EBU 3.5L guide was used and BMW wire advanced to the distal vessel. A 2.5 × 15mm Maverick® balloon (Boston Scientific, Natick, MA, USA) crossed the lesion with difficulty and on inflation, clearly failed to dilate the lesion with the balloon bursting at 14atm. A second attempt at balloon angioplasty was unsuccessful so a 0.9mm X80 excimer laser catheter was advanced to the lesion. Three trains of 60mJ/mm^2 at 40Hz followed by two trains of 80mJ/mm^2 at 80Hz achieved adequate lesion modification to permit balloon dilation with another 2.5 × 15mm balloon. The vessel was stented back to the body of the left main stem using overlapping Taxus®) drug-eluting stents (3.0 × 20; 3.0 × 8; and 4.0 × 12mm;) which were post dilated to high pressure with IVUS guidance to confirm satisfactory stent expansion throughout.

Case 6 (Fig. 34.6D–F)

A 61-year-old gentleman was admitted with unstable angina, unremarkable ECG, and negative troponin. He had suffered an AMI 8 years before, was hypertensive, dyslipidaemic, and type 2 diabetic with a body mass index of 42. Coronary angiography demonstrated a chronically occluded RCA in the proximal vessel with extensive collateralization from the intermediate and distal LAD with the suggestion of a short skip segment. The LAD had moderate–severe proximal disease and a large-calibre intermediate had a severe proximal stenosis. The options for coronary revascularization were discussed with the patient and he decided to undergo an attempt at PCI to the RCA occlusion in the first instance. With a 7F AL0.75 guide in the RCA and a JL4 diagnostic catheter in the LMS bilateral injections were performed. To cross into the occlusion, a Miracle® 6 (Asahi Intecc, Japan) guidewire with over the wire balloon support was required which was exchanged for a Pilot® 150 wire to advance into the distal vessel. The occlusion could not be crossed with either a 1.25 × 15mm or a 0.85 × 10mm balloon. A 0.9mm X80 excimer laser catheter was advanced and after 8 trains of 45mJ/mm^2 at 25Hz the laser catheter advanced to the

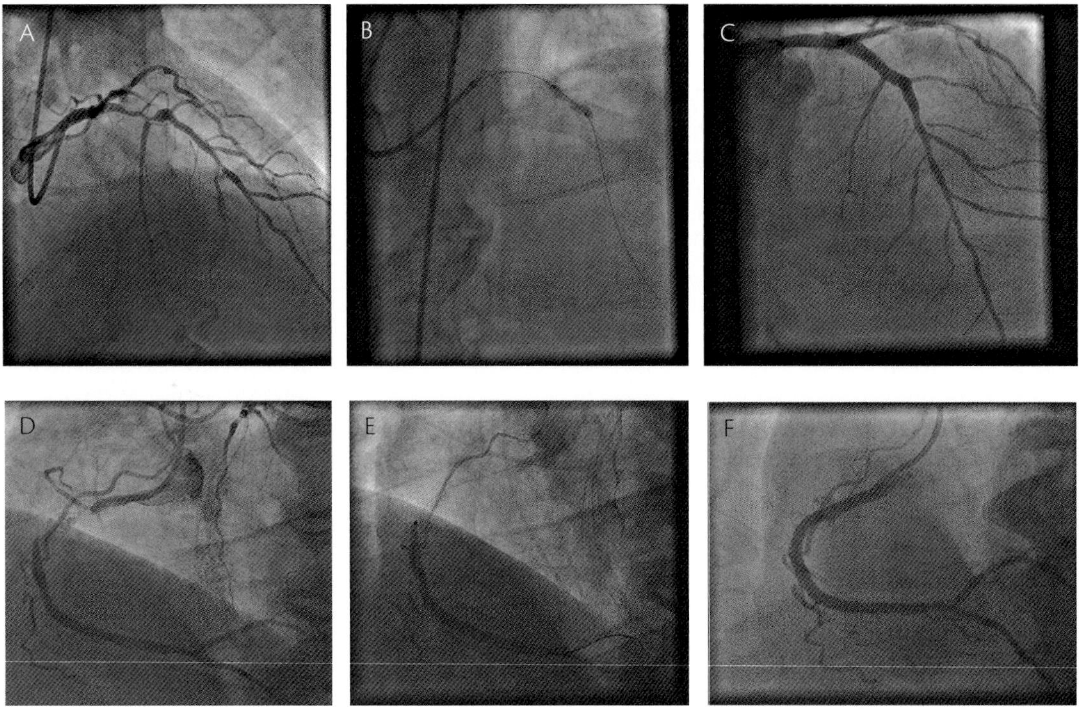

Fig. 34.6 Use 0.9mm ELCA for PCI in non-dilatable coronary lesions (A-C refer to case 5; D-F refer to case 6) - (A) Severe proximal LAD stenosis (B) 2.5x15mm balloon underexpanded (C) Following ELCA and stenting (D) Bilateral injections demonstrating RCA CTO (E) Crossable with guide wire but not any balloon until ELCA had modified lesion (F) Final stent result.

distal vessel. Lower energy was used because of the difficulty in achieving adequate saline flushing with an occluded vessel. The lesion was subsequently pre-dilated and stented using overlapping Taxus® drug-eluting stents (3.5 × 32; and 4.0 × 16mm; which were post dilated to high pressure. An excellent angiographic result was achieved and the patient subsequently had successful PCI to both LAD and intermediate coronary arteries.

In-stent restenosis

In-stent restenosis (ISR) remains a major limitation of PCI following stent implantation with rates of restenosis reported to occur in 10–50% of patients receiving a bare-metal stent[(42)]. ELCA has been shown to be safe and effective in treating ISR[(43)]. However, there is no evidence that ELCA can reduce target lesion revascularization when compared to balloon angioplasty alone[(44)] despite lesions treated with the ELCA having greater lumen gain, more intimal hyperplasia ablation, and a larger cross-sectional area on IVUS in this study.

ELCA has also been compared with rotational atherectomy where both groups underwent adjunctive balloon angioplasty[(45)]. Volumetric IVUS analysis showed significantly greater reduction in intimal hyperplasia volume after rotational atherectomy compared to ELCA because of higher ablation efficiency although this did not translate to improved target lesion revascularization rate (26% in ELCA group vs. 28% in the rotational atherectomy group).

Concerns that using lasers within stents could lead to thermal injury were addressed by Papaioannou and colleagues who evaluated *in vitro* temperature changes during excimer laser activation within stents compared to unstented control vessels[(46)]. A variety of stents deployed in porcine coronary arteries were examined during activation of an eccentric 2.0mm excimer laser catheter and acceptable temperatures changes were observed. In a separate study, excimer laser did not alter stainless-steel stent endurance or liberate any significant material when five types of stainless-steel stents were subjected to 1000 pulses of laser energy from a 2.0mm eccentric excimer laser catheter[(47)].

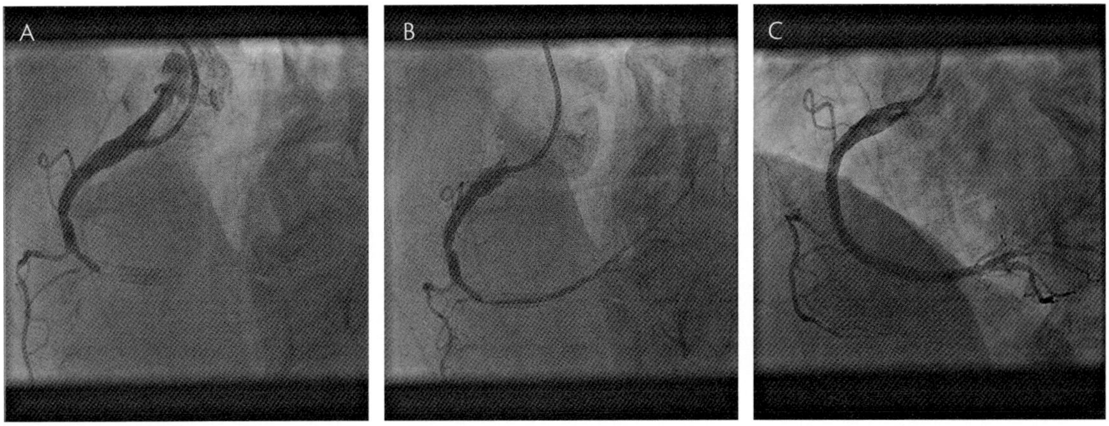

Fig. 34.7 Use of 0.9mm ELCA catheter to treat occlusive in-stent restenosis (A-C refer to case 7) - (A) Set up shot (B) Post ELCA (C) Final stent result.

Case example of ELCA for treatment of in-stent restenosis

Case 7 (Fig. 34.7A–C)

A 76-year-old gentleman underwent elective PCI to occlusive ISR within the mid-RCA. The original procedure had been several years before and precise details of that intervention were not known. He had significant limiting exertional angina with preserved LV systolic function. A 6F AL1 guide catheter was used and the lesion was crossed with a Miracle® 3 guidewire which was then exchanged for a medium support Whisper® wire (Guidant Corporation, Santa Clara, CA, USA). ELCA was performed with a 0.9mm X80 laser catheter and after 7 trains of $60mJ/mm^2$ at 40Hz the vessel was pre-dilated and stented with Cypher®) drug-eluting stents (2.5 ×18; 3.0×33 and 3.5 × 28mm). Stents were post dilated to high pressure with excellent stent expansion on IVUS.

Conclusions

The technological development of the excimer laser catheter and improved, safer delivery techniques have advanced the use of this device in PCI. Not every atherosclerotic lesion requires laser debulking but in certain subgroups there are advantages of using this modality either independent to or as an adjunct to conventional techniques. As coronary interventionalists accept more challenging and complex cases, there may be a greater need to discover well evaluated, safe, alternative therapies that are more efficacious than standard equipment.

References

1. Goldman L, Blaney DJ, Kindel DJ Jr, *et al.* Pathology of the effect of the laser beam on the skin. *Nature* 1963; **197**:912–14.
2. McGuff PE, Bushnell D. Studies of the surgical applications of the laser. *Surgical Forum* 1963; **14**(143):145.
3. Choy DS, Stertzer S, Rotterdam HZ, *et al.* Transluminal laser catheter angioplasty. *Am J Cardiol* 1982; **50**(6): 1206–8.
4. Geschwind HJ, Boussignac G, Teisseire B, *et al.* Conditions for effective Nd-YAG laser angioplasty. *Br Heart J* 1984; **52**:484–9.
5. Ginsburg R, Kim D, Guthaner S, *et al.* Salvage of an ischaemic limb by laser angioplasty: Description of a new technique. *Clin Cardiol* 1984; **7**:54–8.
6. Cook SL, Eigler N, Shefer A, *et al.* Percutaneous excimer laser coronary angioplasty of lesions not ideal for balloon angioplasty. *Circulation* 1991; **84**:632–43.
7. Boulnois JL. Photophysical process in laser tissue interactions. In Ginsburg R, Geschwind HJ (eds). *Primer on Laser Angioplasty*, pp.45–100. New York: Futura, 1992.
8. Welch AJ, Valvano JW, Pearce J, *et al.* Effect of laser radiation on tissue during laser angioplasty. *Lasers Surg Med* 1985; **5**:251–64.
9. Oraevsky AA, Jacques SL, Pettit GH, *et al.* XeCl laser ablation of atherosclerotic aorta: optical properties and energy pathways. *Lasers Surg Med* 1992; **12**:585–97.
10. Topaz O. Plaque removal and thrombus dissolution with the photoacoustic energy of pulsed-wave laser: biotissue interactions and their clinical manifestations. *Cardiology* 1996; **87**(5):384–91.
11. Grundfest WS, Segalowitz J, Laudenslager J. The physical and biological basis for laser angioplasty. In Litvack F (ed). *Coronary Laser Angioplasty*, pp.1–12. Oxford: Blackwell Scientific Publications1992.

12. Bittl JA, Brinker JA, Sanborn TA, *et al.* The changing profile of patient selection, procedural techniques, and outcomes in excimer laser coronary angioplasty. *J Interv Cardiol* 1995; **8**:653–60.
13. Grundfest WS, Litvack F, Forrester JS, *et al.* Laser ablation of human atherosclerotic plaque without adjunt tissue injury. *J Am Coll Cardiol* 1985; **5**:929–33.
14. Deckelbaum LI, Isner JM, Donaldson RF, *et al.* Reduction of laser-induced pathologic tissue injury using pulsed energy delivery. *Am J Cardiol* 1985; **56**(10):662–7.
15. Dahm JB, Kuon E. High-energy eccentric excimer laser angioplasty for debulking diffuse in-stent restenois leads to better acute- and 6-month follow-up results. *J Invas Cardiol* 2000; **12**:335–42.
16. Taylor K, Reiser C. Next generation catheters for excimer laser coronary angioplasty. *Lasers Med Sci* 2001; **16**(2):133–40.
17. Topaz O, Lippincott R, Bellendir J, *et al.* "Optimally spaced" excimer laser coronary catheters: performance analysis. *J Clin Laser Med Surg* 2001; **19**(1):9–14.
18. Bilodeau L, Fretz EB, Taeymans Y, *et al.* Novel use of a high-energy excimer laser catheter for calcified and complex coronary artery lesions. *Catheter Cardiovasc Interv* 2004; **62**(2):155–61.
19. Baumbach A, Haase KK, Rose C, *et al.* Formation of pressure waves during in vitro excimer laser irradiation in whoile blood and the effect of dilution with contrast media and saline. *Lasers Surg Med* 1994; **14**(1):3–6.
20. Tcheng JE, Wells LD, Phillips HR, *et al.* Development of a new technique for reducing pressure pulse generation during 308nm excimer laser coronary angioplasty. *Catheter Cardiovasc Interv* 1995; **34**(3):15–22.
21. Deckelbaum LI, Natatajan MK, Bittl JA, *et al.* Effect of intra-coronary saline infusion on dissection during excimer laser coronary angioplasty: a randomized trial. *J Am Coll Cardiol* 1995; **26**:1264–9.
22. Topaz O, Minisi AJ, Mohanty L, *et al.* In-vivo effect of coronary laser angioplasty on atherosclerotic plaques: histopathologic analysis. *Cardiovasc Pathol* 2001; **10**(5):223–8.
23. Topaz O, Das T, Dahm JB, *et al.* Excimer Laser Revascularisation: Current indications, applications and techniques. *Lasers Med Sci* 2001; **16**:72–7.
24. Holmes D, Reeder GS, Chazzal ZMB, *et al.* Coronary perforation after excimer laser coronary angioplasty: the Excimer Laser Coronary Angioplasty Registry experience. *J Am Coll Cardiol* 1994; **23**:330–335.
25. Baumbach A, Bittl JA, Fleck E, *et al.* Acute complications of excimer laser coronary angioplasty: a detailed analysis of multicenter results. Coinvestigators of the U.S. and European Percutaneous Excimer Laser Coronary Angioplasty (PELCA) Registries. *J Am Coll Cardiol* 1994; **23**:1305–13.
26. Bittl JA. Clinical results with excimer laser coronary angioplasty. *Semin Interv Cardiol* 1996; **1**(2):129–34.
27. Litvack F, Eigler N, Margolis J, *et al.* Percutaneous excimer laser coronary angioplasty: results in the first consecutive 3,000 patients. The ELCA Investigators. *J Am Coll Cardiol* 1994; **23**:323–9.
28. Appelman YE, Piek JJ, Strikwerda S, *et al.* Randomized trial of excimer laser versus balloon angioplasty for treatment of obstructive coronary artery disease. *Lancet* 1996; **347**:79–84.
29. Serruys PW, Hamburger JN, Koolen J, *et al.* Total occlusion trial with angioplasty by using laser guidewire. *Eur Heart J* 2000; **21**:1797–805.
30. Webb JG, Carere RG, Virmani R, *et al.* Retrieval and analysis of particulate debris after saphenous vein graft intervention. *J Am Coll Cardiol* 1999; **34**:468–75.
31. Bittl JA, Sanborn TA, Yardley DE, *et al.* Predictors of outcome of percutaneous excimer laser coronary angioplasty of saphenous vein bypass graft lesions. The Percutaneous Excimer Laser Coronary Angioplasty Registry. *Am J Cardiol* 1994; **74**(2):144–8.
32. Hong MK, Wong SC, Popma JJ. Favourable results of debulking followed by immediate adjunct stent therapy for high risk sapehnous vein graft lesions. *J Am Coll Cardiol* 1996; **27**:179A.
33. Topaz O, Ebersole D, Das T, *et al.* Excimer laser angioplasty in acute myocardial infarction (the CARMEL multicenter trial). *Am J Cardiol* 2004; **93**(6):694–701.
34. Ebersole D, Dahm JB, Das T, *et al.* Excimer Laser Revascularization of Saphenous Vein Grafts in Acute Myocardial Infarction. *J Invas Cardiol* 2004; **16**:177–80.
35. Baim DS, Wahr D, George B, *et al.* Randomized trial of a distal embolic protection device during percutaneous intervention of saphenous vein aorto-coronary bypass grafts. Saphenous vein graft Angioplasty Free of Emboli Randomized (SAFER) Trial Investigators. *Circulation* 2002; **105**(11):1285–90.
36. Keeley EC., Boura JA, Grines CL. Primary angioplasty versus intravenous thrombolytic therapy for acute myocardial infarction: a quantitative review of 23 randomised trials. *Lancet* 2003; **361**:13–20.
37. Topaz O, Minisi AJ, Bernardo NL, McPherson RA, Martin E, Carr SL *et al.* Alterations of platelet aggregation kinetics with ultraviolet laser emission: The "stunned platelet" phenomenon. *Thromb Haemost* 2001; **86**(4):1087–93.
38. Topaz O, Shah R, Mohanty PK, *et al.* Application of excimer laser angioplasty in acute myocardial infarction. *Lasers Surg Med* 2001; **29**:185–92.
39. Ambrosini V, Cioppa A, Salemme L, *et al.* Excimer laser in acute myocardial infarction: single centre experience on 66 patients. *Int J Cardiol* 2008; **127**(1):98–102.
40. Svilaas T, Vlaar PJ, van der Horst IC, *et al.* Thrombus aspiration during primary percutaneous coronary intervention. *NEJM* 2008; **358**(6):557–67.
41. Dörr M, Vogelgesang D, Hummel A, *et al.* Excimer laser thrombus elimination for prevention of distal embolization and no-reflow in patients with acute ST elevation myocardial infarction: results from the randomized LaserAMI study. *Int J Cardiol* 2007; **116**(1):20–6.

42. Lowe H, Oesterle S, Khachigian LM. Coronary in-stent restenosis: current status and future strategies. *J Am Coll Cardiol* 2002; **39**:183–93.
43. Koster R, Hamm CW, Seabra-Gomes R, *et al.* Laser angioplasty of restenosed coronary stents: Results of a multicenter surveillance trial. *J Am Coll Cardiol* 1999; **34**(1):25–32.
44. Mehran R, Mintz GS, Satler LF, *et al.* Treatment of in-stent restenosis with excimer laser coronary angioplasty: mechanisms and results compared to PTCA alone. *Circulation* 1997; **96**(7):2183–9.
45. Mehran R, Dangas G, Mintz GS, *et al.* Treatment of in-stent restenosis with excimer laser coronary angioplasty versus rotational atherectomy: comparative mechanisms and results. *Circulation* 2000; **101**(21):2484–9.
46. Papaioannou T, Yadegar D, Vari S, *et al.* Excimer laser (308nm) recanalisation of in-stent restenosis: Thermal considerations. *Lasers Med Sci* 2001; **16**(2):90–100.
47. Burris N, Lippincott R, Elfe A, *et al.* Effects of 308 nanometer excimer laser energy on 316 L stainless-steel stents: implications for laser atherectomy of in-stent restenosis. *J Invas Cardiol* 2000; **12**(11):555–9.

CHAPTER 35

Cutting balloons and AngioSculpt®

Mike Seddon and Nick Curzen

Introduction

Although percutaneous coronary intervention has revolutionized the treatment of coronary artery disease, it has been limited by acute ischaemic complications and restenosis. It is well recognized that elastic recoil, negative remodelling, and neointimal hyperplasia are the underlying mechanisms of restenosis, with a clear association between the extent of vascular injury sustained and subsequent intimal hyperplasia. The search for a method to dilate an obstructive coronary lesion without invoking this proportional injury response led to the development of a variety of devices designed to excise or modify plaque in order to limit intimal injury. In 1991, Barath and colleagues[1] developed a non-compliant cutting balloon with three or four microblades fixed radially to it. It was hypothesized that the discrete longitudinal incisions created during balloon inflation might improve the success of conventional balloon angioplasty by reducing elastic recoil and minimizing intimal injury, thereby minimizing the subsequent neointimal proliferative response. Theoretically, this effect would allow cutting balloon angioplasty to achieve and maintain a larger lumen diameter using lower balloon inflation pressures and durations than conventional balloon angioplasty. Technology has since progressed rapidly through several stages, with the introduction of intracoronary stents, advances in adjunctive antiplatelet therapies, and the advent of drug-eluting stents. However, the Cutting Balloon®, and the recently approved AngioSculpt® scoring balloon, remain in the armamentarium of the interventional cardiologist today. This chapter summarizes the clinical experience with these devices to date and their place in the current era.

The devices

Cutting Balloon® (Boston Scientific, USA)

The Cutting Balloon® consists of microsurgical stainless steel blades, or atherotomes, 0.28–0.33mm in height by 0.10–0.15mm in width, mounted longitudinally on the outer surface of a non-compliant balloon (Fig. 35.1). Balloon diameters range from 2.0–4.0mm, in 0.25-mm increments. 2.0–3.25-mm balloons incorporate three atherotomes whilst those of 3.5–4.0mm have four atherotomes, with a choice of lengths of 6, 10, or 15mm. When deflated, the balloon is folded in such a way as to shield the blades and protect the vessel from the edges of the atherotomes as the catheter is passed to and from the lesion. On inflation, the atherotomes, which are three to five times sharper than conventional surgical blades, are exposed radially and deliver longitudinal incisions in the plaque and vessel, thereby relieving its hoop stress. A controlled fault line is delivered during dilation to facilitate crack propagation in an orderly fashion. The concept is to cut first and then dilate conventionally, resulting in reduced histological damage outside the cutting area compared to standard balloons (Fig. 35.2). The resultant lumen enlargement occurs due to widening of these initial cuts through balloon inflation.

Since its introduction, the design of the cutting balloon has evolved considerably. First-generation devices incorporated rigid atherotomes, making tortuous vessel negotiation difficult, whilst the catheter shaft was not coated. The second generation Ultra 2® device incorporated: (1) T notches in the atherotome base to increase device flexibility; (2) a smaller catheter shaft with bioslide hydrophilic coating; and (3) a smaller catheter tip to improve crossability and deliverability. The recently

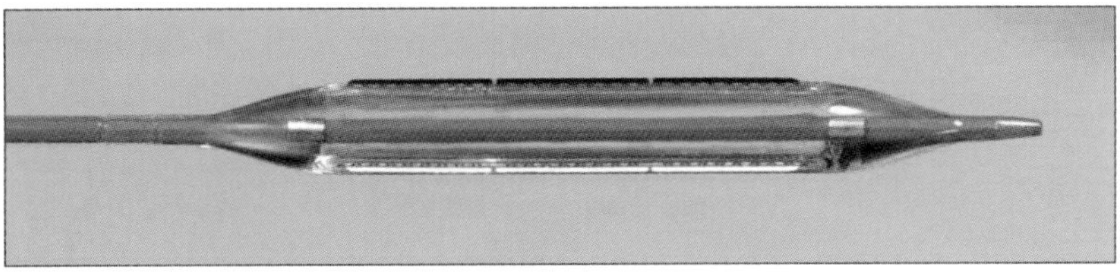

Fig. 35.1 The Cutting Balloon®. The atherotomes, which are mounted longitudinally on the non-compliant nylon balloon, score the plaque allowing controlled dilatation of the lesion.

available Flextome® Cutting Balloon incorporates atherotome flex points every 5mm for further improved flexibility, an improved catheter delivery system, and nylon balloon material with better re-wrap properties and puncture resistance.

Technical considerations

Equipment

The Cutting Balloon® can be delivered via a 6-French (F) guiding catheter over conventional 0.014-inch guide wires, via a monorail delivery system. Good guiding catheter support is necessary to allow delivery of the device due to the stiffness of the balloons, whilst a moderate to extra support guide wire may be helpful.

Sizing

In selecting diameter, the balloon to artery ratio should not exceed 1.1:1.0, so as to avoid deep vascular wall incisions. Device length should be minimized in tortuous anatomy, with re-inflation along the length of the lesion if necessary.

Inflation/deflation

It is important to use slow inflation rates (1 atmosphere every 5s) to ensure that the balloon material unfolds evenly from around the blades, to avoid puncturing the balloon and similar slow deflation rates for optimal balloon re-wrap. Multiple inflations can be performed.

Lesion characteristics

The target lesion should ideally be discrete (<15mm in length) or tubular (10–20mm in length), with a reference vessel diameter of 2.0–4.0mm, in a vessel of limited tortuosity and in a non-angulated lesion segment, with no visible thrombus.

Contraindications

Due to the risk of entanglement, the use of the Cutting Balloon® is contraindicated in situations where the device would be passed through the struts of a previously placed stent. Use of the Cutting Balloon® for a lesion distal to a previously placed stent requires the operator to be certain that the guide wire has passed through the lumen of the stent rather than through a stent cell. In the treatment of a bifurcation lesion, the Cutting Balloon® should only be used in lesion preparation prior to placing a stent.

AngioSculpt® scoring balloon (Angioscore, USA)

More recently, the AngioSculpt® scoring balloon has been approved for use. This device consists of a flexible

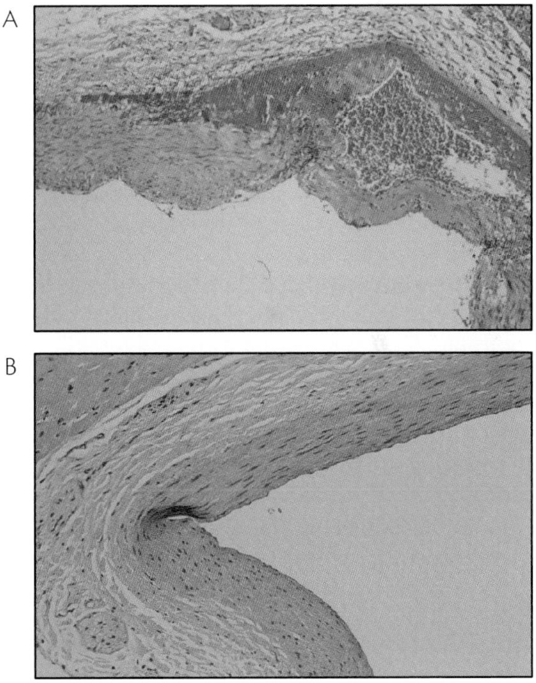

Fig. 35.2 Porcine artery models of the differential acute effects of (A) conventional balloon angioplasty and (B) the Cutting Balloon®, on the vessel wall at 30% over-stretch. Conventional balloons dilate the vessel via fissuring and disruption of the atherosclerotic plaque, dehiscence of the atheroma from the underlying media, and tearing of the intima, By contrast, the Cutting Balloon® scores the plaque by severing the elastic and fibrotic continuity of the vessel wall.

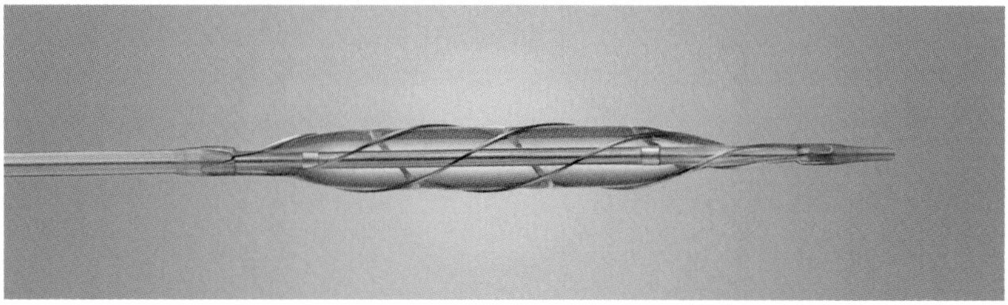

Fig. 35.3 The AngioSculpt® scoring balloon. A flexible nitinol scoring element with three or four rectangular spiral wires is mounted on a conventional semi-compliant nylon balloon. The mechanism of action is similar to that of the cutting balloon. However, the AngioSculpt® has 1.5 times the linear blade length of the Cutting Balloon®.

nitinol scoring element with three or four rectangular spiral wires, approximately 0.13mm in height, mounted on a conventional semi-compliant nylon balloon (Fig. 35.3). Balloon diameters range from 2.0–5.0mm, with a choice of 10, 15, or 20-mm lengths. As with the Cutting Balloon®, the deflated balloon is folded to shield the nitinol wires from the vessel walls. The mechanism of action is similar to that of the Cutting Balloon®. As the balloon inflates, the radial forces are concentrated along the linear cutting surfaces of the nitinol scoring element, allowing a controlled focused force which is equally distributed throughout the surface of the balloon, allowing low-pressure dilatation and avoiding balloon slippage. Once the balloon is deflated, the spiral wires collapse to their original closed configuration. The AngioSculpt® has 1.5 times the linear blade length of the Cutting Balloon®. Balloon diameters ranging from 2.0–3.5mm are compatible with 0.014-inch guide wires, 5F and 6F guiding catheters, whilst 4.0 and 5.0mm diameter balloons are compatible with 0.014- or 0.018-inch guide wires, 6F and 7F guiding catheters. Other technical considerations including sizing of the device, target lesion characteristics, and contraindications are similar to those of the Cutting Balloon®.

Mechanisms of action

Acute lumen gain following conventional balloon angioplasty is achieved by the combined effect of vessel stretching and, to a lesser extent, plaque reduction. During balloon inflation, dilation of the target lesion occurs with a generalized force that is converted to circumferential shear stress because of the artery-balloon geometry, with radial expansion of the vessel. Vessel stretch leads to fissuring and disruption of the atherosclerotic plaque, dehiscence of the atheroma from the underlying media, tearing of the intima, and stretching of the lesser-diseased or non-diseased arterial segment. Furthermore, differential resistance to radial force within the lesion, due to varying degrees of fibrosis or calcification, may result in multiple arcs of dissection.

The acute effect of cutting balloon angioplasty on the vessel wall has been investigated in a number of studies using intravascular ultrasound (IVUS). In the REDUCE (Restenosis reduction by Cutting Balloon evaluation) multi-centre trial, IVUS was performed to compare the extent and mechanisms of acute lumen gain following Cutting Balloon versus conventional balloon angioplasty in 224 patients[(2)]. In non-calcified lesions, the Cutting Balloon® achieved similar luminal dimensions to balloon angioplasty at lower inflation pressures, with increased plaque reduction and a trend towards less vessel expansion. In calcified lesions, acute luminal gain was achieved (as with conventional balloon angioplasty) predominantly by vessel expansion, and was associated with the presence of dissections. Another IVUS study demonstrated a greater contribution of plaque compression (55%) rather than vessel expansion (45%) towards luminal expansion following Cutting Balloon® compared to conventional balloon angioplasty (33% plaque compression, 67% vessel expansion). Importantly, this translated into significantly lower rates of angiographic restenosis (20% vs. 33%, $p < 0.05$) and target lesion revascularization (17% vs. 29%, $p < 0.05$) at 3-month follow-up[(3)]. These studies suggest that cutting balloon angioplasty produces a luminal gain predominantly by compression of plaque rather than vessel expansion and injury. Furthermore, the Cutting Balloon® has been demonstrated to result in less early elastic recoil and early lumen loss at 24h compared to conventional balloon angioplasty [(4)]. Porcine models have demonstrated the AngioSculpt® scoring balloon to induce similar patterns of injury to the Cutting Balloon®, and it is perceived to expand the vessel by the same mechanisms.

Biological response to cutting balloon angioplasty

The strain on the vessel wall following balloon angioplasty triggers a series of cellular and sub-cellular events leading to myointimal proliferation and consequently to restenosis in a substantial proportion of patients. Comparatively, the mechanism of cutting balloon angioplasty leads to a smaller degree of vessel wall injury localized to the area of incisions and sparing the segments in between. Animal experiments have demonstrated that this type of microsurgical incision causes less stretching of the medial smooth muscle cells. Meanwhile, mRNA expression and DNA synthesis of platelet-derived growth factor A (an important mitogen released locally by platelets, in response to tissue trauma, to recruit cells involved in the process of myointimal repair and proliferation) are localized to the incisional segments, in contrast to circumferential vessel wall involvement after conventional balloon angioplasty[5]. In addition, cutting balloon angioplasty appears to induce a lower level of neutrophil activation[6]. This is theoretically advantageous because neutrophil activation can aggravate the endothelial injury, and further stimulate platelets, thus promoting development of intimal hyperplasia and restenosis. Furthermore, lower systemic levels of markers reflective of platelet activation and thrombin formation have been demonstrated following cutting balloon angioplasty compared with conventional balloon angioplasty and stenting[7]. These results suggest that the Cutting Balloon® produces a lower level of localized vascular inflammatory response to the injury it induces than is the case for conventional balloon angioplasty.

De novo coronary lesions

Multiple early case series, as well as small randomized studies suggested the safety and utility of cutting balloon angioplasty, as well as a possible reduction in restenosis in patients treated with cutting balloon compared with balloon angioplasty. The Cutting Balloon Global Randomized Trial was a large multi-centre, randomized trial designed to compare the incidence of restenosis after cutting balloon angioplasty versus conventional balloon angioplasty in the treatment of de novo type A or B lesions up to 20mm in length in native vessels of 2.0–4.0mm in 1238 patients[8]. In contrast to the findings of the preceding smaller series, there were no significant differences between cutting balloon and conventional balloon angioplasty in angiographic or clinical results. The primary endpoint, the 6-month binary angiographic restenosis rate, was 31.4% for cutting balloon and 30.4% for conventional balloon angioplasty, whilst acute procedural success, defined as the attainment of <50% diameter stenosis without in-hospital major adverse cardiac events, was 92.9% for cutting balloon and 94.7% for conventional balloon angioplasty. Five coronary perforations occurred in the cutting balloon arm, and none in the conventional balloon arm. Freedom from target vessel revascularization at nine months was marginally higher in the cutting balloon arm (88.5% vs. 84.6%, $p < 0.05$), whilst there were no significant differences in 9-month major adverse cardiac events. Therefore, the proposed mechanism of controlled dilatation did not translate into a reduction in the rate of angiographic restenosis for the cutting balloon compared with conventional balloon angioplasty in unselective group of patients and lesions. It was concluded that definitive treatment by cutting balloon angioplasty in simple lesions was not superior to conventional balloon angioplasty for the prevention of restenosis, and should be reserved for more complex lesions in which the controlled dilatation of the cutting balloon might provide more advantageous results over conventional balloon angioplasty. Since then, a number of specific clinical applications for the Cutting Balloon® and AngioSculpt® have been described in the literature, as discussed below, including resistant and calcified lesions, aorto-ostial lesions, small vessels, bifurcations, and in-stent restenosis.

Since the advent of intracoronary stents, the role of the plain angioplasty balloon has evolved from that of lesion treatment to lesion preparation. The Cutting Balloon® and AngioSculpt® have recently been re-evaluated in the treatment of de novo lesions in this context. The impact on restenosis of cutting balloon angioplasty prior to bare-metal stenting was evaluated in the REDUCE III prospective randomized multicentre trial[9]. A total of 521 patients with a single target lesion in a native coronary artery less than 4mm in diameter were randomized, of which 260 patients were pre-treated with the Cutting Balloon®, whilst 261 were pre-treated with conventional balloon angioplasty. Sixty-two per cent of the lesions were classified as type B2 or C, and the average vessel diameter was 2.82mm. IVUS-guided procedures were performed in 279 (54%) patients and angiographic guidance was used in the remainder. Post procedure, minimal lumen diameter was significantly greater and percent diameter stenosis was less in the Cutting Balloon® arm, with lower rates of angiographic restenosis (11.8% vs. 19.6%, $p < 0.05$) and less target vessel revascularization (9.6% vs. 15.3%, p <0.05) at 6-month follow-up. However, this result was driven almost entirely by the IVUS-guided Cutting Balloon® group, in which despite similar vessel size and lesion severity, significantly better acute and follow-up results were achieved. It was postulated that IVUS-guidance likely facilitated the use of larger balloons, which favoured the Cutting Balloon® group more by maximizing minimal lumen diameter whilst minimizing vessel injury and risk of complications. It is notable in the modern context that the 6-month restenosis rates in the IVUS-guided Cutting Balloon® group (6.6%) in this study were comparable to those achieved in some drug-eluting stent studies. This study highlighted the importance of optimal lesion preparation and expansion prior to implantation of coronary stents, and this remains an essential component of percutaneous coronary intervention in the drug-eluting stent era. Inadequate stent expansion is recognized as a risk factor for both restenosis and stent thrombosis, yet directly-deployed stents achieve on average only 70% of the diameter and area predicted by their compliance charts[10] and a significant proportion fail to achieve a minimum in-stent luminal area of greater than 5.5mm^2, a consistent predictor of drug-eluting stent failure[11]. In a recent observational, non-randomized study of 299 consecutive de novo lesions larger than 2.5mm, treated with a drug-eluting stent under IVUS guidance, pre-dilatation with the AngioSculpt® balloon resulted in better stent expansion (defined as the ratio of IVUS-measured minimum stent area to the manufacturer's predicted values) compared with either direct stenting or stenting after pre-dilatation with conventional balloon angioplasty (88% vs. 67% and 70% respectively, p <0.001)[12]. Optimal preparation of complex lesions, including calcified lesions, lesions of the left main stem, branch ostial or bifurcation lesions, is even more important in the drug-eluting stent era since these lesions account for an increasing proportion of those tackled by percutaneous coronary intervention.

The Cutting Balloon® and AngioSculpt® in complex lesions

Data on 'real-world' use of the Cutting Balloon® in complex lesion subsets was collected in the Web-Based Cutting Balloon® E-Registry (WINNER)[13], a multicentre, prospective registry of Cutting Balloon® utilization in 52 sites in the United States, reported in 2004. Endpoints included technical success and final residual stenosis, as reported by the operators. Data regarding 868 lesions in 685 patients treated by cutting balloon angioplasty were captured. The results are shown in Table 35.1. In-stent restenosis was an exclusion criterion for the study. In this open registry, the Cutting Balloon® was primarily used in small vessels, bifurcation lesions and ostial/fibrotic lesions with a high degree of technical success and low complication rates.

Table 35.1 Characterization of the use of the Cutting Balloon® in 'real world' settings with respect to lesion subsets, adjunctive stent use and acute procedural outcomes*

Indication	Primary treatment	Prior to planned stent	All lesions
Small vessel	66%	30%	53%
Bifurcation lesion	34%	25%	31%
Ostial/fibrotic lesion	35%	28%	32%
Other (2.0mm–4.0mm)	11%	39%	21%
Device success			
Delivered to lesion	94.2%	96.4%	95%
Dilated lesion	97.4%	96.2%	96.8%
Average residual stenosis	12.8%	3%	N/A
Device safety			
Balloon slippage	0%	0%	0%
Total dissections	9.2%	10.3%	9.7%
Dissection grade C, D, E, F	1.1%	1.2%	1.1%
Perforation	0.4%	0.6%	0.45%

Data from the WINNER Registry, 2004[13].

The U.S. multicentre trial was a multi-centre, non-randomized, single-arm prospective trial, designed to evaluate the use of the AngioSculpt® device in lesion preparation prior to stent implantation in 219 complex lesions in 200 patients enrolled from nine sites[14]. The primary endpoint was procedural success, and clinical follow-up was continued until 14–21 days. Of the 219 lesions, 76% were classified as B2 or C lesions, 35% as moderately or severely calcified, 29% were bifurcations, 13% were ostial lesions, and 16% in-stent restenosis. Average lesion length was 17.8mm, with average reference vessel diameter 2.72mm. Procedural success was achieved in 98.5%. There was no device slippage in de novo or in-stent restenosis lesions. Minor dissections occurred in 13.6% of lesions, all but one resolved after stenting with final TIMI 3 flow in 99%. There were no device-related perforations.

More recently, a large two-centre Israeli registry compiled the clinical experience of the use of the

AngioSculpt® device in 745 lesions in 521 patients for plaque modification prior to stent implantation (predominantly drug-eluting stents)[15]. The primary endpoint was procedural success. The lesions were on average small (2.48mm diameter) and long (19.2mm). 75% were moderately or severely calcified, 53% were B2 or C lesions, 18% were bifurcations and 22% were in-stent restenosis lesions. IVUS was used in the majority of cases (80.1%). In this large series of patients with highly complex disease, the procedural success was 97.9%. Device slippage occurred in only 1.2% of lesions. Significant dissection post-AngioSculpt® was rare (1.5%) and there were no perforations. Long-term follow-up at mean 33 months demonstrated excellent results with a low rate of major adverse cardiac events (7.1%), stent thrombosis (0.9%), and target lesion revascularization (5.9%).

Resistant and calcified lesions

Resistant coronary lesions, due to either calcification or fibrosis within the lesion, remain a challenge for modern percutaneous coronary intervention. Conventional approaches to dilate such lesions with a balloon, including high-pressure inflations, prolonged inflations, balloon oversizing, and the use of non-compliant balloons are often unsuccessful and can lead to plaque shift, balloon rupture, extensive vessel dissection, and even rupture. Meanwhile, high-pressure stent implantation may cause arterial medial disruption, or lipid-core penetration leading to excessive inflammation and neointimal growth. A number of devices, including rotational atherectomy, the Cutting Balloon®, AngioSculpt®, and excimer laser angioplasty have been utilized in resistant lesions with the aim of improving vessel wall compliance and facilitating vessel expansion, either through plaque modification or debulking.

Significant calcification is a strong predictor for decreased success in lesion dilation following balloon angioplasty, whilst calcified lesions make balloon angioplasty unpredictable because of the occurrence of extensive dissection. Furthermore, lesion calcification imposes a rigid obstacle to optimal and symmetrical stent expansion and results in smaller gain compared to non-calcified lesions. Optimal stent expansion reduces restenosis rates, whilst uniform stent expansion in drug-eluting stents ensures maintained integrity of the drug platform and homogenous drug delivery and diffusion into the vessel wall. Importantly, angiography is relatively insensitive for mild or moderate lesion calcification, and frequently underestimates the extent of calcification. By contrast, IVUS is extremely useful in defining plaque geometry, calcification, and complexity. However, if it is not available, fibrocalcific lesions should be suspected if conventional balloons will not expand at 10 atmospheres (Fig. 35.4).

It is now generally accepted that rotational atherectomy is the preferred device for percutaneous treatment of heavily calcified lesions. However, this technique remains technically more difficult, expensive, and is restricted to certain operators in a relatively limited number of centres. By contrast, the Cutting Balloon® and AngioSculpt® use the same technology as conventional balloon angioplasty, require no change in guide wire, no additional operator training, or expensive and technically challenging equipment. Furthermore, calcified lesions may often be amenable to expansion using the Cutting Balloon® or AngioSculpt® after failed conventional balloon expansion (Fig. 35.5). Finally, these devices can be used in heavily calcified lesions after small-burr rotablation (instead of larger burr rotablation) with the goal of minimizing any distal embolization.

By first cutting or scoring the plaque, these devices relieve the hoop stress of the vessel, thereby interrupting the continuity and rigidity imposed by calcium. In the REDUCE trial, an IVUS study comparing mechanisms of lumen enlargement following Cutting Balloon® versus conventional balloon angioplasty in type A and B1 lesions, acute results were favourable for Cutting Balloon® in calcified lesions[2]. However, in that study, calcification was detected on IVUS, and was not even angiographically visible. Karvouni *et al.* evaluated the use of cutting balloon angioplasty in 37 angiographically moderate and severely calcified lesions[16], all of which were classified as B2 or C lesions. Pre-dilatation with conventional balloon angioplasty was performed in 27 lesions. Acute gain following the Cutting Balloon® in predilated lesions was significantly greater than that following conventional balloon predilatation (1.51 vs. 0.78mm, $p < 0.0001$) and was achieved with lower inflation pressures (10.4 vs. 13.2 atmospheres, $p < 0.001$), whilst there was no difference in acute gain achieved by the Cutting Balloon® in pre-dilated and non pre-dilated lesions. However, use of the Cutting Balloon® resulted in more dissections compared to conventional balloon angioplasty in this study, perhaps related to eccentric dilatation and deep vessel injury to the non-calcified part of the vessel wall.

There are also anecdotal reports of the Cutting Balloon® being successful in dilating circumferentially calcified plaque. However, the likelihood of success is lower, and this should be weighed against the risk of perforation.

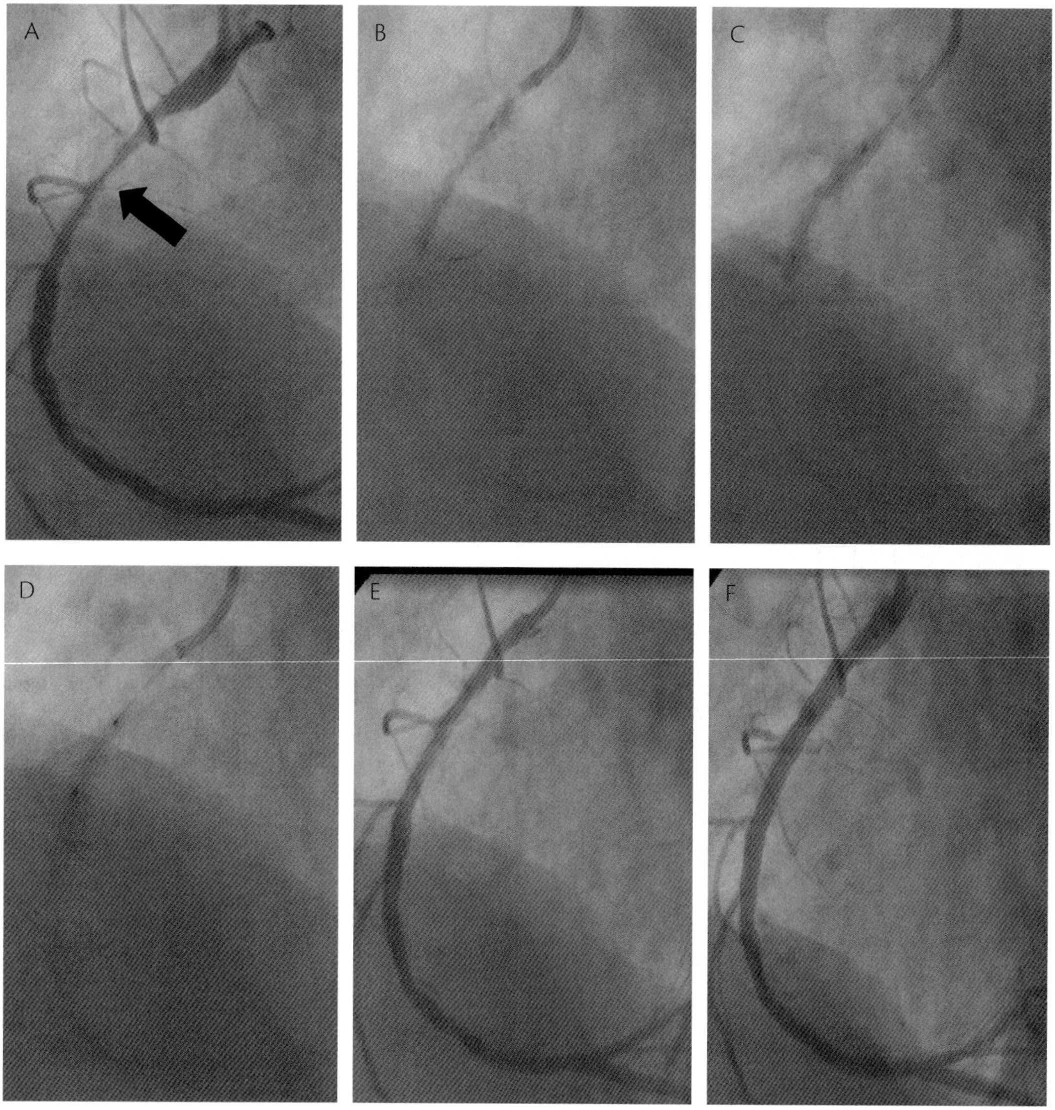

Fig. 35.4 A) Severe resistant lesion in the proximal right coronary artery (black arrow) of an 81-year-old man. Pre-treatment with (B) 2.5 × 20mm and (C) 3.0 × 20mm conventional balloons failed to fully dilate the lesion. D) Dilatation of the lesion with a 2.75 × 10mm Cutting Balloon®. Angiographic result (E) post Cutting Balloon® and (F) after insertion of a 4.0 × 30mm bare-metal stent.

Aorto-ostial lesions

Aorto-ostial lesions are frequently characterized by atherosclerosis, fibrosis, and calcification in the aortic wall, and may be resistant to dilatation by conventional balloon angioplasty despite high-pressure inflations[17]. These properties may affect not only the origins of the native coronary arteries, but also graft insertions at the aorta. Due to the higher concentration of muscle and elastic fibres around the ostium, these lesions also exhibit increased elastic recoil after conventional balloon inflation. Furthermore, aorto-ostial lesions are prone to the phenomenon of 'melon-seeding', whereby ordinary angioplasty balloons slip backwards or forwards through the target lesion. Meanwhile, direct stenting may result in stent underexpansion, malapposition, or embolization distally in ostial disease. The Cutting

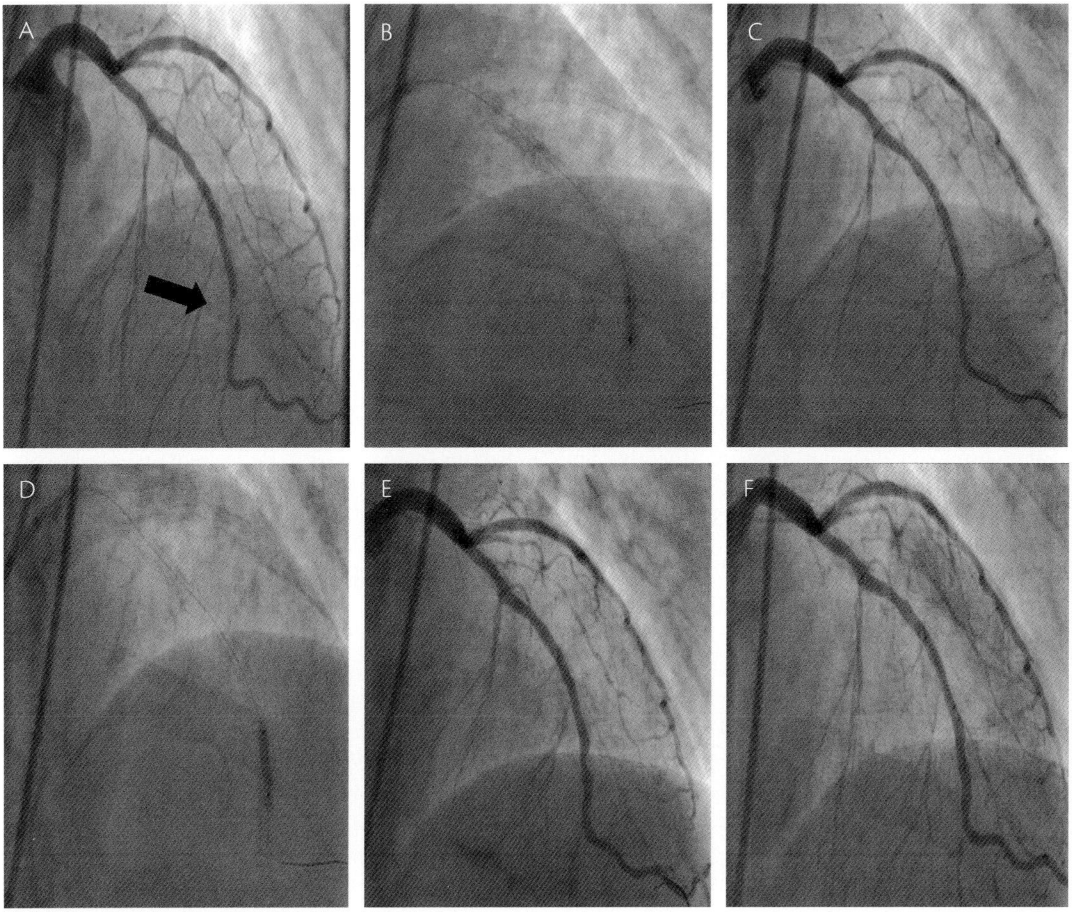

Fig. 35.5 A) Severe resistant lesion (black arrow) in the heavily calcified left anterior descending artery of a 56-year-old woman. Pre-treatment with (B) 2.5 × 9mm conventional balloon failed to fully dilate the lesion, with (C) residual tight stenosis. D) Dilatation of the lesion with a 2.5 × 10mm AngioSculpt®. Angiographic result (E) post AngioSculpt® and (F) after insertion of a 2.25 × 13mm drug-eluting stent, post dilated with a 2.5 × 8mm non-compliant balloon.

Balloon® and AngioSculpt® offer theoretical advantages over conventional balloon angioplasty since they exert a stronger radial force on the vessel wall and are relatively protected against slippage. Kurbaan *et al.*[17]. investigated the use of the Cutting Balloon® in aorto-ostial lesions prior to stent implantation in a small observational study. High-pressure balloon angioplasty (18 atmospheres) led to little change in percent luminal stenosis, which, by contrast, was markedly reduced following use of the Cutting Balloon®. In clinical practice, the Cutting Balloon® and AngioSculpt® are often used to prepare ostial lesions prior to stent insertion (Fig. 35.6). However, there have been no randomized trials to establish the safety or benefits of this technique.

Bifurcation lesions and ostial disease

Bifurcation lesions, which represent up to 20% of the percutaneous coronary intervention caseload, have been consistently associated with: (1) a lower procedural success rate; (2) a relatively high incidence of procedural complications related to plaque shift; (3) ostial recoil; (4) coronary dissection; and (5) restenosis. Consequently, multiple approaches have been developed to prepare and treat these lesions. The Cutting Balloon® and AngioSculpt® offer theoretical advantages in bifurcation lesions by means of targeted vessel trauma, resulting in less damage to the intima, with fewer dissections and less plaque shift. The benefit of

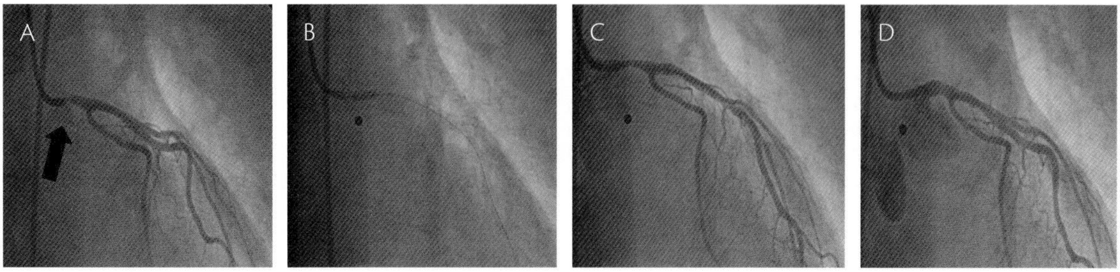

Fig. 35.6 A) Severe ostial lesion of the unprotected left main stem (black arrow) of a 75-year-old man. B) Pre-treatment with a 2.5 × 6mm Cutting Balloon®. Angiographic result (C) post Cutting Balloon® and (D) after insertion of a 4 × 8mm drug-eluting stent.

plaque modification by these devices in bifurcation lesions has been assessed in a number of small studies.

Muramatsu and colleagues compared the results of 39 coronary ostial branch lesions in 37 patients treated by cutting balloon angioplasty with 78 lesions in 74 patients treated by conventional balloon angioplasty[(18)]. The success rate was 94.8% in the cutting balloon group and 84.6% in the conventional balloon angioplasty group (p = ns). Whilst the frequency of intimal dissection was not significantly different between the two groups, all cases of intimal dissection in the cutting balloon group were mild whereas there were many severe intimal dissections following conventional balloon angioplasty. At 5 months follow-up, binary restenosis rates were 43% in the cutting balloon group and 53% following conventional balloon angioplasty (p = ns).

In another retrospective study, the immediate and 3-month follow-up outcome for 87 consecutive bifurcation lesions treated either with conventional balloon angioplasty (37 lesions) or cutting balloon angioplasty (50 lesions) was described[(19)]. This study included lesions in the parent vessel where the side branch originated from the area of stenosis, but the ostium of the side branch itself had minimal or no disease (30%), and true bifurcation lesions with severe stenosis in the parent vessel and the ostium of the side branch (70%). Compared to conventional balloon angioplasty, cutting balloon dilatation was associated with a significant improvement in procedural success (92% vs. 76%, p<0.05), a reduced need for simultaneous or sequential balloon inflations in the side branch (28% vs. 57%, p<0.01), a reduction in the need for bailout stenting (8% vs. 24%, p <0.05), and lower rates of angiographic binary restenosis at 3 months (40% vs. 67%, p <0.05). In the more complex true bifurcation lesions, improved procedural success (94% vs. 75%, p <0.05) and reduced rates of restenosis (44% vs. 77%, p <0.05) were maintained.

The value of the Cutting Balloon® as stand-alone treatment in Duke B and E ostial bifurcation lesions (i.e. Medina 0,1,0 and 0,0,1 respectively) (>70% stenosis involving a diagonal and/or marginal branch >2mm deriving from a non-diseased parent vessel) was assessed in a subgroup analysis within the prospective NICECUT multicentre trial[(20)]. The primary endpoint was the rate of binary stenosis and target lesion revascularization at 6 months; secondary endpoints were procedural success and major adverse cardiac events at 6 months. Sixty-three out of 65 lesions (56 patients) were successfully amenable to treatment with the Cutting Balloon®; 76.9% of patients were successfully treated with Cutting Balloon® as stand-alone procedure, whilst provisional stenting was necessary in 23.1%. Angiographic stenosis was reduced significantly from 86.3% to 7.4% immediately after Cutting Balloon®, and there were no acute complications related to the device. At angiographic follow-up, overall binary stenosis was seen in 23.2% (19.6% side branch, 3.6% parent vessel), target lesion revascularization in 7.7% (6.1% side branch, 1.6% parent vessel), and major adverse cardiac events in 3.6%. In those treated with Cutting Balloon® stand-alone, target lesion revascularization and major adverse cardiac events were 4.0% and 2.0% compared to 20% and 6.7% among those who required stenting. This retrospective subgroup analysis demonstrated that Cutting Balloon® was safe and effective for Duke B and E ostial bifurcation lesions with low plaque burden, and was associated with a low rate of recurrent stenosis. In patients with a Cutting Balloon® stand-alone procedure, ostial obstructive plaque did not adversely affect the parent vessel, and simple single-vessel interventions were carried out solely for the target lesion.

The AngioSculpt® Coronary Bifurcation (AGILITY) study is currently recruiting participants. This trial will evaluate the use of the AngioSculpt® device in patients with de novo coronary artery bifurcation disease involving the ostium of a side branch (medina class 0,0,1) with a simple strategy of AngioSculpt® treatment alone in the side branch, and drug-eluting stent in

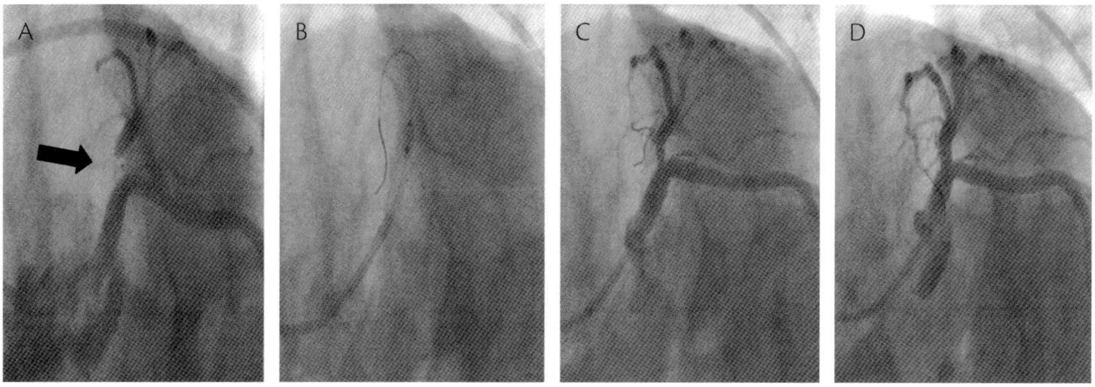

Fig. 35.7 A) Severe ostial lesion of the left anterior descending artery (black arrow) of a 48-year-old man. B) Dilatation of the lesion with a 2.75 × 6mm Cutting Balloon® after pre-treatment with a 2 × 9mm conventional balloon. Angiographic result (C) post Cutting Balloon® and (D) after insertion of a 3.5 × 12mm drug-eluting stent, post-dilated with a 4.0 × 9mm non-compliant balloon.

the main vessel. The study aims to recruit 100 patients, with angiographic follow-up at 9 months, and clinical follow-up at 30 days and 9 months.

Currently, in bifurcation lesions in which there is significant fibrotic plaque at the ostium of a vessel, the use of the Cutting Balloon® or AngioSculpt® as a pre-dilatation strategy before stenting is a reasonable strategy (Fig. 35.7). However, their use in a side branch may be limited by their relatively large profile and reduced flexibility, particularly in angulated bifurcations. Lesions may need pre-dilatation with a conventional balloon before the device will cross into the side branch. Finally, the kissing balloon technique should not be employed using these devices.

Small vessels

Small vessel coronary disease remains a major challenge to revascularization procedures, since often these vessels represent poor targets for coronary artery bypass grafting, and percutaneous coronary interventions are associated with high rates of restenosis. This relates to the fact that the amount of neointimal hyperplasia, and therefore angiographic late luminal loss, following percutaneous coronary intervention is independent of vessel size. Therefore the lumen of the small vessel is compromised earlier, since the cross sectional area is given by πr^2 and the area below which flow can be expected to be compromised is predictable regardless of vessel starting diameter.

The role of the Cutting Balloon® in the treatment of small-vessel disease has been evaluated in a number of small studies. Ergene *et al.*[21] compared the immediate and 6-month follow-up angiographic and clinical outcome of cutting balloon angioplasty (51 lesions in 36 patients) versus conventional balloon angioplasty (47 lesions in 35 patients) in vessels less than 3mm diameter. Procedural success rates were 92% and 97% respectively (p = ns). The immediate post-procedural minimal luminal diameter, residual stenosis and acute gain were similar in both groups, with fewer dissections in the Cutting Balloon® arm. Angiographic binary restenosis at six months was also lower following use of the Cutting Balloon® (27% vs. 47%, $p < 0.05$).

In the single-centre prospective randomized CAPAS trial[22], cutting balloon angioplasty (120 lesions) was compared to conventional balloon angioplasty (128 lesions) in the treatment of type B or C lesions in vessels with reference diameter <3mm. The primary endpoint was 90-day angiographic binary restenosis, with a secondary endpoint of event-free survival at 1 year. Reference diameter was 2.16mm in the Cutting Balloon® group versus 2.18mm in the group treated by conventional balloon angioplasty, with similar pre-procedural percent diameter stenosis. Post-procedural acute vessel gain and residual percent diameter stenosis were similar. However, at 90-day follow-up, angiographic restenosis was significantly lower in the Cutting Balloon® group (25.2% vs. 41.5%, $p < 0.01$) and at 1 year, target lesion revascularization rates were significantly lower than in the conventional balloon angioplasty arm (22.1% vs. 33.9%, $p < 0.05$) suggesting superior angiographic and clinical outcomes for those treated with the Cutting Balloon®.

The effect of cutting balloon angioplasty in vessels less than 3mm diameter has also been evaluated in comparison with both conventional balloon angioplasty and a strategy of gradual and prolonged balloon angioplasty, with cumulative inflation times greater than10min using a perfusion balloon, in a study of 263 patients[23]. The primary endpoint of angiographic binary restenosis at 6 months was lower with gradual and prolonged balloon angioplasty than conventional balloon angioplasty (31.3% vs. 50.6%, $p < 0.05$) with a trend towards lower restenosis rates with cutting balloon angioplasty (32.9%; $p = 0.059$ for cutting balloon vs. conventional balloon angioplasty). This translated into lower rates of target lesion revascularization for both strategies compared to conventional balloon angioplasty (gradual and prolonged balloon angioplasty 20.5% and cutting balloon 20.0% vs. 37.6%, $p < 0.05$ for both).

The results of observational studies and randomized trials comparing bare-metal stents with conventional balloon angioplasty demonstrated that, unlike in larger vessels, bare-metal stents had only modest superiority in reducing restenosis rates. A few studies have compared the effect of the Cutting Balloon® to bare-metal stents in small vessels.

Chung *et al.*[24] evaluated the acute and follow-up results of 61 patients with small branch (<3mm) ostial lesions treated by Cutting Balloon® or bare-metal stent. The stent group achieved greater acute luminal gain, larger minimal lumen diameter, and less percent diameter stenosis. However, at 3-month follow-up, these parameters were equivalent, with less late loss in those treated with the Cutting Balloon®. At 6 months, both angiographic binary restenosis and target lesion revascularization were lower in the Cutting Balloon® group (41% vs. 63% and 29% vs. 53% respectively, $p = 0.05$ for both).

In a larger retrospective study[25] the clinical and angiographic benefits of Cutting Balloon® were compared to both conventional balloon angioplasty and bare-metal stenting in coronary arteries less than 2.5mm in diameter in 327 lesions. At 6-month follow-up, angiographic binary restenosis rates were lower in the Cutting Balloon® arm (31% vs. 46.5% following balloon angioplasty, $p < 0.05$, and vs. 43.9% following implantation of a bare-metal stent, $p = 0.05$). Correspondingly, rates of target lesion revascularization were also lower after Cutting Balloon® than after balloon angioplasty (20.3% vs. 34.7%, $p < 0.05$) but not significantly different to rates following bare-metal stent (27.6%, p = ns). It was concluded that the Cutting Balloon® provided a cost-effective and reasonable approach for the treatment of lesions in small coronary arteries.

In-stent restenosis

Although the incidence of restenosis following conventional balloon angioplasty was markedly reduced by the advent of bare-metal stents, and even further by drug-eluting stents, restenosis—now predominantly in-stent restenosis—remains the major limitation of percutaneous coronary intervention. It represents a significant clinical problem in the form of requirement for further revascularization. The mechanism of in-stent restenosis parallels wound-healing responses, with thrombus deposition and acute inflammation processes in the early phase followed by the smooth muscle cell proliferation. Histologically, in-stent restenotic tissue is composed of a greater proportion of smooth muscle cells, at the expense of macrophage and collagen, compared to restenotic tissue after conventional balloon angioplasty.

Initial management of in-stent restenosis was with conventional balloon angioplasty. However, recurrence rates were unacceptably high, especially in the subgroup of patients with diffuse and/ or severe in-stent restenosis. Debulking techniques including excimer laser angioplasty and directional or rotational atherectomy as well as bare-metal stent-in-stent were proposed as alternative treatment options. However, these techniques did not demonstrate any significant advantage over conventional balloon angioplasty. In particular, whilst repeat stenting with bare-metal stents led to increased acute lumen gain, this was offset by a high late lumen loss. Meanwhile, numerous initial small retrospective studies suggested a benefit for the Cutting Balloon® over conventional balloon angioplasty. There are a number of in-stent restenotic lesion characteristics that make it a favourable lesion subset for use of the Cutting Balloon® or the AngioSculpt® balloon. Due to the slippery surface of the hyperplastic restenotic plaque, conventional balloons tend to slip forward or backwards during inflation into larger segments with lower resistance, so called 'melon seeding'. This effect is reduced by the use of these devices, which are anchored in the plaque by their blades or wires, reducing the likelihood of dissection at the stent edges and injury to vessel wall outside the stented segment. Meanwhile, the framework of the stent protects against perforation in these lesions.

A number of IVUS studies have demonstrated that luminal gain following treatment of in-stent restenosis by conventional balloon angioplasty is due to a combination of extrusion of neointimal tissue through stent struts and additional stent expansion. In comparison, cutting balloon angioplasty for in-stent restenosis has been demonstrated in one study to result in: (1) no increase in total vessel area; (2) a constant stent area; (3) a decrease in plaque area; and (4) an increase in lumen area[26], possibly as a result of a reduction of the plaque by plaque compression and redistribution along the horizontal axis. At a mean follow-up of 5.4 months, the binary restenosis rate was significantly lower in the Cutting Balloon® group compared with the conventional balloon angioplasty group (24% vs. 59%). Correspondingly, mean percent diameter stenosis (36.5% vs. 49.5%) was lower, and minimal lumen area ($4.0mm^2$ vs. $2.5mm^2$) larger in the Cutting Balloon® arm ($p < 0.01$ for both) at follow-up. This predominant mechanism of acute luminal gain by plaque reduction via plaque redistribution following cutting balloon angioplasty was confirmed in another IVUS study of 66 patients and 71 restenotic lesions, which suggested that this plaque reduction accounted for 70% of luminal increase whilst the remainder was due to stent expansion. Favourable IVUS and quantitative coronary angiography results for the Cutting Balloon® were maintained 24h after the procedure[27].

In a matched comparison study of 258 lesions treated for in-stent restenosis[28], four different treatment strategies were compared: (i) cutting balloon angioplasty; (ii) rotational atherectomy; (iii) additional stenting with bare-metal stent;and (iv) conventional balloon angioplasty. Acute lumen gain was significantly higher in the stent group (2.12mm) than the other three strategies which achieved comparable gains (1.70, 1.79, and 1.56mm for Cutting Balloon®, rotational atherectomy and balloon angioplasty respectively). However, the lumen loss at mean follow-up of 11 months was lower for the Cutting Balloon® group (0.63mm vs. 1.30 and 1.36mm for rotational atherectomy and stent respectively, $p < 0.0001$ for both), resulting in a significantly lower restenosis rate (20% vs. 35.9 and 41.4% for rotational atherectomy and stent respectively, $p < 0.05$ for both). By multivariate analysis, cutting balloon angioplasty (odds ratio 0.17) and diffuse in-stent restenosis were identified as predictors of target lesion revascularization.

Two randomized controlled multicentre trials have compared conventional balloon angioplasty with the Cutting Balloon® in the treatment of in-stent restenosis. The RESCUT trial[29] compared the immediate and 7-month results of these two treatments for all types of in-stent restenosis (focal, multifocal, diffuse, and proliferative) in lesions shorter than 25mm. The primary endpoint was angiographic binary restenosis at 7 months. Secondary endpoints included the occurrence of major adverse cardiac events at 30 days and 7 months, the need for target lesion revascularization, and the pattern of restenosis recurrence. In this study, the number of balloons used was significantly lower in the Cutting Balloon® arm, and balloon slippage was less frequent (6.5% vs. 25%, $p < 0.01$). The Cutting Balloon® was shorter, and inflated to lower maximal pressures, with a trend toward a lower need for additional stenting (3.9% vs. 8%, $p = 0.07$) due to a lower frequency of residual stenosis greater than 30% and fewer complex dissections. However, in contrast to previous smaller studies, there were no significant differences between the two approaches regarding any of the pre-defined study endpoints above. Angiographic binary restenosis rates were 29.8% in the Cutting Balloon® arm and 31.4% following conventional balloon angioplasty ($p = ns$), whilst target lesion revascularization rates were 13.5% and 13.1% respectively ($p = ns$).

In the REDUCE II trial, 248 patients with in-stent restenotic lesions were randomized to treatment with the Cutting Balloon®, and 244 to conventional balloon angioplasty. Binary restenosis at 6 months was 24% for cutting balloon and 22% for conventional balloon angioplasty, whilst target lesion revascularization rates were 20% for both groups. This trial did not show any significant difference between cutting balloon and conventional balloon angioplasty in the treatment of in-stent restenosis[30].

Prior to the advent of drug-eluting stents, intracoronary brachytherapy was established as an effective therapy for in-stent restenosis. However, a major limitation was the occurrence of the 'edge effect', i.e. re-restenosis at the margins of the treated area. This was related to geographical miss, a phenomenon that described unintentional balloon injury of the vessel outside the radiation treatment area. Therefore interest developed in the use of the cutting balloon technique prior to intracoronary brachytherapy in the treatment of in-stent restenosis. Theoretically, the cutting balloon would lead to controlled dissection and vessel dilatation without slippage of the balloon, or 'melon-seeding', and therefore a reduction in uncontrolled injury and prevention of geographical miss. In the RENO registry, 166 patients pre-treated with the Cutting Balloon® prior to beta radiation had lower rates of major adverse cardiac events, including target vessel revascularization, at 6 months than a reference group of 712 patients pre-treated with conventional balloon angioplasty (10.2% vs. 16.6%, $p < 0.05$)[31]. However, this was a non-randomized registry study, and in addition, lesion length, vessel diameter, and source distance were different for both groups. Furthermore, other studies have failed to show any superiority of cutting balloon angioplasty over conventional angioplasty prior to intracoronary brachytherapy in terms of either acute results or restenosis rates. Meanwhile, brachytherapy has limited availability, is costly, requires additional training and

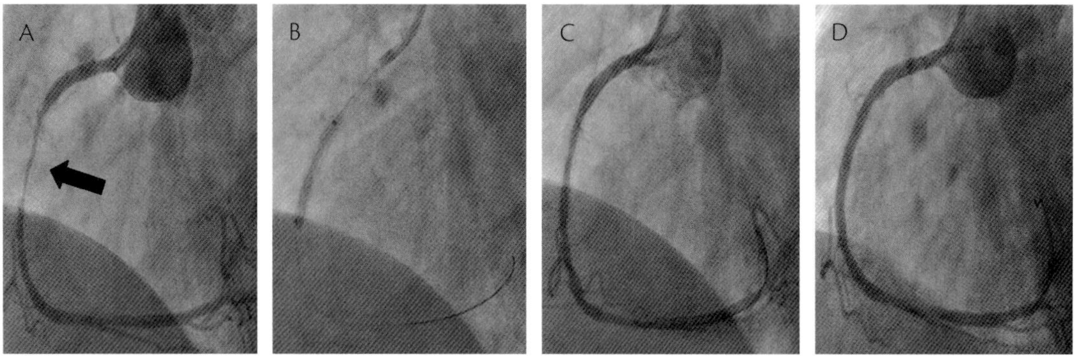

Fig. 35.8 A) Severe diffuse in-stent restenosis in a 2.5 × 24mm drug-eluting stent implanted in the right coronary artery of a 64-year-old woman 5 years previously (black arrow). B) Successful dilatation of the lesion with a 2.5 × 20mm AngioSculpt® after a 2.5 × 15mm conventional balloon slipped forwards and backwards without dilating the lesion. Angiographic results (C) post AngioSculpt® and (D) after insertion of a 3.0 × 30mm drug-eluting stent, post-dilated with a 3.25 × 8mm non-compliant balloon.

personnel, and has now been superseded by drug-eluting stents, which not only avoid all of these issues, but have also been demonstrated to be superior in the treatment of in-stent restenosis[32].

Whilst the implantation of drug-eluting stents has become the widely established treatment for bare-metal in-stent restenosis, their efficacy in complex in-stent restenosis is, as expected, less effective than in focal in-stent restenosis or in de novo lesions. The Cutting Balloon® or AngioSculpt® device can be used in lesion preparation prior to the insertion of a drug-eluting stent to prevent 'melon seeding' and to facilitate optimal stent expansion via maximizing plaque reduction.

Currently, little information is available regarding the best treatment for in-stent restenosis in drug-eluting stents. Most operators favour implanting a second, different, drug-eluting stent. However, the rates of re-restenosis remain high. The use of debulking devices, including the Cutting Balloon® and AngioSculpt®, inside a drug-eluting stent might theoretically disrupt the polymer coating, with the potential adverse effects of exposing elements of the polymer to the systemic circulation, or releasing significant reservoirs of unreleased drug. However, the clinical significance of this remains unknown, and these devices are currently used in this setting in lesion preparation, again to avoid balloon slippage and allow maximal plaque reduction prior to implanting a second drug-eluting stent (Fig. 35.8).

The Focal In-Stent Restenosis After Drug-Eluting Stent (FOCUS) trial is currently recruiting. In this study, patients with focal drug-eluting stent restenosis (lesion length <10mm) with diameter stenosis greater than 50% with documented myocardial ischaemia or symptoms of angina will be randomized in a 1:1 fashion to Cypher® stent (Cordis, USA) versus cutting balloon angioplasty. The primary endpoint will be angiographic binary in-segment restenosis at 9 months, with secondary endpoints of a composite of death, myocardial infarction or target vessel revascularization; stent thrombosis in hospital, at 30 days, 9 months and 1 year; and late lumen loss at 9 months.

The Cutting Balloon® and AngioSculpt® remain important tools for the interventional cardiologist in a variety of these lesion subsets. Common indications for their use in contemporary percutaneous coronary intervention practice are listed in Table 35.2.

Complications

Complications associated with the use of the Cutting Balloon® or AngioSculpt® balloon are infrequent, and include coronary dissection, perforation, spasm, and device entrapment within a vessel or stent (Table 35.3).

Table 35.2 Common indications for the use of the Cutting Balloon® or AngioSculpt® in contemporary percutaneous coronary intervention practice

Lesions resistant to conventional balloon dilatation
Lesions already prepared by conventional balloon that still do not allow stent access
Aorto-ostial and ostial lesions
In-stent restenosis
Resistant lesions within stented segments

Table 35.3 Technical problems and reasons for failure with the Cutting Balloon® or AngioSculpt®

Failure to access resistant lesion
Difficulty sizing balloon to vessel
Device entrapment
Vessel haematoma/dissection/perforation

The risk of coronary dissection may relate to the presence of a number of different factors. Indeed, many of the lesion characteristics for which these devices are indicated, including calcified, eccentric, long, or complex lesions, are associated with a higher risk of coronary dissection in their own right. As with coronary dissections following conventional balloon angioplasty in the current era, assuming a guide wire is (or can be) positioned in the true lumen, dissections following the use of these devices can be treated with the deployment of stents to tack the dissection flap.

Perforations are similarly more common in complex lesions, and particular care must be taken with these devices in calcified or eccentric lesions, or lesions in tortuous vessels, whilst overzealous balloon inflations must be avoided. The appearance of an overexpanded vessel after the use of these devices should raise suspicion of an excessively deep cut and the risk of dissection/ perforation. Management of coronary perforations is no different to that following the use of conventional balloons.

Entrapment of the device during the treatment of in-stent restenosis may occur following the inadvertent passage of the wire through an incompletely apposed stent strut, and if there is any question about the location of the wire, the use of these devices should be avoided. A number of strategies exist to remove an entrapped AngioSculpt® or Cutting Balloon®. Initially, the device should be advanced forward and rotated to unhook a potentially trapped atherotome or wire strut. Other techniques include the use of a second balloon inflated alongside the entrapped device to distort the relationship between the device and the stent, and cautious deep-seating of the guiding catheter into the artery to allow concentrated retraction force. If these manoeuvres are unsuccessful, then surgical removal of the device with coronary artery bypass grafting must be considered.

Future directions

Animal feasibility testing is underway in the development of a paclitaxol-coated AngioSculpt® device. Preliminary results with drug-coated conventional balloons are encouraging, and drug delivery to the vessel wall may be more effective with a scoring element. In the future, this may allow stand-alone therapy in a range of coronary lesions without adjunctive stenting.

Conclusion

The 'average' case in interventional cardiology is now well treated using modern balloon and stent technologies. In a minority of cases, however, additional lesion preparation is of value and the Cutting Balloon® or AngioSculpt® represent valuable options in this category. The potential value of these devices in resistant, restenotic, and ostial disease is well recognized by the experienced operator, despite relatively modest scientific data.

References

1. Barath P, Fishbein MC, Vari S, *et al.* Cutting balloon: a novel approach to percutaneous angioplasty. *Am J Cardiol* 1991; **68**(11):1249–52.
2. Okura H, Hayase M, Shimodozono S, *et al.* Mechanisms of acute lumen gain following cutting balloon angioplasty in calcified and noncalcified lesions: an intravascular ultrasound study. *Catheter Cardiovasc Interv* 2002; **57**(4):429–36.
3. Hara H, Nakamura M, Asahara T, *et al.* Intravascular ultrasonic comparisons of mechanisms of vasodilatation of cutting balloon angioplasty versus conventional balloon angioplasty. *Am J Cardiol* 2002; **89**(11):1253–6.
4. Kawaguchi K, Kondo T, Shumiya T, *et al.* Reduction of early elastic recoil by cutting balloon angioplasty as compared to conventional balloon angioplasty. *J Invasive Cardiol* 2002; **14**(9):515–19.
5. Barath P. Microsurgical Dilatation Concept: Animal Data. *J Invasive Cardiol* 1996; **8**(Suppl A):2A–5A.
6. Inoue T, Sakai Y, Hoshi K, *et al.* Lower expression of neutrophil adhesion molecule indicates less vessel wall injury and might explain lower restenosis rate after cutting balloon angioplasty. *Circulation* 1998; **97**(25):2511–18.
7. Namiki A, Toma H, Nakamura M, *et al.* Hemostatic and fibrinolytic activation is less following cutting balloon angioplasty of the coronary arteries. *Jpn Heart J* 2004; **45**(3):409–17.
8. Mauri L, Bonan R, Weiner BH, *et al.* Cutting balloon angioplasty for the prevention of restenosis: results of the Cutting Balloon Global Randomized Trial. *Am J Cardiol* 2002; **90**(10):1079–83.
9. Ozaki Y, Yamaguchi T, Suzuki T, *et al.* Impact of cutting balloon angioplasty (CBA) prior to bare metal stenting on restenosis. *Circ J* 2007; **71**(1):1–8.
10. de Ribamar Costa J, Mintz GS, Carlier SG, *et al.* Intravascular ultrasonic assessment of stent diameters derived from manufacturer's compliance charts. *Am J Cardiol* 2005; **96**(1):74–8.

11. Hong MK, Mintz GS, Lee CW, *et al.* Intravascular ultrasound predictors of angiographic restenosis after sirolimus-eluting stent implantation. *Eur Heart J* 2006; **27**(11):1305–10.
12. de Ribamar Costa J, Mintz GS, Carlier SG, *et al.* Non randomized comparison of coronary stenting under intravascular ultrasound guidance of direct stenting without predilation versus conventional predilation with a semi-compliant balloon versus predilation with a new scoring balloon. *Am J Cardiol* 2007; **100**(5):812–17.
13. Taniuchi M. The WINNER registry: utilization of cutting balloon device in "real world" settings. *Cathet Cardiovasc Interv* 2004; **62**(1):122 (C-36).
14. Costa RA, Mooney MR, Teirstein PS, *et al.* Final Results from the U.S. multi-center Trial of the AngioSculpt Scoring Balloon Catheter for the Treatment of Complex Coronary Artery Lesions. *Am J Cardiol* 2006; **98**(8 (Suppl)):121M.
15. Grenadier E, Kerner A, Gershony G, *et al.* Optimizing plaque modification in complex lesions utilizing the AngioSculpt device: acute and long term results from a large two-centre registry. *Am J Cardiol* 2008; **102**(8(Suppl 1)):531.
16. Karvouni E, Stankovic G, Albiero R, *et al.* Cutting balloon angioplasty for treatment of calcified coronary lesions. *Catheter Cardiovasc Interv* 2001; **54**(4):473–81.
17. Kurbaan AS, Kelly PA, Sigwart U. Cutting balloon angioplasty and stenting for aorto-ostial lesions. *Heart* 1997; **77**(4):350–2.
18. Muramatsu T, Tsukahara R, Ho M, *et al.* Efficacy of cutting balloon angioplasty for lesions at the ostium of the coronary arteries. *J Invasive Cardiol* 1999; **11**(4):201–6.
19. Takebayashi H, Haruta S, Kohno H, *et al.* Immediate and 3-month follow-up outcome after cutting balloon angioplasty for bifurcation lesions. *J Interv Cardiol* 2004; **17**(1):1–7.
20. Dahm JB, Dörr M, Scholz E, *et al.* Cutting-balloon angioplasty effectively facilitates the interventional procedure and leads to a low rate of recurrent stenosis in ostial bifurcation coronary lesions: A subgroup analysis of the NICECUT multicenter registry. *Int J Cardiol* 2008; **124**(3):345–50.
21. Ergene O, Seyithanoglu BY, Tastan A, *et al.* Comparison of angiographic and clinical outcome after cutting balloon and conventional balloon angioplasty in vessels smaller than 3 mm in diameter: a randomized trial. *J Invasive Cardiol* 1998; **10**(2):70–5.
22. Izumi M, Tsuchikane E, Funamoto M, *et al.* Final results of the CAPAS trial. *Am Heart J* 2001; **142**(5):782–9.
23. Umeda H, Iwase M, Kanda H, *et al.* Promising efficacy of primary gradual and prolonged balloon angioplasty in small coronary arteries: a randomized comparison with cutting balloon angioplasty and conventional balloon angioplasty. *Am Heart J* 2004; **147**(1):E4.
24. Chung CM, Nakamura S, Tanaka K, *et al.* Comparison of cutting balloon vs stenting alone in small branch ostial lesions of native coronary arteries. *Circ J* 2003; **67**(1):21–5.
25. Iijima R, Ikari Y, Wada M, *et al.* Cutting balloon angioplasty is superior to balloon angioplasty or stent implantation for small coronary artery disease. *Coron Artery Dis* 2004; **15**(7):435–40.
26. Muramatsu T, Tsukahara R, Ho M, *et al.* Efficacy of cutting balloon angioplasty for in-stent restenosis: an intravascular ultrasound evaluation. *J Invasive Cardiol* 2001; **13**(6):439–44.
27. Montorsi P, Galli S, Fabbiocchi F, *et al.* Mechanism of cutting balloon angioplasty for in-stent restenosis: an intravascular ultrasound study. *Catheter Cardiovasc Interv* 2002; **56**(2):166–73.
28. Adamian M, Colombo A, Briguori C, *et al.* Cutting balloon angioplasty for the treatment of in-stent restenosis: a matched comparison with rotational atherectomy, additional stent implantation and balloon angioplasty. *J Am Coll Cardiol* 2001; **38**(3):672–9.
29. Albiero R, Silber S, Di Mario C, *et al.* Cutting balloon versus conventional balloon angioplasty for the treatment of in-stent restenosis: results of the restenosis cutting balloon evaluation trial (RESCUT). *J Am Coll Cardiol* 2004; **43**(6):943–9.
30. Suzuki T. REDUCE II Clinical Study. Transcatheter Cardiovascular Therapeutics, 2002.
31. Roguelov C, Eeckhout E, De Benedetti E, *et al.* Clinical outcome following combination of cutting balloon angioplasty and coronary beta-radiation for in-stent restenosis: a report from the RENO registry. *J Invasive Cardiol* 2003; **15**(12):706–9.
32. Mukherjee D, Moliterno DJ. Brachytherapy for in-stent restenosis: a distant second choice to drug-eluting stent placement. *JAMA* 2006; **295**(11):1307–9.

CHAPTER 36

Thrombus extraction in the contemporary management of ST-segment elevation myocardial infarction

Youlan L. Gu and Felix Zijlstra

Background and introduction

ST-segment elevation myocardial infarction (STEMI) is primarily caused by an acute thrombotic event resulting in total occlusion of a coronary artery. The precipitating factor for acute thrombosis is generally the rupture of a coronary atherosclerotic plaque, responsible for approximately 75% of all coronary thrombi leading to myocardial infarction (MI) or death(1). After rupture of the atherosclerotic plaque, fragments of its lipid-rich core are exposed to the arterial lumen. This highly thrombogenic material induces local platelet aggregation, resulting in an early mural thrombus that partially occludes the artery. In time, the formation of a fibrin network causes consolidation of the thrombus. This can be followed by stabilization of the plaque without clinical sequelae, but additional thrombus formation may progress until eventually the whole lumen can be occluded. If occlusion continues for several hours, the ischaemic myocardium becomes irreversibly damaged. The longer this coronary occlusion persists, the worse the clinical outcomes are(2).

Historically, treatment of STEMI has focused on restoring flow in the infarct-related artery by dissolving, compressing, or surgically bypassing the occlusion. In recent years, it is widely accepted that primary percutaneous coronary intervention (PCI) consisting of coronary stenting with or without balloon angioplasty is the preferred reperfusion strategy for STEMI patients(2). This approach is able to restore flow through the epicardial artery in over 90% of patients and is associated with favourable short- and long-term survival(3).

However, reperfusion of the myocardium still remains impaired in over 50% of patients after successful primary PCI, which is a strong predictor of long-term mortality(4,5). Therefore, these suboptimal results of the conventional primary PCI strategy have spurred the development of adjunctive approaches to reperfuse the occluded artery.

One of the causes of impaired myocardial perfusion is the occurrence of embolization of atherothrombotic material from the intracoronary thrombus or the ruptured plaque into the distal circulation. Embolization can occur both spontaneously during plaque rupture or thrombus formation as well as during reperfusion, induced by the intracoronary therapy of balloon angioplasty and stenting, leading to obstruction of the distal microcirculation and impaired reperfusion and myocardial salvage(6). In accordance, angiographically visible embolization of atherothrombotic debris into the distal circulation after primary PCI is present in up to 16% of patients and is associated with impaired myocardial perfusion, larger infarct size, reduced left ventricular function, and increased mortality(7). Furthermore, the incidence of distal embolization is related to the presence and severity of angiographically visible thrombus(8,9).

In recognition of the clinical impact of atherothrombotic embolization, it became attractive to develop mechanical interventions to reduce its occurrence. These devices remove atherothrombotic debris not by compressing but by extracting or entrapping the atherothrombotic material. In the latest guidelines on the management of patients presenting with STEMI, the use of these devices are recommended as adjunctive therapy to primary PCI to improve myocardial perfusion[2].

This chapter focuses on the role of devices to extract thrombus during primary PCI in patients with STEMI. The first section will discuss methods to evaluate thrombus, including visual assessment on coronary angiography, intracoronary imaging modalities, and histopathological analysis. Second, an overview of the types of extraction devices will be provided, divided into distal protection devices, non-manual thrombus aspiration devices, and manual thrombus aspiration catheters. In the following section, the clinical role of these devices will be evaluated in the current strategy of primary PCI in patients with STEMI. Finally, two clinical cases will be presented of patients with STEMI, illustrating the pivotal role of thrombus extraction in the contemporary percutaneous management of STEMI patients. It is neither the scope of this chapter to review the use of mechanical devices in indications other than STEMI, such as in non-ST-segment elevation acute coronary syndromes, nor to review its use in other interventions, such as vein grafts and peripheral arteries.

Table 36.1 TIMI thrombus grading score

TIMI thrombus grade	Definition
0	No angiographic characteristics of thrombus
1	Possible thrombus present, angiographic characteristics such as reduced contrast density, haziness, irregular lesion contour, or a smooth convex 'meniscus' at the site of total occlusion suggestive but not diagnostic of thrombus
2	Definitive thrombus, greatest dimensions ≤1/2 vessel diameter
3	Definitive thrombus, greatest dimensions >1/2 but <2 vessel diameter
4	Definitive thrombus, greatest dimensions ≥2 vessel diameter
5	Total occlusion

Thrombus characterization

Intracoronary imaging

The presence of intracoronary thrombus was first demonstrated invasively by De Wood and colleagues[10], who retrieved thrombus using a Fogarty catheter from the coronary artery of STEMI patients with and without angiographic features of thrombus. Angiographic criteria for the presence of thrombus in a coronary artery were defined by Mabin and colleagues[11] as: 1) the presence of an intraluminal central filling defect or lucency surrounded by contrast material that is seen in multiple projections; 2) absence of calcium within the defect; and 3) persistence of contrast material within the lumen. To assess the severity of the thrombotic lesion, the TIMI (Thrombolysis in Myocardial Infarction) thrombus score is widely adopted in clinical practice and clinical trials[12]. This score ranges from grade 0, representing no presence of angiographic thrombus, to grade 5, representing total occlusion (Table 36.1).

Despite these clear definitions and their use in many important trials assessing intracoronary interventions, these visual estimations underestimate the incidence of thrombus as illustrated by the high retrieval rate of atherothrombotic material when thrombus aspiration is performed[13,14]. In addition, it is impossible to assess thrombus burden on the coronary angiogram in patients presenting with total occlusion of the infarct-related artery. In recent years, several technical advancements have enabled a more objective assessment of thrombus presence and size. These intracoronary imaging modalities include angioscopy, intravascular ultrasound, and optical coherence tomography (OCT). Of these modalities, OCT seems to be most promising, being superior in characterizing the coronary atherosclerotic plaque as well as in identifying thrombus in STEMI patients[15,16]. At least, all of these techniques are better able to identify presence of thrombus in STEMI patients than coronary angiography.

Histopathological analysis

As discussed earlier, the actual rate of retrieved atherothrombotic material by aspiration devices is far higher than can be assessed visually by coronary angiography of the culprit lesion. Similarly, the retrieval rate by distal protection devices is much higher than the incidence of angiographically visible distal embolization[7–9,17].

Atherothrombotic material consists of platelets, erythrocytes, and components of atherosclerotic plaque such as vessel wall fragments, cholesterol crystals, inflammatory cells, and collagen tissue. When platelet aggregation occurs, caused by atherosclerotic plaque rupture, a mural white thrombus is formed first consisting mainly of platelets. During this early phase with intermittent coronary flow, the white thrombus is unstable and easily embolizes into the distal circulation[1,6]. As platelet aggregation continues, the formation of a fibrin

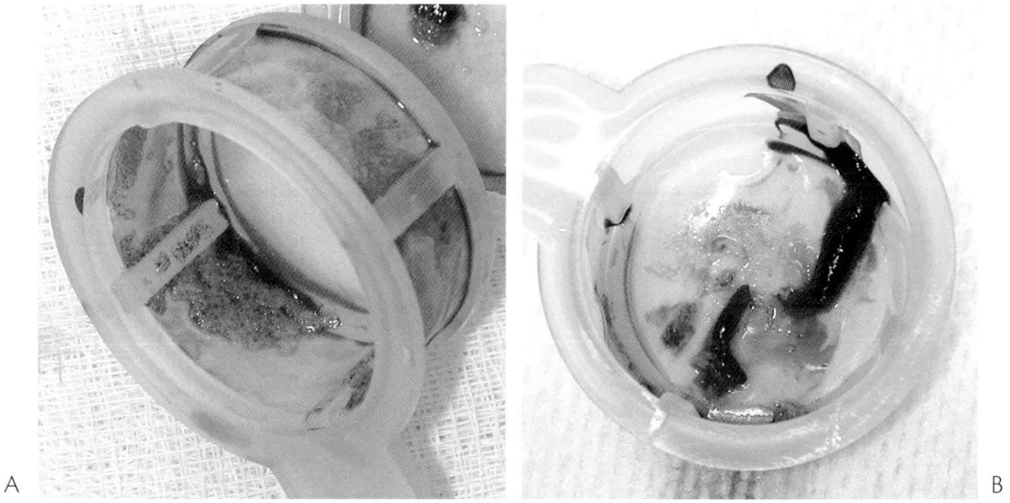

Fig. 36.1 Macroscopical images of retrieved atherothrombotic material showing white (A) and red (B) thrombus.

network causes stabilization of the white platelet-rich thrombus, which may result in total coronary occlusion. When obstruction of coronary flow persists, blood coagulates proximal and distal to the occlusion and causes red thrombus formation, consisting mainly of erythrocytes and inflammatory cells entrapped by a fibrin network[(18)].

Several studies have reported histopathological features of retrieved atherothrombotic material. Macroscopically, the distinction between white and red thrombus can be made on the retrieved atherothrombotic debris (Fig. 36.1), while plaque is only identified on histopathological analysis. Fig. 36.2 shows histopathological examples of white and red thrombus. In a study with manually aspirated atherothrombotic material, the majority consisted of platelets only (68%), mostly smaller than 0.5mm in size, while 15% contained organized layers of erythrocytes that were generally larger (>2.0mm)[(14)]. In 17%, plaque components were identified. In patients with angiographically visible distal embolization after PCI, the histopathological specimens contain erythrocytes more often and are generally larger compared to the specimens of patients without embolization[(8)]. Another feature that has been studied is the age of aspirated atherothrombotic debris. In STEMI patients presenting within 6h of symptom onset, the aspirated atherothrombotic material was at least in part older than 1 day in 51%[(19)], emphasizing that the process of thrombus formation can be initiated long before clinical symptoms occur.

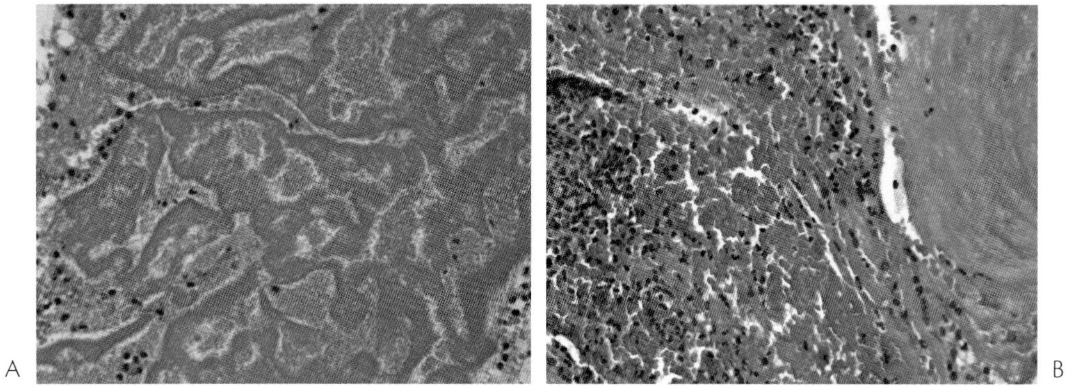

Fig. 36.2 Histopathological images of atherothrombotic material containing platelets only (white thrombus, A) and erythrocytes (red thrombus, B).

Table 36.2 Trials performed with distal protection devices in patients with ST-segment elevation myocardial infarction

Author	Acronym	Year*	No.	Device	Design	Angiography	Primary endpoint	Outcome	FU (days)
Stone[17]	EMERALD	2005	501	GuardWire Plus®	Multi-centre	–	STR, infarct size	–	180
Gick[23]	PROMISE	2005	200	FilterWire-Ex®	Single-centre	Thrombus present, IRA ≥3mm	Flow velocity	–	30
Cura[24]	PREMIAR	2007	140	SpideRX®	Multi-centre	TIMI <3, IRA ≥2.5mm	STR	–	180
Muramatsu[22]	ASPARAGUS	2007	341	GuardWire Plus®	Multi-centre	IRA ≥2.5mm	TIMI flow, cTFC, MBG	+/–	30
Kelbaek[25]	DEDICATION	2008	626	Filter Wire-Ex®	Multi-centre	–	STR	–	30

*Year of publication as full article

cTFC, corrected TIMI frame count; FU, follow-up; IRA, infarct-related artery; MBG, myocardial blush grade; No., number of patients; TIMI, Thrombolysis in Myocardial Infarction; STR, ST-segment resolution.

Not only have studies on thrombus characterization provided insights into the pathophysiology of infarction, but these characteristics may also be useful in the prediction of clinical risk and outcome[20,21]: the age of aspirated thrombus is an independent predictor of long-term mortality in STEMI patients undergoing primary PCI[21].

Types of thrombus extraction devices

Thrombus extraction devices are classified into distal protection devices, non-manual thrombus aspiration devices, and manual thrombus aspiration catheters. An overview of efficacy studies investigating these devices is shown in Tables 36.2–36.4.

Distal protection devices

These devices have an occlusive balloon or non-occlusive filter that is placed distally to the lesion in order to retrieve atherothrombotic material that would otherwise embolize into the distal circulation. The Enhanced Myocardial Efficacy and Recovery by Aspiration of Liberated Debris (EMERALD) trial randomized 501 patients to PCI without or without the GuardWire Plus® System (Medtronic Inc., Santa Rosa, USA), an occlusive balloon device. Distal protection neither reduced infarct size as measured by technetium (Tc) 99m sestamibi imaging, nor did it improve the incidence of complete ST-segment resolution[17]. A Japanese trial confirmed the negative results with the use of an occlusive device[22]. Similar negative results were reported in trials investigating distal filter systems in STEMI patients. The FilterWire-EX® (Boston Scientific Corp., Natick, USA) showed no improvement of coronary flow velocity or infarct size as assessed by magnetic resonance imaging (MRI)[23]. Likewise, the SpideRX® protection device (ev-3, Minneapolis, USA) did not demonstrate improvement of ST-segment resolution as compared to conventional primary PCI[24]. The Drug Elution and Distal Protection in ST-Elevation Myocardial Infarction (DEDICATION) trial, the largest distal protection trial (n = 626) did not show improvement of myocardial perfusion as assessed by ST-segment resolution in patients randomized to the FilterWire-EX® or SpideRX® device[25].

Non-manual thrombus aspiration devices

Non-manual aspiration devices are characterized by fragmentation of atherothrombotic material prior to aspiration or aspiration by means of an external mechanical pump. The X-Sizer® catheter (ev-3, White Bear Lake, USA) is a dual-lumen over-the-wire system that has a helical-shaped cutter at the distal tip of the inner lumen. Driven by a hand-held control unit, this system rotates at 2100rpm once activated, fragmenting and collecting the atherothrombotic debris in a vacuum bottle through the outer lumen. Small- to medium-sized randomized clinical trials have shown that the X-Sizer® system improves electrocardiographic markers of myocardial perfusion and reduces the incidence of angiographically visible distal embolization in comparison to conventional PCI in patients with STEMI[26–28].

Table 36.3 Trials performed with non-manual thrombus aspiration devices in patients with ST-segment elevation myocardial infarction

Author	Acronym	Year*	No	Device	Design	Angiography	Primary endpoint	Outcome	FU (days)
Beran[28]		2002	66	X-Sizer®	Single-centre	Vessel occlusion/ intraluminal filling defect	cTFC	+	30
Napodano[27]		2003	92	X-Sizer®	Single-centre	TIMI ≤2, TS ≥2, and/or ≥70% stenosis, IRA ≥2.5mm	MBG	+	30
Antoniucci[29]		2004	100	AngioJet®	Single-centre	IRA ≥2.5mm	STR	+	30
Lefevre[26]	X AMINE ST	2005	201	X-Sizer®	Multicentre	TIMI 0/1, thrombus present, IRA ≥2.5mm	STR	+	180
Ikari[53]	VAMPIRE	2008	355	TVAC®	Multicentre	IRA 2.5–5mm	Slow/no reflow	+/–	240
Kaltoft[54]		2006	215	Rescue®	Single-centre	–	Myocardial salvage	–	30
Ali[30]	AIMI	2006	480	AngioJet®	Multicentre	IRA >2.0mm	Infarct size	–	30

*Year of publication as full article.

cTFC, corrected TIMI frame count; FU, follow-up; IRA, infarct-related artery; MBG, myocardial blush grade; No, number of patients; TIMI, Thrombolysis in Myocardial Infarction; STR, ST-segment resolution.

A different approach to fragmenting thrombus is used in rheolytic thrombectomy with the AngioJet® catheter (Possis Medical, Inc., Minneapolis, USA). Based on Bernoulli's principle, a piston pump produces a high-pressure saline jet that is ejected against a loop in the distal tip, creating a local low-pressure zone. At the tip, atherothrombotic material is aspirated, fragmented, and removed. Compared with conventional PCI, rheolytic thrombectomy led to a higher rate of ST-segment resolution, better coronary flow, and a smaller infarct size as assessed by Tc 99m sestamibi imaging at 1 month[29]. However, these positive results could not be reproduced in the larger AngioJet Rheolytic Thrombectomy In Patients Undergoing Primary Angioplasty for Acute Myocardial Infarction (AIMI) trial in 480 patients, showing no differences in myocardial

Table 36.4 Trials performed with manual thrombus aspiration devices in patients with ST-segment elevation myocardial infarction

Author	Acronym	Year*	No.	Device	Design	Angiography	Primary endpoint	Outcome	FU (days)
Burzotta[31]	EMEDIA	2005	99	Diver CE	Single-centre	–	MBG, STR	+	30
De Luca[35]		2006	76	Diver CE	Single-centre	TIMI 0/1, thrombus present, successful PCI	LV remodelling	+	180
Silva-Orrego[13]	DEAR-MI	2006	148	Pronto	Single-centre	–	MBG + STR	+	In-hospital
Svilaas[14]	TAPAS	2008	1071	Export	Single-centre	–	MBG	+	30
Chevalier[32]		2008	249	Export	Multicentre	TIMI 0/1	MBG + STR	+	30
Sardella[33]	EXPIRA	2009	175	Export	Single-centre	TIMI ≤1, TS≥3, IRA ≥2.5mm	MBG, STR	+	270

* Year of publication as full article.

FU, follow-up; IRA, infarct-related artery; LV, left ventricular; MBG, myocardial blush grade; No., number of patients; TIMI, Thrombolysis in myocardial infarction; STR, ST-segment resolution.

perfusion as assessed by myocardial blush grade (MBG) and ST-segment resolution[30]. Instead, in patients randomized to rheolytic thrombectomy, infarct size as measured by Tc 99m sestamibi imaging at 14–28 days was even larger (12.5 ± 12.13 vs. 9.8 ± 10.92, p = 0.03). Furthermore, the occurrence of major adverse cardiac events (MACE) at 30 days was higher (6.7 vs. 1.7%, p = 0.01), due to a higher mortality rate in patients treated with the AngioJet® system (4.6 vs. 0.8%, p = 0.02), although no death was directly attributed to the device.

Third, non-manual aspiration catheters aspirate atherothrombotic material through continuous suction of an external vacuum pump. Medium-scaled trials investigating these non-manual aspiration catheters have reported conflicting results in unselected STEMI patients. In 355 patients with STEMI, the TransVascular Aspiration Catheter® (TVAC®, Nipro, Osaka, Japan) was associated with a higher rate of post-procedural MBG 3 in the STEMI group compared to the conventional PCI group (46.0 vs. 20.5%, p <0.001) as well as a reduction in MACE at 8 months (12.9 vs. 20.9%, p <0.05), primarily driven by a reduction in target lesion revascularization. However, a clinical trial in 215 patients using the Rescue® thrombus management system (Boston Scientific Corp./Scimed, Maple Grove, USA) did not report better myocardial salvage estimated by Tc 99m sestamibi imaging in STEMI patients randomized to the Rescue® catheter (13 vs. 18%, p = 0.12). Furthermore, final infarct size was increased in the aspiration versus the conventional group (15 vs. 8%, p = 0.004).

Manual thrombus aspiration catheters

These rapid-exchange manual aspiration catheters have the following common features: 1) they contain two lumens, a smaller guide wire lumen, and a larger one to aspirate atherothrombotic debris; 2) the distal end has a flexible atraumatic tip with one or multiple entry ports; and 3) the larger lumen is connected proximally to a syringe to allow manual suction. Manual thrombus aspiration catheters include the Diver Clot Extraction® (CE) catheter (ev3 Inc, Plymouth, USA), the Pronto® extraction catheter (Vascular Solutions, Minneapolis, USA), the QuickCat Extraction Catheter® (Spectranetics, Colorado Springs, USA) and the Export® aspiration catheter (Medtronic Inc., Santa Rosa, USA).

Several small to medium-sized trials have demonstrated improvement of myocardial perfusion in STEMI patients randomized to manual thrombus aspiration[13,31–33]. In addition, substudies have reported a reduction of microvascular obstruction as assessed by contrast-enhanced MRI with the Export® aspiration catheter[33] and as assessed by myocardial contrast echocardiography with the Diver CE® catheter[34]. Furthermore, De Luca and colleages[35] have reported a lower incidence of left ventricular remodelling in patients with anterior STEMI successfully treated with the Diver CE® catheter.

In concert, improvement of myocardial perfusion was found in the Thrombus Aspiration during Percutaneous Coronary Intervention in Acute Myocardial Infarction Study (TAPAS), the largest trial to date investigating the effect of an adjunctive manual aspiration catheter to the conventional primary PCI strategy[14]. This study was designed to enrol an unselected population of STEMI patients without angiographic in- or exclusion criteria. Therefore, this study randomized 1071 consecutive STEMI patients to treatment with the Export® aspiration catheter or to conventional primary PCI before coronary angiography was performed. In the aspiration group, the catheter was advanced into the infarct-related segment under continuous aspiration to restore antegrade flow prior to stenting. In the conventional PCI group, antegrade flow was established by balloon dilatation. Thrombus aspiration was applicable in 89%. In 73% of these patients, thrombus aspiration resulted in retrieval of atherothrombotic material. Compared to conventional PCI, post-procedural myocardial perfusion was improved in patients randomized to thrombus aspiration as assessed by the occurrence of MBG 0/1 (17.1% vs. 26.3%; RR 0.65; 95% CI 0.51–0.83; p <0.001), complete ST-segment resolution (56.5% vs. 44.2%; RR 1.28; 95% CI 1.13–1.45; p <0.001), as well as absence of persistent ST-segment deviation (53.1% vs. 40.5%; RR 1.31; 95% CI 1.14–1.50; p <0.001). Furthermore, analysis on pre-specified subgroups consistently showed improvement in myocardial perfusion in the aspiration group compared to conventional PCI in all major categories of STEMI patients including gender, age, total ischaemic time, infarct-related vessel, infarct-related segment, pre-procedural TIMI flow, as well as angiographic evidence of thrombus (Fig. 36.3). In contrast to these positive findings, the incidence of angiographically visible distal embolization was not significantly reduced in the thrombus aspiration compared to the conventional PCI group (6.7 vs. 6.0%, p = NS)[8]. Clinical follow-up at 30 days showed no differences between both groups. At 1 year, however, assignment to thrombus aspiration was associated with a reduction of cardiac mortality (3.6% vs. 6.7%; HR 1.93; 95% CI 1.11–3.37; p = 0.020) and the combined endpoint of cardiac mortality or

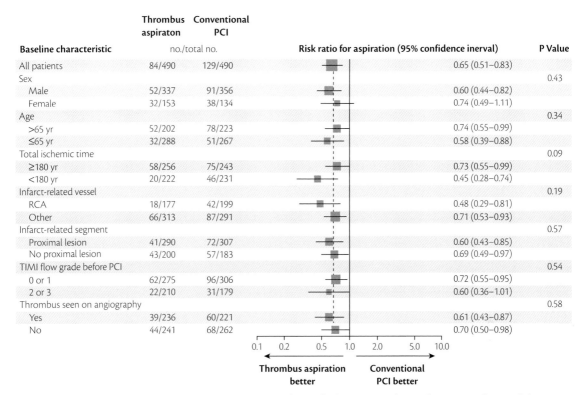

Baseline characteristic	Thrombus aspiraton	Conventional PCI	Risk ratio for aspiration (95% confidence inerval)	P Value
	no./total no.			
All patients	84/490	129/490	0.65 (0.51–0.83)	
Sex				0.43
Male	52/337	91/356	0.60 (0.44–0.82)	
Female	32/153	38/134	0.74 (0.49–1.11)	
Age				0.34
>65 yr	52/202	78/223	0.74 (0.55–0.99)	
≤65 yr	32/288	51/267	0.58 (0.39–0.88)	
Total ischemic time				0.09
≥180 yr	58/256	75/243	0.73 (0.55–0.99)	
<180 yr	20/222	46/231	0.45 (0.28–0.74)	
Infarct-related vessel				0.19
RCA	18/177	42/199	0.48 (0.29–0.81)	
Other	66/313	87/291	0.71 (0.53–0.93)	
Infarct-related segment				0.57
Proximal lesion	41/290	72/307	0.60 (0.43–0.85)	
No proximal lesion	43/200	57/183	0.69 (0.49–0.97)	
TIMI flow grade before PCI				0.54
0 or 1	62/275	96/306	0.72 (0.55–0.95)	
2 or 3	22/210	31/179	0.60 (0.36–1.01)	
Thrombus seen on angiography				0.58
Yes	39/236	60/221	0.61 (0.43–0.87)	
No	44/241	68/262	0.70 (0.50–0.98)	

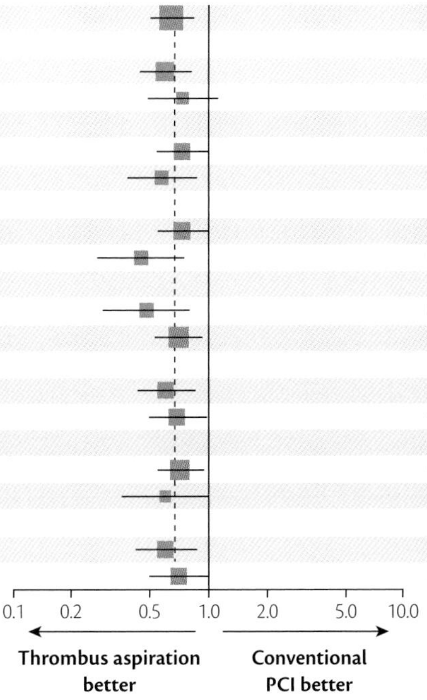

Fig. 36.3 TAPAS subanalysis on pre-specified subgroups: given are risk ratios for the primary endpoint of occurrence of myocardial blush grade 0/1 in the aspiration versus the conventional PCI group. Reproduced with permission from Svilaas T, Vlaar PJ, van der Horst IC, *et al*. Thrombus aspiration during primary percutaneous coronary intervention. *N Engl J Med* 2008; **358**(6):557–67. Copyright © 2008 Massachusetts Medical Society. All rights reserved.

non-fatal reinfarction (5.6% vs. 9.9%; HR 1.81; 95% CI 1.16–2.84; p = 0.009) compared to conventional PCI[(36)]. The Kaplan–Meier curve for the combined end point of cardiac mortality or non-fatal reinfarction is illustrated in Fig. 36.4.

One limitation of this study is the use of functional or surrogate endpoints and the limited statistical power to estimate the magnitude of the clinical benefits. Although TAPAS was not primarily designed to detect differences in clinical outcome, the angiographic and electrocardiographic endpoints used are well accepted and widely used markers of myocardial perfusion in infarction studies that are strongly associated with mortality and MACE. Second, TAPAS represents a single-centre experience. Third, the use of balloon dilatation prior to stenting was left at the operator's discretion as this study was not designed to investigate the impact of predilatation. Therefore, the precise role of predilatation versus direct stenting on myocardial perfusion outcomes is still to be elucidated.

The role of adjunctive thrombus extraction during primary PCI

From the late 1990s, case reports and studies on small patient series showed that thrombus extraction devices were feasible and safe during primary PCI in STEMI patients. Larger efficacy studies followed, reporting mostly positive but also several negative results (see Tables 36.2–36.4). Although these studies were not powered to detect differences in clinical outcomes, they generally used accepted surrogate endpoints to assess myocardial perfusion. Myocardial perfusion can be measured in several ways, of which MBG and ST-segment resolution are widely used and practical methods. These classifications have proven to correlate well with long-term cardiac mortality after primary PCI[(4,5)]. Therefore, in studies using these surrogate endpoints, improvement in myocardial perfusion is expected to translate into clinical benefits.

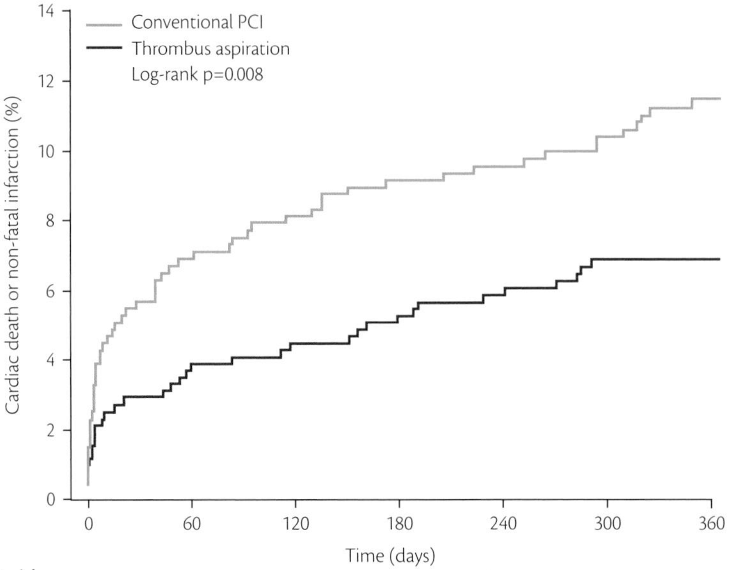

Number at risk

	0	60	120	180	240	300	360
Conventional PCI	536	495	489	484	482	479	472
Thrombus aspiration	535	512	508	504	500	495	494
Total	1071	1007	997	988	982	974	966

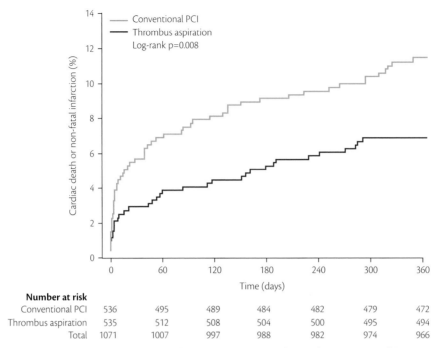

Fig. 36.4 Kaplan–Meier curve for the combined endpoint of cardiac mortality or non-fatal reinfarction at 1-year follow-up in aspiration versus conventional PCI patients in TAPAS. Reproduced with permission from Vlaar PJ, Svilaas T, van der Horst IC, *et al.* Cardiac death and reinfarction after 1 year in the Thrombus Aspiration during Percutaneous coronary intervention in Acute myocardial infarction Study (TAPAS): a 1-year follow-up study. *Lancet* 2008; **371**(9628):1915–20, with permission from Elsevier.

Early meta-analyses on thrombus extraction devices did not report improvement of clinical outcomes at 30 days, although these devices were associated with improved epicardial and myocardial perfusion and a lower incidence of distal embolization(37–39). However, more recent meta-analyses demonstrated that manual thrombus aspiration was associated with a reduction of mortality compared to conventional PCI at 30 days (1.7 vs. 3.1%; OR 0.58; 95% CI 0.34–0.98; p = 0.04)(40) and at a mean follow-up of 6.2 months (2.7 vs. 4.4%; RR 0.63; 95% CI 0.43–0.93; p = 0.018)(41). At present, a beneficial effect of manual thrombus aspiration has been reported on 1-year clinical outcomes in the TAPAS trial as mentioned earlier(36). Furthermore, the very recent pooled Analysis of Trials on ThrombEctomy in acute Myocardial infarction based on individual PatienT data, ATTEMPT has reported similarly that manual thrombus aspiration in particular is associated with improved long-term survival and clinical outcome(42). While heterogeneity among the individual trials should be acknowledged (inclusion criteria, devices, and definitions), there is convincing evidence that manual thrombus aspiration is associated with improved angiographic, electrocardiographic, as well as clinical outcomes.

In contrast to the positive results of manual thrombus aspiration, the other devices do not share the same clinical benefit. While manual thrombus aspiration was associated with a reduction in mortality compared to conventional PCI, non-manual thrombus aspiration was associated with an increase (5.3 vs. 2.8%; RR 1.93; 95% CI 1.00–3.72; p = 0.050) and distal protection devices with a neutral effect on mortality (3.1 vs. 3.4%; RR 0.92; 95% CI 0.60–1.40; p = 0.69)(41).

Table 36.5 summarizes the published meta-analyses on thrombus extraction devices. While filter systems have the theoretical advantage of maintaining antegrade flow through the culprit coronary artery, efficacy studies on neither distal occlusive devices nor filter systems could demonstrate improvement of myocardial perfusion or infarct size. Therefore, there is currently no evidence to recommend the routine use of non-manual thrombus aspiration devices or distal protection devices during primary PCI in STEMI patients. For non-manual devices, the results of a European multicentre study are still to be expected. In this trial,

Table 36.5 Meta-analyses of mechanical adjunctive devices in patients with ST-segment elevation myocardial infarction

Author	Year*	Search period	Included trials (n)	No.	Device	Endpoints	Outcome	FU
Kunadian[38]	2007	Sep 2000–Oct 2005	14	2630	all	mortality/reinfarction	–	30 days
De Luca[37]	2007	Jan 1990–Oct 2006	21	3721	all	TIMI flow	+	30 days
						MBG	+	
						DE	+	
						mortality	–	
Burzotta[39]	2008	Oct 2003–Jun 2006	18	3180	all	mortality/reinfarction	–	≤30 days
						DE	+	
						TIMI flow	+	
						MBG	+	
						STR	+ (for TA)	
De Luca[40]	2008	Jan 1990–May 2008	9	2417	TA	TIMI flow	+	30 days
						MBG	+	
						DE	+	
						mortality/reinfarction	+	
Bavry[41]	2008	Jan 1996–Jun 2008	30	6415	TA (47%)	mortality	+	6.2 months**
					NTA (15%)	mortality	–	4.6 months**
					DPD (38%)	mortality	–	3.7 months**
Burzotta[42]	2009	Oct 2003–Feb 2008	11	2686	TA (68%)	mortality	+	365 days**
					NTA (32%)			

*Year of publication as full article.

**Mean follow-up duration within the subgroup.

DE, distal embolization; DPD, distal protection device; FU, follow-up; MBG, myocardial blush grade; No., number of patients; NTA, non-manual thrombus aspiration; TIMI, Thrombolysis in Myocardial Infarction; STR, ST-segment resolution; TA, manual thrombus aspiration.

500 STEMI patients are randomized to primary PCI with or without aspiration with the AngioJet® system and may provide additional insights into the role of non-manual aspiration in STEMI patients[43]. While distal protection devices are not recommended during primary PCI, they have a class Ia recommendation for use as adjunctive devices during elective PCI of vein grafts[44].

Although the exact patient population in which thrombus aspiration should be performed in clinical practice is not clearly defined, it seems reasonable to attempt aspiration in all patients presenting with STEMI. Angiographic evidence of thrombus should not be a selection criterion for the use of a manual aspiration catheter, as demonstrated in TAPAS. In this study, the benefit of thrombus aspiration on myocardial perfusion was irrespective of angiographic presence of thrombus.

Next to its benefit on clinical outcome, manual thrombus aspiration has several practical advantages. First, these aspiration catheters are effective in crossing, even small, target lesions. On the contrary, the other devices require a more permissive coronary anatomy as non-manual devices can usually target only larger vessels and distal protection devices need a distal landing zone. Second, the clinical applicability of manual aspiration catheters is high. Its use is easy and it does not require much practice to gain clinical experience. Third, manual aspiration catheters are safe, with no clinically manifest major complications reported. An additional advantage is that these catheters are inexpensive, being available in the same price range as balloon catheters. In most cases, thrombus aspiration has resulted in restoration of brisk antegrade flow and predilatation with a balloon catheter is not needed. Although formally it has not been investigated whether the use of thrombus

Table 36.6 Comparison of features of manual thrombus aspiration, non-manual thrombus aspiration, and distal protection devices

Feature	Manual thrombus aspiration	Non-manual thrombus aspiration	Distal protection
Ability to reach target lesion	++	+	+
Effective retrieval	+	+	+
Technical complexity	–	+	+
Complications	–	+	+
Costs	–	++	+(+)

aspiration catheters is cost-effective, it seems clear that their use does not lead to increased costs of the primary PCI strategy. In contrast, the more sophisticated and complex other approaches involve more expenditure, in increased costs of either disposables or additional equipment. These features of the three types of mechanical devices are summarized in Table 36.6.

Several factors may explain why the published studies have produced heterogeneous results. First of all, there is a clear group distinction between the manual aspiration catheters and non-manual and distal protection devices in their clinical performance in routine practice. Although the latter were able to retrieve atherothrombotic debris, this did not unequivocally translate into improvement of myocardial perfusion, infarct size, or clinical outcome. On the contrary, non-manual devices as well as distal protection systems may result in longer and more complex PCI procedures[30] and even major complications such as coronary dissection[28] or an AV fistula[26], negating a possible beneficial effect. Another reason why some studies were negative could be that the devices studied are not fully able to prevent device-induced embolization when wire and/or device cross the lesion. In addition, technical details may influence this risk of embolization. For instance, it is believed that embolization is more easily induced by thrombus aspiration if a distal-to proximal approach is applied, in which aspiration is started after crossing the lesion, than if a proximal-to-distal approach is used, in which the catheter is advanced into the lesion during continuous active aspiration[45]. As the first approach was used in 52% of patients enrolled in the AIMI trial, this may have confounded the results.

Finally, the large negative studies investigating non-manual aspiration devices did not require angiographic selection criteria. While manual aspiration catheters are effective in all patients, these more complex devices may only benefit STEMI patients with a high thrombus burden. Unfortunately, their role in this subset of patients is not well investigated. Therefore, non-manual devices may be indicated in STEMI patients with a large thrombus load in case residual, more organized, thrombus remains after performance of manual thrombus aspiration.

Future perspectives

At present, there is convincing evidence for the superiority of adjunctive manual thrombus aspiration during primary PCI over conventional PCI in removing the source of embolization and in improving myocardial perfusion. Its benefit on clinical outcomes is derived from the 1-year results of the TAPAS trial and from several meta-analyses. Comparisons between individual devices have been sparingly performed[46], with a small-sized study reporting improved angiographic outcomes with the Export® compared to the Diver® catheter[47]. Further research should clarify this issue. In addition, more objective imaging techniques will be adopted in clinical practice to characterize and grade thrombus load. These techniques may also illustrate the other components of the multiple mechanisms by which vessels can become occluded.

Before retrieval of atherothrombotic material was performed in STEMI patients, histopathological analysis could only be performed in post-mortem studies. The knowledge largely derived from these studies, evidently suffering from a selection bias, is expected to be supplemented by analysis of aspiration samples.

An important limitation of thrombus aspiration is its inability to prevent distal embolization that has occurred spontaneously before PCI. Furthermore, distal embolization itself is only one of the causes of impaired myocardial perfusion in patients with STEMI. Several other mechanisms account for this phenomenon, including myocardial reperfusion injury, tissue oedema, capillary leakage, and endothelial dysfunction[48,49]. Therefore, although thrombus aspiration has proven to reduce the risk of atherothrombotic embolization, it neither compensates for these additional mechanisms that impair myocardial perfusion, nor for distal embolization that has occurred prior to intervention. These insights, together with the current knowledge of the histopathology and pathophysiology of thrombotic occlusions, should stimulate the development of adjunctive pharmacological therapies to target these pathways.

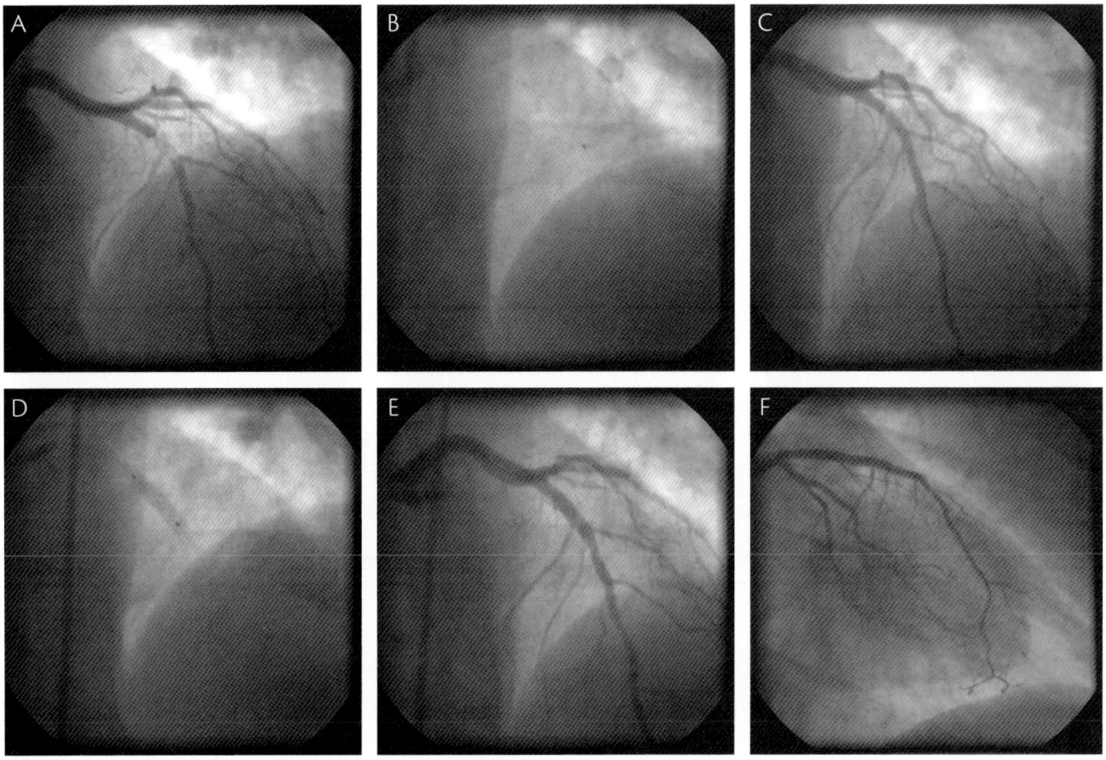

Fig. 36.5 Primary PCI in a patient with subtotal occlusion of the left anterior descending artery with a high thrombus burden.

Last but not least, time to reperfusion remains one of the major predictors of clinical outcome in STEMI. Therefore, efforts to reduce ischaemic time in patients with STEMI are of paramount importance.

Clinical case studies

Case 1

A 61-year old male smoker was referred to the catheterization laboratory within 2h after symptom onset with electrocardiographic evidence of an anterior infarction. Although antegrade flow was present on initial coronary angiography of the left coronary system, subtotal occlusion was observed of the mid left anterior descending (LAD) artery with a large thrombus burden grade 4 (Fig. 36.5A). Coronary angiography of the right coronary system was normal. The initial treatment step was thrombus aspiration in the mid LAD (Fig. 36.5B), leading to aspiration of macroscopically visible white thrombus. On angiography, TIMI 3 flow was restored through the culprit artery and the thrombus burden was successfully reduced to grade 1 (Fig. 36.5C). Finally, after stent deployment (Biotronik PRO-kinetic®, 3.5×15mm, Fig. 36.5D), no thrombus was visible (Fig. 36.5E). At the end of procedure, a dedicated run (30° right anterior oblique view) was performed to allow assessment of TIMI flow and myocardial perfusion, measured both visually using the MBG as well as computerized using the Quantitative Blush Evaluator (QuBE, Fig. 36.5F)[50]. In this patient, optimal reperfusion of both the epicardial artery as well as the myocardium was obtained.

Case 2

An 83-year-old woman was admitted after a sudden onset of chest pain for 6h. The initial coronary angiogram showed single-vessel disease with a distal site of total occlusion in the right coronary artery (RCA) as identified by staining from the test injection (Fig. 36.6A). Thrombus aspiration (Fig. 36.6B) resulted in removal of macroscopically red thrombus. Afterwards, brisk antegrade flow was restored through the culprit lesion without angiographically visible thrombus or a residual stenosis that required stenting. However, distal embolization was visible in the posterolateral branch (Fig. 36.6C). Additional thrombus aspiration was performed in this lesion (Fig. 36.6D), which led to restoration of TIMI 3

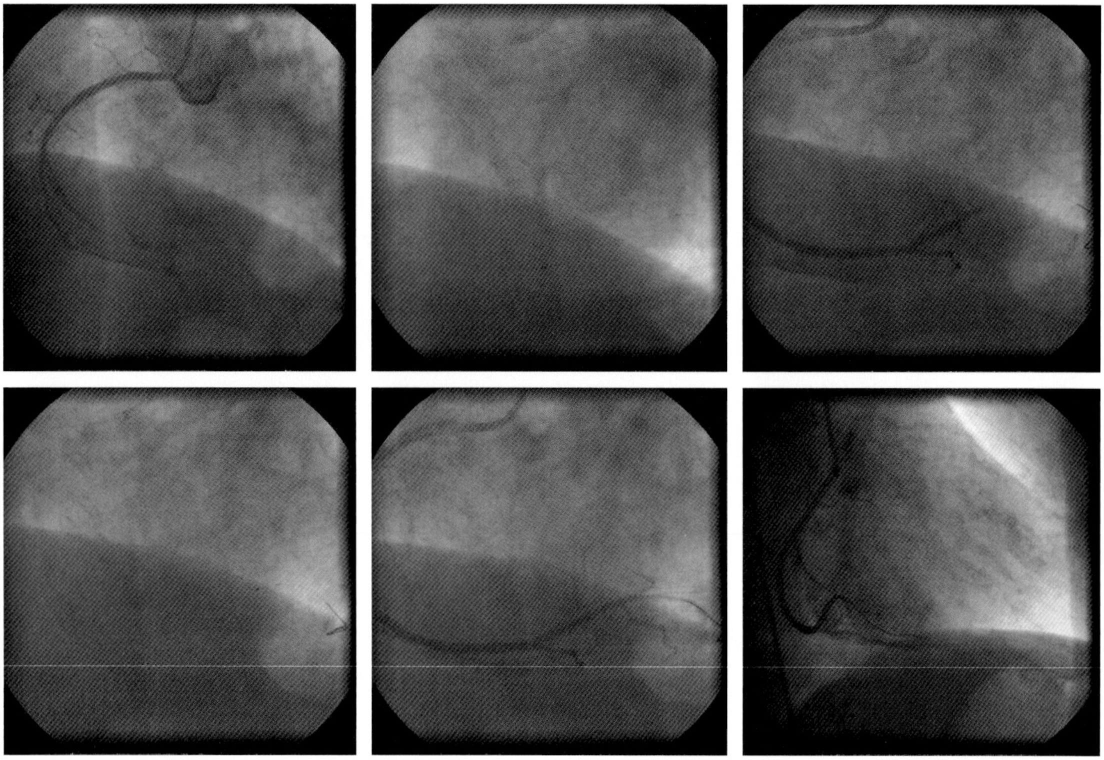

Fig. 36.6 Primary PCI in a patient with total occlusion of the RCA.

flow through the entire, large, RCA (Fig. 36.6E). Without further coronary intervention, optimal myocardial perfusion was achieved (Fig. 36.6F). Thrombus aspiration has been described as a safe and effective definitive treatment in STEMI patients[51,52].

Conclusion

In patients with STEMI, adjunctive manual thrombus aspiration devices during primary PCI are able to protect the distal coronary microvasculature from atherothrombotic embolization and lead to better restoration of myocardial perfusion compared to conventional primary PCI. At present, there is increasing evidence that the use of manual thrombus aspiration is associated with improved long-term survival. Manual thrombus aspiration is safe and easily applicable in a large majority of patients presenting with STEMI. In contradistinction, the routine use of non-manual aspiration and distal protection devices is not recommended.

References

1. Falk E. Coronary thrombosis: pathogenesis and clinical manifestations. *Am J Cardiol* 1991; **68**(7):28B–35B.
2. Van de Werf F, Bax J, Betriu A, *et al.* Management of acute myocardial infarction in patients presenting with persistent ST-segment elevation: the Task Force on the Management of ST-Segment Elevation Acute Myocardial Infarction of the European Society of Cardiology. *Eur Heart J* 2008; **29**(23):2909–45.
3. Keeley EC, Boura JA, Grines CL. Primary angioplasty versus intravenous thrombolytic therapy for acute myocardial infarction: a quantitative review of 23 randomised trials. *Lancet* 2003; **361**(9351):13–20.
4. van't Hof AW, Liem A, de Boer MJ, *et al.* Clinical value of 12-lead electrocardiogram after successful reperfusion therapy for acute myocardial infarction. Zwolle Myocardial infarction Study Group. *Lancet* 1997; **350**(9078):615–19.
5. van't Hof AW, Liem A, Suryapranata H, *et al.* Angiographic assessment of myocardial reperfusion in patients treated with primary angioplasty for acute myocardial infarction: myocardial blush grade. Zwolle Myocardial Infarction Study Group. *Circulation* 1998; **97**(23):2302-6.

6. Topol EJ, Yadav JS. Recognition of the importance of embolization in atherosclerotic vascular disease. *Circulation* 2000; **101**(5):570–80.
7. Henriques JP, Zijlstra F, Ottervanger JP, de Boer MJ, van 't Hof AW, Hoorntje JC, *et al.* Incidence and clinical significance of distal embolization during primary angioplasty for acute myocardial infarction. *Eur Heart J* 2002; **23**(14):1112–17.
8. Fokkema ML, Vlaar PJ, Svilaas T, *et al.* Incidence and clinical consequences of distal embolization on the coronary angiogram after percutaneous coronary intervention for ST-elevation myocardial infarction. *Eur Heart J* 2009; **73**(5):627–35.
9. Napodano M, Ramondo A, Tarantini G, *et al.* Predictors and time-related impact of distal embolization during primary angioplasty. *Eur Heart J* 2009; **30**(3):305–13
10. DeWood MA, Spores J, Notske R, *et al.* Prevalence of total coronary occlusion during the early hours of transmural myocardial infarction. *N Engl J Med* 1980; **303**(16):897–902.
11. Mabin TA, Holmes DR, Jr, Smith HC, *et al.* Intracoronary thrombus: role in coronary occlusion complicating percutaneous transluminal coronary angioplasty. *J Am Coll Cardiol* 1985; **5**(2 Pt 1):198–202.
12. Gibson CM, de Lemos JA, Murphy SA, *et al.* Combination therapy with abciximab reduces angiographically evident thrombus in acute myocardial infarction: a TIMI 14 substudy. *Circulation* 2001; **103**(21):2550–4.
13. Silva-Orrego P, Colombo P, Bigi R, *et al.* Thrombus aspiration before primary angioplasty improves myocardial reperfusion in acute myocardial infarction: the DEAR-MI (Dethrombosis to Enhance Acute Reperfusion in Myocardial Infarction) study. *J Am Coll Cardiol* 2006; **48**(8):1552–9.
14. Svilaas T, Vlaar PJ, van der Horst IC, *et al.* Thrombus aspiration during primary percutaneous coronary intervention. *N Engl J Med* 2008; **358**(6):557–67.
15. Jang IK, Tearney GJ, MacNeill B, *et al.* In vivo characterization of coronary atherosclerotic plaque by use of optical coherence tomography. *Circulation* 2005; **111**(12):1551–5.
16. Kubo T, Imanishi T, Takarada S, *et al.* Assessment of culprit lesion morphology in acute myocardial infarction: ability of optical coherence tomography compared with intravascular ultrasound and coronary angioscopy. *J Am Coll Cardiol* 2007; **50**(10):933–9.
17. Stone GW, Webb J, Cox DA, Brodie BR, *et al.* Distal microcirculatory protection during percutaneous coronary intervention in acute ST-segment elevation myocardial infarction: a randomized controlled trial. *JAMA* 2005; **293**(9):1063–72.
18. Thim T, Hagensen MK, Bentzon JF, Falk E. From vulnerable plaque to atherothrombosis. *J Intern Med* 2008; **263**(5):506–16.
19. Rittersma SZ, van der Wal AC, Koch KT, *et al.* Plaque instability frequently occurs days or weeks before occlusive coronary thrombosis: a pathological thrombectomy study in primary percutaneous coronary intervention. *Circulation* 2005; **111**(9):1160–5.
20. Gu YL, Fokkema ML, Zijlstra F. The emerging role of thrombus aspiration in the management of acute myocardial infarction. *Circulation* 2008; **118**(18):1780–2.
21. Kramer MC, van der Wal AC, Koch KT, *et al.* Presence of older thrombus is an independent predictor of long-term mortality in patients with ST-elevation myocardial infarction treated with thrombus aspiration during primary percutaneous coronary intervention. *Circulation* 2008; **118**(18):1810–16.
22. Muramatsu T, Kozuma K, Tsukahara R, *et al.* Comparison of myocardial perfusion by distal protection before and after primary stenting for acute myocardial infarction: angiographic and clinical results of a randomized controlled trial. *Catheter Cardiovasc Interv* 2007; **70**(5):677–82.
23. Gick M, Jander N, Bestehorn HP, *et al.* Randomized evaluation of the effects of filter-based distal protection on myocardial perfusion and infarct size after primary percutaneous catheter intervention in myocardial infarction with and without ST-segment elevation. *Circulation* 2005; **112**(10):1462–9.
24. Cura FA, Escudero AG, Berrocal D, *et al.* Protection of Distal Embolization in High-Risk Patients with Acute ST-Segment Elevation Myocardial Infarction (PREMIAR). *Am J Cardiol* 2007; **99**(3):357–63.
25. Kelbaek H, Terkelsen CJ, Helqvist S, *et al.* Randomized comparison of distal protection versus conventional treatment in primary percutaneous coronary intervention: the drug elution and distal protection in ST-elevation myocardial infarction (DEDICATION) trial. *J Am Coll Cardiol* 2008; **51**(9):899–905.
26. Lefevre T, Garcia E, Reimers B, *et al.* X-sizer for thrombectomy in acute myocardial infarction improves ST-segment resolution: results of the X-sizer in AMI for negligible embolization and optimal ST resolution (X AMINE ST) trial. *J Am Coll Cardiol* 2005; **46**(2):246–52.
27. Napodano M, Pasquetto G, Sacca S, *et al.* Intracoronary thrombectomy improves myocardial reperfusion in patients undergoing direct angioplasty for acute myocardial infarction. *J Am Coll Cardiol* 2003; **42**(8):1395–402.
28. Beran G, Lang I, Schreiber W, *et al.* Intracoronary thrombectomy with the X-sizer catheter system improves epicardial flow and accelerates ST-segment resolution in patients with acute coronary syndrome: a prospective, randomized, controlled study. *Circulation* 2002; **105**(20):2355–60.
29. Antoniucci D, Valenti R, Migliorini A, *et al.* Comparison of rheolytic thrombectomy before direct infarct artery stenting versus direct stenting alone in patients undergoing percutaneous coronary intervention for acute myocardial infarction. *Am J Cardiol* 2004; **93**(8):1033–5.
30. Ali A, Cox D, Dib N, *et al.* Rheolytic thrombectomy with percutaneous coronary intervention for infarct size

reduction in acute myocardial infarction: 30-day results from a multicenter randomized study. *J Am Coll Cardiol* 2006; **48**(2):244–52.

31. Burzotta F, Trani C, Romagnoli E, *et al.* Manual thrombus-aspiration improves myocardial reperfusion: the randomized evaluation of the effect of mechanical reduction of distal embolization by thrombus-aspiration in primary and rescue angioplasty (REMEDIA) trial. *J Am Coll Cardiol* 2005; **46**(2):371–6.
32. Chevalier B, Gilard M, Lang I, Systematic primary aspiration in acute myocardial percutaneous intervention: a multicentre randomised controlled trial of the export aspiration catheter. *EuroIntervention* 2008;**4**(2):222–8.
33. Sardella G, Mancone M, Bucciarelli-Ducci C, Thrombus Aspiration During Primary Percutaneous Coronary Intervention Improves Myocardial Reperfusion and Reduces Infarct Size The EXPIRA (Thrombectomy With Export Catheter in Infarct-Related Artery During Primary Percutaneous Coronary Intervention) Prospective, Randomized Trial. *J Am Coll Cardiol* 2009; **53**(4):309–15.
34. Galiuto L, Garramone B, Burzotta F, Thrombus aspiration reduces microvascular obstruction after primary coronary intervention: a myocardial contrast echocardiography substudy of the REMEDIA Trial. *J Am Coll Cardiol* 2006; **48**(7):1355–60.
35. De Luca L, Sardella G, Davidson CJ, Impact of intracoronary aspiration thrombectomy during primary angioplasty on left ventricular remodelling in patients with anterior ST elevation myocardial infarction. *Heart* 2006; **92**(7):951–7.
36. Vlaar PJ, Svilaas T, van der Horst IC, *et al.* Cardiac death and reinfarction after 1 year in the Thrombus Aspiration during Percutaneous coronary intervention in Acute myocardial infarction Study (TAPAS): a 1-year follow-up study. *Lancet* 2008; **371**(9628):1915–20.
37. De Luca G, Suryapranata H, Stone GW, *et al.* Adjunctive mechanical devices to prevent distal embolization in patients undergoing mechanical revascularization for acute myocardial infarction: a meta-analysis of randomized trials. *Am Heart J* 2007; **153**(3):343–53.
38. Kunadian B, Dunning J, Vijayalakshmi K, *et al.* Meta-analysis of randomized trials comparing anti-embolic devices with standard PCI for improving myocardial reperfusion in patients with acute myocardial infarction. *Catheter Cardiovasc Interv* 2007; **69**(4):488–96.
39. Burzotta F, Testa L, Giannico F, *et al.* Adjunctive devices in primary or rescue PCI: a meta-analysis of randomized trials. *Int J Cardiol* 2008; **123**(3):313–21.
40. De Luca G, Dudek D, Sardella G, *et al.* Adjunctive manual thrombectomy improves myocardial perfusion and mortality in patients undergoing primary percutaneous coronary intervention for ST-elevation myocardial infarction: a meta-analysis of randomized trials. *Eur Heart J* 2008; **29**(24):3002–10.
41. Bavry AA, Kumbhani DJ, Bhatt DL. Role of adjunctive thrombectomy and embolic protection devices in acute myocardial infarction: a comprehensive meta-analysis of randomized trials. *Eur Heart J* 2008; **29**(24):2989–3001.
42. Burzotta F, De Vita M, Gu YL, *et al.* Clinical impact of thrombectomy in acute ST-elevation myocardial infarction: an individual patient-data pooled analysis of 11 trials. *Eur Heart J.* 2009; **30**(18):2193–203.
43. Antoniucci D. Rheolytic thrombectomy in acute myocardial infarction: the Florence experience and objectives of the multicenter randomized JETSTENT trial. *J Invasive Cardiol* 2006; **18**(Suppl.C):32C–34C.
44. Silber S, Albertsson P, Aviles FF, *et al.* Guidelines for percutaneous coronary interventions. The Task Force for Percutaneous Coronary Interventions of the European Society of Cardiology. *Eur Heart J.* 2005; **26**(8):804–47.
45. Antoniucci D, Valenti R, Migliorini A. Thrombectomy during PCI for acute myocardial infarction: are the randomized controlled trial data relevant to the patients who really need this technique? *Catheter Cardiovasc Interv* 2008; **71**(7):863–9.
46. Vlaar PJ, Svilaas T, Vogelzang M, *et al.* A Comparison of 2 thrombus aspiration devices with histopathological analysis of retrieved material in patients presenting with ST-segment elevation myocardial infarction. *J Am Coll Cardiol Interv* 2009; **1**:258–64.
47. Sardella G, Mancone M, Nguyen BL, *et al.* The effect of thrombectomy on myocardial blush in primary angioplasty: the Randomized Evaluation of Thrombus Aspiration by two thrombectomy devices in acute Myocardial Infarction (RETAMI) trial. *Catheter Cardiovasc Interv* 2008; **71**(1):84–91.
48. Reffelmann T, Kloner RA. The “no-reflow” phenomenon: basic science and clinical correlates. *Heart* 2002; **87**(2):162–8.
49. Eeckhout E, Kern MJ. The coronary no-reflow phenomenon: a review of mechanisms and therapies. *Eur Heart J* 2001; **22**(9):729–39.
50. Vogelzang M, Vlaar PJ, Svilaas T, *et al.* Computer-assisted myocardial blush quantification after percutaneous coronary angioplasty for acute myocardial infarction: a substudy from the TAPAS trial. *Eur Heart J* 2009; **30**(5):594–9.
51. Fokkema ML, Vlaar PJ, Svilaas T. Thrombus aspiration as definitive mechanical intervention for ST-elevation myocardial infarction: a report of five cases. *J Invasive Cardiol* 2008; **20** (5):242–4.
52. Stoel MG, von Birgelen C, Zijlstra F. Aspiration of embolized thrombus during primary percutaneous coronary intervention. *Catheter Cardiovasc Interv* 2009; **73**(6).
53. Ikari Y, Sakurada M, Kozuma K, *et al.* Upfront thrombus aspiration in primary coronary intervention for patients with ST-segment elevation acute myocardial infarction: report of the VAMPIRE (VAcuuM asPIration thrombus REmoval) trial. *J Am Coll Cardiol Cardiovasc Interv.* 2008; **1**(4):424–31.
54. Kaltoft A, Bøttcher M, Nielsen SS, *et al.* Routine thrombectomy in percutaneous coronary intervention for acute ST-segment-elevation myocardial infarction: a randomized, controlled trial. *Circulation.* 2006; **114**(1):40–7.

CHAPTER 37

Distal protection

William J. van Gaal and Adrian P. Banning

Introduction

Percutaneous coronary intervention (PCI) aims to restore normal epicardial flow and improve microvascular perfusion to the vascular bed beyond the obstructive coronary stenosis. In the setting of elective PCI, the goal is to achieve this without injury to the distal myocardium, whilst in acute coronary syndromes, namely acute ST elevation myocardial infarction (STEMI), the goal is restore epicardial patency and microvascular perfusion as quickly as possible to limit the extent of irreversibly injured (necrotic) myocardium. The pathophysiology of distal injury in these clinical scenarios differs, and thus protection of the myocardium in the elective and acute setting requires different approaches.

The concept of distal protection was initially trialled during vein graft PCI. Vein grafts are large capacious conduits with large volumes of plaque. The concept that a basket placed downstream on the wire might catch plaque liberated during balloon expansion was the subject of a number of landmark studies proving in concept that this approach might be beneficial in these specific patients. A number of different devices have evolved and their use is considered routine in most centres when vein grafts are being treated.

Whether downstream injury is important in patients with stable angina undergoing elective PCI has been debated for many years. However it is now clear that this process can cause injury to the distal myocardium which is detected as a post-procedural elevation of cardiac enzymes. The incidence of injury varies and the mechanisms of injury can also vary. Recently, peri-procedural myocardial necrosis in elective patients (with normal baseline cardiac enzymes) has been arbitrarily defined by any post-procedural rise in cardiac enzymes above the 99th percentile upper reference limit (URL)[1]. Increases in biomarkers greater than 3×99th percentile URL define peri-procedural myocardial infarction[1]. The distinction between necrosis and infarction is inevitably arbitrary as both represent irreversibly injured myocardium which is destined ultimately to become scar.

In elective PCI, the most frequent mechanisms of injury are side-branch occlusion and/or distal embolization[2]. In these elective PCI patients, injury to the distal vascular bed may manifest as a reduction in coronary flow or more subtly as a reduction in the corrected TIMI frame count or myocardial blush grade. When reduced coronary flow is particularly evident following intervention it is referred to as 'coronary no-reflow' which is defined as inadequate myocardial perfusion of a given coronary segment without angiographic evidence of mechanical vessel obstruction[3]. In the cardiac catheterization laboratory, this coronary no-reflow is visualized angiographically as a reduction in TIMI flow grade, and it may be accompanied by chest pain, electrocardiographic changes with ST segment shift, and possible haemodynamic compromise. Coronary no-reflow and injury to the distal microvascular bed are inexorably linked, and thus protection of the distal vascular bed is primarily aimed at the prevention and treatment of no-reflow.

In the setting of primary PCI for acute STEMI, injury to the distal vascular bed has already occurred and is ongoing. Further damage will occur with ongoing delays in reperfusion, and can also occur during PCI due to a combination of ischaemia/reperfusion injury and/or distal embolization. In the setting of STEMI, the pathophysiologic processes of no-reflow begin at the time of vessel occlusion, develop further during the ischaemic period and then paradoxically increase during reperfusion. During the coronary occlusive period, studies utilizing microscopy have demonstrated endothelial damage with intraluminal protrusions which may plug the capillary lumen within the anatomic zone of no-reflow[3]. Cellular oedema ensues with compression of the capillary lumen[4,5], and plugs of platelet and/or fibrin thrombi cause microvascular occlusion[6].

Following cessation of prolonged epicardial occlusion, reperfusion can result in structural changes to the microvasculature and lead to expansion of no-reflow zones despite restoration of epicardial flow[7,8]. This is due in part to an exacerbation of tissue oedema, as well as leucocyte plugging[9,10] and free radical production[11]. Distal embolization is common during PCI in patients with acute STEMI, and usually occurs after stenting. The burden of distal embolization during primary PCI for STEMI is associated with no-reflow and poor recovery of left ventricular function[12]. Clinically, the development of angiographic no-reflow following revascularization therapy for STEMI has been associated with worse outcomes, including cardiac death[13–18]. The prevention and successful treatment of no-reflow can improve blood and drug delivery to necrotic areas, aid healing and collateral development, and reduce infarct size, and thus the management of no-reflow in the cardiac catheterization laboratory has important prognostic implications.

The incidence of peri-procedural myocardial injury is dependent on definition. A recent meta-analysis of 7578 patients undergoing PCI for stable or unstable angina with normal baseline troponin values demonstrated troponin elevation in 28.7%. Using the new universal definition[1], 14.5% of patients sustain a PCI-related myocardial infarction[19]. Importantly, PCI-related myocardial infarction was associated with an increased risk of death, myocardial infarction, and reintervention. Certain angiographic criteria are predictive of no-reflow. Thrombus rich lesions predict no-reflow in the setting of primary PCI[20,21], which probably reflects an increased risk of distal embolization resulting in microvascular plugging. Patients with acute STEMI involving the right coronary artery are also appear to be at higher risk of distal embolization[22].

Protection of the distal vascular bed during PCI can be divided broadly into pharmacotherapy and mechanical devices. Pharmacotherapy is aimed primarily at the platelet, as well as coronary vasodilation to improve microvascular perfusion. Mechanical therapy is aimed at removal of thrombus and prevention of downstream embolization of thrombus and other debris into the microvasculature.

Embolic protection devices

Prevention of distal embolization is challenging and requires careful operator technique, particularly when crossing a complex lesion with coronary guide wires and other devices. Ideally, embolic protection devices should be in place for the entirety of the procedure, and prior to any balloon inflation; however in practice, low-pressure inflation using a small-diameter compliant balloon is often necessary to allow passage of the device. An alternative, if available, is to use a small laser fibre (for example, 1.4mm) to safely create a lumen sufficient to allow passage of the device (see Chapter 34). In particular high-risk settings, embolic protection devices are effective at reducing the amount of embolic debris reaching the microvasculature, as shown by studies capturing liberated debris during PCI[23–25]. Several embolic protection devices are approved, and are based primarily on two principles. The first is balloon occlusion to arrest antegrade flow followed by aspiration, and secondly is the filter-based 'basket' type devices which capture liberated debris as it flows downstream. Balloon occlusive devices arrest antegrade flow during PCI, and allow for aspiration of embolic debris after intervention and before the occlusive balloon is deflated, thereby preventing any liberated debris from reaching the distal microvascular bed. Filter-based devices allow for antegrade flow during PCI and are designed to trap liberated debris during PCI. A special purpose sheath acts as a basket retrieval system to remove the filter with captured debris *in situ*. Selection of which embolic protection device to use will depend on operator familiarity, availability, and lesion location. The latter is perhaps the most important consideration, as both distal and proximal protection devices require suitable landing zones for the device, and as such, certain lesions are more suitable for particular devices. Meticulous technique is necessary during procedures using embolic protection, as improper use is associated with less efficient capture of embolic material. This was demonstrated with the FilterWire EX® system (Boston Scientific Corp., Natick, MA, USA) during the first trials of the device[26], in which embolic debris could bypass the filter if not positioned properly, although subsequent design modifications have since improved vessel wall apposition and minimized the chance of debris bypassing the filter basket.

Distal balloon occlusive devices

The PercuSurge GuardWire® device (Medtronic, Santa Rosa, CA, USA) was the first distal protection device used in clinical practice. The device is a distal balloon occlusive protection system which arrests antegrade coronary flow and allows for aspiration of any plaque debris generated during PCI. The device consists of a pentatetrafluoroethane balloon at the tip of a 0.014-inch hollow nitinol (nickel titanium ally) tube, an inflation

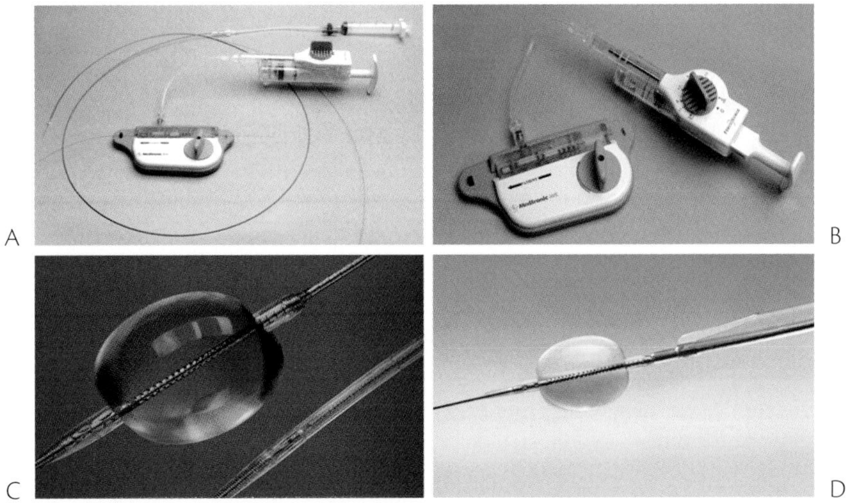

Fig. 37.1 The GuardWire® embolic protection system. The GuardWire® embolic protection system consists of four major components: the GuardWire® balloon occlusion wire (C and D), the Export® aspiration catheter (A and D), and an inflation system consisting of the EZ Adaptor® device and EZ Flator® inflation device (A and B). The GuardWire® embolic protection balloon has a radiopaque coil tip that may be shaped in the same way you would a standard angioplasty wire. An introducer tool is provided to help advance the wire through the haemostatic valve on the guiding catheter without damaging the wire tip. Once the GuardWire® balloon occlusion wire tip is properly positioned distal to the lesion, insert the wire into the EZ Adaptor® device (bottom left, panel B), and turn the adaptor knob clockwise. Briefly pull negative with the EZ Flator® device handle to remove any small amounts of air that may have been introduced when loading the wire into the introducer. Return the handle to the neutral position and dial on the EZ Flator® device to the desired size for occluding the vessel. Confirm that the vessel is occluded by injecting a small amount of contrast. There should not be any flow in the vessel. If the balloon is not occlusive, turn the dial to the next higher setting, which will increase the balloon size by 0.5mm. Once the vessel is occluded, turn the gray knob on the Adaptor® counterclockwise and remove the wire from the EZ Adaptor® device. Perform the intervention being sure to stabilize the wire during all catheter exchanges. The inflated balloon is intended to gently occlude the vessel, and is not intended to act as an anchor. Prior to deflating the balloon, aspirate any debris that may have been created during the intervention. Load the Export® aspiration catheter onto the GuardWire® balloon occlusion wire. Advance the catheter up to the inflated GuardWire® occlusion balloon (D). You will see the marker band on the distal end of the Export® aspiration catheter approach the balloon marker band (the two markers will not actually meet). Initiate aspiration by turning the stopcock open to the aspiration syringe. Allow the catheter to sit just proximal to the balloon whilst aspirating for a few seconds. Then slowly withdraw the catheter through the vein graft while continuing to aspirate. It is recommended to aspirate the vessel twice to ensure complete debris removal. Once the vessel has been aspirated, reinsert the GuardWire® balloon occlusion wire into the EZ Adaptor® device. Turn the grey knob on the Adaptor® clockwise between the two markers. Make certain the dial on the EZ Flator® inflation device is turned back to zero and pull back on the deflation handle, then lock the handle in the negative position. Allow the balloon to fully deflate, and then return the EZ Flator® device handle to the neutral position. Turn the grey adaptor knob counterclockwise until it stops and the jaws are open, and then remove the wire.

device and microseal adaptor (Fig. 37.1). After advancing the wire across the lesion, the compliant balloon is inflated and contrast injected to ensure that antegrade coronary flow has been completely arrested. If not, the balloon is inflated further until flow in the vessel is completely occluded. The microseal is then closed using the adaptor, and the adaptor removed from the wire so that balloons and stents may be placed over the wire to perform PCI. Following lesion treatment, the stagnant column of blood in the vessel is aspirated using the Export® (Medtronic, Santa Rosa, CA, USA) aspiration catheter over the GuardWire® to retrieve any debris generated during the procedure. The GuardWire® is then reinserted into the adapter and the microseal opened so that the occlusive balloon may be deflated. The GuardWire® balloon is then deflated to restore normal antegrade coronary flow. In order to reduce the time of balloon occlusion and thereby minimize ischaemia, the treatment catheter should be loaded to the tip of the guiding catheter prior to inflation of the occlusive balloon. Likewise, the GuardWire® should be loaded into the adapter during the aspiration sequence so that the occlusive balloon may be deflated as soon as aspiration is complete.

The TriActiv® system (Kensey Nash, Exton, PA, USA) is another distal balloon occlusive protection system which works using a similar principle. The TriActiv® system differs in that it employs the use of a flush catheter to infuse saline following intervention, with the overflow, blood, and debris extracted through the guiding catheter.

Purported advantages of distal occlusion balloons for distal embolic protection are that they allow for more complete capture of embolic debris, whereas filter-based devices may allow for debris to bypass either through fenestrations or alongside the device. In addition, soluble factors liberated during PCI may contribute to distal injury, and will potentially be aspirated along with physical debris when using balloon occlusive devices. Thus balloon occlusion devices may offer protection not only against physical debris but soluble factors as well. Distal balloon occlusive devices have the lowest lesion crossing profile of embolic protection devices to date, with crossing profiles ranging from approximately 0.026 inches. Thus these devices may be easier to use when crossing tight lesions; however in practice, distal occlusion balloon embolic protection requires greater procedural complexity than their distal filter counterparts. Other disadvantages of these devices include the potential for ischaemic myocardial damage due to prolonged interruption of antegrade flow. Distal balloon occlusive devices therefore require a more timely approach to PCI than with other devices which allow continued blood supply to the distal vascular bed. Also, direct trauma from the inflated balloon may cause local vessel wall injury, and care should be taken only to inflate the balloon to the amount required to arrest antegrade flow. Any branches proximal to the deployed occlusion balloon may be subject to emboli, and an important principle of distal protection devices is to place them proximal to any major bifurcations. Balloon placement assumes that there is an adequate landing site distal to the lesion, and proximal to any major bifurcation. Incomplete aspiration of the stagnant debris is another potential limitation of balloon occlusive devices. Perhaps one of the biggest disadvantages of these devices is the lack of visibility during PCI, given that antegrade flow has been arrested, and contrast injection cannot be used to guide PCI.

Distal filter-based devices

Distal filter-based embolic protection devices employ the use of a fenestrated basket deployed distal to the treated lesion prior to intervention. Due to the porous nature of filter-based distal protection devices, they offer certain advantages over occlusive balloon devices, including better visualization of the lesion during PCI, and allowing for perfusion of the distal vascular bed during the period of embolic protection. Among their disadvantages, the most significant may be incomplete protection of the vascular bed, not only from embolic debris, but also soluble vasoactive substances released during PCI which may pass through the filter into the microcirculation[27].

The FilterWire EX® device was the first such device available. The latest generation device (FilterWire EZ®) contains a nitinol loop supporting the filter which floats free from the shaft allowing for better apposition to the vessel wall and thus the potential for better myocardial protection (Fig. 37.2A,B). It has a 3.2F crossing profile, and comes in lengths of 190cm and 300cm, and basket sizes of 3.5mm and 5.5mm. Vessels suitable for use of the FilterWire® are those that are <5.5cm in diameter, have at least a 1 inch gap between the lesion and anastomosis (or branches), and have a relatively straight landing zone of 2cm for the filter basket (Fig. 37.3). The FilterWire® system consists of a flexible mesh filter mounted on its own coronary guide wire. Prior to crossing the lesion, the filter basket is placed in heparinized saline and retracted into its monorail sheath to allow the device to cross the lesion. Care should be taken to remove any trapped air prior to use. Using a supplied plastic introducer sheath, the FilterWire® is used to cross the lesion and when the basket is in a suitable landing zone, the monorail sheath is removed, thus deploying the filter basket. Two orthogonal views should be obtained to ensure adequate deployment of the basket. Care should be taken to fix the FilterWire® during intervention so that the basket does not move. Once the intervention is complete, a special purpose sheath is used to pass over the basket, trapping any contents (Fig. 37.4). The system is then removed. In cases where the basket contains considerable angiographically visible debris, the sheath should only partly cover the basket so as not to cause extrusion of any contents which may subsequently embolize the distal microvasculature (Fig. 37.2D, example shown using SpiderRX® [ev3 Inc., Plymouth, Minnesota]).

The SpiderRX® is another filter-based distal protection device which allows for operator choice of coronary guidewire to cross the lesion. The filter-basket is then delivered using a low-profile monorail exchange system designed to improve deliverability. The newer generation SpiderFX® device is more flexible with improved deliverability, and comes in 3, 4, 5, and 6mm sizes (Fig. 37.2C–F).

The Defender® (Medtronic, Santa Rosa, California) embolic protection device is another 6F compatible filter based distal protection device on a 0.014-inch 180cm guidewire. The Defender® is mounted to the

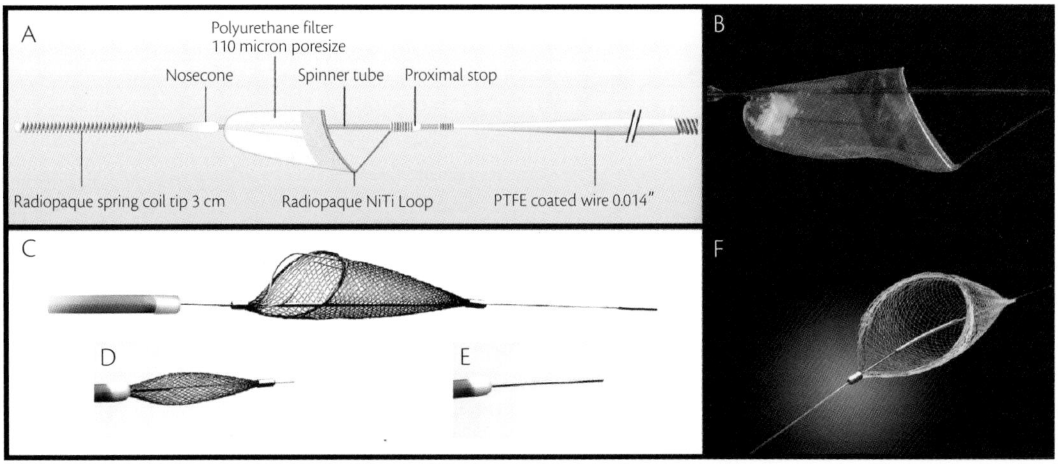

Fig. 37.2 The FilterWire® and Spider FX® systems. The newer generation FilterWire EZ® device contains a nitinol loop which suspends the filter basket free from the spinner tube (A). This allows for better apposition to the vessel wall with improved embolic protection. A photomicrograph of the device is pictured (B) demonstrating embolic debris captured from a saphenous vein graft. The SpiderRX® device is shown fully deployed (C). The basket is partially retracted within the recovery sheath, and the device can be withdrawn as is when significant amounts of thrombus are present to avoid 'spillage' of contents (D). The basket is fully retracted within the recovery sheath (E). The newer-generation SpiderFX® has a simplified monorail delivery system and is more flexible allowing for improved deliverability (F).

core wire between two stops allowing the filter basket to move independently on the wire (rotation and horizontal movement). The system has a filter transition segment that provides a smooth transition from the delivery sheath to the spring wire. The Defender® basket is made up of 24 strands loaded with platinum, providing four large proximal openings, and pores of 100 microns. The distal tip of the wire is coated with silicone, and the delivery profile is 2.2F. The four proximal openings are 1400–2100 microns in size depending on the size of the filter, which is available in 3.5, 4.5, 5.5, and 6.5mm sizes (Fig. 37.5).

The main advantage of distal filtration over balloon occlusive devices is that they allow for continuous antegrade flow. Contrast injections are therefore able to proceed in normal fashion, and myocardial ischaemia during embolic protection is less likely than with balloon occlusive devices. In general, distal filter-based protection devices are easier to use, and reduce procedural complexity. Disadvantages of distal filter-based embolic protection devices include the possibility of clogging the filter with debris, and thereby causing 'filter no-reflow'[28]. If considerable debris is present it may overload the basket and pass into the distal microvasculature upon removal of the filter device. Likewise, incomplete apposition of the filter against the vessel wall may allow particulate matter to bypass the device. Another theoretical disadvantage of these devices is their porous nature, which may allow for any soluble vasoactive substances to pass through the filter and

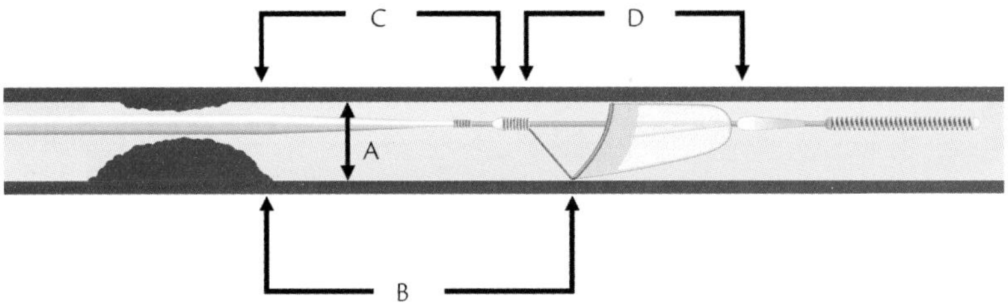

Fig. 37.3 Landing zone requirement for the FilterWire®. (A) The radiopaque nitinol loop accommodates 3.5–5.5mm vessels. (B) There should be at least 2.5cm from the lesion to the anastomosis for saphenous vein graft applications, and (C) the loop of the filter should be placed ≥1.5cm distal to the distal edge of the lesion. (D) The nitinol loop requires a 2-cm segment of relatively straight vessel.

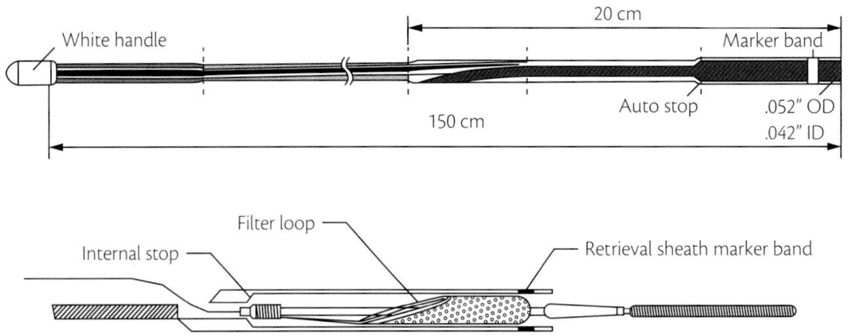

Fig. 37.4 FilterWire® retrieval system. Remove the EZ® Retrieval Sheath from its packaging coil grasping it by the white proximal handle. Flush the EZ® Retrieval Sheath with heparinized saline. Advance the retrieval sheath over the protection wire past any deployed stent up to the proximal end of the filter loop. Gently and slowly retract the protection wire and filter loop back into the retrieval sheath until resistance is felt. Observe the entire retrieval procedure under fluoroscopic imaging. The distal edge of the collapsed filter loop should align with, or be proximal to, the sheath marker band. Slowly and carefully retract the entire system until the tip of the retrieval sheath is adjacent to the tip of the guiding catheter or guiding sheath. If there is any resistance, retract the guiding catheter or guiding sheath and FilterWire EZ® system together. This is done in case there is a large amount of embolic material captured in the filter that may not fit inside the guiding catheter or guiding sheath.

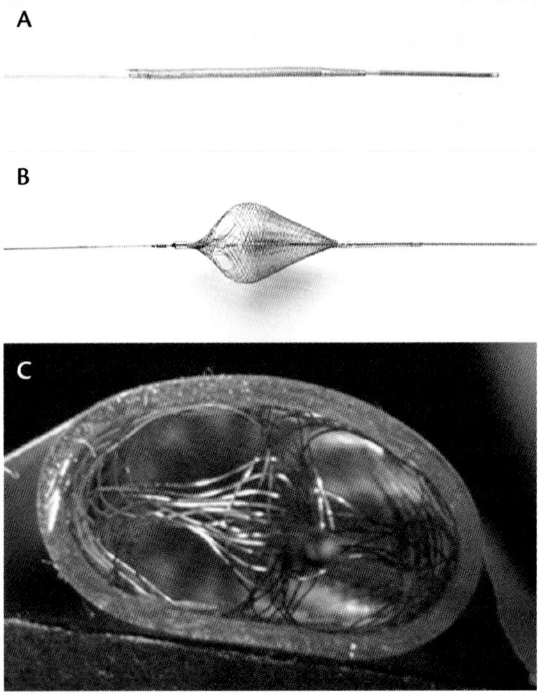

Fig. 37.5 The Defender® embolic protection device. The Defender® filter device has a very low crossing profile of (A). The basket is made up of 24 strands loaded with platinum providing pores of 100 microns (B). The device has 4 large proximal openings of 1400–2100 microns depending on the size of the filter (C), which is available in 3.5, 4.5, 5.5, and 6.5mm sizes.

exert their effect on the distal vascular bed. In general, these devices have a pore size of approximately 80–100 microns, and therefore could allow smaller debris particles to bypass through the system, although particulate matter of this size may have little clinical consequence. One significant disadvantage of these devices is their larger crossing profile compared with distal balloon occlusive devices, and this can cause difficulty with lesion crossing. Because they are bulkier, distal embolization is more likely to occur when crossing the lesion and pre-dilatation is more often required with these devices to allow passage of the filter.

Proximal balloon occlusive devices

The basic principle of proximal occlusion devices is to occlude the vessel proximal to the target lesion, therefore suspending antegrade flow during target vessel PCI. The goal is to prevent the distal release of both particulate debris and vasoactive substances. Like distal occlusive devices, the stagnant column of blood must be suctioned to remove any particulate matter and/or soluble humoral factors before antegrade flow is restored at the completion of PCI. Some vessels are also not suitable for distal protection systems due to the lack of an appropriate 'landing zone' for the device, either due to tortuosity, plaque disease, or both.

The Proxis® device (St. Jude Medical, Minneapolis, MN, USA) is a proximal balloon occlusive protection

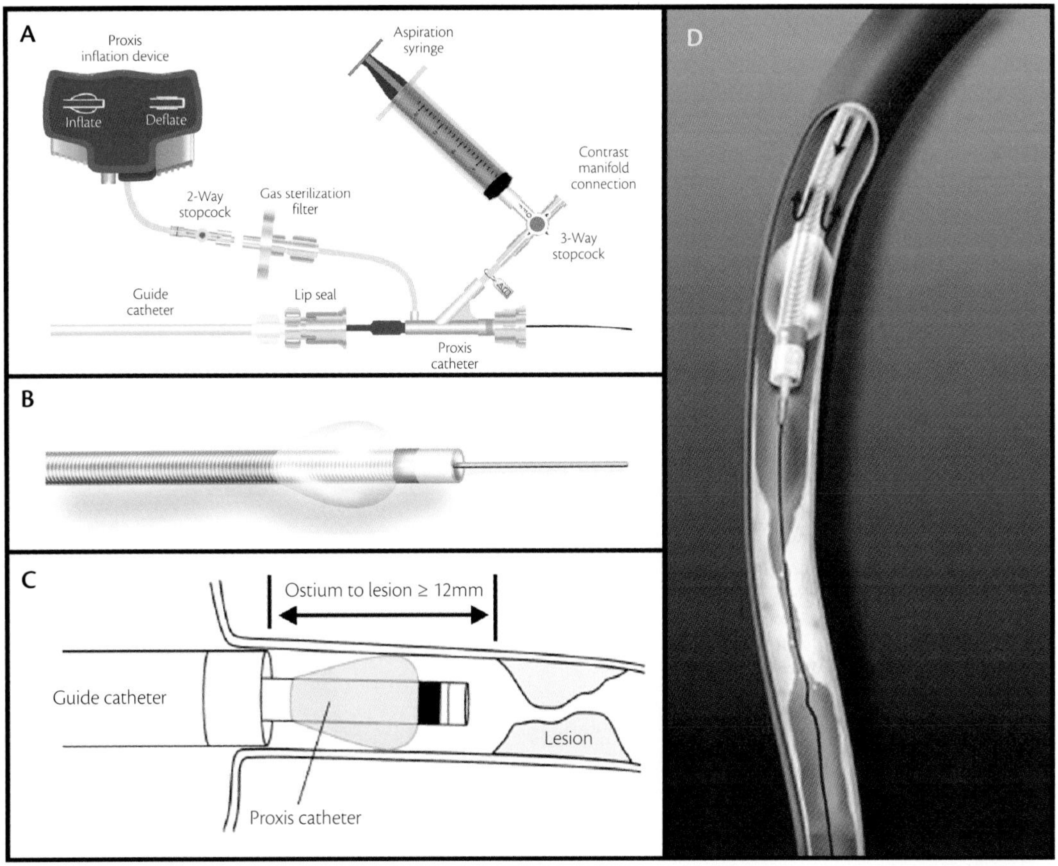

Fig. 37.6 The Proxis® device. The proximal end of the Proxis® catheter has a built-in standard Y-adapter configuration (haemostasis valve for device entry and a Luer connection for aspiration) and an additional Luer connection for the inflation device. The catheter is connected to an automated carbon dioxide inflation device. A 20-cc evacuation syringe with a 3-way stopcock is provided for the removal of blood, thrombus and embolic debris (A). The Proxis® Catheter is a sheath with a single working lumen and vessel sealing balloon 3mm from its tip (B). Landing zone requirements for the Proxis® catheter include at least 12mm from the tip of the guiding catheter to the lesion (C). Once deployed, PCI is undertaken through the Proxis® catheter with the balloon inflated (D).

system which has demonstrated similar efficacy to distal protection systems (Fig. 37.6)[29]. The device consists of a catheter with a low pressure, urethane occlusive sealing balloon at its tip. The catheter itself is a wound stainless steel coil, and the entire shaft and balloon is hydrophilic. Prior to intervention, the Proxis® catheter is inserted through the guide catheter and extends into the coronary vessel. The balloon is inflated with carbon dioxide using a push button inflation device which automatically inflates the sealing balloon to the ideal pressure (2–3 atmospheres). The intervention is then performed in the absence of antegrade flow, and upon completion, the stagnant column of blood is suctioned to remove any debris.

The main advantage of proximal protection devices is the fact that they offer embolic protection prior to any device passing across the target lesion, thus reducing the risk of mechanical distal embolization compared with distal devices which must first cross the lesion prior to being deployed. Theoretically, proximal occlusive devices also have the advantage of protecting side branches distal to the target lesion. Since the procedure is performed through the Proxis® catheter, the operator can gain additional support which provides for greater pushability and trackability. Potential disadvantages may include the presence of collateral flow allowing 'washout' of debris prior to balloon deflation and ischaemia during balloon occlusion.

Other embolic protection devices

Other devices aimed at protecting the distal microvascular bed include aspiration and rheolytic thrombectomy devices. These devices are designed to remove thrombus which may be present prior to PCI, and are of particular use in acute coronary syndromes and STEMI. Simple aspiration devices have been shown to improve outcomes and reduce infarct size following primary angioplasty for acute STEMI[30,31], and are now standard of care in many centres performing primary angioplasty. These devices are described further in Chapters 16 and 36.

Local plaque trapping devices that trap all potentially embolic debris against the vessel wall at the treatment site present another technique for the prevention of distal embolization. Conventional stents liberate large amounts of debris when deployed in SVGs, which was the rationale for stents covered with microporous polytetrafluoroethylene (PTFE), such as those used to treat coronary perforations, which could also serve as a form of 'local filter' during SVG interventions. Examples include the Graftmaster® (Abbott Vascular) and Symbiot® (Boston Scientific) stents. Early trials however showed no reduction in acute MACE and an increase in late occlusion with covered as opposed to bare metal stents, and no covered stents have clinical evidence to support a role in reducing distal embolization during SVG intervention[32–34]. Covered stents thus do not have approval status for their use in saphenous vein graft (SVG) intervention in lieu of other embolic protection strategies, in contrast to their approval for use in the treatment of life-threatening perforations. Other local plaque-trapping approaches are under study include a nitinol stent in which the structural nitinol elements are covered by an integral nitinol mesh. These devices are currently undergoing clinical trials, and have shown promise in pilot human testing, particularly in the setting of SVG and primary PCI.

Clinical settings

Saphenous vein graft PCI

Distal embolization of material is particularly problematic during SVG intervention as the plaque is very bulky and has a lower thrombus content than native coronary plaque. Distal embolization may be clinically and angiographically silent, or may present as a major reductions in coronary flow causing no-reflow and haemodynamic compromise.

During SVG PCI, distal embolization has proven to be virtually universal and can occur regardless of lesion characteristics or procedural technique[24]. Despite the universality of distal embolization during SVG intervention[23,25], only 15–20% of patients experience major adverse cardiac events (MACE), in the absence of embolic protection[35]. Unfortunately no clinical, angiographic or procedural variables can predict which patients undergoing SVG PCI are likely to obtain the most benefit from embolic protection, nor which grafts will liberate the greatest amount debris[24,36]. Even the most benign looking vein grafts have the potential to liberate significant amounts of debris during PCI (Fig. 37.7). As such, some form of embolic protection for all SVG procedures is recommend where feasible, regardless of graft age, degeneracy or appearance.

In the literature three exceptions have been suggested to this rule mandating protection for all grafts. Firstly, PCI of vein grafts <3 years old are associated with less bulky disease and a reduced incidence of distal embolization and no-reflow[37,38]. Secondly, ostial SVG lesions are subject to sheer stress which may create more fibrotic lesions[39], and likewise, the hyperplastic lesions of in-stent restenosis are relatively stable and less prone to cause distal embolization and subsequent no-reflow[40,41]. In our opinion consideration should always been given to protection where it can be performed safely even in these circumstances.

Early studies of the GuardWire® device demonstrated that considerable amounts of debris were retrieved following SVG PCI, including cholesterol crystals, fibrin, and lipid-rich macrophages[25]. The first randomized study of embolic protection versus no embolic protection for SVG PCI was the SVG Angioplasty Free of Emboli Randomised (SAFER) study[35]. This large study demonstrated a 42% relative risk reduction in 30-day MACE using the GuardWire® device, driven mainly by a reduction in no-reflow (3% vs. 9%) and myocardial infarction (8.6% vs. 14.7%). The TriActiv® system has demonstrated non-inferiority to both the GuardWire® and FilterWire® devices in the setting of SVG PCI[42].

Data for the efficacy of distal filter-based protection devices comes from the FilterWire EX Randomised Evaluation (FIRE) trial which demonstrated the non-inferiority of the FilterWire EX® device compared with the GuardWire® device in a large randomized study of SVG PCI[43]. In this study of 651 patients undergoing SVG PCI, the primary endpoint of death, myocardial infarction, or target vessel revascularization at 30 days occurred in 9.9% of the FilterWire EX® patients and 11.6% of GuardWire® patients (p for superiority = 0.53, p for non-inferiority = 0.0008). Device success was similar in both groups, defined as the ability to deliver,

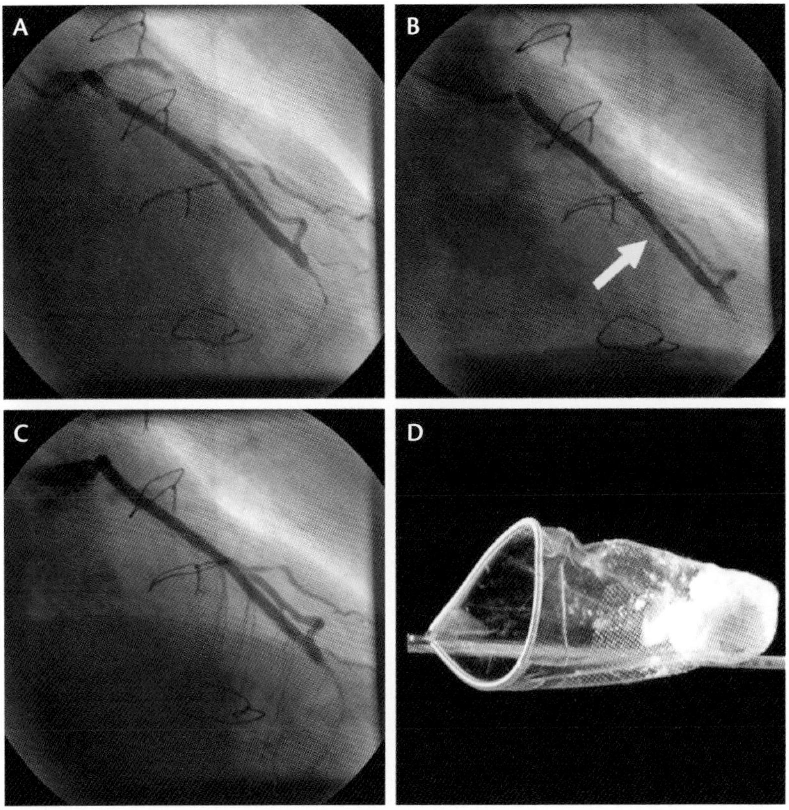

Fig. 37.7 An innocuous appearing lesion in the proximal portion of a saphenous vein graft (A). Following placement of a FilterWire EX®, the lesion is direct stented. Embolized material can be seen as a mobile filling defect in the filter basket (yellow arrow) (B). After removal of the FilterWire®, there is TIMI 3 flow with good distal run off (C). The FilterWire® contains a significant amount of embolized material (D).

deploy, and remove the device, and to maintain vessel occlusion in the case of the GuardWire®. Post-procedural measures of epicardial flow and angiographic complications were similar, although bailout IIb/IIIa inhibitors were required more frequently in the GuardWire® group (0.0% versus 1.5%, p = 0.03). The SpiderRX® device has also proved non-inferior to currently available distal protection systems in the setting of SVG PCI[44].

The Proxis® system was evaluated in the FASTER (Feasibility And Safety Trial for its embolic protection device during transluminal intervention in coronary vessels: a European Registry) trial. This showed that retrograde blood flow can be achieved during proximal occlusion and that the device can be safely used in both SVG and native-vessel PCI[45]. The PROXIMAL (Proximal Protection during SVG Intervention using the Proxis Embolic Protection System: A Randomised, Prospective, Multicentre Clinical Trial) study compared the Proxis® device to distal protection systems, including the GuardWire® and FilterWire® systems. This study demonstrated an equally high device success rate of 95.4% for the Proxis® device, with clinical success in 90.5% of patients. The primary composite endpoint of death, myocardial infarction, or target vessel revascularization at 30 days by intention to treat analysis occurred in 9.2% of Proxis® patients versus 10.0% of controls (p,for non-inferiority = 0.0061). The authors concluded that using proximal embolic protection whenever possible during treatment of diseased SVG produced outcomes similar to those with distal embolic protection.

A discussion of myocardial protection during PCI would not be complete without consideration of pharmacotherapy. Multiple studies (EPIC, EPILOG, IMPACT-II, EPISTENT and PURSUIT) have evaluated the adjunctive use of glycoprotein IIb/IIIa inhibition for patients undergoing SVG PCI[46–50]. Whilst the EPIC investigators did find a reduction in the rate of distal embolization with the use of IIb/IIIa inhibition, no clinical benefit was identified[51]. In a pooled analysis of these five studies incorporating 605 patients with complete follow-up, no clinical benefit for IIb/IIIa inhibition in patients undergoing SVG PCI was detected; however there was a 6% absolute increase in the occurrence of both minor and major bleeding episodes for patients in the treatment group[52]. Two retrospective studies including a total of 1880 SVG PCI procedures have found similar results[53,54]. The largest of these from the Cleveland Clinic Foundation, Ohio, found no benefit of glycoprotein IIb/IIIa inhibition with or without the combined use of a distal protection device[54]. A recent post hoc analysis of the FIRE trial however demonstrated that glycoprotein IIb/IIIa inhibition was associated with superior FilterWire® (but not GuardWire®) performance, including better preservation of flow through the filter, reduced procedural ischaemia, and reduced occurrence of abrupt closure, no-reflow, and distal embolization[55].

Data on other pharmacologic agents aimed at protecting the myocardium for patients undergoing SVG PCI are limited. In a retrospective study of 143 consecutive patients who underwent SVG PCI, the incidence of no-reflow was not different in patients who received intragraft adenosine prior to PCI[56]. In the small randomized VAPOR study of 22 patients, 200mcg of intragraft verapamil, however, had a significant beneficial effect with no-reflow occurring in none of the patients in the treatment group and one-third of patients in the control group[57].

In a recently published registry of 83 consecutive SVG interventions performed without distal embolic protection, intragraft nicardipine (200–300mcg) resulted in excellent angiographic and clinical outcomes[58]. The incidence of no-reflow was only 2/83 (2.4%) and in-hospital MACE was 3/83 (3.6%). Although no control group was available for comparison, the results compare favourably with historical controls of SVG PCI performed without distal protection, where the occurrence of no-reflow is as high as 15%[18,59], and MACE occurs in 15–20%[35]. The rationale for use of nicardipine comes from studies which demonstrate a sharp rise in soluble vasoconstrictors during SVG PCI which challenge the hypothesis of distal embolization (and hence use of embolic protection) as the primary event in no-reflow[60]. The ease of use and cost-effective nature of intragraft nicardipine compared with embolic protection devices presents a promising development in the percutaneous management of SVG disease. A randomized head-to-head comparison with embolic protection is required to assess for non-inferiority (or superiority) of nicardipine before its use can be recommended in place of mechanical protection.

Currently there is no solid evidence from randomized trials to support the use adjunctive pharmacology for the prevention of myocardial injury during SVG PCI, although the use of IIb/IIIa inhibitors may be safe in the setting of distal protection with filter-based devices, particularly in the presence of significant thrombus. Distal embolization of friable plaque contents is common during SVG PCI, and may be the predominate mechanism of myocardial injury which would explain the greater success of embolic protection devices compared with pharmacologic approaches in studies to date. However, adverse events still occur in approximately 10% of patients even with the use of these devices, emphasizing the need for further research into complementary pharmacologic approaches which may enhance the safety of intervention in these high-risk patients.

Native vessel PCI

Primary PCI is a very effective treatment strategy for patients with acute STEMI, and achieves normal epicardial flow in the vast majority of patients. However, even when normal epicardial flow (TIMI grade 3) is restored, microvascular perfusion is often abnormal when assessed by myocardial perfusion blush grade, and these patients sustain larger infarcts and have a worse prognosis[61]. This is mostly due to the presence of significant ischaemia/reperfusion injury which obstructs the microvasculature, but further injury due to distal embolization is important, as patients who experience a transient reduction in TIMI flow during primary PCI have significantly higher 6-month mortality compared with those who do not (31% vs. 3%)[62] The concept that distal embolization is likely to be important in primary PCI has resulted in many studies, but no randomized study of embolic protection in native coronary arteries has demonstrated a clinical benefit for their use.

Studies using the GuardWire® distal embolic protection system as adjunctive treatment during rescue or primary PCI for acute STEMI demonstrated improved coronary perfusion post-procedure[63,64]. However these findings were not supported by the large randomized Enhanced Myocardial Efficacy and Removal by Aspiration of Liberated Debris (EMERALD) study, which was unable to demonstrate any improvement in coronary microvascular flow, reperfusion success, infarct size, or event-free survival in patients undergoing primary PCI with distal balloon protection despite capture of embolic debris in 73% of patients in the treatment group[65]. Furthermore, the potential for harm was present, with fluoroscopy and procedural times significantly increased by 5min and 25min respectively, and a delay in door to first balloon inflation of 21min in the GuardWire® group.

Initial results with filter-based protection in native coronary arteries were encouraging, particularly with the FilterWire® system which was shown to improve angiographic measures of reperfusion for patients with acute STEMI undergoing primary PCI[66]. However the larger randomised Protection Devices in PCI-Treatment of Myocardial Infarction for Salvage of Endangered Myocardium (PROMISE) study of the same device was unable to demonstrate a benefit in the primary endpoint of coronary flow reserve. Likewise, no benefit was seen in TIMI flow, myocardial blush grade, or 30-day mortality[67]. The FilterWire® system used in the Treatment of an Acute Myocardial Infarction for Embolic Protection (FLAME) trial examined the ability of the second generation FilterWire EZ® device to capture embolic debris compared with either aspiration alone using the Export® or Rescue® catheter, or in combination with aspiration. It showed that the combined approach of filter protection and aspiration was significantly more efficient at capturing embolic debris (70% versus 15% for FilterWire EZ® only and 11% for aspiration only). Despite the encouraging results seen in the combined group with respect to capture of embolic debris, no effect on infarct size or clinical benefit was demonstrable[68].

The Protection of Distal Embolisation in High-Risk Patients with Acute Myocardial Infarction (PREMIAR) study evaluated the SpiderRX® filter system in native vessel PCI for high-risk patients with STEMI[69]. The primary endpoint was ST-segment resolution, while secondary endpoints included MACE, TIMI blush score, corrected TIMI frame count, distal embolization, and no-reflow. No differences in the primary or secondary endpoints were found. Likewise, no differences in MACE were seen at 30 days or 6 months following the procedure.

Proximal protection devices offer theoretical advantages over distal protection including the ability to protect the distal vascular bed without first crossing the lesion with a bulky device which may itself cause distal embolization, and the inclusion of side-branch protection. Registry data including over 200 patients treated for acute STEMI with primary PCI has shown that the Proxis® embolic protection device appears safe and effective in capturing debris, however no prospective randomized controlled trials have been performed to date[70], and no randomized controlled trials have assessed the Proxis® or other proximal occlusion devices in STEMI.

A recent meta-analysis has confirmed that whilst adjunctive devices for primary PCI reduce distal embolization and improve final myocardial blush grade, they have no impact on clinical outcomes[71]. It may be that embolic protection devices for all patients undergoing native vessel PCI for acute STEMI is the wrong approach, and reserving these devices for patients with significant thrombotic burden is probably more appropriate.

These disappointing data contrast with the benefit of simple aspiration devices, which have been shown to improve clinical outcomes and reduce infarct size following primary angioplasty for acute STEMI[30,31]. Aspiration devices are designed to physically remove intracoronary thrombus and therefore reduce the potential for embolization following balloon inflation. The large (n = 1071) randomized Thrombus Aspiration during Primary Percutaneous Coronary Intervention in Acute Myocardial Infarction Study (TAPAS) using the Export® catheter, thrombus aspiration prior to direct stenting for primary PCI was shown to improve myocardial blush post-procedure and ST segment resolution compared with standard pre-dilatation and stenting[31], and at 1 year follow-up there was a significant reduction in cardiac death and myocardial infarction[72]. As such, thrombus aspiration prior to stenting in primary PCI is now routine care in many centres performing primary PCI.

In the setting of elective PCI of native coronary arteries, distal embolization of plaque contents is reflected by elevation of CK and troponin[73–76]. There is a direct relationship not only between peri-procedural infarct size and absolute troponin elevation in elective native vessel PCI, but also between reduction in plaque volume following PCI and peri-procedural myocardial injury[2,77]. No-reflow during native vessel PCI occurs in 0.6–2.0% of all comers[18,78], however it is much more frequent in patients with acute STEMI compared with non-infarct patients (11.5% vs. 1.5%)[78]. Patients with acute coronary syndromes involving the right coronary artery (RCA) may be at higher risk of distal embolization during PCI[22] but there is no data to demonstrate clinical benefit in any endpoint from using distal protection during elective or urgent PCI in native coronaries.

In contrast to SVG PCI, there is considerable evidence for pharmacotherapy over the use of mechanical devices, in particular for IIb/IIIa inhibitors, in protecting the myocardium and improving angiographic and clinical outcomes. There is evidence that the beneficial effects of glycoprotein IIb/IIIa inhibition are mediated by improved microvascular perfusion, and the results of abciximab with respect to hard clinical endpoints including mortality strongly favour its use as standard of care in patients undergoing primary PCI for acute STEMI, particularly for those at higher risk[79,80].

Conclusion

Use of distal protection should be considered standard when treating vein graft disease and there are a number of devices which are equally effective. There are currently no data to support routine use of distal protection in routine cases or primary PCI but with best medical therapy and thrombus aspiration some patients still do not achieve normal restoration of epicardial flow. These patients may represent a subset of patients who could benefit from the use of improved embolic protection devices in the future.

References

1. Thygesen K, Alpert JS, White HD, *et al.* Joint ESC/ACCF/AHA/WHF Task Force for the Redefinition of Myocardial Infarction. Universal definition of myocardial infarction. *Circulation* 2007; **116**:2634–53.
2. Porto I, Selvanayagam JB, van Gaal WJ, *et al.* Plaque volume and occurrence and location of periprocedural myocardial necrosis after percutaneous coronary intervention: insights from delayed-enhancement magnetic resonance imaging, thrombolysis in myocardial infarction myocardial perfusion grade analysis, and intravascular ultrasound. *Circulation* 2006; **114**:662–9.
3. Kloner RA, Ganote CE, Jennings RB. The "no-reflow" phenomenon after temporary coronary occlusion in the dog. *J Clin Invest* 1974; **54**:1496–508.
4. Manciet LH, Poole DC, McDonagh PF, *et al.* Microvascular compression during myocardial ischemia: mechanistic basis for no-reflow phenomenon. *Am J Physiol* 1994; **266**:H1541–50.
5. Gavin JB, Thomson RW, Humphrey SM, *et al.* Changes in vascular morphology associated with the no-reflow phenomenon in ischaemic myocardium. *Virchows Arch A Pathol Anat Histopathol* 1983; **399**:325–32.
6. Seydoux C, Goy JJ, Davies G. Platelet and neutrophil imaging techniques in the investigation of the response to thrombolytic therapy and the no-reflow phenomenon. *Am Heart J* 1993; **125**:1142–7.
7. Ambrosio G, Weisman HF, Mannisi JA, Becker LC. Progressive impairment of regional myocardial perfusion after initial restoration of postischemic blood flow. *Circulation* 1989; **80**:1846–61.
8. Hickey MJ, Hurley JV, Morrison WA. Temporal and spatial relationship between no-reflow phenomenon and postischemic necrosis in skeletal muscle. *Am J Physiol* 1996; **271**:H1277–86.
9. Engler RL, Schmid-Schonbein GW, Pavelec RS. Leukocyte capillary plugging in myocardial ischemia and reperfusion in the dog. *Am J Pathol* 1983; **111**:98–111.
10. Sheridan FM, Cole PG, Ramage D. Leukocyte adhesion to the coronary microvasculature during ischemia and reperfusion in an in vivo canine model. *Circulation* 1996; **93**:1784–7.
11. Engler RL, Dahlgren MD, Morris DD, Peterson MA, Schmid-Schonbein GW. Role of leukocytes in response to acute myocardial ischemia and reflow in dogs. *Am J Physiol* 1986; **251**:H314–23.
12. Okamura A, Ito H, Iwakura K, *et al.* Clinical implications of distal embolization during coronary interventional procedures in patients with acute myocardial infarction: Quantitative study with Doppler guidewire. *J Am Coll Cardiol Interv* 2008; **1**:268–76.
13. Aiello EA, Jabr RI, Cole WC. Arrhythmia and delayed recovery of cardiac action potential during reperfusion after ischemia. Role of oxygen radical-induced no-reflow phenomenon. *Circ Res* 1995; **77**:153–62.
14. Ito H, Maruyama A, Iwakura K, *et al.* Clinical implications of the 'no reflow' phenomenon. A predictor of complications and left ventricular remodeling in reperfused anterior wall myocardial infarction. *Circulation* 1996; **93**:223–8.
15. Morishima I, Sone T, Mokuno S, *et al.* Clinical significance of no-reflow phenomenon observed on angiography after successful treatment of acute myocardial infarction with percutaneous transluminal coronary angioplasty. *Am Heart J* 1995; **130**:239–43.
16. Morishima I, Sone T, Okumura K, *et al.* Angiographic no-reflow phenomenon as a predictor of adverse long-term outcome in patients treated with percutaneous transluminal coronary angioplasty for first acute myocardial infarction. *J Am Coll Cardiol* 2000; **36**:1202–9.
17. Gerber BL, Rochitte CE, Melin JA, *et al.* Microvascular obstruction and left ventricular remodeling early after acute myocardial infarction. *Circulation* 2000; **101**:2734–41.
18. Abbo KM, Dooris M, Glazier S, *et al.* Features and outcome of no-reflow after percutaneous coronary intervention. *Am J Cardiol* 1995; **75**:778–82.
19. Testa L, van Gaal WJ, Biondi Zoccai GG, *et al.* Myocardial infarction after percutaneous coronary intervention: a meta-analysis of troponin elevation applying the new universal definition. *QJM* 2009; **102**(6):369–78.
20. Yip HK, Chen MC, Chang HW, *et al.* Angiographic morphologic features of infarct-related arteries and timely reperfusion in acute myocardial infarction: predictors of slow-flow and no-reflow phenomenon. *Chest* 2002; **122**:1322–32.
21. Hara M, Saikawa T, Tsunematsu Y, *et al.* Predicting no-reflow based on angiographic features of lesions in patients with acute myocardial infarction. *J Atheroscler Thromb* 2005; **12**:315–21.
22. Napodano M. Predictors of distal embolization during direct angioplasty for acute myocardial infarction. Presented at The 16th Annual Transcatheter Cardiovascular Therapeutics; October 16–21, Washington, DC, 2005.
23. Popma JJ, Cox N, Hauptmann KE, *et al.* Initial clinical experience with distal protection using the FilterWire in patients undergoing coronary artery and saphenous vein graft percutaneous intervention. *Catheter Cardiovasc Interv* 2002; **57**:125–34.

24. van Gaal WJ, Choudhury RP, Porto I, *et al.* Prediction of distal embolization during percutaneous coronary intervention in saphenous vein grafts. *Am J Cardiol* 2007; **99**:603–6.
25. Webb JG, Carere RG, Virmani R, *et al.* Retrieval and analysis of particulate debris after saphenous vein graft intervention. *J Am Coll Cardiol* 1999; **34**:468–75.
26. Stone GW, Rogers C, Ramee S, *et al.* Distal filter protection during saphenous vein graft stenting: technical and clinical correlates of efficacy. *J Am Coll Cardiol* 2002; **40**:1882–8.
27. Leineweber K, Bose D, Vogelsang M, *et al.* Intense vasoconstriction in response to aspirate from stented saphenous vein aortocoronary bypass grafts. *J Am Coll Cardiol* 2006; **47**:981–6.
28. Porto I, Choudhury RP, Pillay P, *et al.* Filter no reflow during percutaneous coronary interventions using the Filterwire distal protection device. *Int J Cardiol* 2006; **109**:53–8.
29. Rogers C. A prospective randomized comparison of proximal and distal protection in patients with diseased saphenous vein grafts. Presented at The 16th Annual Transcatheter Cardiovascular Therapeutics; October 16 – 21, Washington, DC, 2005.
30. Silva-Orrego P, Colombo P, Bigi R, *et al.* Thrombus aspiration before primary angioplasty improves myocardial reperfusion in acute myocardial infarction: the DEAR-MI (Dethrombosis to Enhance Acute Reperfusion in Myocardial Infarction) study. *J Am Coll Cardiol* 2006; **48**:1552–9.
31. Svilaas T, Vlaar PJ, van der Horst IC, *et al.* Thrombus aspiration during primary percutaneous coronary intervention. *N Engl J Med* 2008; **358**:557–67.
32. Schachinger V, Hamm CW, Munzel T, *et al.* A randomized trial of polytetrafluoroethylene-membrane-covered stents compared with conventional stents in aortocoronary saphenous vein grafts. *J Am Coll Cardiol* 2003; **42**:1360–9.
33. Stankovic G, Colombo A, Presbitero P, *et al.* Randomized evaluation of polytetrafluoroethylene-covered stent in saphenous vein grafts: the Randomized Evaluation of polytetrafluoroethylene COVERed stent in Saphenous vein grafts (RECOVERS) Trial. *Circulation* 2003; **108**:37–42.
34. Blackman DJ, Choudhury RP, Banning AP, *et al.* Failure of the Symbiot PTFE-covered stent to reduce distal embolization during percutaneous coronary intervention in saphenous vein grafts. *J Invasive Cardiol* 2005; **17**:609–12.
35. Baim DS, Wahr D, George B, *et al.* Randomized trial of a distal embolic protection device during percutaneous intervention of saphenous vein aorto-coronary bypass grafts. *Circulation* 2002; **105**:1285–90.
36. Giugliano GR, Kuntz RE, Popma JJ, *et al.* Determinants of 30-day adverse events following saphenous vein graft intervention with and without a distal occlusion embolic protection device. *Am J Cardiol* 2005; **95**:173–7.
37. Kalan JM, Roberts WC. Morphologic findings in saphenous veins used as coronary arterial bypass conduits for longer than 1 year: necropsy analysis of 53 patients, 123 saphenous veins, and 1865 five-millimeter segments of veins. *Am Heart J* 1990; **119**:1164–84.
38. Neitzel GF, Barboriak JJ, Pintar K, *et al.* Atherosclerosis in aortocoronary bypass grafts. Morphologic study and risk factor analysis 6 to 12 years after surgery. *Arteriosclerosis* 1986; **6**:594–600.
39. Saltissi S, Webb-Peploe MM, Coltart DJ. Effect of variation in coronary artery anatomy on distribution of stenotic lesions. *Br Heart J* 1979; **42**:186–91.
40. Assali AR, Sdringola S, Moustapha A, *et al.* Percutaneous intervention in saphenous venous grafts: in-stent restenosis lesions are safer than de novo lesions. *J Invasive Cardiol* 2001; **13**:446–50.
41. Ashby DT, Dangas G, Aymong EA, *et al.* Effect of percutaneous coronary interventions for in-stent restenosis in degenerated saphenous vein grafts without distal embolic protection. *J Am Coll Cardiol.* 2003; **41**:749–52.
42. Carrozza J, Joseph P, Mumma M, *et al.* Randomized evaluation of the TriActiv Balloon-Protection Flush and Extraction System for the treatment of saphenous vein graft disease. *J Am Coll Cardiol* 2005; **46**:1677–83.
43. Stone GW, Rogers C, Hermiller J, *et al.* Randomized comparison of distal protection with a filter-based catheter and a balloon occlusion and aspiration system during percutaneous intervention of diseased saphenous vein aorto-coronary bypass grafts. *Circulation* 2003; **108**:548–53.
44. Dixon R. SPIDER: Saphenous vein protection in a distal embolic protection randomized trial. Presented at The 16th Annual Transcatheter Cardiovascular Therapeutics; October 16 – 21, Washington, DC, 2005.
45. Sievert H, Wahr DW, Schuler G, *et al.* Effectiveness and safety of the Proxis system in demonstrating retrograde coronary blood flow during proximal occlusion and in capturing embolic material. *Am J Cardiol* 2004; **94**:1134–9.
46. The EPIC Investigators. Use of a monoclonal antibody directed against the platelet glycoprotein IIb/IIIa receptor in high-risk coronary angioplasty. *N Engl J Med* 1994; **330**:956–61.
47. The EPILOG Investigators. Platelet glycoprotein IIb/IIIa receptor blockade and low-dose heparin during percutaneous coronary revascularization. *N Engl J Med* 1997; **336**:1689–97.
48. The IMPACT-II Investigators. Randomised placebo-controlled trial of effect of eptifibatide on complications of percutaneous coronary intervention: IMPACT-II. *Lancet* 1997; **349**:1422–8.
49. Topol EJ. Randomised placebo-controlled and balloon-angioplasty-controlled trial to assess safety of coronary stenting with use of platelet glycoprotein-IIb/IIIa blockade. *Lancet* 1998; **352**:87–92.

50. The PURSUIT Trial Investigators. Inhibition of platelet glycoprotein IIb/IIIa with eptifibatide in patients with acute coronary syndromes. *N Engl J Med* 1998; **339**:436–43.
51. Mak K-H, Challapalli R, Eisenberg MJ, *et al.* Effect of platelet glycoprotein IIb/IIIa receptor inhibition on distal embolization during percutaneous revascularization of aortocoronary saphenous vein grafts. *Am J Cardiol* 1997; **80**:985–8.
52. Roffi M, Mukherjee D, Chew DP, *et al.* Lack of benefit from intravenous platelet glycoprotein IIb/IIIa receptor inhibition as adjunctive treatment for percutaneous interventions of aortocoronary bypass grafts: a pooled analysis of five randomized clinical trials. *Circulation* 2002; **106**:3063–7.
53. Mathew V, Grill DE, Scott CG, *et al.* The influence of abciximab use on clinical outcome after aortocoronary vein graft interventions. *J Am Coll Cardiol* 1999; **34**:1163–9.
54. Karha J, Gurm HS, Rajagopal V, *et al.* Use of platelet glycoprotein IIb/IIIa inhibitors in saphenous vein graft percutaneous coronary intervention and clinical outcomes. *Am J Cardiol* 2006; **98**:906–10.
55. Jonas M, Stone GW, Mehran R, *et al.* Platelet glycoprotein IIb/IIIa receptor inhibition as adjunctive treatment during saphenous vein graft stenting: differential effects after randomization to occlusion or filter-based embolic protection. *Eur Heart J* 2006; **27**:920–8.
56. Sdringola S, Assali A, Ghani M, *et al.* Adenosine use during aortocoronary vein graft interventions reverses but does not prevent the slow-no reflow phenomenon. *Catheter Cardiovasc Interv* 2000; **51**:394–9.
57. Michaels AD, Appleby M, Otten MH, *et al.* Pretreatment with intragraft verapamil prior to percutaneous coronary intervention of saphenous vein graft lesions: results of the randomized, controlled vasodilator prevention on no-reflow (VAPOR) trial. *J Invasive Cardiol* 2002; **14**:299–302.
58. Fischell TA, Subraya RG, Ashraf K, Perry B, Haller S. Pharmacologic distal protection using prophylactic, intragraft nicardipine to prevent no-reflow and non-Q-wave myocardial infarction during elective saphenous vein graft intervention. *J Invasive Cardiol* 2007; **19**:58–62.
59. Resnic FS, Wainstein M, Lee MK, *et al.* No-reflow is an independent predictor of death and myocardial infarction after percutaneous coronary intervention. *Am Heart J* 2003; **145**:42–6.
60. Salloum J, Tharpe C, Vaughan D, Zhao DX. Release and elimination of soluble vasoactive factors during percutaneous coronary intervention of saphenous vein grafts: analysis using the PercuSurge GuardWire distal protection device. *J Invasive Cardiol* 2005; **17**:575–9.
61. Henriques JPS, Zijlstra F, van't Hof AWJ, *et al.* Angiographic assessment of reperfusion in acute myocardial infarction by myocardial blush grade. *Circulation* 2003; **107**:2115–19.
62. Mehta RH, Harjai KJ, Boura J, *et al.* Prognostic significance of transient no-reflow during primary percutaneous coronary intervention for ST-elevation acute myocardial infarction. *Am J Cardiol* 2003; **92**:1445–7.
63. Nakamura T, Kubo N, Seki Y, *et al.* Effects of a distal protection device during primary stenting in patients with acute anterior myocardial infarction. *Circ J* 2004; **68**:763–8.
64. Yip H-K, Wu C-J, Chang H-W, *et al.* Effect of the PercuSurge GuardWire device on the integrity of microvasculature and clinical outcomes during primary transradial coronary intervention in acute myocardial infarction. *Am J* Cardiol 2003; **92**:1331–5.
65. Stone GW, Webb J, Cox DA, *et al.* Distal microcirculatory protection during percutaneous coronary intervention in acute ST-segment elevation myocardial infarction: a randomized controlled trial. *JAMA* 2005; **293**:1063–72.
66. Limbruno U, Micheli A, De Carlo M, *et al.* Mechanical prevention of distal embolization during primary angioplasty: safety, feasibility, and impact on myocardial reperfusion. *Circulation* 2003; **108**:171–6.
67. Gick M, Jander N, Bestehorn H-P, *et al.* Randomized evaluation of the effects of filter-based distal protection on myocardial perfusion and infarct size after primary percutaneous catheter intervention in myocardial infarction with and without ST-segment elevation. *Circulation* 2005; **112**:1462–9.
68. Hermiller J, Cox D, Barbeau G, *et al.* Distal filter embolic protection in AMI – The FLAME Registry. Presented at The 16th Annual Transcatheter Cardiovascular Therapeutics; October 16–21, Washington, DC, 2005.
69. Cura FA, Escudero AG, Berrocal D, *et al.* Protection of Distal Embolization in High-Risk Patients with Acute ST-Segment Elevation Myocardial Infarction (PREMIAR). *Am J Cardiol* 2007; **99**:357–63.
70. Koch K. Proximal aspiration in AMI introduced: The Proxis registry. Presented at The 16th Annual Transcatheter Cardiovascular Therapeutics; October 16–21, Washington, DC, 2005.
71. Burzotta F, Testa L, Giannico F, *et al.* Adjunctive devices in primary or rescue PCI: A meta-analysis of randomized trials. *Int J Cardiol* 2008: **123**(3):313–21.
72. Vlaar PJ, Svilaas T, van der Horst IC, *et al.* Cardiac death and reinfarction after 1 year in the Thrombus Aspiration during Percutaneous coronary intervention in Acute myocardial infarction Study (TAPAS): a 1-year follow-up study. *Lancet* 2008; **371**:1915–20.
73. Abdelmeguid AE, Topol EJ, Whitlow PL, *et al.* Significance of mild transient release of creatine kinase–mb fraction after percutaneous coronary interventions. *Circulation* 1996; **94**:1528–36.
74. Califf RM, Abdelmeguid AE, Kuntz RE, *et al.* Myonecrosis after revascularization procedures. *J Am Coll Cardiol* 1998; **31**:241–51.
75. Herrmann J, Haude M, Lerman A, *et al.* Abnormal coronary flow velocity reserve after coronary intervention is associated with cardiac marker elevation. *Circulation* 2001; **103**:2339–45.

76. Mehran R, Dangas G, Mintz GS, *et al.* Atherosclerotic plaque burden and CK-MB enzyme elevation after coronary interventions: intravascular ultrasound study of 2256 patients. *Circulation* 2000; **101**:604–10.
77. Selvanayagam JB, Porto I, Channon K, *et al.* Troponin elevation after percutaneous coronary intervention directly represents the extent of irreversible myocardial injury: insights from cardiovascular magnetic resonance imaging. *Circulation* 2005; **111**:1027–32.
78. Piana RN, Paik GY, Moscucci M, *et al.* Incidence and treatment of 'no-reflow' after percutaneous coronary intervention. *Circulation* 1994; **89**:2514–8.
79. De Luca G, Suryapranata H, Stone GW, *et al.* Abciximab as adjunctive therapy to reperfusion in acute ST-segment elevation myocardial infarction: a meta-analysis of randomized trials. *JAMA* 2005; **293**:1759–65.
80. De Luca G, Suryapranata H, Stone GW, *et al.* Relationship between patient's risk profile and benefits in mortality from adjunctive abciximab to mechanical revascularization for ST-segment elevation myocardial infarction: a meta-regression analysis of randomized trials. *J Am Coll Cardiol* 2006; **47**:685–6.

SECTION 8

Non-coronary percutaneous interventions

CHAPTER 38

Percutaneous device closure of atrial septal defect and patent foramen ovale

Patrick A. Calvert, Bushra S. Rana, and David Hildick-Smith

Introduction

Structural heart disease interventions look set to form an increasing proportion of the interventional cardiologist's workload. Device closure of atrial septal connections, both patent foramen ovale (PFO) and atrial septal defect (ASD), are the most commonly performed adult structural interventional procedure in the United Kingdom, with 793 PFO and 573 ASD closure procedures performed in adults in 2007[(1)]. Device closure of ASDs and PFOs are elegant procedures which combine technical and imaging skills with a detailed understanding of cardiac anatomy. More importantly, they also provide tangible clinical benefits to patients.

Embryology and anatomy

Development of the atrial septum in utero

The cardiac septa form between the 27th and 37th days post conception[(2)]. At the end of the 4th week a thin band of tissue (shaded dark blue in Fig. 38.1) grows from the cranial aspect of the common atria towards the endocardial cushion (green in Fig. 38.1) which is developing in the common atrioventricular canal. The gap between the primum septum and the endocardial cushion is the ostium primum (Fig. 38.1A). Before the ostium primum is closed by the primum septum, a series of fenestrations form in the middle of the primum septum (Fig. 38.1B). These coalesce to form the ostium secundum (Fig. 38.1C).

At the same time the secundum septum forms (shaded pink in Fig. 38.1C and D). The secundum septum is not a true septum, rather, it is an invagination of the atrial wall. This is important, as penetration of the atrial septum through the secundum septum will actually be exiting the heart into the pericardial space, risking tamponade. The secundum septum is probably generated by differential growth of the atria walls[(2)]. The secundum septum forms a thick crescent-shaped peripheral margin to the ovale fossa and the thin primum septum lines the floor of the ovale fossa.

During embryological development, the overlapping atrial septa progressively fuse. However, a section, usually anterosuperior, remains patent. This permits blood to bypass the lungs and flow directly from the right to the left atrium. At birth, the increase in left atrial pressures causes rightward deviation of the septum primum, pushing it against the septum secundum. These septa then fuse in the majority of people. Failure of the atrial septa to fuse results in a PFO. Failure of the ostium secundum to close can be due to excessive resorption of the primum septum or deficient growth of the secundum septum such that the two septa do not overlap. This is termed an ostium secundum ASD. Failure of closure of the ostium primum is due to failure of the endocardial cushion to fuse and is termed ostium primum ASD.

Anatomy of atrial septal defects

Ostium secundum ASDs represent 60–70% of ASDs. Ostium primum ASDs (15–20% of ASDs) are often associated with mitral regurgitation secondary to an anterior leaflet cleft. Sinus venosus defects (5–15% of ASDs) are nearly always associated with anomalous pulmonary venous drain. Unroofed coronary sinus is a

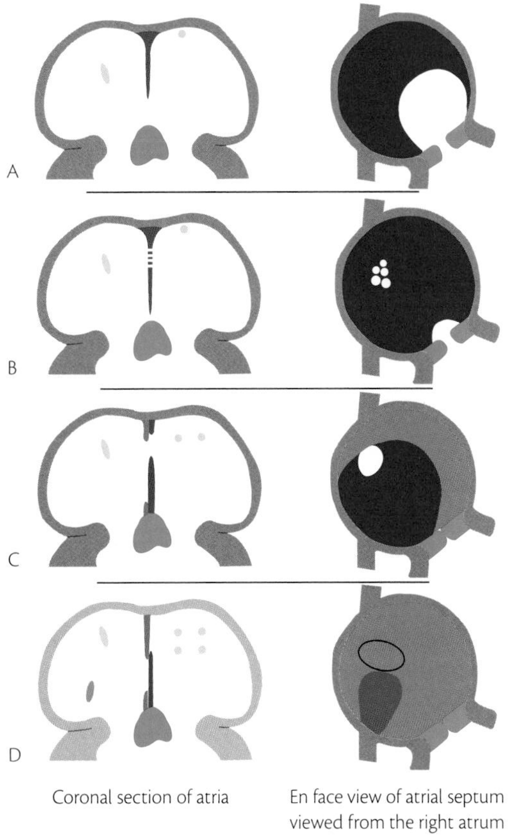

Fig. 38.1 Development of the atrial septum. Fig. 38.1A shows development of the primum septum (dark blue) growing form the cranial margin of the atria towards the endocardial cushion (green) to fill the ostium primum which lies between these two structures. In Fig. 38.2B the ostium primum has been almost totally obliterated. During this phase fenestrations start to form in the centre of the septum primum which coalesce to form the ostium secundum (Fig. 38.1C). The secundum septum (pink) is seen forming in Fig. 38.1C and D by invagination of the atrial wall and therefore is not a true septum. Fig. 38.1D shows the atrial septum just before birth with the black circle representing the tunnel like communication between the right and left atria known as the patent foramen ovale. This tunnel closes in the majority of people after birth.

rare cause of left-to-right shunt. Ostium secundum ASDs are the only type that can be successfully closed percutaneously. The position of the various types of atrial level shunts are displayed in Fig. 38.2.

The anatomy of the atrial septum and therefore of secundum ASDs is highly variable and must be accurately delineated prior to any attempt at closure. In some patients the invagination of tissue that forms the secundum septum almost meets centrally leaving a very small oval fossa. In other patients, the secundum septum only forms a limited rim leaving a large oval fossa lined by the primum septum. The failure of overlap of the two septa can occur at any part of the oval fossa but often lies anterosuperiorly, close to where the tunnel of the PFO tends to be. Secundum ASDs can be multiple (Fig. 38.3B) or indeed fenestrated, resulting in numerous tiny shunts or fenestrations (Fig. 38.3D). Occasionally the primum septum is aneurysmal and billows according to the pressure differential between the two atria (Fig. 38.3C). Cabanes defined an atrial septal aneurysm as one that can deviate 10mm in either direction from the midline[3]. Aneurysmal atrial septa are associated with fenestrated ASDs or larger PFOs and are therefore associated with an apparent higher risk of recurrent stroke[4].

Anatomy of a patent foramen ovale

Failure of overlap of the primum and secundum septa results in an ostium secundum ASD. However, if the septa do overlap but fail to fuse, this results in a tunnel or flap known as a PFO. The anatomy and position of this tunnel is highly variable and will determine the best device to achieve closure or indeed if device closure is feasible. A typical PFO tunnel is represented schematically in Fig. 38.4, shaded in dark green. The PFO is usually in an anterosuperior position close to the aortic valve. There is a clear overlap zone (dark green in Fig. 38.4) with openings at the right and left atrial ends of the tunnel. As shown in Fig. 38.4, the tunnel is often shorter in its central portion and devices that can self-centre will do so in the shortest tunnel zone.

Variation can occur with tunnel position, size, length, and shape. The degree of adherence of the two septa in the walls of the tunnel also varies. Some tunnels are long and tightly stuck down (Fig. 38.5A). Other tunnels are poorly adherent and the primum septum can retract right back such that the overlap is lost and a 'functional' secundum ASD is created. If the two septa are held apart by some structure or ridge in the walls of the tunnel, or by septation of the septum primum in its attachment, then it will be more difficult to oppose the septa and bring about closure with a device—in effect 'fixed splitting' of the atrial septa (Fig. 38.5D).

Indications for closure

Closure of atrial septal defects for shunt-related symptoms

Natural history of atrial septal defects

ASDs account for approximately 10% of congenital cardiac defects and 22–40% of congenital heart disease in adults[5]. They are general well tolerated in the first

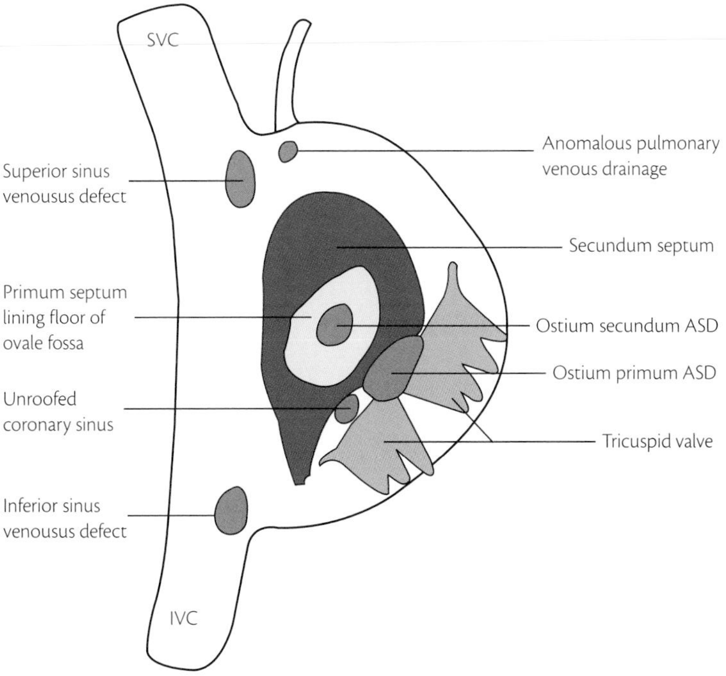

Fig. 38.2 Schematic of the atrial septum viewed from the right atrium demonstrating the positions of various atrial level shunts.

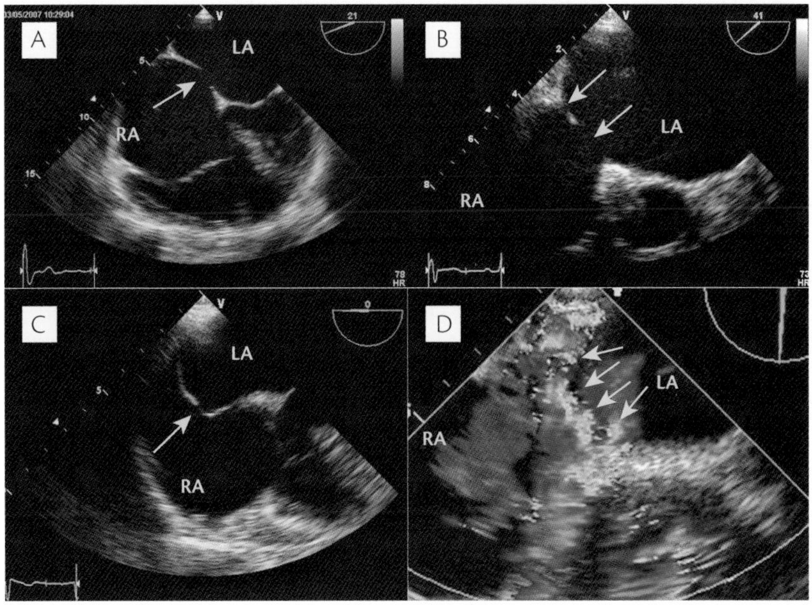

Fig. 38.3 Transoesophageal images of ASDs marked by arrow. A) Single ASD B) Two ASDs (arrows) C) Aneurysmal primum septum with secumdum ASD and D) Fenestrated primum septum with multiple secundum ASDs seen on with colour Doppler (LA = left atrium, RA = right atrium).

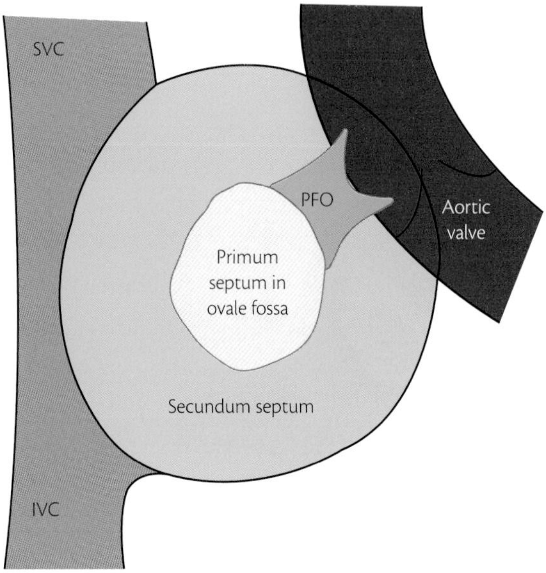

Fig. 38.4 Schematic of the atrial septum as viewed from the right atrium showing typical PFO anatomy.

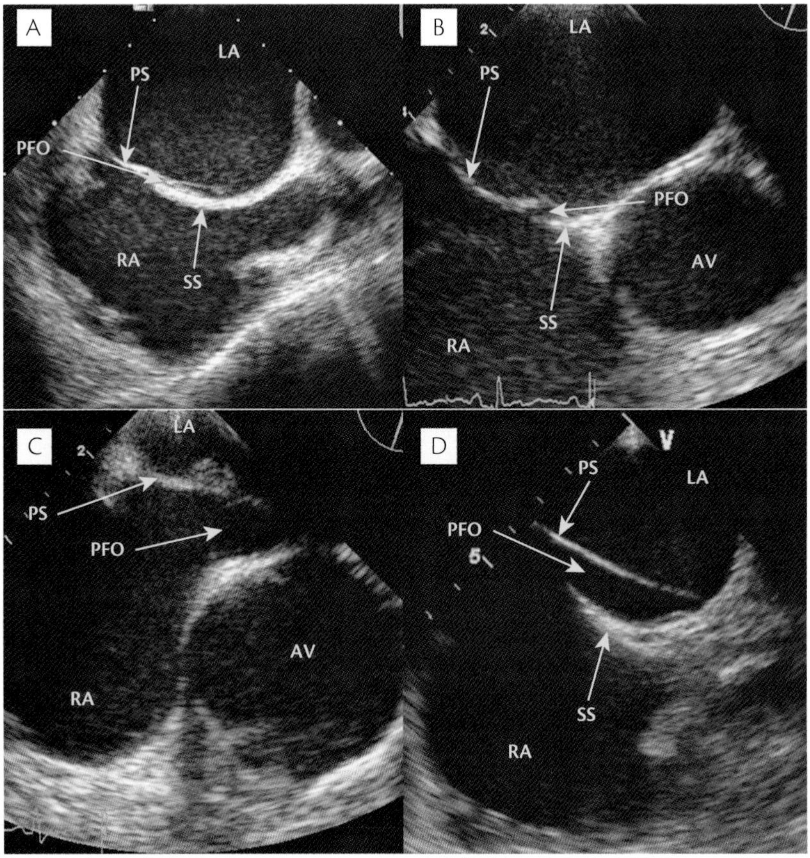

Fig. 38.5 A) Long tunnel PFO. B) Short tunnel PFO. C) PFO with spontaneous retraction of the primum septum. D) Fixed splitting of the septa in the tunnel. (LA = left atrium, RA = right atrium, AV = aortic valve, PS = primum septum, SS = secundum septum, PFO = patent foramen ovale) .

two decades[6]. Presentation depends upon the magnitude of the left-to-right shunt. Effort dyspnoea is seen in 30% of patients by the third decade and more than 75% of patients by the fifth decade[6]. Atrial arrhythmias (atrial fibrillation and flutter) are common and are secondary to atrial dilatation. Clinical examination may reveal fixed splitting of the second heart sound coupled with a pulmonary flow murmur[7]. The classically described electrocardiogram of an ASD is right bundle branch block (RBBB) and axis deviation (right for secundum and left for primum). These changes are thought to be due to right-sided volume overload[8]. The presence of these electrocardiographic changes improved diagnostic sensitivity and specificity of haemodynamically significant ASDs[9].

Knowledge of the mortality rates of patients with uncorrected ASDs is based largely on an often quoted paper from 1970[6]. The author calculated mortality rates from a retrospective cohort and from an autopsy series and appeared to achieve good agreement between the two methods. The mortality rates for the first to the seventh decades were: 0.6%, 0.7%, 2.7%, 4.5%, 5.4%, and 7.5% respectively. The mean age of death was 37.5 ± 4.5 years with three-quarters dying by age 50 years. Although this paper is imperfect, no better understanding of the natural history of ASD will be published due to the widespread surgical and percutaneous correction of this defect.

Evidence supporting surgical closure of atrial septal defects

The first attempted closure of an ASD was reported as early as 1948[10]. This involved externally suturing the septum through the right atrial wall and was only partial successful. Due to the relative simplicity of the procedure, closure of an ASD was the first ever open heart operation, perform in 1952 by F. John Lewis[11].

Several retrospective surgical series have been reported throughout the decades[12, 13] which suggested that the results were best if correction was performed within the first two decades. The outcome of those who had surgical ASD closure after 40 years old was specifically examined in a non-randomized retrospective series of 179 consecutive ASD patients who had corrective surgery or medical (non-corrective) management[14]. Despite the study design and with the exception of age, there were no significant differences between baseline demographics of the two cohorts. Multivariable analysis demonstrated that surgical correction of ASD was associated with a relative risk of death = 0.31 ($p = 0.02$) as compared to non-corrective treatment.

Further support for the closure of ASDs in adults was provided by Attie and colleagues who prospectively randomized 521 patients over 40 years old to surgical or medical (non-corrective) management[15]. After a median follow-up of 7.3 years, the combined primary endpoint of major adverse cardiovascular event was nearly twice as frequent in the non-corrected than the surgical group (univariable hazard ratio (HR) = 1.99 (confidence interval [CI] 1.2–3.2, $p < 0.005$), multivariable HR = 1.85 (CI 1.1–3.2). Although there was no significant overall mortality difference with univariable analysis, multivariable analysis revealed a significant excess of deaths on the medical group (HR = 4.1, $p < 0.001$).

Evidence supporting percutaneous closure of atrial septal defect

Experimental closure of ASDs have been reported as early as 1974[16] with clinical application from 1976[17]. Despite initial low complication rates, the large 23F delivery sheath limited widespread uptake of the device. In 1990, Rome and colleagues published a series of 40 ASDs that had been closed using various modifications of the Rahskind patent ductus arteriosus (PDA) closure device[18]. The beauty of this device was that it could be delivered through an 11F venous catheter. The Rashkind device had a single umbrella on the right atrial side and hooks to anchor on the left atrial side. These hooks prevented self-centring and after two modifications the double umbrella device was born. This basic design format was to form the basis of most future ASD closure devices.

In 1997, Masura and colleagues published the first in man experience of a new device known as the Amplatzer® Septal Occluder (AGA Medical Corp., Golden Valley, MN, USA)[19]. This device consisted of a weave of a nickel titanium alloy (nitinol) that can be fashioned to return to a particular conformation after deformation, so called memory metal. This innovation permitted the device to be elongated to fit within a 12F deliver catheter and then reconform in the heart to a double-disc shape that achieved a high closure rate of the ASD (24 out of 30 patients had complete closure on day 1). This, combined with ease of use and the ability to recapture and redeploy the device means the Amplatzer® Septal Occluder remains popular.

Percutaneous device closure of secundum ASD with Amplatzer® Septal Occluder was compared to surgical closure in a multicentred non-randomized trial of 596 patients[20]. The authors commented that enrolment was 'largely prospective' and that the method of closure was determined by physician and patient preference.

This non-randomized enrolment resulted in some significant baseline demographic differences between the device and surgical groups in particular age (mean age of device patients 18.1 ± 19.3 years versus, mean age of surgical patients 5.9 ± 6.2 years). Importantly there was no significant difference between the sizes of the ASDs in both groups. 442 patients had device closure and 154 patients had surgical closure of their ASD. The primary efficacy endpoint of successful closure (no leak greater than small, no embolization, no reintervention) at 12 months was not significantly different between the two groups (device group 98.5% vs. surgical group 100%, $p > 0.05$). However, the complication rate (device group 7.2% vs. surgical group 24%; $p < 0.001$) and the mean length of hospital stay (device group 1.0 ± 0.3 days vs. surgical group 3.4 ± 1.2 days; $p < 0.001$) where both greater in the surgical group. No deaths were reported in either group.

Device safety

A wide range of devices have now been developed which are capable of closing secundum ASDs, each with their own safety data. However, the Amplatzer® Septal Occluder remains one of the most commonly used devices and a 'world experience' of safety data was published in 2001[21]. This paper reported the 3-year complication rates on 3535 patients who had ASD closure with this device. Excluding 75 patients, in whom the device could not be deployed, the authors claimed a 100% closure rate at 3 months and at 3 years as defined by a residual shunt that is no more than small. Major and minor complications occurred in 0.3% and 2.8% of cases respectively. Although no deaths were reported in this series, a small number of deaths have been reported which may in part be related to oversizing of the device[22–24]. Major complications include stroke, air embolization, death, cardiac tamponade, device erosion or embolization, and bleeding. Minor complications include arrhythmia and bruising.

Which atrial septal defects should we close?

When a secundum ASD is being considered for closure for shunt alone, there is much debate as to the thresholds which should prompt closure. As for all procedures this should be a balance of risk between intervention and surveillance. The physician (and surgeon) should explain the published data relevant to the patient and make an individual decision in conjunction with the patient.

The natural history paper by Campbell from 1970 suggests a rather grim prognosis; however, no information is given in this paper regarding the size of the shunt or of the ASDs of the patients included[6]. Although there are no trials directly comparing device closure with surveillance (this would have been unethical in light of the surgical data) we do know that mortality and morbidity are reduced with surgical closure of ASDs[14,15]. We also know that device closure is as effective as surgery with lower complications rates[20]. In the surgical studies the entry criteria was shunt greater than or equal to 1.5 and 1.7 respectively[14,15]. The trial comparing device versus surgical closure included patients with shunt greater than or equal to 1.5 or presence of right ventricular volume loading[20]. This trial also included patients with minimal shunt who had dyspnoea, arrhythmia, or transient ischaemic attack (TIA).

It may be deduced that patients with shunts less than 1.5 and without right ventricular volume loading or symptoms may be safely left unclosed. However, the correlation between the shunt and ASD size is, at best, fair ($r = 0.76$) and shunt size can vary widely in large ASDs[25]. The correlation between echocardiographic and catheter measured shunt is better ($r = 0.85$)[26].

Furthermore, patients may not appreciate their lifelong limitations until there ASD is closed. This is support by a study that examined the maximal oxygen uptake (VO_2max) and ventricular dimension before and after ASD closure in NHYA Class I (asymptomatic) and NHYA II patients[27]. Both groups had significant improvements in VO_2max and right ventricular dimension with 35 out of 37 patients being asymptomatic after closure versus 17 out of 35 prior to closure.

Cryptogenic stroke and systemic embolus

Paradoxical embolus

The cause of stroke remains unidentified in up to 40% of patients[28]. These so-called cryptogenic strokes or TIA should have clinical and imaging evidence of brain ischaemia or infarction. Other sources of thromboemboli need to be determined with imaging of the heart, head, and neck vessels.

A proposed mechanism for cryptogenic stroke is that of paradoxical embolus, which is a thrombus passing from the system venous to the systemic arterial circulation via a communication in the heart, in particular a PFO. As fanciful as this explanation sounds, the concomitant diagnosis of systemic venous thrombosis and cryptogenic stroke is far from rare. A study that identified the deep venous thrombosis (DVT) rates of stroke victims using magnetic resonance venography showed that DVT was more common in patients with cryptogenic stroke than stroke of known origin (20% vs. 4%, $p < 0.03$), as were PFOs (61% vs. 19%)[29]. Although this

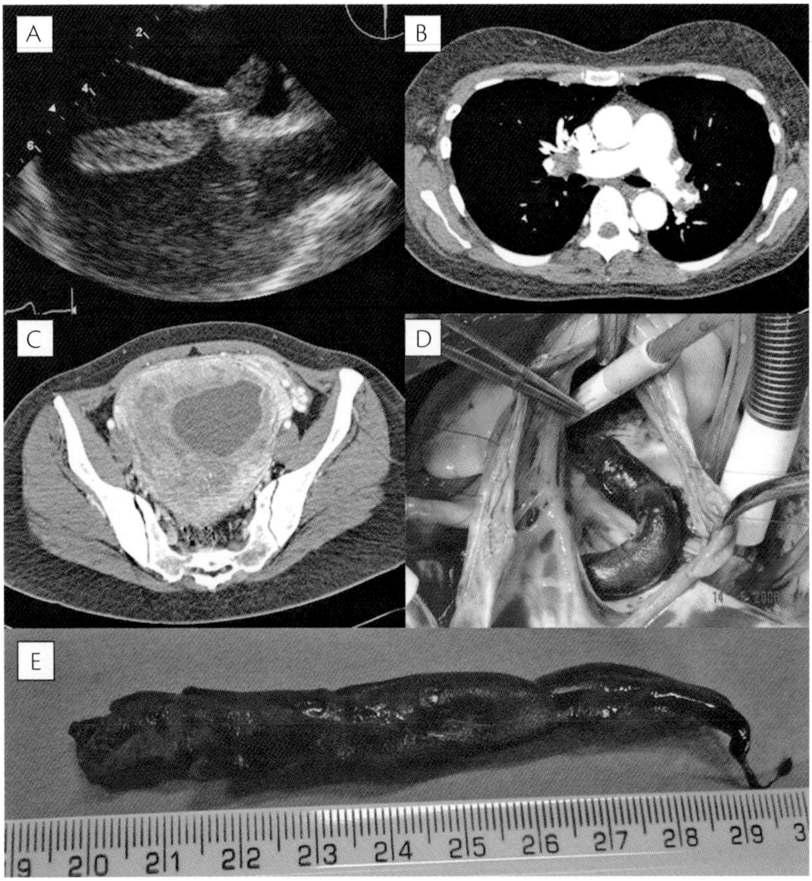

Fig. 38.6 A) TOE of paradoxical embolus lodged in PFO. B) Pulmonary emboli in main pulmonary arteries. C) Multi-fibroid uterus lying upon clot-laden femoral veins seen on CT. D) Paradoxical embolus seen in the right atrium at surgery. E) Excised paradoxical embolus against a centimetre scale[30].

does not prove the mechanism, many case reports of thrombus caught in a PFO (impending paradoxical emboli) provide compelling evidence[30–33].

The term paradoxical embolus was coined in 1881 when Zahn described a branched thrombus from a uterine vein caught in a PFO at post mortem[34]. Fig. 38.6 demonstrates a large paradoxical embolus found in a 47-year-old woman who had presented with dyspnoea and syncope proceeded by a week of bed rest due to a sprained ankle. The images show multiple bilateral DVTs and pulmonary emboli (PEs) seen on CT (Figs. 38.6C and B) and a large multifibroid uterus compressing the common iliac veins (Fig. 38.6C). The paradoxical embolus is seen on transoesophageal echo, intraoperatively, and excised (Fig. 38.6A, D, and E respectively). The patient made a good recovery following surgical embolectomy and PFO closure[30].

An alternative proposed mechanism for the involvement of PFO in thrombus formation relates to the relatively static column of blood that is often seen in long tunnel PFOs prompting thrombus formation *in situ*. However, the commonly reported occurrence of DVTs and PEs with impending paradoxical emboli supports the former theory, and the low rate of peri-procedural stroke at the time of transcatheter closure of PFOs militates against this explanation.

The association between cryptogenic stroke and patent foramen ovale

There are many studies supporting an association between cryptogenic stroke and PFO[3,4,35–40]. These studies also support an association between cryptogenic stroke and atrial septal aneurysm (ASA) as defined by an excursion of greater than 10mm in either direction. A large meta-analysis by Overell compared cryptogenic stroke with strokes of known causes and found odds ratios for PFO = 3.16 (95% CI 2.30–4.35) (22 studies); for ASA = 3.65 (95% CI 1.34–9.97) (five studies); and for PFO plus ASA = 23.26 (95% CI 5.24–103.20) (two studies)[4]. The association was strongest for those less than 55 years of age. However, Handke specifically examined the relationship in the over 55 years age group and again found a strong association between cryptogenic stroke and PFO[40].

Device closure of patent foramen ovale

The first reported series of device closure of a PFO was in 1992[41]. Bridges and colleagues closed 36 PFOs with a double-umbrella device for presumed paradoxical embolus with no serious complications. At a mean follow up of 8.4 months, all but one patient had no or trivial leak and there were no recurrent events.

The literature on device closure of PFO for cryptogenic stroke has largely been driven by uncontrolled registry data designed to assess safety and feasibility rather than efficacy[42–47]. Khairy attempted to make sense of the existing data with a meta-analysis in 2003[48]. The authors found that the 1-year recurrence rate of neurological event was 0–4.9% for device closure (1335 patients in 10 studies) versus 3.8–12% for medical therapy (895 patients in six studies). However, significant baseline differences prevented the authors from concluding that device closure was superior to medical therapy.

The retrospective cases series by Windecker and colleagues remains the primary evidence to date, supporting closure of PFO in cryptogenic stroke[49]. They identified all patients with cryptogenic stroke and PFO who were admitted to the Bern University Stroke Unit over a 6.5-year period. One hundred and fifty patients had device closure of their PFO and 158 had medical therapy which consisted of warfarin, aspirin, or clopidogrel. Patients who had device closure were more likely to have suffered more than one stroke (risk ratio = 1.68, $p = 0.03$) and also had a larger right-to-left shunt ($p<0.001$). After 4 years of follow-up, percutaneous PFO closure resulted in a non-significant trend toward risk reduction of death, stroke, or TIA combined (8.5% vs. 24.3%; $p = 0.05$; 95% CI 0.23–1.01). It is notable that during the first 2 years there was no apparent benefit, presumably indicating that the potential benefit was cancelled out by procedural or post-procedural adverse events.

It is also noteworthy that the centre did not use intraoperative echocardiographic guidance of the procedure and complete closure of PFO was only gained in 81% of patients. Accordingly, patients with complete PFO occlusion after device closure had a significantly lower risk of recurrent stroke or TIA than medically treated patients (6.5% vs. 22.2%; $p = 0.04$). Similarly, patients with more than one cerebrovascular event at baseline, had a significantly lower risk of recurrent stroke or TIA after percutaneous PFO closure than medically treated patients (7.3% vs. 33.2%; $p = 0.01$).

Prospective randomized controlled trials comparing device closure of PFO versus medical treatment of cryptogenic stroke are in progress but have been dogged by slow recruitment. The CLOSURE 1 trial sponsored by NMT Medical completed enrolment in August 2008 with 900 patients recruited[50]. AGA Medical Corporation is running two similar trials. The US trial is called RESPECT and continues to recruit. Recruitment to the 'OUS' trial (PC Trial) has recently halted at 410 recruits. W. L. Gore and Associates commenced the Gore REDUCE trial in 2008.

Systemic arterial emboli

Systemic arterial embolization of paradoxical embolus to limbs and gut are described in the literature[31–33]. However, due to the large cerebral blood supply which arises proximally from the aorta, and the extreme sensitivity of the end-organ in question, such paradoxical emboli tend to manifest as cerebral ischaemia or infarction.

Decompression illness

Diving related decompression illness

The ambient increased pressures encountered during diving lead to super-saturation of tissues with nitrogen. Pressure increases by one atmosphere per 10m of dive depth, therefore tissue will contain a four times greater concentration of nitrogen at a depth of 40m than at the surface. During ascent, the reduction in ambient pressure means that nitrogen comes out of solution to form bubbles. Nucleation of bubbles occurs both in the venous blood and in tissue. If an ascent is appropriate, then nitrogen bubbles are safely filtered out by pulmonary capillary diffusion. However, rapid ascents may result in the pulmonary filter being overwhelming and nitrogen bubbles appearing in the systemic arterial circulation. The nitrogen follows the concentration gradient from the supersaturated tissue to the bubbles. This results in enlargement of bubbles, tissue trauma, and vessel occlusion with the resulting neurological deficits and rashes which forms part of the syndrome known as decompression illness.

If any right-to-left shunt is present then the filter of the lungs is additionally bypassed. Such syndromes do not occur when a large positive bubbles contrast study is performed at normal atmospheric pressure because the nitrogen again follows the concentration gradient which is now reversed from the bubbles to the unsaturated tissue and the bubbles dissipate.

The presence of a large PFO is associated with some forms of decompression illness[51,52]. Studies have demonstrated that decompression illness following a non-provocative dive is more likely to be associated with a shunt than those who suffer it after a provocative dive[52–54]. A blinded case–control study examined the shunt size in 100 consecutive divers with neurological decompression illness to 123 case controls[55]. A large or medium shunt was seen with Valsalva manoeuvre in 52% of cases and 12.2 % of controls (p <0.001). Furthermore, the severity and duration of a decompression illness event appears to be related to the size of the PFO[56].

Transcatheter closure of ASD to prevent decompression illness was first reported in 1996[57]. Professional divers who have suffered from decompression illness should be referred to a physician with a specialist interest in diving medicine. If it is felt that the symptoms are consistent with shunt-related decompression illness and they have a PFO then they may be considered for device closure after informing the patient of the available data. There has not yet been any prospective randomized controlled trials examining the efficacy of PFO closure in preventing decompression illness.

Subatmospheric decompression illness

High altitude pilots and astronauts have also been reported to suffer decompression illness upon moving from atmospheric to subatmospheric pressures[58,59].

Conditions with inconsistent evidence for closure

Migraine with aura

Migraines affect approximately 13% of the population aged between 20–64 years old[60] with 36% preceded by aura[61]. Migraine with aura is associated with PFO and other causes of right-to-left shunting[62]. It is hypothesized that a blood-borne substance which would ordinarily be filtered out by the lungs is delivered to the cerebral circulation via the shunt. However, the triggering mechanism of migraines is unknown and this theory remains unproven.

Patients who have PFO closed for non-migraine indication have reported an improvement of their migraine symptoms[55,63–65]. However, these are retrospective non-randomized studies. Furthermore, migraine frequency is influenced by placebo effect.

These points were addressed in a prospective randomized sham-controlled study called the MIST trial[66]. One hundred and sixty-three patients with migraine with aura and a moderate or large right-to-left shunt on bubble contrast echo study were randomized to PFO closure or a sham procedure in which the patient was anaesthetized and a skin incision was made in the groin. The ambitious primary endpoint was headache cessation 6 months post randomization, based on patient diaries. The authors found no significant difference between the treatment and control groups for the primary or secondary endpoints which assessed the frequency and severity of migraines during the first 3 months. Post hoc analysis revealed that once two extreme outliers were removed, there was a significant reduction in the median total headache days with PFO closure (p = 0.027).

The MIST trial has pioneered a robust study design for PFO closure trials. However, the ambitious primary endpoint was not reached perhaps in part due to underpowering and therefore the scientific question remains unanswered. The trial has, however, raised a number of further questions which will be addressed in future studies.

Atrial right-to-left shunting causing significant hypoxia despite normal pulmonary artery pressures

Significant hypoxia due to atrial right-to-left shunting in the absence of pulmonary hypertension is rare but has been reported[67–74]. Two principal mechanisms have been proposed. Firstly, an alteration of the normal cardiac haemodynamics exists such that there is a right-to-left pressure gradient across the atrial septum in the absence of pulmonary hypertension. This can be induced by right ventricular infarction, tricuspid regurgitation, and mechanical ventilation especially with positive pulmonary end-expiratory pressure[69]. A second theory relates to preferential streaming of deoxygenated blood from the inferior vena cava (IVC) through a PFO or ASD. This is often due to an overdeveloped Eustachian valve[75,76] but may be due to a change in the orientation of the atrial septum such that it lies in line with flow from the IVC. This may result, for example, from aortic root dilatation[76–78]. In a case series of 11 patients, all but one of the patients who had successful closure of their PFO or ASD had a significant improvement in arterial oxygenation[69].

Platypnoea orthodeoxia is a term used to describe a subset of these patients who suffer dyspnoea and desaturation in the upright position. These patients have often had pulmonary surgery or have significant lung disease. However the shunt is atrial not pulmonary[67] and the desaturation stops after closure of the shunt[70,71].

Obstructive sleep apnoea (OSA) is a condition where patients are rendered apnoeic due to upper airways obstruction and can have a serious impact on quality of life. Patients with OSA have a higher incidence of PFO[79]. Patients with OSA appear to have desaturations that are out or proportion to the degree of hypoventilation[80,81]. Furthermore OSA patients with PFOs have more frequent desaturations[82]. So far no studies have been done to determine the effect of closing PFOs in these patients, though there are sporadic case reports.

Transient global amnesia

PFO has been found in increased frequency in those with transient global amnesia (TGA) than in control patients (55% vs. 27%, $p < 0.01$)[83]. Similarly to migraines, the mechanism of TGA remains unexplained and little data regarding its claimed link with PFOs exist.

Pre-procedure investigations

Atrial septal defects

Once the diagnosis of an ASD is suspected, investigations must be undertaken to determine the type and anatomy of the ASD and look for other associated cardiac anomalies. Echocardiography can, in most instances, provide all the anatomical information required.

The atrial septum is a posterior cardiac structure and therefore is better imaged by a transoesophageal echocardiography (TOE) than transthoracic echocardiography (TTE). Nonetheless, the transthoracic echocardiogram can give good views of the atrial septum, especially subcostal, parasternal short axis, and 'off-axis' four-chamber views (Fig. 38.7A). Transthoracic images also give important general cardiac anatomy and are better at determining left and right ventricular size and function as well as atrial sizes. The shunt can be calculated by measuring the annular dimension and velocity time integral at the aortic and pulmonary valves. An estimate of pulmonary artery pressure is also important.

The oesophagus lies immediately posterior to the left atrium and therefore TOE gives exquisite views of the atrial septum. The type and the position of the ASD is determined by scanning inferiorly and superiorly with the probe in multiple multiplane angles. The rims of the ASD must be sufficient to stabilize any device although partial rim deficiency does not exclude the possibility of device closure. The relationship between the ASD and its surrounding structures must be determined to ensure that there is enough distance such that the device does not compromise these structures, in particular, caval veins, mitral valve, and coronary sinus. It is also important to ensure that the atria are large enough to accommodate any device needed to close the ASD.

Other associated cardiac anomalies must be excluded, especially anomalous pulmonary venous drainage. The inferior atrial septum can be difficult to image with TOE and it is important to ensure that there is an inferior rim between the ASD and the IVC. If there is true rim deficiency inferiorly, then this is in fact an inferior sinus venosus defect rather than a secundum ASD and device closure should not be attempted. If there is any doubt, then cardiac magnetic resonance or computed tomographic scanning should be performed. Intracardiac echocardiography (ICE) also images the inferior septum very well but this is an invasive and expensive technique.

Cardiac catheterization is no longer mandated but can be used to confirm the echo findings by measuring chamber pressures, oxygen saturation, and shunt calculation. There should be a step-up in oxygen saturation from the right atrium to the right ventricle. Coronary angiography is only indicated if the patient has ischaemic symptoms.

Patent foramen ovale

Patients with PFO usually have normal cardiac anatomy and this is established for certain using TTE and TOE as explained earlier. The indication for most PFO closures is cryptogenic stroke and therefore the main focus is looking for a cardiac source of embolus as well as determining if there is a PFO capable of right-to-left shunting. Investigations to prove the stroke is cryptogenic such as scanning of the head and neck vessels should be undertaken prior to looking for a PFO.

Other cardiac sources of embolus

Atrial fibrillation is a strong risk factor for stroke. If present it may be associated with spontaneous contrast or even thrombus in the left atrial appendage which is best seen on TOE. The combination of atrial fibrillation and a previous stroke is a firm indication for warfarin[84] and there is no evidence to suggest that closure of a PFO will reduce the embolic risk further. Such findings are particular common in mitral stenosis. An impaired and dilated left ventricle of any cause increased the risk of thromboembolism, especially left ventricular aneurysms and thrombus. Thromboembolic stroke secondary to non-compaction has been reported[85,86], however, the true risk is not known. Atheroma of the ascending aorta and aortic arch may be visualized on both TTE and TOE.

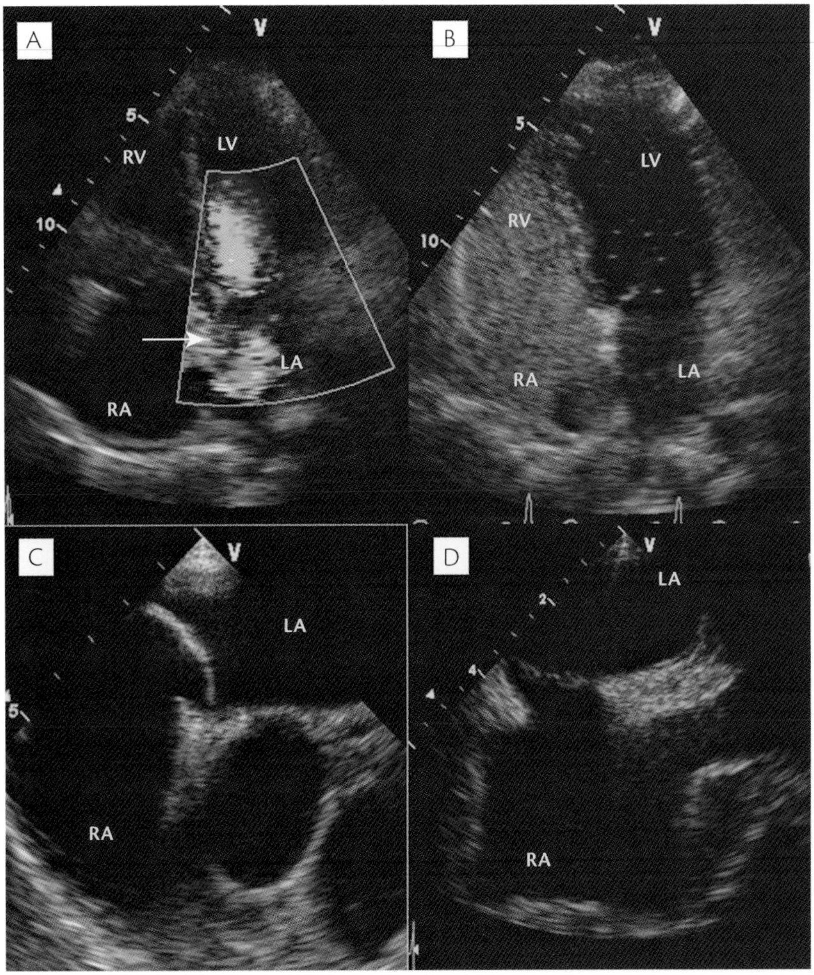

Fig. 38.7 A) TTE four-chamber view with colour flow (red) across ASD (arrow). B) TTE bubble study with right heart opacified with bubble contrast and some bubbles crossing into the left atrium and ventricle. C) Right-to-left bowing of the primum septum on release of the Valsalva manoeuvre seen on TOE. D) Thick secundum septum seen on TOE. (LA = left atrium, RA = right atrium, LV = left ventricle, RV = right ventricle)

Right-to-left shunting of PFO

Bubble contrast echocardiography

For a PFO to be diagnosed you must demonstrate its ability to transmit blood (or bubbles) from the right to the left atrium. The tunnel of a PFO is usually closed by the left atrial pressure exceeding that of the right atrium. Therefore, in order to allow the tunnel to open you need to perform haemodynamic manoeuvres that allow the right atrial pressure to transiently exceed the left atrial pressure. The most effective way of doing this is a Valsalva manoeuvre which increases intrathoracic pressure and therefore reduces venous return to the right atrium. Since the lungs and the left atrium are intrathoracic, this manoeuvre does not affect the pressure gradient responsible for left atrial filling. Upon release of the Valsalva manoeuvre, the blood pooled in the IVC rushes into the right atrium and you get a transient pressure gradient across the atrial septum from right to left. This can be seen on TOE as the atrial septum bouncing from right to left (Fig. 38.7C). This may also be generated by asking the patient to sniff or by deep palpation of the liver.

Since most TOE examinations in the United Kingdom are performed under sedation, it is easier for the patient to perform these haemodynamic manoeuvres during a TTE rather than a TOE. This study requires an experiences sonographer and a high-end machine capable of recording long video loops.

A large-bore cannula is inserted in a large left antecubital fossa vein. Two 10-mL Luer lock syringes and a three-way tap are used to agitate 9mL of saline with 1ml of air until the bubbles form a fine and uniform suspension.

Some operators believe that drawing 2mL of blood to the saline potentiates the air suspension. Once a clear four-chamber view is achieved, the bubble/saline suspension is drawn into one of the 10-mL syringes and the excess air is expelled. The suspension is rapidly injected into the cannula whilst the patient simultaneously performs a Valsalva manoeuvre. Once the bubbles are seen to fill the whole of the right atrium the Valsalva should be released and bubbles should appear in the left atrium if a PFO opens (Fig. 38.7B). Providing the quality of haemodynamic manoeuvre is good, this should be performed at rest, after Valsalva (twice), with cough and with sniff.

Distinguishing an atrial from a pulmonary shunt can be difficult on echocardiography alone and may require magnetic resonance imaging of the lungs. However, bubbles from an atrial shunt should appear in the left heart within three cardiac cycles[36,87]. Various classification schemes have been proposed to standardize the grading of the size of the shunt, although none are, as yet, predominant.

If the bubble study is positive, a TOE is necessary to define the anatomy of the shunt. Although haemodynamic manoeuvres may be better performed at TTE, it is not until you see the atrial septum bouncing from right to left that you know that the manoeuvres have been adequate to rule out a PFO. This is usually better seen on TOE and for this reason we would recommend a TOE bubble study in those with negative TTE bubble studies in whom the index of suspicion is high. Liver palpation or simpler manoeuvres such as sniffing combined with lighter sedation usually yields the desired septal bounce from right to left. If necessary, TOE probe mobilization can induce gentle retching.

TOE should be used to define the tunnel anatomy and determine whether both ends of the tunnel are patent. The maximum size of the right and left atrial openings both at rest and on provocation should be measured to determine device size. Equally, the length of the tunnel and the degree of retraction of the primum septum at rest and on provocation is also important in determining the correct device.

The length of the atrial septum must be measured to ensure that the atria can accommodate the chosen device. Measurements must also be made to ensure that the surrounding structures (caval veins, mitral valve, and coronary sinus) will not be compromised by the device.

The way in which the chosen device will sit should be anticipated. Fixed splitting of the primum and secundum septa is unlikely to results in closure even after balloon modification of the tunnel. Devices will conform poorly if the secundum septum is very thick and untapered (see Fig. 38.7D). Furthermore, fixed-waist devices cope poorly with long tunnels.

Transcranial Doppler

Transcranial Doppler uses ultrasound to quantify the number of bubbles that reaches the cerebral circulation. It is a highly sensitive technique, and possibly more sensitive than is clinically useful. Also, it does not discriminate between cardiac and pulmonary shunts[37].

The procedure and the devices

The procedure (Figs. 38.8 and 38.9)

Procedural imaging is recommended. Some operators have developed a method of screening out the simpler PFOs and closing them with fluoroscopic guidance alone and this may be possible in up to 70% cases[88]. However, despite careful pre-procedural imaging and the presence of stand-by ICE it can be difficult to predict certain complications such as thrombus formation and device malposition.

Procedural imaging can be done with either TOE or ICE. Both can be done as day cases[7]. ICE is an 8F (110cm) or 10F (90cm) steerable probe which is introduced into the femoral vein and passed up to the right atrium. Its proximity to the atrial septum permits high scanning frequencies which generates high resolution but can sometimes limit the field of view, especially in a small right atrium. ICE images the inferior atrial septum better than TOE. In experienced hands, both provide flexible and detailed imaging of the relevant anatomy. The major disadvantages of ICE are that it is invasive and is itself a potential source of complications. It is also costly as, in the United Kingdom, it is single use only.

Patients are usually pre-medicated with 300mg of aspirin and clopidogrel although evidence to support this regimen is lacking. Access is gained in the right femoral vein with a short sheath and 100IU/kg of heparin is injected intravenously. The ASD or PFO is then crossed using an exchange length standard weight 0.035-inch guide wire in a multipurpose 1 (MPA1) diagnostic catheter. This is often easier with 20° of left anterior oblique angulation (LAO 20) on X-ray screening. Some operators prefer an extra-stiff weight guide wire as this provides better support but it is also more likely to traumatize left atrial structures and should be handled with caution. Before entering the heart echo should be used to exclude pericardial effusion (baseline measurement) and left atrial appendage thrombus.

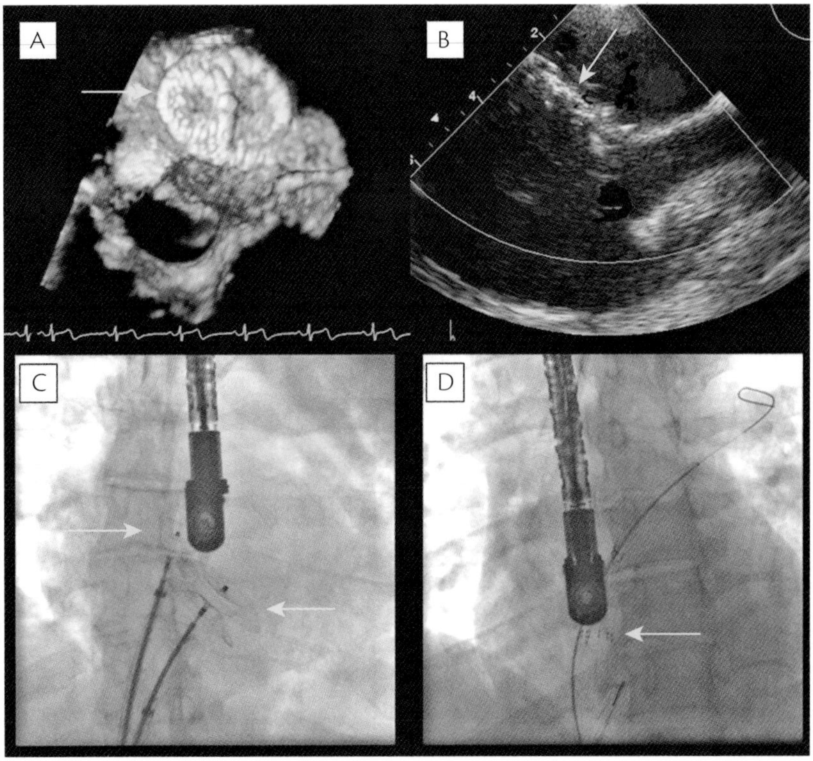

Fig. 38.8 A) 30mm Amplatzer® Cribriform Occluder (arrow) seen on three-dimensional TOE. B) Final echo result of a Solysafe® device (arrow). C) Simultaneous deployment of a 12mm and a 22mm Amplatzer® Septal Occluder (arrow). D) Solysafe® device (arrow) before conformation on its 0.018-inch nitinol guidewire.

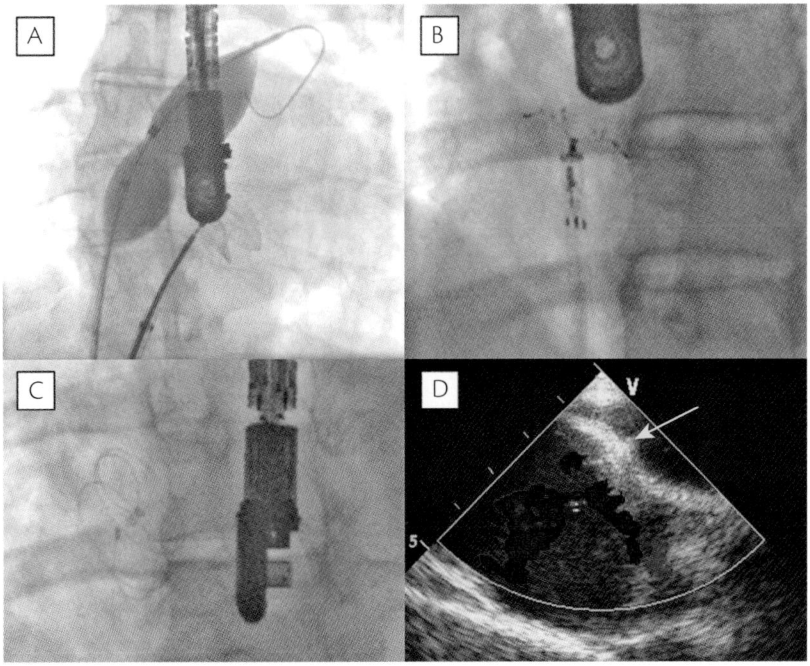

Fig. 38.9 A) Balloon sizing a residual leak after deployment of 22mm Amplatzer® Septal Occluder. B) BioSTAR® device with left atrial disc deployed but right atrial disc still in the delivery sheath. C) Final result of HELEX® septal Occluder. D) Final result of Premere® PFO Closure System on TOE (arrow).

The echo should be used to help guide crossing of the correct ASD (in the case of multiple ASDs) or to enter the right atrial opening of the tunnel (for PFOs). If the catheter can be inserted into the right atrial end of a PFO but the 'J'-tipped guide wire does not cross, the soft end of a straight-tipped wire can be used with caution. If this does not work, then a hydrophilic wire (e.g. Terumo®) can be used but with extreme caution as they can dissect tissue plans. Sometimes the MPA1 is not supportive enough to direct the guide wire into the right atrial opening of the tunnel. If so, a transseptal sheath can be used to direct the wire into the tunnel. At no time should any force be used to cross the PFO with a wire.

Sometimes the anatomy of a PFO tunnel is such that even a hydrophilic wire will not cross but bubbles will. Most operators would abandon the procedure at this point. If you are convinced that there are bubbles shunting from right to left, through a PFO and you are still unable to cross it, an argument could be been made in favour of a transseptal puncture in order to facilitate device delivery. This is a controversial strategy. More usually there is doubt over the bubbles or the position of the shunt and the procedure is abandoned.

Once in the left atrium, the catheter tends to enter the left atrial appendage. This should be avoided as this thin-walled structure is easily ruptured. Draw the catheter back 2cm, rotated 45° clockwise (so the catheter tip moves more posteriorly) and then advance the catheter or wire into the left upper pulmonary vein. This position will give stability to the delivery sheath and device.

Meanwhile, the retraction of the primum septum with the guide wire in the tunnel should be assessed on echo. Retraction often results in a shortening of the tunnel and therefore the anatomy of the tunnel must be reassessed. Most operators choose to balloon size the PFO although the information it gives may be derived from echo measurements alone. Despite the use of compliant material, balloon sizing inevitably results in some tearing of adhesions between the primum and secundum septa. In the case of a long tunnel PFO, this may be desirable as it tends to shorten the tunnel making it more suitable for a fixed waist device. However, aggressive balloon sizing may convert a long tunnel with tethered left atrial opening (suitable for the variable waist Premere® device [St Jude Medical]), into to a shorter tunnel that now has a left atrial opening too wide for a Premere® but that is not short enough for a fixed waist device.

There are multiple methods of choosing the correct device to close an ASD which involve 2-D echo measurements ± colour flow doppler ± balloon sizing ± a formula adjustment for flimsy edges. Balloon sizing of ASDs has become less popular because of the belief that it may result in oversizing of devices which may be associated with device erosions[24]. However, the colour map 'stop-flow' technique gently palpates the edges of the defect and allows accurate measurement of the effective defect. In the absence of balloon sizing, the ASD should be measured in orthogonal planes using 2-D with or without colour (colour flow doppler tends to over-estimate ASD size relative to 2-D echo alone. An unpublished formula developed by Dr Evelyn Lee measures the ASDs on 2-D TOE (without colour) in two orthogonal planes. The average of the measurement is multiplied by 1.2 for firm ASD rims, 1.3 if there are floppy rims and 1.25 for those in between. Other formulae also exist that avoids balloon sizing ASDs.

If balloon sizing is performed then anatomical two- or three-dimensional assessment should be repeated to ensure that there has been no significant change in measurements post-balloon dilatation.

Once the device is chosen, the femoral venous sheath should be exchanged for an appropriate transseptal delivery sheath whilst maintaining the exchange wire in the left upper pulmonary vein. Once in position, great care must be taken to de-air the sheath. This is usually done by dropping the sheath tip below the level of the heart to remove the air and then injecting saline to eject the column of blood to reduce the risk of thrombus formation. Sometimes the atrial septum lies almost parallel to the IVC. This can results in deployment difficulties. In such cases a three-dimensionally shaped sheath such as the Hausdorf® (Cook, Bloomington, IN, USA) sheath or a steerable transseptal sheath, designed for pulmonary vein isolation, may be used.

Some devices come pre-mounted on their delivery catheter. All devices must be de-aired carefully which is best done underwater. Similarly, the device is best introduced into the delivery sheath underwater to reduce the risk of air embolism.

The catheter is advanced to the tip if the delivery sheath which lies in the left atrium. The left atrial disc or anchor is deployed and then the sheath and catheter are drawn back until the left atrial disc lies tightly on the atrial septum. The right atrial disc is then deployed, often by being unsheathed. For all of the manufacturers, the devices can still be recovered at this point although only some devices can be redeployed. The echo should now be closely examined to ensure that both discs are in the appropriate position and apposed to the atrial septum. A small residual shunt is common at this point and is acceptable assuming that there is no device malposition. A small shunt is often related to tension on the delivery catheter or cable. It should also be ensured that there is no encroachment of the major structures such as the caval veins, mitral valve, and coronary sinus. Some devices can be pushed or pulled to ensure that they do not embolize. All of the devices have slightly different mechanisms and these will be discussed in the next section.

Once satisfied that all post-deployment checks are satisfactory, then the device can be released. If there are any doubts about deployment then the device should be removed prior to deployment as recapturing the device with a snare is challenging. Finally, the pericardium should be re-checked for an effusion.

It may take up to 6 months before the endothelium has grown over the device. During this period there is a risk of thrombus formation on the device. Patients are usually therefore advised to take 75mg of aspirin and clopidogrel for 6 months although there are no data to support this. There is also a small risk of endocarditis during this period. Device closure of a PFO for cryptogenic stroke reduces but does not abolish the risk of recurrent events, therefore such patients usually continue aspirin 75mg for life.

The optimal follow-up regimen has not been determined. However, the patients should have a transthoracic bubble contrast study and clinical follow up at 6 months as a minimum to ensure closure.

The devices

There are too many ASD and PFO closure devices to review all of them. Therefore, we will review the major manufacturers only.

AGA Medical Corporation

This company manufactures a range of closure devices based on a nickel/titanium alloy weave called nitinol. This alloy has the ability to return to its original conformation after deformation—so called 'memory metal'. They produce a range of devices in various sizes including the Amplatzer® PFO Occluder (Fig. 38.10E), Amplatzer® Septal Occluder (for ASDs), and the Amplatzer® Cribriform Occluder (for fenestrated ASDs). Although all of the devices have a fixed waist, the flexibility of the nitinol permits some conformation to longer tunnels. The device is also strong and will self-centre in the shortest tunnel region. All of the devices have an established track record with a good safety profile and are easy to use. AGA devices are relatively strong and erosions have been reported with a frequency of 0.3% which may be related to device oversizing[22].

NMT Medical, Inc.

Various iterations of the NMT medical closure devices include CardioSEAL®, STARflex®, and BioSTAR® (Fig. 38.10B). The latest device, BioSTAR®, is licensed in Europe for closure of PFOs and secundum ASDs less than 17mm. BioSTAR® is a double umbrella device consisting of two heparin-coated porcine collagen patches on a MP35N alloy framework. The collagen is highly biocompatible and ultimately is absorbed into the endocardium leaving only the framework. The device has a self-centring mechanism consisting of nitinol microsprings. Biostar® has a fixed waist but the jointed framework does permit some conformation to longer tunnels. The device comes in 23mm, 28mm, and 33mm sizes, and has excellent 6-month complete closure data[89]. STARflex® is the predecessor to BioSTAR® and is identical except that the collagen patches are instead made from Dacron®. Safety data shows a low erosion/perforation rate of 0.05%[22] Thrombus has been detected on the device in six out of 220 patients at 30 days[90]. NMT are in the process of developing a fully absorbable device which is currently called BioTREK®.

W.L Gore & Associates, Inc.

The HELEX® septal occluder is composed of a circumferential helical nitinol support frame covered with an ePTFE membrane (Fig. 38.10A). This elegant device is soft and low profile causing minimal disruption to the surrounding tissues. The device is licensed in Europe for closure of PFOs and ASDs less than 17mm and comes in five sizes between 15–35mm. This device is not self-centring and has a fixed waist although the nitinol frame permits it to conform a little to longer tunnels. In one study, embolization of the device occurred in three out of 220 prior to discharge[90].

St Jude Medical

The Premere™ PFO Closure System is the only variable waist device and is theoretically well suited to closure of long tunnel PFOs (Fig. 38.10F). It is not suitable for closure of ASDs or larger PFOs. The left atrial anchor, which is bare and made from nitinol, is attached to the right atrial anchor, which is cover by a polyester patch, by a polyester thread. Once the device is deployed, the thread can be locked at a length that is suitable for the PFO tunnel. This device has a favourable safety profile but long-term data is lacking[42].

Swissimpant®

The Solysafe® device is licensed in Europe for closure of PFO and ASDs up to 30mm (Fig. 38.10C). This device consists of two polyester patches attached to

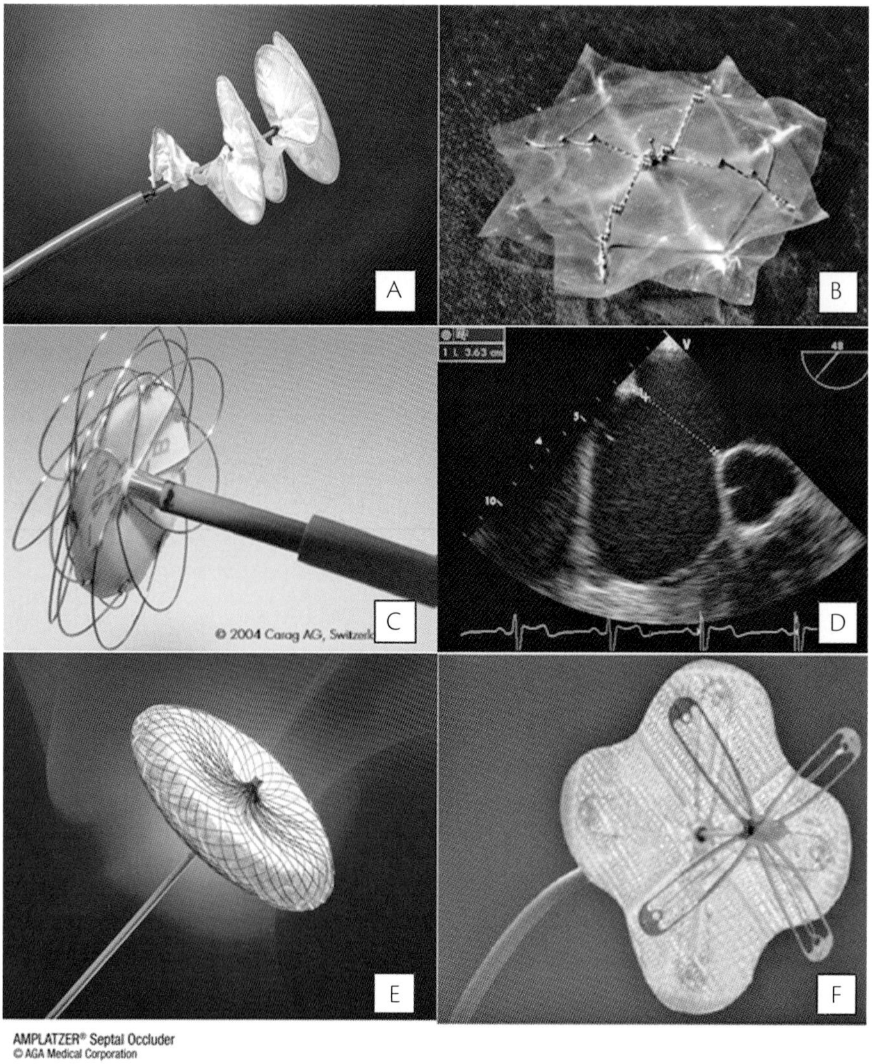

Fig. 38.10 A) HELEX® septal Occluder (image provided by W.L. Gore & Associates). B) BioSTAR® (image provided by NMT Medical). C) Solysafe® device (image provided by Swissimplant). D) Large ASD with deficient rims. E) Amplater® PFO Occluder (image provided by AGA Medical). F) Premere® PFO Closure System (image provided by St Jude Medical).

eight phynox wires by platinum iridium markers. This device is delivered in an 'over-the-wire' manner similar to an angioplasty balloon and no sheath is necessary. This reduces the risk of air and thromboembolism. The left and right atrial discs are conformed once the device is across the atrial septum by moving two attached catheters. This device can be completely locked and released, whilst remaining on the guide wire and still be recaptured. This is a strong, self-centring device but appears to conform to a lower profile than the AGA devices. It has a fixed waist with limited conformation to long PFO tunnels. It has a favourable safety profile but long-term data are lacking[(47)].

Other devices

Many other manufactures exist. One of the more novel systems is the PFx® Closure System (Cierra Inc., Redwood City, CA, USA) which used radiofrequency energy to close the tunnel, thus avoiding the need for a device. Early results suggest that this system is effective in smaller PFOs[(91)]. Other devices include the Flatstent® (Coherex Medical Inc.) which uses a small intra-tunnel device to close the PFO [92] and a suture based system [93,94].

Acknowledgements

Len M Shapiro and Evelyn M Lee. Papworth Hospital NHS Foundation Trust, Cambridge, UK.

References

1. Ludman P. BCIS National Audit Data. Presented at Crewe Sept 2008. http://www.bcis.org.uk/resources/documents/BCIS%20Audit%20web.pdf 2008.
2. Sadler TW. *Langman's Medical Embryology*, 6th edn. Balitmore: Williams and Wilkins, 1990.
3. Cabanes L, Mas JL, Cohen A, *et al.* Atrial septal aneurysm and patent foramen ovale as risk factors for cryptogenic stroke in patients less than 55 years of age. A study using transesophageal echocardiography. *Stroke* 1993; **24**(12):1865–73.
4. Overell JR, Bone I, Lees KR. Interatrial septal abnormalities and stroke: a meta-analysis of case-control studies. *Neurology* 2000; **55**(8):1172–9.
5. Bedford DE. The anatomical types of atrial septal defect. Their incidence and clinical diagnosis. *Am J Cardiol* 1960; **6**:568–74.
6. Campbell M. Natural history of atrial septal defect. *Br Heart J* 1970; **32**(6):820–6.
7. Calvert PA, Klein AA. Anaesthesia for percutaneous closure of atrial septal defects. *Contin Educ Anaest, Crit Care Pain* 2008; **8**:16–20.
8. Sung RJ, Tamer DM, Agha AS, *et al.* Etiology of the electrocardiographic pattern of "incomplete right bundle branch block" in atrial septal defect: an electrophysiologic study. *J Pediatr* 1975; **87**(6 PT 2):1182–6.
9. Zufelt K, Rosenberg HC, Li MD, *et al.* The electrocardiogram and the secundum atrial septal defect: a reexamination in the era of echocardiography. *Can J Cardiol* 1998; **14**(2):227–32.
10. Murray G. Closure of defects in cardiac septa. *Ann Surg* 1948; **128**(4):843–53.
11. Lewis FG TM. Closure of atrial septal defects with the aid of hypothermia: experimental accomplishments with the report of one successful case. *Surgery* ; **33**:52–9.
12. Tsuchioka H, Iyomasa Y, Kakihara R, *et al.* Effects of corrective surgery on natural history of atrial septal defect of secundum type. *Jpn Circ J* 1981; **45**(2):249–59.
13. Matsuki H, Yagihara T, Hamaji M, *et al.* [Evaluation of surgery of atrial septal defect in 83 cases]. *Nippon Kyobu Geka Gakkai Zasshi* 1974; **22**(5):436–7.
14. Konstantinides S, Geibel A, Olschewski M, *et al.* A comparison of surgical and medical therapy for atrial septal defect in adults. *N Engl J Med* 1995; **333**(8):469–73.
15. Attie F, Rosas M, Granados N, *et al.* Surgical treatment for secundum atrial septal defects in patients >40 years old. A randomized clinical trial. *J Am Coll Cardiol* 2001; **38**(7):2035–42.
16. King TD, Mills NL. Nonoperative closure of atrial septal defects. *Surgery* 1974; **75**(3):383–8.
17. King TD, Thompson SL, Steiner C, *et al.* Secundum atrial septal defect. Nonoperative closure during cardiac catheterization. *JAMA* 1976; **235**(23):2506–9.
18. Rome JJ, Keane JF, Perry SB, *et al.* Double-umbrella closure of atrial defects. Initial clinical applications. *Circulation* 1990; **82**(3):751–8.
19. Masura J, Gavora P, Formanek A, *et al.* Transcatheter closure of secundum atrial septal defects using the new self-centering amplatzer septal occluder: initial human experience. *Cathet Cardiovasc Diagn* 1997; **42**(4):388–93.
20. Du ZD, Hijazi ZM, Kleinman CS, *et al.* Comparison between transcatheter and surgical closure of secundum atrial septal defect in children and adults: results of a multicenter nonrandomized trial. *J Am Coll Cardiol* 2002; **39**(11):1836–44.
21. Omeish A, Hijazi ZM. Transcatheter closure of atrial septal defects in children & adults using the Amplatzer Septal Occluder. *J Interv Cardiol* 2001; **14**(1):37–44.
22. Delaney JW, Li JS, Rhodes JF. Major complications associated with transcatheter atrial septal occluder implantation: a review of the medical literature and the manufacturer and user facility device experience (MAUDE) database. *Congenit Heart Dis* 2007; **2**(4):256–64.
23. Divekar A, Gaamangwe T, Shaikh N, *et al.* Cardiac perforation after device closure of atrial septal defects with the Amplatzer septal occluder. *J Am Coll Cardiol* 2005; **45**(8):1213–8.
24. Amin Z, Hijazi ZM, Bass JL, *et al.* Erosion of Amplatzer septal occluder device after closure of secundum atrial septal defects: review of registry of complications and recommendations to minimize future risk. *Catheter Cardiovasc Interv* 2004; **63**(4):496–502.
25. Chen C, Kremer P, Schroeder E, *et al.* Usefulness of anatomic parameters derived from two-dimensional echocardiography for estimating magnitude of left to right shunt in patients with atrial septal defect. *Clin Cardiol* 1987; **10**(6):316–21.
26. Vanzetto G, Rossignol AM, Hadjian O, *et al.* [Measurement by Doppler echocardiography of the ratio of pulmonary/systemic flow rates in atrial septal defects. Apropos of 15 cases]. *Ann Cardiol Angeiol (Paris)* 1992; **41**(5):287–94.
27. Brochu MC, Baril JF, Dore A, Borrel E, Contard M, Machecourt J, Improvement in exercise capacity in asymptomatic and mildly symptomatic adults after atrial septal defect percutaneous closure. *Circulation* 2002; **106**(14):1821–6.
28. Sacco RL, Ellenberg JH, Mohr JP, *et al.* Infarcts of undetermined cause: the NINCDS Stroke Data Bank. *Ann Neurol* 1989; **25**(4):382–90.
29. Cramer SC, Rordorf G, Maki JH, *et al.* Increased pelvic vein thrombi in cryptogenic stroke: results of the Paradoxical Emboli from Large Veins in Ischemic Stroke (PELVIS) study. *Stroke* 2004; **35**(1):46–50.

30. Choong CK, Calvert PA, Falter F, *et al.* Life-threatening impending paradoxical embolus caught "red-handed": successful management by multidisciplinary team approach. *J Thorac Cardiovasc Surg* 2008; **136**(2):527–528 e8.
31. Kim RJ, Girardi LN. "Lots of clots": multiple thromboemboli including a huge paradoxical embolus in a 29-year-old man. *Int J Cardiol* 2008; **129**(2):e50–2.
32. Madani H, Ransom PA. Paradoxical embolus illustrating speed of action of recombinant tissue plasminogen activator in massive pulmonary embolism. *Emerg Med J* 2007; **24**(6):441.
33. Ahmed S, Sadiq A, Siddiqui AK, *et al.* Paradoxical arterial emboli causing acute limb ischemia in a patient with essential thrombocytosis. *Am J Med Sci* 2003; **326**(3):156–8.
34. Zahn F. *Med Suisse Romande* 1881; **1**:227.
35. Lechat P, Mas JL, Lascault G, *et al.* Prevalence of patent foramen ovale in patients with stroke. *N Engl J Med* 1988; **318**(18):1148–52.
36. Webster MW, Chancellor AM, Smith HJ, *et al.* Patent foramen ovale in young stroke patients. *Lancet* 1988; **2**(8601):11–2.
37. Job FP, Ringelstein EB, Grafen Y, *et al.* Comparison of transcranial contrast Doppler sonography and transesophageal contrast echocardiography for the detection of patent foramen ovale in young stroke patients. *Am J Cardiol* 1994; **74**(4):381–4.
38. Di Tullio M, Sacco RL, Gopal A, *et al.* Patent foramen ovale as a risk factor for cryptogenic stroke. *Ann Intern Med* 1992; **117**(6):461–5.
39. Yeung M, Khan KA, Shuaib A. Transcranial Doppler ultrasonography in the detection of venous to arterial shunting in acute stroke and transient ischaemic attacks. *J Neurol Neurosurg Psychiatry* 1996; **61**(5):445–9.
40. Handke M, Harloff A, Olschewski M, *et al.* Patent foramen ovale and cryptogenic stroke in older patients. *N Engl J Med* 2007; **357**(22):2262–8.
41. Bridges ND, Hellenbrand W, Latson L, *et al.* Transcatheter closure of patent foramen ovale after presumed paradoxical embolism. *Circulation* 1992; **86**(6):1902–8.
42. Buscheck F, Sievert H, Kleber F, *et al.* Patent foramen ovale using the Premere device: the results of the CLOSEUP trial. *J Interv Cardiol* 2006; **19**(4):328–33.
43. Luermans JG, Post MC, Schrader R, *et al.* Outcome after percutaneous closure of a patent foramen ovale using the Intrasept device: a multi-centre study. *Catheter Cardiovasc Interv* 2008; **71**(6):822–8.
44. Bruch L, Parsi A, Grad MO, *et al.* Transcatheter closure of interatrial communications for secondary prevention of paradoxical embolism: single-center experience. *Circulation* 2002; **105**(24):2845–8.
45. Braun MU, Fassbender D, Schoen SP, *et al.* Transcatheter closure of patent foramen ovale in patients with cerebral ischemia. *J Am Coll Cardiol* 2002; **39**(12): 2019–25.
46. Ende DJ, Chopra PS, Rao PS. Transcatheter closure of atrial septal defect or patent foramen ovale with the buttoned device for prevention of recurrence of paradoxic embolism. *Am J Cardiol* 1996; **78**(2):233–6.
47. Ewert P, Soderberg B, Dahnert I, *et al.* ASD and PFO closure with the Solysafe septal occluder - results of a prospective multicenter pilot study. *Catheter Cardiovasc Interv* 2008; **71**(3):398–402.
48. Khairy P, O'Donnell CP, Landzberg MJ. Transcatheter closure versus medical therapy of patent foramen ovale and presumed paradoxical thromboemboli: a systematic review. *Ann Intern Med* 2003; **139**(9):753–60.
49. Windecker S, Wahl A, Nedeltchev K, *et al.* Comparison of medical treatment with percutaneous closure of patent foramen ovale in patients with cryptogenic stroke. *J Am Coll Cardiol* 2004; **44**(4):750–8.
50. NMT. Press Release. http://www.snl.com/irweblinkx/file.aspx?IID=4148066&FID=6801157. 2008.
51. Moon RE, Camporesi EM, Kisslo JA. Patent foramen ovale and decompression sickness in divers. *Lancet* 1989; **1**(8637):513–4.
52. Wilmshurst PT, Byrne JC, Webb-Peploe MM. Relation between interatrial shunts and decompression sickness in divers. *Lancet* 1989; **2**(8675):1302–6.
53. Wilmshurst PT, Byrne JC, Webb-Peploe MM. Neurological decompression sickness. *Lancet* 1989; **1**(8640):731.
54. Wilmshurst PT, Byrne JC, Webb-Peploe MM. Relation between interatrial shunts and decompression sickness in divers. In Sterk W, Geeraedts L (eds) *EUBS 1990 Proceedings*, pp.147–53. London: European Undersea Biomedical Society, 1990.
55. Wilmshurst P, Bryson P. Relationship between the clinical features of neurological decompression illness and its causes. *Clin Sci (Lond)* 2000; **99**(1):65–75.
56. Torti SR, Billinger M, Schwerzmann M, *et al.* Risk of decompression illness among 230 divers in relation to the presence and size of patent foramen ovale. *Eur Heart J* 2004; **25**(12):1014–20.
57. Wilmshurst P, Walsh K, Morrison L. Transcatheter occlusion of foramen ovale with a button device after neurological decompression illness in professional divers. *Lancet* 1996; **348**(9029):752–3.
58. Bendrick GA, Ainscough MJ, Pilmanis AA, *et al.* Prevalence of decompression sickness among U-2 pilots. *Aviat Space Environ Med* 1996; **67**(3):199–206.
59. Conkin J, Bedahl SR, Van Liew HD. A computerized databank of decompression sickness incidence in altitude chambers. *Aviat Space Environ Med* 1992; **63**(9):819–24.
60. Lipton RB, Liberman JN, Kolodner KB, *et al.* Migraine headache disability and health-related quality-of-life: a population-based case-control study from England. *Cephalalgia* 2003; **23**(6):441–50.
61. Lipton RB, Stewart WF, Diamond S, *et al.* Prevalence and burden of migraine in the United States: data

from the American Migraine Study II. *Headache* 2001; **41**(7):646–57.

62. Anzola GP, Magoni M, Guindani M, *et al.* Potential source of cerebral embolism in migraine with aura: a transcranial Doppler study. *Neurology* 1999; **52**(8):1622–5.
63. Morandi E, Anzola GP, Angeli S, *et al.* Transcatheter closure of patent foramen ovale: a new migraine treatment? *J Interv Cardiol* 2003; **16**(1):39–42.
64. Anzola GP, Frisoni GB, Morandi E, *et al.* Shunt-associated migraine responds favorably to atrial septal repair: a case-control study. *Stroke* 2006; **37**(2):430–4.
65. Wilmshurst PT, Nightingale S, Walsh KP, *et al.* Effect on migraine of closure of cardiac right-to-left shunts to prevent recurrence of decompression illness or stroke or for haemodynamic reasons. *Lancet* 2000; **356**(9242): 1648–51.
66. Dowson A, Mullen MJ, Peatfield R, *et al.* Migraine Intervention With STARFlex Technology (MIST) trial: a prospective, multicenter, double-blind, sham-controlled trial to evaluate the effectiveness of patent foramen ovale closure with STARFlex septal repair implant to resolve refractory migraine headache. *Circulation* 2008; **117**(11):1397–404.
67. Seward JB, Hayes DL, Smith HC, *et al.* Platypnea-orthodeoxia: clinical profile, diagnostic workup, management, and report of seven cases. *Mayo Clin Proc* 1984; **59**(4):221–31.
68. Smeenk FW, Postmus PE. Interatrial right-to-left shunting developing after pulmonary resection in the absence of elevated right-sided heart pressures. Review of the literature. *Chest* 1993; **103**(2):528–31.
69. Godart F, Rey C, Prat A, *et al.* Atrial right-to-left shunting causing severe hypoxaemia despite normal right-sided pressures. Report of 11 consecutive cases corrected by percutaneous closure. *Eur Heart J* 2000; **21**(6):483–9.
70. Bakris NC, Siddiqi AJ, Fraser CD, Jr, *et al.* Right-to-left interatrial shunt after pneumonectomy. *Ann Thorac Surg* 1997; **63**(1):198–201.
71. Murray KD, Kalanges LK, Weiland JE, *et al.* Platypnea-orthodeoxia: an unusual indication for surgical closure of a patent foramen ovale. *J Card Surg* 1991; **6**(1):62–7.
72. Dear WE, Chen P, Barasch E, *et al.* Sixty-eight-year-old woman with intermittent hypoxemia. *Circulation* 1995; **91**(8):2284–9.
73. Davidson A, Chandrasekaran K, Guida L, *et al.* Enhancement of hypoxemia by atrial shunting in cystic fibrosis. *Chest* 1990; **98**(3):543–5.
74. Herregods MC, Timmermans C, Frans E, *et al.* Diagnostic value of transesophageal echocardiography in platypnea. *J Am Soc Echocardiogr* 1993; **6**(6):624–7.
75. Gallaher ME, Sperling DR, Gwinn JL, *et al.* Functional Drainage Of The Inferior Vena Cava Into The Left Atrium—Three Cases. *Am J Cardiol* 1963; **12**:561–6.
76. Thomas JD, Tabakin BS, Ittleman FP. Atrial septal defect with right to left shunt despite normal pulmonary artery pressure. *J Am Coll Cardiol* 1987; **9**(1):221–4.
77. Laybourn KA, Martin ET, Cooper RA, *et al.* Platypnea and orthodeoxia: shunting associated with an aortic aneurysm. *J Thorac Cardiovasc Surg* 1997; **113**(5):955–6.
78. Landzberg MJ, Sloss LJ, Faherty CE, *et al.* Orthodeoxia-platypnea due to intracardiac shunting--relief with transcatheter double umbrella closure. *Cathet Cardiovasc Diagn* 1995; **36**(3):247–50.
79. Shanoudy H, Soliman A, Raggi P, *et al.* Prevalence of patent foramen ovale and its contribution to hypoxemia in patients with obstructive sleep apnea. *Chest* 1998; **113**(1):91–6.
80. Bradley TD, Martinez D, Rutherford R, *et al.* Physiological determinants of nocturnal arterial oxygenation in patients with obstructive sleep apnea. *J Appl Physiol* 1985; **59**(5):1364–8.
81. Appelberg J, Nordahl G, Janson C. Lung volume and its correlation to nocturnal apnoea and desaturation. *Respir Med* 2000; **94**(3):233–9.
82. Johansson MC, Eriksson P, Peker Y, *et al.* The influence of patent foramen ovale on oxygen desaturation in obstructive sleep apnoea. *Eur Respir J* 2007; **29**(1):149–55.
83. Klotzsch C, Sliwka U, Berlit P, *et al.* An increased frequency of patent foramen ovale in patients with transient global amnesia. Analysis of 53 consecutive patients. *Arch Neurol* 1996; **53**(6):504–8.
84. Hart RG, Pearce LA, Koudstaal PJ. Transient ischemic attacks in patients with atrial fibrillation: implications for secondary prevention: the European Atrial Fibrillation Trial and Stroke Prevention in Atrial Fibrillation III trial. *Stroke* 2004; **35**(4):948–51.
85. Ker J, Van Der Merwe C. Isolated left ventricular non-compaction as a cause of thrombo-embolic stroke: a case report and review. *Cardiovasc J S Afr* 2006; **17**(3):146–7.
86. Vijayvergiya R, Jha A, Panda SN, *et al.* Biventricular non-compaction - The rare cause of stroke in a young boy. *Int J Cardiol* 2008; **129**(3):e84–e85.
87. Van Camp G, Schulze D, Cosyns B, *et al.* Relation between patent foramen ovale and unexplained stroke. *Am J Cardiol* 1993; **71**(7):596–8.
88. Hildick-Smith D, Behan M, Haworth P, *et al.* Patent foramen ovale closure without echocardiographic control: use of "standby" intracardiac ultrasound. *JACC Cardiovasc Interv* 2008; **1**(4):387–91.
89. Mullen MJ, Hildick-Smith D, De Giovanni JV, *et al.* BioSTAR Evaluation STudy (BEST): a prospective, multicenter, phase I clinical trial to evaluate the feasibility, efficacy, and safety of the BioSTAR bioabsorbable septal repair implant for the closure of atrial-level shunts. *Circulation* 2006; **114**(18):1962–7.
90. Taaffe M, Fischer E, Baranowski A, *et al.* Comparison of three patent foramen ovale closure devices in a randomized trial (Amplatzer versus CardioSEAL-STARflex versus Helex occluder). *Am J Cardiol* 2008; **101**(9):1353–8.

91. Sievert H, Ruygrok P, Salkeld M, *et al.* Transcatheter closure of patent foramen ovale with radiofrequency: Acute and intermediate term results in 144 patients. *Catheter Cardiovasc Interv* 2008; **71**(7):921–6.
92. Reiffenstein I, Majunke N, Wunderlich N, *et al.* Percutaneous closure of patent foramen ovale with a novel FlatStent. *Expert Rev Med* Devices 2008; **5**(4):419–25.
93. Ruiz CE, Kipshidze N, Chiam PT, *et al.* Feasibility of patent foramen ovale closure with no-device left behind: first-in-man percutaneous suture closure. *Catheter Cardiovasc Interv* 2008; **71**(7):921–6.
94. Majunke N, Baranowski A, Zimmermann W, *et al.* A suture not always the ideal solution: Problems encountered in developing a suture-based PFO closure technique. *Catheter Cardiovasc Interv* 2009; **73**(3):376–82.

CHAPTER 39

Transcatheter aortic valve replacement

John G. Webb and Fabian Nietlispach

Background

Aortic stenosis (AS) is the most common valvular heart disease for which patients undergo valve replacement. Although the condition may develop in mid-life in association with a congenitally bicuspid valve, AS is for the most part a disease of the elderly, as demonstrated by a recent community-based study in the United States which reported a prevalence in those older than 75 years of age of 4.6%[(1)]. Medically treated severe symptomatic AS has been associated with predictable clinical deterioration and a poor survival, reportedly averaging 2–3 years after the onset of symptoms[(2–6)].

Surgical management of aortic stenosis

There is a large body of evidence suggesting that surgical aortic valve replacement (AVR) can result in clinical improvement and improves survival in patients with symptomatic AS[(2,3,5)]. Nonetheless, recent European and American studies report that 30–60% of elderly patients with symptomatic severe aortic valve stenosis do not undergo AVR[(6–9)]. To some degree lower than recommended rates of surgical AVR reflect a combination of both perception and reality. Surgical AVR requires a general anaesthetic, sternotomy, aortotomy, and cardiopulmonary bypass. While well tolerated and relatively low risk in many patients, this is not the case in others[(10–13)]. Common comorbidities such as advanced age, cerebrovascular, aortic, pulmonary, renal, hepatic disease, as well as left ventricular dysfunction and coronary disease increase surgical risk[(6,8)]. Debility and frailty, although both difficult to quantify and often the result of chronic AS, are increasingly recognized as risk factors for poor outcomes.

Transcatheter aortic valve replacement

Aortic balloon valvuloplasty was first developed in the 1980s as a percutaneous therapeutic option for AS. Although sometimes helpful, benefit is generally modest at best, always short-lived, and prognosis is not altered[(14–16)]. After initial enthusiasm, aortic balloon valvuloplasty has played a relatively minor role in palliation and bridging to definitive therapy. More recently valvuloplasty has found a major new role as a component of transcatheter valve implantation.

The concept of transcatheter valve implantation can be traced to 1992 when Anderson in Denmark reported transarterial implantation of a stent-mounted valve in a porcine model[(17)]. Subsequently several groups pursued development of a practical transcatheter procedure. A decade passed before the first percutaneous aortic valve implantation was accomplished by Cribier in France[(18)]. Initial implants utilized an antegrade delivery technique with femoral vein access followed by a transseptal puncture to allow passage through the left atrium, mitral valve, and left ventricle. This technique, while often successful, was difficult to reproduce and complications were common. Nevertheless, feasibility and the potential for clinical benefit was established[(19)]. Subsequently the development of a reproducible transarterial procedure in Vancouver in 2005[20] and a transapical procedure in Vancouver and Leipzig the following year spurred further enthusiasm[(21–25)]. The prototypic Anderson valve and currently available valves are shown in Fig. 39.1.

Current valves

The first-generation Cribier-Edwards® valve (Edwards Lifesciences Inc, Irvine, CA, USA) consisted of a stainless

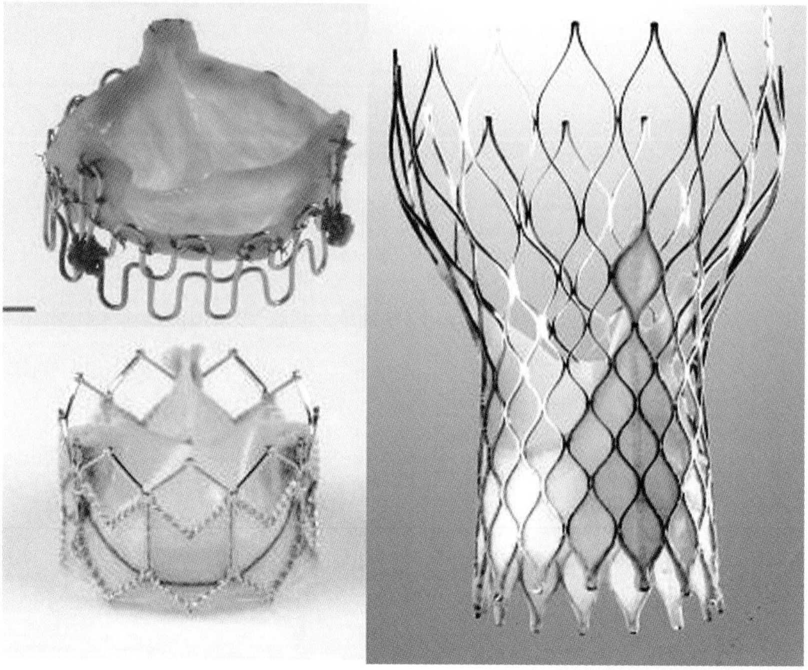

Fig. 39.1 Prototype Anderson valve (top left). Edwards SAPIEN XT®valve (bottom left). CoreValve® prosthesis (right).

steel balloon-expandable stent frame to which were sewn equine pericardial leaflets. A synthetic fabric cuff was attached to the ventricular end of the stent so as to provide an external seal[18–20]. This first-generation device was subsequently replaced by the Edwards SAPIEN® valve, incorporating more durable bovine pericardial leaflets and a larger sealing cuff[26]. The third-generation SAPIEN XT® valve utilizes a redesigned cobalt chromium alloy frame to allow thinner, yet stronger struts and enable the use of new low-profile delivery systems[27]. All measure approximately 14–16mm in length when expanded and are intended to be crimped onto a balloon catheter, which when inflated expands the prosthesis and displaces the native valve as shown in Fig. 39.2. The initial transvenous cases utilized a standard valvuloplasty balloon[18,19]. A reproducible transarterial procedure became possible with the development of a deflectable RetroFlex® catheter[20], followed by RetroFlex® 2 which incorporated a retractable nosecone[27], and RetroFlex® 3 with a fixed nosecone incorporated into the balloon[27] as shown in Fig. 39.3. The most recent iteration, Novaflex, facilitates a reduction in delivery profile from 22F to 24F down to 18F to 19F, greatly enhancing deliverability.

The CoreValve ReValving System® (CoreValve Inc, Irvine, CA, USA) incorporates a nitinol alloy frame (see Fig. 39.1). The self-expanding tubular frame is constrained within a delivery sheath, which is advanced to the left ventricle. As the sheath is withdrawn the frame expands to assume its predetermined shape. The lower portion of the frame with its sealing cuff is positioned within the aortic annulus displacing the native leaflets. The middle portion contains a trileaflet porcine pericardial valve and is tapered to avoid contact with the coronary ostia. The upper portion extends above the coronaries to anchor the prosthesis against the ascending aorta. This valve has seen several iterative versions with a progressive reduction in delivery profile from 25F[28,29] down to the current 18F system (Fig. 39.3)[30–32].

The successes and deficiencies of early transcatheter valve and delivery systems have led to the development of a number of newer percutaneous valves currently or imminently in human trials such as the Lotus® Sadra valve, Direct Flow® valve[33,34], Heart Leaflet Technologies® valve, and Embracer® valve (Fig. 39.4). Most attempt to improve deliverability, reduce paravalvular regurgitation or facilitate positioning, repositioning. and even removal.

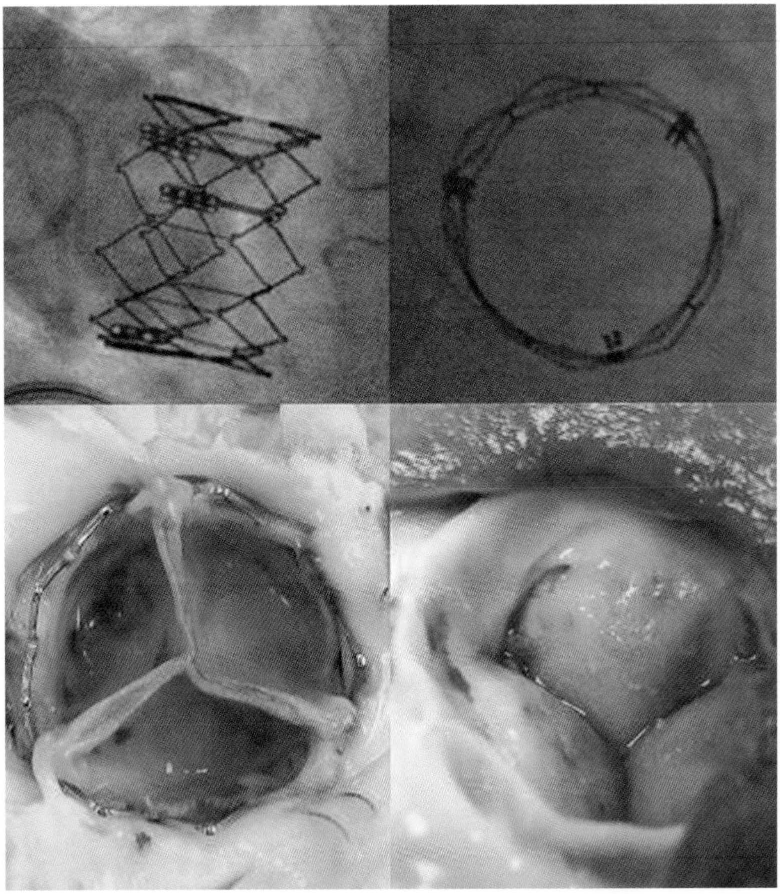

Fig. 39.2 Top: fluoroscopic images of Edwards SAPIEN XT® valve implant. Bottom. Sheep implant at 20 weeks.

Transcatheter aortic valve replacement procedures in general

Procedures can be performed in a cardiac catheterization laboratory or hybrid operating room. The need for excellent fluoroscopic imaging argues against performing procedures in a standard cardiac operating room with substandard fluoroscopy. Valve implantation and the potential need for arterial repair argue for a greater level of sterility than can be obtained in the average catheterization laboratory.

Although transarterial procedures can be done under conscious sedation, a general anaesthetic and intubation may often be necessary and is often preferred to increase patient safety and comfort or to facilitate transoesophageal echocardiography. Transapical procedures are almost always done under general anaesthetic, although rarely a spinal may be considered in a patient with respiratory compromise.

Rarely ischaemic left ventricular dysfunction may require femoro-femoral or TandemHeart® cardiopulmonary support to complete a procedure successfully. An interdisciplinary team including interventional cardiologist, cardiac surgeon, vascular surgeon, cardiac anaesthesia, perfusionists, and skilled nursing[35] are fundamental to a successful transcatheter programme.

Patients are generally pre-medicated with aspirin, clopidogrel, and prophylactic antibiotics. Heparin is administered during the procedure. Procedures can be performed with conscious sedation, although general anaesthesia with intubation is often utilized[36]. Central venous access from the neck and a radial arterial line may be useful in higher-risk patients. Radiolucent defibrillation pads are placed on the chest. Patients, if intubated, are typically extubated rapidly, typically on the table after a transarterial procedure or in the postoperative care unit after transapical access. Intensive care

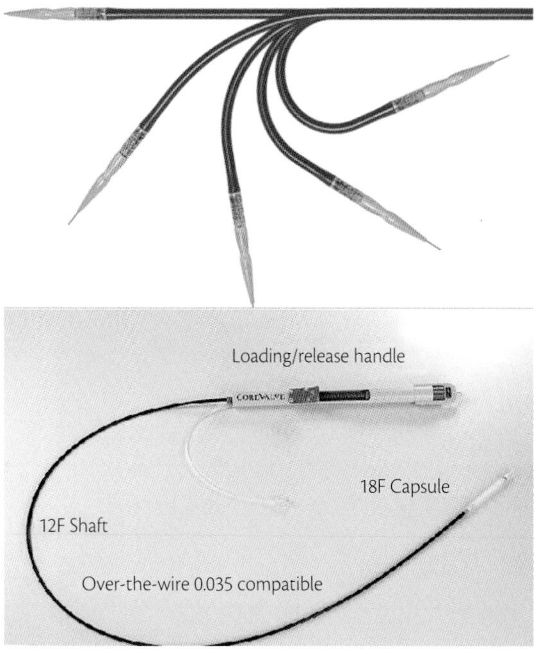

Fig. 39.3 RetroFlex 3® delivery system (top). CoreValve ReValving System® (bottom).

unit observation is common for a day, followed by early mobilization and a period of telemetry[37].

Transarterial procedure

Sheaths are typically placed in two arteries and one vein. Currently a temporary pacing lead is placed into the right ventricle, most often from the femoral vein. This allows for burst pacing during valvuloplasty or valve deployment and for backup pacing should atrioventricular block develop. A pigtail catheter is placed from a femoral or radial artery into the aortic root to allow contrast aortography and assist in accurate positioning of the prosthesis. A large sheath for introduction of the prosthetic valve is typically placed in the larger, straighter, less calcified of the two femoral arteries. Alternatively surgical arterial access can be achieved utilizing the axillary, or retroperitoneal iliac arteries or even the ascending aorta, although experience with these approaches is limited at this time[38,39].

After arterial access is achieved the aortic valve is crossed with a straight or hydrophilic guide wire in combination with an appropriately angled catheter

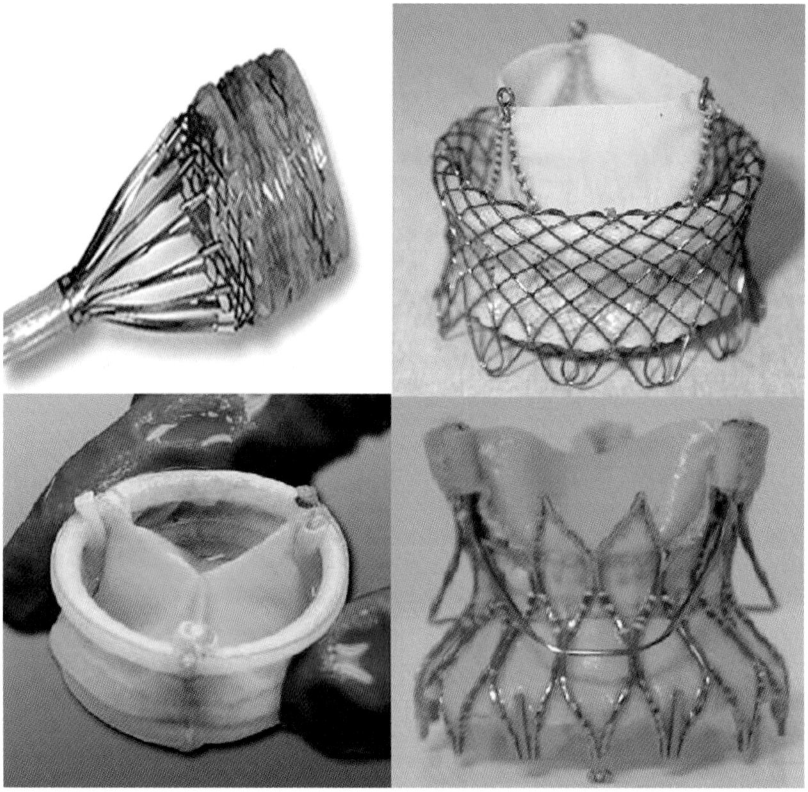

Fig. 39.4 Clockwise from top left: Lotus valve® Heart Leaflet Technologies valve. Direct Flow® valve. Embracer® valve.

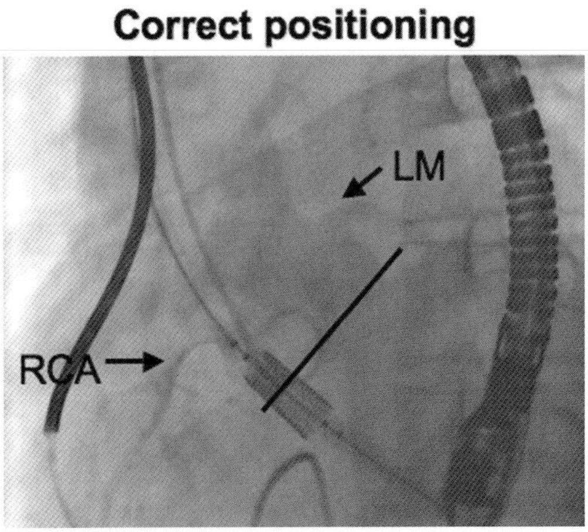

Fig. 39.5 Positioning of the Edwards SAPIEN® valve. Aortic contrast injection using a pigtail catheter in the aortic root shows correct positioning. With deployment the valve will typically move slightly towards the aorta.

(e.g. Amplatz left 1 or 2, Judkins right,or multipurpose). A stiff exchange length J-curve guidewire is advanced through the catheter and positioned securely well into the ventricle. Balloon valvuloplasty is routinely performed, generally with burst ventricular pacing to reduce transvalvular blood flow and cardiac motion during dilation[40]. Pre-dilation of the native valve facilitates subsequent insertion and positioning of the prosthesis.

The valve delivery catheter is advanced over a guidewire across the stenotic valve and positioned utilizing fluoroscopic imaging (Fig. 39.5). Transoesophageal imaging may be helpful, although use varies[41]. Balloon-expandable valves (e.g. SAPIEN®) are deployed by rapid balloon inflation and deflation during rapid burst pacing[20,26]. Self-expandable valves (e.g. CoreValve®) are currently deployed by withdrawing a constraining sheath[30,31]. Newer valves may well have other, more unique deployment mechanisms.

Early in the transarterial experience a surgical cutdown was routinely utilized to place, or at least remove, the large 22–25F internal diameter sheaths required. With increasing experience and technical improvements allowing the use of smaller sheaths, percutaneous access and closure is rapidly becoming the norm[42,43]. Preclosure techniques (Fig. 39.6) currently require placement of one or more percutaneous suture devices at the beginning of the procedure (e.g. Prostar XL® 10F or Proglide® 6F, Abbott Laboratories, Abbott Park, IL, USA).

Transapical procedure

Left ventricular access was developed as a more direct route of access to the aortic valve than the venous and arterial approaches. The apex of the left ventricle is readily accessible through an anterolateral intercostal thoracotomy[22,44]. Epicardial wires or a right ventricular transvenous lead are placed to allow burst pacing for balloon inflation or backup pacing for heart block. Pledgeted sutures are placed in a non-fatty portion of the apical left ventricle which is then punctured with a standard arterial needle. A sheath is placed in the left ventricle and a guidewire is advanced across the aortic valve. Standard balloon valvuloplasty is performed.

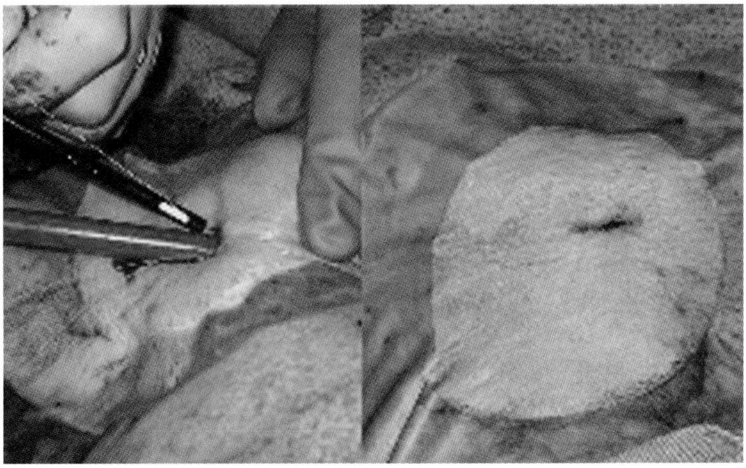

Fig. 39.6 Percutaneous closure of the puncture site following removal of a 24F sheath.

A large sheath, currently 26F, is placed over the wire through the apex into the left ventricle through which is introduced an Edwards balloon-expandable valve mounted on an Ascendra® delivery catheter (Edwards Lifesciences, Irvine, CA, USA). The balloon is inflated expanding and deploying the valve while burst pacing is utilized to reduce transvalvular flow and cardiac motion.

Although transapical implantation of the CoreValve® device has been performed in small number of patients the current device is not ideally suited for this approach and transapical implantation is not currently being pursued[45]. More recently human trials have been initiated with the Embracer® System (Ventor Technologies, Israel). This self-expanding nitinol frame device incorporates three aortic elements which assist in commissural alignment, positioning at the level of the leaflets, and axial fixation.

Transapical access offers several potential advantages over a transarterial approach[44,46]. The risks of arterial injury are minimized. Passage of a bulky prosthesis across the stenotic native valve is easier from the ventricle than the aorta. It may be easier to ensure coaxial positioning and prosthesis movement may be less. However, all patients receive a thoracotomy, chest tube, and general anaesthesia. There may be problems with post-procedural chest discomfort and respiratory compromise, non-coaxial sheath/annulus alignment, injury to mitral chordae, apical tears and bleeding, and apical pseudoaneurysms. Patient selection requires balancing these advantages and disadvantages.

Clinical outcomes

In the initial report of transarterial valve implantation in 17 high-risk patients procedural success was 78% and 30-day mortality was 11%[20]. However with technical improvements and experience outcomes continued to improve. In a subsequent publication 30-day mortality fell to 3.6% in the second half of this continued single-centre Vancouver experience[47], comparing favourably with estimates of surgical 30-day mortality (STS 8.7%, logistic EuroSCORE 25.0%).

Preliminary information is available from a number of transarterial registries utilizing the Edwards Lifesciences balloon-expandable valve. In the first European transarterial trial 30-day mortality was 13.2% (REVIVE, 106 patients). This was followed by the first American trial with a mortality of 7.3% (REVIVAL II, 55 patients). In a subsequent European trial mortality was 8.3% (PARTNER EU, 60 patients), followed by a European post-marketing registry with a mortality of 6.4% (SOURCE, 204 patients). By way of placing this in perspective, logistic EuroSCORE estimates of surgical mortality were 28.9%, 34.1%, 24.6%, and 26.4%, respectively.

Preliminary 30-day mortality rates are available for a number of, as yet, unpublished transapical registries as well. In the initial American experience in the REVIVE II trial, 30-day mortality was 17.6% (40 patients)[48]. In the initial European experience mortality was 14.9% (TRAVERSE, 168 patients), followed by a second European trial at 18.6% (PARTNER EU, 70 patients), and a post-CE mark registry at 9.4% (SOURCE, 173 patients). For comparison, logistic EuroSCORE estimates of surgical mortality were 35.5%, 26.9%, 33.8%, and 29.4% respectively. In 50 high-risk (logistic EuroSCORE 27.6%) and 25 very high-risk patients (logistic EuroSCORE 39%) from Leipzig, 30-day mortality was 8% for the high-risk and 12% for the very high-risk population[49].

Similar improving results have been documented with the transarterial CoreValve® experience. Initial procedures in India were associated with poor clinical outcomes. Subsequently Grube in Siegburg reported 25 high-risk patients in whom implantation was successful in 88% with an in-hospital mortality of 20%. This was followed by a multicentre report of 86 cases, in which implantation was successful in 88% of patients with a 30-day mortality of 12% (logistic EuroSCORE 23.4%)[28–31]. In a more recent single-centre report of 30 patients in which exclusively the third-generation CoreValve® was used, 30-day mortality was 7%[50]. Interim analysis of the 646-patient CoreValve® 18F post-CE mark surveillance registry reported a 30-day mortality of 8%[32]. As yet unpublished data from the same registry with 1243 patients reportedly shows a 30-day mortality of 6.7% (logistic EuroSCORE 22.9%).

Although such registry data is encouraging, direct randomized comparison with conservative management and conventional surgery will be needed for appropriate perspective. The ongoing large multicentre North American PARTNER trial completed enrolment and compares the Edwards SAPIEN® valve to medical management in non-surgical patients and to surgery in high-risk surgical candidates. Both transarterial and transapical approaches will be evaluated with a primary endpoint of 1 year mortality and multiple secondary endpoint analyses. This study will likely have a major impact on defining the role of transcatheter AVR for years to come[51].

Valve function

The haemodynamic characteristics of current transcatheter valves compare favourably to surgical valves.

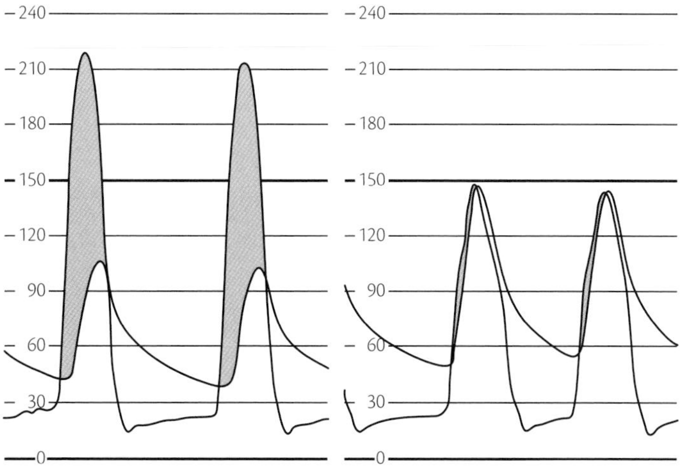

Fig. 39.7 Aortic transvalvular gradient before and after transcatheter aortic valve replacement

Post-procedural gradients are typically <10mmHg (Fig. 39.7) with valve areas ranging from 1.5–1.8cm depending on prosthesis size[20,26,30,32,47,52,53]. *In vitro* evaluation suggests that valve orifice areas are larger than comparable surgical valves; presumably due the absence of a bulky sewing ring. Clinical case-match analyses document transcatheter valve areas superior to current surgical prostheses, particularly in patients with smaller aortic roots where patient–prosthesis mismatch appears uncommon[54].

Significant valvular regurgitation is rare following successful transcatheter AVR. However, paravalvular regurgitation is ubiquitous, at least with currently available devices. For the most part this is relatively mild and well tolerated. Clinical haemolysis has not been reported. However, more severe leaks may occasionally result in chronic congestive failure or rarely with acute severe hypotension at the time of implantation.

Most severe paravalvular leaks can be attributed to: 1) undersizing; 2) underexpansion; 3) positioning the sealing cuff below; or 4) above, the plane of the annulus. To minimize paravalvular regurgitation it is common practice to oversize stent valves by 10–20% to improve apposition to the native annulus. There is little that can be done about an undersized prosthesis once implanted other than medical management or conversion to open surgical AVR. Successful percutaneous leak closure has not been reported in this setting. The best approach is prevention with accurate measurement of the native annulus and selection of an appropriately oversized prosthesis. If underexpansion is suspected, dilation with a slightly oversized balloon may be of benefit. However, expansion is ultimately limited by the size of the non-distensible sealing cuff and the use of oversized balloons may result in deformation of the valve frame, damage to the leaflets, or dislodgement. If the prosthesis is implanted with its sealing cuff too aortic or too ventricular implantation of a second overlapping prosthesis so as to extend the seal in the desired direction can be very effective (Fig. 39.8).

Valve durability

Transcatheter valves are required to undergo the same rigorous testing as surgically implanted valves. Accelerated wear testing demonstrates *in vitro* durability well in excess of 10 years and late structural valve failure has not been reported to date. However, clinical follow-up remains limited, with only anecdotal reports out to 5 years. Concerns remain that leaflet durability may be compromised by the use of newer materials and untested design elements, damage due to compression or catheter trauma, asymmetric frame expansion, suboptimal leaflet coaptation, and other factors.

It appears likely that the durability of transcatheter valves will exceed that of some surgical valves, but fall short of others. However, it can be argued that the importance of durability bears a direct relationship to patient longevity and the implications of late valve failure. Current valves appear sufficiently durable to provide benefit in the mostly elderly patients currently considered candidates[47]. Repeat 'valve in valve' implants appear likely to prove a common way of managing late valve failure when this occurs[55,56]. The feasibility of

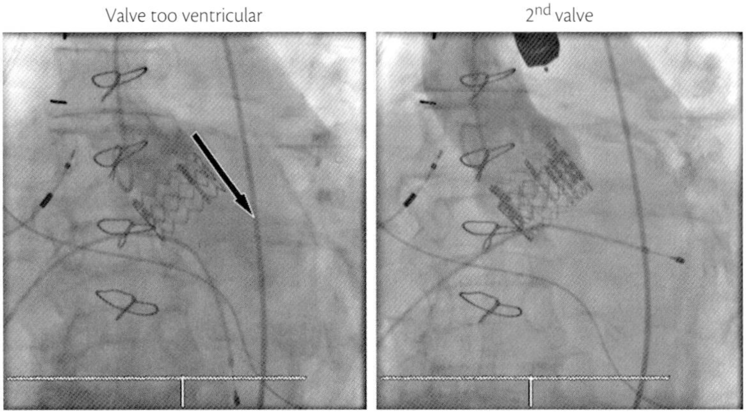

Fig. 39.8 Left: an Edwards SAPIEN® valve was implanted 'too low' and was associated with hypotension with a very low diastolic pressure. Aortography and transoesophageal echocardiography confirmed severe paravalvular regurgitation. Right: a second 'valve-in-valve' implant positioned slightly 'higher' provided effective sealing with clinical improvement.

implanting transcatheter valves in failed aortic and pulmonary surgical prostheses, as well as in tricuspid and mitral prostheses (personal experience), has been demonstrated. Similarly transcatheter valve implantation within previously placed malfunctioning transcatheter valves has been found effective (Fig. 39.9). Although hopeful, the full implications of a valve-in-valve strategy remain unknown[57].

Indications for TAVR

European Society of Cardiology, American College of Cardiology, and American Heart Association guidelines for management of severe aortic stenosis specify symptoms, left ventricular dysfunction, or concomitant non-aortic cardiac surgery as class I indications for surgical valve replacement[2,5,58]. It seems reasonable to expect that these criteria represent a rational starting point for considering the appropriateness of transcatheter AVR as well.

Currently, surgical AVR remains the therapy of choice for symptomatic aortic stenosis due to a long and established history of improved outcomes and durability. In the absence of greater experience, transcatheter AVR should be considered only in patients for whom the risks of surgical morbidity or mortality are high. This raises the question of how surgical risk is estimated. A number of models have been developed to estimate surgical risk. Logistic EuroSCORE estimates of a 30-day mortality exceeding 20% or Society of Thoracic Surgeons (STS) estimates exceeding 10% have been widely used to determine high surgical risk (http://www.euroscore.org and http://www.sts.org). Unfortunately these models commonly overestimate risk in patients in whom comorbities are accounted for in the model used. They may on the other hand underestimate risk in patients with many important comorbidities such as porcelain aorta, multi-valve disease, frailty etc. which are not taken into account in the specific model. Nor do these models adequately account for morbidity, functional recovery of the effects of surgical expertise. Although useful in a general way, for decisions on an individual

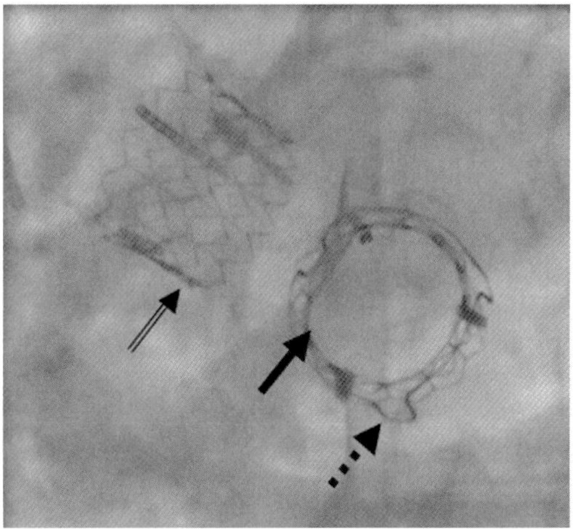

Fig. 39.9 A patient with aortic stenosis and a regurgitant mitral surgical bioprosthesis underwent single stage transapical double valve implantation. An Edwards SAPIEN® valve can be seen in the aortic position (double line arrow) and a valve-in-valve implant (solid arrow) in the mitral surgical prosthesis (dotted arrow).

patient the opinion of an experienced surgeon is often the best estimate of risk[59–61].

Pre-procedural assessment

A careful history, physical examination and routine laboratory investigations to exclude anaemia, bleeding diathesis, and renal dysfunction are necessary. A transthoracic echocardiogram is needed to confirm aortic stenosis severity and to assess left ventricular function, hypertrophy, subaortic obstruction, thrombus, other valve disease, and, importantly, annular diameter. Coronary angiography is necessary to assess the possible need for revascularization. We typically couple this with an ascending and descending aortogram with visualization of both iliac and femoral arteries. CT imaging of the descending aorta and access arteries is an alternative or adjunct. A full surgical consultation is necessary. Subsequently patients should be reviewed together by cardiologists, surgeons, and other professionals with a consensus determination of relative risks and benefits.

Access assessment

Since arterial dissection and perforation are major causes of morbidity and mortality complicating transarterial AVR, detailed arterial assessment of the femoral and iliac arteries is mandatory. The diameter of current transarterial valve delivery systems requires careful assessment of the arterial system right from the site of femoral access, through the iliac artery, to the aorta.

The 18F, 20F, 22F, and 24F sheaths utilized have external diameters of ~6mm, 7mm, 8mm, and 9mm respectively. Since the femoral artery is somewhat compliant it is typically possible to safely pass a sheath through a slightly smaller artery. However if an oversized sheath is left in contact with a very tight artery for too long the two may become adherent, with the possibility of arterial avulsion at the time of sheath removal with haemodynamic collapse.

Although normal arteries are compliant this may not be the case in the presence of atheroma, calcification, and tortuosity leading to perforation or dissection at the time of sheath insertion. Abdominal aortography with imaging of the femoral and iliac arteries bilaterally is often utilized and is best done with a calibrated catheter to allow precise measurement. More important than average femoral and iliac arterial diameters is appreciation of the minimum diameter of the artery the sheath must traverse. Many groups favour or utilize adjunctive multislice CT angiography to assess lumen size and tortuosity, with non-contrast imaging to assess calcification. Even severe calcification is not necessarily a contraindication to transarterial access in the presence of an adequate lumen. However, dense calcification can be a significant problem in combination with a borderline lumen, particularly if circumferential.

Assessment of the aortic root

Although the size of the aortic annulus can be readily measured at the time of open heart surgery a non-invasive assessment is needed prior to transcatheter AVR. The annulus is an ill-defined concept as much as a structure, but for practical purposes extends from the left ventricular outflow tract to the crown-like attachments of the leaflets[62]. Echocardiography is the current standard for measurement[41,63]. The diameter of the aortic annulus is typically measured from a parasternal long-axis view at the level of the basal insertion of the valve leaflets. Measurements made at the level of the left ventricular outflow tract may over- or underestimate annular diameter and should not be accepted as a substitute. Measurements not made at the very basal insertion of the leaflets tend to overestimate the annular diameter, as the leaflet attachments rise into the sinuses in a crown-like manner[62]. When transthoracic imaging is suboptimal or measurements are borderline transoesophageal echocardiography in the mid-oesophageal long-axis view may provide more accurate estimation of annulus diameter[41].

Multislice CT can also be used for annulus sizing[37,64,65]. Three-dimensional imaging reveals the annulus to be an elliptical structure and enables estimation of both a greater and lesser diameter in contrast to echocardiography which typically allows measurement only in a sagittal plane. Although there may be intrinsic advantages to CT measurements, clinical correlates have been less well standardized at this time. CT may also allow measurement of the diameter of the aortic root, sinotubular junction, and ascending aorta which may be of value.

Annulus size is an important determinant of prosthesis selection and patient exclusion as current transcatheter valves are limited in terms of available sizes. Balloon-expandable valves should be slightly larger in diameter than the native annulus to minimize paravalvular leaks and provide secure seating. Similarly, the self-expanding valve must be oversized to allow continued radial force. The 23mm Edwards SAPIEN® valve is recommended for annular diameters of 18–22mm and the 26mm valve for diameters of 21–25mm. The 26mm CoreValve® is recommended for annular diameters of 0–23mm and the 29mm valve for diameters of 23–27mm. In addition an ascending aorta diameter ≤43mm is considered necessary for the CoreValve® device to allow for supracoronary fixation.

Coronary disease

Concomitant coronary disease is common in the setting of aortic stenosis. In the presence of coronary disease, bypass would typically be performed at the time of surgical AVR. However, transcatheter AVR represents not only a therapy but an alternate strategy, in which percutaneous coronary intervention may be performed before, during or after AVR, or held in abeyance and applied later if needed. Consequently comparisons of transcatheter AVR in patients with coronary disease and isolated surgical AVR are problematic.

Early experience suggests that the majority of patients who are currently considered candidates for valve implantation do well with conservative management of coronary disease[47,66]. Angina typically improves after AVR alone. However angioplasty may be indicated in preparation for transcatheter AVR in the presence of acute coronary syndromes, where a large amount of potentially ischaemic myocardium may increase the risk of valve implantation, or where long-term benefit from revascularization is anticipated[67].

Coronary obstruction as a consequence of transcatheter AVR is a unique concern. This generally occurs when a bulky native leaflet is displaced over the left main coronary ostium (Fig. 39.10) [20,68,69]. Predisposing factors include: 1) a low lying coronary ostium (<10–12mm from the basal leaflet insertion to coronary ostium); 2) bulky native leaflets; 3) shallow (as opposed to deep) sinuses leaving little room for the native leaflets. All can be assessed by echo, aortography, and CT and can be further assessed during valvuloplasty or even further by aortic root injection during valvuloplasty[69].

The risk of coronary ostial obstruction may vary with the specific type of transcatheter prosthesis, although this remains to be definitively evaluated. Coronary obstruction has most often been identified with tubular balloon-expandable valves and typically presents as ST elevation and hypotension immediately following valve implantation. Immediate institution of cardiopulmonary support may be necessary and successful management has generally required either emergency bypass or stenting[68,69].

Complications of transcatheter aortic valve replacement

Vascular injury (perforation, dissection, thrombosis) is currently the most important complication associated with transarterial AVR and has been the major predictor of procedural mortality. Delivery systems with a diameter of 18–24F are placed through sheaths with much larger outer diameters of 7–9mm. Many patients will have smaller femoral arteries, often in combination with atheroma, calcification, or tortuosity. Careful screening of the femoral and iliac arteries with aortography and multislice CT is the best way to avoid vascular injury, morbidity, and mortality. Familiarity with ilio-femoral intervention and the ready availability of occlusion balloons and large vessel covered stents is necessary to mitigate this risk[70].

Hypotension is common and predictable during transcatheter AVR as a consequence of the limited cardiac

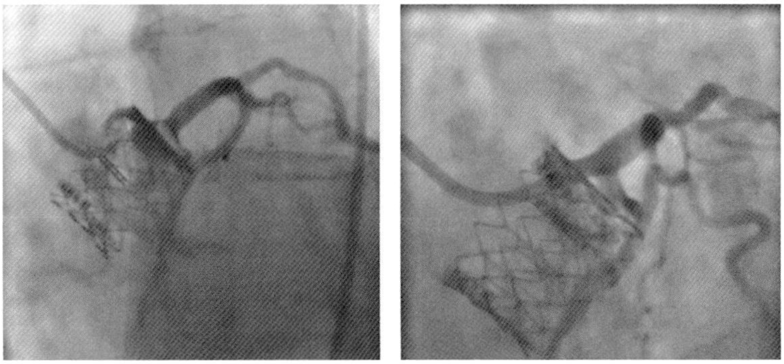

Fig. 39.10 Left: cardiogenic shock developed immediately after transcatheter AVR requiring institution of cardiopulmonary support. Aortography shows that a native leaflet has been displaced obstructing the left main ostium. Right: stenting through the valve frame into the left coronary restored haemodynamic stability. The patient remains well.

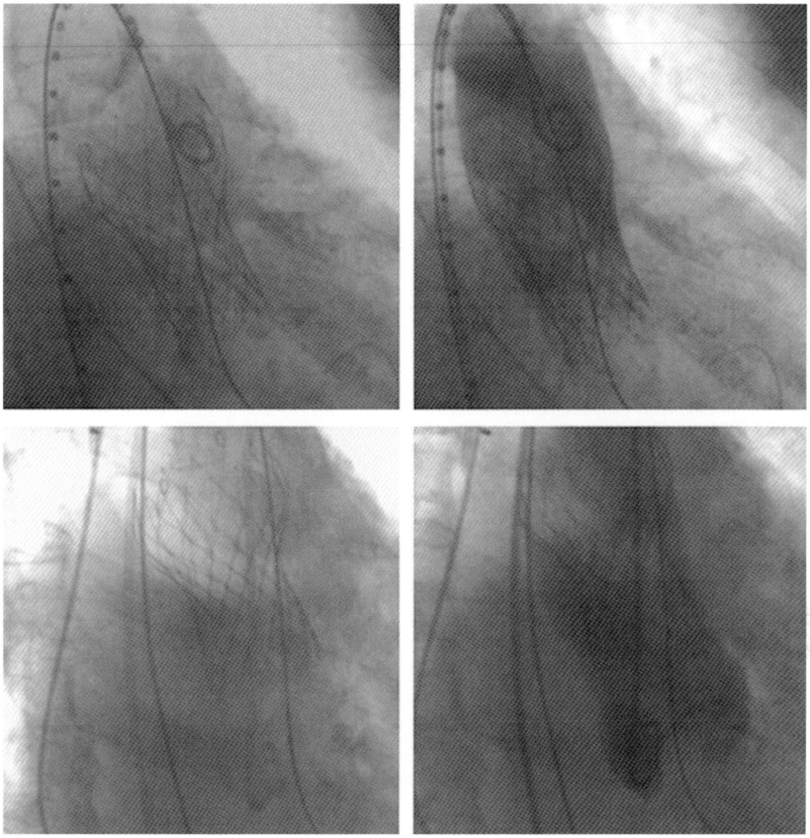

Fig. 39.11 Top: CoreValve® correctly positioned. The inflow of the prosthesis is fixed in the left ventricular outflow tract. The outflow is fixed against the supracoronary aortic wall. Bottom: CoreValve® positioned too aortic due to movement during deployment. Courtesy of Christoph Kaiser, MD, University Hospital Basel, Switzerland.

reserve in the setting of aortic stenosis. Predisposing factors include: 1) reduced coronary perfusion pressure due to pharmacologic/anaesthetic medications or vagal-induced vasodilation, blood loss, or bradycardia; 2) increased myocardial oxygen demands due to tachycardia induced by chronotropic medications, pacing, or catheter-induced extrasystoles; 3) blood loss and anaemia; 4) acute aortic valve dysfunction due to catheter interference or leaflet injury; 5) acute mitral valve dysfunction due to catheter interference, chordal injury or tethering in the presence of left ventricular ischaemia or dilation. Avoidance requires minimizing ischaemic stress during valve implantation and the judicious use of volume expansion and pressors as required.

In addition, sudden and unexpected hypotension may occur. In addition to the above considerations attention must be turned to the possibility of: 1) perforation of the aorta, iliac, or femoral arteries; 2) cardiac perforation due to catheter, wire, or pacemaker lead injury or due to transapical apical access problems; 3) aortic annulus rupture due to balloon dilation; 4) a profound vagal stimulus due to annular dilation; 5) acute, severe prosthetic regurgitation due to positioning/sizing errors; and 6) coronary occlusion. Successful management requires prompt recognition, pharmacologic support, and volume expansion. On occasion rapid institution of cardiopulmonary support may be necessary as the majority of these complications are salvageable if appropriately addressed[71].

Valve malposition, where the prosthesis is implanted somewhere other than the aortic annulus, occurs uncommonly but remains a problem (Fig. 39.11). Accurate positioning depends on careful attention to procedural technique but also to pre-implantation planning (Fig. 39.12). If the prosthesis is positioned within the native valve but the sealing cuff does not appose the annulus adequately a second overlapping prosthesis may be considered. If the prosthesis

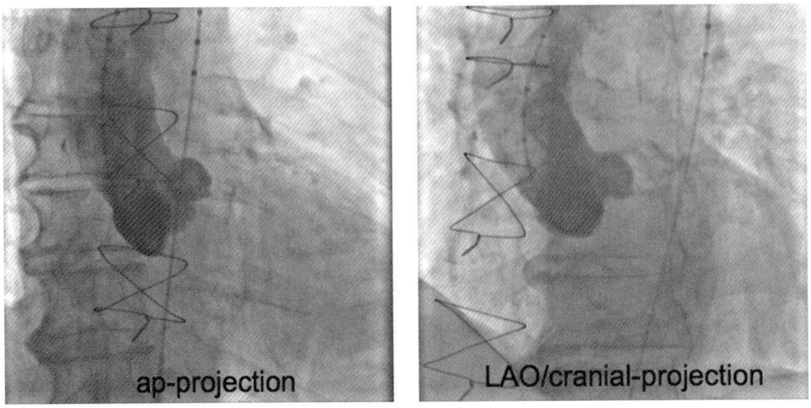

Fig. 39.12 Left: angiographic imaging perpendicular to the valve plane shows three symmetrical leaflets. This view would be well suited to accurate positioning of a transcatheter valve. Right: aortography shows only two leaflets indicating that the fluoroscopic imaging plane is not perpendicular to the valve.

extends into the ventricle, interfering with mitral or ventricular function, then surgery may be necessary. If the prosthesis is deployed in the aorta then so long as fixation is adequate and important side branches are not jeopardized it may be left in place[72,73].

Valve embolization is a concern with prosthetic stent valves. Primarily this is an issue with shorter valves with a single point of fixation such as the Edwards SAPIEN® and unlikely with longer valves such as the CoreValve® device which has a secondary point of fixation in the ascending aorta. Embolization appears to occur when the prosthesis is deployed above the plane of the annulus and occurs at or immediate after deployment. Management has been extensively reviewed elsewhere[71,73]. Briefly this involves maintaining wire position and utilizing the partially inflated delivery balloon to reposition and fix the prosthesis in the more distal aorta where it can be left *in situ* (Fig. 39.13).

Stroke rates vary widely from 0–10%[30,43,71,74]. Available data from the Edwards transarterial series show stroke rates falling to 3.3% (PARTNER EU) and 3.4% (SOURCE) and from the transapical series down to 3% (TRAVERSE), 1.4% (PARTNER EU), 0.6% (SOURCE). Similarly CoreValve® stroke rates have reportedly fallen to approximately 2% in recent reports[30–32]. Undoubtedly the true incidence of cerebral emboli may be higher than clinically apparent.

Stroke is generally attributable to embolization from the native valve or from the aortic arch. Early data suggests that the risk of embolic stroke may be lower with transapical, as opposed to transarterial access[47, 49], and lower with later generation low profile, atraumatic transarterial delivery systems and with increasing experience[27,30,32]. Screening the ascending aorta for friable atheroma is an obvious preventative measure that has not been widely utilized.

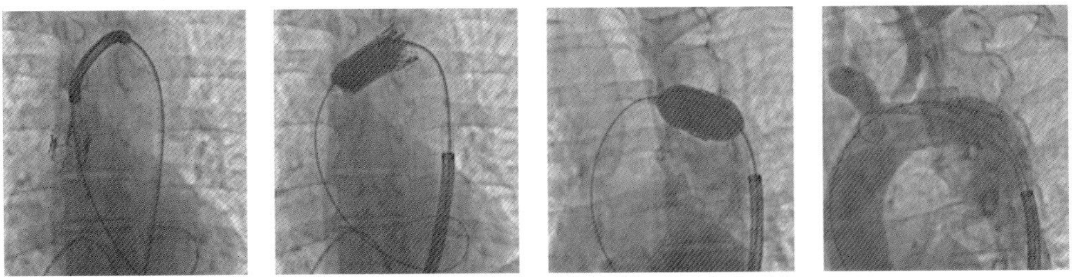

Fig. 39.13 Valve embolization. A Cribier–Edwards valve was deployed too aortic and was immediately discharged into the aorta. A partially inflated balloon was utilized to withdraw the valve and fix it in the transverse aorta. The patient remains well.

Atrioventricular block occurs as a common complication of surgical AVR due to the proximity of the aortic valve and His bundle. Similarly heart block can occur as a consequence of transcatheter AVR, presumably due to pressure effects[75, 76]. Block generally occurs immediately, although delayed block has been observed. Most centres continue electrocardiographic monitoring for 48h after implantation, although others continue monitoring for up to 1 week[44, 75, 76]. Predisposing factors may include pre-existing conduction abnormalities (particularly right bundle branch block), prosthesis oversizing, extension of the prosthesis into the outflow tract adjacent to the subvalvular septum, and continued radial expansion with self-expanding prostheses. The incidence of pacemaker implantation appears to vary from 5–25%, depending on the valve type implanted and on local practice.

The future

An increasing role for transcatheter AVR appears certain. New valves, delivery systems, and strategies will likely improve outcomes and widen the population of patients who are potential candidates. While benefits may be large, risks are also large and neither durability nor late implications of this therapy are known. A cautious, measured approach to dissemination, training, and patient selection seems prudent[77–79].

Disclosures

Dr. Webb is a consultant to Edwards Lifesciences, Irvine, California, USA. Dr. F. Nietlispach receives an unrestricted grant from the Cardiovascular Research Foundation, Basel, Switzerland.

References

1. Nkomo VT, Gardin JM, Skelton TN, *et al.* Burden of valvular heart diseases: a population-based study. *Lancet* 2006; **368**:1005–11.
2. Bonow RO, Carabello BA, Chatterjee K, *et al.* 2008 Focused Update Incorporated Into the ACC/AHA 2006 Guidelines for the Management of Patients With Valvular Heart Disease: A Report of the American College of Cardiology/American Heart Association Task Force on Practice Guidelines (Writing Committee to Revise the 1998 Guidelines for the Management of Patients With Valvular Heart Disease) Endorsed by the Society of Cardiovascular Anesthesiologists, Society for Cardiovascular Angiography and Interventions, and Society of Thoracic Surgeons. *J Am Coll Cardiol* 2008; **52**(13):e1–e142.
3. Bonow RO, Carabello BA, Kanu C, *et al.* ACC/AHA 2006 guidelines for the management of patients with valvular heart disease: a report of the American College of Cardiology/American Heart Association Task Force on Practice Guidelines. Circulation 2006; 114:e84–231.
4. Rahimtoola SH. Valvular heart disease: a perspective on the asymptomatic patient with severe valvular aortic stenosis. *Eur Heart J* 2008; **29**:1783–90.
5. Vahanian A, Baumgartner H, Bax J, *et al.* Guidelines on the management of valvular heart disease; the task force on the management of valvular heart disease fo the European Society of Cardiology. *Eur Heart J* 2007; **28**:230–68.
6. Bach DS CN, Deeb M,. Unoperated patients with severe aortic stenosis. *J Am Coll Cardiol* 2007; **50**:2018–19.
7. Iung B, Baron G, Butchart EG, *et al.* A prospective survey of patients with valvular heart disease in Europe: The Euro Heart Valve Survey on Valvular Disease. *Eur Heart J* 2003; **24**:1231–43.
8. Iung B, Cachier A, Baron G, *et al.* Decision-making in elderly patients with severe aortic stenosis: why are so many denied surgery? *Eur Heart Journal* 2005; **26**:2714–20.
9. Charlson E, Legedza ATR, Hamel MB. Decision-making and outcomes in severe symptomatic aortic stenosis. *J Heart Valve Dis* 2006; **15**:312–21.
10. Ngaage DL, Cowen ME, Griffin S, *et al.* Are initial valve operations still high-risk in the current era? J *Heart Valve Dis* 2008; **17**:227–32.
11. Bossone E, Di Benedetto G, Frigola A, *et al.* Valve surgery in octogenarians: in-hospital and long-term outcomes. *Can J Cardiol* 2007; **23**:223–7.
12. Bouma BJ, van den Brink RB, Zwinderman K, *et al.* Which elderly patients with severe aortic stenosis benefit from surgical treatment? An aid to clinical decision making? *J Heart Valve Dis* 2004; **13**:374–81.
13. Vadarajian P, Kapoor N, Bansal RC, *et al.* Survival in elderly patients with severe aortic stenosis is dramatically improved by aortic valve replacement: results from a cohort of 277 patients aged >80 years. *Eur J Cardiothor Surg* 2006; **30**:722–7.
14. Pedersen WR, Klaassen PH, Boisjolie CR, *et al.* Feasibility of transcatheter intervention for severe aortic stenosis in patients > or = 90 years of age: aortic valvuloplasty revisited. *Cathet Cardiovasc Interv* 2007; **70**:149–54.
15. Otto CM, Mickel MC, Kennedy JW, *et al.* Three-year outcome after balloon aortic valvuloplasty: insights into prognosis of valvular aortic stenosis. *Circulation* 1994; **89**:642–50.
16. Shareghi S, Rasouli L, Shavelle DM, *et al.* Current results of balloon aortic valvuloplasty in high-risk patients. *J Invasive Cardiol* 2007; **19**:1–5.
17. Andersen HR, Knudsen LL, Hasenkam JM. Transluminal implantation of artificial heart valves. Description of a new expandable aortic valve and initial results with implantation by catheter technique in closed chest pigs. *Eur Heart J* 1992; **13**:704–8.

18. Cribier A, Eltchaninoff H, Bash A, *et al.* Percutaneous transcatheter implantation of an aortic valve prosthesis for calcific aortic stenosis: first human case description. *Circulation* 2002; **106**:3006–8.
19. Cribier A, Eltchaninoff H, Tron C, *et al.* Early experience with percutaneous transcatheter implantation of heart valve prosthesis for the treatment of end-stage inoperable patients with calcific aortic stenosis. *J Am Coll Cardiol* 2004; **43**:698–703.
20. Webb JG, Chandavimol M, Thompson C, *et al.* Percutaneous aortic valve implantation retrograde from the femoral artery. *Circulation* 2006; **113**:842–50.
21. Ye J, Cheung A, Lichtenstein SV, *et al.* Transapical aortic valve implantation in humans. *J Thorac Cardiovasc Surg* 2006; **131**(5):1194–6.
22. Lichtenstein SV, Cheung A, Ye J, *et al.* Transapical transcatheter aortic valve implantation in man. *Circulation* 2006; **114**:591–6.
23. Walther T, Dewey T, Wimmer-Greinecker G, *et al.* Transapical approach for sutureless stent-fixed aortic valve implantation: experimental results. *Eur J Cardiothorac Surg* 2007; **29**:703–8.
24. Walther T, Falk V, Borger MA, *et al.* Minimally invasive transapical beating heart aortic valve implantation – proof of concept. *Eur J Cardiothorac Surg* 2007; **31**:9–15.
25. Walther T, Simon P, Dewey T, *et al.* Transapical minimally invasive aortic valve implantation. Multicenter experience. *Circulation* 2007; **116**(suppl I):I-240–I-245.
26. Webb JG, Pasupati SJ, Humphries K, *et al.* Percutaneous transarterial aortic valve replacement in selected high risk patients with aortic stenosis. *Circulation* 2007; **116**:755–63.
27. Webb JG AL, Masson JB, Al Bugami S, *et al.* A new transcatheter aortic valve and percutaneous valve delivery system. *J Am Coll Cardiol* 2009; **53**(20):1855–8.
28. Grube E, Laborde JC, Zickmann B, *et al.* First report on a human percutaneous transluminal implantation of a self-expanding valve prosthesis for interventional treatment of aortic valve stenosis. *Catheter Cardiovasc Interv* 2005; **66**:465–9.
29. Grube E, Laborde JC, Gerckens U, *et al.* Percutaneous implantation of the CoreValve self-expanding valve prosthesis in high-risk patients with aortic valve disease: the Siegburg first-in-man study. *Circulation* 2006; **114**(15):1616–24.
30. Grube E, Buellesfeld, L, Mueller, R, *et al.* Progress and current status of percutaneous aortic valve replacement: results of three device generations of the CoreValve revalving system. *Circ Cardiovasc Intervent* 2008; **1**:167–75.
31. Grube E, Schuler G, Buellesfeld L, *et al.* Percutaneous aortic valve replacement for severe aortic stenosis in high-risk patients using the second and current third generation self-expanding CoreValve prosthesis: device success and 30day outcome. *J Am Coll Cardiol* 2007; **50**:69–76.
32. Piazza N, Grube E, Gerckens U, *et al.* Procedural and 30-day outcomes following transcatheter aortic valve implantation using the third generation (18Fr) CoreValve ReValving System: results from the multicentre, expanded evaluation registry 1-year following CE mark approval. *EuroIntervention* 2008; **4**:242–9.
33. Low RI, Bolling SF, Yeo KK, *et al.* Direct flow medical percutaneous aortic valve: proof of concept. *EuroIntervention* 2008; **4**:256–61.
34. Schofer J, Schluter M, Treede H, *et al.* Retrograde transarterial implantation of a nonmetallic aortic valve prosthesis in high-surgical-risk patients with severe aortic stenosis. A first-in-man feasibility and safety study. *Circ Cardiovasc Interv* 2008; **1**:126–33.
35. Lauck S, MacKay M, Galte C, *et al.* A new treatment option for the treatment of aortic stenosis: percutaneous aortic valve replacement. *Crit Care Nurse* 2008; **28**:40–51.
36. Ree RM BJ, Schwarz SKW. Case series: anesthesia for retrograde percutaneous aortic valve replacement – experience with the first 40 patients. *Can J Anesth* 2008; **55**:761–8.
37. Tops LF Wood DA, Delgado V, *et al.* Noninvasive evaluation of the aortic root with multislice computed tomography: implications for transcatheter aortic valve replacement. *J Am Coll Cardiol Imaging* 2008; **1**:321–30.
38. Ruge H, Lange R, Bleiziffer S, *et al.* First successful aortic valve implantation with the CoreValve ReValving System via a right subclavian artery access: a case report. *Heart Surgery Forum* 2008; **11**:E323–E324.
39. Bauernschmitt R, Schreiber C, Bleiziffer S, *et al.* Transcatheter aortic valve implantation through the ascending aorta: an alternative option for no-access patients. *Heart Surgery Forum* 2009; **12**:E63–E64.
40. Webb JG, Pasupati S, Achtem L, *et al.* Rapid pacing to facilitate transcatheter prosthetic heart valve implantation. *Catheter Cardiovasc Interv* 2006; **68**:199–204.
41. Moss RR, Ivens E, Pasupati S, *et al.* Echocardiography and percutaneous aortic valve implantation. *J Am Coll Cardiol Imaging* 2008; **1**:15–24.
42. De Jaegere P, van Dijk C, Laborde JC, *et al.* True percutaneous implantation of the CoreValve aortic valve prosthesis by the combined use of ultrasound guided vascular access, Prostar XL and the TandemHeart. *Eurointervention* 2007; **2**:500–5.
43. Webb JG. Percutaneous aortic valve replacement will be a common treatment for aortic valve disease. *J Am Coll Cardiol Interv* 2008; **1**:122–6.
44. Walther T, Dewey T, Borger MA, *et al.* Transapical aortic valve implantation: step by step. *Ann Thorac Surg* 2008; **87**:276–83.
45. Lange R, Schreiber C, Gotz W, *et al.* First successful transapical aortic valve implantation with the CoreValve Revalving System: a case report. *Heart Surgery Forum* 2007; **10**:E478–E479.
46. Webb JG. The shortest way to the heart. *Cathet Cardiovasc Interv* 2008; **71**(7):920.

47. Webb JG, Altwegg L, Boone RH, *et al.* Transcatheter aortic valve implantation. Impact on clinical and valve-related outcomes. *Circulation* 2009; **119**(23):3009–16.
48. Svensson LG, Dewey T, Kapadia S, *et al.* United States feasibility study of transcatheter insertion of a stented aortic valve by the left ventricular apex. *Ann Thorac Surg* 2008; **86**:46–55.
49. Walther T, Falk V, Kempfert J, *et al.* Transapical minimally invasive aortic valve implantation; the initial 50 patients. *Eur J Cardiothorac Surg* 2008; **33**:983–8.
50. Tamburino C, Capodanno D, Mul EM, *et al.* Procedural success and 30-day clinical outcomes after percutaneous aortic valve replacement using current third-generation self-expanding CoreValve prosthesis. *J Invasive Cardiol* 2009; **21**:93–8.
51. Zuckerman BD, Saperstien W, Swain JA. The FDA role in the development of percutaneous valve technology. *EuroInterv* 2007; Supplement A:A75–A78.
52. Cribier A, Eltchaninoff H, Tron C, *et al.* Treatment of calcific aortic stenosis with the percutaneous heart valve. Mid-term follow-up from the initial feasibility studies: The French experience. *J Am Coll Cardiol* 2006; **47**:1214 –23.
53. Cribier A, Eltchaninoff H, Tron C, *et al.* Percutaneous implantation of aortic valve prosthesis in patients with calcific aortic stenosis: technical advances, clinical results and future strategies. *J Invasive Cardiol* 2006; **19**:S88–S96.
54. Clavel MA, Webb JG, Pibarot P, *et al.* Comparison of the hemodynamic performance of percutaneous and surgical bioprostheses for the treatment of severe aortic stenosis. *J Am Coll Cardiol* 2009; **53**(20):1883–91.
55. Webb JG. Transcatheter valve in valve implants for failed prosthetic valves. *Cathet Cardiovasc Interven* 2007; **70**:765–6.
56. Walther T Kempfert J, Borger MA, *et al.* Human minimally invasive off-pump valve-in-a-valve implantation. *Ann Thorac Surg* 2008; **85**:1072–3.
57. Webb JG. Transcatheter valve in valve implants for failed prosthetic valves. *Catheter Cardiovasc Interv* 2007; **70**(5):765–6.
58. Bonow RO CB, Chatterjee K, de Leon AC, *et al.* ACC/AHA 2006 practice guidelines for the management of patients with valvular heart disease: executive summary. *J Am Coll Cardiol* 2006; **48**:598–675.
59. Osswald BR, Gegouskov V, Badowcki-Zyla D, *et al.* Overestimation of aortic valve replacement risk by EuroSCORE: implications for percutaneous valve replacement. *Eur Heart J* 2009; **30**:74–80.
60. Brown ML Shaff HV, Sarano ME, *et al.* Is the European System for Cardiac Operative Risk Evaluation model valid for estimating the operative risk of patients considered for percutaneous aortic valve replacement? *J Thorac Cardiovasc Surg* 2008; **136**:566–71.
61. Dewey TM, Brown D, Ryan WH, *et al.* Reliability of risk algorithms in predicting early and late operative outcomes in high-risk patients undergoing aortic valve replacement. *J Thorac Cardiovasc Surg* 2008; **135**:180–7.
62. Piazza N, de Jaegere PP, Serrrys P, *et al.* Anatomy of the aortic valvar complex and its implications for percutaneous implantation of the aortic valve. *Circulation* 2008; **1**:74–81.
63. De Jaegere P, Piazza N, Galema TW, *et al.* Early echocardiographic evaluation following percutaneous implantation with the self-expanding CoreValve ReValving System aortic valve bioprosthesis. *EuroInterv* 2008; **4**:351–7.
64. Wood DA, Mayo JR, Tops LF, *et al.* The role of multislice computed tomography in the assessment of transcatheter aortic valve replacement. *Am J Cardiol* 2007; **100**(Suppl 8A):75L.
65. Leipsic J WD, Manders D, *et al.* The evolving role of multidetector computed tomography in transcatheter aortic valve replacement: a radiologist's perspective. *Am J Radiol* 2009; **193**(3):W214–9.
66. Webb JG. Strategies in the management of coronary artery disease and transcatheter aortic valve implantation. *Cathet Cardiovasc Interv* 2009; **73**:68.
67. Piazza N SP, de Jaegere PP, Serruys P. Feasibility of complex coronary intervention in combination with percutaneous aortic valve implantation in patients with aortic stenosis using percutaneous left ventricular assist device (TandemHeart). *Cathet Cardiovasc Interv* 2009; **73**:161–6.
68. Kapadia S, Svensson LG, Tuzcu EM. Successful percutaneous management of left main trunk occlusion during percutaneous aortic valve replacement. *Cathet Cardiovasc Interv* 2009; **73**(7):966–72.
69. Webb JG. Coronary obstruction due to transcatheter valve implantation. *Catheter Cardiovasc Interv* 2009; **73**(7):973.
70. Masson JB WJ. Endovascular balloon occlusion for catheter-induced large arterial perforation in the catheterization laboratory. *Cathet Cardiovasc Interv* 2009; **73**:514–18.
71. Masson JB, Kovac J, Schuler G, *et al.* Transcatheter aortic valve implantation: review of the nature, management and avoidance of procedural complications. *JACC Cardiovasc Intervt* 2009; **2**(9):811–20
72. Piazza N SC, de Jaegere PPT, Serrrys PW. Implantation of two self-expanding aortic bioprosthetic valves during the same procedure-insights into valve-in-valve implantantation ("Russian doll concept"). *Cathet Cardiovasc Interv* 2009; **73**:530–9.
73. Al Ali AM Atlwegg L, Horlick EM, *et al.* Prevention and management of transcatheter balloon-expandable aortic valve malposition. *Cathet Cardiovasc Interv* 2008; **72**:573–8.
74. Vahanian A, Palacios IF. Percutaneous approaches to valvular disease. *Circulation* 2004; **109**:1572–9.
75. Sinhal A, Pasupati S, Humphries K, *et al.* Atrioventricular block after transcatheter aortic valve implantation. *J Am Coll Cardiol Intervent* 2008; **1**:304–9.

76. Piazza N, Onuma Y, Jesserun E, *et al.* Early and persistent intraventricular conduction abnormalities and requirements for pacemaking after percutaneous replacement of the aortic valve. *JACC Cardiovasc Interv* 2008; **1**:310–16.
77. Vassiliades TA, Jr, Block PC, Cohn LH, *et al.* The clinical development of percutaneous heart valve technology: a position statement of the Society of Thoracic Surgeons (STS), the American Association for Thoracic Surgery (AATS), and the Society for Cardiovascular Angiography and Interventions (SCAI) Endorsed by the American College of Cardiology Foundation (ACCF) and the American Heart Association (AHA). *J Am Coll Cardiol* 2005; **45**:1554–60.
78. Rosengart TK Feldman T, Borger MA, *et al.* Percutaneous and Minimally Invasive Valve Procedures. A Scientific Statement From the American Heart Association Council on Cardiovascular Surgery and Anesthesia, Council on Clinical Cardiology, Functional Genomics and Translational Biology Interdisciplinary Working Group, and Quality of Care and Outcomes Research Interdisciplinary Working Group. *Circulation* 2008; **117**(13):1750–67.
79. Vahanian A Alfieri O, Al-Attar N, *et al.* Transcatheter valve implantation for patients with aortic stenosis: a position statement from the European Association of Cardio-Thoracic Surgery (EACTS) and the European Society of Cardiology (ESC), in collaboration with the European Association of Percutaneous Cardiovascular Interventions (EAPCI). *Eur Heart J* 2008; **29**(11):1463–70.

CHAPTER 40

Mitral balloon valvuloplasty

Alec Vahanian, Dominique Himbert, Eric Brochet, Grégory Ducrocq, and Bernard Iung

Although the prevalence of rheumatic fever has greatly decreased in Western countries, mitral stenosis (MS) still results in significant morbidity and mortality worldwide[1]. The treatment of MS has been revolutionized since the development of balloon mitral valvuloplasty (BMV). Until the first publication by Inoue[2] in 1984, surgery was the only treatment for patients with mitral stenosis. Since then, the technique has evolved considerably. A large number of patients with varied conditions[3] have now been treated worldwide, enabling us to assess the efficacy and risk of the technique, and long-term results make us better able to select the most appropriate candidates for treatment using this method.

Mechanisms

BMV acts in the same way as surgical commissurotomy by opening the fused commissures, suggesting that BMV will share the same good long-term results of the technique, which is known to provide good results up to 20 years in patients with favourable characteristics[4]. BMV is of little or no help in cases of restricted valvular mobility caused by valve fibrosis or severe subvalvular disease.

Technique

The techniques and devices used for BMV have varied over time and from group to group.

Approaches

The retrograde technique without transseptal catheterization[5] has been used with good results, but its use is now very limited.

The transvenous or antegrade approach is most widely used. Transseptal catheterization is the first step of the procedure and one of the most crucial[6].

Transseptal puncture is usually performed using a Brockenbrough needle and a dilator which is most often that of the Mullins sheath.

The following steps should be taken:

- A 5F pigtail is positioned retrogradely from the femoral artery to the right coronary sinus for identification of the aorta and systemic pressure monitoring
- Percutaneous access is via a puncture of the right femoral vein as this offers a direct approach from the inferior vena cava to the interatrial septum at the fossa ovalis. In very rare cases, transseptal catheterization has been performed using a transjugular or transhepatic approach[7]
- A 0.032-inch J-tipped guide wire is advanced into the superior vena cava, up to the origin of the left innominate vein, in anteroposterior view
- The catheter is advanced over the guide wire into the superior vena cava and the guide wire is removed
- The Brockenbrough needle is connected to a pressure line, which is continuously flushed, and is inserted into the dilator just inside the distal end under fluoroscopic guidance. When the needle reaches the desired position inside the catheter the flush is stopped and pressure is continuously monitored
- Initially, the tip of the catheter is orientated towards the right shoulder of the patient in anteroposterior view. Then, under continuous fluoroscopic and pressure monitoring, both catheter and needle are withdrawn downwards and rotated counterclockwise

until contact with the septum is felt. Whatever the method used, the proximal arrow and the tip of the needle have a posteromedial position, looking from bottom to top in anteroposterior view. The angle is chosen according to the size of the left atrium (LA) (4 o'clock in normal size and up to 6 in a large atrium). In anteroposterior view, the correct position of the tip of the needle is usually mid way between the pigtail and the right atrial border in the horizontal axis and slightly below the horizontal line at the level of the pigtail. It is recommended to use a complementary view to provide further information on the orientation of the needle in the anteroposterior axis before puncturing the septum. This could be a lateral view with a target zone at the mid-part of the line between the pigtail and the spina, or right anterior oblique 30° with a target zone vertically in the middle of the line between the pigtail and the spina and below a horizontal line at the level of the pigtail (Fig. 40.1). For BMV using the Inoue technique, the preferred site for the transseptal puncture is usually slightly lower than the fossa ovale if the LA is severely enlarged

- Before puncturing the interatrial septum, the following parameters should be checked: right atrial pressure tracing, correct position, and tactile contact with the septum. If these criteria are fulfilled, the needle can be advanced
- Entry into the LA is indicated by changes in the pressure tracing. The dilator should be advanced only when assurance is obtained that the needle has crossed the septum. When both the needle and the catheter have crossed the septum, the needle is withdrawn while applying a counterclockwise rotation to the proximal part in order to orientate the catheter towards the mitral valve. LA pressure is then recorded.

The procedure is performed under fluoroscopic guidance with several views, ideally using biplane fluoroscopy. Additional right atrial angiography has been proposed to better locate the puncture site, but today this has been largely replaced by echographic monitoring using either transoesophageal[8] or intracardiac[9] approaches.

Both echocardiographic techniques provide excellent imaging of the interatrial septum, which is useful to guide the orientation of the needle in the fossa ovale, to show proper positioning and to monitor the crossing of the septum and its tenting. Echocardiography is a useful adjunct in the early part of the operator's experience. The drawbacks are the need for anaesthesia, or at least analgesia, in most patients when transoesophageal echocardiography (TEE) is performed, and the cost of the devices as regards intracardiac echocardiography. The recent introduction of real time three-dimensional (3D) transoesophageal echocardiography further improves imaging of the septum. In experienced teams, echocardiographic guidance is restricted to cases where there are known difficulties, such as severe thoracic deformity, or when unexpected difficulties occur.

Finally, transthoracic echographic guidance is seldom used because it is difficult to perform at the same time

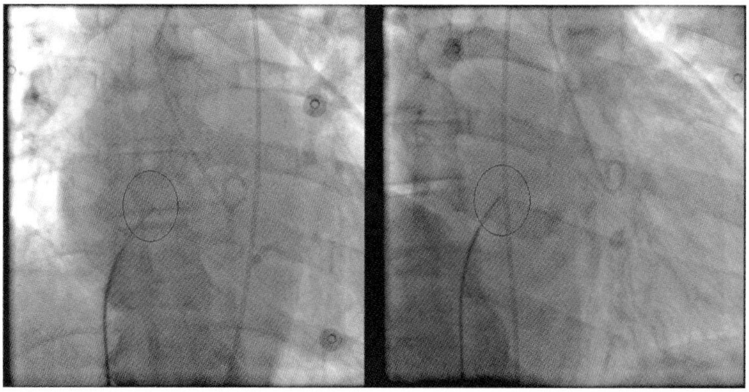

A B

Fig. 40.1 Transseptal puncture. A) Anterior posterior view. The catheter and needle are at the level of the fossa ovale, below and lateral to the pigtail catheter which is positioned on the aortic cusps. B) Right anterior oblique view 30°. The catheter and the needle are below and posterior to the pigtail catheter, around mid-distance between the spina and the pig-tail catheter.

as fluoroscopic imaging. However, it could be helpful in experienced hands.

Devices

With regards to the balloons themselves, the double balloon technique and its variant, the multi-track balloons, are very seldom used and exclusively in developing countries where the economic constraints lead to reuse of the balloons. The metallic commissurotome has been abandoned.

The Inoue technique was the first one described[2] and wide experience has now been acquired by a number of groups worldwide. The data currently available suggests that the Inoue technique eases the procedure and has equivalent efficacy and lower risk than the other techniques. In fact, the Inoue technique has already become the most popular in the world, having been used in more than 10 000 patients. The stepwise technique under echocardiographic guidance certainly allows the best use of the mechanical properties of the Inoue balloon and therefore optimizes the results[10].

The Inoue balloon, composed of nylon and rubber micromesh, is self-positioning and pressure-extensible. It is large (24–30mm in diameter) and has a low profile (4.5mm). The balloon has three distinct parts, each with a specific elasticity, enabling them to be inflated sequentially. This sequence allows fast, stable positioning across the valve. There are four sizes of the Inoue balloon (24, 26, 28, and 30mm); and each is pressure-dependent, so its diameter can be varied by up to 4mm as required by circumstances.

The main steps are as follows:

- Balloon size is chosen in accordance with the patient's height (26mm in very small patients or infants, 28mm in patients less than 1.60m, and 30mm in patients taller than 1.6m)
- After transseptal catheterization, the Inoue guide wire, which is a stiff guide wire with a soft curved tip, is introduced into the left atrium through the transseptal catheter which is then withdrawn. This should be done in AP view and care should be taken to avoid pushing the guide wire into the left atrial appendage (Fig. 40.2)
- The femoral entry site and the atrial septum are dilated using the Inoue dilator (14F) over the guide wire. Several passages are performed until less resistance is felt at the level of the septum and the groin (Fig. 40.3)

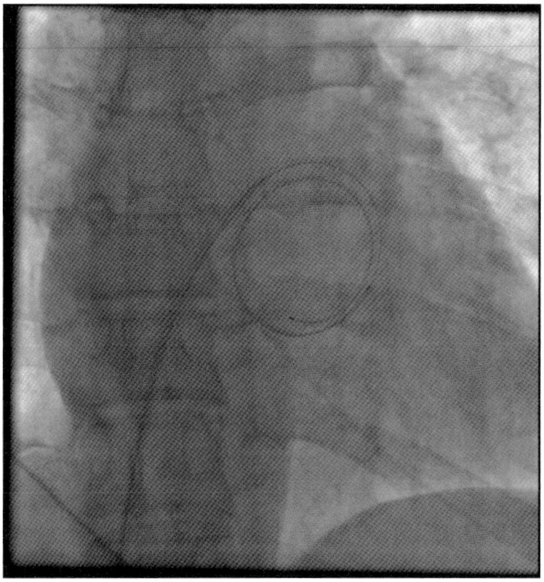

Fig. 40.2 BMV using the Inoue technique Step 1. The Inoue guide wire is introduced into the left atrium through the transseptal catheter (AP view).

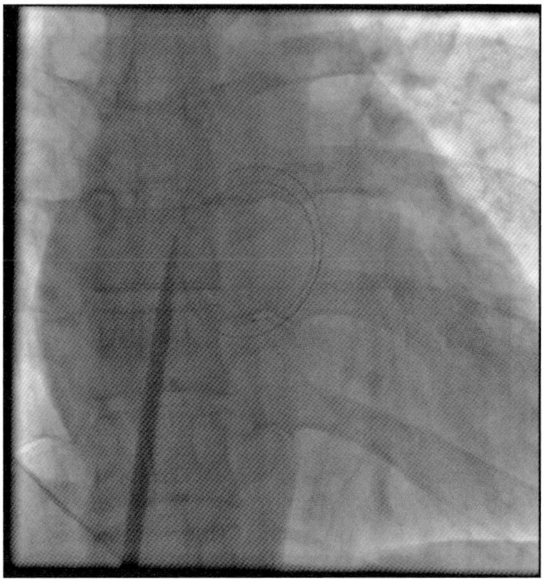

Fig. 40.3 BMV using the Inoue technique Step 2. The Inoue balloon dilator is used to dilate the interatrial septum over the guidewire (AP view).

- After withdrawal of the dilator, the Inoue balloon, which is slenderized using a stretching tube, is introduced into the left atrium. If resistance is felt at any level, excessive pressure should be avoided to avoid impairment of the tip of the Inoue balloon, and alternative techniques should be used. If resistance occurs at the level of the femoral entry site despite adequate dilatation it is advisable to use a 16F sheath (Cook) and to introduce the balloon through it. If resistance occurs at the level of the interatrial septum it could be dilated using an 8F peripheral angioplasty balloon
- When the Inoue balloon is positioned into the left atrium, the guide wire and the stretching tube are withdrawn, which shortens the balloon
- After careful flushing, the stylet is introduced into the balloon catheter to direct it through the mitral valve. When the stylet has reached the distal part of the balloon, the fluoroscopy arm, which was until then in AP, should be turned to RAO 30
- The balloon is inflated sequentially
- Firstly, the distal portion is inflated with 1 or 2mL of a diluted contrast medium and acts as a floating balloon catheter to cross the mitral valve. Crossing of the valve needs simultaneous manipulation of the stylet, which is gently pulled and turned counterclockwise, and of the balloon, which is gently pushed forward. Several attempts could be necessary using different orientations of the tip of the balloon. In cases where the atrium is very large, or if the transseptal puncture is too anterior, the 'Loop technique' may be necessary (Fig. 40.4). If the crossing of the mitral valve is not possible using this technique it

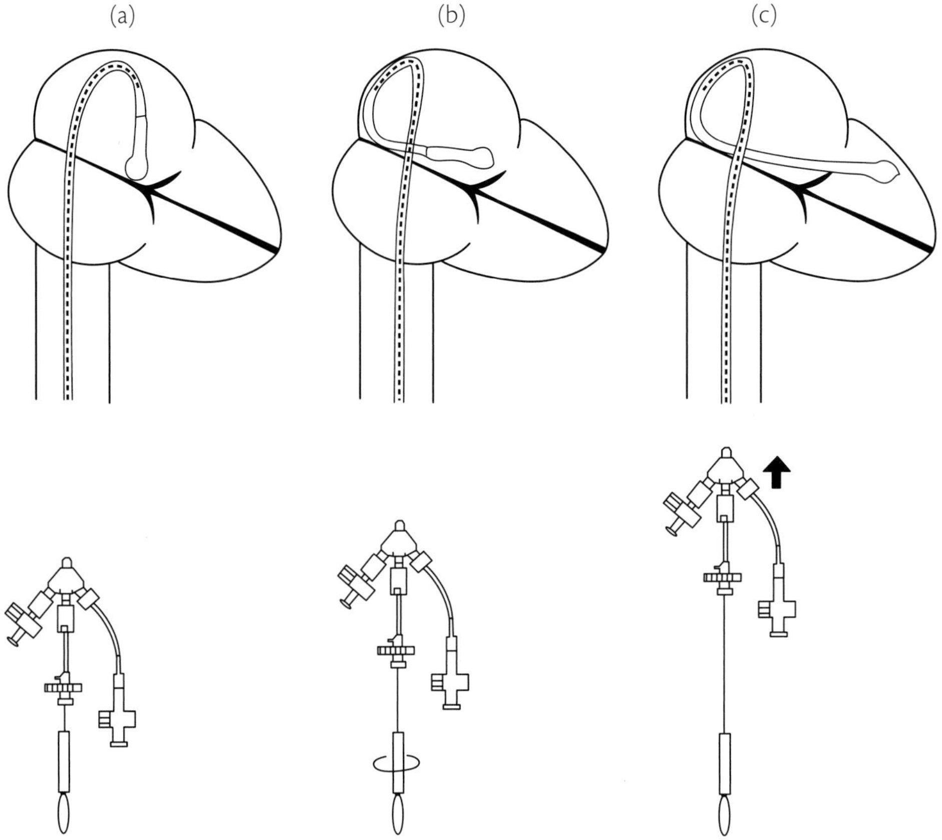

Fig. 40.4 BMV using the Inoue technique Step 3. Crossing of the mitral valve using the loop technique A large loop is created in the distal par of the balloon. The stylet tip is withdrawn to a point at 5cm from the tip of the balloon. The stylet is rotated clockwise. Only the balloon is advanced, which causes the catheter to form a loop in the left atrium and facilitate entry in the left ventricle. After the balloon has crossed the mitral orifice the balloon is withdrawn slowly to break the loop in the catheter in the left atrium and complete the inflation of the balloon.

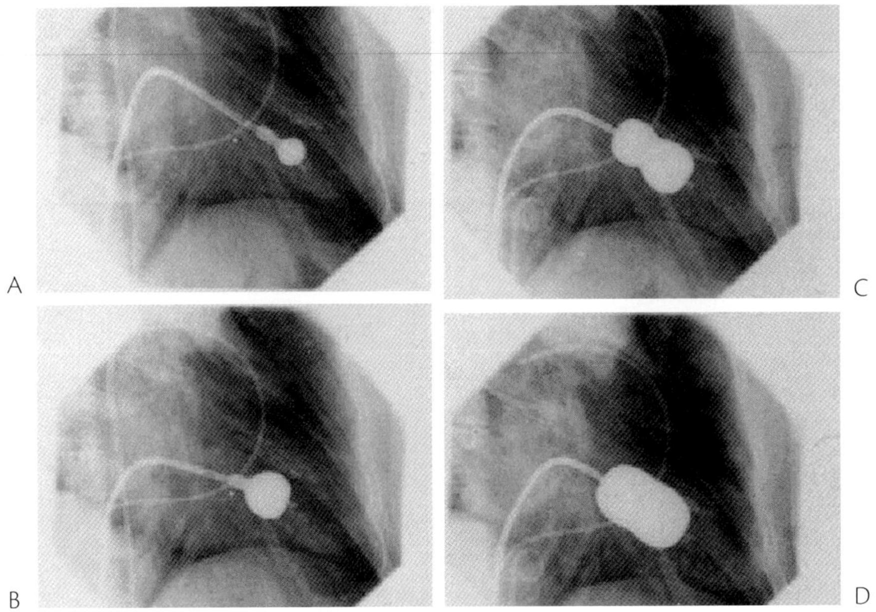

Fig. 40.5 BMV using the Inoue technique. The four sequences of inflation of the Inoue balloon catheter (RAO 30° view). A) Inflation of the distal portion of the balloon, which is thereafter pulled back and anchored at the mitral valve. B) Subsequent inflation of the proximal and middle portions of the balloon. At full inflation, the waist of the balloon in its midportion has disappeared. Reproduced from Topol EJ. *Textbook of Interventional Cardiology*, 5th edn. Philadelphia, PA: W.B. Saunders, 2007 with permission of Elsevier.

may be necessary to redo the transseptal puncture in a slightly higher position and more posteriorly

- When the balloon has crossed the mitral valve and is floating into the ventricular cavity, the distal part is further inflated, and the balloon is pulled back to anchor at the level of the valve. The inflation is pursued, leading to inflation of the proximal and medium part of the balloon. When the balloon has a bone shape, the smaller diameter being at the level of the mitral orifice, full inflation is performed. Then the balloon is rapidly deflated and withdrawn into the LA (Fig. 40.5). The total inflation/deflation time is less than 5s. The stylet is withdrawn and the balloon is flushed.

Heparin, usually 3000–5000IU, is administered after the first balloon inflation, ideally when echocardiographic examination has eliminated the presence of pericardial effusion.

Although echocardiography may be difficult to perform in the catheterization laboratory for logistical reasons, it provides essential information on the course of the mitral opening, which is of utmost importance when using the stepwise Inoue technique, and also enables detection of early complications such as a pericardial haemorrhage or severe mitral regurgitation. The accuracy of measurements of the mean mitral gradient during BMV is low because it is dependent on the loading conditions and cardiac output. It can be helpful in patients in sinus rhythm and stable condition, while it is of little help in those in atrial fibrillation and low output. Therefore, the measurement of valve area using planimetry from two-dimensional (2D) echocardiography appears to be the method of choice when it is technically feasible. Colour Doppler assessment is the method of choice for sequential evaluation of the changes in the degree of regurgitation. Commissural opening can be assessed by 2D echocardiography, or even better using 3D imaging[11] in the short-axis view.

The first inflation is performed 4mm below the maximal balloon size, and the balloon size is increased in steps of 1mm each. If mitral regurgitation has not increased >1/4, and the valve area is less than $1cm^2/m^2$ of body surface area, the balloon is re-advanced across the valve[5] and BMV is repeated with a balloon diameter increased by 1mm (Fig. 40.6).

The following criteria have been proposed for the desired endpoint of the procedure: 1) mitral valve area of more than $1cm^2/m^2$ of body surface area; 2) complete opening of at least one commissure (Fig. 40.7); or

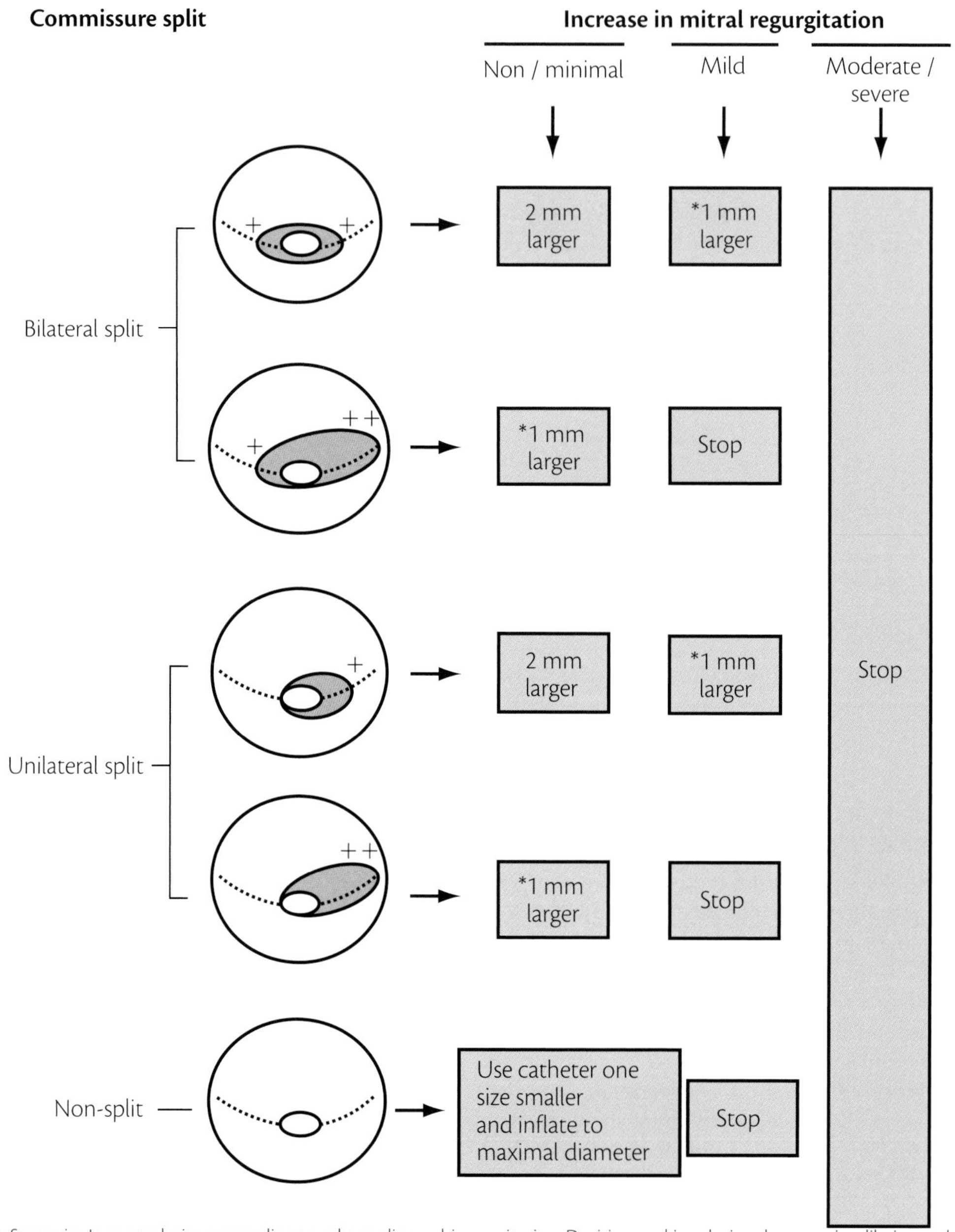

Fig. 40.6 Step-wise Inoue technique according to echocardiographic monitoring. Decision-making during the stepwise dilation technique based on echocardiographic findings after each balloon dilation. +, incomplete split; ++, complete split; *, stop in cases of severely diseased valve or age older than 65 years. Reproduced from Topol EJ. *Textbook of Interventional Cardiology*, 5th edn. Philadelphia, PA: W.B. Saunders, 2007 with permission of Elsevier.

3) appearance or increment of regurgitation of more than 1/4. It is vital that the strategy be tailored to the individual circumstances, taking into account clinical factors together with anatomic factors and the cumulative data of peri-procedural monitoring. For example, balloon size, increments of size, and expected final valve area are smaller in patients where surgery would be at high risk such as the elderly or pregnant women; in the presence of initially tight MS, extensive valve and subvalvular disease, and nodular commissural calcification.

When the results are judged to be satisfactory, the Inoue guide wire and stretching tube are introduced

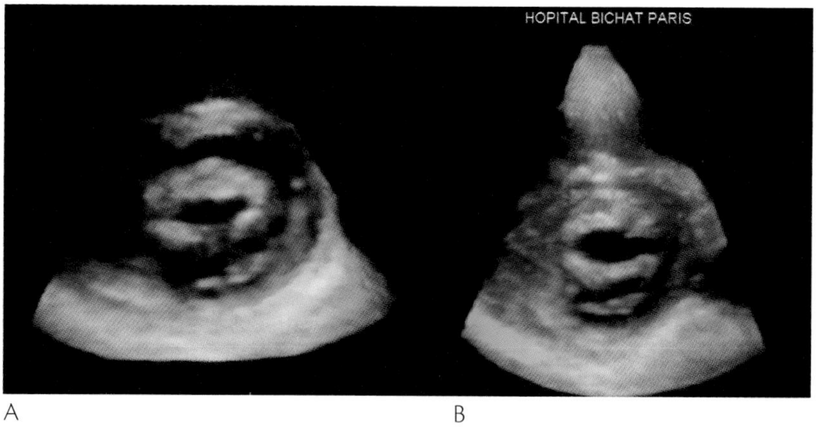

Fig. 40.7 3D echocardiography before and after BMV—short axis view. A) Mitral stenosis with bicommissural fusion before BMV. B) Splitting of both commissures after BMV.

again in AP view. At this time it is crucial to avoid pushing the guide wire into the appendage. Then the balloon is slenderized and pulled back down to the femoral entry site. It is recommended that only the coiled portion of the guide wire remains outside the distal end of the balloon during the pullback.

After the procedure, the most accurate evaluation of valve area is achieved by echocardiography(12). To allow for the slight loss during the first 24h, this should be performed 1–2 days after BMV, when the valve area may be evaluated by planimetry or from the continuity equation method because the half-pressure time is reputed invalid just after BMV because of acute compliance changes. Finally, the degree of regurgitation may be assessed by colour Doppler flow. In current practice, the use of TEE after BMV is limited to patients with severe mitral regurgitation to evaluate the mechanisms or, in case of doubt, the degree of post procedural mitral regurgitation.

Even though the considerable simplification resulting from the use of the Inoue balloon may lead to a false sense of security when applying the technique, BMV clearly should be restricted to teams that have extensive experience with transseptal catheterization and are able to perform an adequate number of procedures(13). The interventionists who perform BMV must also be able to perform emergency pericardiocentesis.

Immediate results

Haemodynamics

BMV usually provides more than a 100% increase in valve area with a final valve area around 1.7–2cm^2(13–16). This improvement in valve function results in an immediate decrease in left atrial pressure and a slight increase in cardiac index. A gradual decrease in pulmonary arterial pressure and pulmonary vascular resistance is observed.

BMV has a beneficial effect on exercise capacity. In addition, studies have shown that this technique improves left atrial and left atrial appendage pump function.

Failures

The failure rates range from 1–17%(2,3,15–17). Failure is often due to an inability to puncture the atrial septum or position the balloon correctly across the valve. Most failures occur early in the investigator's experience. Failures can also be due to unfavourable anatomy, such as severe atrial or predominant subvalvular stenosis.

Complications

Large series(13–18) enable assessment of the risks of the technique.

Haemopericardium may be related to transseptal catheterization or to left ventricular perforation by the guide wires or balloons. Its incidence varies from 0.5–12%. Haemopericardium usually has immediate clinical consequences resulting in tamponade and should always be suspected when hypotension occurs during BMV. Haemopericardium related to the transseptal puncture mostly occurs when the operator is less experienced. Unfavourable patient characteristics such as severe atrial enlargement or severe thoracic deformity also increase risk. With the Inoue technique the risk of left ventricular perforation by the balloon is virtually eliminated. If haemopericardium is suspected, echocardiography should be performed urgently before deterioration occurs. This stresses the importance of the immediate availability of echocardiography when performing BMV. Haemopericardium requires immediate pericardiocentesis, ideally performed under echocardiographic guidance after reversal of anticoagulation.

If this is successful, BMV can be re-attempted and the patient should be closely monitored. In most cases haemopericardium due to transseptal catheterization can be managed by pericardiocentesis, especially when it results from only an incorrect puncture by the transseptal needle. To minimize the incidence of this, complication training is of course crucial. In addition, BMV should not be performed in patients with bleeding disorders, in particular those with too high anticoagulation. Transseptal catheterization should not be performed if the INR is >1.2. In patients receiving intravenous heparin it should be discontinued 4h before the procedure and can be restarted 2h after. Vitamin K should not be given before the procedure in patients who are at high risk for left atrial thrombosis, and BMV should be delayed until a satisfactory level of coagulability is reached. To further increase safety the absence of haemopericardium could be verified using echocardiography before administrating heparin.

Embolism may be due to a thrombus that was pre-existing, mostly in the left atrial appendage, or which developed during the procedure due to air leaking from the balloon. Very rarely, it may be due to calcium. Embolism is encountered in 0.5–5% of cases. Cerebral embolism usually results in a stroke. Coronary embolism leads to transient ST segment elevation in inferior leads, which is well tolerated when it is due to microbubbles of air that can occur when using the Inoue balloon and which will resolve spontaneously. The treatment of cerebral embolism should be in collaboration with a stroke centre. Cerebral imaging should be performed on an emergency basis to rule out haemorrhage, and intra-arterial fibrinolytic therapy should be administered early in the absence of contraindication. In the case of persistent ST segment elevation, coronary angiography should be performed. If a coronary occlusion is present, coronary angioplasty can be performed, while thrombo-aspiration could be an attractive alternative. Although the incidence of embolism is low, its potential consequences are severe, and all possible precautions should be taken to prevent it. In particular, transoesophageal echocardiography should be performed a few days prior to intervention to rule out the presence of intra atrial thrombosis. The occurrence of air embolism may be decreased by careful venting of the Inoue balloon before use and finally repeated inflations in saline water to flush the last bubbles of air.

Severe mitral regurgitation is rare but represents an ever-present risk. Surgical findings[18] have shown that it is most often related to non-commissural leaflet tearing, which could be associated with chordal rupture. In these cases, one or both commissures are often too tightly fused to be split. Severe mitral regurgitation may also be due to excessive commissural splitting, or in very rare cases, rupture of a papillary muscle. The frequency of severe mitral regurgitation ranges from 2–19%. As mitral regurgitation is usually initially well tolerated, surgery can be performed on a scheduled basis. The precise timing of intervention should be based on functional tolerance and surgical risk. Subsequent surgical treatment is usually necessary because the prognosis of patients with severe mitral regurgitation is usually poor, with secondary objective deterioration and a lack of symptom alleviation. In most cases, valve replacement is required because of the severity of the underlying valve disease. Conservative surgery has been successfully performed in cases of less severe valve deformity. The majority of cases of severe mitral regurgitation occur in patients with unfavourable anatomy. However, the occurrence of severe mitral regurgitation remains largely unpredictable for a given patient and its development depends more on the distribution of morphologic changes than on their severity. The available data suggests, but does not prove, that the stepwise Inoue technique combined with echocardiographic monitoring is likely to decrease the incidence of severe regurgitation, even if it does not eliminate it.

Although urgent surgery (within 24h) is seldom needed for complications (<1%), it may be required for massive haemopericardium resulting from left ventricular perforation intractable to treatment by pericardiocentesis. According to circumstances, this could be drainage of the pericardial effusion alone or could also include valve surgery. Less frequently, severe mitral regurgitation, leading to haemodynamic collapse or refractory pulmonary oedema may necessitate emergency surgery with the support of an intra-aortic balloon pump en route to the operating room. The exact arrangement for surgical backup varies from institution to institution, according to the severity of the condition being treated and the experience of the cardiologic and surgical teams.

The main causes of death are massive haemopericardium or the poor condition of the patient. The latter is often a factor in end-stage patients, such as elderly patients where BMV is attempted as a palliative procedure or in emergency cases where it is performed in patients in pulmonary oedema or, very occasionally, in cardiogenic shock. The fatality rate ranges from 0–3%. The decrease in fatality is related to the experience of the team in BMV, the availability of rescue surgery, and also to the selection of the patients.

The clinical importance of interatrial shunting was largely overemphasized in the early days of BMV. These shunts are usually small and without consequence since most of them will disappear on follow-up after successful BMV due to a reduced interatrial pressure gradient. In rare circumstances, right-to-left shunts may occur in patients with severe pulmonary hypertension when BMV is not successful and this may lead to hypoxemia. The frequency of interatrial shunts varies from 10–90% depending on the technique used for detection. Surgery has been very seldom necessary because of inter atrial shunting. On the other hand, if surgery is needed for unsuccessful BMV or restenosis, the interatrial septum should be looked at and septal tears sutured at the time of surgery. To our knowledge, no cases of percutaneous closure of such defects have been reported, and such a procedure is unlikely to be successful because the interatrial shunts are not due to defects similar to patent foramen ovale or congenital atrial septal defects but to longitudinal tears. The use of the Inoue technique has significantly decreased the incidence of this complication in comparison with other techniques. To further decrease the magnitude of the problem it is necessary to fully slenderize the Inoue balloon before withdrawal and also to pull the guide wire, leaving only the soft part of it exteriorized when withdrawing the balloon across the interatrial septum in order to avoid an 'effect', which may occur if the stiff part of the guide wire is out of the tip of the balloon during the manoeuvre.

Atrial fibrillation rarely occurs during the procedure. When it does, it is usually transient and resolves within a few hours under medical treatment. In rare cases, it requires electric countershock a few days after.

The incidence of transient, complete heart block is rare (<1%) and exceptionally requires the implantation of a permanent pacemaker.

Vascular complications are the exception when using the antegrade or transvenous approach. In teams experienced in transseptal catheterization, left heart catheterization may be avoided to simplify the procedure and further reduce the incidence of vascular complication as well as shortening the duration of hospital stay.

Endocarditis is extremely rare and does not justify prophylaxis before the procedure. The risk is higher when balloons are reused, which occurs in many centres in developing countries. The same holds to be true for transmissible infections such as hepatitis or AIDS.

Predictors of immediate results

Evaluation of immediate results is mainly based on haemodynamic criteria. The definition of good immediate results varies from series to series. The definition usually employed is a final valve area larger than 1.5cm^2 without mitral regurgitation greater than 2/4.

It is now agreed that the prediction of results is multifactorial[14,19–21]. In addition to morphological factors, preoperative variables such as age, history of surgical commissurotomy, functional class, small mitral valve area, presence of mitral regurgitation before valvuloplasty, sinus rhythm, pulmonary artery pressure, presence of severe tricuspid regurgitation, and procedural factors such as balloon size are all independent predictors of the immediate results. The identification of these variables has enabled predictive models to be developed with a high sensitivity of prediction. Nevertheless, the specificity is low, indicating insufficient prediction of poor immediate results. This low specificity is particularly true in regard to the lack of accurate prediction of severe mitral regurgitation.

Mid-term results

We are now able to analyse follow-up data up to 17 years[21–26].

In clinical terms, which are the most widely used, the overall mid-term results of valvuloplasty are satisfactory. Prediction of long-term results is also multifactorial, based on clinical variables such as age; valve anatomy as assessed by echocardiography scores, factors related to the evolutive stage of the disease, (i.e. higher New York Heart Association [NYHA] class before valvuloplasty); history of previous commissurotomy; severe tricuspid regurgitation; cardiomegaly; atrial fibrillation; high pulmonary vascular resistance; and the results of the procedure. The identification of these predictors provides important information for patient selection and is relevant to follow-up: Patients who have good immediate results but who are at high risk of further events must be carefully followed-up to detect deterioration and to allow timely intervention. Awareness of these predictors explains the discrepancies in the follow-up results from reports that included patients with different characteristics: late results are clearly less satisfactory in North American or European series (event-free survival: 33–56% after 10–12 years[21,24]) where patients are older and frequently have severe valve deformities, than in studies from developing countries, where the patients studied have more favourable characteristics, and up to 77% event-free survival after 17 years[22].

If BMV is initially successful, survival rates are excellent, the need for secondary surgery is infrequent, and functional improvement occurs in most cases. Ultrasound techniques are ideally suited for serially assessing the results of the procedure, whereas serial haemodynamic data is more difficult to obtain and less satisfactory because of overestimation of the valve area immediately after the procedure. With 2D echocardiography or the Doppler technique, the improvement in valve function is stable in most cases.

Restenosis following BMV has generally been defined by a loss of more than 50% of the initial gain with a valve area less than 1.5cm^2. After successful BMV, the incidence of restenosis is usually low, between 2–40%, at time intervals ranging from 3–10 years. Age, mitral valve area after BMV, and anatomy are considered predictors of restenosis, but it must be stressed that the small number of series reporting patients with restenosis and the limited duration of follow-up preclude any definite conclusion in this regard[25].

The possibility of repeating valvuloplasty in cases of recurrent mitral stenosis is one of the potentials of this non-surgical procedure. Repeated valvuloplasty can be proposed if recurrent stenosis leads to symptoms, occurs several years after an initially successful procedure, and the predominant mechanism of restenosis is commissural refusion. At the moment, despite the fact that repeat BMV represents 10–30% of the total number of BMV only a few series are available on revalvuloplasty[27,28]. They report good immediate and mid-term outcomes in patients with favourable characteristics. Although the results are less favourable in patients presenting with worse characteristics, repeat valvuloplasty has a palliative role if the patients are not surgical candidates.

When the immediate results are unsatisfactory, mid-term functional results are usually poor. The prognosis of patients with severe mitral regurgitation after surgical commissurotomy or BMV is usually poor, with a lack of symptom alleviation and secondary objective deterioration. Surgical treatment is usually necessary during the following months.

In cases of an insufficient initial opening, delayed surgery is usually performed when the extra-cardiac condition allows it. Here, valve replacement is necessary in almost all cases because of the unfavourable valve anatomy responsible for the poor initial results.

Follow-up studies using sequential echocardiography have shown that despite numerous individual variations, the degree of mitral regurgitation on the whole remains stable, or slightly decreases during follow-up. Atrial septal defects are likely to close later in most cases because of a reduced interatrial pressure gradient. The persistence of shunts is related to their magnitude or to unsatisfactory relief of the valve obstruction.

The low incidence of embolism during follow-up, the progressive decrease in intensity or disappearance of spontaneous echocardiographic contrast, and the improved left atrial function after BMV suggest a beneficial effect of the procedure on left atrial blood stasis, from which a lower risk of thromboembolism may be expected[29]. Finally, there is no direct evidence that BMV reduces the incidence of atrial fibrillation, even if it has a favourable influence on the predictors of atrial fibrillation (e.g. atrial size or degree of obstruction), which seems to indicate that this is indeed the case[30].

Selection of patients

The selection of candidates for BMV should follow the following steps:

1. Assessment of the severity

Intervention should be performed only in patients with significant MS, i.e. valve area<1.5cm^2. In patients with only mild mitral stenosis (valve area >1.5cm^2) the risks of BMV probably outweigh the benefits, and these patients can usually be well managed by medical treatment.

BMV can occasionally be performed in patients with a slightly larger valve area who have a large body surface area and an objective functional limitation.

2. Exclusion of contraindications

Contraindications to transseptal catheterization, and therefore to BMV, include suspected left atrial thrombosis, severe hemorrhagic disorder, and severe cardiothoracic deformity.

The current guidelines consider a thrombus localized in the LA as a contraindication[31]. This recommendation is self-evident if the thrombus is free-floating or is situated in the left atrial cavity. This also applies when it is located on the interatrial septum. When the thrombus is located in the left atrial appendage, and if the patient is clinically stable, anticoagulant therapy can be given for 2–6 months[32], and BMV can be attempted if a new transoesophageal examination shows that the thrombus has disappeared.

Other contraindications for BMV include more than mild mitral regurgitation, severe calcification, absence of commissural fusion, combined severe aortic valve disease, and severe tricuspid stenosis and regurgitation, or coronary disease requiring bypass surgery.

On the other hand, coexisting moderate aortic valve disease and functional tricuspid regurgitation are not considered as contraindications for the technique.

3. Assessment of the feasibility of BMV

Echocardiographic assessment allows the classification of patients into anatomic groups with a view to predicting the results. Most investigators use the Wilkins score[19] (Table 40.1), whereas others[14] use a more general assessment of valve anatomy (Table 40.2). Controversy exists regarding the most effective echocardiography

Table 40.1 Anatomic classification of the mitral valve (Massachusetts General Hospital, Boston)

Leaflet mobility
Highly mobile valve with restriction of only the leaflet tips
Mid-portion and base of leaflets have reduced mobility
Valve leaflets move forward during diastole mainly at the base
No or minimal forward movement of the leaflets during diastole
Valvular thickening
Leaflets near normal (4–5mm)
Mid-leaflet thickening, marked thickening of the margins
Thickening extends through the entire leaflets (5–8mm)
Marked thickening of all leaflet tissue (>8–10mm)
Subvalvular thickening
Minimal thickening of chordal structures just below the valve
Thickening of chordae extending up to one-third of chordal length
Thickening extending to the distal third of the chordae
Extensive thickening and shortening of all chordae extending down to the papillary muscle
Valvular calcification
Single area of increased echocardiographic brightness
Scattered areas of brightness confined to leaflet margins
Brightness extending into the mid-portion of leaflets
Extensive brightness through most of the leaflet tissue

Adapted from Abascal V, Wilkins GT, O'Shea JP, *et al* Prediction of successful outcome in 130 patients undergoing percutaneous balloon mitral valvotomy. *Circulation* 1990; **82**:448–56.

scoring system in the prediction of results of mitral valvuloplasty. In fact, none of the scores available today have been shown to be superior to the others; and all echocardiographic classifications have the same limitations: 1) reproducibility is difficult, as the scores are only semi-quantitative; 2) lesions may be underestimated, especially with regards to the assessment of subvalvular disease; and 3) the use of scores describing the degree of overall valve deformity may not identify localized changes in specific portions of the valve apparatus (leaflets, commissures), which may increase the risk of severe mitral regurgitation. Therefore, we can only recommend the use of the system with which one is most familiar and at ease. More recently, scores that take into account the uneven distribution of the anatomic deformities of the leaflets or the commissural area have been developed. The preliminary results of these scores are promising but disputed, so further studies are needed to determine their exact value[33].

Table 40.2 Anatomic classification of the mitral valve (Bichat Hospital, Paris)

Echocardiographic group	Mitral valve anatomy
1	Pliable non-calcified anterior mitral leaflet and mild subvalvular disease (i.e. thin chordae ≥10mm long)
2	Pliable non-calcified anterior mitral leaflet and severe subvalvular disease (i.e. thickened chordae <10mm long)
3	Calcification of mitral valve of any extent, as assessed by fluoroscopy, whatever the state of subvalvular apparatus

Adapted from Iung B, Cormier B, Ducimetiere P, *et al.* Immediate results of percutaneous mitral commissurotomy. *Circulation* 1996; **94**:2124–30.

4. Evaluation of the functional status and extra cardiac condition

Usually, symptoms appear gradually over years and patients frequently adapt their level of functional capacity and deny dyspnoea despite objective effort limitation. Bicycle ergometry may provide a useful objective assessment of functional capacity in patients whose symptoms are equivocal. Exercise echocardiography may also be used to assess the evolution of mitral gradient and pulmonary pressure in patients with doubtful symptoms. However, the added value for decision making has to be further defined.

In symptomatic patients (Fig. 40.8)

BMV is the procedure of choice for patients at high risk or when surgery is contraindicated, or in patients with favourable characteristics. As regards high-risk patients, preliminary series have suggested that BMV can be performed safely and effectively in patients with severe pulmonary hypertension[34].

In Western countries, many patients with MS have concomitant non-cardiac disease, which may also increase the risk of surgery[1]. In elderly patients, BMV results in moderate but significant improvement in valve function at an acceptable risk, although subsequent functional deterioration is frequent[35,36]. Therefore, BMV is a valid, if only palliative, treatment for these patients, in particular when the alternative of surgery carries a high risk because of age, comorbidities, and the evolutive stage of the disease.

BMV can be performed as a life-saving procedure in critically ill patients[37], as the sole treatment when there is an absolute contraindication to surgery, or as a 'bridge' to surgery in other cases. In this context dramatic

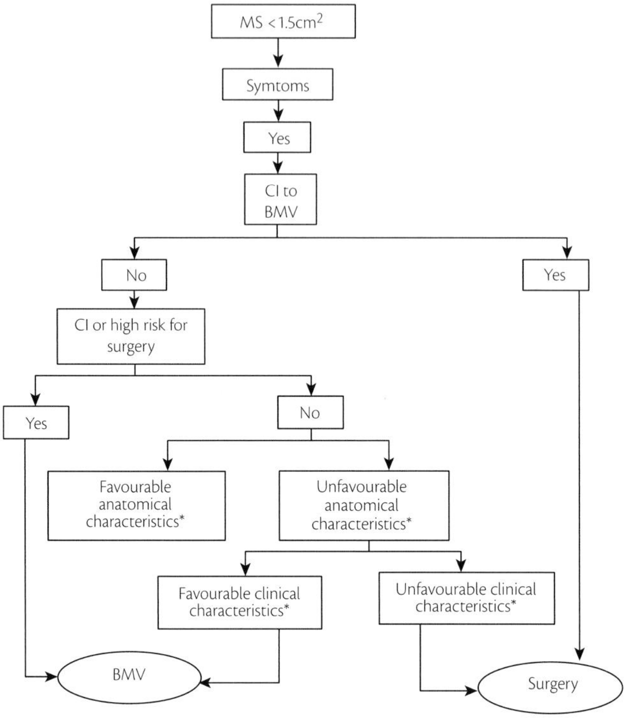

Fig. 40.8 Management of severe symptomatic mitral stenosis (adapted from ESC Guidelines). BMV, balloon mitral valvuloplasty; CI, contraindication; MS, mitral stenosis. *Favourable characteristics for BMV can be defined by the absence of several of the following:
- Clinical characteristics: old age, history of commissurotomy, NYHA class IV, atrial fibrillation, severe pulmonary hypertension
- Anatomical characteristics: echo score>8, Cormier score 3 (calcification of mitral valve of any extent, as assessed by fluoroscopy), very small mitral valve area, severe tricuspid regurgitation.

improvement has been observed in young patients, but the outcome is very bad in elderly patients presenting with 'end-stage' disease who would probably be better treated conservatively.

BMV appears to be the procedure of choice in young adults with good anatomy—that is, pliable valves and only moderate subvalvular disease. Several studies have compared surgical commissurotomy with BMV, mostly in patients with favourable characteristics. They consistently showed that valvuloplasty is at least comparable to surgical commissurotomy as regards short- and mid-term follow-up up to 7 years[38]. In addition, if restenosis occurs, patients treated by valvuloplasty could undergo repeat balloon catheterization or surgery without the difficulties and inherent risks resulting from pericardial adhesions and chest wall scarring[39].

In practice, in Europe BMV has virtually replaced surgical commissurotomy[1].

Much remains to be done to define the indications for patients with unfavourable anatomy, who are more common in Western countries. For this group, some advocate immediate surgery because of the less satisfying results of valvuloplasty, whereas others prefer BMV as an initial treatment for selected candidates, reserving the use of surgery for cases of failure or late deterioration[40,41]. Unfortunately, no randomized studies are available for these patients, and a comparison of the results of BMV with those of surgical series is difficult because of differences in the patients involved and the fact that the surgical alternative is usually valve replacement, since open commissurotomy is now very seldom performed, in particular in such cases. Valve replacement has its drawbacks: operative mortality, particularly in the elderly, and prosthesis-related complications whose cumulative incidence worsens the outcome, particularly in young patients who are most exposed to the risk of long-term deterioration. The indications in this subgroup of patients must take into account its heterogeneity with respect to anatomy and clinical status. In this group of patients, an individualistic approach allows for the multifactorial nature of prediction. Current opinion is that surgery can be considered the treatment of choice in patients with bicommissural or heavy calcification. On the other hand, BMV can be attempted as a first approach in patients with extensive lesions of the subvalvular apparatus or moderate or unicommissural calcification, even more so if the clinical status argues in favour of it. Surgery should be considered reasonably early if the results are unsatisfactory or if there is secondary deterioration.

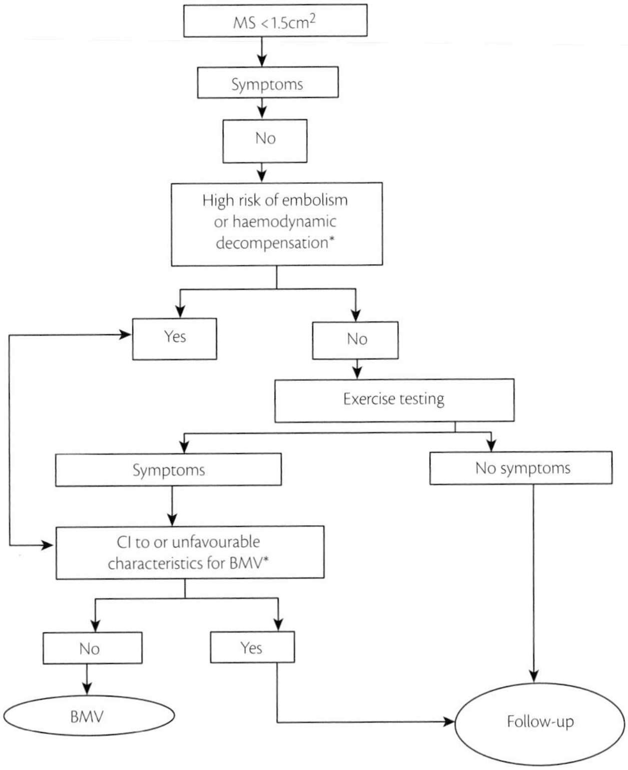

Fig. 40.9 Management of severe asymptomatic mitral stenosis (adapted from ESC Guidelines). BMV, balloon mitral valvuloplasty; CI, contraindication; MS, mitral stenosis. *Favourable characteristics for BMV can be defined by the absence of several of the following:
- Clinical characteristics: old age, history of commissurotomy, NYHA class IV, atrial fibrillation, severe pulmonary hypertension:
- Anatomical characteristics: echo score >8, Cormier score 3 (calcification of mitral valve of any extent, as assessed by fluoroscopy), very small mitral valve area, severe tricuspid regurgitation.

In asymptomatic patients (Fig. 40.9)

In these patients the alternatives are medical treatment or BMV. Because of the small but definite risk inherent in BMV, truly asymptomatic patients are not usually candidates for the procedure, except in the following cases: increased risk of thromboembolism (previous history of embolism, dense spontaneous contrast in the LA, or, to a lesser extent, recent or paroxysmal atrial fibrillation); risk of haemodynamic decompensation (systolic pulmonary pressure >50mmHg at rest; need for major extra-cardiac surgery; or finally, to allow pregnancy. In these cases, BMV should be performed in patients with favourable characteristics and by experienced operators.

Applications of balloon mitral commissurotomy in special patient groups

After surgical commissurotomy

This category of patients is of interest because recurrent MS is becoming more frequent than primary MS in Western countries, and because reoperation in this context is associated with a higher risk of morbidity and mortality, requiring valve replacement in most cases[42]. BMV is feasible in this setting and significantly improves valve function. On the whole, the results are good, even if slightly less satisfactory than those obtained in patients without previous commissurotomy. This can probably be attributed to less favourable characteristics observed in patients previously subjected to operation. These encouraging preliminary data suggest that BMV may well postpone reoperation in selected patients with restenosis after commissurotomy. The indications for BMC in this subgroup of patients are similar to those for 'primary BMV', but echocardiographic examination must exclude any patients in whom restenosis is mainly due to valve rigidity without significant commissural refusion. The latter mechanism is often responsible for the exceptional cases of MS that develop in patients who have undergone mitral ring annuloplasty for the correction of mitral regurgitation.

During pregnancy

During pregnancy, surgery carries a substantial risk of fetal mortality and morbidity, especially if extra-corporeal circulation is required. The experience reported in the literature on BMV during pregnancy is limited to a few hundred patients, but suggests the following: from a technical point of view, during the last weeks of pregnancy (>20 weeks), which was when BMV was performed in most cases, the procedure may be more difficult because of the enlarged uterus. All measures should be taken to shorten the procedure. Contrast injection should be avoided to avoid the risk of hypothyroidy for the fetus. The aim should be to allow for a safe delivery, which is usually possible if valve area is over 1.5cm^2, and one should not excessively increase balloon size at the risk of creating severe mitral regurgitation with its inherent risks. The procedure is effective and results in normal delivery in most cases. As regards radiation exposure, BMV is safe for the fetus, provided that protection is given using a shield that completely surrounds the patient's abdomen and that the procedure is performed after the 20th week. Preliminary series have shown satisfactory development in the infants over 5–10 years follow-up[(43)]. Nevertheless, one must bear in mind that, in addition to radiation, BMV carries the potential risk of complications that require urgent surgery. These data suggest that BMV can be a useful technique in the treatment of pregnant patients with MS and refractory heart failure despite medical treatment.

Conclusions

Due to the good results that have been obtained with BMV, it now has an important role in the treatment of mitral stenosis, and has virtually replaced surgical commissurotomy. Finally, when treating mitral stenosis, BMV and valve replacement must be considered not as rivals but as complementary techniques, each applicable at the appropriate stage of the disease.

References

1. Iung B, Baron G, Butchart EG, *et al.* A prospective survey of patients with valvular heart disease in Europe: the Euro Heart Survey on valvular heart disease. *Eur Heart J*, 2003; **13**:1231–43.
2. Inoue K, Owaki T, Nakamura T, *et al.* (Clinical application of transvenous mitral commissurotomy by a new balloon catheter. *J Thorac Cardiovasc Surg* 1984; **87**:394–402.
3. Marijon E, Iung B, Mocumbi, *et al.* What are the differences in presentation of candidates for percutaneous mitral commissurotomy across the world and do they influence the results of the procedure? *Arch Cardiovasc Dis* 2008; **101**(10):611–17.
4. Hickey MS, Blackstone EH, Kirklin JW, *et al.* Outcome probabilities and life history after surgical mitral commissurotomy: implications for balloon commissurotomy. *J Am Coll Cardiol* 1991; **17**:29–42.
5. Stefanadis C, Stratos C, Lambrou S, *et al.* Retrograde nontransseptal balloon mitral valvuloplasty: immediate results and intermediate long-term outcome in 441 cases-a multi-centre experience. *J Am Coll Cardiol* 1998; **32**:1009–16.
6. Babaliaros VC, Green JT, Lerakis S, *et al.* Emerming applications for transseptal left heart catheterization. *J Am Coll Cardiol* 2008; **22**:2116–22.
7. Joseph G, Chandy S, George P, *et al.* Evaluation of a simplified transseptal mitral valvuloplasty technique using over-the-wire single balloons and complementary femoral and jugular venous approaches in 1,407 consecutive patients. *J Invasive Cardiol* 2005; **17**:132–8.
8. Park SH, Kim MA, Hyon MS. The advantages of on-line transesophageal echocardiography guide during percutaneous balloon mitral valvuloplasty. *J Am Soc Echocardiogr* 2000; **13**:26–34.
9. Liang KW, Fu YC, Lee WL, *et al.* Intra-cardiac echocardiography guided trans-septal puncture in patients with dilated left atrium undergoing percutaneous transvenous mitral commissurotomy. *Int J Cardiol* 2007; **117**:418–21.
10. Vahanian A, Cormier B, Iung B. Percutaneous transvenous mitral commissurotomy using the Inoue balloon: international experience. *Cathet Cardiovasc Diagn* 1994; **2**:8–15.
11. Messika-Zeitoun D, Brochet E, Holmin C, *et al.* Three-dimensional evaluation of the mitral valve area and commissural opening before and after percutaneous mitral commissurotomy in patients with mitral stenosis. *Eur Heart J* 2007; **28**:72
12. Palacios I. What is the gold standard to measure mitral valve area post mitral balloon valvuloplasty ? *Cathet Cardiovasc Diagn* 1994; **33**:315–16.
13. Iung B, Nicoud-Houel A, Fondard O, *et al.* Temporal trends in percutaneous mitral commissurotomy over a 15-year period. *Eur Heart J* 2004; **25**:702–8.
14. Iung B, Cormier B, Ducimetiere P, *et al.* Immediate results of percutaneous mitral commissurotomy. *Circulation* 1996; **94**:2124–30.
15. Chen CR, Cheng TO. Percutaneous balloon mitral valvuloplasty by the Inoue technique: a multicenter study of 4832 patients in China. *Am Heart J* 1995; **129**:1197–202.
16. Arora R, Kalra GS, Singh S, *et al.* Percutaneous transvenous mitral commissurotomy: immediate and long-term follow-up results. *Cathet Cardiovasc Interv* 2002; **55**:450–6.
17. Harrison KJ, Wilson JS, Hearne SE, *et al.* Complications related to percutaneous transvenous mitral commissurotomy. *Cathet Cardiovasc Diagn* 1994; **2**: 52–60.
18. Varma PK, Theodore S, Neema PK, *et al.* Emergency surgery after percutaneous transmitral commissurotomy: operative versus echocardiographic findings, mechanisms of complications, and outcomes. *J Thorac Cardiovasc* Surg 2005; **130**:772–6.

19. Abascal V, Wilkins GT, O'Shea JP, *et al.* Prediction of successful outcome in 130 patients undergoing percutaneous balloon mitral valvotomy. *Circulation* 1990; **82**:448–56.
20. Hernandez R, Macaya C, Benuelos C, *et al.* Predictors, mechanisms and outcome of severe mitral regurgitation complicating percutaneous mitral valvotomy with the Inoue balloon. *Am J Cardiol* 1993; **70**:1169–74.
21. Palacios IF, Sanchez PL, Harrell LC, *et al.* Which patients benefit from percutaneous mitral balloon valvuloplasty? Pre-valvuloplasty and post-valvuloplasty variables that predict long-term outcome. *Circulation* 2002; **105**:1465–71.
22. Fawzy ME, Shoukri M, Al Buraiki J, *et al.* Seventeen years' clinical and echocardiographic follow up of mitral balloon valvuloplasty in 520 patients, and predictors of long-term outcome. *J Heart Valve Dis* 2007; **16**:454–60.
23. Kang DH, Park SW, Song JK, *et al.* Long-term clinical and echocardiographic outcome of percutaneous mitral valvuloplasty: randomized comparison of Inoue and double-balloon techniques. *J Am Coll Cardiol* 2000; **35**:169–75.
24. Iung B, Garbarz E, Michaud P, *et al.* Late results of percutaneous mitral commissurotomy in a series of 1024 patients: analysis of late clinical deterioration: frequency, anatomic findings, and predictive factors. *Circulation* 1999; **99**:3272–8.
25. Wang A, Krasuski RA, Warner JJ, *et al.* Serial echocardiographic evaluation of restenosis after successful percutaneous mitral commissurotomy. *J Am Coll Cardiol* 2002; **39**:328–34.
26. Langerveld J, Thijs Plokker HW, Ernst SMPG, *et al.* Predictors of clinical events or restenosis during follow-up after percutaneous mitral balloon valvotomy. *Eur Heart J* 1999; **20**:519–26.
27. Iung B, Garbarz E, Michaud P, *et al.* Immediate and mid-term results of repeat percutaneous mitral commissurotomy for restenosis following earlier percutaneous mitral commissurotomy. *Eur Heart J* 2000; **21**:1683–90.
28. Fawzy ME, Hassan W, Shoukri M, *et al.* Immediate and long-term results of mitral balloon valvotomy for restenosis following previous surgical or balloon mitral commissurotomy. *Am J Cardiol* 2005; **96**:971–5.
29. Chiang CW, Lo SK, Ko YS, *et al.* Predictors of systemic embolism in patients with mitral stenosis. A prospective study. *Ann Intern Med* 1998; **128**:885–9.
30. Langerveld J, Van Hemel NM, Kelder JC, *et al.* Long-term follow-up of cardiac rhythm after percutaneous mitral balloon valvotomy. Does atrial fibrillation persist? *Eurospace* 2003; **5**:47–53.
31. Vahanian A, Baumgartner H, Bax J, *et al.* Guidelines on the management of valvular heart disease. *Eur Heart J* 2007; **28**:230–68.
32. Silaruks S, Thinkhamrop B, Kiatchoosakun S, *et al.* Resolution of left atrial thrombus after 6 months of anticoagulation in candidates for percutaneous transvenous mitral commissurotomy. *Ann Intern Med* 2004; **140**:101–5.
33. Padial LR, Abascal VM, Moreno PR, *et al.* Echocardiography can predict the development of severe mitral regurgitation after percutaneous mitral valvulotomy by the Inoue technique. *Am J Cardiol* 1999; **83**:1210–13.
34. Maoqin S, Guoxiang H, Zhiyuan S, *et al.* The clinical and hemodynamic results of mitral balloon valvuloplasty for patients with mitral stenosis complicated by severe pulmonary hypertension. *Eur J Intern Med* 2005; **16**:413–18.
35. Sutaria N, Elder AT, Shaw TRD. Long term outcome of percutaneous mitral balloon valvotomy in patients aged 70 and over. *Heart* 2000; **83**:433–8.
36. Iung B, Cormier B, Farah B, *et al.* Percutaneous mitral commissurotomy in the elderly. *Eur Heart J* 1995; **16**:1092–9.
37. Vahanian A, Iung B, Nallet O. Percutaneous valvuloplasty in cardiogenic shock. In Hasdai D, Berger P, Battler A, et al. (eds) *Cardiogenic Shock: Diagnosis and Treatment*, pp.181–93. Hew Jersey, Humana Press Inc, 2002
38. Ben Fahrat M, Ayari M, Maatouk F. Percutaneous balloon versus surgical closed and open mitral commissurotomy: seven-year follow-up results of a randomized trial. *Circulation* 1998; **97**:245–50.
39. Gamra H, Betbout F, Ben Hamda K, *et al.* Balloon mitral commissurotomy in juvenile rheumatic mitral stenosis: a ten-year clinical and echocardiographic actuarial results. *Eur Heart J* 2003; **24**:1349–56.
40. Hildick-Smith DJR, Taylor GJ, *et al.* Inoue balloon mitral valvuloplasty: long-term clinical and echocardiographic follow-up of a predominantly unfavorable population. *Eur Heart J* 2000; **21**:1691–8.
41. Iung B, Garbarz E, Doutrelant L, *et al.* Late results of percutaneous mitral commissurotomy for calcific mitral stenosis. *Am J Cardiol* 2000; **85**:1308–14.
42. Iung B, Garbarz E, Michaud P, *et al.* Percutaneous mitral commissurotomy for restenosis after surgical commissurotomy: late efficacy and implications for patient selection. *J Am Coll Cardiol* 2000; **35**:1295–2.
43. Sivadasanpillai H, Srinivasan A, Sivasubramoniam S, *et al.* Long-term outcome of patients undergoing balloon mitral valvotomy in pregnancy. *Am J Cardiol* 2005: **95**:1504–6.

CHAPTER 41

Alcohol septal ablation for obstructive hypertrophic cardiomyopathy

Charles Knight and Saidi A. Mohiddin

Introduction

Hypertrophic cardiomyopathy (HCM) is a genetic disease occurring in approximately one in 500–1000 of the general population[1,2]. HCM is often undiagnosed or misdiagnosed, and asymptomatic cases are often unrecognized. Asymmetric left ventricular (LV) hypertrophy (LVH) most often develops during the period of rapid body growth of adolescence, but it may be present in childhood or, rarely, before birth. Progressive LVH after age 20 is uncommon, but initial diagnosis even in old age is not. The hypertrophy predominantly involves the LV, and is often more marked than in any other cardiac disease. Hypertrophy may involve the right ventricle (RV), and an atrial myopathy may be progressive (left atrial enlargement [LA) and increased risks of atrial fibrillation [AF]). RV and LA involvement may be secondary to the LV disease, and/or a primary consequence of the basic molecular defect. The LVH represents hypertrophy and hyperplasia of several cell types, including cardiac myocytes, fibroblasts, and smooth muscle cells, along with excessive collagen and matrix deposition, and abnormalities of the microvasculature[3]. The normal parallel arrangement of myocytes is often disturbed (fibre disarray).

The first descriptions of hypertrophic cardiomyopathy HCM) are often attributed to Teare in the late 1950s[4]. In the following half century, what was considered a rare clinical entity, associated with a dire prognosis, is increasingly understood as a group of myocardial diseases with surprisingly heterogeneous genetic causes and phenotypic expressions. A benign outcome is frequently the more common clinical course. Important events in HCM research include: 1) the development of therapies reducing LV outflow obstruction; 2) the beginning of an understanding of the genetic basis of hereditary LVH; 3) the development of cardiac imaging providing both diagnostic and prognostic information; and 4) the development of strategies addressing risks of sudden death.

Further advances will require: 1) a better understanding of symptom development, including improved detection/management of 'diastolic failure', myocardial ischaemia, and myocardial fibrosis; 2) an ability to make more precise predictions of clinical events, particularly of sudden death, thromboembolic disease, and systolic impairment; 3) an unravelling of the cellular processes leading from mutation to disease, novel pharmacological therapies may follow; 4) randomized clinical trials to evaluate existing and future clinical intervention.

Clinical practice addresses three needs: 1) assessing and treating the symptomatic patient; 2) assessing and addressing prognostic risks; and 3) genetic counselling, family screening, and mutation detection (genetic testing). Symptoms due to HCM will often have a striking variation in severity when patients may describe good and bad days, exacerbation of symptoms following large meals and an intolerance of dehydration or a hot climate. Chest pain, with a quality similar to angina pectoris but often developing at rest, dyspnoea, palpitations, dizziness, pre/syncope, and fatigue are the common complaints. Although the relief of LV outflow obstruction (LVOTO) by alcohol septal ablation (ASA) for the management of symptomatic HCM is the focus of this chapter, we will first describe some of the more important features of HCM in order that this procedure can be placed in the context of a complex cardiac condition.

HCM comprises several cardiac diseases

HCM is diagnosed on the basis of morphologic abnormalities, requiring the demonstration of a criterion magnitude of LVH unexplained by another cause of LVH[5,6]. This definition encounters difficulties when LVH accompanies other cardiovascular or muscle disease, and when a genetic abnormality associated with familial HCM is identified in individuals with mild or no LVH.

Heterogeneity is a striking feature of HCM, and is evident from morphologic, clinical, prognostic, and molecular perspectives. For example, any sarcomeric mutation associated with HCM can result in a variety of disease phenotypes or no LVH all. Clinical phenotypes remain disconnected from the causes of HCM presumably because powerful (unidentified) factors modify the end result of mutant gene expression[7]. The utility of attempts to classify HCM into different types of disease are discussed in the following sections.

Morphological classification

Early investigators determined that LVH varied in magnitude and its distribution in the LV[8]. Asymmetric septal hypertrophy (ASH) describes the most commonly observed distribution of hypertrophy in the LV septum. Approximately one-quarter of HCM patients with ASH develop dynamic LVOTO as a consequence of systolic anterior movement (SAM) of the mitral valve leaflets towards the basal septum (obstructive HCM)[9]. More unusual morphologic variants include mid-cavity obstructive HCM, apical (or Japanese) HCM, and dilated-phase or 'burnt-out' HCM (Fig. 41.1). Finally, tissue characterization promises to be cardiac magnetic resonance (CMR) imaging's 'killer application' (Fig. 41.1). The detection of myocardial scarring by delayed enhancement following gadolinium enhancement (DGE) may prove both diagnostically and prognostically powerful.

Pathophysiological classification

The physiologic abnormalities and symptoms associated with HCM correlate poorly with morphology. Arrhythmia risk, abnormal myocardial relaxation/compliance, and ischaemia can be demonstrated in patients with severe/mild LVH, unobstructed/obstructed, high/low risk and in symptomatic/asymptomatic patients. Furthermore, physiologic disturbances may contribute to the evolution of symptoms in the absence of obvious changes in LV morphology.

Although making objective measurements of physiologic abnormalities has proven difficult, we increasingly refer to restrictive or diastolic failure HCM, dilated phase HCM, ischaemic HCM, HCM with associated atrial myopathy, and pro-arrhythmic HCM. The development of therapy tailored to abnormal physiology provides motivation; for example, assessing the potential benefit of renin–angiotensin–aldosterone system (RAAS) blockade for restrictive disease.

Genetic classification

Despite the identification of mutant genetic causes of HCM, genetic classifications have proven to be of limited clinical utility. Mutations in sarcomeric genes are the commonest causes of HCM, accounting for 50–60% of cases in tertiary referral populations[10,11]. Sarcomeric genes code for the components of the cardiomyocyte's sarcomeres—the basic contractile unit of cardiac muscle. Although HCM is sometimes referred to as a disease of the sarcomere, non-sarcomeric genetic causes are recognized and include genes encoding components of systems regulating or producing ATP. Indeed, perturbed energy metabolism may comprise a common pathway towards the development of LVH that is shared by several causes of hypertrophy[12].

The clinical utility of a genetic diagnosis is limited: 1) a genetic cause for HCM is not found in approximately 40% of patients[10,11]; 2) there are many different mutations, most of which are very rare or even unique to a family[13]; and (3) there is a poor correlation between genotype and phenotype, even within a single pedigree. A reasonable genotype–phenotype correlation is described for only a few of the many hundreds of mutations thus far detected. This includes sudden death risk, AF, mid cavity disease, and associated conduction disease[14–17].

Molecular or motor function classification

The development of a classification scheme derived from a mechanistic understanding of the molecular dysfunction due to mutant protein expression remains an attractive goal. It stands to reason that the functional consequences of a mutation correspond to the severity of the resulting cardiac disease. At present, no studies associate bench-top assays of mutant protein function with any aspect of clinical outcome[18–20]. Some researchers have proposed that 'gain of function' mutations cause LVH and that DCM results from 'loss of function' mutations[21]. However, parameters of *in vitro* acto-myosin interaction bear no relation to the resulting phenotype[20].

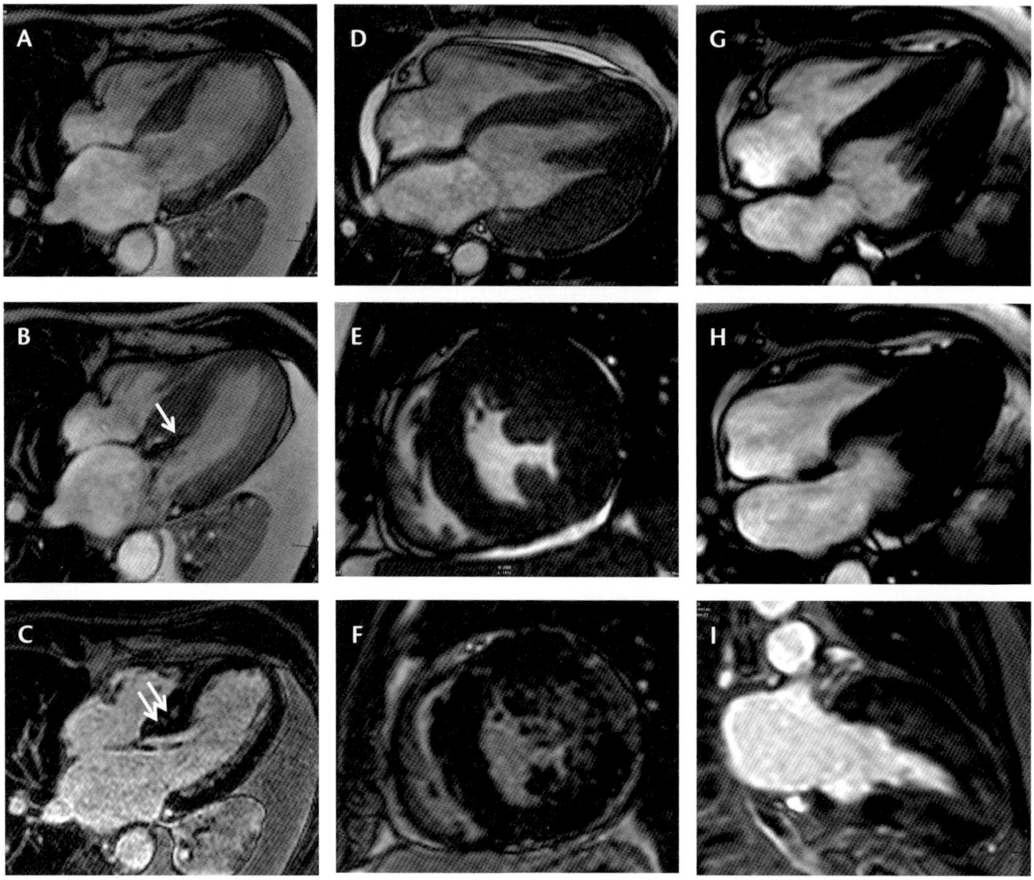

Fig. 41.1 Examples of HCM morphological variants and delayed gadolinium enhancement demonstrated with CMR imaging. A, B, C) Asymmetric septal hypertrophy (ASH) with four-chamber views demonstrating cardiac morphology at end diastole (A), end systole (B), and delayed enhancement. The systolic frame demonstrates SAM with complete septal contact (arrow) resulting in LVOTO and MR. Delayed enhancement following gadolinium infusion (DGE) is seen in the basal septum (double arrows). A unilateral pleural effusion and collapse of the left lung is also seen. D, E, F) Reversed ASH seen in four-chamber (D) and basal short-axis (E) views. There is extensive patchy DGE in the hypertrophied basal anterolateral segment. G, H, I) The uncommon apical variant of HCM. The four-chamber views demonstrate the distal LVH and small end-diastolic cavitary volumes (D) and the systolic obliteration of the distal two-thirds of the LV cavity. DGE is extensive, and was demonstrated in all LV segments (I). Images courtesy of the London Chest CMR unit (M. Westwood, C. Davies, and A. Mathur)

Clinical classification

A pragmatic clinical approach divides HCM into symptomatic and asymptomatic disease, into obstructive and non-obstructive HCM, and into categories of estimated risk of sudden death from arrhythmia or stroke. In these schemes, morphologic features (for example, the LVH magnitude, LA involvement, LV dilatation), clinical variables (prior clinical events, family history, and results of routine cardiac testing such as exercise testing), and occasionally the precise genetic cause (for example, the detection of a 'malignant' mutation) are helpful in predicting clinical outcome. This approach is based on the few clinical interventions currently available, and is how indications for invasive treatment of LVOTO are considered (Fig. 41.2).

Risks of premature death

Several studies have identified that HCM is the commonest cause of sudden death (SD) in the young, usually defined as death occurring within 24h of the onset of symptoms in individuals under the age of 45 years. Differences in reported SD risk are partly due to the

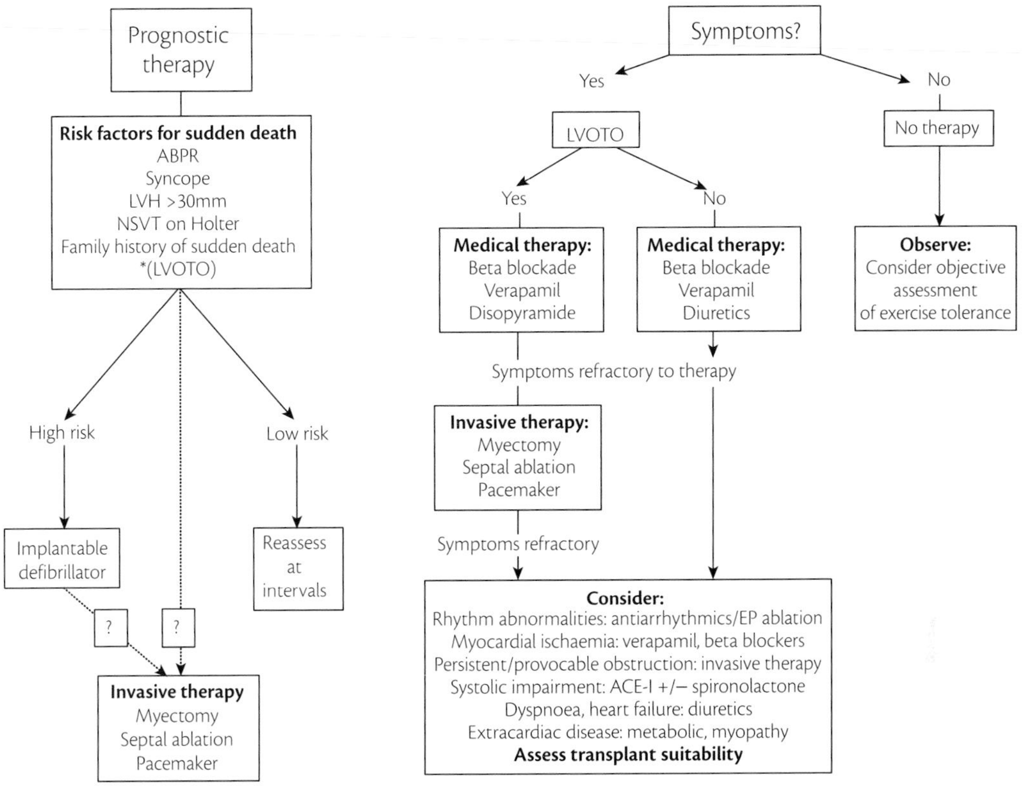

Fig. 41.2 Management of symptoms and sudden death risk in HCM patients: Decision-making tree or therapeutic cascades consider prognostic and symptomatic indications for intervention. At present, the presence of LVOTO is only considered important in symptomatic HCM. *LVOTO is an independent risk factor for poor prognosis, and future indications for either ICD therapy or ASA might consider one or both of these interventions in asymptomatic individuals with obstruction. ABPR, abnormal blood pressure response to exercise; LVH, LV hypertrophy; LVOTO, LV outflow tract obstruction; NSVT, non-sustained ventricular tachycardia.

provenance of the cohort studied; annual mortality in tertiary centre cohorts is greater than that in studies of 'community-based' patients[22]. An annual risk for death in relatively unselected HCM patients is likely to be 0.1–1% per year, rising to 2% or even higher in certain groups, such as in symptomatic patients or when HCM presents in children[23–27]. Few studies adequately differentiate between cause of SD—including ventricular arrhythmia, heart failure-related death (with arrhythmia as a frequent terminal event), and stroke. A number of studies have associated certain clinical features with poorer prognosis (Table 41.1); when considered individually, each has a poor positive predictive performance.

In a retrospective analysis of 368 HCM patients, risk factor accumulation identified patients at high SD risk[28]. Even though implantable cardioverter defibrillator (ICD) implantation recommendations are made on the basis of the results, this study (and most others) did not adequately address cause of death. Similarly, no trials examine efficacy of prognostic intervention (ICDs, anticoagulation or heart failure medication). The sizeable fraction of patients in the retrospective ICD studies (discussed in a later section) with only one risk factor yet who receive appropriate shocks also attests to the limitations in current risk management. For enhanced risk stratification, the relative contributions to death from arrhythmia, stroke, and heart failure from these and other risk factors will need to be defined. Finally, although LVOTO (see 'Additional indications for invasive therapy' section) is established as an indicator of poor prognosis, it is not known whether its abolition will improve outcome.

Ventricular arrhythmia

A consensus document prepared for the AHA, ACC and ESC unequivocally recommends ICD implantation for secondary prevention of arrhythmic SD[6].

Table 41.1 Conventional and candidate risk factors for predicting premature death in HCM

Established risk factors	Candidate risk factors
Cardiac arrest†	Atrial fibrillation
Sustained VT†	Left atrial enlargement
Non-sustained VT*	Myocardial ischaemia
Family history of premature SD*	DGE imaging
Unexplained syncope*	'Malignant' mutation
LV wall thickness ≥30mm*	Environmental**
Abnormal exercise BP*	
LVOTO	
LV dilation	

†Implantable cardioverter defibrillator (ICD) indicated for secondary prevention; *'Major' risk factors used in summation to risk stratify for the purposes of primary prevention ICD implantation(77).
**Environmental refers to common situations that may increase risk, for example hypertension, competitive sports, recreational drug taking.
BP, blood pressure; DGE, delayed gadolinium enhancement; LV, left ventricular; LVOTO, left ventricular outflow obstruction; SD, sudden death; VT, ventricular tachycardia.
Modified from Maron BJ, McKenna WJ, Danielson GK, *et al.* American College of Cardiology/European Society of Cardiology clinical expert consensus document on hypertrophic cardiomyopathy. A report of the American College of Cardiology Foundation Task Force on Clinical Expert Consensus Documents and the European Society of Cardiology Committee for Practice Guidelines. *J Am Coll Cardiol* 2003; **42**:1687–713.

ICD implantation for primary prevention has a Class 2a indication (level of evidence C) in patients with one or more 'major' risk factor for SD (see Table 41.1). In other words, many but not all experts would recommend ICD implantation at this level of perceived risk. No prospective studies examine accuracy of risk prediction or success of intervention. Retrospective studies describe high intervention rates in patients receiving ICDs for primary prevention, but also frequent complications (including inappropriate shocks in one-quarter)[29–31]. Finally, as the risk factor profiles of those patients receiving appropriate ICD discharges were no different from those not shocked, our ability to stratify risk remains severely limited. In one study, one-third of the patients shocked appropriately had only a single 'major' risk factor[31].

Thromboembolic events

Stroke risk in HCM increases with advancing age and is associated with a progressive LA myopathy; increasing LA size, depressed LA systolic function, and higher prevalence of AF. Approximately 2% of HCM patients per year develop AF, associated with an odds ratio of 18 for stroke (compared with HCM without AF)[32]. Anticoagulation is considered for severe LA enlargement (>50mm) even without evidence of AF; impairment of LA contractile and capacitance function may contribute to stroke risk and there is a reasonable likelihood that undetected PAF is present (or will soon develop).

Systolic left ventricular failure

Although symptoms of congestive heart failure are common (often attributed to diastolic abnormalities), development of progressive LV systolic impairment, relative LV dilatation is not. Approximately 10% enter this phase of the disease, sometime termed end-stage (ES) disease[32,33]. LV chamber sizes in ES disease may be in a control population's normal range are best appreciated relative to the smaller 'normal' dimensions in an HCM population.

ES disease is associated with higher risks of adverse events, including mortality/transplant rates of approximately 10% per annum[32,33]. ES disease is invariably associated with DGE; serial CMR imaging with detailed assessment of LV volumes and quantification of DGE may have a role in the early detection of ES disease[34–36]. Interventions of proven prognostic benefit in systolic heart failure have not been specifically examined in ES HCM; however, similar indications for pharmacological and device therapy are generally assumed.

Obstruction and mitral regurgitation

In one-quarter of HCM patients, almost exclusively where the LVH has an ASH distribution, mitral–septal contact in systole can result in dynamic LVOTO. This systolic anterior motion (SAM) of the mitral valve also interrupts leaflet coaptation producing a variable degree of mitral regurgitation (MR). Echocardiography with Doppler or cardiac catheterization best estimates LVOTO gradients; CMR can provide more accurate quantification of septal wall thickness, systolic function, and image myocardial scar (see Fig. 41.1). Cardiac catheterization using an end-hole catheter in the LV can demonstrate the sub-aortic nature of the intra-cavitary obstruction (Fig. 41.3). Obstructive HCM is often associated with symptoms, particularly on effort or following provocation (after large meals, vasodilators, postural change). LVOTO is also associated with a poorer prognosis[37–39].

In symptomatic individuals, pharmacological treatment with beta-blockade, verapamil, or disopyramide (alone or in combination) may reduce measured

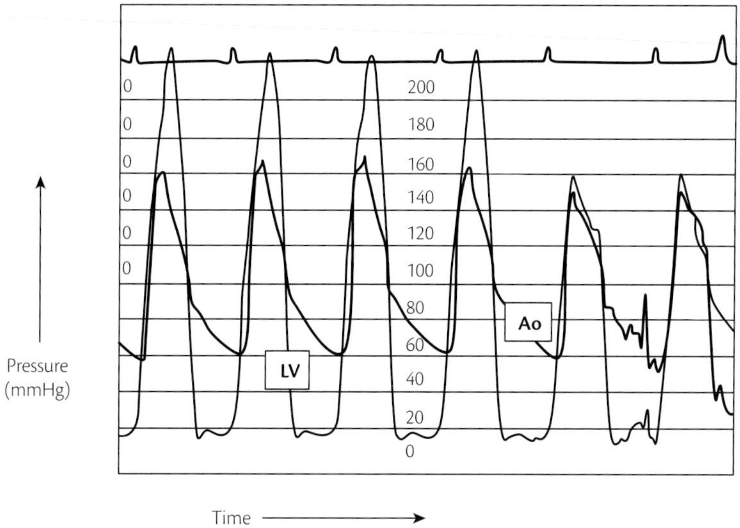

Fig. 41.3 Sub-aortic LVOTO in HCM: simultaneous LV and aortic pressures are measured and demonstrate the sub-aortic nature of LVOTO caused by SAM. A 6F end-hole catheter is used for LV pressure measurement, and is compared with the pressure measurement transduced from the side-arm of the 8F femoral sheath. A resting LVOTP gradient of 60mmHg is measured; following provocation, a gradient of nearly 200mmHg was demonstrated. Following ablation with 1mL of alcohol, the resting gradient was acutely abolished and the provoked gradient reduced to 40mmHg. Ao, aortic pressure; LV, left ventricular pressure.

outflow gradients and symptoms. Invasive reduction of LVOTO is indicated if symptoms in patients with LVOTO resulting from SAM persist despite maximum pharmacological treatment (see Fig. 41.2). The premise of all LVOTO therapies is that outflow obstruction and MR contribute to symptoms; the relatively poor correlation between both LVOTO magnitude and MR with symptom status probably reflects the additional and variable importance to symptoms of myocardial ischaemia, impaired LV filling, small stroke volumes, and arrhythmia.

The determinants of SAM are uncertain; is there a 'pull' or 'push' force on the mitral apparatus? The conventional understanding is that the anterior leaflet is pulled towards the LVOTO as the result of the Venturi effect produced as systolic flow accelerates across the convexity of the ventricular surface of the anterior mitral leaflet. The resulting negative pressure lifts the anterior leaflet away from the posterior leaflet and towards the septum. Alternatively, as the result of distorted LV geometry, the systolic effort pushes the mitral leaflets towards the LVOT(40). This uncertainty contributes to the vigorous debate concerning the preferred invasive treatment modality.

Following the initial description of ASA in 1995(41–43), it has become the most commonly-chosen treatment option for LVOTO reduction. More ASA procedures than operations have now been performed despite the passage of more than 50 years since surgical LV septal myectomy (LVM) was first developed(44). The debate concerning the relative merits of ASA and LVM is not informed by any randomized studies. The only randomized trials addressing drug-refractory symptomatic LVOTO treatment options examine dual chamber (DDD) pacing(45,46). DDD, ASA, and LVMM, have all been subject to the contrary opinions of enthusiasts and detractors. A fourth option, mitral valve replacement, is considered only in the presence of other indications for mitral valve replacement.

Surgical myectomy

In the 1960s, a surgical approach to resect the subaortic ventricular septum through the retracted aortic valve at aortotomy was developed(44). The Morrow procedure or LVM is still considered the 'gold standard' treatment by several influential opinions. Modern surgical results are impressive, with low operative mortality, substantial symptom improvement, increased exercise tolerance, and perhaps an improved prognosis(47–51). While few doubt the potential benefits of LVM, its designation as 'gold standard' is not supported by randomized trial data or contemporary real-world practice. Additionally, published results are from the few centres with considerable experience where complication rates are low. Complications include aortic incompetence, heart block, ventricular septal defects, and all the complications of open-heart surgery. Surgical techniques are clearly superior when more complex anatomic problems are to be addressed, for example if the subvalvar apparatus is abnormal or there is coexisting mid-cavity obstruction[51].

Pacemaker therapy

Pacing therapy (DDD) with right ventricular pre-excitation reduces LVOTO acutely and chronically[52–54]. This effect is likely to be the result of (paradoxical) septal movement away from the direction of SAM, but a negatively inotropic effect may also contribute. Apical RV lead placement and carefully chosen paced A–V intervals are important for successful therapy. In M-PATHY, a prospective double-blind study with a cross-over design, 3 months of active pacing was compared with placebo pacing[46]. No benefits of active pacing were demonstrated over an apparently large placebo effect. The haemodynamic and symptomatic benefits of pacing are reported to be progressive throughout the first 6 months following implantation and persist after cessation of pacing[55]. Potential bias from crossover treatment effects and type 2 error due to the abbreviated duration of therapy may have contributed to both the failure to demonstrate treatment benefit and the substantial placebo effect apparent. Significant haemodynamic and symptomatic improvement after DDD pacing were demonstrated in the larger randomized double-blinded PIC study[45,54].

Potential adverse effects on LV systolic and diastolic function of chronic RV pacing[56,57], the equivocal trial data, and the development of ASA have resulted in the relegation of pacing to a poor third choice. Nonetheless, pacing therapy has low complication rates compared with ASA and LVMM, and the use rate of ICD implantation in HCM patients is increasing where almost all devices are dual chamber systems (to minimize inappropriate shocks in patients capable of achieving high sinus rates). A therapeutic trial of pacing therapy in ICD patients with symptomatic LVOTO may prove reasonable before ASA or LVM. Pacing-ICD therapy will also increase safety following ASA or LVM.

Alcohol septal ablation

ASA's rapid acceptance has undoubtedly been influenced by the convictions of proponents and a greater willingness of patients for less invasive procedures. In the non-randomized and uncontrolled studies now available, ASA substantially reduces LVOT gradient, increases blood pressure, improves symptoms, increases exercise tolerance, and leads to desirable changes in cardiac anatomy and physiology[58–66]. These include reduced LV filling pressure, abolition or attenuation of MR, smaller LA size, improved coronary flow reserve, and reduction in LVH. Early concerns regarding arrhythmogenicity of the 'infarct' scar are not supported by data, but the potential for long-term complications cannot be dismissed[67,68]. The major complication in contemporary ASA cohorts remains complete heart block, and permanent pacing is required in approximately 10% of treated patients[58,60–62,69,70]. However, it should be noted that despite ASA's comparative youth, the number of patient treatment years must now exceed that of LVM. ASA has evolved such that its procedural mortality and efficacy are similar to that of LVM. The vigorous debate in the HCM community regarding the relative merits of the established 'gold standard' of LVM and the de-facto 'gold standard' of ASA will only be settled following large randomized trials[6,47,60,71–73]. Until such time, a pragmatic clinician must surely accept that both procedures have intrinsic merit and that choosing between them will involve considerations such as patient choice, availability of either procedure, and individual patient characteristics such as patient comorbidity and disease morphology.

Additional indications for invasive therapy

Provoked LVOTO

LVOTO worsens if end-diastolic LV volumes are reduced (postural change, dehydration, vasodilatation, post-prandially etc.) or if inotropy is increased (after ventricular extrasystoles, exertion). A systolic murmur apparent on standing from a squat is strongly suggestive of provoked LVOTO, as are symptoms of postural presyncope and an intolerance of extrasystoles. Labile LVOTO may be missed if echocardiographic or invasive studies do not include techniques to provoke SAM. Most studies (LVM, DDD, and ASA) include patients with provokable LVOTO, and symptomatic benefits are demonstrated.

The Valsalva manoeuvre and exercise can be used to demonstrate provokable LVOTO, though Valsalva detects fewer patients with provoked LVOTO than exercise studies[74]. Pharmacological agents used to demonstrate provokable LVOTO include amyl nitrate, sublingual glycerin trinitrate and intravenous isoproterenol. Dobutamine is not recommended as it can provoke LVOTO in normal hearts[75]. The Brokenborough effect following ventricular extrasystoles can demonstrate provokable LVOTO in the catheter laboratory, either through the irritant effects of manipulating a catheter in the ventricle, or by paced extrasystoles. Paced extrasystoles (a premature paced ventricular extrasystole every few cardiac cycles) are particularly useful for monitoring the magnitude of provokable LVOTO during ASA.

Mitral valve abnormalities and mid-cavity obstruction

Benign structural abnormalities of the mitral valve are common in HCM[76]. More important abnormalities include anomalous insertions of the papillary muscles/chordae onto the mitral leaflets or septum, and displacement of the papillary muscles[76,77]. Surgery is the treatment of choice if significant structural mitral abnormalities coexist with SAM, but the MR of SAM should be abolished or improve following successful ASA.

Pronounced papillary muscle hypertrophy may result in the uncommon and poorly understood mid-cavity (mid-ventricular) variant[78,79]. Mid-cavity obstruction can coexist with LVOTO, or can become apparent after successful LVOTO treatment[80]. Monomorphic VT, uncommon in HCM, is frequently associated with a distal LV aneurysm resulting from mid-cavity obstruction. The detection of monomorphic VT should prompt a search for apical abnormalities that may not be apparent on standard echo views (Fig. 41.4).

Several groups report that pacing[81], ASA[82], and surgery[78] can reduce mid-cavity gradients. However, although mid-cavity disease is often associated with drug-refractory symptoms, it is not yet understood why

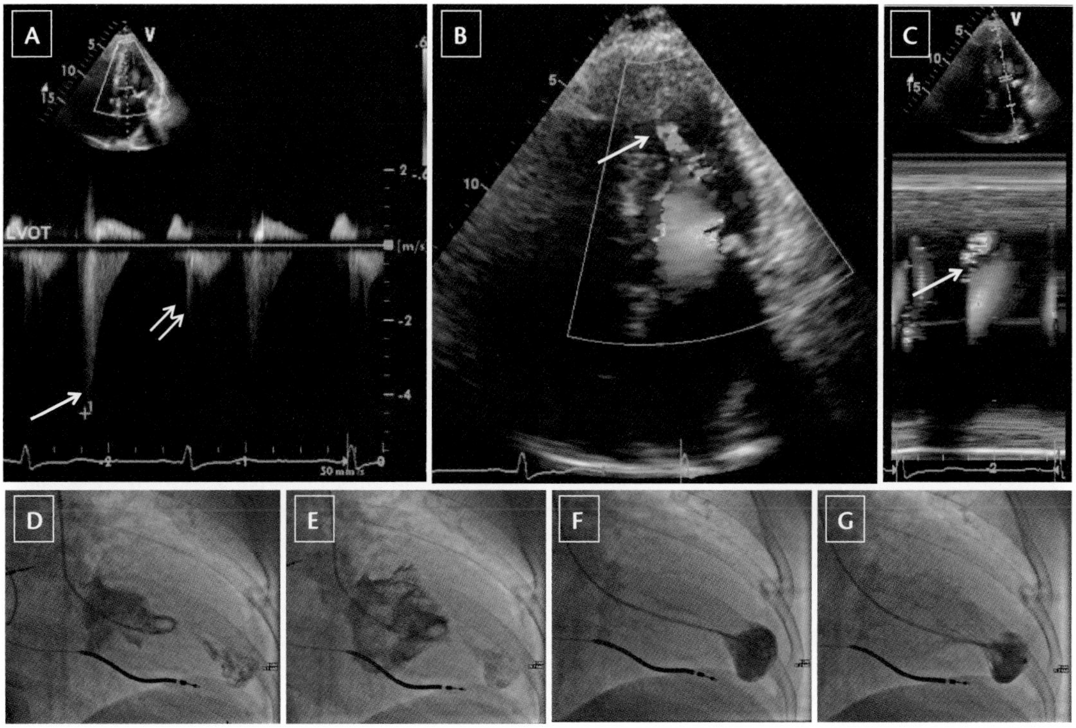

Fig. 41.4 Echocardiographic and angiographic findings in the rare variant of mid cavity obstructive HCM. This patient, in her 50s was referred for consideration of alcohol septal ablation. Doppler studies were initially interpreted as demonstrating an outflow gradient of approximately 70mmHg (A). A more careful examination of Doppler signals reveals that the high velocity signal is in early diastole (arrow), and the systolic outflow velocity is normal (double arrow). The location and timing in the cardiac cycle of this high velocity Doppler signal (arrow) are demonstrated in a four-chamber view (B) and in colour M-mode (C). The presence of an apical aneurysm, undetected by echocardiography, is demonstrated on the LV angiograms (D–G). In systolic frames (D and F), it can be seen that the apical and the proximal LV are disconnected by mid-ventricular obliteration. In early diastole (E and G) and with relief of the mid ventricular obstruction, the high pressure apical cavity empties into the relaxing proximal LV generating the high Doppler velocities.

symptoms develop or if gradient reduction improves these.

Asymptomatic LVOTO

A fundamental understanding in cardiology is that MR and aortic stenosis are associated with increased risks of heart failure and sudden death, even in asymptomatic patients. Are LVOTO and MR in obstructive HCM independently associated with worse prognosis, including risks of SD, AF, pulmonary hypertension, and ES disease? Retrospective studies report that LVOTO is independently associated with greater risks of death[(37–39)]. These reports include important differences concerning mode of death (heart failure or arrhythmic), the importance of LVOTO as a binary or continuous risk factor, and the significance of symptom status.

In a retrospective study of 1101 patients, those with LVOTO (resting gradient >30mmHg) had a relative risk (RR) of death of 1.6. LVOTO was dichotomous; risk did not increase with increments of LVOTO above 30mmHg[(38)]. Death was most often related to heart failure or stroke rather than from arrhythmic SD. In half as many patients, Autore and colleagues report that LVOTO predicted cardiovascular death best in asymptomatic patients (RR 2.4)[(39)]. In patients with functional class III or IV, symptom status, and not LVOTO, was a powerful predictor (RR 7.9). Elliott and colleagues also report reduced survival in patients with LVOTO[(37)]. In this study, LVOTO confers an incremental risk, with an RR of 1.24 per 20mmHg of LVOTO (for all-cause death and transplantation). A very low SD risk in the least symptomatic leads the authors to conclude that septal reduction therapy in the asymptomatic is not indicated for the prevention of SD.

At present, symptom relief is the only indication for invasive LVOTO reduction. Long-term consequences on cardiac structure and function of chronic LVOTO and MR may include progressive atrial enlargement and AF, pulmonary hypertension and LV systolic impairment. Furthermore, LVOTO reduction leads to modest LVH regression remote from the ablated myocardium, suggesting that some of the LVH develops in response to afterload, in addition to the 'primary' hypertrophy[(63,64)]. Future approaches to LVOTO may include prognostic indications and treatment protocols may resemble those for the management of asymptomatic and symptomatic structural valve disease. Finally, HCM is a complex syndrome where several mechanisms are responsible for symptoms. A patient with successful LVOTO reduction still has HCM, and remains subject to symptom limitation, disease progression and SD risk.

Alcohol septal ablation: patient selection and procedural details

Patient selection

Appropriate patient selection maximizes the likelihood of benefit from LVOTO reduction. ASA is currently indicated only when patients remain significantly symptomatic despite maximal medical therapy, and when LVOTO of sufficient magnitude is demonstrated. A convention is to regard a resting LVOT gradient of >30mmHG or a provoked gradient of >60mmHg as thresholds. While these thresholds do not account for MR severity (and its contribution to symptoms), they emphasize an understanding that symptom development is multifactorial; abolition of mild obstruction is unlikely to be of symptomatic benefit. Importantly, a patient must be counselled that the procedure is offered for symptom relief and not prognostic benefit. The physician must not regard an outflow gradient as the sole indication for ASA.

Avoiding complications

Theoretical risk of a ventricular septal defect following ASA mean that relatively mild septal thickness (<15mm) is a relative contraindication; this complication is reported following LVM, but is rare in the large ASA series. Mitral valve abnormalities, coexisting mid-cavity obstruction, unsuitable septal perforator anatomy, and significant coronary disease favour LVM. Conduction block requiring permanent pacing is more frequent following ASA if conduction disease is evident before the procedure[(83–85)]. As heart block may develop days or longer following patient discharge, it may be prudent to consider pacemaker implantation (and therapeutic trial of DDD pacing for LVOTO reduction) prior to ASA in high-risk patients. In patients with high-risk features for heart block, 87% required permanent pacing after ASA[(69)] (Table 41.2). This might be the preferred strategy in, for example, elderly female patients with left bundle branch block. Similarly, patients with pre-existing conduction delay or with prolonged intra-procedural complete heart block should have prolonged in-patient assessment with temporary wire support for up to 6 days[(85)]. Smaller volumes of alcohol (typically 1–2mL) injected slowly over minutes rather than as a bolus are also associated with reduced risks of heart block[58,73,86].

ASA procedure

The technique aims to selectively ablate the basal septal myocardium adjacent to the location of SAM-septal

Table 41.2 Risk factors for the development of complete heart block requiring permanent pacing[83,85]

Risk factor	Odds ratio
Female	4.3
Bolus ethanol	51
>1 septal	4.6
Prior LBBB	39
Prior 1° HB	14
Increasing age	
Intra-procedural CHB	

CHB, complete HB; HB, heart block; LBBB, left bundle branch block.

contact by injection of absolute alcohol into an isolated septal perforator artery. The procedure is usually accomplished under local anaesthesia and with conscious sedation. The administration of sedation is usually delayed until after baseline assessments of the (dynamic) LVOTO have been completed.

Heart block during or following the procedure is common, and a temporary pacing wire is routinely inserted. If monitoring of the LVOT gradient at the time of ablation is desired, catheters are simultaneously placed into both the LV and left main coronary. For uncomplicated procedures, a single femoral arterial sheath for the left coronary guide may suffice. After the guiding catheter is selectively engaged, a 0.014-inch guide wire is advanced into a proximal septal branch of the left anterior descending (LAD) artery. The first septal artery is usually selected (Fig. 41.5), and a short (approximately 10mm) 'over-the-wire' (OTW) balloon introduced into the branch. The lumen of this device

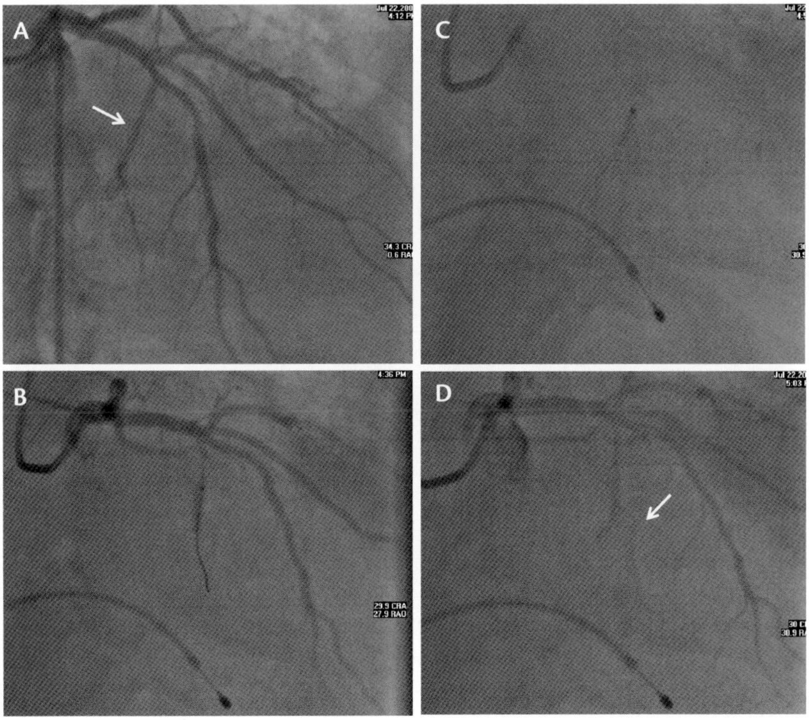

Fig. 41.5 Various stages of the procedure are illustrated in these panels. A cranial view of the left anterior descending shows a large proximal septal perforator artery (A). The OTW is inflated after placement in the perforator (B), and the isolation of the distal perforator and its branches is demonstrated after angiographic dye is injected through the central bore of the balloon's shaft (C). After the slow infusion of ethanol, the balloon is left inflated for about 5min. Angiography following this often demonstrates angiographic amputation of the septal artery (D), frequently with biphasic flow at the septal stump.

provides the route for selective delivery of angiographic contrast, echo contrast, and ultimately alcohol into the septal artery. Over-sizing balloon diameter is prudent; perforator artery barotrauma is relatively unimportant as the balloon's role is to isolate the distal vessel and prevent reflux of ethanol into the epicardial vessel.

The balloon is positioned under flouroscopy to ensure it is entirely within the septal branch before it is inflated and the guide wire removed. A small volume of angiographic contrast injected through the lumen of the OTW balloon ensures that the (distal) septal artery is isolated from the LAD. Echocardiographic contrast (e.g. Optison®, Amersham Health, United Kingdom) injected through the lumen indicates the myocardial territory subtended by the selected septal artery. Transthoracic echocardiography is usually of sufficient quality (transoesophageal echo may be necessary in some cases) to demonstrate that the contrast agent reaches only the target myocardium. The target lies adjacent and just distal to the point of mitral–septal contact and is best seen from the apical four-chamber view. The RV free wall, LV apex, and papillary muscles may on occasion be supplied by proximal septal vessels and several echo views should be used to ensure contrast enhancement is confined to the target area.

Multiple injections of contrast and several echocardiographic views may be needed before the three-dimensional distribution of the contrast within the basal septum is fully appreciated. Ablation should not proceed if contrast does not enter into the desired target area or if contrast is not confined to the basal septum. An alternative septal artery may be investigated. Ablation may proceed if echocardiographic localization is supportive. Intravenous analgesia is administered (the alcohol can cause intense, transient discomfort), and 1–2mL of absolute alcohol are administered slowly through the lumen of the OTW balloon, with the balloon remaining inflated for a further 5min. The echocardiographic gradient is usually markedly reduced, though this acute effect is likely to reflect myocardial stunning and may not accurately reflect the long-term outcome. The LVOT gradient may increase in the days following the procedure, to fall again over a period of weeks as septal remodelling occurs[87]. Importantly, although the LVOTO is often acutely abolished or markedly reduced, this is not pursued. Reduction in basal septal mass is the treatment aim, and is achieved in the longer term following remodelling of the ablated myocardium. The acute effects include disruption of myocytes, the microvasculature and lead to scar formation (Fig. 41.6).

Complications and procedural failure

Serious complications were uncommon in a systematic review[58]. Early (30-day) mortality was 1.5% with a late mortality of 0.5%. Ventricular fibrillation in the peri-operative period occurred in 2.2%, LAD dissection in 1.8%, and pericardial effusion in 0.6%. As the review considers trials early in the evolution of the technique and cohorts often too frail for surgery, these data may reflect an overestimation of risk and an underestimation of benefit.

Minor damage to the conducting system is common with right bundle branch block and first-degree atrioventricular (AV) block each developing in about 50% of patients[58]. The temporary pacing wire should be left in place for at least 24h in uncomplicated patients. In some centres, beta-blockers or verapamil are prescribed to test AV conduction prior to removal of the temporary wire. Complete heart block can occur up to several days following ASA and in-patient monitoring for 5–7 days is recommended. Permanent complete heart block requiring device implantation was necessary in 10% of the patients included in the systemic review[58]. The need for permanent pacing is more likely in female patients, if more than one septal artery is treated, with more rapid injections of alcohol, and when there is pre-existing conducting system disease (especially left bundle branch block)[83–85].

Procedural failure can be considered in terms of either insufficient LVOTO reduction, or persistence of symptoms despite LVOTO abolition. In the former, further intervention utilizing any of the three modalities may be considered. In the systematic analysis, ASA was repeated in 6.6% of patients and 1.9% went on to septal myectomy[58]. The persistence of significant symptoms despite LVOTO abolition (by ASA, DDD, or LVM) is possibly important in about 10–20% of patients and illustrates the importance of appropriate patient selection and the complexity of the disease.

Conclusions

ASA is established as the most frequently used modality in the contemporary management of drug-refractory symptomatic HCM associated with LVOTO. While ASA is undoubtedly efficacious, is relatively safe, and is minimally invasive, outcomes from randomized trials are not yet available and many experts still consider surgical approaches as the 'gold standard'. For the present, patients must be counselled that choices between ASA and surgery (and pacing) are made on the basis of considerations other than proven differences in

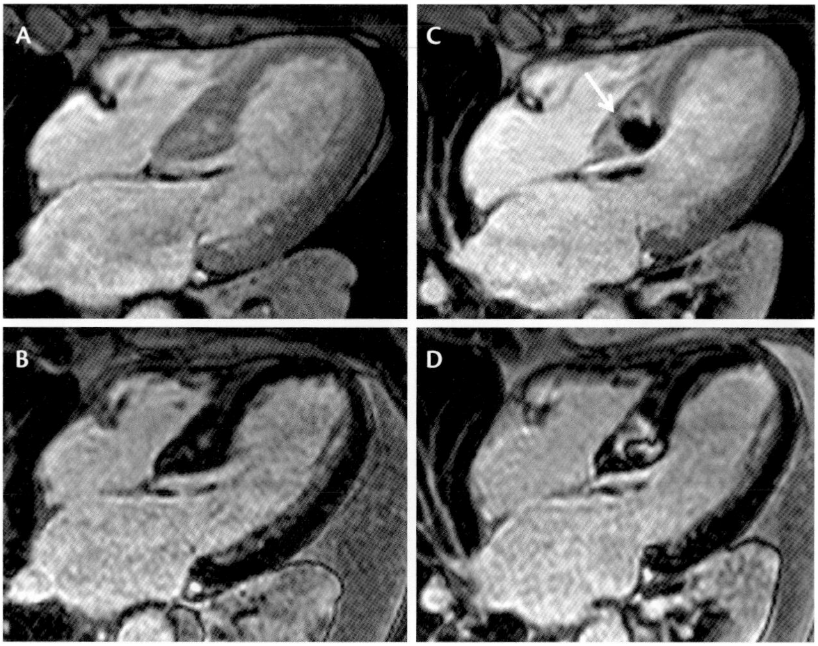

Fig. 41.6 Imaging with CMR clearly illustrates the accuracy and the limited extent of the myocardial lesion following ASA. These images are obtained on the day of the ASA procedure (A, B) and 3 days following (C, D) in the patient with obstructive HCM, also shown in Fig. 41.1. (A) and (C) illustrate early enhancement of the myocardium following gadolinium infusion; in (C) the arrow indicates disruption of microvascular flow to a well-defined myocardial volume in the basal septum caused by the ablative effects of alcohol. (B) and (D) demonstrate DGE patterns and also confirm that the ablative effects of the alcohol are confined to the region of the basal septum adjacent to the point of contact with SAM. Over weeks, there will be resolution of the associated myocardial oedema, remodelling of the basal septum, and a degree of reduction in the LVH in more distant myocardial segments. Images courtesy of the London Chest CMR unit (M. Westwood, C. Davies, and A. Mathur)

outcome. Surgery has a clear advantage in patients with complex LV anatomy, but ASA is less invasive and provides very similar results to surgery in most patients with symptomatic LVOTO. Pacing may warrant a therapeutic trial in patients with additional indications for ICD implantation. Finally, if LVOTO reduction is demonstrated to improve prognosis in asymptomatic patients, it will be even more important to compare these three therapeutic modalities in prospective randomized trials.

References

1. Maron BJ, Gardin JM, Flack JM, *et al.* Prevalence of hypertrophic cardiomyopathy in a general population of young adults. Echocardiographic analysis of 4111 subjects in the CARDIA Study. Coronary Artery Risk Development in (Young) Adults. *Circulation* 1995; **92**:785–9.
2. Fananapazir L, Epstein ND. Prevalence of hypertrophic cardiomyopathy and limitations of screening methods. *Circulation* 1995; **92**:700–4.
3. Hughes SE. The pathology of hypertrophic cardiomyopathy. *Histopathology* 2004; **44**:412–27.
4. Goodwin JF, Hollman A, Cleland WP, *et al.* Obstructive cardiomyopathy simulating aortic stenosis. *Br Heart J* 1960; **22**:403–14.
5. Elliott P, McKenna WJ. Hypertrophic cardiomyopathy. *Lancet* 2004; **363**:1881–91.
6. Maron BJ, McKenna WJ, Danielson GK, *et al.* American College of Cardiology/European Society of Cardiology clinical expert consensus document on hypertrophic cardiomyopathy. A report of the American College of Cardiology Foundation Task Force on Clinical Expert Consensus Documents and the European Society of Cardiology Committee for Practice Guidelines. *J Am Coll Cardiol* 2003; **42**:1687–713.
7. Tardiff JC. Sarcomeric proteins and familial hypertrophic cardiomyopathy: linking mutations in structural proteins to complex cardiovascular phenotypes. *Heart Fail Rev* 2005; **10**:237–48.
8. Tsoutsman T, Lam L, Semsarian C. Genes, calcium and modifying factors in hypertrophic cardiomyopathy. *Clin Exp Pharmacol Physiol* 2006; **33**:139–45.

9. Ommen SR, Shah PM, Tajik AJ. Left ventricular outflow tract obstruction in hypertrophic cardiomyopathy: past, present and future. *Heart* 2008; **94**:1276–81.
10. Girolami F, Olivotto I, Passerini I, *et al.* A molecular screening strategy based on beta-myosin heavy chain, cardiac myosin binding protein C and troponin T genes in Italian patients with hypertrophic cardiomyopathy. *J Cardiovasc Med (Hagerstown)* 2006; **7**:601–7.
11. Richard P, Charron P, Carrier L, *et al.* Hypertrophic cardiomyopathy: distribution of disease genes, spectrum of mutations, and implications for a molecular diagnosis strategy. *Circulation* 2003; **107**:2227–32.
12. Ashrafian H, Redwood C, Blair E, *et al.* Hypertrophic cardiomyopathy: a paradigm for myocardial energy depletion. *Trends Genet* 2003; **19**:263–8.
13. Mohiddin SA, Begley DA, McLam E, *et al.* Utility of genetic screening in hypertrophic cardiomyopathy: prevalence and significance of novel and double (homozygous and heterozygous) beta-myosin mutations. *Genet Test* 2003; **7**:21–7.
14. Gollob MH, Green MS, Tang AS, *et al.* Identification of a gene responsible for familial Wolff–Parkinson–White syndrome. *N Engl J Med* 2001; **344**:1823–31.
15. Gruver EJ, Fatkin D, Dodds GA, *et al.* Familial hypertrophic cardiomyopathy and atrial fibrillation caused by Arg663His beta-cardiac myosin heavy chain mutation. *Am J Cardiol.* 1999; **83**:13H–18H.
16. Poetter K, Jiang H, Hassanzadeh S, *et al.* Mutations in either the essential or regulatory light chains of myosin are associated with a rare myopathy in human heart and skeletal muscle. *Nat Genet* 1996; **13**:63–9.
17. Epstein ND, Cohn GM, Cyran F, *et al.* Differences in clinical expression of hypertrophic cardiomyopathy associated with two distinct mutations in the beta-myosin heavy chain gene. A 908Leu----Val mutation and a 403Arg----Gln mutation. *Circulation* 1992; **86**:345–52.
18. Alpert NR, Brosseau C, Federico A, *et al.* Molecular mechanics of mouse cardiac myosin isoforms. *Am J Physiol Heart Circ Physiol* 2002; **283**:H1446–54.
19. Keller DI, Coirault C, Rau T, *et al.* Human homozygous R403W mutant cardiac myosin presents disproportionate enhancement of mechanical and enzymatic properties. *J Mol Cell Cardiol* 2004; **36**:355–62.
20. Palmiter KA, Tyska MJ, Haeberle JR, *et al.* R403Q and L908V mutant beta-cardiac myosin from patients with familial hypertrophic cardiomyopathy exhibit enhanced mechanical performance at the single molecule level. *J Muscle Res Cell Motil* 2000; **21**:609–20.
21. Seidman JG, Seidman C. The genetic basis for cardiomyopathy: from mutation identification to mechanistic paradigms. *Cell* 2001; **104**:557–67.
22. Maron BJ, Casey SA, Poliac LC, *et al.* Clinical course of hypertrophic cardiomyopathy in a regional United States cohort. *JAMA* 1999; **281**:650–5.
23. Maron BJ, Fananapazir L. Sudden cardiac death in hypertrophic cardiomyopathy. *Circulation* 1992; **85**:I57–63.
24. Cecchi F, Olivotto I, Montereggi A, *et al.* Hypertrophic cardiomyopathy in Tuscany: clinical course and outcome in an unselected regional population. *J Am Coll Cardiol* 1995; **26**:1529–36.
25. Elliott PM, Gimeno JR, Thaman R, *et al.* Historical trends in reported survival rates in patients with hypertrophic cardiomyopathy. *Heart* 2006; **92**:785–91.
26. Takagi E, Yamakado T, Nakano T. Prognosis of completely asymptomatic adult patients with hypertrophic cardiomyopathy. *J Am Coll Cardiol* 1999; **33**:206–11.
27. Eriksson MJ, Sonnenberg B, Woo A, *et al.* Long-term outcome in patients with apical hypertrophic cardiomyopathy. *J Am Coll Cardiol* 2002; **39**:638–45.
28. Elliott PM, Poloniecki J, Dickie S, *et al.* Sudden death in hypertrophic cardiomyopathy: identification of high risk patients. *J Am Coll Cardiol* 2000; **36**:2212–18.
29. Maron BJ, Shen WK, Link MS, *et al.* Efficacy of implantable cardioverter-defibrillators for the prevention of sudden death in patients with hypertrophic cardiomyopathy. *N Engl J Med* 2000; **342**:365–73.
30. Begley DA, Mohiddin SA, Tripodi D, *et al.* Efficacy of implantable cardioverter defibrillator therapy for primary and secondary prevention of sudden cardiac death in hypertrophic cardiomyopathy. *Pacing Clin Electrophysiol* 2003; **26**:1887–96.
31. Maron BJ, Spirito P, Shen WK, *et al.* Implantable cardioverter-defibrillators and prevention of sudden cardiac death in hypertrophic cardiomyopathy. *JAMA* 2007; **298**:405–12.
32. Olivotto I, Cecchi F, Casey SA, *et al.* Impact of atrial fibrillation on the clinical course of hypertrophic cardiomyopathy. *Circulation* 2001; **104**:2517–24.
33. Harris KM, Spirito P, Maron MS, *et al.* Prevalence, clinical profile, and significance of left ventricular remodeling in the end-stage phase of hypertrophic cardiomyopathy. *Circulation* 2006; **114**:216–25.
34. Dumont CA, Monserrat L, Soler R, *et al.* [Clinical significance of late gadolinium enhancement on cardiovascular magnetic resonance in patients with hypertrophic cardiomyopathy]. *Rev Esp Cardiol* 2007; **60**:15–23.
35. Moon JC, McKenna WJ, McCrohon JA, *et al.* Toward clinical risk assessment in hypertrophic cardiomyopathy with gadolinium cardiovascular magnetic resonance. *J Am Coll Cardiol* 2003; **41**:1561–7.
36. Popovic ZB, Kwon DH, Mishra M, *et al.* Association between regional ventricular function and myocardial fibrosis in hypertrophic cardiomyopathy assessed by speckle tracking echocardiography and delayed hyperenhancement magnetic resonance imaging. *J Am Soc Echocardiogr* 2008; **21**:1299–305.
37. Elliott PM, Gimeno JR, Tome MT, *et al.* Left ventricular outflow tract obstruction and sudden death risk in patients with hypertrophic cardiomyopathy. *Eur Heart J* 2006; **27**:1933–41.

38. Maron MS, Olivotto I, Betocchi S, *et al.* Effect of left ventricular outflow tract obstruction on clinical outcome in hypertrophic cardiomyopathy. *N Engl J Med* 2003; **348**:295–303.
39. Autore C, Bernabo P, Barilla CS, *et al.* The prognostic importance of left ventricular outflow obstruction in hypertrophic cardiomyopathy varies in relation to the severity of symptoms. *J Am Coll Cardiol* 2005; **45**:1076–80.
40. Sherrid MV, Chaudhry FA, Swistel DG. Obstructive hypertrophic cardiomyopathy: echocardiography, pathophysiology, and the continuing evolution of surgery for obstruction. *Ann Thorac Surg* 2003; **75**:620–32.
41. Sigwart U. Non-surgical myocardial reduction for hypertrophic obstructive cardiomyopathy. *Lancet* 1995; **346**:211–14.
42. Knight C, Kurbaan AS, Seggewiss H, *et al.* Nonsurgical septal reduction for hypertrophic obstructive cardiomyopathy: outcome in the first series of patients. *Circulation* 1997; **95**:2075–81.
43. Knight C, Sigwart U. Non-surgical ablation of the ventricular septum for the treatment of hypertrophic cardiomyopathy. *Heart* 1996; **76**:92.
44. Morrow AG, Fogarty TJ, Hannah H, *et al.* Techniques, and the results of preoperative and postoperative clinical and hemodynamic assessments. *Circulation* 1968; **37**:589–96.
45. Kappenberger LJ, Linde C, Jeanrenaud X, *et al.* Clinical progress after randomized on/off pacemaker treatment for hypertrophic obstructive cardiomyopathy. Pacing in Cardiomyopathy (PIC) Study Group. *Europace* 1999; **1**:77–84.
46. Maron BJ, Nishimura RA, McKenna WJ, *et al.* Assessment of permanent dual-chamber pacing as a treatment for drug-refractory symptomatic patients with obstructive hypertrophic cardiomyopathy. A randomized, double-blind, crossover study (M-PATHY). *Circulation* 1999; **99**:2927–33.
47. Maron BJ, Dearani JA, Ommen SR, *et al.* The case for surgery in obstructive hypertrophic cardiomyopathy. *J Am Coll Cardiol* 2004; **44**:2044–53.
48. Stone CD, Hennein HA, McIntosh CL, *et al.* The results of operation in patients with hypertrophic cardiomyopathy and pulmonary hypertension. *J Thorac Cardiovasc Surg* 1990; **100**:343–51; discussion 352.
49. Valeti US, Nishimura RA, Holmes DR, *et al.* Comparison of surgical septal myectomy and alcohol septal ablation with cardiac magnetic resonance imaging in patients with hypertrophic obstructive cardiomyopathy. *J Am Coll Cardiol* 2007; **49**:350–7.
50. McLeod CJ, Ommen SR, Ackerman MJ, *et al.* Surgical septal myectomy decreases the risk for appropriate implantable cardioverter defibrillator discharge in obstructive hypertrophic cardiomyopathy. *Eur Heart J* 2007; **28**(21):2583–8.
51. Minakata K, Dearani JA, Nishimura RA, *et al.* Extended septal myectomy for hypertrophic obstructive cardiomyopathy with anomalous mitral papillary muscles or chordae. *J Thorac Cardiovasc Surg* 2004; 127:481–19.
52. Gilligan DM. Dual-chamber pacing in hypertrophic cardiomyopathy. *Curr Cardiol Rep* 2000; **2**:154–9.
53. Topilski I, Sherez J, Keren G, *et al.* Long-term effects of dual-chamber pacing with periodic echocardiographic evaluation of optimal atrioventricular delay in patients with hypertrophic cardiomyopathy >50 years of age. *Am J Cardiol* 2006; **97**:1769–75.
54. Gadler F, Linde C, Daubert C, *et al.* Significant improvement of quality of life following atrioventricular synchronous pacing in patients with hypertrophic obstructive cardiomyopathy. Data from 1 year of follow-up. PIC study group. Pacing In Cardiomyopathy. *Eur Heart J* 1999; **20**:1044–50.
55. Fananapazir L, Epstein ND, Curiel RV, *et al.* Long-term results of dual-chamber (DDD) pacing in obstructive hypertrophic cardiomyopathy. Evidence for progressive symptomatic and hemodynamic improvement and reduction of left ventricular hypertrophy. *Circulation* 1994; **90**:2731–42.
56. Wilkoff BL, Cook JR, Epstein AE, *et al.* Dual-chamber pacing or ventricular backup pacing in patients with an implantable defibrillator: the Dual Chamber and VVI Implantable Defibrillator (DAVID) Trial. *JAMA* 2002; **288**:3115–23.
57. Nishimura RA, Hayes DL, Ilstrup DM, *et al.* Effect of dual-chamber pacing on systolic and diastolic function in patients with hypertrophic cardiomyopathy. Acute Doppler echocardiographic and catheterization hemodynamic study. *J Am Coll Cardiol* 1996; **27**:421–30.
58. Alam M, Dokainish H, Lakkis N. Alcohol septal ablation for hypertrophic obstructive cardiomyopathy: a systematic review of published studies. *J Interv Cardiol* 2006; **19**:319–27.
59. Jaber WA, Yang EH, Nishimura RA, *et al.* Immediate improvement in coronary flow reserve after alcohol septal ablation in patients with hypertrophic obstructive cardiomyopathy. *Heart* 2009; **95**(7):564–9.
60. Sorajja P, Valeti U, Nishimura RA, *et al.* Outcome of alcohol septal ablation for obstructive hypertrophic cardiomyopathy. *Circulation* 2008; **118**:131–9.
61. Fernandes VL, Nagueh SF, Wang W, *et al.* A prospective follow-up of alcohol septal ablation for symptomatic hypertrophic obstructive cardiomyopathy – the Baylor experience (1996-2002). *Clin Cardiol* 2005; **28**:124–30.
62. Fernandes VL, Nielsen C, Nagueh S.F, *et al.* Follow-up of alcohol septal ablation for symptomatic hypertrophic obstructive cardiomyopathy. *JACC: Cardiovasc Interv* 2008; **1**:561–570.
63. van Dockum WG, Beek AM, ten Cate FJ, *et al.* Early onset and progression of left ventricular remodeling after alcohol septal ablation in hypertrophic obstructive cardiomyopathy. *Circulation* 2005; **111**:2503–8.
64. van Dockum WG, Kuijer JP, Gotte MJ, *et al.* Septal ablation in hypertrophic obstructive cardiomyopathy improves systolic myocardial function in the lateral (free) wall: a follow-up study using CMR tissue tagging and 3D strain analysis. *Eur Heart J* 2006; **27**:2833–9.

65. Hage FG, Karakus G, Luke WD, Jr, *et al.* Effect of alcohol-induced septal ablation on left atrial volume and ejection fraction assessed by real time three-dimensional transthoracic echocardiography in patients with hypertrophic cardiomyopathy. *Echocardiography* 2008; **25**:784–9.
66. Meliga E, Steendijk P, Valgimigli M, *et al.* Effects of percutaneous transluminal septal myocardial ablation for obstructive hypertrophic cardiomyopathy on systolic and diastolic left ventricular function assessed by pressure-volume loops. *Am J Cardiol* 2008; **101**:1179–84.
67. Cuoco FA, Spencer WH, 3rd, Fernandes VL, *et al.* Implantable cardioverter-defibrillator therapy for primary prevention of sudden death after alcohol septal ablation of hypertrophic cardiomyopathy. *J Am Coll Cardiol* 2008; **52**:1718–23.
68. Guo H, Wang P, Xing Y, *et al.* Delayed electrocardiographic changes after percutaneous transluminal septal myocardial ablation in hypertrophic obstructive cardiomyopathy. *J Electrocardiol* 2007; **40**:356 e1–6.
69. Faber L, Welge D, Fassbender D, *et al.* Percutaneous septal ablation for symptomatic hypertrophic obstructive cardiomyopathy: managing the risk of procedure-related AV conduction disturbances. *Int J Cardiol* 2007; **119**:163–7.
70. Faber L, Welge D, Fassbender D, *et al.* One-year follow-up of percutaneous septal ablation for symptomatic hypertrophic obstructive cardiomyopathy in 312 patients: predictors of hemodynamic and clinical response. *Clin Res Cardiol* 2007; **96**:864–73.
71. Firoozi S, Elliott PM, Sharma S, *et al.* Septal myotomy-myectomy and transcoronary septal alcohol ablation in hypertrophic obstructive cardiomyopathy. A comparison of clinical, haemodynamic and exercise outcomes. *Eur Heart J* 2002; **23**:1617–24.
72. Olivotto I, Ommen SR, Maron MS, *et al.* Surgical myectomy versus alcohol septal ablation for obstructive hypertrophic cardiomyopathy. Will there ever be a randomized trial? *J Am Coll Cardiol* 2007; **50**:831–4.
73. Nagueh SF, Ommen SR, Lakkis NM, *et al.* Comparison of ethanol septal reduction therapy with surgical myectomy for the treatment of hypertrophic obstructive cardiomyopathy. *J Am Coll Cardiol* 2001; **38**:1701–6.
74. Maron MS, Olivotto I, Zenovich AG, *et al.* Hypertrophic cardiomyopathy is predominantly a disease of left ventricular outflow tract obstruction. *Circulation* 2006; **114**:2232–9.
75. Pellikka PA, Oh JK, Bailey KR, *et al.* Dynamic intraventricular obstruction during dobutamine stress echocardiography. A new observation. *Circulation* 1992; **86**:1429–32.
76. Klues HG, Maron BJ, Dollar AL, *et al.* Diversity of structural mitral valve alterations in hypertrophic cardiomyopathy. *Circulation* 1992; **85**:1651–60.
77. Maron BJ, Nishimura RA, Danielson GK. Pitfalls in clinical recognition and a novel operative approach for hypertrophic cardiomyopathy with severe outflow obstruction due to anomalous papillary muscle. *Circulation* 1998; **98**:2505–8.
78. Cecchi F, Olivotto I, Nistri S, *et al.* Midventricular obstruction and clinical decision-making in obstructive hypertrophic cardiomyopathy. *Herz* 2006; **31**:871–6.
79. Maron MS, Finley JJ, Bos JM, *et al.* Prevalence, clinical significance, and natural history of left ventricular apical aneurysms in hypertrophic cardiomyopathy. *Circulation* 2008; **118**:1541–9.
80. Minakata K, Dearani JA, Schaff HV, *et al.* Mechanisms for recurrent left ventricular outflow tract obstruction after septal myectomy for obstructive hypertrophic cardiomyopathy. *Ann Thorac Surg* 2005; **80**:851–6.
81. Begley D, Mohiddin S, Fananapazir L. Dual chamber pacemaker therapy for mid-cavity obstructive hypertrophic cardiomyopathy. *Pacing Clin Electrophysiol* 2001; **24**:1639–44.
82. Seggewiss H, Faber L. Percutaneous septal ablation for hypertrophic cardiomyopathy and mid-ventricular obstruction. *Eur J Echocardiogr* 2000; **1**:277–80.
83. Chang SM, Nagueh SF, Spencer WH, 3rd, *et al.* Complete heart block: determinants and clinical impact in patients with hypertrophic obstructive cardiomyopathy undergoing nonsurgical septal reduction therapy. *J Am Coll Cardiol* 2003; **42**:296–300.
84. El-Jack SS, Nasif M, Blake JW, *et al.* Predictors of complete heart block after alcohol septal ablation for hypertrophic cardiomyopathy and the timing of pacemaker implantation. *J Interv Cardiol* 2007; **20**:73–6.
85. Lawrenz T, Lieder F, Bartelsmeier M, *et al.* Predictors of complete heart block after transcoronary ablation of septal hypertrophy: results of a prospective electrophysiological investigation in 172 patients with hypertrophic obstructive cardiomyopathy. *J Am Coll Cardiol* 2007; **49**:2356–63.
86. Veselka J, Duchonova R, Prochazkova S, *et al.* Effects of varying ethanol dosing in percutaneous septal ablation for obstructive hypertrophic cardiomyopathy on early hemodynamic changes. *Am J Cardiol* 2005; **95**:675–8.
87. Veselka J, Duchonova R, Prochazkova S, *et al.* The biphasic course of changes of left ventricular outflow gradient after alcohol septal ablation for hypertrophic obstructive cardiomyopathy. *Kardiol Pol* 2004; **60**:133–6; discussion 137.

CHAPTER 42

Carotid artery stenting

Iqbal Malik

Introduction

'Primum non nocere'... first not to harm

Stroke is the third leading cause of death in the developed world. Internal carotid artery (ICA) stenosis is a major correctable cause of ischaemic stroke, the risk being related to the degree of stenosis and the presence of recent symptoms. Carotid endarterectomy (CEA) has become the preferred method of treatment for patients with asymptomatic or symptomatic high-grade ICA stenosis, supplanting medical therapy alone. In coronary disease, the increasing use of percutaneous coronary intervention (PCI) has reduced the need for coronary artery bypass surgery (CABG). Unlike coronary stenting, where immediate relief of anginal symptoms can justify the procedure, carotid intervention is not usually done for haemodynamic or flow indications, but to reduce future emboli. For significant (greater than 50% angiographic) ICA stenosis, carotid artery stenting (CAS) is a reasonable alternative to CEA, but its true place is as yet undecided, and awaits the conclusion of several ongoing randomized trials.

Background

Stroke is defined as a rapidly developing episode of focal loss of cerebral function for more than 24h, with no apparent cause other than being of vascular origin. There are 5–10 million stroke deaths/year worldwide, making it the third commonest cause of death, responsible for 7% of all deaths in the Western world[1,2].

Given that 20% of strokes are fatal and 50% of survivors have permanent disability, prevention is better than cure. Although seen as a disease of the older person, 25% of strokes occur in patients under the age of 65 years.

The risk factors for stroke are similar to those for coronary heart disease (CHD). Whilst smoking and diabetes form the bulk of modifiable risk for CHD, hypertension and atrial fibrillation are associated with the largest relative risk for stroke (Table 42.1). Alcohol excess produces differential risks of CHD and stroke, with moderate intake increasing stroke risk more than CHD risk. However, it is ICA stenosis that provides a correctable risk factor that is unique to stroke. Although over 80% of strokes are ischaemic, it is perhaps only 5% that are related to ICA stenosis[3].

Treatment options both for primary and secondary prevention are optimal medical therapy, CEA, or CAS. This chapter assesses the role of CAS in the treatment of ICA stenosis. Acute treatment of stroke, with thrombolysis or catheter-based interventions, although of considerable interest, are discussed elsewhere[4].

History

Atherosclerosis of the carotid bifurcation was suggested as a risk factor for stroke over 50 years ago[5]. It has been incriminated in causing symptoms such as amaurosis fugax (retinal embolism, transient ischaemic attack [TIA] (lasting <24h) and hemispheric stroke (lasting >24h).

Optimal medical therapy

Adequate blood pressure (BP) control, smoking cessation, and the detection and treatment of atrial fibrillation are basic requirements in both primary and secondary prevention (see Table 42.1).

Stroke risk rises with systolic BP above 115mmHg. Most guidelines suggest keeping the systolic BP <140mmHg in all, and <130mmHg in higher risk groups such as diabetic patients. Combining data from over 160 000 patients in randomized trials, the type of drug used appears less important than achieving BP control[6].

For patients in atrial fibrillation, the National Institute for Health and Clinical Excellence (NICE) guidelines clearly specify when warfarin therapy is warranted. Use of the CHAD2 score incorporating age, diabetes, hypertension, a history of congestive cardiac failure, and stroke/TIA, allows risk stratification to either aspirin

Table 42.1 Risk factors for stroke*

Risk factor	Relative risk	Estimated prevalence	Population attributable risk
Hypertension	1.4–4.0	20–60%	49–62%
Hypercholesterolaemia	1.0–2.0	6–40%	18–20%
Smoking	1.5–2.5	20–40%	12%
Atrial fibrillation	1.5–18.0	0.5–9%	9%
Heavy alcohol consumption	1.0–3.0	5–30%	5%

*Data from Gorelick *et al.*[144] and the AHA guidelines[145].

or warfarin therapy[7]. In those who have already had ischaemic stroke, all patients should be considered for warfarin therapy (http://guidance.nice.org.uk/CG36). There is no evidence for the use of warfarin or heparin outside the setting of atrial fibrillation.

Aspirin is validated therapy in stroke management[8]. Dipyridamole in combination with aspirin does appear to have some benefit and is currently the standard antiplatelet regimen for secondary prevention[9,10]. The use of clopidogrel on top of aspirin was tested in the MATCH trial and no benefit was found with the combination[11], whilst the PRoFESS trial also failed to show that clopidogrel monotherapy was better or worse than aspirin plus sustained release dipyridamole[12].

Lipid levels have a less firm association with stroke than with CHD. However, most trials have consistently shown the benefits of statin therapy on stroke as well as CHD reduction[13,14].

Carotid endarterectomy

Surgery for the treatment of atherosclerotic ICA stenosis was developed in the 1950s by Eastcott in the UK, and DeBakey in the USA[15,16]. Following this, CEA became a popular procedure amongst vascular surgeons well before the publication of randomized controlled trial data, and increased even further after these trials were reported[17–19].

Carotid artery stent

The role of CAS in non-atherosclerotic disease is reviewed elsewhere and will not be discussed in this chapter[20]. The report of first carotid angioplasty was published in 1983[21], with stenting becoming more popular in the early 1990s[22,23]. Given that embolic complications can result from such intervention, distal protection devices (DPDs) were developed in a primitive form in 1987[24]. It has really been the development of usable embolic protection devices in recent years that has lead to the rapid growth of CAS[25].

Patient selection

Three major patient groups need to be considered for carotid intervention: 1) the patient with symptomatic ICA stenosis; 2) one with an asymptomatic stenosis; and 3) finally the asymptomatic patient with one or two ICA stenoses detected prior to major cardiac surgery, a group known to be at high risk of perioperative stroke.

To answer the question of which treatment choice best suits each group, the development of PCI for single-vessel and multivessel coronary disease after the advent of CABG already provides a route map for collecting the evidence base. CABG was shown to be superior to medical therapy alone in multivessel disease[26]; then PCI was shown to be equivalent to surgery in terms of medium-term survival in most patient groups[27,28]. We need to consider how best medical therapy has been supplemented by CEA, and then if CAS has matched or superseded the results of CEA.

Symptomatic carotid stenosis

Three trials have addressed the benefit of the treatment of symptomatic ICA stenosis. The Veterans Administration (VA) trial was terminated early due to publication of the results of the other two[29–33] (see Table 42.2).

Table 42.2 Trials in symptomatic internal carotid artery stenosis: medical therapy versus carotid endarterectomy

Trial (year)	% stenosis	Time from CVA/TIA	30-day operative risk (CVA/death)	F/u period ipsilateral CVA/death	Medical Rx	CEA
NASCET[29]N = 659 (1991)	>70% Angiographic	<120 days	6.5%	5 years	28%	13%
NASCET[32]N = 858 (1998)	50–69% Angiographic	<120 days	6.7%	5 years	22.2%	15.7%
NASCET[32]N = 1368 (1998)	0–49% Angiographic	<120 days	6.7%	5 years	18.7%	14.9%
ECST[33]N = 3024 (1998)	>70–99% Duplex	<6 months	7.5%	3 years	26.5%	14.9%

CEA, carotid endarterectomy; CVA, cerebrovascular accident; F/u, follow-up; TIA, transient ischaemic attack.

The VA Carotid Endarterectomy Trial for Symptomatic Stenosis studied 190 symptomatic patients with carotid stenosis 50% or greater, randomized into medical or surgical therapy. At a mean follow-up of 11.9 months there was a significant reduction in stroke or crescendo TIA in patients who underwent CEA (7.7% vs. 19.4%). The relative risk reduction was 60% ($p = 0.011$). Due to early termination, it was underpowered to confirm the results[30].

The North American Symptomatic Carotid Endarterectomy Trial (NASCET) randomized 2885 patients with 30–99% ICA stenosis at angiography and recent stroke (CVA) or TIA to medical therapy or CEA. In patients with 70–99% stenosis, operation reduced 2-year ipsilateral CVA risk from 26% to 9% (relative risk reduction 65%) and combined major CVA and death rates from 13.1% to 2.5% (relative risk reduction 81%)[29]. In those with 50–69% stenosis, 5-year ipsilateral CVA risk was reduced from 22.2% to 15.7% (relative risk reduction 29%)[32]. There was no benefit in patients with stenosis <50%, although this group still had an event rate of 15–19% at 2 years, suggesting medical therapy also needed to be improved.

The European Carotid Surgery Trial (ECST) randomized 3024 patients with symptomatic ICA stenosis in a similar manner, using duplex ultrasound criteria of >60% stenosis[31,33]. In patients with 70–99% stenosis, at 3 years, risk of ipsilateral CVA was reduced from 16.8% to 10.3% (relative risk reduction 39%). Risk of major stroke or death was reduced from 11% to 6% (relative risk reduction 45%). There was no benefit in patients with <70% duplex stenosis.

A duplex stenosis of 70–75% equates to an angiographic stenosis of approximately 50%, providing consistency of evidence of benefit in symptomatic patients within the two completed trials. A meta-analysis of these trials suggested most benefit in men, those under 75 years, and those treated within 2 weeks of symptoms[34].

So, for symptomatic patients, a duplex stenosis of >70% should be treated to improve prognosis. American guidelines suggest that the surgeon should have <6% peri-procedural CVA and death rates for the procedure to be worthwhile[35]. If surgical event rates are too high, then the benefits in the long term are lost due to perioperative events. In addition to stroke and death, myocardial infarction (MI) can occur during and after CEA. However, the more common complications are of haematoma formation, and cranial nerve palsies, including damage to the recurrent laryngeal nerve, with the consequent effect on speech.

Asymptomatic carotid stenosis

The value of CEA in asymptomatic ICA stenosis is less clear. It has been recognized that stroke can occur for other reasons even if a carotid stenosis is present[36,37].

Screening for asymptomatic ICA stenosis

A recent US document has summarized the evidence base for screening for ICA stenosis[38]. Screening can be performed with physical examination or carotid ultrasound. Although physical examination (the presence of a bruit) makes a carotid stenosis more likely both its sensitivity and specificity are less than 50%. As for any screening strategy, to be worthwhile, it has to reduce the endpoint (in this case stroke rate), be able to detect the disease accurately, and not cause harm.

The most important risk factor for future stroke is a previous stroke, and thus a duplex scan is performed in almost all patients with hemispheric symptoms. The presence of heart disease doubles the risk for ICA stenosis[39]. Thus targeted screening in patients with peripheral vascular disease, coronary disease, or stroke may be of benefit[40]. On the other hand, the population prevalence of significant ICA stenosis appears to be <1% even over the age of 65[38]. Thus there appears to be little evidence for population screening for carotid disease to reduce stroke.

Trials in asymptomatic patients

Three small initial trials failed to show a benefit, but may have been underpowered to do so[41–43]. However, there are now two larger trials which have shown positive results[44,45] (Table 42.3).

The Asymptomatic Carotid Atherosclerosis Study (ACAS) studied 1662 patients under the age of 80 years with greater than 60% ultrasound stenosis, randomizing them to CEA or medical therapy[44]. At 5 years, the risk of ipsilateral CVA or death was reduced from 11% to 5.1% by CEA ($p = 0.004$). The value of the procedure in women was not proven.

The Asymptomatic Carotid Surgery Trial (ACST) randomized 3120 patients, and again used greater than 60% stenosis on ultrasound as the entry criterion, and showed that after 5 years, ipsilateral CVA or death rate was reduced from 11.8% to 6.4% by CEA($p < 0.001$)[45].

So, in asymptomatic patients, a duplex stenosis of more than 60% could be treated, if the patient is male, less than 80 years old, and has a good chance of living for 5 years. Since the benefit was mainly in those with greater than 75% duplex stenosis, this is a more robust cut-off to use, matching an angiographic stenosis of 50% by NASCET criteria (Fig. 42.1).

Table 42.3 Trials in asymptomatic internal carotid artery stenosis: medical therapy versus carotid endarterectomy. The CASANOVA trial was criticized for a large cross-over to surgery in the medical arm, whilst the VACS trial had a very high event rate in both arms at 5 years

Trial (year)	% stenosis	30-day operative risk (CVA/death)	F/u period ipsilateral CVA/death	Medical Rx	CEA	Relative risk reduction
CASANOVA[41] N = 334 (1991)	>50% Angiographic	3.2%	3 years	10.7%	11.3%	0.94 (0.57–1.98)
VACS[42] N = 444 (1993)	>50% Angiographic	4.7%	5 years	44.2%	41.2%	0.92 (0.69–1.22)
ACAS[44] N = 1662 (1995)	>60% Angiographic	2.3%	5 years	11%	5.1%	0.53 (0.22–0.72)
ACST[45] N = 3120 (2004)	>60% Angiographic	3.1%	5 years	11.8%	6.4%	0.46

CEA, carotid endarterectomy; CVA, cerebrovascular accident; F/u, follow-up.

It should be recalled that the background event rate is <less than 2% stroke risk per year, which would be reduced to 1% by the procedure. This compares well with the risk reductions offered by lipid-lowering therapy, or the benefit of clopidogrel over aspirin in patients with vascular disease[46,47]. Based on these trials, US guidelines suggest that the surgeon should have a less than 3% peri-procedural CVA and death rate for asymptomatic patients for the procedure to be useful (see Table 42.3)[35].

In addition, the risk of intervention in patients outside trials should not be underestimated. A study of event rates after CEA suggested that although mortality was 0.1% in the ACAS trial and 0.6% in NASCET, outside of the trial patients, the NASCET hospitals had a mortality for CEA of 1.4%, whilst low volume non-trial hospitals had a mortality of 2.5%[48]. In addition, when looking at neurological event rates, self-reporting of data to national registries is flawed. Full assessment by a neurologist both before and after helps to detect all events that may have occurred and has been shown to elevate reported event rates[49]. There has to be certainty that the operator is able to deliver measurable low event rates (<3% death/stroke rate at 30 days) if an asymptomatic patient is to gain benefit.

Pre-cardiac surgery

In addition to a 1–2% morality rate, the average risk of stroke after CABG is about 2%. Risk factors include age, recent symptoms of cerebrovascular disease, and presence of a carotid bruit. Patients with asymptomatic ICA stenoses face enhancing this risk further[50]. About 8% of patients undergoing CABG have a significant (>50%) ICA stenosis[51]. A tight (>80%) stenosis was found in 4%, with bilateral tight disease or a tight stenosis plus an occlusion in 0.5%[52]. The calculated stroke risk for an asymptomatic patient with unilateral stenosis is 3%, for bilateral stenosis 5.2%, and for a stenosis with a contralateral occlusion is 11%. In symptomatic patients the stroke rate is at least 8%. CABG mortality is also increased in the presence of ICA stenosis to 4.4%[53].

However, whether carotid intervention is beneficial in some or all these cases is controversial, since the intervention itself can carry a higher risk in the presence of severe cardiac disease[54]. A systematic review of

NASCET (% stenosis)	ECST (% stenosis)
30	65
40	70
50	75
60	80
70	85
80	91
90	97

A

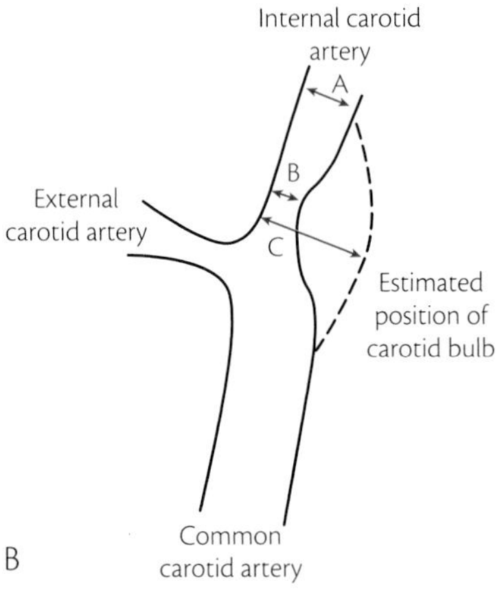

B

Fig. 42.1 A) Comparison of measurement of ICA stenosis using NASCET (angiographic) or ECST (Duplex ultrasound) criteria. Data from Rothwell *et al.*[149]. B) NASCET = $\frac{A-B}{C}$ ECST= $\frac{C-B}{C}$

Table 42.4 Carotid intervention in patients awaiting CABG*

Strategy	Number of cases	Operative death rate	30-day death/ any stroke	30-day death/ any stroke/MI
Synchronous CEA and CABG—pre bypass	5386	4.5%	8.2%	11.5%
Synchronous CEA and CABG—on bypass	844	4.7%	8.1%	9.5%
Synchronous CEA and off-pump CABG	324	1.5%	2.2%	3.6%
Staged CEA then CABG	917	3.9%	6.1%	10.2%
Staged CABG then CEA	302	2.0%	7.3%	5.0%
CAS then CABG	760	5.5%	9.1%	9.4%

*Adapted from Naylor *et al.*[56]. Note that the data sets are not directly comparable.
CABG, coronary artery bypass graft; CAS, carotid artery stent; CEA, carotid endarterectomy; MI, myocardial infarction.

nearly 9000 patients has suggested that the strategy of simultaneous or staged CEA plus CABG carries a combined risk of death, MI, or stroke of 10–12%[55]. There is some evidence that synchronous CEA with off-pump surgery might have lower risk than on-pump surgery, but these reports may well reflect publication bias and selection of lower risk cases for off-pump surgery[56] (Table 42.4).

Systematic review of the data from 277 patients in six retrospective studies on CAS in conjunction with CABG has suggested that the death/stroke/MI event rate is also about 12%, with a combined stroke rate of 6%, and a death rate post CABG of 4.1%[57]. The patients waited about 1 month post CAS to have CABG. There were six deaths (2.2%), all due to coronary events, in this waiting period. Given that these event rates are similar to those without any carotid intervention, it is hard to argue for CAS, at least for unilateral stenosis or bilateral disease without occlusion. In an updated review of patients requiring CABG, the rate of death/MI/CVA was 9.4% by 30 days post CABG, with mortality 5.5%[56]. Performing CAS and then operating within 48h did not appear to influence outcome, suggesting that delaying the CABG may not be necessary, although this was based on small numbers of patients.

Screening for carotid stenosis prior to cardiac surgery thus remains useful despite the lack of data on intervention, as knowledge of the risk of stroke will guide therapy. Carotid duplex scanning provides the most accessible screening tool. Treatment will only ever result in the prevention of about 40% of strokes as the effects of crossclamping with aortic atheroma, atrial fibrillation, and other factors will remain[58]. If intervention is needed, CAS appears equivalent to CEA performed with CABG, but the data on off-pump surgery to reduce stroke risk need to be explored further. In this situation of combined carotid and coronary disease, consideration might be given to a strategy of PCI instead for CABG, rather than trying to intervene on the asymptomatic carotid stenosis.

The restenotic lesion—after CEA

When discussing the treatment of restenotic lesions in the ICA, the data is limited. Restenosis in the first few years after CEA or CAS tends to be due to intimal hyperplasia. In later years, the pathology tends to be indistinguishable from atherosclerosis[59–61].

Data on the incidence after CEA suggests a restenosis rate of up to 14%[59,62] but with neurological event rates of only 1–5%. Data from the ACAS study suggests that most of the recurrence is within the first 18 months (7.6%) with a further 1.9% up to 5 years of follow-up[63]. Detection is with surveillance duplex scanning, undertaken at 6-monthly intervals for the first 2 years, and then annually. There has been a vogue to treat both symptomatic restenosis (which seems justified just as it is for first-time de novo ICA lesions), but also high grade (>80%) restenosis. Data to provide an evidence base for this latter approach are lacking. If intervention is planned, both repeat CEA, first reported in 1976[64], and CAS[65] have been performed. CEA reoperation carries higher risks that the first procedure for wound haematoma, transient cranial nerve injuries, but probably not stroke[61]. In 116 reoperations, 19.6% had cranial nerve injuries compared to 9% in the CAVATAS trial[61,66]. Thus there is some consensus that CAS (if available) be the treatment of choice in restenosis after CEA[67].

Trials of CAS versus CEA

The explosion in use of PCI has in part been the result of trials showing equivalent death and MI rates comparing

Table 42.5 Possible indication to perform CAS rather than CEA*

Condition	Details
High medical comorbidity	◆ Age >80 ◆ Coronary disease (CAD) with acute myocardial infarction <4 weeks ago ◆ CAD with CABG <6 months ago ◆ Congestive cardiac failure ◆ Dialysis-dependant renal failure ◆ Chronic airways disease (FEV1 <1L) ◆ Uncontrolled diabetes mellitus
Local surgical factors	◆ Restenosis after endarterectomy (CEA) ◆ Radiation-induced carotid stenosis ◆ Anatomically high ICA stenosis (above C2) ◆ Prior neck scarring or surgery ◆ Contralateral recurrent laryngeal nerve (RLN) injury ◆ Contralateral ICA occlusion

CABG, coronary artery bypass graft; CAD, coronary artery disease; CAS, carotid artery stent; CEA, carotid endarterectomy; FEV1, forced expiratory volume in 1s.
Adapted from Veith et al. [67].

CABG and PCI. It was seen as unethical to try to show PCI was better than medical therapy when CABG had become a validated treatment for CAD[27,28]. In a similar way, trials of CAS versus medical therapy are unlikely to be performed, at least in symptomatic patients. Thus, ongoing trials need to confirm that CEA and CAS are equivalent if CAS is to become the default treatment for ICA stenosis. There are patients, however, who have been shown to be at elevated operative risk, and who might benefit more from a percutaneous approach if risks were shown to be lower[68–70] (Table 42.5).

CEA carries risks, including CVA, surgical haematoma, cranial nerve injury and, of course, risks related to anaesthesia[71]. These risks in real-life practice are higher than those reported in the trials, both due to selection of lower risk patients for trials, and indeed selection of operators, since the best and largest volume operators often participate in these studies[48]. Development of local anaesthetic CEA has not been proven to reduce these risks as assessed by the revised Cochrane review in 2008. The death rate, for example, was about 1.3% in both groups[72].

The same operator volume-dependency has also been seen for CAS, with early cases having a higher complication rate than later ones: the so called 'learning curve'[73]. Even in early experience of 528 cases of CAS from Roubin *et al.*[73] however, the relative safety of CAS became clear. Despite 83% of the symptomatic patients being ineligible for CEA by NASCET criteria due to comorbidity, 30-day CVA and death rates were 7.4%, comparable to the CEA arm of the NASCET trial[29].

Symptomatic carotid stenosis

There are now several published randomized trials of CAS versus CEA. Very early trials were stopped because of high event rates in the CAS arm[74–76]. More recent trials, 2001 onwards, are summarized in Table 42.6.

The Carotid and Vertebral Artery Transluminal Angioplasty Study (CAVATAS) randomized 504 patients with symptomatic ICA stenosis to balloon angioplasty (only 26% got a stent) or CEA[66]. This showed that 30-day stroke and death rates were equivalent in both arms at 9%, but that haematomas and cranial nerve injuries were higher in the CEA arm. Although it was argued that the perioperative risk was higher than expected in the CEA arm, these were experienced surgeons who had participated in previous trials, and in fact it was CAS, which was a novel procedure still, without the use of DPDs, that should have been at a disadvantage.

The Stenting and Angioplasty with Protection in Patients at High Risk for Endarterectomy (SAPPHIRE) study was the first trial to compare modern CAS with use of DPDs with CEA[77]. All patients were considered high risk (see Table 42.5). A total of 723 patients were enrolled with >50% symptomatic or >80% asymptomatic angiographic stenosis of the ICA. Of these, 307 were randomized to CAS or CEA. However, 409 were considered unsuitable for CEA and were put in the CAS registry, whilst only seven patients were considered unsuitable for CAS, and were placed in the CEA registry. All CAS procedures were done with the AngioGuard® DPD and Precise® stent (Cordis, Johnson and Johnson). The combined outcome of 30-day stroke and death rate was seen in 4.8% for CAS versus 5.6% for CEA (p = ns). More interestingly, the rate in the CAS registry was only 3%. MI was defined as rise of creatinine kinase twice the upper limit of normal. Although the MI rate was 0% in the stent arm versus 1.2% after CEA, this was also not significant. However, the primary endpoint of the study (30-day combined death/CVA/MI) occurred in 5.8% of the CAS group versus 12.6% of the CEA group ($p = 0.047$). The same trend was seen in asymptomatic and symptomatic patients, and was maintained at 1 year.

The EVA-3S trial was conducted only in France and was stopped early due to a high event rate in the CAS arm[78,79]. The 30-day death/stroke rate was 9.6% for CAS and 3.9% for CEA. The reason for the high event

Table 42.6 Trials of symptomatic ICA stenosis: CAS versus CEA

Trial (year)	% stenosis	Time from CVA/TIA	Operative risk (CVA/death)	30-day CVA/death/MI	F/u	F/u period CVA/death
CAVATAS[66,146] N = 505 (2001)	Mean 86%	<1 year	CAS 10% CEA 9.9% (ns)	CAS 10% CEA 10.7% (ns)	8 years	CAS 11.3% CEA 8.6% (ns) (ipsilateral stroke data only)
CARESS[147] N = 439 (2003)	Sympt >50% Asympt >80%	68% asymptomatic	CAS 2.1% CEA 3.6% (ns)	CAS 2.1% CEA 4.4 % (ns)	1year	CAS 10% CEA 13.6% (ns)
SAPPHIRE[77] N = 334 (2004)	Sympt >50% Asympt >80%	Sympt + asympt	CAS 4.8% CEA 5.6%	CAS 4.8% CEA 9.8% (p = 0.09)	3 years	CAS 24.6% CEA 26.2% –
EVA-3S[78,79] N = 527 (2006)	>60%	<4 months	CAS 9.6% CEA 3.9%	–	4 years	CAS 11% CEA 6.2% (p = 0.03)
SPACE[80,81] N = 1183 (2006)	>70%	<180 days	CAS 6.84% CEA 6.34% (ns)	–	2 years	CAS 9% CEA 8% (ns)
ICSS[87] N = 1713 (2009)	>50%	<1 year	CAS 7.4% CEA 3.4% (p <0.001)	CAS 7.4% CEA 4% (p = 0.004)	TBA	TBA

CAS, carotid artery stent; CEA, carotid endarterectomy; CVA, cerebrovascular accident; F/u, follow-up; MI, myocardial infarction; ns, not significant; TBA, to be announced.

rate in the stent arm (the same as in CAVATAS, incidentally) was investigated, but could not be linked to patient characteristics, operator volume, or other factors.

The SPACE trial was designed as a non-inferiority trial, and was stopped early after 1200 patients as it was felt that enough patients would not be recruited to reach its primary endpoint[80,81]. The death/stroke rate at 30 days was 7.7% for CAS and 6.5% for CEA. The wide confidence intervals meant that no conclusions could be drawn from it, but it certainly failed to confirm the non-inferiority of CAS compared to CEA. Again similar results were seen at 2 years.

The Acculink for Revascularisation in High-Risk Patients (ARCHER) Registry further examined the role of CAS with DPDs. High risk was defined as in SAPPHIRE or any of the following: two-vessel coronary disease, uncontrolled diabetes mellitus, and dialysis dependence. Combined death/CVA/MI rate at 30 days was 8.3%, similar to that in the SAPPHIRE Registry[82].

Several meta-analyses have recently tried to combine the results[83–85]. The latest of these suggests that CEA and CAS are equivalent in terms of death and MI rates (within a error range of ± 2%) but that no comment could be made on stroke due to lack of sufficient data[85]. The difficulty in comparing these two treatments is highlighted by the fact that the benefits of CEA over medical therapy were based on 3202 strokes and deaths[34] whilst conclusions about the relative merits of CEA and CAS are being made on a total of 210 strokes and deaths[84] (Fig. 42.2).

The results of further ongoing trials are therefore awaited. For symptomatic patients, the Carotid REvascularisarion Endarterectomy vs Stent (CREST) Trial (http://www.cresttrial.org) will target >50% (>70% on duplex) ICA stenosis within 180 days of a cerebrovascular event, but also include asymptomatic patients with greater than 60% angiographic stenosis (70% on duplex)[86]. Planned enrolment is 2500 patients.

The International Carotid Stent or Surgery (ICSS) Trial (http//www.cavatas.com) has recently presented data for symptomatic patients in Europe, North America, and Australia[87]. It provides the largest cohort to date of symptomatic patients treated with either modality and in conjunction with an updated meta-analysis will help to guide the future of CAS. Full results are not yet available, but at the European Stroke Meeting

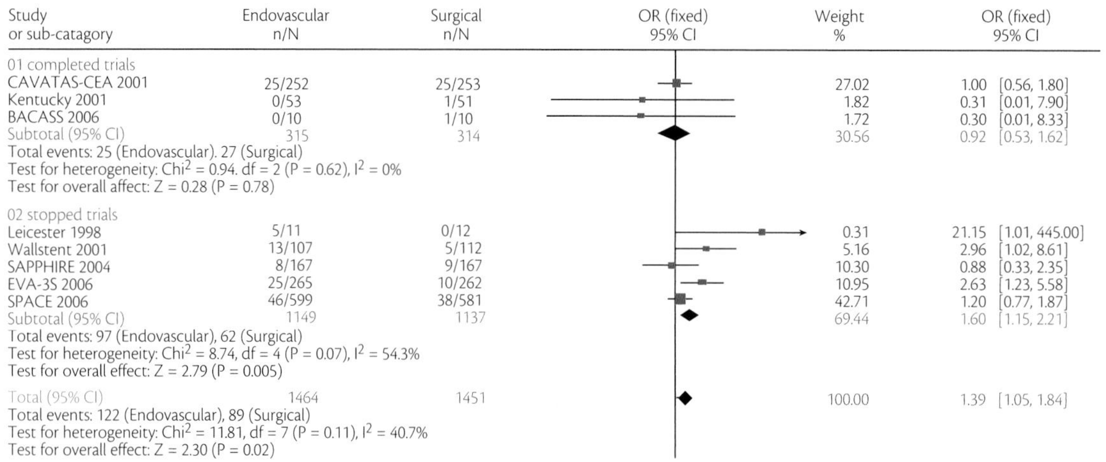

Fig. 42.2 Meta-analysis of trials of CEA versus CAS. Data from Ederle J, Featherstone RL, Brown MM. Percutaneous transluminal angioplasty and stenting for carotid artery stenosis. *Cochrane Database Syst Rev* 2007; **4**:CD000515. Copyright © 2009 The Cochrane Collaboration.

in 2009, results appeared in favour of CEA over CAS, at least in centres performing fewer than 50 CAS procedures per year. The rate of stroke or death at 30 days was 7.4% for CAS versus 3.4% for CEA (risk ratio 2.1, p <0.001), driven mainly by a higher rate of non-disabling stroke in the CAS arm[(88)].

Asymptomatic carotid stenosis

For asymptomatic patients, the Asymptomatic Carotid Surgery Trial-2 (ACST-2) and the Carotid Stenting versus Surgery of Severe Carotid Artery Disease and Stroke Prevention in Asymptomatic Patients (ACT-1) trials have begun recruitment, but will not report for several years[(89)]. The Transatlantic Asymptomatic Carotid Intervention Trial (TACIT) also hopes to provide answers to the question of whether medical therapy is in fact as good as CEA or CAS in asymptomatic patients (Table 42.7).

The restenotic lesion-after CAS

Stents reduce restenosis compared to balloon angioplasty in the ICA. In the CAVATAS trial, up to 8 years follow-up, restenosis (>70%) for CEA was 14%, for CAS was 17%, but with angioplasty without stent was 34%[(90)]. The rate of >80% restenosis has been estimated at 6.4% at 5 years of follow-up in registry data[(91,92)]. This would not matter if restenosis was always asymptomatic. The CAVATAS data suggests that restenosis >50% does carry some risk—the rate of ipsilateral vascular events in follow-up was 10.7% if there was no restenosis versus 22.7% with restenosis (p = 0.02).

Table 42.7 Ongoing trials of asymptomatic ICA stenosis: CAS versus CEA

Trial	% stenosis	CEA:CAS	30-day risk (CVA/death/MI)	FU	Endpoint ipsilateral stroke
CREST N = 1100	Sympt >50% Asympt >60%	1:1	–	4 years	–
ACT 1 N = 1540	>80%	1:3	–	1 year	–
TACIT N = 2400	>70%	1:1:1 Medical arm also	–	3 years	–
ACST-2 N = 5000	>70%	1:1	–	5 years	–

Restenosis occurs more often if the stent was placed for a restenotic lesion, and in patients with diabetes[93]. Progression to occlusion in in-stent restenosis is more likely if the restenosis is diffuse and extending outside of the stent.

It has been suggested that 6-monthly duplex scans be utilized for follow-up after CAS[94]. Detection of restenosis remains an issue. Placing a stent alters the fluid dynamics in the carotid artery, making velocity criteria for stenosis that exist for native ICA stenosis invalid. The stent struts make two-dimensional imaging difficult. Angiographic validation studies have suggested very variable cut-off recommended for peak systolic velocities in the ICA. (This area is reviewed in Lal *et al.*[94,95]) Suspicion of high-grade (>70%) stenosis should lead to computed tomography (CT) angiogram confirmation, or invasive angiography, although of course this carries a risk of complications.

For symptomatic stenosis, repeat intervention seems appropriate as for restenosis post CEA and native ICA disease. For asymptomatic restenosis, data to confirm the benefits of reintervention are lacking. If cerebral blood supply is felt to be jeopardized by restenosis, perhaps because of poor collaterals in the circle of Willis, then repeat intervention may be more justified. Both balloon angioplasty with or without stent[96,97] and CEA[98] have been used, but the CEA is more challenging as the original stent has to be removed.

Key investigations

Carotid duplex scanning

Due to ease of access, the carotid duplex ultrasound scan has become the screening tool of choice (Fig. 42.3). Two meta-analyses have suggested its sensitivity at detecting an ICA stenosis of 70–99% on invasive angiography was 86–90% with specificity 87–94%[99,100]. There is considerable skill involved in performing and interpreting the scan, however, and trust has to be developed with the ultrasonographer. Repeat scans at different institutions can produce widely varying results[100]. It should include two-dimensional measurements, but also velocity measurements in assessing stenosis in the carotid bulb and both higher and lower in the carotid circulation. In addition, flow in the vertebral artery is assessed. Attempts have been made to try to improve plaque characterization, and these may develop further with the advent of virtual histology. There is some data to suggest that plaque morphology predicts outcome after intervention, although greater experience and use of proximal protection devices might significantly diminish this risk[101,102].

Invasive angiography

Selective angiography for assessing ICA stenosis carries a risk of TIA and CVA, and so is now rarely performed except in those with inconclusive non-invasive results (Fig. 42.4). The risks are higher in those with highly significant (>90%) stenoses and permanent (>7 days) neurological deficit can occur in up to 2.5% of cases[103]. Using arch aortography and digital subtraction and intravenous contrast, non-selective images can be obtained to allow measurement of stenosis. However, these methods have not been widely validated[104].

Magnetic resonance angiography

Access to magnetic resonance angiography (MRA) is limited in the UK, but can produce excellent images of the aortic arch, great vessels, and intra-cerebral vasculature (Fig. 42.5A). Decisions on treatment may be swayed by the presence or absence of intracerebral collaterals from the circle of Willis. However, pseudostenoses can result from movement artefact. If combined with MRI brain imaging, this may become the best investigation after carotid duplex screening (Fig. 42.5B).

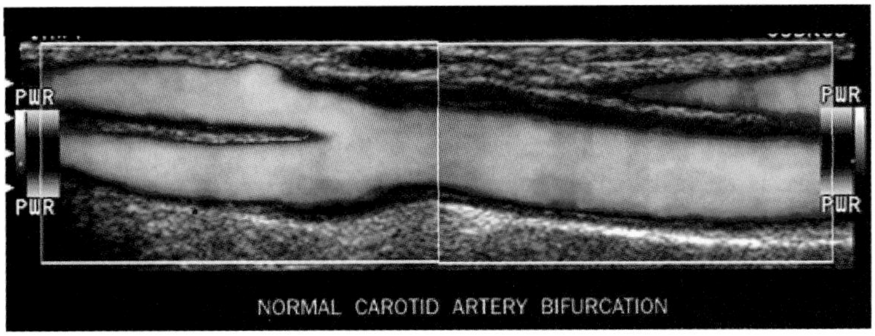

Fig. 42.3 Carotid duplex scanning.

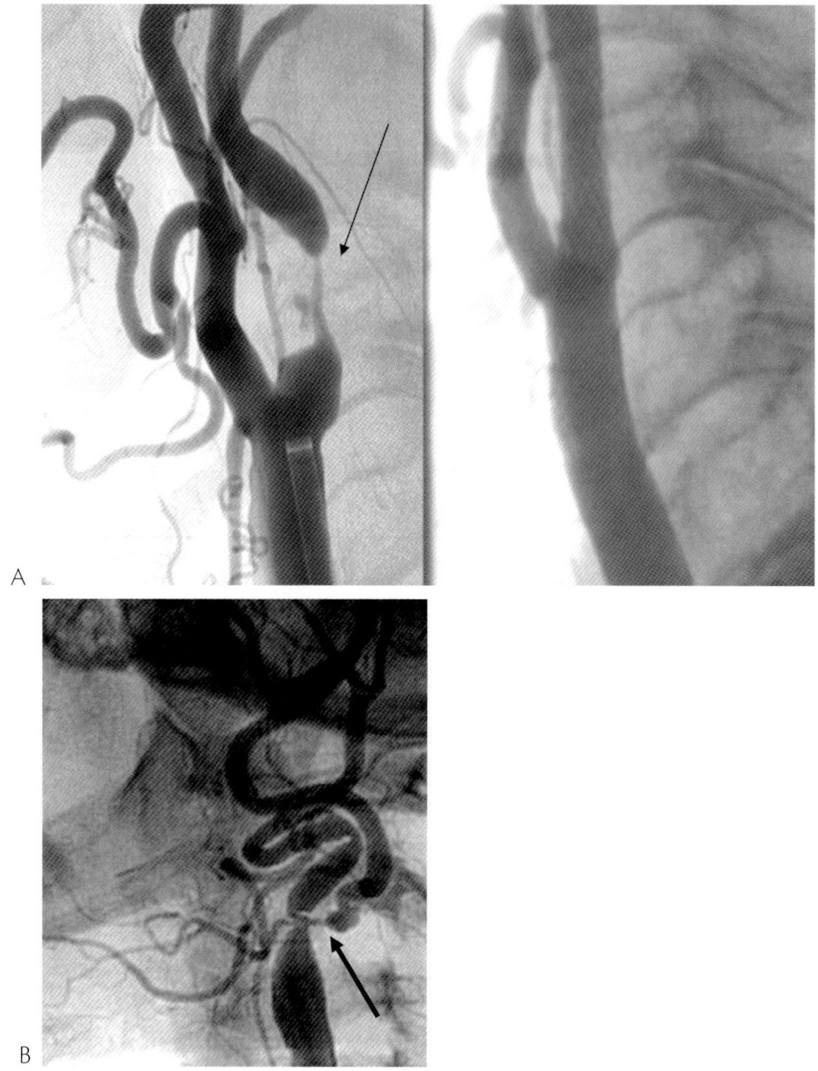

Fig. 42.4 A) Invasive carotid angiography with digital subtraction showing a tight ICA stenosis (before and after stenting). B) Invasive angiogram of an ICA stenosis not favourable for stenting.

CT angiography

With the advent of multislice CT, detailed imaging of the arch and great vessels can be achieved (Fig. 42.6). In addition, the intracerebral circulation can be imaged. Invasive angiography remains as the gold standard, but image quality is rapidly improving allowing accurate assessment of the stenosis, as well as plaque composition. Sensitivity for a 70–99% ICA stenosis is rated at 85% and specificity at 92%(105). The main limitations of CT compared to MRI scanning is that brain imaging is less detailed, and, of course, the radiation dose. As for invasive angiography, the percent stenosis needs to be calculated with reference to the distal diameter of the ICA (NASCET measurement), although, given that the cross-section of the ICA stenosis is available, the equivalent to the duplex stenosis (ECST measurement) can also be assessed(106) (see Fig. 42.1).

Summary of imaging techniques

The ever increasing number of methods for assessment of carotid stenosis has led to controversy about the gold standard. Good quality comparative studies are lacking(104). As the major trials have used duplex scanning or intra-arterial invasive angiography, new techniques will need to be validated against these until they too have been used to independently select patients for

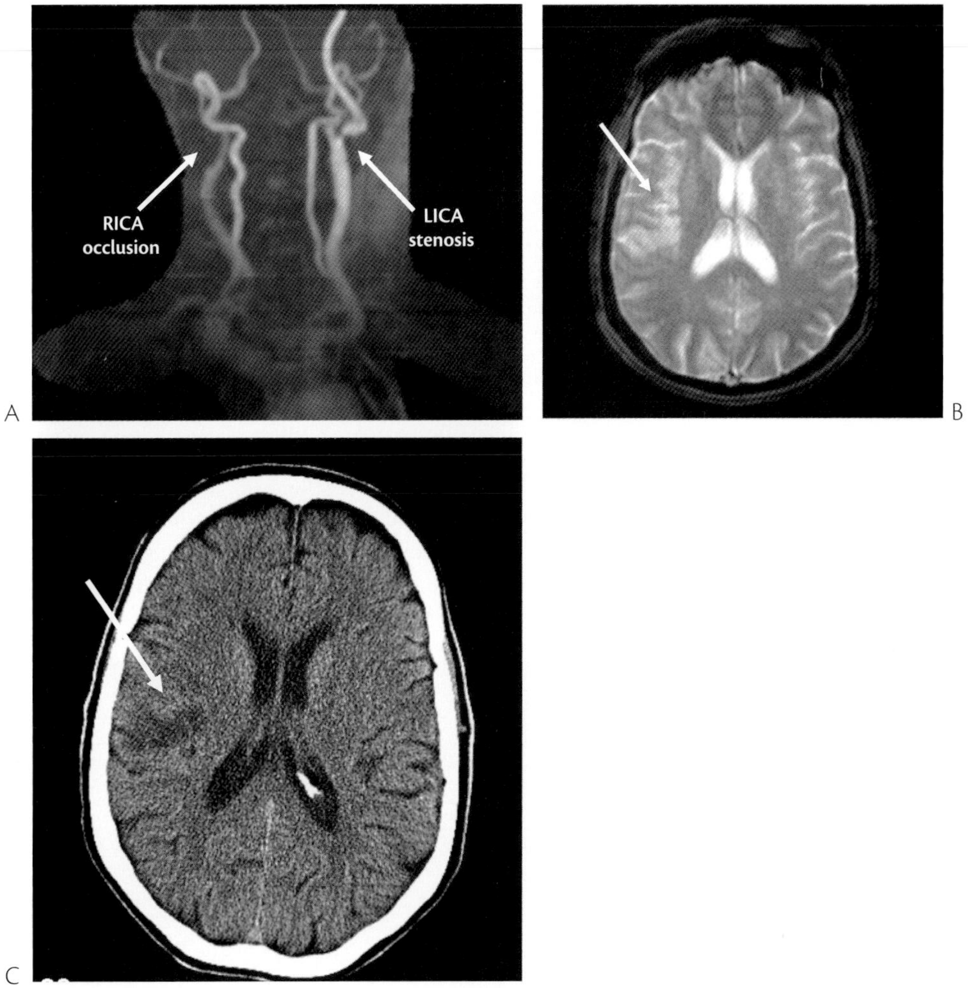

Fig. 42.5 A) MRA of carotid arteries: LICA stenosis. RICA occluded. B) MRI showing right middle cerebral artery infarct (arrow). The imaging is clearer than on CT scanning (panel C). C) CT scan of right middle cerebral artery infarct (arrow). The imaging is not as clear as on the MRI scan (panel B).

intervention with proven improvement in outcome. Units will vary as to which technique to rely upon, but duplex scanning will remain the best method of initial assessment, being non-invasive, repeatable, and hopefully reproducible. Knowledge of the anatomy and lesion type assist in making the final decision between stenting and surgery as both are thought to be associated with elevated risk during CAS[101,102,107].

Technique for CAS

Planning and pre-treatment

Once the patient has been reviewed by the multidisciplinary team (MDT), and accepted for stenting, the imaging should be reviewed again by the interventionalist performing the case. Knowledge of the anatomy of the peripheral access vessels (usually femoral), arch, and cervical vessels allows appropriate planning. With the advent of simulators allowing case scenarios, a virtual procedure might be performed in high-risk cases to assess equipment choices[108](Fig. 42.7).

Preoperative medication

The patient should be adequately hydrated as with all vascular catheterization procedures, and renal protection given if there is known renal dysfunction. Use of N-acetyl-cysteine (NAC) is still controversial, but is usually given at 600mg bd starting the day before

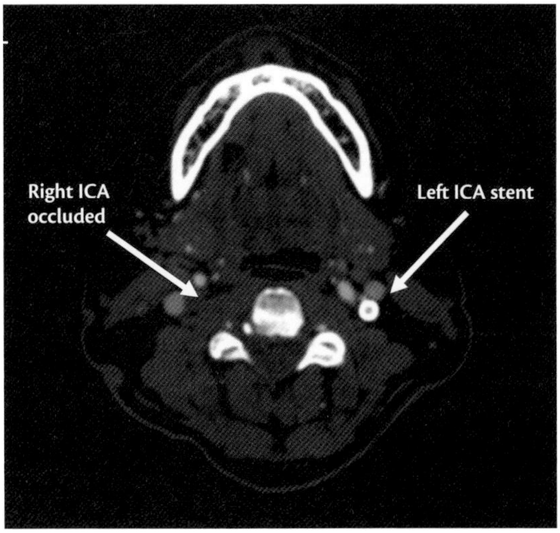

Fig. 42.6 CT angiogram of a left ICA stent. Image quality is improved with multislice scanning.

the procedure[109]. Aspirin and clopidogrel need to be initiated at least 24h prior to the procedure. A loading dose of 300mg of each is given if the patient is not on them regularly, with 75 once daily thereafter. Antihypertensive medication is reviewed, and the beta-blocker stopped for the day of the procedure. The aim is to have a systolic pressure between 120–180mmHg at the start of the procedure, given that perioperative hypotension can occur.

Perioperative medication

Unfractionated heparin (UFH) is administered, prior to attempting to cannulate the common carotid, artery at a dose of 70–100U/kg. The activated clotting time (ACT) should be maintained at 250–300s. If the procedure is prolonged for >1h, then the ACT should be rechecked and more heparin given if required.

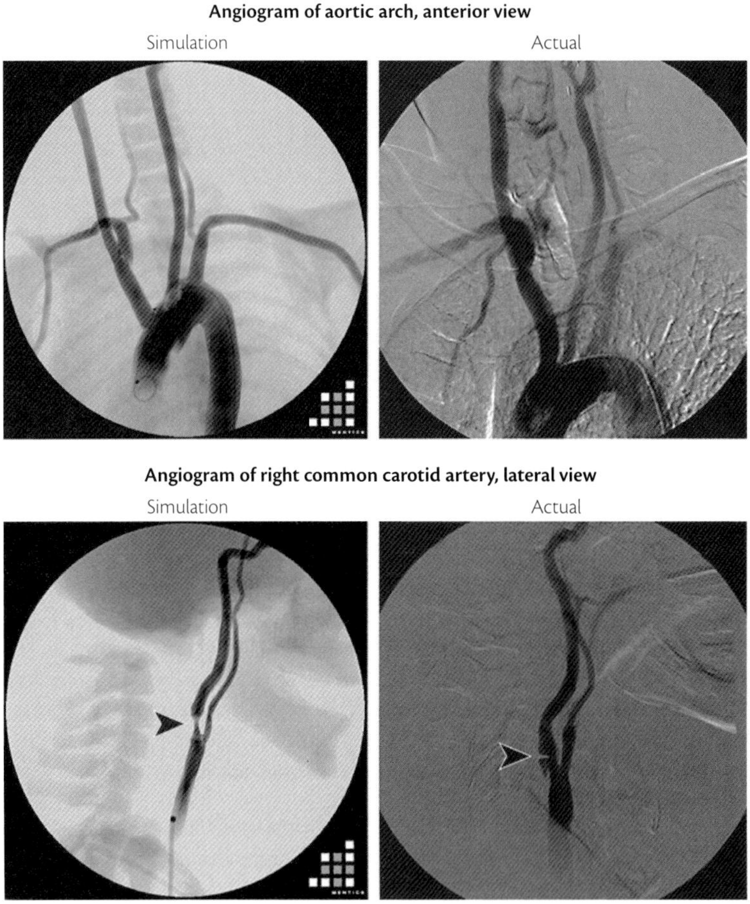

Fig. 42.7 Virtual reality simulation of real-life scenario. Reproduced with permission from Cates CU, Patel AD, Nicholson WJ. Use of virtual reality simulation for mission rehearsal for carotid stenting. *JAMA* 2007; **297**(3):265–6.

Although data is limited, if heparin cannot be tolerated, bivalirudin (Angiomax®, The Medicines Company, USA) provides an alternative. A bolus of 0.75mg/kg is followed by 1.75mg/kg/h infusion for the duration of the procedure[110,111].

Use of adjunctive pharmacology has improved outcomes in PCI. Data in CAS suggests that use of DPDs gives greater benefit than use of glycoprotein IIb/IIIa agents, and in large series, no benefit from these agents has yet been shown[112,113].There is a danger of haemorrhagic transformation if embolic stroke occurs with these agents on board. However, they may find a place *in addition* to DPDs to reduce platelet aggregation within the filter device, and when an obvious thrombotic complication has occurred[112,114].

Gaining a stable working platform

The patient should be comfortable with a head cushion to maintain a stable position. There should be electrocardiographic and haemodynamic monitoring attached as bradycardia and hypotension are not uncommon during the procedure. An intravenous line should be available and functional. In some laboratories, the patient is given a noise-making device in the contralateral hand to the ICA being treated, to provide an audio clue to neurological decline during the procedure. This is usually supplemented by communication with the patient during the case to assess speech and cognitive function, and sedation is thus kept to a minimum.

A standard technique should be employed to gain familiarity with the approach. Although radial access CAS was first described in 1999, and has been suggested as feasible, the femoral approach—to increase catheter support, and allow larger stents to be placed—remains the standard approach[115–117]. Direct cervical access to the common carotid artery with subsequent percutaneous completion has also been tried, but requires surgical expertise[118].

Femoral access is gained with a Seldinger technique and a 6–8F sheath. A 5F pigtail catheter is used to perform a non-selective arch aortogram if this has not been done as part of the work-up. Once the origin of the great arteries has been visualized, a 5F diagnostic guide catheter is used to gain access to the innominate artery (if treating the right ICA) or left common carotid artery (CCA) in the left anterior oblique (LAO) position (see Fig. 42.8) Problems arise with a bovine origin of the left CCA (take-off from innominate artery) or origin of the innominate artery from the earlier part of the ascending aorta (a type III arch).

Once the CCA is intubated, images are taken of the carotid stenosis in two planes to define the severity of the stenosis and the best image to separate the origin of the external carotid artery (ECA). This might require lateral, LAO, anteroposterior (AP), or right anterior oblique (RAO) projection. In addition, lateral and AP projections of the intracerebral vessels are taken to compare to run-off at the end in case of complications.

A 0.035-inch 190cm Terumo® guide wire is used to help advance the 5F diagnostic catheter into the ECA. This is made easier if road mapping is available. Care needs to be taken to avoid inadvertently crossing the ICA stenosis with the Terumo® wire. The 5F catheter is then advanced into the ECA, and the Terumo® wire exchanged for an 0.035-inch 300cm stiff Amplatzer wire. This allows the support needed to pass either a sheath or a guide catheter into the CCA. Most commonly, the procedure in the hands of radiologists involves a long sheath as the conduit, whilst cardiologists prefer a 7F or 8F guide catheter. Care needs to be taken not to perforate a branch of the ECA with the stiff wire. The stiff wire is then withdrawn and an image or road map of the lesion taken to allow easy passage of the angioplasty wire or embolic protection device (DPD).

An alternative to a guide catheter is to use a shuttle sheath, which may be preloaded on the diagnostic 5F-glide catheter. Once entry into the ECA is achieved with the glide catheter, the 6F or 7F 90-cm sheath is again positioned in the CCA below the carotid bifurcation, taking care not to disturb the ICA stenosis with the introducer.

The image intensifier is now positioned to image the lesion and the ICA at least to the base of the skull and allow an embolic protection device to be placed.

Protection or not?

Micro-embolization is thought to be the major cause of perioperative neurological complications during CAS[119]. Transcranial Doppler measurements suggest that without distal protection, the incidence of micro-embolization is higher with CAS than CEA[120]. Thus prevention of distal embolization would seem logical.

This can be achieved with distal filter devices, distal occlusion devices, or proximal occlusion devices. (For a full review of this subject see Boisiers *et al.*[121]) (Table 42.8). Most cardiologists are likely to prefer distal protection filters due to their familiarity with them. Large-scale trials comparing outcomes with and without distal protection are lacking, but registry data suggests that some form of protection device should be

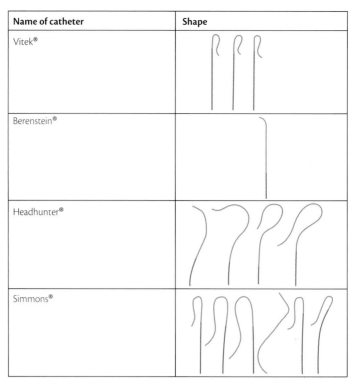

Name of catheter	Shape
Vitek®	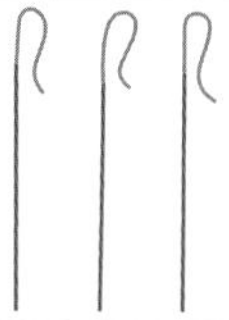
Berenstein®	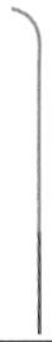
Headhunter®	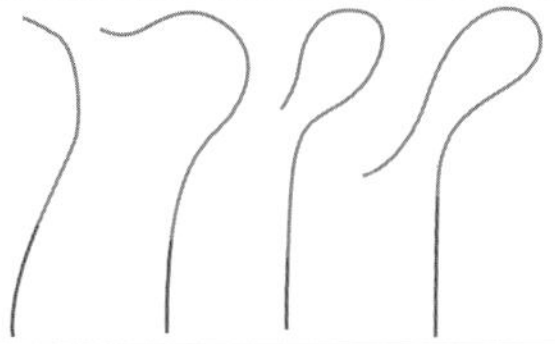
Simmons®	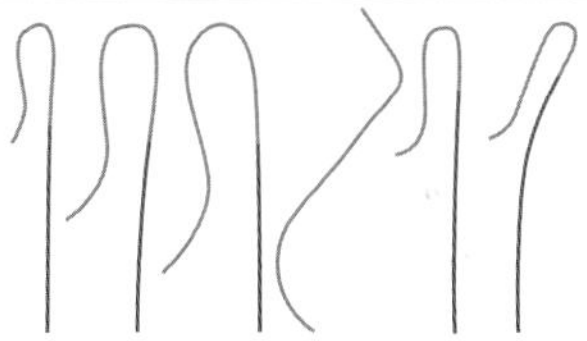

Fig. 42.8 Diagnostic catheters used to intubate the great vessels.

used in most cases. Event rates (30-day stroke and death) in symptomatic patients having CAS in the pre-protection era were 6.7% versus 2.82% in the modern age[122]. For asymptomatic patients, rates were 3.97% and 1.75% respectively.

Distal balloon occlusion requires crossing the ICA lesion with the device, inflation of a low-pressure balloon to block the passage of debris distally during CAS, and removal of debris by aspiration in the ICA prior to the end of the procedure[24]. Because blood flow is interrupted, the patient may become restless due to cerebral hypoperfusion if collateral circulation in the brain is not adequate. If hypoperfusion occurs, the balloon can be temporarily deflated, but of course that risks distal embolization. Therefore, the CAS procedure must be completed within a few minutes. An additional problem with this technique is that angiographic images cannot be taken during the procedure as dye will preferentially pass into the external carotid artery during balloon occlusion of the ICA.

Filter DPDs use 80–100-micron filters inserted via the guide catheter or sheath, and deployed beyond the ICA stenosis. Several types exist, some mounted on a wire, whilst others pass over a guide wire that has already crossed the lesion. The blood flow is maintained, and so the procedure is better tolerated. In addition, repeated contrast images can be obtained. However, movement of the device can result in spasm or even dissection of the ICA, and if apposition around the circumference of the vessel wall is not perfect, debris can still pass upwards to the brain. The device is re-captured after the CAS procedure and withdrawn through the stent to remove the debris that has been caught. These devices would be favoured if pre-procedure assessment suggested an incomplete circle of Willis, and hence poor collateral circulation (Fig. 42.9).

The third device involves the proximal occlusion of the CCA and the ECA[123,124]. A large catheter with an extension arm for the ECA is advanced into the CCA. Occlusion balloons mounted on the catheter are inflated in the CCA and then the ECA. This creates a negative pressure in the ICA and should allow the collaterals in the circle of Willis to produce reverse flow or at least no forward flow, thus preventing distal embolization into the ICA. The problems highlighted with distal balloon occlusion, regarding cerebral perfusion and imaging,

Table 42.8 Advantage and disadvantages of embolic protection devices used for CAS procedures

Technique	Advantages	Disadvantages
Balloon occlusion:		
◆ Percusurge® (Medtronic) ◆ Twin-one® (Minavasys)	◆ Can be used in patients with low cardiac output ◆ No embolic debris if used correctly	◆ Requires lesion to be crossed without protection to deliver device ◆ Maximum vessel size 6mm ◆ Can lead to cerebral hypoperfusion ◆ No flow of contrast, so imaging difficult ◆ Risk of trauma to ICA with movement of the filter
Distal filter:		
◆ Angioguard® (Cordis) ◆ Accunet® (Guidant) ◆ EZ-Filter® (Boston) ◆ Interceptor® (Medtronic) ◆ NeuroShield® (Abbott) ◆ Spider Rx® (EV-3) ◆ FibreNet® (Lumen Biomedical)	◆ Maintain anterograde perfusion ◆ Allow imaging whilst in use	◆ Requires lesion to be crossed without protection to deliver device (device crossing profile up to 3.9F) ◆ Filter may clog or get overloaded ◆ Can be difficult to retrieve in tortuous vessels ◆ Maximum size 8mm ◆ Risk of trauma to ICA with movement of the filter
Proximal occlusion:		
◆ Parodi® (Arteria) ◆ MOMA® (Invotec)	◆ Can be used in large vessels ◆ No need to cross ICA lesion prior to protection ◆ No embolic debris if used correctly	◆ Can lead to cerebral hypoperfusion ◆ Large sheath size in femoral artery (10F or 11F) ◆ Requires disease-free ECA

ECA, external carotid artery; ICA, internal carotid artery.

also exist with this technique, but the lesion does not need to be crossed, making it useful if the lesion is felt to be particularly thrombus laden or high risk. Once the stent procedure is completed aspiration is performed to clear debris from the ICA prior to device removal. These devices are larger, up to 10F, and so may not suitable for patients with peripheral vascular disease.

Possible complications with the use of DPDs include difficulty in deploying the device in the distal ICA, effectiveness of emboli capture, vessel injury by the device, and problems with retrieval[127]. Although one small study using MRI scanning has suggested less debris passes to the brain with proximal occlusion devices, patient factors, operator experience, and perhaps the choice of stent are likely to be more relevant[126,127].

In summary, data on whether to use devices is not yet categorical, although registry data favour their use[128]. The choice of device, if any, needs to be made on the anatomy of the lesion and operator experience with the equipment.

Balloon and stent

Once the DPD is in place, if the lesion is tight, with less than a 2mm diameter, or looks calcified, the predilatation with a 3mm × 20mm balloon is recommended. Rapid exchange systems are usually preferred over over-the-wire systems for ease of use and wire stability. Direct stenting may be performed for less severe stenoses. It is vital to give atropine 600mcg prior to balloon inflation. Failure to do so will result in bradycardia and hypotension which can be difficult to manage and may be prolonged.

Which stent?

The choice of stent depends on the characteristics of the lesion and the shape of the vessel. Self-expanding stents have an inherent ability to expand, minimizing the concern about stent collapse if carotid palpation is performed after stenting.

It is important to become familiar with a few stents and how they perform rather than use a large range.

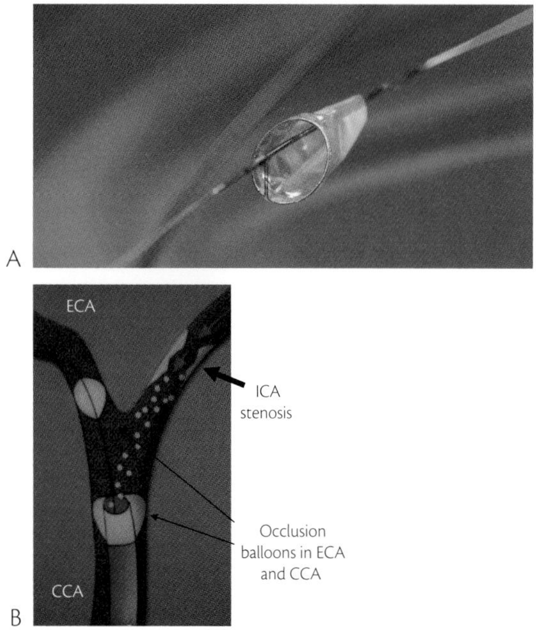

Fig. 42.9 Cerebral protection devices. A) The EZ® (Boston Scientific Inc, USA) filter wire distal protection device B) MOMA® (Invatec, Italy) proximal protection device—reversed flow. CCA common carotid artery, ECA external carotid artery.

Most important is to ensure the stent is large enough to expand into the ICA and, as the lesion usually extends into the CCA, the CCA also. Most stents shorten as they expand, and so adequate length of stent is important. Unlike the coronary, stent length has not been linked to restenosis, and so a 20–30mm length is often taken to avoid geographical miss. The stent can be positioned using bony markers, a reference image on a second screen or using road mapping.

Once the stent is in place, post-dilatation is usually required to allow the stenosis to be reduced to <20–30%. A 5-mm balloon is usually adequate. There appears to be no need to go for 0% as one might for the coronary, and high pressure, large-balloon inflation may lead to unnecessary additional risk by causing more embolization and haemodynamic change related to activation of the carotid baroreceptors.

An angiogram is done to confirm the final result in two planes, and to ensure the DPD has not caused any injury to the distal ICA (see Fig. 42.4). If flow is slow, but there is no obvious cause, it might be due to a full filter. The filter can be removed, or a device such as an export catheter can be used to remove some of the debris from the filter. Once the result is acceptable, the DPD is then recovered and some final shots of the result taken via the guide catheter. If there is no neurological deficit, then in many instances, repeat intracranial images are not taken, in order to reduce contrast load.

Table 42.9 Summary of technique to perform carotid artery stenting in standard cases*

Pre-treated with aspirin and clopidogrel
Transfemoral 8F sheath placed via Seldinger technique
0.035-inch wire to reach aortic arch
Aortogram to assess take-off of great vessels
Heparin given to achieve ACT 250–300
5F Vitek® or other catheter to selectively cannulate IA or left CCA (no wire)
Imaging to visualize stenosis and origin of ECA
0.035-in coated Terumo® guide wire to advance catheter into ECA
Exchange inside catheter for long 0.035-in stiff Amplatzer wire 3
Place 8F guide catheter (or sheath) into CCA 2cm below bifurcation
Remove stiff wire
Cross lesion with DPD on 0.014-inch wire and deploy device 2–3cm above lesion in ICA
Predilate if needed with 3 × 20mm balloon—essential to give 600mcg of atropine prior to this
Place self-expanding stent in position and release
Post-dilate to achieve <20% residual stenosis
Retrieve DPD
Remove guide catheter/sheath and use closure device to seal femoral puncture
Continue aspirin and clopidogrel 4 weeks

ACT, activated clotting time; CCA, common carotid artery; DPD, distal protection device; ECA, external carotid artery; IA, innominate artery; ICA, internal carotid artery.
*Modified from Hobson *et al.*[148]

The catheters are removed, sheath removed, and the femoral puncture site sealed with a closure device to allow the patient to sit up more rapidly (Table 42.9).

Material, cell structure, and flexibility (Table 42.10)

All current stents are made either of nitinol (nickel–titanium alloy) or stainless steel (cobalt alloy). The nitinol stents have a thermal memory and expand as they reach body temperature. Stainless steel stents recoil from their compressed state similar to a coiled spring. The other feature to consider is whether the design is closed cell (where all possible adjacent contact points

Table 42.10 Types of carotid stent*

Stent	Design	Material	Max. free-cell area (mm^2)
Carotid Wallstent® (Boston Scientific)	Closed cell Self tapering	Stainless steel Woven tube	1.08
NexStent® (Boston Scientific)	Closed cell Self tapering	Nitinol sheet	4.70
X-Act® (Abbot Vascular)	Closed cell Straight or taper	Nitinol tube	2.74
Acculink® (Abbot Vascular)	Open cell Straight or taper	Nitinol tube	11.48
Exponent RX® (Medtronic)	Open cell Self tapering	Nitinol tube	6.51
Precise® (Cordis)	Open cell Self taper	Nitinol tube	5.89
Protégé RX® (EV3)	Open cell Straight or taper	Nitinol tube	10.71
CrystalloIdeale® (Invatec)	Closed cell Tapered	Nitinol tube	Variable along stent

*Adapted from Boisiers *et al.*[121]

on a stent are sealed together), or open cell (where not all junction points are fused).

A closed-cell design will improve lesion coverage if a lot of debris is expected, but will not be as flexible as an open-cell design. There is some evidence to suggest lower embolization rates with closed-cell designs[128,129]. It has been suggested that a better measure of coverage is the maximum gap between stent struts. This variation in free-cell area may explain the variability of results between stents seen in some registries[129].

A stainless steel stent (Carotid Wallstent®, Boston Scientific, USA) is likely to have more radial strength, but will not be as conformable as a nitinol stent (e.g. Precise® stent, Cordis, or Acculink®, Guidant). In very tortuous vessels, the ICA can become kinked after placing the Wallstent®.

The role for tapered stents (designed to be smaller in the ICA section than the CCA section) is not clear (e.g. Acculink (R), Guidant (R), USA). It appears that stenting across the ECA origin does not matter clinically. Since many ICA stenoses extend into the carotid bifurcation, the norm is to stent into the CCA from the ICA.

Postoperative care

The patient needs monitoring, including neurological observations every 15min for 2h, and needs to remain in the high-dependency unit for 12h to ensure that these observations, and the arterial access site, are managed properly. Although CAS can be performed as a day-case procedure, there is a small but persistent incidence of late complications. Neurological review prior to discharge is good practice. The preoperative antihypertensive medication often needs to be reduced prior to discharge. Aspirin and clopidogrel at 75mg od each, need to be continued for 1 month, after which aspirin is continued long-term. If the patient was previously on dual aspirin and persantin therapy, this is restarted at 1 month. If warfarin is needed for atrial fibrillation, this is again restarted at 1 month. Warfarin required for other reasons (e.g. metal valves) will need to be reinitiated early, but there will be an increased bleeding risk.

Complications and management

General complication common to all percutaneous vascular procedures, such as femoral puncture complications, and bradycardia will be dealt with elsewhere. This section will focus on those related to CAS specifically.

Hypotension

Hypotension can occur if preparation of the patient is not adequate. Patients on extensive antihypertensive medication may see a permanent reduction in therapy, the effect is so profound and prolonged. Some data suggest that mild degrees of hypotension are not associated with adverse outcome and can occur in over 50% of cases[130], but it is best avoided[131]. If hypotension does occur, then it may be corrected with hydration, and increasing heart rate with atropine. Vasopressors can be used to maintain BP above 100 systolic, but are rarely needed beyond 24h.

Hypertension

Hypertension might be related to a need to micturate, and the patient should be asked. In addition, withdrawal of antihypertensive medication preoperatively may be the cause. It is best managed conservatively, but there is an association with hyperperfusion syndrome. If persistent, a glyceryl trinitrate infusion can be used to reduce the pressure below 180mmHg systolic[132].

Perforation of ECA

If a leak is seen on angiography, then it is at a rate of at least 3mL/min[133]. It is usually related to wire manipulation in ECA, especially if the stiff wire has passed into a very small distal branch. It should be noted that it can occur after sheath removal and should be checked for on the finishing angiogram. It can cause substantial swelling in the subglottic area, and may need intubation. To reduce blood loss, management may include: (1) reversal of heparin, and (2) there may be a need to embolize—with a coil, glue, or foam[134].

Vessel rupture

Although rare, high-pressure balloon inflation in calcified lesions may cause ICA rupture. This is usually managed conservatively, although covered stents may be useful in this setting[135].

Spasm

Manipulation with the wire, and in particular distal filter devices, can result in spasm of the ICA. This usually resolves after removal of the device. The administration of 100–200mcg of isosorbide dinitrate will usually resolve it if treatment is required.

Neurological

The most dreaded complications are neurological. No DPD is 100% efficient in catching debris, and in addition, there is an incidence of late embolic stroke after the DPD is removed, in the first 7 days post-procedure. This is presumably generated by detachment of a mobile piece of atheroma. Late events are usually managed conservatively once bleeding has been excluded. Large CVAs occurring during the procedure should prompt intracerebral angiography to exclude acute occlusion due to embolism. The role of thrombolysis in this situation is not defined, and catheter and wire-based fragmentation of the debris may be warranted. This requires a high degree of neurointerventional skill, and the availability of appropriate equipment.

Hyperperfusion syndrome

Cerebral hyperperfusion can be found in more than 50% of cases, if accurately measured. The hyperperfusion syndrome occurs in a small number of cases (up to 3%, with intracranial bleeding in up to 1.3%). Unilateral headache, fits, and focal neurological deficit not related to ischaemia are the classic triad of clinical manifestations. It is thought that increased cerebral perfusion after intervention (CEA and CAS) overwhelms cerebral autoregulation. Intracerebral bleeding can be catastrophic. For this reason, bilateral procedures should be avoided and BP control should be achieved prior to carotid intervention. Mortality rates of more than 50% have been reported, with few surviving without neurological sequelae[132].

The ideal training programme

Training in invasive coronary procedures comes from didactic lectures, followed by an apprenticeship. This is now supplemented with formal direct observation of procedural skills (DOPS) as well as the testing of ability to make appropriate clinical decisions with the help of colleagues and the involvement of the patient (mini-CEX). With the advent of improved computer simulation, inroads are being made in allowing practice for each step of the procedure.

Coronary intervention has become increasingly safe over the years and also occurs in volumes that allows hands-on training to occur. CAS is presently done in selected centres. The volume of cases is substantially lower, reducing training opportunities, whilst the risks of the procedure are considerably higher. Thankfully, simulation programmes for CAS are increasingly available and realistic. There are at least four commercial endovascular simulators available. Nearly all VR simulators have integrated patient monitoring, drug administration, and responsiveness to physiological disturbances during the endovascular procedure. In addition, the occurrence of complications can now be included[136].

Thus, similar to the aviation industry, the ideal training programme would involve:

- Didactic learning.
- Scenario-based case review.
- Hands on simulator training.
- Direct observation of real-life procedures with an experienced operator.
- Assessment of all cases with a MDT of neurologists, radiologists, vascular surgeons, and interventionalists.
- Proctorship with appropriate case selection.
- Independent operation.
- Detailed case review and audit.

It is essential to move training outside the interventional suite and standardize technical skills training and assessment in order to minimize surgical errors[137]. Though further work is required to validate the simulators, experienced interventionalists in CAS (>50 CAS procedures) have confirmed that the simulated CAS procedure is a realistic interpretation of the actual procedure (face validity). It has been suggested that endovascular therapists should all train on this model prior to performing CAS in real patients[138]. Task analysis needs to be done to identify during which task or step of the CAS procedure most errors are made. The outcomes of both the task analysis and weighting of the errors should enhance the metrics currently available and might assist designers of future simulators[139].

CAS is generally performed by individuals who already possess advanced endovascular skills. Nevertheless these physicians also exhibit a learning curve during CAS procedures[110].The performance during a virtual CAS procedure improved after a 2-day course. The intervention post-course was not only carried out quicker with less radiation, but more importantly, catheter handling errors and spasms of the ICA occurred less frequently[140,141]. The ability to 'practise the case' on a simulator with 'patient-specific data' has been called mission or procedure rehearsal. This will be the next phase of simulation[108].

Simulation-based training is unlikely to replace real-life experience though it may be an adjunct to teach and improve basic and advanced endovascular technical skills with the hope of shortening the learning curve on patients.

Conclusion

CEA is not as invasive as CABG surgery, whilst CAS carries higher risks than PCI, since the brain is more unforgiving than the myocardium. However, the move towards the development of less invasive treatments is unrelenting and with the appropriate training, many interventionalists will be able to perform CAS safely.

It is important to pay attention to initial patient selection and appropriate investigation. This is best done in the context of a MDT. Careful selection of technique to be employed, choice of equipment, and meticulous preoperative, perioperativ,e and postoperative care is vital to ensure that the procedure is performed at lowest possible risk. Careful liaison with the MDT allows clinical governance and audit to be transparent and honest.

The evidence base comparing CAS to CEA is enlarging, with both registry and trial data. There is a position of clinical equipoise in low-risk patients, but for patients with high operative risk, if an intervention is definitely warranted, CAS may be a reasonable alternative if local event rates match that achieved by the vascular surgeons for CEA[142,143].

Disclosures

Dr Malik is part of the EVEResT (European Virtual Research Endovascular RESearch Team) and is on the steering committee of the ICSS trial.

References

1. Kung HC, Hoyert DL, Xu J, *et al.* Deaths: final data for 2005. *Natl Vital Stat Rep* 2008; **56**(10):1–120.
2. Health Development Agency. Health Update: Coronary Heart Disease and Stroke. London: Health Development Agency, 2000.
3. Adams HP, Jr, Bendixen BH, Kappelle LJ, *et al.* Classification of subtype of acute ischemic stroke. Definitions for use in a multicenter clinical trial. TOAST. Trial of Org 10172 in Acute Stroke Treatment. *Stroke* 1993; **24**(1):35–41.
4. NICE. Stroke: Diagnosis and initial management of acute stroke and transient ischaemic attack (TIA). London: NICE, 2008.
5. Fischer CM, Gore I, Okabe N, *et al.* Atherosclerosis of the carotid and vertebral arteries: extracranial and intracranial. *J Neuropath Exp Neurol* 1965; **24**:455–76.
6. Turnbull F. Blood Pressure Lowering Treatment Trialists' Collaboration. Effects of different blood-pressure-lowering regimens on major cardiovascular events: results of prospectively-designed overviews of randomised trials. *Lancet* 2003; **362**(9395):1527–35.
7. Gage BF, Waterman AD, Shannon W, *et al.* Validation of clinical classification schemes for predicting stroke; results from the National Registry of Atrial Fibrillation. *JAMA* 2001; **285**:2864–70.
8. Collaborative overview of randomised trials of antiplatelet therapy – I: Prevention of death, myocardial infarction, and stroke by prolonged antiplatelet therapy in various categories of patients. Antiplatelet Trialists' Collaboration [published erratum appears in BMJ 1994; 308(6943):1540]. *BMJ* 1994; **308**(6921):81–106.
9. Vane JR, Meade TW. Second European Stroke Prevention Study (ESPS 2): clinical and pharmacological implications. *J Neurol Sci* 1997; **145**(2):123–5.
10. Halkes PH, van Gijn J, Kappelle LJ, *et al.* Aspirin plus dipyridamole versus aspirin alone after cerebral ischaemia of arterial origin (ESPRIT): randomised controlled trial. *Lancet* 2006; **367**(9523):1665–73.
11. Diener HC, Bogousslavsky J, Brass LM, *et al.* Aspirin and clopidogrel compared with clopidogrel alone after recent ischaemic stroke or transient ischaemic attack in high-risk patients (MATCH): randomised, double-blind, placebo-controlled trial. *Lancet* 2004; **364**(9431):331–7.
12. Sacco RL, Diener HC, Yusuf S, *et al.* Aspirin and extended-release dipyridamole versus clopidogrel for recurrent stroke. *N Engl J Med* 2008; **359**(12):1238–51.
13. Baigent C, Keech A, Kearney PM, *et al.* Efficacy and safety of cholesterol-lowering treatment: prospective meta-analysis of data from 90,056 participants in 14 randomised trials of statins. *Lancet* 2005; **366**(9493):1267–78.
14. The Stroke Prevention by Aggressive Reduction in Cholesterol Levels (SPARCL) Investigators. High-Dose Atorvastatin after Stroke or Transient Ischemic Attack. *N Engl J Med* 2006; **355**(6):549–59.

15. Eastcott HH, Pickering GW, Rob CG. Reconstruction of internal carotid artery in a patient with intermittent attacks of hemiplegia. *Lancet* 1954; **267**(6846):994–6.
16. DeBakey ME. Successful carotid endarterectomy for cerebrovascular insufficiency. Nineteen-year follow-up. *JAMA* 1975; **233**(10):1083–5.
17. Tu JV, Hannan EL, Anderson GM, *et al.* The fall and rise of carotid endarterectomy in the United States and Canada. *N Engl J Med* 1998; **339**(20):1441–7.
18. Gillum RF. Epidemiology of Carotid Endarterectomy and Cerebral Arteriography in the United States. *Stroke* 1995; **26**(9):1724–8.
19. Murie JA. Carotid endarterectomy in Great Britain and Ireland: practice between 1984 and 1992. *Br J Surg* 1994; **81**(6):827–31.
20. DuBose J, Recinos G, Teixeira PG, *et al.* Endovascular stenting for the treatment of traumatic internal carotid injuries: expanding experience. *J Trauma* 2008; **65**(6):1561–6.
21. Bockenheimer SA, Mathias K. Percutaneous transluminal angioplasty in arteriosclerotic internal carotid artery stenosis. *AJNR Am J Neuroradiol* 1983; **4**(3):791–2.
22. Diethrich EB, Ndiaye M, Reid DB. Stenting in the carotid artery: initial experience in 110 patients. *J Endovasc Surg* 1996; **3**(1):42–62.
23. Yadav JS, Roubin GS, Iyer S, *et al.* Elective stenting of the extracranial carotid arteries. *Circulation* 1997; **95**(2):376–81.
24. Theron J, Raymond J, Casasco A, *et al.* Percutaneous angioplasty of atherosclerotic and postsurgical stenosis of carotid arteries. *AJNR Am J Neuroradiol* 1987; **8**(3):495–500.
25. Wholey MH, Wu WC. Current status in cervical carotid artery stent placement. *J Cardiovasc Surg (Torino)* 2009; **50**(1):29–37.
26. Bonow RO, Epstein SE. Indications for coronary artery bypass surgery in patients with chronic angina pectoris: implications of the multicenter randomized trials. *Circulation* 1985; **72**(6 Pt 2):V23–V30.
27. Daemen J, Boersma E, Flather M, *et al.* Long-term safety and efficacy of percutaneous coronary intervention with stenting and coronary artery bypass surgery for multivessel coronary artery disease: a meta-analysis with 5-year patient-level data from the ARTS, ERACI-II, MASS-II, and SoS trials. *Circulation* 2008; **118**(11):1146–54.
28. Takagi H, Kawai N, Umemoto T. Meta-analysis of four randomized controlled trials on long-term outcomes of coronary artery bypass grafting versus percutaneous coronary intervention with stenting for multivessel coronary artery disease. *Am J Cardiol* 2008; **101**(9):1259–62.
29. Beneficial effect of carotid endarterectomy in symptomatic patients with high-grade carotid stenosis. North American Symptomatic Carotid Endarterectomy Trial Collaborators. *N Engl J Med* 1991; **325**(7):445–53.
30. Mayberg MR, Wilson SE, Yatsu F, *et al.* Carotid endarterectomy and prevention of cerebral ischemia in symptomatic carotid stenosis. Veterans Affairs Cooperative Studies Program 309 Trialist Group. *JAMA* 1991; **266**(23):3289–94.
31. MRC European Carotid Surgery Trial: interim results for symptomatic patients with severe (70–99%) or with mild (0–29%) carotid stenosis. European Carotid Surgery Trialists' Collaborative Group. *Lancet* 1991; **337**(8752):1235–43.
32. Barnett HJ, Taylor DW, Eliasziw M, *et al.* Benefit of carotid endarterectomy in patients with symptomatic moderate or severe stenosis. North American Symptomatic Carotid Endarterectomy Trial Collaborators. *N Engl J Med* 1998; **339**(20):1415–25.
33. Randomised trial of endarterectomy for recently symptomatic carotid stenosis: final results of the MRC European Carotid Surgery Trial (ECST). *Lancet* 1998; **351**(9113):1379–87.
34. Rothwell PM, Eliasziw M, Gutnikov SA, *et al.* Analysis of pooled data from the randomised controlled trials of endarterectomy for symptomatic carotid stenosis. *Lancet* 2003; **361**(9352):107–16.
35. Moore WS, Barnett HJ, Beebe HG, *et al.* Guidelines for carotid endarterectomy. A multidisciplinary consensus statement from the Ad Hoc Committee, American Heart Association. *Circulation* 1995; **91**(2):566–79.
36. Barnett HJ, Gunton RW, Eliasziw M, *et al.* Causes and severity of ischemic stroke in patients with internal carotid artery stenosis. *JAMA* 2000; **283**(11):1429–36.
37. Inzitari D, Eliasziw M, Gates P, *et al.* The causes and risk of stroke in patients with asymptomatic internal-carotid-artery stenosis. North American Symptomatic Carotid Endarterectomy Trial Collaborators. *N Engl J Med* 2000; **342**(23):1693–700.
38. Wolff T, Guirguis-Blake J, Miller T, *et al.* Screening for carotid artery stenosis: an update of the evidence for the U.S. Preventive Services Task Force. *Ann Intern Med* 2007; **147**(12):860–70.
39. Rockman CB, Jacobowitz GR, Gagne PJ, *et al.* Focused screening for occult carotid artery disease: patients with known heart disease are at high risk. *J Vasc Surg* 2004; **39**(1):44–51.
40. Cina CS, Safar HA, Maggisano R, *et al.* Prevalence and progression of internal carotid artery stenosis in patients with peripheral arterial occlusive disease. *J Vasc Surg* 2002; **36**(1):75–82.
41. Carotid surgery versus medical therapy in asymptomatic carotid stenosis. The CASANOVA Study Group. *Stroke* 1991; **22**(10):1229–35.
42. Hobson RW, Weiss DG, Fields WS, *et al.* Efficacy of carotid endarterectomy for asymptomatic carotid stenosis. The Veterans Affairs Cooperative Study Group. *N Engl J Med* 1993; **328**(4):221–7.

43. Results of a randomized controlled trial of carotid endarterectomy for asymptomatic carotid stenosis. Mayo Asymptomatic Carotid Endarterectomy Study Group. *Mayo Clin Proc* 1992; **67**(6):513–18.
44. Endarterectomy for asymptomatic carotid artery stenosis. Executive Committee for the Asymptomatic Carotid Atherosclerosis Study. *JAMA* 1995; **273**(18):1421–8.
45. Halliday A, Mansfield A, Marro J, *et al.* Prevention of disabling and fatal strokes by successful carotid endarterectomy in patients without recent neurological symptoms: randomised controlled trial. *Lancet* 2004; **363**(9420):1491–502.
46. Simes J. Long-term effectiveness and safety of pravastatin in 9014 patients with coronary heart disease and average cholesterol concentrations: the LIPID trial follow-up. *Lancet* 2002; **359**(9315):1379–87.
47. A randomised, blinded, trial of clopidogrel versus aspirin in patients at risk of ischaemic events (CAPRIE). CAPRIE Steering Committee. *Lancet* 1996; **348**(9038):1329–39.
48. Wennberg DE, Lucas FL, Birkmeyer JD, *et al.* Variation in Carotid Endarterectomy Mortality in the Medicare Population: Trial Hospitals, Volume, and Patient Characteristics. *JAMA* 1998; **279**(16):1278–81.
49. Theiss W, Hermanek P, Mathias K, *et al.* Pro-CAS: a prospective registry of carotid angioplasty and stenting. *Stroke* 2004; **35**(9):2134–9.
50. Brener BJ, Brief DK, Alpert J, *et al.* The risk of stroke in patients with asymptomatic carotid stenosis undergoing cardiac surgery: a follow-up study. *J Vasc Surg* 1987; **5**(2):269–79.
51. Huh J, Wall MJ, Jr, Soltero ER. Treatment of combined coronary and carotid artery disease. *Curr Opin Cardiol* 2003; **18**(6):447–53.
52. Naylor AR, Mehta Z, Rothwell PM, *et al.* Carotid artery disease and stroke during coronary artery bypass: a critical review of the literature. *Eur J Vasc Endovasc Surg* 2002; **23**(4):283–294.
53. Das SK, Brow TD, Pepper J. Continuing controversy in the management of concomitant coronary and carotid disease: an overview. *Int J Cardiol* 2000; **74**(1):47–65.
54. Durand DJ, Perler BA, Roseborough GS, *et al.* Mandatory versus selective preoperative carotid screening: a retrospective analysis. *Ann Thorac Surg* 2004; **78**(1):159–66.
55. Naylor AR, Cuffe RL, Rothwell PM, *et al.* A systematic review of outcomes following staged and synchronous carotid endarterectomy and coronary artery bypass. *Eur J Vasc Endovasc Surg* 2003; **25**(5):380–9.
56. Fareed KR, Rothwell PM, Mehta Z, *et al.* Synchronous carotid endarterectomy and off-pump coronary bypass: an updated, systematic review of early outcomes. *Eur J Vasc Endovasc Surg* 2009; **37**(4):375–8.
57. Guzman LA, Costa MA, Angiolillo DJ, *et al.* A systematic review of outcomes in patients with staged carotid artery stenting and coronary artery bypass graft surgery. *Stroke* 2008; **39**(2):361–5.
58. Goto T, Baba T, Yoshitake A, *et al.* Craniocervical and aortic atherosclerosis as neurologic risk factors in coronary surgery. *Ann Thorac Surg* 2000; **69**(3):834–40.
59. Lattimer CR, Burnand KG. Recurrent carotid stenosis after carotid endarterectomy. *Br J Surg* 1997; **84**(9):1206–19.
60. Sterpetti AV, Schultz RD, Feldhaus RJ, *et al.* Natural history of recurrent carotid artery disease. *Surg Gynecol Obstet* 1989; **168**(3):217–23.
61. Bartlett FF, Rapp JH, Goldstone J, *et al.* Recurrent carotid stenosis: operative strategy and late results. *J Vasc Surg* 1987; **5**(3):452–6.
62. Healy DA, Zierler RE, Nicholls SC, *et al.* Long-term follow-up and clinical outcome of carotid restenosis. *J Vasc Surg* 1989; **10**(6):662–8.
63. Moore WS, Kempczinski RF, Nelson JJ, *et al.* Recurrent carotid stenosis : results of the asymptomatic carotid atherosclerosis study. *Stroke* 1998; **29**(10):2018–25.
64. Stoney RJ, String ST. Recurrent carotid stenosis. *Surgery* 1976; **80**(6):705–710.
65. Hobson RW, Goldstein JE, Jamil Z, *et al.* Carotid restenosis: operative and endovascular management. *J Vasc Surg* 1999; **29**(2):228–35.
66. Endovascular versus surgical treatment in patients with carotid stenosis in the Carotid and Vertebral Artery Transluminal Angioplasty Study (CAVATAS): a randomised trial. *Lancet* 2001; **357**(9270):1729–37.
67. Veith FJ, Amor M, Ohki T, *et al.* Current status of carotid bifurcation angioplasty and stenting based on a consensus of opinion leaders. *J Vasc Surg* 2001; **33**(2 Suppl):S111–S116.
68. McCarthy WJ, Wang R, Pearce WH, *et al.* Carotid endarterectomy with an occluded contralateral carotid artery. *Am J Surg* 1993; **166**(2):168–71.
69. Rothwell PM, Slattery J, Warlow CP. Clinical and angiographic predictors of stroke and death from carotid endarterectomy: systematic review. *BMJ* 1997; **315**(7122):1571–7.
70. Borger MA, Fremes SE, Weisel RD, *et al.* Coronary bypass and carotid endarterectomy: does a combined approach increase risk? A metaanalysis. *Ann Thorac Surg* 1999; **68**(1):14–20.
71. Paciaroni M, Eliasziw M, Kappelle LJ, *et al.* Medical complications associated with carotid endarterectomy. North American Symptomatic Carotid Endarterectomy Trial (NASCET). *Stroke* 1999; **30**(9):1759–63.
72. Rerkasem K, Rothwell PM. Local versus general anaesthesia for carotid endarterectomy. *Cochrane Database Syst Rev* 2008; **4**:CD000126.
73. Roubin GS, New G, Iyer SS, *et al.* Immediate and late clinical outcomes of carotid artery stenting in patients with symptomatic and asymptomatic carotid artery stenosis: a 5-year prospective analysis. *Circulation* 2001; **103**(4):532–7.
74. Alberts MJ. Results of a Prospective Multicentre Randomised Trial of carotid artery stenting vs carotid endarterectomy. *Stroke* 2001; **32**: 325.

75. Brooks WH, McClure RR, Jones MR, *et al.* Carotid angioplasty and stenting versus carotid endarterectomy: randomized trial in a community hospital. *J Am Coll Cardiol* 2001; **38**(6):1589–95.
76. Naylor AR, Bolia A, Abbott RJ, *et al.* Randomized study of carotid angioplasty and stenting versus carotid endarterectomy: a stopped trial. *J Vasc Surg* 1998; **28**(2):326–34.
77. Yadav JS, Wholey MH, Kuntz RE, *et al.* Protected carotid-artery stenting versus endarterectomy in high-risk patients. *N Engl J Med* 2004; **351**(15):1493–501.
78. Mas JL, Chatellier G, Beyssen B, *et al.* Endarterectomy versus stenting in patients with symptomatic severe carotid stenosis. *N Engl J Med* 2006; **355**(16):1660–71.
79. Mas JL, Trinquart L, Leys D, *et al.* Endarterectomy Versus Angioplasty in Patients with Symptomatic Severe Carotid Stenosis (EVA-3S) trial: results up to 4 years from a randomised, multicentre trial. *Lancet Neurol* 2008; **7**(10):885–92.
80. Ringleb PA, Allenberg J, Bruckmann H, *et al.* 30 day results from the SPACE trial of stent-protected angioplasty versus carotid endarterectomy in symptomatic patients: a randomised non-inferiority trial. *Lancet* 2006; **368**(9543):1239–47.
81. Eckstein HH, Ringleb P, Allenberg JR, *et al.* Results of the Stent-Protected Angioplasty versus Carotid Endarterectomy (SPACE) study to treat symptomatic stenoses at 2 years: a multinational, prospective, randomised trial. *Lancet Neurol* 2008; **7**(10):893–902.
82. Gray WA, Hopkins LN, Yadav S, *et al.* Protected carotid stenting in high-surgical-risk patients: the ARCHeR results. *J Vasc Surg* 2006; **44**(2):258–68.
83. Ringleb PA, Chatellier G, Hacke W, *et al.* Safety of endovascular treatment of carotid artery stenosis compared with surgical treatment: a meta-analysis. *J Vasc Surg* 2008; **47**(2):350–5.
84. Ederle J, Featherstone RL, Brown MM. Percutaneous transluminal angioplasty and stenting for carotid artery stenosis. *Cochrane Database Syst Rev* 2007; **4**:CD000515.
85. Murad MH, Flynn DN, Elamin MB, *et al.* Endarterectomy vs stenting for carotid artery stenosis: a systematic review and meta-analysis. *J Vasc Surg* 2008; **48**(2):487–93.
86. Hobson RW. Update on the Carotid Revascularization Endarterectomy versus Stent Trial (CREST) protocol. *J Am Coll Surg* 2002; **194**(1 Suppl):S9–14.
87. Featherstone RL, Brown MM, Coward LJ. International carotid stenting study: protocol for a randomised clinical trial comparing carotid stenting with endarterectomy in symptomatic carotid artery stenosis. *Cerebrovasc Dis* 2004; **18**(1):69–74.
88. http://www.ion.ucl.ac.uk/cavatas_icss/downloads/FirstResultsofICSS.pdf
89a. Asymptomatic Carotid Surgery Study-2. http://www.acst.org.uk. 2008.
89b. Asymptomatic Carotid Trial (ACT-1). http://www.act1trial.com.
90. McCabe DJ, Pereira AC, Clifton A, et al. Restenosis after carotid angioplasty, stenting, or endarterectomy in the Carotid and Vertebral Artery Transluminal Angioplasty Study (CAVATAS). Stroke 2005; 36(2):281–6.
91. Lal BK, Hobson RW, Goldstein J, *et al.* In-stent recurrent stenosis after carotid artery stenting: life table analysis and clinical relevance. *J Vasc Surg* 2003; **38**(6):1162–8.
92. Bosiers M, Peeters P, Deloose K, *et al.* Does carotid artery stenting work on the long run: 5-year results in high-volume centers (ELOCAS Registry). *J Cardiovasc Surg (Torino)* 2005; **46**(3):241–7.
93. Lal BK, Kaperonis EA, Cuadra S, *et al.* Patterns of in-stent restenosis after carotid artery stenting: classification and implications for long-term outcome. *J Vasc Surg* 2007; **46**(5):833–40.
94. Lal BK. Recurrent carotid stenosis after CEA and CAS: diagnosis and management. *Semin Vasc Surg* 2007; **20**(4):259–66.
95. Lal BK, Hobson RW, Tofighi B, *et al.* Duplex ultrasound velocity criteria for the stented carotid artery. *J Vasc Surg* 2008; **47**(1):63–73.
96. Zhou W, Lin PH, Bush RL, *et al.* Management of in-sent restenosis after carotid artery stenting in high-risk patients. *J Vasc Surg* 2006; **43**(2):305–12.
97. Setacci C, De Donato G, Setacci F, *et al.* In-stent restenosis after carotid angioplasty and stenting: a challenge for the vascular surgeon. *Eur J Vasc Endovasc Surg* 2005; **29**(6):601–7.
98. Akin E, Knobloch K, Pichlmaier M, *et al.* Instent restenosis after carotid stenting necessitating open carotid surgical repair. *Eur J Cardiothorac Surg* 2004; **26**(2):442–3.
99. Nederkoorn PJ, van der GY, Hunink MG. Duplex ultrasound and magnetic resonance angiography compared with digital subtraction angiography in carotid artery stenosis: a systematic review. *Stroke* 2003; **34**(5):1324–32.
100. Jahromi AS, Cina CS, Liu Y, *et al.* Sensitivity and specificity of color duplex ultrasound measurement in the estimation of internal carotid artery stenosis: a systematic review and meta-analysis. *J Vasc Surg* 2005; **41**(6):962–72.
101. Biasi GM, Froio A, Diethrich EB, *et al.* Carotid plaque echolucency increases the risk of stroke in carotid stenting: the Imaging in Carotid Angioplasty and Risk of Stroke (ICAROS) study. *Circulation* 2004; **110**(6):756–62.
102. Reiter M, Bucek RA, Effenberger I, *et al.* Plaque Echolucency Is Not Associated With the Risk of Stroke in Carotid Stenting. *Stroke* 2006; **37**(9):2378–80.
103. Davies KN, Humphrey PR. Complications of cerebral angiography in patients with symptomatic carotid territory ischaemia screened by carotid ultrasound. *J Neurol Neurosurg Psychiatry* 1993; **56**(9):967–72.
104. Rothwell PM, Pendlebury ST, Wardlaw J, *et al.* Critical appraisal of the design and reporting of studies of

imaging and measurement of carotid stenosis. *Stroke* 2000; **31**(6):1444–50.

105. Koelemay MJ, Nederkoorn PJ, Reitsma JB, *et al.* Systematic review of computed tomographic angiography for assessment of carotid artery disease. *Stroke* 2004; **35**(10):2306–12.
106. Rothwell PM, Gibson RJ, Slattery J, *et al.* Prognostic value and reproducibility of measurements of carotid stenosis. A comparison of three methods on 1001 angiograms. European Carotid Surgery Trialists' Collaborative Group. *Stroke* 1994; **25**(12):2440–4.
107. Faggioli GL, Ferri M, Freyrie A, *et al.* Aortic arch anomalies are associated with increased risk of neurological events in carotid stent procedures. *Eur J Vasc Endovasc Surg* 2007; **33**(4):436–41.
108. Cates CU, Patel AD, Nicholson WJ. Use of virtual reality simulation for mission rehearsal for carotid stenting. *JAMA* 2007; **297**(3):265–6.
109. Pucelikova T, Dangas G, Mehran R. Contrast-induced nephropathy. *Catheter Cardiovasc Interv* 2008; **71**(1):62–72.
110. Lin PH, Bush RL, Peden EK, *et al.* Carotid artery stenting with neuroprotection: assessing the learning curve and treatment outcome. *Am J Surg* 2005; **190**(6):850–7.
111. MacLean AA, Peña CS, Katzen BT. Bivalirudin in peripheral interventions. *Tech Vasc Interv Radiol* 2006; **9**(2):80–3.
112. Ho DS, Wang Y, Chui M, *et al.* Intracarotid abciximab injection to abort impending ischemic stroke during carotid angioplasty. *Cerebrovasc Dis* 2001; **11**(4):300–4.
113. Zahn R, Ischinger T, Hochadel M, *et al.* Glycoprotein IIb/IIIa antagonists during carotid artery stenting: results from the carotid artery stenting (CAS) registry of the Arbeitsgemeinschaft Leitende Kardiologische Krankenhausarzte (ALKK). *Clin Res Cardiol* 2007; **96**(10):730–7.
114. Arab D, Yahia AM, Qureshi AI. Use of intravenous abciximab as adjunctive therapy for carotid angioplasty and stent placement. *Int J Cardiovasc Intervent* 2003; **5**(2):61–6.
115. Castriota F, Cremonesi A, Manetti R, *et al.* Carotid stenting using radial artery access. *J Endovasc Surg* 1999; **6**(4):385–6.
116. Folmar J, Sachar R, Mann T. Transradial approach for carotid artery stenting: a feasibility study. *Catheter Cardiovasc Interv* 2007; **69**(3):355–61.
117. Pinter L, Cagiannos C, Ruzsa Z, *et al.* Report on initial experience with transradial access for carotid artery stenting. *J Vasc Surg* 2007; **45**(6):1136–41.
118. Feldtman RW, Buckley CJ, Bohannon WT. How I do it: cervical access for carotid artery stenting. *Am J Surg* 2006; **192**(6):779–81.
119. Ohki T, Marin ML, Lyon RT, *et al.* Ex vivo human carotid artery bifurcation stenting: correlation of lesion characteristics with embolic potential. *J Vasc Surg* 1998; **27**(3):463–71.
120. Jordan WD, Jr, Voellinger DC, Doblar DD, *et al.* Microemboli detected by transcranial Doppler monitoring in patients during carotid angioplasty versus carotid endarterectomy. *Cardiovasc Surg* 1999; **7**(1):33–8.
121. Bosiers M, Deloose K, Verbist J, *et al.* What practical factors guide the choice of stent and protection device during carotid angioplasty? *Eur J Vasc Endovasc Surg* 2008; **35**(6):637–43.
122. Wholey MH, Al Mubarek N, Wholey MH. Updated review of the global carotid artery stent registry. *Catheter Cardiovasc Interv* 2003; **60**(2):259–66.
123. Lo CH, Doblas M, Criado E. Advantages and indications of transcervical carotid artery stenting with carotid flow reversal. *J Cardiovasc Surg (Torino)* 2005; **46**(3):229–39.
124. Reimers B, Sievert H, Schuler GC, *et al.* Proximal endovascular flow blockage for cerebral protection during carotid artery stenting: results from a prospective multicenter registry. *J Endovasc Ther* 2005; **12**(2):156–65.
125. Ohki T, Veith FJ. Critical analysis of distal protection devices. *Semin Vasc Surg* 2003; **16**(4):317–25.
126. El Koussy M, Schroth G, Do DD, *et al.* Periprocedural embolic events related to carotid artery stenting detected by diffusion-weighted MRI: comparison between proximal and distal embolus protection devices. *J Endovasc Ther* 2007; **14**(3):293–303.
127. Bosiers M, Deloose K, Verbist J, *et al.* The impact of embolic protection device and stent design on the outcome of CAS. *Perspect Vasc Surg Endovasc Ther* 2008; **20**(3):272–9.
128. Jansen O, Fiehler J, Hartmann M, *et al.* Protection or nonprotection in carotid stent angioplasty. the influence of interventional techniques on outcome data from the SPACE trial. *Stroke* 2009; **40**(3):841–6.
129. Bosiers M, De Donato G, Deloose K, *et al.* Does free cell area influence the outcome in carotid artery stenting? *Eur J Vasc Endovasc Surg* 2007; **33**(2):135–41.
130. Cieri E, De Rango P, Maccaroni MR, *et al.* Is haemodynamic depression during carotid stenting a predictor of peri-procedural complications? *Eur J Vasc Endovasc Surg* 2008; **35**(4):399–404.
131. Qureshi AI, Luft AR, Sharma M, *et al.* Frequency and determinants of postprocedural hemodynamic instability after carotid angioplasty and stenting. *Stroke* 1999; **30**(10):2086–93.
132. Coutts SB, Hill MD, Hu WY. Hyperperfusion syndrome: toward a stricter definition. *Neurosurgery* 2003; **53**(5):1053–8.
133. Berjljung L, Hjorth S, Svendler CA, *et al.* Angiography in acute gastrointestinal bleeding. *Surg Gynecol Obstet* 1977; **145**(4):501–3.
134. Ecker RD, Guidot CA, Hanel RA, *et al.* Perforation of external carotid artery branch arteries during endoluminal carotid revascularization procedures:

consequences and management. *J Invasive Cardiol* 2005; **17**(6):292–5.

135. Broadbent LP, Moran CJ, Cross DT, III, *et al.* Management of ruptures complicating angioplasty and stenting of supraaortic arteries: report of two cases and a review of the literature. *AJNR Am J Neuroradiol* 2003; **24**(10):2057–61.
136. Tsang JS, Naughton PA, Leong S, *et al.* Virtual reality simulation in endovascular surgical training. *Surgeon* 2008; **6**(4):214–20.
137. Scott DJ, Dunnington GL. The new ACS/APDS Skills Curriculum: moving the learning curve out of the operating room. *J Gastrointest Surg* 2008; **12**(2):213–21.
138. Van Herzeele I, Aggarwal R, Choong A, *et al.* Virtual reality simulation objectively differentiates level of carotid stent experience in experienced interventionalists. *J Vasc Surg* 2007; **46**(5):855–63.
139. Dawson S, Gould DA. Procedural simulation's developing role in medicine. *Lancet* 2007; **369**(9574):1671–73.
140. Van Herzeele I, Aggarwal R, Neequaye S, *et al.* Experienced endovascular interventionalists objectively improve their skills by attending carotid artery stent training courses. *Eur J Vasc Endovasc Surg* 2008; **35**(5):541–50.
141. Katzen BT, Criado FJ, Ramee SR, *et al.* Carotid artery stenting with emboli protection surveillance study: thirty-day results of the CASES-PMS study. *Catheter Cardiovasc Interv* 2007; **70**(2):316–23.
142. Freedman B. Equipoise and the ethics of clinical research. *N Engl J Med* 1987; **317**(3):141–5.
143. Coward LJ, Featherstone RL, Brown MM. Safety and efficacy of endovascular treatment of carotid artery stenosis compared with carotid endarterectomy: a Cochrane systematic review of the randomized evidence. *Stroke* 2005; **36**(4):905–11.
144. Gorelick PB. Stroke prevention: windows of opportunity and failed expectations? A discussion of modifiable cardiovascular risk factors and a prevention proposal. *Neuroepidemiology* 1997; **16**(4):163–73.
145. Goldstein LB, Adams R, Alberts MJ, *et al.* Primary Prevention of Ischemic Stroke: A Guideline From the American Heart Association/American Stroke Association Stroke Council: Cosponsored by the Atherosclerotic Peripheral Vascular Disease Interdisciplinary Working Group; Cardiovascular Nursing Council; Clinical Cardiology Council; Nutrition, Physical Activity, and Metabolism Council; and the Quality of Care and Outcomes Research Interdisciplinary Working Group: The American Academy of Neurology affirms the value of this guideline. *Stroke* 2006; **37**(6):1583–633.
146. Coward LJ, McCabe DJ, Ederle J, *et al.* Long-term outcome after angioplasty and stenting for symptomatic vertebral artery stenosis compared with medical treatment in the Carotid And Vertebral Artery Transluminal Angioplasty Study (CAVATAS): a randomized trial. *Stroke* 2007; **38**(5):1526–30.
147. Carotid Revascularization Using Endarterectomy or Stenting Systems (CaRESS) phase I clinical trial: 1-year results. *J Vasc Surg* 2005; **42**(2):213–219.
148. Hobson RW, Lal BK, Chakhtoura E, *et al.* Carotid artery stenting: analysis of data for 105 patients at high risk. *J Vasc Surg* 2003; **37**(6):1234–9.
149. Rothwell PM, Gibson RJ, Slattery J, *et al.* Equivalence of measurements of carotid stenosis. A comparison of three methods on 1001 angiograms. European Carotid Surgery Trialists' Collaborative Group. *Stroke* 1994; **25**(12):2435–9.

Index